CAMPBELL-WALSH

Urology

Tenth Edition Review

CAMPBELL-WALSH

Urology

Tenth Edition Review

EDITORS

W. Scott McDougal, MD, MA (Hon)
Professor of Urology
Harvard Medical School;
Chief, Urology
Massachusetts General Hospital
Boston, Massachusetts

Alan J. Wein, MD, PhD (Hon)
Professor and Chair, Division of Urology
University of Pennsylvania School of Medicine
University of Pennsylvania Health System
Philadelphia, Pennsylvania

Louis R. Kavoussi, MD, MBA
Chairman and Waldbaum-Gardner Distinguished
    Professor of Urology
Smith Institute for Urology
Hofstra North Shore–LIJ School of Medicine
Long Island, New York

Andrew C. Novick, MD
Chairman, Glickman Urological Institute
Cleveland Clinic Foundation
Professor of Surgery
Cleveland Clinic Lerner College of Medicine of Case
    Western Reserve University
Cleveland, Ohio

Alan W. Partin, MD, PhD
Professor and Director of Urology
Johns Hopkins School of Medicine
Baltimore, Maryland

Craig A. Peters, MD, FACS, FAAP
Chief, Division of Surgical Innovation, Technology,
    and Translation
Principle Investigator, Sheikh Zayed Institute for
    Pediatric Surgical Innovation
Children's National Medical Center
Washington, DC;
Professor of Urology
University of Virginia
Charlottesville, Virginia

Parvati Ramchandani, MD
Professor of Radiology and Surgery
Section Chief, Genitourinary Radiology
University of Pennsylvania School of Medicine
Philadelphia, Pennyslvania

ELSEVIER
SAUNDERS

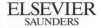

1600 John F. Kennedy Blvd.
Ste 1800
Philadelphia, PA 19103-2899

CAMPBELL-WALSH UROLOGY TENTH EDITION REVIEW   ISBN: 978-1-4377-2393-9

Notices

Knowledge and best practice in this field are constantly changing. As new research and experience broaden our understanding, changes in research methods, professional practices, or medical treatment may become necessary.

Practitioners and researchers must always rely on their own experience and knowledge in evaluating and using any information, methods, compounds, or experiments described herein. In using such information or methods they should be mindful of their own safety and the safety of others, including parties for whom they have a professional responsibility.

With respect to any drug or pharmaceutical products identified, readers are advised to check the most current information provided (i) on procedures featured or (ii) by the manufacturer of each product to be administered, to verify the recommended dose or formula, the method and duration of administration, and contraindications. It is the responsibility of practitioners, relying on their own experience and knowledge of their patients, to make diagnoses, to determine dosages and the best treatment for each individual patient, and to take all appropriate safety precautions.

To the fullest extent of the law, neither the Publisher nor the authors, contributors, or editors, assume any liability for any injury and/or damage to persons or property as a matter of products liability, negligence or otherwise, or from any use or operation of any methods, products, instructions, or ideas contained in the material herein.

Library of Congress Cataloging-in-Publication Data
Campbell-Walsh urology tenth edition review / editors, W. Scott McDougal ... [et al.].—10th ed.
       p. ; cm.
    Urology tenth edition review
    Companion v. to: Campbell-Walsh urology. 10th ed. / editor-in-chief, Alan J. Wein ; editors, Louis R. Kavoussi ... [et al.]. c2012.
    ISBN 978-1-4377-2393-9 (pbk. : alk. paper)
    1. Urology—Examinations, questions, etc.   I. McDougal, W. Scott (William Scott), 1942–
II. Campbell-Walsh urology.   III. Title: Urology tenth edition review.
    [DNLM: 1. Female Urogenital Diseases—Problems and Exercises.   2. Male Urogenital Diseases—Problems and Exercises.   3. Urology—methods—Problems and Exercises. WJ 18.2]
    RC871.C33 2012 Suppl.
    616.60076—dc23
                                                                    2011014986

Acquisitions Editor: Stefanie Jewell-Thomas
Senior Developmental Editor: Maureen Iannuzzi
Publishing Services Manager: Patricia Tannian
Senior Project Manager: Kristine Feeherty
Design Direction: Lou Forgione

Printed in China

Last digit is the print number: 9   8   7   6   5   4   3   2

Robert Abouassaly, MD, MSc

Assistant Professor, Department of Urology
Case Western Reserve University School of Medicine;
Urologic Oncologist
Urologic Institute
University Hospitals Case Medical Center
Cleveland, Ohio

Paul Abrams, MD

Professor, Department of Urology
Bristol Urologic Institute
Southmead Hospital
Bristol, United Kingdom

Mark C. Adams, MD, FAAP

Professor, Department of Urology and Pediatrics
Vanderbilt University Medical Center;
Division of Pediatric Urology
Monroe Carell Jr. Children's Hospital at Vanderbilt
Nashville, Tennessee

Ashok Agarwal, PhD

Professor of Surgery
Department of Urology
Case Western Reserve University;
Director of Andrology
Director, Center for Reproductive Medicine
Department of Urology
Cleveland Clinic
Cleveland, Ohio

Mohamad E. Allaf, MD

Associate Professor, Departments of Urology, Oncology,
   and Biomedical Engineering
Johns Hopkins Medical Institutions;
Director of Minimally Invasive and Robotic Surgery
Johns Hopkins Hospital
Baltimore, Maryland

James Kyle Anderson, MD

Assistant Professor, Department of Urologic Surgery
University of Minnesota;
Staff Urologist, Department of Urologic Surgery
VA Medical Center
Minneapolis, Minnesota

Karl-Erik Andersson, MD, PhD

Professor, Department of Urology
Wake Forest University School of Medicine;
Professor, Institute for Regenerative Medicine
Wake Forest University Baptist Medical Center
Winston Salem, North Carolina

Kenneth W. Angermeier, MD

Associate Professor
Center for Genitourinary Reconstruction
Glickman Urological and Kidney Institute
Cleveland Clinic
Cleveland, Ohio

Emmanuel S. Antonarakis, MD

Assistant Professor of Oncology
Department of Medical Oncology
Johns Hopkins University;
Attending Physician, Department of Medical Oncology
Sidney Kimmel Comprehensive Cancer Center at John Hopkins
Baltimore, Maryland

Dean G. Assimos, MD

Professor of Surgical Sciences
Department of Urology
Wake Forest University School of Medicine;
Attending Physician, Department of Urology
Wake Forest University Baptist Medical Center
Winston-Salem, North Carolina

Anthony Atala, MD

W. Boyce Professor and Chair
Department of Urology
Wake Forest University School of Medicine;
Director, Wake Forest Institute for Regenerative Medicine
Winston Salem, North Carolina

Darius J. Bägli, MDCM, FRCSC, FAAP, FACS

Professor, Department of Surgery
Division of Urology and Institute of Medical Science
University of Toronto;
Senior Attending Urologist
Associate Surgeon-in-Chief
The Hospital for Sick Children;
Director of Urology Research
Senior Associate Scientist
Division of Developmental and Stem Cell Biology
The Hospital for Sick Children Research Institute
Toronto, Ontario, Canada

John Maynard Barry, MD

Professor Emeritus of Surgery
Divisions of Urology and Abdominal Organ Transplantation
The Oregon Health and Science University;
Staff Surgeon
University Hospital and Doenbecher Children's Hospital;
Consultant, Surgery
Veterans Affairs Medical Center
Portland, Oregon

Julia Spencer Barthold, MD

Professor of Urology and Pediatrics
Jefferson Medical College at Thomas Jefferson University
Philadelphia, Pennsylvania;
Associate Chief and Head of Urology Research Laboratory
Department of Surgery/Urology
Nemours/Alfred I. DuPont Hospital for Children;
Head, Urology Laboratory
Nemours Biomedical Research
Wilmington, Delaware

Stuart B. Bauer, MD

Professor of Surgery (Urology)
Harvard Medical School;
Senior Associate in Urology
Children's Hospital Boston
Boston, Massachusetts

Clair J. Beard, MD

Director, Testicular Cancer Center
Department of Radiation Oncology
Dana-Farber Cancer Institute and Brigham and Women's
   Hospital
Boston, Massachusetts

Arie S. Belldegrun, MD

Roy and Carol Doumani Chair in Urologic Oncology
Professor and Chief, Urologic Oncology
Director, Institute of Urologic Oncology
David Geffen School of Medicine at UCLA;
Department of Urology
Ronald Reagan UCLA Medical Center
Los Angeles, California

Mitchell C. Benson, MD

Herbert & Florence Irving and George F. Cahill Professor
   and Chair
Department of Urology
Columbia University College of Physicians and Surgeons;
Urologist-in-Chief, Department of Urology
New York-Presbyterian Hospital, Columbia University
   Medical Center
New York, New York

Brian M. Benway, MD

Assistant Professor, Department of Surgery
Division of Urologic Surgery
Washington University School of Medicine
St. Louis, Missouri

Ryan Kent Berglund, MD

Assistant Professor of Surgery
Glickman Urologic and Kidney Institute
Cleveland Clinic Lerner College of Medicine at Case Western
   Reserve University
Cleveland Clinic
Cleveland, Ohio

David M. Berman, MD, PhD

Associate Professor, Departments of Pathology, Oncology,
   and Urology
Johns Hopkins University School of Medicine;
Attending Pathologist
Johns Hopkins Hospital
Baltimore, Maryland

Sam B. Bhayani, MD

Associate Professor of Urology
Department of Surgery
Washington University School of Medicine
St. Louis, Missouri

Jay Todd Bishoff, MD, FACS

Clinical Professor of Surgery
Department of Urology
University of Utah School of Medicine;
Director, Intermountain Urological Institute
Intermountain Healthcare;
Director, Department of Urology
LDS Hospital
Salt Lake City, Utah;
Director, Department of Urology
Intermountain Medical Center
Murray, Utah

Michael L. Blute, Sr., MD

Professor, Department of Surgery
Mary C. DeFeudis Chair, Cancer Care and Research
University of Massachusetts Memorial Medical School;
Director, Cancer Center of Excellence
Interim Chief, Department of Urology
UMass Memorial Medical Center
Worcester, Massachusetts

Joseph G. Borer, MD

Assistant Professor, Department of Surgery
Harvard Medical School;
Assistant in Urology
Department of Urology
Children's Hospital Boston
Boston, Massachusetts

George J. Bosl, MD

Professor, Department of Medicine
Weill Cornell Medical College;
Chair, Department of Medicine
Memorial Sloan-Kettering Cancer Center
New York, New York

Charles B. Brendler, MD

Clinical Professor, Department of Surgery
Division of Urology
University of Chicago Medical Center
Chicago, Illinois;
Vice Chairman, Research and Development
Department of Surgery
North Shore University Health System
Evanston, Illinois

Gregory A. Broderick, MD

Professor, Department of Urology
Mayo Clinic College of Medicine;
Consultant, Department of Urology
Mayo Clinic
Jacksonville, Florida

James D. Brooks, MD

Associate Professor, Department of Urology
Stanford University School of Medicine
Stanford, California

Arthur L. Burnett, MD, MBA, FACS

Patrick C. Walsh Professor of Urology
Department of Urology
Johns Hopkins Medical Institutions
Baltimore, Maryland

Jeffrey A. Cadeddu, MD

Professor, Departments of Urology and Radiology
University of Texas Southwestern Medical Center
Dallas, Texas

Anthony A. Caldamone, MD, MMS, FAAP, FACS

Professor of Surgery (Urology) and Pediatrics
Division of Urology
Warren Alpert Medical School of Brown University
Rhode Island Hospital;
Head of Pediatric Urology
Hasbro Children's Hospital
Providence, Rhode Island

Steven C. Campbell, MD, PhD

Professor of Surgery
Department of Urology
Cleveland Clinic Lerner of College of Medicine at Case
   Western Reserve University;
Professor of Surgery
Director, Urology Residency Program
Vice Chairman, Urology
Center for Urologic Oncology
Cleveland Clinic
Cleveland, Ohio

Douglas A. Canning, MD

Professor, Department of Urology
University of Pennsylvania School of Medicine;
Director, Division of Pediatric Urology
The Children's Hospital of Philadelphia
Philadelphia, Pennsylvania

Michael A. Carducci, MD

AEGON Professor in Prostate Cancer Research
Departments of Oncology and Urology
Sidney Kimmel Comprehensive Cancer Center at Johns Hopkins
Baltimore, Maryland

Michael C. Carr, MD, PhD

Associate Professor, Department of Urology
University of Pennsylvania School of Medicine;
Attending Surgeon, Division of Pediatric Urology
The Children's Hospital of Philadelphia
Philadelphia, Pennsylvania

Peter R. Carroll, MD, MPH

Professor and Chair, Department of Urology
University of California, San Francisco
UCSF Medical Center
San Francisco, California

Herbert Ballentine Carter, MD

Professor, Departments of Urology and Oncology
Johns Hopkins School of Medicine
Baltimore, Maryland

Anthony J. Casale, MD

Professor and Chairman, Department of Urology
University of Louisville;
Chief of Urology
Kosair Children's Hospital;
Chief of Urology and Surgery (Urology)
University of Louisville Hospital
Louisville, Kentucky

Pasquale Casale, MD

Assistant Professor, Department of Urology
University of Pennsylvania School of Medicine;
Attending Surgeon, Division of Pediatric Urology
The Children's Hospital of Philadelphia
Philadelphia, Pennsylvania

William J. Catalona, MD

Professor, Department of Urology
Northwestern University Feinberg School of Medicine;
Director, Clinical Prostate Cancer Program
Robert H. Lurie Comprehensive Cancer Center
Northwestern Memorial Hospital
Chicago, Illinois

R. Duane Cespedes, MD

Associate Professor, Department of Urology
Johns Hopkins School of Medicine;
Co-Director, Women's Center for Pelvic Health
James Buchanan Brady Urological Institute
Johns Hopkins Medical Institutions
Baltimore, Maryland

Michael B. Chancellor, MD

Clinical Professor, Department of Urology
Oakland University William Beaumont School of Medicine;
Director, Neurourology Program
William Beaumont Hospital
Royal Oak, Michigan

Christopher R. Chapple, MD, FRCS (Urol), FEBU

Honorary Professor, Faculty of Health and Wellbeing
Sheffield Hallam University;
Honorary Senior Lecturer of Urology
University of Sheffield;
Consultant Urological Surgeon
Department of Urology
Sheffield Teaching Hospitals NHS Foundation Trust
Sheffield, United Kingdom;
Adjunct Secretary General for Education
European Association of Urology
Arnhem, The Netherlands

Christopher J. Chermansky, MD

Assistant Professor, Department of Urology
Louisiana State University Health Sciences Center New Orleans
  School of Medicine
New Orleans, Louisiana

Robert L. Chevalier, MD

Harrison Professor of Pediatrics
Department of Pediatrics
University of Virginia;
Pediatric Nephrologist
University of Virginia Health System
Charlottesville, Virginia

George K. Chow, MD

Assistant Professor, Department of Urology
Consultant in Urology
Mayo Clinic
Rochester, Minnesota

Jeanne S. Chow, MD

Assistant Professor, Department of Radiology
Harvard Medical School;
Pediatric Radiologist
Children's Hospital Boston
Boston, Massachusetts

Benjamin I. Chung, MD

Assistant Professor, Department of Urology
Stanford University School of Medicine;
Director, Laparoscopic and Minimally Invasive Urologic Surgery
Department of Urology
Stanford Hospital and Clinics
Stanford, California

Ralph V. Clayman, MD

Dean, University of California, Irvine School of Medicine
Professor, Department of Urology
University of California, Irvine;
Professor, Department of Urology
UC Irvine Medical Center
Orange, California
Professor, Department of Urology
Long Beach Veterans Administration Hospital
Long Beach, California

Michael Joseph Conlin, MD, FACS

Associate Professor of Urology
Department of Surgery
Oregon Health & Science University
Portland, Oregon

Raymond A. Costabile, MD

Senior Associate Dean for Clinical Strategy
Professor, Department of Urology
University of Virginia
Charlottesville, Virginia

Paul L. Crispen, MD

Assistant Professor, Department of Surgery
Division of Urology
University of Kentucky
Lexington, Kentucky

Juanita M. Crook, MD, FRCPC

Professor, Department of Radiation Oncology
University of British Columbia;
Active Medical Staff
Department of Radiation Oncology
Kelowna General Hospital;
Radiation Oncologist
British Columbia Cancer Agency
Kelowna, British Columbia, Canada

Douglas M. Dahl, MD

Assistant Professor of Surgery (Urology)
Harvard Medical School;
Associate Urologist
Massachusetts General Hospital
Boston, Massachusetts

Anthony V. D'Amico, MD, PhD

Professor and Chief, Genitourinary Radiation Oncology
Brigham and Women's Hospital and Dana-Farber
  Cancer Institute
Boston, Massachusetts

John W. Davis, MD

Assistant Professor, Department of Urology
University of Texas MD Anderson Cancer Center
Houston, Texas

G. Joel DeCastro, MD, MPH

Assistant Professor, Department of Urology
Columbia University College of Physicians and Surgeons
New York, New York

John D. Denstedt, MD, FRCSC, FACS

Richard Ivey Professor and Chair, Department of Surgery
Schulich School of Medicine & Dentistry
The University of Western Ontario
Richard Ivey Professor and Chair, Division of Urology
Department of Surgery
London Health Sciences Centre and St. Joseph's Health
  Care London
London, Ontario, Canada

Theodore L. DeWeese, MD

Professor and Chair, Department of Radiation Oncology
    and Molecular Radiation Sciences
Johns Hopkins University School of Medicine;
Radiation Oncologist-in-Chief
Johns Hopkins Hospital and Health System
Baltimore, Maryland

David Andrew Diamond, MD

Associate Professor of Surgery (Urology)
Harvard Medical School;
Senior Associate in Urology
Department of Urology
Children's Hospital Boston
Boston, Massachusetts

Roger R. Dmochowski, MD, FACS

Professor of Urologic Surgery
Vanderbilt University School of Medicine;
Director, Vanderbilt Continence Center
Director, Vanderbilt Female Reconstructive Fellowship
Executive Physician, Safety
Vanderbilt University Hospital
Nashville, Tennessee

Leo R. Doumanian, MD

Assistant Professor, Department of Urology
Temple University School of Medicine
Philadelphia, Pennsylvania

Marcus Drake, DM, MA, FRCS (Urol)

Senior Lecturer in Urology
School of Clinical Sciences
University of Bristol;
Consultant Surgeon
Urology Department
Southmead Hospital
Bristol, United Kingdom

Branden Duffey, DO

Endourology Fellow
Department of Urology
University of Minnesota and University of Minnesota
    Medical Center
Minneapolis, Minnesota

Daniel D. Dugi III, MD

Assistant Professor, Department of Urology
Oregon Health & Science University
Portland, Oregon

James A. Eastham, MD

Chief, Urology Service
Department of Surgery
Memorial Sloan-Kettering Cancer Center
New York, New York

Louis Eichel, MD

Clinical Assistant Professor, Department of Urology
University of Rochester Medical Center;
Director, Minimally Invasive Surgery
Center For Urology
Rochester, New York

Mario A. Eisenberger, MD

R. Dale Hughes Professor of Oncology and Urology
Johns Hopkins University and The Johns Hopkins Hospital
Baltimore, Maryland

Jonathan I. Epstein, MD

Reinhard Professor of Urological Pathology
Departments of Pathology, Urology, and Oncology
Johns Hopkins Medical Institutions;
Director, Surgical Pathology
Department of Pathology
Johns Hopkins Hospital
Baltimore, Maryland

Carlos R. Estrada, Jr., MD

Assistant Professor, Department of Surgery
Harvard Medical School;
Assistant in Urology
Department of Urology
Children's Hospital Boston
Boston, Massachusetts

Robert L. Fairchild, PhD

Professor, Department of Molecular Medicine
Cleveland Clinic;
Professor, Department of Pathology
Case Western Reserve University School of Medicine
Cleveland, Ohio

Amr Fergany, MD, PhD

Staff Sections of Oncology, Minimally Invasive Surgery,
    and Robotics
Glickman Urological and Kidney Institute
Cleveland Clinic
Cleveland, Ohio

Michael N. Ferrandino, MD

Assistant Professor, Department of Surgery
Division of Urology
Duke University and Duke University Medical Center
Durham, North Carolina

Lynne R. Ferrari, MD

Associate Professor, Department of Anethesia
Harvard Medical School;
Medical Director, Preoperative Services and Operating Rooms
Chief, Division of Perioperative Anesthesia
Department of Anethesiology, Perioperative, and Pain
    Management
Children's Hospital Boston
Boston, Massachusetts

James H. Finke, PhD

Professor of Molecular Medicine
Department of Pathology
Case Western Reserve University School of Medicine;
Professor of Immunology
Joint-Appointment, Glickman Urological Institute and Taussig
  Cancer Institute
Cleveland Clinic
Cleveland, Ohio

John M. Fitzpatrick, MCh, FRCSI

Professor and Chairman, Department of Surgery
University College Dublin;
Professor of Surgery and Consultant Urologist
Department of Urology
Mater Misericordiae University Hospital
Dublin, Ireland

Robert C. Flanigan, MD

Albert J. Jr. and Claire R. Speh Professor and Chair
Department of Urology
Loyola University Medical Center and Stritch School of
  Medicine;
Professor, Department of Urology
Loyola University Health System
Maywood, Illinois

Stuart M. Flechner, MD, FACS

Professor, Department of Surgery
Cleveland Clinic Lerner College of Medicine at Case Western
  Reserve University;
Director of Clinical Research
Section of Renal Transplantation
Glickman Urological and Kidney Institute
Cleveland Clinic
Cleveland, Ohio

Tara Lee Frenkl, MD, MPH

Clinical Associate, Department of Surgery
Division of Urology
University of Pennyslvania Medical Center
Philadelphia, Pennsylvania

Dominic C. Frimberger, MD

Associate Professor, Department of Urology
University of Oklahoma Health Sciences Center;
Department of Urology
Children's Hospital and Presbyterian Hospital
Oklahoma City, Oklahoma

Pat F. Fulgham, MD, DABU, FACS

Clinical Professor, Department of Urology
University of Texas Southwestern Medical School;
Surgical Director, Oncology Services
Texas Health Presbyterian Dallas
Dallas, Texas

John P. Gearhart, MD

Professor and Director
Division of Pediatric Urology
Johns Hopkins University School of Medicine
Baltimore, Maryland

Glenn S. Gerber, MD

Associate Professor of Surgery/Urology
University of Chicago Pritzker School of Medicine;
Director, Endourology
University of Chicago Medical Center
Chicago, Illinois

Jason L. Gerboc, DO

Staff Urologist
Department of Urology
Wilford Hall Medical Center
Lackland Air Force Base, Texas

Robert H. Getzenberg, PhD

The Donald S. Coffey Professor of Urology, Pharmacology,
  and Molecular Sciences
Department of Urology
Johns Hopkins University School of Medicine;
Director, James Buchanan Brady Urological Institute
Johns Hopkins Hospital
Baltimore, Maryland

Islam A. Ghoneim, MD, PhD

Staff, Urology Department
Cairo University
Cairo, Egypt;
Fellow, Department of Urology
Glickman Urologic and Kidney Institute
Cleveland Clinic
Cleveland, Ohio

Inderbir S. Gill, MD, MCh

Professor and Chairman, Department of Urology
Keck School of Medicine
University of Southern California;
Director, USC Institute of Urology
Los Angeles, California

Timothy D. Gilligan, MD, MS

Director, Late Effects Clinic
Program Director, Hematology/Oncology Fellowship
Department of Solid Tumor Oncology
Taussig Cancer Institute;
Deputy Editor, Cleveland Clinic Journal of Medicine
Cleveland Clinic
Cleveland, Ohio

David A. Goldfarb, MD

Professor of Surgery
Department of Urology
Cleveland Clinic Lerner College of Medicine at Case Western
    Reserve University;
Surgical Director, Renal Transplantaton
Department of Urology
Glickman Urological and Kidney Institute
Cleveland Clinic
Cleveland, Ohio

Marc Goldstein, MD, DSc (Hon)

Matthew P. Hardy Distinguished Professor, Urology and
    Reproductive Medicine
Weill Cornell Medical College;
Surgeon-in Chief, Male Reproductive Medicine and Surgery
Attending Urologist, Department of Urology
New York-Presbyterian Hospital, Weill Cornell Medical Center;
Senior Scientist, Center for Biomedical Reseach
The Population Council
New York, New York

Leonard G. Gomella, MD, FACS

Chairman, Department of Urology
The Bernard W. Godwin Jr. Professor of Prostate Cancer
Jefferson Medical College at Thomas Jefferson University;
Associate Director, Kimmel Cancer Center;
Director, Kimmel Cancer Center Network;
Chairman, Department of Urology
Thomas Jefferson University Hospital
Philadelphia, Pennsylvania

Mark L. Gonzalgo, MD, PhD

Associate Professor, Department of Urology
Stanford University School of Medicine
Stanford, California

Thomas J. Guzzo, MD, MPH

Assistant Professor of Urology
Department of Surgery, Division of Urology
University of Pennsylvania School of Medicine
Philadelphia, Pennsylvania

Ethan J. Halpern, MD, MSCE

Professor, Departments of Radiology and Urology
Jefferson Medical College at Thomas Jefferson University
Philadelphia, Pennsylvania

Misop Han, MD, MS

Associate Professor, Department of Urology
Johns Hopkins University School of Medicine;
Staff Surgeon, Department of Urology
Johns Hopkins Medical Institutions
Baltimore, Maryland

Philip M. Hanno, MD, MPH

Professor of Urology
Department of Surgery
University of Pennsylvania School of Medicine;
Attending Urologist, Department of Surgery
Hospital of the University of Pennsylvania and the Veterans
    Administration Medical Center
Philadelphia, Pennsylvania

Harry W. Herr, MD

Professor, Department of Urology
Weill Cornell Medical College;
Attending Surgeon, Department of Urology
Memorial Sloan-Kettering Cancer Center
New York, New York

Sender Herschorn, MDCM, FRCSC

Professor and Chairman, Division of Urology
Martin Barkin Chair, Urological Research
University of Toronto;
Attending Urologist, Division of Urology
Sunnybrook Health Sciences Centre
Toronto, Ontario, Canada

Thomas H.S. Hsu, MD

Director of Laparoscopic, Robotic, and Minimally Invasive
    Urologic Surgery
Northern California Kaiser Permanente Medical Center
Santa Clara, California

Mark Hurwitz, MD

Department of Radiation Oncology
Harvard Medical School;
Director, Regional Program Development
Department of Radiation Oncology
Dana-Farber/Brigham and Women's Cancer Center
Boston, Massachusetts

Douglas A. Husmann, MD

Professor and Chair, Department of Urology
Mayo Clinic
Rochester, Minnesota

Thomas W. Jarrett, MD

Professor and Chairman, Department of Urology
George Washington University School of Medicine
Washington, DC

J. Stephen Jones, MD, MBA

Professor of Surgery
Department of Urology
Cleveland Clinic Lerner College of Medicine at Case Western
    Reserve University;
Chairman, Department of Regional Urology
Glickman Urological and Kidney Institute
Cleveland Clinic
Cleveland, Ohio

Gerald H. Jordan, MD, FACS, FAAP (Hon), FRCS (Hon)

Professor, Department of Urology
Eastern Virginia Medical School;
Urology of Virginia
Norfolk, Virginia

David B. Joseph, MD, FACS, FAAP

Professor, Department of Surgery
Chief, Pediatric Urology
University of Alabama at Birmingham;
Beverly P. Head Endowed Chair in Pediatric Urology
Children's Hospital
Birmingham, Alabama

Martin Kaefer, MD, FAAP, FACS

Professor, Department of Urology
Division of Pediatric Urology
Indiana University School of Medicine
Indianapolis, Indiana

Jihad H. Kaouk, MD

Professor, Department of Surgery
Cleveland Clinic Learner College of Medicine;
Director, Laparoscopic and Robotic Surgery
Department of Urology
Cleveland Clinic
Cleveland, Ohio

Irving D. Kaplan, MD

Assistant Professor, Department of Radiation Oncology
Harvard Medical School;
Staff Radiation Therapist
Beth Israel Deaconess Medical Center
Boston, Massachusetts

Louis R. Kavoussi, MD, MBA

Chairman and Waldbaum-Gardner Distinguished Professor of Urology
Smith Institute for Urology
Hofstra North Shore–LIJ School of Medicine
Long Island, New York

Parviz K. Kavoussi, MD

Andrology Fellow
Department of Urology
University of Virginia
Charlottesville, Virginia;
Andrologist/Urologist
Austin Fertility & Reproductive Medicine
Austin, Texas

Patrick A. Kenney, MD

Clinical Associate, Department of Urology
Tufts University School of Medicine
Boston, Massachusetts;
Chief Resident, Institute of Urology
Lahey Clinic
Burlington, Massachusetts

Antoine E. Khoury, MD, FRCSC, FAAP

Professor, Department of Urology
Chief, Pediatric Urology
University of California, Irvine;
Medical Director, Pediatric Urology
Children's Hospital of Orange County;
Chief, Pediatric Urology
UCI Medical Center
Orange, California

Roger Sinclair Kirby, MD, MA, FRCS

Professor, Department of Urology
University of London;
The Prostate Centre
London, United Kingdom

Eric A. Klein, MD

Professor, Department of Surgery
Cleveland Clinic Lerner College of Medicine at Case Western Reserve University;
Chairman, Glickman Urological and Kidney Institute
Cleveland Clinic
Cleveland, Ohio

Kathleen C. Kobashi, MD

Associate Clinical Professor, Department of Urology
University of Washington School of Medicine;
Head, Section of Urology and Renal Transplantation
Department of Surgery
Virginia Mason Medical Center
Seattle, Washington

Michael O. Koch, MD

Chairman and John P. Donohue Professor
Department of Urology
Indiana University School of Medicine
Indianapolis, Indiana

John N. Krieger, MD

Professor, Department of Urology
University of Washington School of Medicine;
Chief, Department of Urology
VA Puget Sound Health Care System;
Attending Surgeon, Department of Urology
University of Washington Medical Center and Harborview Medical Center
Seattle, Washington

Bradley P. Kropp, MD, FAAP

Professor and Vice Chairman, Department of Urology
Chief, Pediatric Urology
University of Oklahoma Health Science Center
Oklahoma City, Oklahoma

Alexander Kutikov, MD

Assistant Professor of Urologic Oncology
Department of Surgical Oncology
Fox Chase Cancer Center
Philadelphia, Pennsylvania

Sarah M. Lambert, MD

Assistant Professor, Department of Surgery
The University of Pennsylvania;
Staff Urologist, Department of Surgery
The Children's Hospital of Philadelphia
Philadelphia, Pennsylvania

Raymond S. Lance, MD

The Paul F. Schellhammer Professor of Cancer Research
Associate Professor, Departments of Urology and Microbiology
  and Cancer Biology
Eastern Virginia Medical School;
Sentara Norfolk General Hospital
Sentara Medical Group—Urology of Virginia
Norfolk, Virginia

Brian R. Lane, MD, PhD

Clinical Associate Professor, Department of Surgery
Michigan State University;
Attending Physician, Department of Urology
Spectrum Health Hospital System
Grand Rapids, Michigan

William A. Larchian, MD

Associate Professor, Department of Surgery
Case Western Reserve University School of Medicine;
Center for Urologic Oncology
Urological Institute
University Hospitals Case Medical Center
Cleveland, Ohio

Richard S. Lee, MD

Assistant Professor of Surgery (Urology)
Harvard Medical School;
Assistant in Urology
Children's Hospital Boston
Boston, Massachusetts

Herbert Lepor, MD

Professor and Martin Spatz Chairman, Department of Urology
Professor of Pharmacology
New York University School of Medicine;
Director, Urology
NYU Langone Medical Center
New York, New York

Seth P. Lerner, MD, FACS

Professor, Department of Urology
Baylor College of Medicine;
Medical Staff, Department of Urology
The Methodist, St. Luke's Episcopal Hospital and Ben Taub
  General Hospital
Houston, Texas

John A. Libertino, MD

Professor, Department of Urology
Tufts University School of Medicine
Boston, Massachusetts;
Chair, Institute of Urology
Director, Sopltia Gordon Cancer Center
Lahey Clinic Medical Center
Burlington, Massachusetts

W. Marston Linehan, MD

Chief, Urologic Oncology Branch
National Cancer Institute;
Physician-in-Chief, Urologic Surgery
Clinical Research Center
National Institutes of Health
Bethesda, Maryland

James E. Lingeman, MD

Volunteer Clinical Professor, Department of Urology
Indiana University School of Medicine
Indianapolis, Indiana

Richard Edward Link, MD, PhD

Associate Professor, Department of Urology
Director, Division of Minimally Invasive Surgery
Scott Department of Urology
Baylor College of Medicine
Houston, Texas

Mark S. Litwin, MD, MPH

Professor of Urology and Health Services
UCLA School of Medicine and Public Health
University of California, Los Angeles
Los Angeles, California

Stacy Loeb, MD

Resident, Department of Urology
James Buchanan Brady Urological Institute
Johns Hopkins Medical Institutions
Baltimore, Maryland

Yair Lotan, MD

Associate Professor, Department of Urology
University of Texas Southwestern Medical Center
Dallas, Texas

Tom F. Lue, MD, ScD (Hon), FACS

Professor and Vice Chairman
Department of Urology
University of California, San Francisco
San Francisco, California

Dawn Lee MacLellan, MD, FRCSC

Assistant Professor, Departments of Urology, Surgery,
  and Pathology
Izaak Walton Killam Health Centre
Dalhousie University
Halifax, Nova Scotia, Canada

Stanley Bruce Malkowicz, MD
Co-Director, Urologic Oncology
Department of Urology
University of Pennsylvania
Philadelphia, Pennsylvania

Vitaly Margulis, MD
Assistant Professor, Department of Urology
The University of Texas Southwestern Medical Center
Dallas, Texas

Surena F. Matin, MD
Associate Professor, Department of Urology
The University of Texas MD Anderson Cancer Center
Houston, Texas

Ranjiv I. Mathews, MD
Associate Professor, Pediatric Urology
James Buchanan Brady Urological Institute
Johns Hopkins Medical Institutions
Baltimore, Maryland

Brian R. Matlaga, MD, MPH
Associate Professor, Department of Urology
Johns Hopkins University School of Medicine;
Director, Stone Disease
James Buchanan Brady Urological Institute
Baltimore, Maryland

Steven D. Mawhorter, MD, DTM&H
Associate Professor, Department of Medicine
Cleveland Clinic Lerner College of Medicine at Case Western
  Reserve University;
Staff Physician, Infectious Disease
Cleveland Clinic
Cleveland, Ohio

Kurt A. McCammon, MD, FACS
Assistant Professor and Chairman, Department of Urology
Eastern Virginia Medical School;
Chief, Department of Urology
Sentara Norfolk General Hospital;
Urology of Virginia
Norfolk, Virginia

W. Scott McDougal, MD, MA (Hon)
Professor of Urology
Harvard Medical School;
Chief, Urology
Massachusetts General Hospital
Boston, Massachusetts

Elspeth M. McDougall, MD, FRCSC, MHPE
Professor of Urology
Associate Dean of Continuing and Simulation
  Medical Education
Director, Minimally Invasive Surgery Education Center
University of California, Irvine
Irvine, California;
Chair, Office of Education
American Urological Association
Linthicum, Maryland

James M. McKiernan, MD
John and Irene Given Associate Professor of Urology
Department of Urology
Columbia University College of Physicians and Surgeons;
Associate Attending Urologist
New York-Presbyterian Hospital, Columbia University
  Medical Center
New York, New York

Alan W. McMahon, MD
Associate Professor, Department of Medicine
University of Alberta
Edmonton, Alberta, Canada

Thomas Anthony McNicholas, MBBS, FRCS, FEBU
Visiting Professor, Faculty of Health and Human Services
University of Hertfordshire;
Consultant Urological Surgeon
Department of Urology
Lister Hospital
Hertfordshire, United Kingdom;
Honorary Senior Lecturer
Institute of Urology
University College London
London, United Kingdom

Alan Keith Meeker, PhD, MA
Assistant Professor, Departments of Pathology, Urology,
  and Oncology
Johns Hopkins University School of Medicine
Baltimore, Maryland

Cathy Mendelsohn, PhD
Associate Professor, Departments of Urology, Pathology,
  and Genetics and Development
Columbia University College of Physicians and Surgeons
New York, New York

Carlos E. Méndez-Probst, MD
Fellow in Endourology
Department of Surgey
Schulisch School of Medicine and Dentistry
The University of Western Ontario and St. Joseph's Health
  Care London
London, Ontario, Canada

Maxwell V. Meng, MD

Associate Professor, Department of Urology
University of California, San Francisco
San Francisco, California

David C. Miller, MD, MPH

Assistant Professor, Department of Urology
University of Michigan Medical School
Ann Arbor, Michigan

Ian Milsom, MD, PhD

Professor, Department of Obstetrics and Gynecology
Institute of Clinical Sciences
Sahlgrenska Academy at Gothenburg University;
Consultant Gynecologist
Sahlgrenska University Hospital
Gothenburg, Sweden

Manoj Monga, MD, FACS

Professor, Department of Surgery
The Cleveland Clinic Lerner College of Medicine at Case
    Western Reserve University;
Director, Steven Streem Center for Endourology & Stone Disease
Glickman Urological Institute
Cleveland Clinic
Cleveland, Ohio

Drogo K. Montague, MD

Professor, Department of Surgery
Cleveland Clinic Lerner College of Medicine at Case Western
    Reserve University;
Director, Center for Genitourinary Reconstruction
Glickman Urological and Kidney Institute
Cleveland Clinic
Cleveland, Ohio

Courtenay Kathryn Moore, MD

Assistant Professor, Department of Surgery
Cleveland Clinic Lerner College of Medicine at Case Western
    Reserve University;
Staff Physcian
Glickman Urological and Kidney Institute
Cleveland Clinic
Cleveland, Ohio

Alvaro Morales, MD, FACS, FRCS

Professor, Department of Urology
Director, Centre for Applied Urological Research
Queen's University;
Attending, Department of Urology
Kingston General Hospital and the Hotel Dieu Hospital
Kingston, Ontario, Canada

Allen F. Morey, MD, FACS

Professor and Paul C. Peters MD Chair of Urology
Department of Urology
University of Texas Southwestern Medical Center;
Chief, Urology Service
Parkland Health and Hospital System
Dallas, Texas

Michael J. Morris, MD

Assistant Professor, Department of Medicine
Weill Cornell Medical College;
Assistant Member, Genitourinary Oncology Service
Department of Medicine
Memorial Sloan-Kettering Cancer Center
New York, New York

John P. Mulhall, MD, MSc (Anat)

Professor, Department of Urology
Weill Cornell Medical College;
Director, Sexual and Reproductive Medicine
Department of Urology Service
Memorial Sloan-Kettering Cancer Center
New York, New York

Stephen Y. Nakada, MD

David T. Uehling Professor and Chairman
Department of Urology
University of Wisconsin, Madison;
Professor and Chairman, Department of Urology
University of Wisconsin Hospital and Clinics
Madison, Wisconsin

Joel B. Nelson, MD

Frederic N. Schwentker Professor and Chairman
Department of Urology
University of Pittsburgh School of Medicine;
Chairman, Department of Surgery
UPMC Shadyside Hospital
Pittsburgh, Pennsylvania

J. Curtis Nickel, MD, FRCSC

Professor, Department of Urology
Queen's University;
Staff Urologist
Kingston General Hospital;
Canada Institute of Health Research Tier One
Canada Research Chair in Urologic Pain and Inflammation
Kingston, Ontario, Canada

Victor W. Nitti, MD

Professor and Vice Chairman, Department of Urology
New York University School of Medicine;
Attending Physician, Department of Urology
NYU Langone Medical Center
New York, New York

†Andrew C. Novick, MD

Chairman, Glickman Urological Institute
Cleveland Clinic Foundation
Professor of Surgery
Cleveland Clinic Lerner College of Medicine of Case Western
    Reserve University
Cleveland, Ohio

†Deceased.

Michael C. Ost, MD

Associate Professor, Department of Urology
University of Pittsburgh School of Medicine;
Associate Professor, Department of Urology
Children's Hospital of Pittsburgh
Magee-Women's Hospital
University of Pittsburgh Medical Center
Pittsburgh, Pennsylvania

Priya Padmanabhan, MD, MPH

Assistant Professor, Department of Urology
The University of Kansas Medical Center
Kansas City, Kansas

Jeffrey S. Palmer, MD, FACS, FAAP

Associate Professor of Surgery
Cleveland Clinic Lerner College of Medicine at Case Western
   Reserve University
Cleveland, Ohio

Lane S. Palmer, MD, FAAP, FACS

Clinical Professor, Department of Urology
Albert Einstein College of Medicine
Bronx, New York;
Chief, Department of Pediatric Urology
Cohen Children's Medical Center of New York
North Shore–Long Island Jewish Health System
New Hyde Park, New York

John M. Park, MD

Cheng-Yang Chang Professor of Pediatric Urology
Department of Urology
University of Michigan Medical School;
The University of Michigan Health System
Ann Arbor, Michigan

Alan W. Partin, MD, PhD

Professor and Director of Urology
Johns Hopkins School of Medicine
Baltimore, Maryland

Christopher K. Payne, MD

Associate Professor, Department of Urology (and Gynecology,
   by courtesy)
Stanford University School of Medicine;
Director, Female Urology & Neurourology
Stanford University Medical Center
Stanford, California

Margaret S. Pearle, MD, PhD

Professor, Departments of Urology and Internal Medicine
University of Texas Southwestern Medical Center
Dallas, Texas

Craig A. Peters, MD, FACS, FAAP

Chief, Division of Surgical Innovation, Technology,
   and Translation
Principle Investigator, Sheikh Zayed Institute for Pediatric
   Surgical Innovation
Children's National Medical Center
Washington, DC;
Professor of Urology
University of Virginia
Charlottesville, Virginia

Andrew C. Peterson, MD, FACS

Associate Professor of Urology
Department of Surgery
Duke University
Durham, North Carolina

Curtis A. Pettaway, MD

Professor, Departments of Urology and Cancer Biology
The University of Texas MD Anderson Cancer Center
Houston, Texas

Paul K. Pietrow, MD

Director, Minimally Invasive Surgery
Hudson Valley Urology, PC
Poughkeepsie, New York

Louis Leon Pisters, MD

Professor, Department of Urology
Surgical Staff, Department of Urology
University of Texas MD Anderson Cancer Center
Houston, Texas

Elizabeth A. Platz, ScD, MPH

Professor, Department of Epidemiology
Johns Hopkins University Bloomberg School of Public Health
Baltimore, Maryland

Emilio D. Poggio, MD

Associate Professor of Medicine, Nephrology, and Hypertension
Cleveland Clinic Lerner College of Medicine at Case Western
   Reserve University;
Director, Renal Function Laboratory
Glickman Urological and Kidney Institute
Cleveland Clinic
Cleveland, Ohio

John C. Pope IV, MD

Associate Professor, Departments of Urology, Surgery,
   and Pediatrics
Vanderbilt University Medical Center;
Associate Professor, Pediatric Urology
Monroe Carell Jr. Children's Hospital at Vanderbilt
Nashville, Tennessee

Jeannette M. Potts, MD

Director, Pelvic Pain Center and Alternative Urological Therapies
Urological Institute
Case Western Reserve University;
University Hospitals of Cleveland
Cleveland, Ohio

Glenn M. Preminger, MD

Professor of Urologic Surgery
Director, Duke Comprehensive Kidney Stone Center
Duke University Medical Center
Durham, North Carolina

John C. Rabets, MD

Department of Urology
Glickman Urological and Kidney Institute
Cleveland Clinic
Cleveland, Ohio

Raymond Robert Rackley, MD

Professor, Department of Surgery
Cleveland Clinic Lerner College of Medicine at Case Western
    Reserve University;
Staff, Center for Pelvic Health and Recontructive Surgery
Glickman Urological and Kidney Institute;
Director, Urothelial Biology Laboratory
Department of Cancer Biology
Lerner Research Institute
Cleveland Clinic
Cleveland, Ohio

Hassan Razvi, MD, FRCSC

Professor and Chairman, Division of Urology
Department of Surgery
Schulich School of Medicine and Dentistry
University of Western Ontario;
Chief, Division of Urology
St. Joseph's Hospital and London Health Sciences Centre
London, Ontario, Canada

Neil M. Resnick, MD

Thomas Detre Endowed Professor of Medicine
Department of Medicine
University of Pittsburgh School of Medicine;
Chief, Division of Geriatric Medicine and Gerontology
Department of Medicine;
Associate Director, Institute on Aging
University of Pittsburgh Medical Center
Pittsburgh, Pennsylvania

Lee Richstone, MD

Assistant Professor, Department of Urology
Hofstra–North Shore LIJ School of Medicine;
Director, Laparoscopic and Robotic Surgery
The Smith Institute for Urology
The North Shore University Hospital (NSUH)
New Hyde Park, New York;
Assistant Professor, Department of Urology
The Albert Einstein College of Medicine
New York, New York

Richard C. Rink, MD, FACS, FAAP

Robert A. Gameh Professor of Pediatric Urologic Research
Department of Pediatric Urology
Indiana University School of Medicine;
Chief, Pediatric Urology
Riley Hospital for Children
Indianapolis, Indiana

Michael L. Ritchey, MD, FAAP, FACS

Professor, Department of Urology
Mayo Clinic College of Medicine
Scottsdale, Arizona;
Chief, Department of Surgery
Phoenix Children's Hospital
Phoenix, Arizona

Ronald Rodriguez, MD, PhD

Associate Professor, Department of Urology
Johns Hopkins University School of Medicine
Baltimore, Maryland

Claus G. Roehrborn, MD

Professor and Chairman, Department of Urology
University of Texas Southwestern Medical School;
Attending Urologist
University Hospital UT Southwestern Medical Center
Parkland Health and Hospital System
VA Medical Center
Dallas, Texas

Eric S. Rovner, MD

Professor, Department of Urology
Medical University of South Carolina;
Attending Staff, Department of Urology
Medical University Hospital
Charleston, South Carolina

Edmund Sabanegh, Jr., MD

Chairman, Department of Urology
Cleveland Clinic
Cleveland, Ohio

Arthur I. Sagalowsky, MD

Professor and Dr. Paul Peters Chair in Urology in Memory of
    Rumsey and Louis Strickland
Department of Urology
Chief, Urology Oncology
University of Texas Southwestern Medical Center;
Department of Urology
Zale Lipshy University Medical Center
St. Paul University Medical Center
Dallas, Texas

Richard A. Santucci, MD

Clinical Professor, Department of Urology
Michigan State College of Osteopathic Medicine;
Specialist-in-Chief, Department of Urology
The Detroit Medical Center
Detroit, Michigan

Peter T. Scardino, MD, FACS

Attending Urologist
New York-Presbyterian Hospital, Weill Cornell Medical Center;
The David H. Koch Chair, Department of Surgery
Memorial Sloan-Kettering Cancer Center
New York, New York

Harriette Miles Scarpero, MD

Associated Urologists
St. Thomas Hospital
Nashville, Tennessee

Anthony J. Schaeffer, MD

Chairman and Herman L. Kretschmer Professor
Department of Urology
Northwestern University Feinberg School of Medicine;
Chairman, Department of Urology
Northwestern Memorial Hospital
Chicago, Illinois

Edward M. Schaeffer, MD, PhD

Associate Professor, Department of Urology
John Hopkins University;
James Buchanan Brady Urological Institute
John Hopkins Medical Institutions
Baltimore, Maryland

Howard I. Scher, MD

Professor, Department of Medicine
Weill Cornell Medical College;
Chief, Genitourinary Oncology Service
Department of Medicine
Memorial Sloan-Kettering Cancer Center
New York, New York

Douglas S. Scherr, MD

The Ronald Stanton Clinical Scholar in Urology
Associate Professor, Department of Urology
Weill Cornell Medical College;
Associate Professor of Urology, Department of Urology
New York-Presbyterian Hospital
New York, New York

Richard N. Schlussel, MD

Assistant Professor, Department of Urology
Columbia University College of Physicians and Surgeons;
Associate Director, Pediatric Urology
Morgan Stanley Children's Hospital of New York-Presbyterian
New York, New York

Francis X. Schneck, MD

Associate Professor, Department of Urology
University of Pittsburgh Medical Center;
Clinical Director, Department of Pediatric Urology
Children's Hospital of Pittsburgh
Pittsburgh, Pennsylvania

Michael J. Schwartz, MD

Assistant Professor, Department of Urology
Hofstra North Shore–LIJ School of Medicine
Hempstead, New York;
Attending Physician
Arthur Smith Institute for Urology;
North Shore University Hospital
New Hyde Park, New York;
Long Island Jewish Hospital
Manhasset, New York

Robert C. Shamberger, MD

Robert E. Gross Professor, Department of Surgery
Harvard Medical School;
Chief, Department of Surgery
Children's Hospital Boston
Boston, Massachusetts

Ellen Shapiro, MD

Professor, Department of Urology
New York University School of Medicine;
Director, Pediatric Urology
NYU Langone Medical Center
New York, New York

David S. Sharp, MD

Assistant Professor, Department of Urology
Ohio State University Medical Center;
Attending Physician, Department of Urology
James Cancer Hospital and Solove Research Institute
Columbus, Ohio

Joel Sheinfeld, MD

Professor, Department of Urology
Weill Cornell Medical College;
Deputy Chief, Department of Urology
Memorial Sloan-Kettering Cancer Center
New York, New York

Linda Marie Dairiki Shortliffe, MD

Stanley McCormick Memorial Professor and Chair of Urology
Department of Urology
Stanford University School of Medicine;
Chief, Department of Urology
Stanford University Medical Center;
Chief, Pediatric Urology
Lucile Salter Packard Children's Hospital
Stanford, California

Daniel A. Shoskes, MD, MSc, FRCSC

Professor, Department of Urology
Cleveland Clinic Lerner College of Medicine at Case Western
    Reserve University;
Director, Novick Center for Clinical and Translational Research
Glickman Urological and Kidney Institute
Cleveland Clinic
Cleveland, Ohio

Jennifer D.Y. Sihoe, MD, BMBS, BMedSci (Hons), FRCSEd (Paed), FHKAM (Surg)

Honorary Clinical Assistant Professor
Department of Surgery
The Chinese University of Hong Kong;
Associate Consultant
Divisions of Pediatric Surgery and Pediatric Urology
Prince of Wales Hospital
Hong Kong

Iqbal Singh, MCh (Urology), DNB (Genitourinary Surgery), MS, DNB

Professor of Urology
Department of Surgery
University of Delhi College of Medical Sciences;
Senior Consultant Urologist
Department of Surgery
UCMS and Guru Teg Bahadur Hospital
Delhi, India;
Formerly Clinical Instructor (Fellow)
Department of Urology
Wake Forest University School of Medicine and WFUMC and
 Baptist Medical Center
Winston-Salem, North Carolina

Donald G. Skinner, MD

Professor and Chair *(Retired)*
Department of Urology
Keck School of Medicine
University of Southern California;
USC Norris Comprehensive Cancer Center
Los Angeles, California

Eila C. Skinner, MD

Professor of Clinical Urology
Department of Urology
Keck School of Medicine
University of Southern California;
Attending Physician, Department of Urology
USC University Hospital and Norris Comprehensive
 Cancer Center
LAC + USC Medical Center
Los Angeles, California

Joseph A. Smith, Jr., MD

Professor and Chairman, Department of Urologic Surgery
Vanderbilt University Medical Center
Nashville, Tennessee

Warren T. Snodgrass, MD

Professor, Department of Urology
University of Texas Southwestern Medical Center;
Chief, Pediatric Urology
Children's Medical Center Dallas
Dallas, Texas

Graham Sommer, MD

Professor of Radiology
Division of Diagnostic Radiology
Stanford University School of Medicine
Stanford, California

Ramaprasad Srinivasan, MD, PhD

Senior Staff Clinician, Department of Urologic Oncology
National Cancer Institute
National Institutes of Health
Bethesda, Maryland

[†]John P. Stein, MD

Associate Professor, Department of Urology
Keck School of Medicine
University of Southern California;
USC Norris Comprehensive Cancer Center
Los Angeles, California

Andrew J. Stephenson, MD, FACS, FRCSC

Associate Professor, Department of Urology
Cleveland Clinic Lerner College of Medicine at Case Western
 Reserve University;
Director, Center for Urologic Oncology
Glickman Urological and Kidney Institute
Cleveland Clinic
Cleveland, Ohio

Cora N. Sternberg, MD, FACP

Chief, Department of Medical Oncology
San Camillo Forlanini Hospital
Rome, Italy

Jack W. Strandhoy, PhD

Professor, Deparment of Physiology and Pharmacology
Wake Forest University School of Medicine
Winston-Salem, North Carolina

Li-Ming Su, MD

David A. Cofrin Professor of Urology
Associate Chairman of Clinical Affairs
Department of Urology
University of Florida College of Medicine
Gainesville, Florida

Stasa D. Tadic, MD, MS

Assistant Professor, Department of Medicine
Division of Geriatric Medicine and Gerontology
University of Pittsburgh School of Medicine;
Attending Physician, Department of Medicine
Division of Geriatric Medicine and Gerontology
University of Pittsburgh Medical Center
Pittsburgh, Pennsylvania

[†]Deceased.

Ian M. Thompson, Jr., MD

Director, Cancer Therapy and Research Center
Professor, Department of Urology
University of Texas Health Science Center at San Antonio
San Antonio, Texas

Joanna Maya Togami, MD

Clinical Assistant Professor, Department of Urology
Louisiana State University School of Medicine;
Senior Staff Urologist, Department of Urology
Ochsner Medical Center
New Orleans, Louisiana

Edouard J. Trabulsi, MD, FACS

Associate Professor, Department of Surgery
Jefferson Medical College at Thomas Jefferson University;
Associate Professor, Department of Urology
Co-Director, Jefferson Prostate Diagnostic Center
Kimmel Cancer Center
Thomas Jefferson University Hospital
Philadelphia, Pennsylvania

Howard Trachtman, MD

Professor, Department of Pediatrics
Albert Einstein College of Medicine
Bronx, New York;
Chief, Division of Nephrology
Department of Pediatrics
Cohen Children's Medical Center of New York
New Hyde Park, New York;
Investigator
Feinstein Institute for Medical Research
Manhasset, New York

Paul J. Turek, MD, FACS, FRSM

Director, The Turek Clinic;
Attending Physician, Department of Urology
California Pacific Medical Center;
Founder, Clinic by the Bay Volunteer Medical Clinic
San Francisco, California

Robert G. Uzzo, MD

G. Willing Pepper Chair, Department of Surgery
Professor of Urologic Oncology
Department of Surgical Oncology
Fox Chase Cancer Center
Philadelphia, Pennsylvania

Sandip P. Vasavada, MD

Associate Professor of Surgery (Urology)
Cleveland Clinic Lerner College of Medicine at Case Western
    Reserve University;
Center for Female Pelvic Medicine and Genitourinary
    Reconstructive Surgery
Glickman Urological and Kidney Institute
Cleveland Clinic
Cleveland, Ohio

Robert W. Veltri, PhD

Associate Professor, Departments of Urology and Oncology
Johns Hopkins School of Medicine;
James Buchanan Brady Urological Institute
Johns Hopkins Medical Institutions
Baltimore, Maryland

Manish A. Vira, MD

Director, Fellowship Program in Urologic Oncology
Assistant Professor of Urology
Hofstra North Shore LIJ School of Medicine
North Shore Long Island Jewish Health System
New Hyde Part, New York

Patrick C. Walsh, MD

University Distinguished Service Professor of Urology
Department of Urology
Johns Hopkins University School of Medicine;
James Buchanan Brady Urological Institute
John Hopkins Medical Institutions;
Department of Urology
Johns Hopkins Hospital
Baltimore, Maryland

Thomas J. Walsh, MD, MS

Assistant Professor, Department of Urology
University of Washington School of Medicine
Seattle, Washington

Alan J. Wein, MD, PhD (Hon)

Professor and Chair, Division of Urology
University of Pennsylvania Health System
Philadelphia, Pennsylvania

Robert M. Weiss, MD

Donald Gutherie Professor, Department of Surgery
Division of Urology
Yale University School of Medicine;
Chief, Division of Urology
Department of Surgery
Yale-New Haven Hospital
New Haven, Connecticut

Hunter Wessells, MD, FACS

Professor and Nelson Chair, Department of Urology
University of Washington School of Medicine
Seattle, Washington

Wesley M. White, MD

Director, Laparoscopic and Robotic Urologic Surgery
Department of Urology
The University of Tennessee Medical Center, Knoxville
Knoxville, Tennessee

Jack Christian Winters, MD

Chairman, Department of Urology
H. Eustis Reilly Professor of Urology and Gynecology
Louisiana State University School of Medicine;
Fellowship Director, Female Pelvic Medicine and Reconstructive
  Surgery
Department of Urology and Gynecology
Louisiana State University Health Sciences Center
New Orleans, Louisiana

J. Stuart Wolf, Jr., MD, FACS

The David A. Bloom Professor of Urology
Director, Division of Endourology
Department of Urology
University of Michigan Health System
Ann Arbor, Michigan

Christopher G. Wood, MD

Professor and Deputy Chairman
Department of Urology
The University of Texas MD Anderson Cancer Center
Houston, Texas

David P. Wood, Jr., MD

The George F. and Sandra G. Valassis Professor of Urology
University of Michigan Medical School;
Chief, Urologic Oncology
Department of Urology
University of Michigan Hospital
Ann Arbor, Michigan

John R. Woodard, MD

Clinical Professor of Urology (Retired)
Director, Pediatric Urology (Retired)
Emory University School of Medicine;
Chief of Urology (Retired)
Henrietta Egleston Hospital for Children
Atlanta, Georgia

Chad Wotkowicz, MD

Senior Staff, Department of Urology
Lahey Clinic
Burlington, Massachusetts

Subbarao V. Yalla, MD

Professor of Surgery (Urology)
Harvard Medical School;
Urologist, Surgical Service
Brigham and Women's Hospital
VA Boston Healthcare System
Boston, Massachusetts;
Urologist, Surgical Service
Togus VA Medical Center
Augusta, Maine

C.K. Yeung, MD

Honorary Clinical Professor in Paediatric Surgery &
  Paediatric Urology
Chinese University of Hong Kong;
Chief of Paediatric Surgery & Paediatric Urology
Union Hospital
Hong Kong

Naoki Yoshimura, MD, PhD

Professor, Department of Urology
University of Pittsburgh School of Medicine
Pittsburgh, Pennsylvania

Richard N. Yu, MD, PhD

Instructor in Surgery (Urology)
Harvard Medical School;
Department of Urology
Children's Hospital Boston
Boston, Massachusetts

HOW TO USE THIS STUDY GUIDE

The questions pertaining to each chapter are meant to review the material presented in the chapter, not as a substitute for reading it. Important points covered in the chapter that were not addressed by the questions are noted at the end of each study guide section in the Additional Study Points. Many of the questions are written for teaching purposes and are not meant to mimic those found in standardized tests; therefore, the formats used for some questions, such as "True/False," "All of the following are true EXCEPT," and "More than one answer may be correct," are not acceptable for standardized tests but are very good for reviewing the chapter. Finally, the imaging and pathology questions are included to make the guide comprehensive. The intent of the Study Guide is to provide the reader with a thorough review of each chapter.

W. Scott McDougal, MD, MA (Hon)

A WORD FROM THE PUBLISHER

This edition of the *Campbell-Walsh Urology Review* includes complimentary access to an Expert Consult online version. In addition to allowing access to the full text online, it also includes a test module to allow you to work through the content in an interactive environment. The questions are available in both a challenging Study Mode and a timed Assessment Mode.

Answers, rationales, and scores are presented in both modes of review.

To access your interactive self-assessment questions, please follow the activation instructions on the inside cover of this book. Once you have logged onto the book's website, select "Review Questions" on the site header to begin.

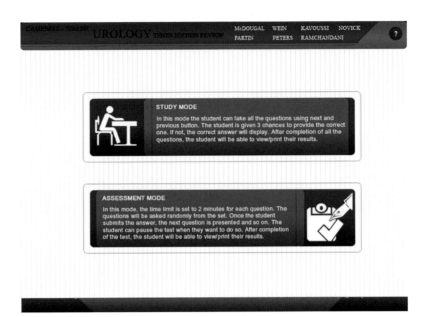

Choose Study Mode to work through questions at your own pace or Assessment Mode for a timed examination simulation.

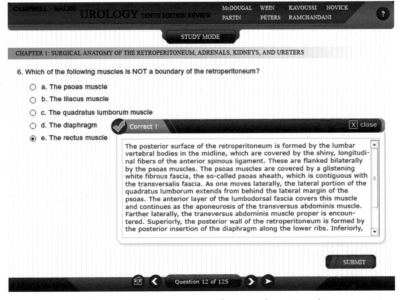

Review each correct answer with a complete rationale.

Contents

SECTION XVII

PEDIATRIC UROLOGY

CAMPBELL-WALSH

Urology

Tenth Edition Review

Anatomy

Surgical Anatomy of the Retroperitoneum, Adrenals, Kidneys, and Ureters

James Kyle Anderson, MD ● Jeffrey A. Cadeddu, MD

QUESTIONS

1. The lumbodorsal fascia originates from the:
   a. latissimus dorsi muscle.
   b. lower rib cage posteriorly.
   c. lumbar vertebrae.
   d. iliac crest.
   e. rectus sheath.

2. The lumbodorsal fascia consists of:
   a. a single layer.
   b. two distinct layers.
   c. three distinct layers.
   d. four distinct layers.
   e. five distinct layers.

3. The lumbodorsal fascia is contiguous anteriorly with the:
   a. transversalis fascia.
   b. aponeurosis of the transversus abdominis muscle.
   c. internal oblique fascia.
   d. external oblique fascia.
   e. rectus sheath.

4. The dorsal lumbotomy incision to expose the kidney:
   a. requires incision of the latissimus dorsi muscle.
   b. requires incision of the quadratus lumborum muscle.
   c. splits the lumbodorsal fascia horizontally from posterior to anterior.
   d. splits the lumbodorsal fascia vertically without incising muscle.
   e. requires excision of the 12th rib.

5. The psoas major muscle:
   a. flexes the thigh at the hip.
   b. extends the thigh at the hip.
   c. adducts the thigh at the hip.
   d. abducts the thigh at the hip.
   e. assists in full contraction of the diaphragm.

6. Which of the following muscles is NOT a boundary of the retroperitoneum?
   a. The psoas muscle
   b. The iliacus muscle
   c. The quadratus lumborum muscle
   d. The diaphragm
   e. The rectus muscle

7. In a subcostal flank approach to the kidney, which of the following may be incised to increase upward mobility of the 12th rib?
   a. The intercostal muscles between the 11th and 12th ribs
   b. The latissimus dorsi muscle
   c. The lumbodorsal fascia
   d. The quadratus lumborum muscle
   e. The costovertebral ligament

8. The first arterial branch(es) from the abdominal aorta is(are):
   a. the paired renal arteries.
   b. the right adrenal artery.
   c. the inferior phrenic artery.
   d. the hepatic artery.
   e. the superior mesenteric artery.

9. Which of the following arteries branches from the celiac arterial trunk?
   a. The left gastric artery
   b. The right gastric artery
   c. The pancreaticoduodenal artery
   d. The superior mesenteric artery
   e. The inferior phrenic arteries

10. The renal arteries typically branch from the abdominal aorta at the level of the:
    a. 12th thoracic vertebral body.
    b. 1st lumbar vertebral body.
    c. 2nd lumbar vertebral body.
    d. 3rd lumbar vertebral body.
    e. 4th lumbar vertebral body.

11. The testicular arteries most commonly originate from the:
    a. renal arteries.
    b. adrenal arteries.
    c. abdominal aorta above the superior mesenteric artery.
    d. abdominal aorta below the renal arteries.
    e. common iliac arteries.

12. A 20-year-old man is undergoing retroperitoneal dissection for a testicular germ cell tumor. The inferior mesenteric artery is divided during reflection of the intestines to expose the retroperitoneum. This can be expected to result in:
    a. ischemia of the descending colon.
    b. ischemia of the sigmoid colon.
    c. ischemia of the rectum.
    d. ischemia of the transverse colon.
    e. none of the above.

13. Which of the following vessels drain(s) into the inferior vena cava?
    a. Renal veins
    b. Superior mesenteric vein
    c. Inferior mesenteric vein
    d. Splenic vein
    e. All of the above

14. The left gonadal vein typically drains into the:
    a. anterior aspect of the inferior vena cava.
    b. left lateral aspect of the inferior vena cava.
    c. inferior aspect of the left renal vein.
    d. left adrenal vein.
    e. inferior aspect of the common iliac vein.

15. The left renal vein crosses the abdominal aorta:
    a. anteriorly, just above the superior mesenteric artery.
    b. anteriorly, just below the superior mesenteric artery.
    c. posteriorly, at the level of the superior mesenteric artery.
    d. anteriorly, just below the inferior mesenteric artery.
    e. anteriorly, just above the inferior mesenteric artery.

16. Which of the following vessels commonly drains into the left renal vein?
    a. The left adrenal vein
    b. The second lumbar vein
    c. The left internal spermatic vein
    d. All of the above
    e. None of the above

17. On a CT scan, a male patient is found to have enlarged lymph nodes along the abdominal aorta between the left renal hilum and the inferior mesenteric artery. Sites of malignancy that would commonly drain directly to these lymph nodes would NOT include the:
    a. colon.
    b. left kidney.
    c. left testis.
    d. left renal pelvis.
    e. bladder.

18. Lymph flow in the lumbar lymphatic chains of the retroperitoneum proceeds:
    a. in a cephalad direction.
    b. in a cephalad direction and from right to left.
    c. in a cephalad direction and from left to right.
    d. caudally.
    e. caudally and from left to right.

19. The cisterna chyli is typically located at approximately the level of the first lumbar vertebral body:
    a. posterior to the inferior vena cava.
    b. posterior to the aorta.
    c. closely approximated to the posterior surface of the right adrenal gland.
    d. associated with the superior mesenteric artery.
    e. posterior to the right renal hilum.

20. The primary lymph node drainage site for the right testis is the:
    a. superficial right inguinal lymph nodes.
    b. deep right inguinal lymph nodes.
    c. right common iliac lymph nodes.
    d. lymph nodes at the right renal hilum.
    e. interaortocaval lumbar lymph nodes.

21. The lumbar sympathetic chains:
    a. run vertically in the retroperitoneum, medial to the psoas muscles.
    b. contain numerous sympathetic ganglia.
    c. are closely associated with the lumbar blood vessels.
    d. contain postganglionic sympathetic neurons supplying the lower extremities.
    e. do all of the above.

22. Disruption of which sympathetic nervous plexus on the anterior abdominal aorta during retroperitoneal dissection will likely cause loss of seminal emission?
    a. Celiac plexus
    b. Renal plexus
    c. Superior mesenteric plexus
    d. Superior hypogastric plexus
    e. All of the above

23. In the lateral abdominal wall, the iliohypogastric nerve will be found coursing in the plane:
    a. deep to the transversalis fascia.
    b. between the transversalis fascia and the transversus abdominis muscle.
    c. between the transversus abdominis and internal oblique muscles.
    d. between the internal oblique and external oblique muscles.
    e. superficial to the external oblique muscle.

24. The cremaster muscle is innervated by the:
    a. ilioinguinal nerve.
    b. iliohypogastric nerve.
    c. obturator nerve.
    d. genital branch of the genitofemoral nerve.
    e. femoral branch of the genitofemoral nerve.

25. In the retroperitoneum, where can the genitofemoral nerve be found?
    a. Posterior to the psoas muscle
    b. On the anterior surface of the psoas muscle
    c. Lateral to the psoas muscle
    d. Medial to the psoas muscle
    e. The genitofemoral nerve is not typically found in the retroperitoneum.

26. The descending duodenum:
    a. lies within the retroperitoneum.
    b. receives the common bile duct.
    c. lies lateral to the head of the pancreas.
    d. lies anterior to the right renal hilum.
    e. does all of the above.

27. The posterior surface of the tail of the pancreas is closely associated with:
    a. the splenic artery.
    b. the splenic vein.
    c. the upper pole of the left kidney.
    d. the left adrenal gland.
    e. all of the above.

28. In cases of renal ectopia, the ipsilateral adrenal gland is typically:
    a. absent.
    b. found in its normal anatomic position in the upper retroperitoneum.
    c. found in association with the contralateral adrenal gland.
    d. found closely applied to the superior pole of the ectopic kidney.
    e. found closely associated with the ipsilateral renal artery.

29. In cases of unilateral renal agenesis, the ipsilateral adrenal gland is commonly:
    a. absent.
    b. found in its normal anatomic position in the upper retroperitoneum.
    c. found in association with the contralateral adrenal gland.
    d. found just inside the ipsilateral internal inguinal ring.
    e. found in an ectopic, intrathoracic location.

30. Which of the following statements is NOT true?
    a. The right renal vein is much shorter than the left renal vein.
    b. The right adrenal vein is much shorter than the left adrenal vein.
    c. The right kidney is typically located lower in the retroperitoneum than the left kidney.
    d. The right adrenal gland is typically located lower in the retroperitoneum than the left adrenal gland.
    e. Both c and d

31. As one proceeds outward from the adrenal medulla, the three separate functional layers of the adrenal cortex are, in correct order:
    a. zona reticularis, zona fasciculata, and zona glomerulosa.
    b. zona fasciculata, zona reticularis, and zona glomerulosa.
    c. zona glomerulosa, zona fasciculata, and zona reticularis.
    d. zona glomerulosa, zona reticularis, and zona fasciculata.
    e. zona reticularis, zona glomerulosa, and zona fasciculata.

32. Which of the following statements is (are) NOT true?
    a. The adrenal medulla produces catecholamines in response to stimulation from the sympathetic nervous system.
    b. The zona glomerulosa produces aldosterone in response to angiotensin II.
    c. The zona reticularis of the adrenal cortex produces androgens in response to luteinizing hormone (LH).
    d. The zona fasciculate of the adrenal cortex produces glucocorticoids in response to adrenocorticotropic hormone (ACTH).
    e. Both b and c

33. The adrenal arteries are branches from:
    a. the aorta.
    b. the inferior phrenic arteries.
    c. the renal arteries.
    d. the celiac arterial trunk.
    e. a, b, and c.

34. The kidney produces:
    a. renin.
    b. angiotensin.
    c. erythropoietin.
    d. both a and c.
    e. a, b, and c.

35. The normal kidney in an average-sized adult man weighs approximately:
    a. 1200 g.
    b. 600 g.
    c. 300 g.
    d. 150 g.
    e. 50 g.

36. Persistent fetal lobation identified in the kidney of an adult patient:
    a. indicates the presence of a congenital renal disorder.
    b. indicates childhood renal injury due to infection.
    c. is observed only with long-standing obstructive uropathy.
    d. is normal.
    e. is never seen.

37. The upper pole of the kidney lies anterior to:
    a. the 12th rib.
    b. the diaphragm.
    c. the pleura.
    d. all of the above.
    e. none of the above.

38. Which of the following statements regarding the typical anatomic positioning of the kidney is TRUE?
    a. The lower pole of the kidney lies more anterior than the upper pole.
    b. The lower pole of the kidney lies more lateral than the upper pole.

c. The medial aspect of the kidney lies more anterior than its lateral aspect.

d. The anterior renal calyces lie lateral to the posterior renal calyces.

e. All of the above.

39. During left radical nephrectomy performed via a transabdominal approach, excessive traction on which of the following structures might be expected to produce a significant injury to the spleen?

a. Left adrenal gland

b. Splenorenal ligament

c. Splenocolic ligament

d. Both b and c

e. a, b, and c

40. Gerota fascia envelops and contains:

a. the adrenal gland.

b. the kidney.

c. the ureter.

d. the gonadal vessels.

e. all of the above.

41. After blunt trauma to the right kidney, with a major laceration to the renal parenchyma and ongoing hemorrhage, the expanding hematoma contained within Gerota fascia will tend to extend:

a. across the midline into Gerota fascia surrounding the left (contralateral) kidney.

b. downward into the pelvis.

c. upward into the thorax.

d. anterolaterally, deep to the transversalis fascia.

e. anterolaterally, between the peritoneum and transversalis fascia.

42. Proceeding from posterior to anterior, the structures encountered in the renal hilum are, in correct order, the:

a. renal artery, renal vein, and renal pelvis.

b. renal pelvis, renal artery, and renal vein.

c. renal pelvis, renal vein, and renal artery.

d. renal vein, renal artery, and renal pelvis.

e. renal artery, renal pelvis, and renal vein.

43. The first branch segmental artery from the main renal artery is typically the:

a. apical anterior segmental artery.

b. lower anterior segmental artery.

c. posterior segmental artery.

d. upper anterior segmental artery.

e. middle anterior segmental artery.

44. During pyeloplasty, the posterior segmental renal artery is inadvertently divided. This will produce:

a. no effect on the kidney.

b. ischemic loss of a large posterior segment of the renal parenchyma.

c. ischemic loss of a small posterior segment of the renal parenchyma.

d. ischemic loss of a segment of upper pole renal parenchyma.

e. ischemic loss of a segment of lower pole renal parenchyma.

45. The sequential branches of the renal artery are, in order, the:

a. segmental, interlobar, arcuate, interlobular, and afferent arteriole.

b. segmental, interlobular, arcuate, interlobar, and afferent arteriole.

c. segmental, subsegmental, interlobar, interlobular, arcuate, and afferent arteriole.

d. segmental, arcuate, interlobar, interlobular, and afferent arteriole.

e. segmental, interlobar, interlobular, arcuate, and afferent arteriole.

46. During pyeloplasty, a large anterior segmental renal vein is inadvertently torn and subsequently ligated to control hemorrhage. This will produce:

a. no effect on the kidney.

b. segmental renal venous congestion and chronic pain.

c. ischemic loss of a large anterior segment of the renal parenchyma.

d. ischemic loss of a small anterior segment of the renal parenchyma.

e. ischemic loss of a segment of lower pole renal parenchyma.

47. Which of the following vessels commonly drains into the right renal vein?

a. The right adrenal vein

b. The second lumbar vein

c. The right gonadal vein

d. All of the above

e. None of the above

48. The most common renal vascular anomaly is a:

a. supernumerary left renal artery.

b. supernumerary right renal artery.

c. supernumerary left renal vein coursing anterior to the aorta.

d. supernumerary left renal vein coursing posterior to the aorta.

e. supernumerary right renal vein.

49. After involvement of lymph nodes directly at the renal hilum, the primary lymph node drainage site for the left kidney is:

a. the left lateral para-aortic lymph nodes.

b. the interaortocaval lymph nodes.

c. the right paracaval lymph nodes.

d. the left retrocrural lymph nodes.

e. all of the above.

50. In a typical human kidney, there are approximately how many renal papillae and corresponding minor calyces?

a. 3 to 5

b. 7 to 9

c. 11 to 12

d. 14 to 15

e. 17 to 18

51. A compound renal papilla and calyx:
    a. is protective against ascending infection.
    b. is least common at the upper pole of the kidney.
    c. is a rare finding.
    d. is commonly associated with formation of kidney stones.
    e. is none of the above.

52. The ureteral smooth muscle consists of:
    a. a single layer of longitudinally oriented muscle bundles.
    b. a single layer of circular and obliquely oriented muscle bundles.
    c. a single layer of randomly oriented muscle bundles.
    d. two layers—an inner layer of longitudinal muscle and an outer layer of circular and oblique muscle.
    e. two layers—an inner layer of circular and oblique muscle and an outer layer of longitudinal muscle.

53. The ureter receives its blood supply from the:
    a. renal artery.
    b. aorta.
    c. common iliac artery.
    d. gonadal artery.
    e. all of the above.

54. An invasive transitional cell carcinoma is diagnosed in the left proximal ureter, at the level of the third lumbar vertebral body. The primary site of potential nodal metastases from this lesion will be the:
    a. left para-aortic lymph nodes.
    b. interaortocaval lymph nodes.
    c. left common iliac lymph nodes.
    d. lymph nodes at the left renal hilum.
    e. left external iliac lymph nodes.

55. During surgical dissection, the ureter can be identified as it enters the pelvis:
    a. at the aortic bifurcation.
    b. crossing the superior border of the sacrum.
    c. crossing the common iliac artery at the branching of the internal iliac artery.
    d. crossing the uterine artery.
    e. at the internal inguinal ring.

56. A young man with right-sided abdominal pain is diagnosed with right hydroureteronephrosis by renal ultrasonography. Which of the following inflammatory processes might impinge on the right ureter and cause obstruction?
    a. Acute appendicitis
    b. Crohn ileitis
    c. Perforated cecal carcinoma
    d. All of the above
    e. None of the above

57. Narrowing of the ureteral luminal caliber naturally occurs at:
    a. the ureteropelvic junction.
    b. the crossing of the iliac vessels.
    c. the ureterovesical junction.
    d. all of the above.
    e. none of the above.

58. Sympathetic nerve input to the kidney typically travels through:
    a. the celiac plexus.
    b. the superior mesenteric plexus.
    c. the superior hypogastric plexus.
    d. the inferior hypogastric plexus.
    e. none of the above.

59. Ureteral peristalsis requires:
    a. intact sympathetic input.
    b. intact parasympathetic input.
    c. both sympathetic and parasympathetic input.
    d. intact spinal cord.
    e. intrinsic smooth muscle pacemakers in the renal collecting system.

60. The pain caused by an obstructing ureteral stone:
    a. is primarily related to distention of the collecting system above the stone.
    b. is transmitted via nerves from the eighth thoracic through the second lumbar spinal segments.
    c. may be referred over the somatic distribution of the subcostal, iliohypogastric, or ilioinguinal nerves.
    d. may be referred over the distribution of the genitofemoral nerve.
    e. is all of the above.

ANSWERS

1. **c. lumbar vertebrae.** The lumbodorsal fascia originates from the lumbar vertebrae.
2. **c. three distinct layers.** There are three distinct layers of the lumbodorsal fascia.
3. **b. aponeurosis of the transversus abdominis muscle.** All three layers of the lumbodorsal fascia join to form a single thick aponeurosis lateral to the quadratus lumborum muscle before extending further anterolaterally, where they are contiguous with the aponeurosis of the transversus abdominis muscle.
4. **d. splits the lumbodorsal fascia vertically without incising muscle.** A vertical incision that parallels the lateral borders of the sacrospinalis and quadratus lumborum can be made through this lumbodorsal fascia, posteromedial to the first transverse muscle fibers of the transversus abdominis muscle, to gain surgical access to the retroperitoneum and kidney without cutting muscle (the so-called lumbodorsal approach, or dorsal lumbotomy) (see Fig. 1–7 in *Campbell-Walsh Urology, 10th Edition*).
5. **a. flexes the thigh at the hip.** The psoas major joins the iliacus muscle, which originates broadly over the inner aspect of the iliac wing of the pelvis, to become the iliopsoas and insert on the lesser trochanter of the femur and flex the thigh at the hip.
6. **e. The rectus muscle.** The posterior surface of the retroperitoneum is formed by the lumbar vertebral bodies in the midline, which are covered by the shiny, longitudinal fibers of the anterior spinous ligament. These are flanked bilaterally by the psoas muscles. The psoas muscles are covered by a glistening white fibrous fascia, the so-called psoas sheath, which is contiguous with the transversalis fascia. As one moves laterally, the lateral portion of the quadratus lumborum extends from behind the lateral

margin of the psoas. The anterior layer of the lumbodorsal fascia covers this muscle and continues as the aponeurosis of the transversus abdominis muscle. Farther laterally, the transversus abdominis muscle proper is encountered. Superiorly, the posterior wall of the retroperitoneum is formed by the posterior insertion of the diaphragm along the lower ribs. Inferiorly, below the level of the iliac crest, the iliopsoas muscle forms the posterior confine of the retroperitoneum.

7. **e. The costovertebral ligament.** The costovertebral, or lumbodorsal, ligament is a strong fascial attachment between the inferior margin of the 12th rib and the transverse processes of the first and second lumbar vertebrae (see Fig. 1–5 in *Campbell-Walsh Urology, 10th Edition*). It is encountered only in posterior approaches to the kidney and can be incised to produce greater mobility of the 12th rib and provide greater exposure and access to the structures of the upper retroperitoneum.

8. **c. the inferior phrenic arteries.** The first abdominal branches of the aorta are the paired inferior phrenic arteries.

9. **a. The left gastric artery.** The short celiac arterial trunk trifurcates into common hepatic, left gastric, and splenic branches.

10. **c. 2nd lumbar vertebral body.** Usually overlying the second lumbar vertebral body, but subject to considerable variation, the paired renal arteries emanate laterally from the aorta.

11. **d. abdominal aorta below the renal arteries.** The paired gonadal arteries arise from the anterolateral aorta—in atypical cases, from a single anterior trunk—at a level somewhat below the renal vessels.

12. **e. none of the above.** The inferior mesenteric artery, especially in younger individuals without atherosclerotic occlusive arterial disease, can almost always be sacrificed without complication.

13. **a. Renal veins.** Inferior mesenteric, superior mesenteric, and splenic veins join to form the portal vein and drain proximally into the liver rather than directly into the inferior vena cava.

14. **c. inferior aspect of the left renal vein.** The left gonadal vein usually enters the inferior aspect of the left renal vein.

15. **b. anteriorly, just below the superior mesenteric artery.** The left renal vein crosses the aorta anteriorly below the takeoff of the superior mesenteric artery.

16. **d. All of the above.** The left renal vein commonly receives a lumbar vein (usually the second lumbar) on its posterior aspect. In addition, the left gonadal vein typically drains into its inferior margin and the left adrenal vein into its superior margin.

17. **e. bladder.** These lumbar nodal chains are extraregional or secondary drainage sites for any metastatic process arising from the lower pelvis.

18. **b. in a cephalad direction and from right to left.** It is important that most of the lateral flow between ascending lymphatics moves from right to left ascending lumbar trunks.

19. **b. posterior to the aorta.** The structure known as the cisterna chyli truly lies within the thorax, posterior to the aorta or slightly to the right, in a retrocrural position, usually anterior to the first or second lumbar vertebral body.

20. **e. interaortocaval lumbar lymph nodes.** The right testis drains primarily to the interaortocaval region.

21. **e. do all of the above.** The sympathetic trunks course vertically along the anterolateral aspect of the spinal column, in the retroperitoneum lying within the groove between the medial aspect of the ipsilateral psoas muscle and the spine, in some cases covered by the psoas. The lumbar arteries and veins, coursing posteriorly, are closely associated with the sympathetic trunks, crossing them perpendicularly and at times proceeding directly through split portions of the sympathetic chain. The lumbar sympathetic trunks contain variable numbers of ganglia of variable size and position. Some of the preganglionic fibers of the sympathetic trunks synapse within these ganglia with postganglionic sympathetic neurons supplying the body wall and lower extremities.

22. **d. Superior hypogastric plexus.** At the lower extent of the abdominal aorta, much of the sympathetic input to the pelvic urinary organs and genital tract travels through the superior hypogastric plexus, which lies on the aorta anterior to its bifurcation and extends inferiorly on the anterior surface of the fifth lumbar vertebra. This plexus is contiguous bilaterally with inferior hypogastric plexuses, which extend into the pelvis. Disruption of the sympathetic nerve fibers that travel through these plexuses during retroperitoneal dissection can cause loss of seminal vesicle emission and/or failure of bladder neck closure, which results in retrograde ejaculation.

23. **c. between the transversus abdominis and internal oblique muscles.** The iliohypogastric nerve and the ilioinguinal nerve originate together as a common extension from the first lumbar spinal nerve before splitting. These somatic nerves cross the anterior or inner surface of the quadratus lumborum muscle before piercing the transversus abdominis muscle and continuing their course between this and the internal oblique muscle.

24. **d. genital branch of the genitofemoral nerve.** The genital branch of the genitofemoral nerve supplies the cremaster and dartos muscles.

25. **b. On the anterior surface of the psoas muscle.** The genitofemoral nerve lies directly atop and parallels the psoas muscle throughout most of its retroperitoneal course.

26. **e. does all of the above.** The second (descending) part of the duodenum descends vertically, directly anterior to the right renal hilum, and thus is intimately related on its posterior aspect to the medial margin of the right kidney, right renal vessels, renal pelvis, ureteropelvic junction, and often the upper right ureter. The common bile duct also lies posterior to and drains into this part of the duodenum. Directly medial and intimately related to the descending duodenum lies the head of the pancreas.

27. **e. all of the above.** The tail of the pancreas on the left is related posteriorly to the left adrenal gland and upper portion of the left kidney. The splenic vein runs directly posterior to the pancreas, and the splenic artery runs just superior to the vein.

28. **b. found in its normal anatomic position in the upper retroperitoneum.** In cases of renal ectopia, the adrenal gland is usually found in approximately its normal anatomic position.

29. **b. found in its normal anatomic position in the upper retroperitoneum.** In cases of renal agenesis, the adrenal gland on the involved side is typically present.

30. **d. The right adrenal gland is typically located lower in the retroperitoneum than is the left**

adrenal gland. The right adrenal tends to lie more superiorly in the retroperitoneum than does the left adrenal.

31. **a. zona reticularis, zona fasciculata, and zona glomerulosa.** Three cell layers can be identified in the adrenal cortex. The outermost layer is the zona glomerulosa, which produces aldosterone in response to stimulation by the renin-angiotensin system. Centripetally located are the zona fasciculata and zona reticularis, which produce glucocorticoids and sex steroids, respectively.

32. **c. The zona reticularis of the adrenal cortex produces androgens in response to luteinizing hormone (LH).** The function of production of sex steroids by the zona reticularis is regulated by pituitary release of adrenocorticotropic hormone (ACTH).

33. **e. a, b, and c. Multiple small arteries supply each adrenal gland.** (See Fig. 1–21 in *Campbell-Walsh Urology, 10th Edition.*) These are branch vessels, which can be traced to three major arterial sources for each gland: (1) superior branches from the inferior phrenic artery, (2) middle branches directly from the aorta, and (3) inferior branches from the ipsilateral renal artery (see Fig. 1–10 in *Campbell-Walsh Urology, 10th Edition*).

34. **d. both a and c.** The kidneys play a central role in fluid, electrolyte, and acid-base balance in humans, but they also have important endocrine functions, known to include vitamin D metabolism and the production of both renin and erythropoietin.

35. **d. 150 g.** The normal kidney in the adult male weighs approximately 150 g.

36. **d. is a normal variant.** It is neither unusual nor abnormal to see persistence of some degree of fetal lobation throughout adult life.

37. **d. all of the above.** The diaphragm covers roughly the upper third or upper pole of each kidney. With the diaphragm travels the pleural reflection, and thus any direct approach to the upper portion of the kidney, whether percutaneous or open surgical, risks entering the pleural space. The 12th rib on either side crosses the kidney at approximately the lower extent of the diaphragm.

38. **e. All of the above.** In part as a result of the contour of the psoas muscle, the lower pole of either kidney lies farther from the midline than does the upper pole, so the upper poles tilt medially at a slight angle (see Fig. 1–25 in *Campbell-Walsh Urology, 10th Edition*). Similarly, the kidneys do not lie in a simple coronal plane, but the lower pole of the kidney is pushed slightly more anterior than the upper pole. The medial aspect of each kidney is rotated anteriorly on a longitudinal axis at an angle of about 30 degrees from the true coronal plane, with the renal vessels and pelvis exiting the hilum medially in a relatively anterior direction (see Figs. 1–11 and 1–25 in *Campbell-Walsh Urology, 10th Edition*). Typically, two longitudinal rows of renal pyramids in the midkidney and corresponding minor calyces, roughly perpendicular to one another, extend anteriorly and posteriorly. The anterior calyces extend laterally in a coronal plane, whereas the posterior calyces extend posteriorly in a sagittal plane.

39. **d. Both b and c.** There is typically a peritoneal extension between the perirenal fascia covering the upper pole of the left kidney and the inferior splenic capsule, called the splenorenal, or lienorenal, ligament. Just as with the adjacent and often contiguous splenocolic ligamentous attachment, care must be taken not to exert undue tension on the splenorenal ligament during operative procedures on the left kidney, to avoid inadvertent tearing of the spleen (see Fig. 1–26 in *Campbell-Walsh Urology, 10th Edition*).

40. **e. all of the above.** The kidneys and associated adrenal glands are surrounded by varying degrees of perirenal or perinephric fat, and these together are loosely enclosed by the perirenal fascia, commonly called Gerota fascia (see Figs. 1–7 and 1–27 to 1–29 in *Campbell-Walsh Urology, 10th Edition*). Inferiorly, Gerota fascia remains an open potential space, containing the ureter and gonadal vessels on either side.

41. **b. downward into the pelvis.** When very large, such collections can and do extend into the pelvis, following the potential space where Gerota fascia does not fuse inferiorly.

42. **b. renal pelvis, renal artery, and renal vein.** The renal vein lies most anteriorly, and behind it lies the artery. Both normally lie anterior to the urinary collecting system, that is, the renal pelvis.

43. **c. posterior segmental artery.** The main renal artery typically divides into four or more segmental vessels, with five branches most commonly described (see Figs. 1–30 and 1–31 in *Campbell-Walsh Urology, 10th Edition*). The first and most constant segmental division is a posterior branch.

44. **b. ischemic loss of a large posterior segment of the renal parenchyma.** The posterior segmental artery usually exits the main renal artery before it enters the renal hilum and proceeds posteriorly to the renal pelvis to supply a large posterior segment of the kidney. The main renal artery and each segmental artery, as well as their multiple succeeding branch arteries, are all "end arteries," without anastomosis or collateral circulation, and occlusion of any of these vessels produces ischemia and infarction of the corresponding renal parenchyma that it supplies.

45. **a. segmental, interlobar, arcuate, interlobular, and afferent arteriole.** The segmental arteries course through the renal sinus and branch further into lobar arteries, which divide again and enter the renal parenchyma as interlobar arteries (see Fig. 1–32 in *Campbell-Walsh Urology, 10th Edition*). The interlobar arteries branch into arcuate arteries, which arc parallel to the renal contour along the corticomedullary junction. The arcuate arteries, in turn, produce multiple radial arterial branches, the interlobular arteries. These have multiple side branches, which are the afferent arterioles to the glomeruli.

46. **a. no effect on the kidney.** Unlike the renal arteries, none of which communicate, the renal parenchymal veins anastomose freely.

47. **e. None of the above.** The right renal vein is short (2 to 4 cm) and enters the right lateral aspect of the inferior vena cava directly, usually without receiving other venous branches.

48. **a. a supernumerary left renal artery.** The most common variation is the occurrence of supernumerary renal arteries. These supernumerary arteries usually arise from the lateral aorta, occur perhaps slightly more often on the left than on the right, and may enter the renal hilum or directly into the parenchyma of one of the poles of the kidney.

49. **a. the left lateral para-aortic lymph nodes.** From the left kidney, the lymphatic trunks then drain primarily into the left lateral para-aortic lymph nodes including nodes anterior and posterior to the aorta, from a level below the inferior mesenteric artery to the diaphragm.

50. **b. 7 to 9.** The renal papillae may number as few as 4 or as many as 18, but 7 to 9 are present in the typical kidney.

51. **e. is none of the above.** A compound renal papilla and calyx often occurs at the renal poles. The compound papillae are of physiologic significance in that their configuration permits urinary reflux into the renal parenchyma with sufficient back pressure, also allowing bacterial reflux into the kidney in the presence of infected urine (see Fig. 1–39 in *Campbell-Walsh Urology, 10th Edition*). Renal parenchymal scarring secondary to infection is typically most severe overlying such compound papillae.

52. **d. two layers—an inner layer of longitudinal muscle and an outer layer of circular and oblique muscle.** Smooth muscle covers the renal calyces, renal pelvis, and ureter. In the ureter, this muscle can usually be divided into an inner layer of longitudinally coursing muscle bundles and an outer layer of circular and oblique muscle.

53. **e. all of the above.** The ureter receives its blood supply from multiple feeding arterial branches along its course. In the retroperitoneum, the ureter may receive branches from the renal artery, gonadal artery, abdominal aorta, and common iliac artery.

54. **a. left para-aortic lymph nodes.** In the abdomen, the left para-aortic lymph nodes form the primary drainage sites for the left ureter.

55. **c. crossing the common iliac artery at the branching of the internal iliac artery.** The ureter is related posteriorly to the psoas muscle throughout its retroperitoneal course, crossing the iliac vessels to enter the pelvis at approximately the bifurcation of the common iliac artery into internal and external iliac arteries (see Fig. 1–1 in *Campbell-Walsh Urology, 10th Edition*).

56. **d. All of the above.** Anteriorly, the right ureter is related to the terminal ileum, cecum, appendix, and ascending colon and their mesenteries.

57. **d. all of the above.** The ureter is not of uniform caliber, with three distinct narrowings normally present along its course (see Fig. 1–46 in *Campbell-Walsh Urology, 10th Edition*). The first of these is the ureteropelvic junction, the second is the crossing of the iliac vessels, and the third is the ureterovesical junction in the pelvis.

58. **a. the celiac plexus.** The kidneys receive preganglionic sympathetic input from the eighth thoracic through the first lumbar spinal segments. Postganglionic fibers arise primarily from the celiac and aorticorenal ganglia.

59. **e. intrinsic smooth muscle pacemakers in the renal collecting system.** Normal ureteral peristalsis does not require outside autonomic input but rather originates and is propagated from intrinsic smooth muscle pacemaker sites located in the minor calyces of the renal collecting system.

60. **e. is all of the above.** Pain fibers leave the kidney, renal pelvis, and ureter, traveling with the sympathetic nerves. They are primarily stimulated by nociceptors sensitive to increased tension (distention) in the renal capsule, renal collecting system, or ureter. The resulting visceral pain is felt directly and is referred to somatic distributions that correspond to the spinal segments providing the sympathetic distribution to the kidney and ureter (eighth thoracic through second lumbar segments). Pain and reflex muscle spasm are typically produced over the distributions of the subcostal, iliohypogastric, ilioinguinal, and/or genitofemoral nerves.

Additional Study Points

1. The psoas minor muscle is present in about half the population; it lies medial to the psoas major, and its tendon is useful to secure the bladder for a psoas hitch operation.
2. The gonadal arteries may be ligated without detrimental effect.
3. The lumbar veins communicate with the azygous venous system on the right side and the hemizygous venous system on the left. This provides a collateral route of venous drainage to the heart when the vena cava is occluded with thrombus or tumor. It is important to remember that lumbar veins connect posteriorly with renal veins and may be injured during dissection of the renal vein. Occasionally lumbar veins drain into the right renal vein, and frequently they drain into the left renal vein.
4. The right adrenal vein is short, located posterior laterally.
5. Gerota fascia extends across the midline medially to fuse with the contralateral side. It envelopes the adrenal superiorly and is open inferiorly.
6. Renal arteries are end arteries; therefore occlusion results in infarction to the segment that the artery supplies.
7. There are 2 million glomeruli.
8. Lower pole arteries on the right tend to cross anterior to the inferior vena cava. Lower pole arteries on either side generally cross anterior to the collecting system.
9. Arterial branches to the abdominal ureter approach from a medial direction, whereas arterial branches to the pelvic ureter approach from a lateral direction.
10. Lymphatic drainage to the ureter parallels the arterial supply.
11. Renal pain fibers are stimulated by tension and direct mucosal irritation. They travel with the sympathetic nerves.

chapter
2

Anatomy of the Lower Urinary Tract and Male Genitalia

Benjamin I. Chung, MD ● Graham Sommer, MD ● James D. Brooks, MD

QUESTIONS

1. The greater and lesser sciatic foramina are separated by the:
   a. sacrotuberous ligament.
   b. Cooper (pectineal) ligament.
   c. arcuate line.
   d. sacrospinous ligament.
   e. piriformis muscle.

2. During inguinal incisions, the vessels invariably encountered in Camper fascia are the:
   a. superficial inferior epigastric artery and vein.
   b. superficial circumflex iliac artery and vein.
   c. external pudendal artery and vein.
   d. gonadal artery and veins.
   e. accessory obturator vein.

3. Rupture of the penile urethra at the junction of the penis and scrotum can result in urinary extravasation into all of the following structures EXCEPT the:
   a. anterior abdominal wall up to the clavicles.
   b. scrotum.
   c. penis, deep to the dartos fascia.
   d. perineum in a "butterfly" pattern.
   e. buttock.

4. During inguinal hernia repair in a male patient, injury of the ilioinguinal nerve in the canal will most likely produce:
   a. anesthesia over the dorsum of the penis.
   b. anesthesia over the pubis and scrotum and loss of cremasteric contraction.
   c. anesthesia over the pubis and anterior scrotum only.
   d. anesthesia over the anterior and medial thigh.
   e. anesthesia over the pubis only.

5. A child has dense scarring after failed extravesical reimplantation. The landmark that can assist in locating the ureter in the pelvis is the:
   a. obturator nerve; the ureter will be medial to it.
   b. obliterated umbilical artery; the ureter will be found lateral to it.

   c. obliterated umbilical artery; the ureter will be found medial to it.
   d. external iliac artery; the ureter crosses it to reach the pelvis.
   e. vas deferens; the ureter will pass anterior to it.

6. The levator ani attaches to all of the following EXCEPT the:
   a. perineal body.
   b. pubis.
   c. coccyx.
   d. vagina.
   e. arcus tendineus fascia pelvis.

7. Accessory obturator veins (from the external iliac artery) and accessory obturator arteries (from the inferior epigastric artery) are encountered in:
   a. 50% and 25% of patients, respectively.
   b. 5% and 50% of patients, respectively.
   c. 50% and 75% of patients, respectively.
   d. 25% and 50% of patients, respectively.
   e. 25% and 5% of patients, respectively.

8. A retractor blade has rested on the psoas muscle during a prolonged procedure, resulting in a femoral nerve palsy. Postoperatively, the patient will experience:
   a. inability to flex the hip and numbness over the anterior thigh.
   b. inability to flex the knee and numbness over the thigh.
   c. numbness over the anterior thigh only.
   d. inability to extend the knee and numbness over the anterior thigh.
   e. inability to flex the knee only.

9. Autonomic nerves contributing to the pelvic plexus include the:
   a. superior hypogastric nerves from the para-aortic plexuses.
   b. pelvic sympathetic trunks.
   c. pelvic parasympathetic neurons from the sacral spinal cord.
   d. a and c only.
   e. a, b, and c.

10. To preserve the vascular supply to the ureter, incisions in the peritoneum should be made:
    a. medially in the abdomen and laterally in the pelvis.
    b. laterally in the abdomen and medially in the pelvis.
    c. always medial to the ureter.
    d. always lateral to the ureter.
    e. directly over the ureter.

11. Relative to the ureter, the uterine vessels are found:
    a. laterally.
    b. posteriorly.
    c. anteriorly.
    d. medially.
    e. running together in a common sheath.

12. All of the following features of the ureterovesical junction cooperate to prevent vesicoureteral reflux EXCEPT:
    a. fixation of the ureter to the superficial trigone.
    b. sphincteric closure of the ureteral orifice.
    c. detrusor backing.
    d. telescoping of the bladder outward over the ureter.
    e. passive closure of the intramural ureter caused by bladder filling.

13. In contrast to that of the male, the female bladder neck:
    a. has extensive adrenergic innervation.
    b. has a thickened middle smooth muscle layer.
    c. is largely responsible for urinary continence.
    d. is surrounded by type I (slow-twitch) fibers.
    e. has longitudinal smooth muscle fibers that extend to the external meatus.

14. Which of the following statements about the trigone is TRUE?
    a. Epithelium is thicker than the rest of the bladder and densely adherent.
    b. Superficial smooth muscle is a continuation of Waldeyer sheath.
    c. Smooth muscle enlarges to form thick fascicles.
    d. Smooth muscle of the ureter forms the interureteric ridge (Mercier bar).
    e. When the bladder empties, the trigone is thrown into thick folds.

15. During a perineal prostatectomy, the muscle that must be divided to gain access to the apex of the prostate is the:
    a. rectourethralis.
    b. internal anal sphincter.
    c. perineal body.
    d. external anal sphincter.
    e. puboanalis.

16. Arterial supply to the bladder includes:
    a. the superior vesical artery.
    b. the inferior vesical artery.
    c. the obturator artery
    d. the uterine artery.
    e. all of the above.

17. The ducts of which of the following prostatic zones drain into the preprostatic urethra?
    a. Periurethral glands
    b. Central zone
    c. Transition zone
    d. Peripheral zone
    e. a and c

18. Benign prostatic hyperplasia (BPH) may arise from the:
    a. periurethral glands.
    b. central zone.
    c. transition zone.
    d. peripheral zone.
    e. a and c.

19. In BPH, blood supply to the adenoma arises from the:
    a. superior vesical artery.
    b. urethral arteries extending down the urethra from the bladder neck.
    c. capsular arteries that arise laterally.
    d. dorsal venous complex.
    e. neurovascular bundle.

20. Which of the following statements concerning the striated urethral sphincter is TRUE?
    a. It is composed of type I (slow-twitch) and type II (fast-twitch) fibers.
    b. It is bounded above by the superior fascia.
    c. It receives motor blanches from the dorsal nerve of the penis.
    d. It is shaped like a signet ring and is 2 to 2.5 cm in length.
    e. It is densely supplied with proprioceptive muscle spindles.

21. The seminal vesicle:
    a. is normally palpable in a rectal examination.
    b. is a lateral outpouching of the prostate (central zone).
    c. contracts in response to excitatory efferents from the sacral parasympathetic nerves.
    d. is medial to the vas deferens.
    e. stores sperm.

22. From medial to lateral, the segments of the fallopian tube are:
    a. uterine, ampulla, infundibulum, isthmus, fimbriae.
    b. uterine, ampulla, isthmus, infundibulum, fimbriae.
    c. uterine, isthmus, ampulla, infundibulum, fimbriae.
    d. uterine, infundibulum, ampulla, isthmus, fimbriae.
    e. uterine, isthmus, infundibulum, ampulla, fimbriae.

23. The peritoneum may be accessed transvaginally through the:
    a. posterior fornix.
    b. anterior fornix.
    c. rectovaginal septum.
    d. lateral fornices.
    e. vesicovaginal space.

24. To avoid denervation of the striated urethral sphincter, incisions through the vaginal wall to enter the retropubic space should be made:
    a. perpendicular to the urethra.
    b. over the urethra.
    c. close to the lateral margins of the urethra.
    d. cephalad to the bladder neck.
    e. far lateral in the vaginal wall, parallel to the urethra.

25. When the endopelvic fascia lateral to the prostate and puboprostatic ligaments is opened, vessels are commonly encountered that pierce the levator ani to join the periprostatic plexus laterally. These vessels are communicating branches from the:
    a. pampiniform plexus of veins.
    b. dorsal vein of the penis.
    c. internal pudendal veins.
    d. external pudendal veins.
    e. accessory obturator veins.

26. Lymphatic drainage from the prostate flows to the:
    a. external iliac and common iliac nodes.
    b. internal iliac and obturator nodes.
    c. para-aortic nodes.
    d. internal iliac and inguinal nodes.
    e. perirectal and common iliac nodes.

27. The first branch of the pudendal nerve in the perineum is the:
    a. dorsal nerve of the penis.
    b. inferior rectal nerve(s).
    c. perineal nerve.
    d. posterior femoral cutaneous branches.
    e. posterior scrotal branches.

28. After fracture of the penis (disruption of the tunica albuginea), if Buck fascia remains intact, the hematoma will be visible in the:
    a. perineum in a butterfly pattern.
    b. penis and scrotum only.
    c. penis, scrotum, and perineum and tracking up the anterior abdominal wall.
    d. shaft of the penis only.
    e. shaft and glans of the penis.

29. The skin of the penile shaft and foreskin can be elevated as a rotational flap supplied by the:
    a. dorsal artery of the penis.
    b. superficial inferior epigastric vessels.
    c. gonadal vessels.
    d. external pudendal vessels.
    e. several branches of the perineal vessels.

30. The dartos layer of smooth muscle and fascia in the scrotum is continuous with:
    a. the dartos layer of the penis.
    b. Colles fascia.
    c. Scarpa fascia.

    d. Buck fascia.
    e. a, b, and c.

31. The cremaster muscle is supplied by the:
    a. ilioinguinal nerve.
    b. genital branch of the genitofemoral nerve.
    c. femoral branch of the genitofemoral nerve.
    d. terminal branches of the subcostal nerve (T12).
    e. iliohypogastric nerve.

32. Lymphatic drainage from the bulbar urethra travels:
    a. through perianal nodes to reach the pelvis.
    b. directly to the deep pelvic lymph nodes.
    c. through the superficial and deep inguinal lymph nodes.
    d. to prepubic nodes.
    e. to para-aortic lymph nodes along with testicular drainage.

33. In their course from the seminiferous tubule to the epididymis, sperm pass through, in order:
    a. straight tubules, efferent ductules, rete testis.
    b. rete testis, straight tubules, efferent ductules.
    c. efferent ductules, rete testis, straight tubules.
    d. straight tubules, rete testis, efferent ductules.
    e. rete testis, efferent ductules, straight tubules.

34. The testicular artery may be ligated without sacrificing the testis because of collateral circulation from:
    a. vasal and cremasteric arteries.
    b. external pudendal and vasal arteries.
    c. external pudendal, vasal, and cremasteric arteries.
    d. numerous anastomotic branches from the scrotal arteries.
    e. cremasteric and external pudendal arteries.

35. To avoid damage to subtunical testicular vessels, biopsy of the testis should be performed at the:
    a. lower pole of the testis.
    b. anterior upper pole directly opposite the testicular mesentery.
    c. medial surface of the lower pole.
    d. lateral surface of the lower pole.
    e. lateral or medial surface of the upper pole.

36. Which layers of the scrotum and testicular tunics usually need to be débrided in patients with Fournier gangrene?
    a. The scrotal skin only
    b. The scrotal skin and dartos layer
    c. The scrotal skin, dartos layer, and external spermatic fascia
    d. The scrotal skin, dartos layer, and external cremasteric and internal spermatic fasciae, leaving the tunica vaginalis intact
    e. All tissues including the tunica vaginalis

37. A Martius (labial fat pad) rotational flap used in the repair of a vesicovaginal fistula receives blood supply from the:
    a. terminal branches of the internal pudendal artery and vein.
    b. superficial inferior epigastric vessels.
    c. inferior epigastric vessels.

d. accessory pudendal vessels.

e. external pudendal vessels.

38. Lymphatic drainage from the bladder passes through the:

    a. external iliac lymph nodes.

    b. obturator and internal iliac lymph nodes.

    c. internal and common iliac lymph nodes.

    d. common iliac, periureteral, and para-aortic lymph nodes.

    e. a, b, and c.

39. To preserve potency during a radical cystectomy, ligation of the lateral and posterior vascular pedicles is best carried out:

    a. close to their origin from the internal iliac vessels.

    b. near the bladder.

    c. from beneath the bladder after rotating the prostate cephalad.

    d. as they cross the ureter.

    e. lateral to the rectum.

ANSWERS

1. **d. sacrospinous ligament.** The sacrospinous ligament separates the greater and lesser sciatic foramina.

2. **a. superficial inferior epigastric artery and vein.** The superficial inferior epigastric vessels are encountered during inguinal incisions and can cause troublesome bleeding during placement of pelvic laparoscopic ports.

3. **e. buttock.** Blood and urine can accumulate in the scrotum and penis deep to the dartos fascia after an anterior urethral injury. In the perineum, their spread is limited by the fusions of Colles fascia to the ischiopubic rami laterally and to the posterior edge of the perineal membrane; the resulting hematoma is therefore butterfly shaped. These processes will not extend down the leg or into the buttock, but they can freely travel up the anterior abdominal wall deep to Scarpa fascia to the clavicles and around the flank to the back.

4. **c. anesthesia over the pubis and anterior scrotum only.** The ilioinguinal nerve (L1) passes through the internal oblique muscle to enter the inguinal canal laterally. It travels anterior to the cord and exits the external ring to provide sensation to the mons pubis and anterior scrotum or labia majora.

5. **c. obliterated umbilical artery; the ureter will be found medial to it.** The obliterated umbilical artery in the medial umbilical fold serves as an important landmark for the surgeon. It can be traced to its origin from the internal iliac artery to locate the ureter, which lies on its medial side.

6. **e. arcus tendineus fascia pelvis.** The tendinous arc of the levator ani serves as the origin of the muscles of the pelvic diaphragm: pubococcygeus and iliococcygeus. The muscle bordering this hiatus has been referred to as "pubovisceral" because it provides a sling for (pubourethralis, puborectalis), inserts directly into (pubovaginalis, puboanalis, levator prostatae), or inserts into a structure intimately associated with the pelvic viscera. The coccygeus muscle extends from the sacrospinous ligament to the lateral border of the sacrum and coccyx to complete the pelvic diaphragm.

7. **a. 50% and 25% of patients, respectively.** In half of patients, one or more accessory obturator veins drain into the underside of the external iliac vein and can easily be torn during lymphadenectomy. In 25% of people, an accessory obturator artery arises from the inferior epigastric artery and runs medial to the femoral vein to reach the obturator canal.

8. **d. inability to extend the knee and numbness over the anterior thigh.** The femoral nerve (L2, L3, L4) supplies sensation to the anterior thigh and motor innervation to the extensors of the knee.

9. **e. a, b, and c.** The presynaptic sympathetic cell bodies reach the pelvic plexus by two pathways: (1) the superior hypogastric plexus and (2) the pelvic continuation of the sympathetic trunks. Presynaptic parasympathetic innervation arises from the intermediolateral cell column of the sacral cord.

10. **b. laterally in the abdomen and medially in the pelvis.** Blood supply to the pelvic ureter enters laterally; thus the pelvic peritoneum should be incised only medial to the ureter.

11. **c. anteriorly.** In women, the ureter first runs posterior to the ovary, then turns medially to run deep to the base of the broad ligament before entering a loose connective tissue tunnel through the substance of the cardinal ligament.

12. **b. sphincteric closure of the ureteral orifice.** The intravesical portion of the ureter lies immediately beneath the bladder urothelium and is therefore quite pliant; it is backed by a strong plate of detrusor muscle. With bladder filling, this arrangement is thought to result in passive occlusion of the ureter, like a flap valve.

13. **e. has longitudinal smooth muscle fibers that extend to the external meatus.** At the female bladder neck, the inner longitudinal fibers converge radially to pass downward as the inner longitudinal layer of the urethra. The middle circular layer does not appear to be as robust as that of the male. The female bladder neck differs strikingly from the male in possessing little adrenergic innervation.

14. **d. Smooth muscle of the ureter forms the interureteric ridge (Mercier bar).** Fibers from each ureter meet to form a triangular sheet of muscle that extends from the two ureteral orifices to the internal urethra meatus. The edges of this muscular sheet are thickened between the ureteral orifices (the interureteric crest, or Mercier bar) and between the ureters and the internal urethral meatus (Bell muscle).

15. **a. rectourethralis.** When approached from below, these fibers of the rectourethralis muscle are 2 to 10 mm thick and must be divided to gain access to the prostate.

16. **e. all of the above.** In addition to the vesical branches, the bladder may be supplied by any adjacent artery arising from the internal iliac artery.

17. **a. Periurethral glands.** At its midpoint, the urethra turns approximately 35 degrees anteriorly, but this angulation can vary from 0 to 90 degrees (see Figs. 2–27, 2–31, and 2–36 in *Campbell-Walsh Urology, 10th Edition*). This angle divides the prostatic urethra into proximal (preprostatic) and distal (prostatic) segments, which are functionally and anatomically discrete. Small periurethral glands, lacking periglandular smooth muscle, extend between the fibers of the longitudinal smooth muscle to be enclosed by the preprostatic sphincter.

18. **e. a and c.** The periurethral glands can contribute significantly to prostatic volume in older men as one of the sites of origin of BPH. The transition zone commonly gives rise to BPH.

19. **b. urethral arteries extending down the urethra from the bladder neck.** The urethral arteries penetrate the prostatovesical junction posterolaterally and travel inward, perpendicular to the urethra. They approach the bladder neck in the 1- to 5-o'clock and 7- to 11-o'clock positions, with the largest branches located posteriorly. They then turn caudally, parallel to the urethra, to supply it, the periurethral glands, and the transition zone. Thus in BPH, these arteries provide the principal blood supply of the adenoma.

20. **d. It is shaped like a signet ring and is 2 to 2.5 cm in length.** The membranous urethra spans on average 2 to 2.5 cm (range: 1.2 to 5 cm). It is surrounded by the striated (external) urethral sphincter, which is often incorrectly depicted as a flat sheet of muscle sandwiched between two layers of fasciae. The striated sphincter is actually shaped like a signet ring, broad at its base and narrowing as it passes through the urogenital hiatus of the levator ani to meet the apex of the prostate.

21. **c. contracts in response to excitatory efferents from the sacral parasympathetic nerves.** Innervation arises from the pelvic plexus, with major excitatory efferents contributed by the (sympathetic) hypogastric nerves.

22. **c. uterine, isthmus, ampulla, infundibulum, fimbriae.** The tubes are divided into four segments: uterine, isthmus, ampulla, and infundibulum, which is crowned by the fimbriae.

23. **a. posterior fornix.** Because the apex of the vagina is covered with the peritoneum of the rectouterine pouch, the peritoneal cavity may be accessed through the posterior fornix.

24. **e. far lateral in the vaginal wall, parallel to the urethra.** Somatic and autonomic nerves to the urethra travel on the lateral walls of the vagina near the urethra. During transvaginal incontinence surgery, the anterior vaginal wall should be incised laterally to avoid these nerves and prevent type III urinary incontinence.

25. **c. internal pudendal veins.** The internal pudendal veins communicate freely with the dorsal vein complex by piercing the levator ani. These communicating vessels enter the pelvic venous plexus on the lateral surface of the prostate and are a common, often unexpected, source of bleeding during apical dissection of the prostate.

26. **b. internal iliac and obturator nodes.** Lymphatic drainage is primarily to the obturator and internal iliac nodes.

27. **a. dorsal nerve of the penis.** The pudendal nerve follows the vessels in their course through the perineum (see Fig. 2–47 in *Campbell-Walsh Urology, 10th Edition*). Its first branch, the dorsal nerve of the penis, travels ventral to the main pudendal trunk in the Alcock canal.

28. **d. shaft of the penis only.** Bleeding from a tear in the corporal bodies (e.g., penile fracture) is usually contained within the Buck fascia, and ecchymosis is limited to the penile shaft.

29. **d. external pudendal vessels.** The blood supply of the skin of the penile shaft is independent of the erectile bodies and is derived from the external pudendal branches of the femoral vessels.

30. **e. a, b, and c.** The dartos layer of smooth muscle is continuous with Colles fascia, Scarpa fascia, and the dartos fascia of the penis.

31. **b. genital branch of the genitofemoral nerve.** The genital branch of the genitofemoral nerve follows the cord through the inguinal canal, supplies the cremaster muscle, and supplies sensation to the anterior scrotum.

32. **c. through the superficial and deep inguinal lymph nodes.** The penis, scrotum, and perineum drain into the inguinal lymph nodes. These nodes can be divided into superficial groups and deep groups.

33. **d. straight tubules, rete testis, efferent ductules.** Septa form 200 to 300 cone-shaped lobules, each containing one or more convoluted seminiferous tubules. Each tubule is U-shaped and has a stretched length of nearly 1 m. Interstitial (Leydig) cells lie in the loose tissue surrounding the tubules and are responsible for testosterone production. Toward the apices of the lobules, the seminiferous tubules become straight (tubuli recti) and enter the mediastinum testis to form an anastomosing network of tubules lined by flattened epithelium. This network, known as the rete testis, forms 12 to 20 efferent ductules and passes into the largest portion of epididymis, the caput.

34. **a. vasal and cremasteric arteries.** A rich arterial anastomosis occurs at the head of the epididymis, between the testicular and capital arteries, and at the tail between the testicular, epididymal, cremasteric, and vasal arteries.

35. **e. lateral or medial surface of the upper pole.** The testicular arteries enter the mediastinum and ramify in the tunica vasculosa, principally in the anterior, medial, and lateral portions of the lower pole and the anterior segment of the upper pole (see Fig. 2–52 in *Campbell-Walsh Urology, 10th Edition*). Thus placement of a traction suture through the lower pole tunica albuginea risks damaging these important superficial vessels and devascularizing the testis. Testicular biopsy should be carried out in the medial or lateral surface of the upper pole, where the risk of vascular injury is minimal.

36. **b. The scrotal skin and dartos layer.** The external, cremasteric, and internal spermatic fasciae are embryologically distinct from the scrotal and dartos layers and have their own blood and nerve supplies. It is uncommon for them to be involved in the necrotic process in Fournier gangrene; therefore they can be spared. (*Editor's comment:* In practice in patients with Fournier gangrene, all scrotal tissue is debrided to the tunica vaginalis.)

37. **e. external pudendal vessels.** The labial fat pads receive blood supply from the external pudendal branches of the femoral vessels.

38. **e. a, b, and c.** The bulk of the lymphatic drainage passes to the external iliac lymph nodes. Some anterior and lateral drainage may go through the obturator and internal iliac nodes, and portions of the bladder base and trigone may drain into the internal and common iliac groups. Complete lymph node dissection during radical cystectomy should encompass all of these lymph node groups.

39. **b. near the bladder.** The bladder vasculature pierces the pelvic autonomic plexuses near the origin of the arteries from the internal iliac arteries. Ligation of these vessels proximally will injure the pelvic autonomic nervous plexuses. Ligation is best carried out near the bladder to avoid nerve damage.

Additional Study Points

1. Scarpa fascia on the abdomen forms a distinct layer and is continuous with Colles fascia of the perineum.
2. The internal oblique and transversalis abdominis fasciae fuse to form the conjoint tendon. The conjoint tendon reinforces the posterior wall of the inguinal canal.
3. There are three important components of the pelvic fasciae: (1) puboprostatic ligaments—in the female they inert on the proximal third of the urethra; (2) arcus tendineus fascia, which extends from the puboprostatic ligament to the ischial spine; and (3) lateral and posterior vesicle ligaments. In the female they are called the *cardinal* and *uterosacral ligaments*.
4. The superior vesicle artery arises from the proximal portion of the obliterated umbilical artery. The latter may be used to find the superior vesicle artery.
5. The male bladder neck receives abundant sympathetic innervation. The female bladder neck receives little sympathetic innervation.
6. The apex of the prostate is continuous with the striated urethra sphincter.
7. The prostate is composed of 70% glandular elements and 30% fibromuscular stroma.
8. The peripheral zone of the prostate has the bulk of prostatic glandular tissue; 70% of adenocarcinomas arise in this zone.
9. Clinically, the prostate has two lateral lobes and a median lobe; however, these do not correspond to distinct anatomic zones in the prostate. They are merely used as clinical guides when endoscopically viewing the prostatic urethra.
10. The blood supply to the prostate enters at the 4 and 8 o'clock positions. It is important to understand this in open prostatectomy when securing hemostasis.
11. Although lymphatic drainage for the prostate is primarily to the obturator and internal iliac nodes, it may drain directly to the presacral and external iliac nodes.
12. Denonvilliers fascia separates the prostate from the rectum.
13. Scrotal lymphatics do not cross the median raphae. Lymphatics from the shaft of the penis cross the midline extensively.

Clinical Decision Making

Evaluation of the Urologic Patient: History, Physical Examination, and Urinalysis

Glenn S. Gerber, MD ● Charles B. Brendler, MD

QUESTIONS

1. What causes the pain associated with a stone in the ureter?
   a. Obstruction of urine flow with distention of the renal capsule
   b. Irritation of the ureteral mucosa by the stone
   c. Excessive ureteral peristalsis in response to the obstructing stone
   d. Irritation of the intramural ureter
   e. Urinary extravasation from a ruptured calyceal fornix

2. What is the most common cause of gross hematuria in a patient older than 50 years of age?
   a. Renal calculi
   b. Infection
   c. Bladder cancer
   d. Benign prostatic hyperplasia
   e. Trauma

3. What is the most common cause of pain associated with gross hematuria?
   a. Simultaneous passage of a kidney stone
   b. Ureteral obstruction due to blood clots
   c. Urinary tract malignancy
   d. Prostatic inflammation
   e. Prostatic enlargement

4. All of the following are typical lower urinary tract symptoms associated with benign prostatic hyperplasia EXCEPT:
   a. urgency.
   b. frequency.
   c. nocturia.
   d. dysuria.
   e. weak urinary stream.

5. What is the most common cause of continuous incontinence (loss of urine at all times and in all positions)?
   a. Enterovesical fistula
   b. Noncompliant bladder
   c. Detrusor hyperreflexia
   d. Vesicovaginal fistula
   e. Sphincteric incompetence

6. All of the following are potential causes of anejaculation EXCEPT:
   a. sympathetic denervation.
   b. pharmacologic agents.
   c. bladder neck and prostatic surgery.
   d. androgen deficiency.
   e. cerebrovascular accidents.

7. What percentage of patients with multiple sclerosis will present with urinary symptoms as the first manifestation of the disease?
   a. 1%
   b. 5%
   c. 10%
   d. 15%
   e. 20%

8. What important information is gained from pelvic bimanual examination that cannot be obtained from radiologic evaluation?
   a. Presence of bladder mass
   b. Invasion of bladder cancer into perivesical fat
   c. Presence of bladder calculi
   d. Presence of associated pathologic lesion in female adnexal structures
   e. Mobility/fixation of pelvic organs

9. With what disease is priapism primarily associated?
   a. Peyronie disease
   b. Sickle cell anemia
   c. Parkinson disease
   d. Organic depression
   e. Leukemia

10. What is the most common cause of cloudy urine?
    a. Bacterial cystitis
    b. Urine overgrowth with yeast
    c. Phosphaturia

d. Alkaline urine

e. Significant proteinuria

11. Conditions that decrease urine specific gravity include all of the following EXCEPT:

    a. increased fluid intake.

    b. use of diuretics.

    c. decreased renal concentrating ability.

    d. dehydration.

    e. diabetes insipidus.

12. Urine osmolality usually varies between:

    a. 10 and 200 mOsm/L.

    b. 50 and 500 mOsm/L.

    c. 50 and 1200 mOsm/L.

    d. 100 and 1000 mOsm/L.

    e. 100 and 1500 mOsm/L.

13. Elevated ascorbic acid levels in the urine may lead to false-negative results on a urine dipstick test for which of the following?

    a. Glucose

    b. Hemoglobin

    c. Myoglobin

    d. Red blood cells

    e. Leukocytes

14. Hematuria is distinguished from hemoglobinuria or myoglobinuria by:

    a. dipstick testing.

    b. the simultaneous presence of significant leukocytes.

    c. microscopic presence of erythrocytes.

    d. examination of serum.

    e. evaluation of hematocrit.

15. The presence of one positive dipstick reading for hematuria is associated with significant urologic pathologic findings on subsequent testing in what percentage of patients?

    a. 2%

    b. 10%

    c. 25%

    d. 50%

    e. 75%

16. The most common cause of glomerular hematuria is:

    a. transitional cell carcinoma.

    b. nephritic syndrome.

    c. Berger disease (IgA nephropathy).

    d. poststreptococcal glomerulonephritis.

    e. Goodpasture syndrome.

17. The most common cause of proteinuria is:

    a. Fanconi syndrome.

    b. excessive glomerular permeability due to primary glomerular disease.

    c. failure of adequate tubular reabsorption.

    d. overflow proteinuria due to increased plasma concentration of immunoglobulins.

    e. diabetes.

18. Transient proteinuria may be due to all of the following EXCEPT:

    a. exercise.

    b. fever.

    c. emotional stress.

    d. congestive heart failure.

    e. ureteroscopy.

19. Glucose will be detected in the urine when the serum level is above:

    a. 75 mg/dL.

    b. 100 mg/dL.

    c. 150 mg/dL.

    d. 180 mg/dL.

    e. 225 mg/dL.

20. The specificity of dipstick nitrite testing for bacteriuria is:

    a. 20%.

    b. 40%.

    c. 60%.

    d. 80%.

    e. >90%.

21. All of the following are microscopic features of squamous epithelial cells EXCEPT:

    a. large size.

    b. small central nucleus.

    c. irregular cytoplasm.

    d. presence in clumps.

    e. fine granularity in the cytoplasm.

22. The number of bacteria per high-power microscopic field that correspond to colony counts of 100,000/mL is:

    a. 1.

    b. 3.

    c. 5.

    d. 10.

    e. 20.

23. Pain in the flaccid penis is usually due to:

    a. Peyronie disease.

    b. bladder or urethral inflammation.

    c. priapism.

    d. calculi impacted in the distal ureter.

    e. hydrocele.

24. Chronic scrotal pain is most often due to:

    a. testicular torsion.

    b. trauma.

    c. cryptorchidism.

    d. hydrocele.

    e. orchitis.

25. Terminal hematuria (at the end of the urinary stream) is usually due to:

    a. bladder neck or prostatic inflammation.

    b. bladder cancer.

    c. kidney stones.

d. bladder calculi.

e. urethral stricture disease.

26. Enuresis is present in what percentage of children at age 5 years?

a. 5%

b. 15%

c. 25%

d. 50%

e. 75%

27. All of the following in the medical history suggest that erectile dysfunction is more likely due to organic rather than psychogenic causes EXCEPT:

a. sudden onset.

b. peripheral vascular disease.

c. absence of nocturnal erections.

d. diabetes mellitus.

e. inability to achieve adequate erections in a variety of circumstances.

28. All of the following should be routinely performed in men with hematospermia EXCEPT:

a. cystoscopy.

b. digital rectal examination.

c. serum prostate-specific antigen (PSA) level.

d. genital examination.

e. urinalysis.

29. Pneumaturia may be due to all of the following EXCEPT:

a. diverticulitis.

b. colon cancer.

c. recent urinary tract instrumentation.

d. inflammatory bowel disease.

e. ectopic ureter.

30. Which of the following disorders may commonly lead to irritative voiding symptoms?

a. Parkinson disease

b. Renal cell carcinoma

c. Bladder diverticula

d. Prostate cancer

e. Testicular torsion

ANSWERS

1. **a. Obstruction of urine flow with distention of the renal capsule.** Pain is usually caused by acute distention of the renal capsule, usually from inflammation or obstruction.

2. **c. Bladder cancer.** The most common cause of gross hematuria in a patient older than age 50 years is bladder cancer.

3. **b. Ureteral obstruction due to blood clots.** Pain in association with hematuria usually results from upper urinary tract hematuria with obstruction of the ureters with clots.

4. **d. dysuria.** Dysuria is painful urination that is usually caused by inflammation.

5. **d. vesicovaginal fistula.** Continuous incontinence is most commonly due to a urinary tract fistula that bypasses the urethral sphincter.

6. **e. cerebrovascular accidents.** Anejaculation may result from several causes: (1) androgen deficiency, (2) sympathetic denervation, (3) pharmacologic agents, and (4) bladder neck and prostatic surgery.

7. **b. 5%.** In fact, 5% of patients with previously undiagnosed multiple sclerosis present with urinary symptoms as the first manifestation of the disease.

8. **e. Mobility/fixation of pelvic organs.** In addition to defining areas of induration, the bimanual examination allows the examiner to assess the mobility of the bladder; such information cannot be obtained by radiologic techniques such as CT and MRI, which convey static images.

9. **b. Sickle cell anemia.** Priapism occurs most commonly in patients with sickle cell disease but can also occur in those with advanced malignancy, coagulation disorders, and pulmonary disease, as well as in many patients without an obvious cause.

10. **c. Phosphaturia.** Cloudy urine is most commonly caused by phosphates in the urine.

11. **d. dehydration.** Conditions that decrease specific gravity include (1) increased fluid intake, (2) diuretics, (3) decreased renal concentrating ability, and (4) diabetes insipidus.

12. **c. 50 and 1200 mOsm/L.** Osmolality is a measure of the amount of material dissolved in the urine and usually varies between 50 and 1200 mOsm/L.

13. **a. Glucose.** False-negative results for glucose and bilirubin may be seen in the presence of elevated ascorbic acid concentrations in the urine.

14. **c. microscopic presence of erythrocytes.** Hematuria can be distinguished from hemoglobinuria and myoglobinuria by microscopic examination of the centrifuged urine; the presence of a large number of erythrocytes establishes the diagnosis of hematuria.

15. **c. 25%.** Investigators at the University of Wisconsin found that 26% of adults who had at least one positive dipstick reading for hematuria were subsequently found to have significant urologic pathologic findings.

16. **c. Berger disease (IgA nephropathy).** IgA nephropathy, or Berger disease, is the most common cause of glomerular hematuria, accounting for about 30% of cases.

17. **b. excessive glomerular permeability due to primary glomerular disease.** Glomerular proteinuria is the most common type of proteinuria and results from increased glomerular capillary permeability to protein, especially albumin. Glomerular proteinuria occurs in any of the primary glomerular diseases such as IgA nephropathy or in glomerulopathy associated with systemic illness such as diabetes mellitus.

18. **e. ureteroscopy.** Transient proteinuria occurs commonly, especially in the pediatric population, and usually resolves spontaneously within a few days. It may result from fever, exercise, or emotional stress. In older patients, transient proteinuria may be due to congestive heart failure.

19. **d. 180 mg/dL.** This so-called renal threshold corresponds to a serum glucose level of about 180 mg/dL; above this level, glucose will be detected in the urine.

20. **e. >90%.** The specificity of the nitrite dipstick test for detecting bacteriuria is greater than 90%.

21. **d. presence in clumps.** Squamous epithelial cells are large, have a central small nucleus about the size of an erythrocyte, and have an irregular cytoplasm with fine granularity.

22. **c. 5.** Therefore 5 bacteria per high-power field reflect colony counts of about 100,000/mL.
23. **b. bladder or urethral inflammation.** Pain in the flaccid penis is usually secondary to inflammation in the bladder or urethra, with referred pain that is experienced maximally at the urethral meatus.
24. **d. hydrocele.** Chronic scrotal pain is usually related to noninflammatory conditions such as a hydrocele or varicocele, and the pain is usually characterized as a dull, heavy sensation that does not radiate.
25. **a. bladder neck or prostatic inflammation.** Terminal hematuria occurs at the end of micturition and is usually secondary to inflammation in the area of the bladder neck or prostatic urethra.
26. **b. 15%.** Enuresis refers to urinary incontinence that occurs during sleep. It occurs normally in children up to 3 years of age but persists in about 15% of children at age 5 and about 1% of children at age 15.
27. **a. sudden onset.** A careful history will often determine whether the problem is primarily psychogenic or organic. In men with psychogenic impotence, the condition frequently develops rather quickly secondary to a precipitating event such as marital stress or change or loss of a sexual partner.
28. **a. cystoscopy.** A genital and rectal examination should be done to exclude the presence of tuberculosis, a PSA assessment and digital rectal examination should be done to exclude prostatic carcinoma, and a urinary cytologic assessment should be done to exclude the possibility of transitional cell carcinoma of the prostate.
29. **e. ectopic ureter. Pneumaturia is the passage of gas in the urine.** In patients who have not recently had urinary tract instrumentation or a urethral catheter placed, this is almost always due to a fistula between the intestine and bladder. Common causes include diverticulitis, carcinoma of the sigmoid colon, and regional enteritis (Crohn disease).
30. **a. Parkinson disease.** The second important example of nonspecific lower urinary tract symptoms that may occur secondary to a variety of neurologic conditions is irritative symptoms resulting from neurologic disease such as cerebrovascular accident, diabetes mellitus, and Parkinson disease.

Additional Study Points

1. See Table 3–1 in *Campbell-Walsh Urology, 10th edition* for the International Prostate Symptom Score.
2. I-PSS score: 0 to 7 mild symptoms, 8 to 19 moderate symptoms, 20 to 35 severe symptoms.
3. Renal pain radiates from the flank anteriorly to the respective lower quadrant and may be referred to the testis, labium, or medial aspect of the thigh. The pain is colicky (fluctuates).
4. Patients with slowly progressive urinary obstruction with bladder distention often have no pain despite residual volumes in excess of a liter.
5. Pain of prostatic origin is poorly localized.
6. Scrotal pain may be primary or referred. Pain referred to the testicle originates in the retroperitoneum, ureter, or kidney.
7. Hematuria, particularly in adults, should be regarded as a symptom of malignancy until proven otherwise.
8. Normally adults arise no more than twice a night to void.
9. Postvoid dribbling: Urine escapes into the bulbar urethra and then leaks at the end micturition. This may be alleviated by perineal pressure following voiding.
10. Those who present with microscopic hematuria and irritative voiding symptoms should be suspected of having carcinoma in situ until proven otherwise.
11. Continuous incontinence is most commonly due to ectopic ureter, urinary tract fistula, or totally incompetent sphincter.
12. Hematospermia almost always resolves spontaneously and is rarely associated with any significant urologic pathology.
13. When urinary obstruction is associated with fever and chills, it should be regarded as a urologic emergency.
14. It is always worthwhile to obtain the previous operative report in patients who are to be operated on.
15. If the patient is uncircumcised, the foreskin must be retracted for inspection of the glans.
16. The testes are normally 6 cm in length and 4 cm in width.
17. If one obtains a stool guaiac test (hemoccult) as a screen for colon cancer, two subsequent stool specimens must be obtained for an adequate test. If the hemoccult is positive, the patient should be on a red meat–free diet for 3 days before collection of three specimens.
18. A male urologist should always perform a female pelvic examination with a female nurse in attendance.
19. The bulbo cavernosus reflex tests the integrity of this spinal cord reflex involving S2 to S4.
20. A positive dipstick for blood in the urine indicates hematuria, hemoglobinuria, or myoglobinuria. Hematuria is distinguished from hemoglobinuria and myoglobinuria by microscopic examination of the centrifuged urine and identification of red blood cells.
21. Hematuria of nephrologic origin is frequently associated with proteinuria.
22. Anticoagulation at normal therapeutic levels does not predispose patients to hematuria.
23. The most accurate method to diagnosis urinary tract infection is by microscopic examination of the urine and identifying pyuria and bacteria. This is confirmed by urine culture.

4

Urinary Tract Imaging: Basic Principles

Pat F. Fulgham, MD, DABU, FACS ● Jay Todd Bishoff, MD, FACS

QUESTIONS

1. The measure of the potential adverse health effects of ionizing radiation in (Sv) is known as:
   a. radiation exposure.
   b. absorbed dose.
   c. equivalent dose.
   d. effective dose.
   e. relative radiation levels.

2. The relative radiation level associated with an abdominal CT without and with contrast is:
   a. none.
   b. minimal: <0.1 mSv.
   c. low: 0.1 to 1.0 mSv.
   d. moderate: 1 to 10 mSv.
   e. high: 10 to 100 mSv.

3. The most important risk of exposure to ionizing radiation is:
   a. induction of malignancy.
   b. alopecia.
   c. cataracts.
   d. diarrhea.
   e. skin irritation.

4. Bladder filling may precipitate autonomic dysreflexia in patients with a spinal cord injury above:
   a. S2.
   b. L4.
   c. T10.
   d. T12.
   e. T6.

5. Radiation exposure diminishes proportionally to the square of the distance from the radiation source. An exposure of 9 mSv at 1 foot from the source would be how much at 3 feet from the source?
   a. 0.09 mSv
   b. 1 mSv
   c. 3 mSv
   d. 9 mSv
   e. 27 mSv

6. The maximum excursion of a wave above and below the baseline is known as its:
   a. wavelength.
   b. frequency.
   c. period.
   d. cycle.
   e. amplitude.

7. The artifact that occurs when an ultrasound wave strikes an interface at a critical angle and is refracted with limited reflection is:
   a. reverberation artifact.
   b. increased thru-transmission artifact.
   c. edging artifact.
   d. comet-tail artifact.
   e. aliasing artifact.

8. Which ultrasound mode allows for detection and characterization of the velocity and direction of motion?
   a. Harmonic scanning
   b. Color Doppler
   c. Power Doppler
   d. Spatial compounding
   e. Gray-scale ultrasonography

9. If the kidney is less echogenic than the liver, it is described as:
   a. hyperechoic.
   b. hypoechoic.
   c. isoechoic.
   d. anechoic.
   e. echogenic.

10. The sonographic hallmark of testicular torsion is:
    a. the "blue dot" sign.
    b. epididymal edema.
    c. paratesticular fluid.

d. increased epididymal blood flow.

e. absence of intratesticular blood flow.

11. Type 2 diabetics on oral metformin biguanide hyperglycemic therapy are at risk for developing biguanide lactic acidosis after exposure to intravascular radiologic contrast media if they:

a. discontinue metformin 48 hours before the study.

b. have severe renal insufficiency and take metformin the day of the study.

c. are given a saline injection while taking metformin.

d. have normal kidney function and fail to stop metformin 48 hours before the study.

e. decrease metformin dose and increase other antihyperglycemic agents on the day of the study.

12. All of the following are true EXCEPT:

a. patients with a history of asthma are at greater risk of having an adverse reaction to contrast media.

b. severe allergic reactions are not dose dependent.

c. hyperosmolar contrast media are more likely to cause contrast reactions than are iso-osmolar agents.

d. the mechanism of action associated with severe idiosyncratic anaphylactoid reactions is an IgE antibody reaction to the contrast media.

e. severe cardiac disease is a risk factor for having an adverse reaction to contrast media.

13. After rapidly assessing airway, breathing, and circulation, the medical treatment of choice for a severe, life-threatening adverse drug reaction following exposure to contrast media is:

a. subcutaneous injection of epinephrine 0.5 mg of 1:10,000 epinephrine.

b. intravenous injection of 100 mg of methylprednisone.

c. 0.01 mg/kg of epinephrine (1:10,000 concentration) intramuscularly in the lateral thigh.

d. intravenous diphenhydramine 50 mg.

e. 0.01 mg/kg of epinephrine (1:1000 concentration) intramuscularly in the lateral thigh.

14. Which of the following is not a risk factor for developing contrast-induced nephropathy (CIN)?

a. Type 2 diabetes mellitus

b. Dehydration

c. Hypertension

d. Ventricular ejection fraction <50%

e. Chronic kidney disease (glomerular filtration rate [GFR] <60 mL/min)

15. Research supports all of the following strategies for the prevention of CIN EXCEPT:

a. hydration with intravenous normal saline 1 mL/kg/hr for 6 hours after the contrast study.

b. intravenous 5% dextrose with water and sodium bicarbonate 154 mEq/L for 1 hour before the procedure.

c. intravenous furosemide 20 mg immediately following contrast study.

d. use of iso-osmolar or low-osmolar contrast media.

e. N-acetylcysteine 600 mg twice daily for two doses before and two doses after the study.

16. Nephrogenic systemic fibrosis (NSF) is:

a. a rare genetic condition exacerbated by the use of gadolinium-based contrast media (GBCM).

b. immediately evident after exposure to gadolinium in 10% of exposed patients.

c. fibrosis of the skin, subcutaneous tissue, and skeletal muscle seen in patients with chronic hypertension exposed to gadolinium contrast media.

d. not seen in patients with GFR greater than 60 mL/min/1.73 m^2.

e. mainly seen in dialysis patients exposed to gadolinium contrast media.

17. When a renal mass is seen on MRI, the most important characteristic indicating the presence of a malignancy is:

a. increase in signal intensity greater than 15% with gadolinium contrast media.

b. bright on T1 weight images.

c. dark in T2 weight images.

d. calcium deposits in the wall or base of the lesion.

e. high fat signal on T1-weighted images.

18. All of the following adrenal lesions are bright on T2-weighted images EXCEPT:

a. pheochromocytoma.

b. aldosterone-producing adenoma.

c. metastasis from renal cell carcinoma.

d. primary adrenal cortical carcinoma.

e. metastasis from malignant breast cancer.

19. During a diuretic renal scintigraphy

a. the diuretic is administered approximately 2 minutes after peak activity is seen in the collecting system.

b. T½ of greater than 14 minutes is consistent with obstruction.

c. 99m Tc-DMSA is the most sensitive for obstruction and determination of GFR.

d. intestinal or gallbladder activity should never be seen with 99m Tc-MAG3.

e. a T½ of less than 10 minutes is consistent with a nonobstructed system.

20. Positron emission tomography (PET):

a. has a higher diagnostic accuracy than CT for seminoma and nonseminoma testis cancer following chemotherapy.

b. is sensitive and specific for detection of postchemotherapy teratoma.

c. can be used with high positive predictive value within 2 weeks of completion of chemotherapy for bulky lymph adenopathy.

d. has greater predictive value of primary disease in metastatic urothelial carcinoma than MRI.

e. is able to detect local or systemic recurrence of prostate cancer in the majority of patients with prostate-specific antigen recurrence.

ANSWERS

1. **d. effective dose.** Although radiation exposure, absorbed dose, and equivalent dose all describe energy created in or absorbed by human tissue during diagnostic imaging studies, only effective dose reflects the biologic risk associated with that absorbed energy and is the correct answer. Various imaging studies can be categorized as having minimal, low, medium, or high potential for biologic risk, and these categorizations are known as the relative radiation levels for each test.

2. **e. high: 10 to 100 mSv.** Abdominal CT scanning with contrast usually involves multiple exposures for three separate phases: a precontrast phase, a postinjection phase, and a delayed phase. The result is often more than 200 individual images. Therefore the relative radiation level associated with abdominal CT scanning is high.

3. **a. induction of malignancy.** Although all of the other answers given are deterministic results of radiation exposure, it is the induction of a secondary malignancy that is the greatest potential risk to patients and radiology personnel.

4. **e. T6.** It is important to know that bladder distention associated with a static cystogram or voiding cystourethrogram may precipitate autonomic dysreflexia in certain patients. The level of spinal cord involvement above which autonomic dysreflexia is most likely to occur is T6.

5. **b. 1 mSv.** The rapid diminution in radiation exposure with increasing distance from the radiation source is based on the inverse square law (formula exposure = $1/\text{distance}^2$). If the radiation exposure at 1 foot from the source is 9 mSv, then at 3 feet from the source the exposure would be 1 mSv.

6. **e. amplitude.** In ultrasound physics it is crucial to understand the concept of amplitude. The amplitude of an ultrasound wave represents its relative energy state, and it is the amplitude of the returning sound wave that determines the pixel brightness to be displayed on a monitor during real-time gray-scale imaging.

7. **c. edging artefact.** Echo reflection is the primary mechanism whereby sound waves are returned to a transducer. It is important to understand how the angle of insonation affects the reflection and refraction of sound waves. There is a critical angle at which waves will travel along an interface rather than being returned to the probe. When this angle is encountered it provides a dark or hypoechoic "shadow" called an "edging artifact." A reverberation artifact is one caused by multiple transits of a sound wave between the transducer and the reflecting object. Increased thru-transmission artifact is caused by decreased attenuation of sound waves as they travel through a fluid-filled structure. Comet tail artifact is seen as the result of the interaction between sound waves and fluid and gas filled structures such as the bowel. Aliasing artifact is seen with Doppler ultrasonography.

8. **b. Color Doppler.** Doppler ultrasonography is important for evaluating motion and flow. The critical difference between color Doppler and power Doppler is that color Doppler is able to evaluate both flow velocity and direction. Power Doppler evaluates integrated amplitude of the returning sound waves. Although gray-scale ultrasonography does permit the evaluation of motion, it does not permit the characterization of velocity or direction. Harmonic scanning and spatial compounding are modes which allow the selective evaluation of, or combination of, reflected frequencies in ways which improve image quality.

9. **b. hypoechoic.** In describing ultrasound images it is important to use correct terminology. Descriptive terms involving echogenicity are relative terms. A hyperechoic or hypoechoic structure is being described in relation to the echogenicity of a reference standard. In most cases, the reference standard is the liver. In the adult, the normal kidney is hypoechoic relative to the normal liver in approximately 75% of patients.

10. **e. absence of intratesticular blood flow.** The absence of intratesticular blood flow is the classic sonographic finding in testicular torsion. However, there are many documented cases of some preserved intratesticular blood flow even in cases with significant torsion. Therefore testicular torsion remains a clinical diagnosis. Epididymal edema, paratesticular fluid, and increased epididymal blood flow may be seen with testicular torsion but may also be seen with other clinical conditions. The blue dot sign is a classic physical finding in torsion of the appendix testis.

11. **b. have severe renal insufficiency and take metformin the day of the study.** Patients with type 2 diabetes mellitus on metformin oral biguanide hyperglycemic therapy may have an accumulation of the drug after administering intravascular radiological contrast medium (IRCM), resulting in biguanide lactic acidosis presenting with vomiting, diarrhea, and somnolence. This condition is fatal in approximately 50% of cases (Wiholm, 1993).* Biguanide lactic acidosis is rare in patients with normal renal function. Consequently in patients with normal renal function and no known comorbidities, there is no need to discontinue metformin before IRCM use, nor is there a need to check creatinine following the imaging study.

12. **d. The mechanism of action associated with severe idiosyncratic anaphylactoid (IA) reactions is an IgE antibody reaction to the contrast media.** The exact mechanism of IA reactions is not known but is believed to be a combination of systemic effects. IA reactions have not been shown to result from a true IgE antibody immunologic reaction to the contrast media (Dawson, 1999). At least four mechanisms may play a role in IA reactions: (1) release of vasoactive substances including histamine; (2) activation of physiologic cascades including complement, kinin, coagulation, and fibrinolytic systems; (3) inhibition of enzymes including cholinesterase which may cause prolonged vagal stimulation; (4) the patient's own anxiety and fear of the actual procedure. IA reactions are not dose dependent. Severe reactions have been reported after only 1 mL injected at the beginning of the procedure and have also occurred after completion of a full dose despite no reaction to the initial test dose (Nelson, 1988; American College of Radiology, 1999; Thomsen, 1999).

13. **e. 0.01 mg/kg of epinephrine (1 : 1000 concentration) intramuscularly in the lateral thigh.** Rapid administration of epinephrine is the treatment of choice for severe contrast reactions. Current guidelines recommend immediate delivery of 0.01 mg/kg of body

---

*Sources referenced can be found in *Campbell-Walsh Urology, 10th Edition,* on the Expert Consult website.

weight to a maximum of 0.5 mg of 1 : 1000 concentration of epinephrine, injected intramuscularly in the lateral thigh as first-line treatment. Subcutaneous injection is much less effective. Intravenous injection can be given with more dilute concentration and must be given slowly (ACR Guidelines, 2008; Lightfoot, 2009).

14. **d. Ventricular ejection fraction less than 50%.** The most common patient-related risk factors resulting in CIN include chronic kidney disease (creatinine clearance <60 mL/min), diabetes mellitus, dehydration, congestive heart failure, age, hypertension, low hematocrit, and ventricular ejection fraction less than 40%. The patients at highest risk for developing CIN are those with both diabetes *and* preexisting renal insufficiency. The most common non–patient-related causes are high osmolar contrast agents, ionic contrast, increased contrast viscosity, and large contrast volume infused (Pannu, 2006).

15. **c. intravenous furosemide 20 mg immediately following contrast study.** The summary of the meta-analysis for the prevention of CIN after contrast media use supports using hydration, bicarbonate, iso- or lo-osmolar contrast media, and N-acetylcysteine. In one review article N-acetylcysteine was determined to be more protective than hydration alone. Furosemide was found to increase the risk of developing CIN. (Pannu, 2006; Kelly, 2008).

16. **d. not seen in patients with GFR greater than 60 mL/min/1.73 m^2.** Patients with a GFR less than 30 mL/min/1.73 m^2 not on chronic dialysis are the most difficult patient population in terms of choosing imaging modality. They are at risk for CIN if exposed to iodinated contrast media for CT imaging and are also at significant risk of developing NSF if exposed to GBCM during MRI. Recent data suggest that the risk of NSF may be greatest in patients with a GFR of less than 15 mL/min/1.73 m^2 and much less in patients with GFRs that are higher. Patients with severe chronic kidney disease have a 1% to 7% chance of developing NSF after GBCM MRI (Kanal, 2008).

17. **a. increase in signal intensity greater than 15% with gadolinium contrast.** The most important characteristic of a solid neoplasm is the presence of enhancement. MRI enhancement is evaluated by comparing nonenhanced T1-weighted images to gadolinium-enhanced T1-weighted images. Any detectable lesion is assessed for measurable increase in signal intensity after gadolinium contrast administration. If the lesion is brighter on the postcontrast image and increases in signal intensity by more than 15%, it is declared enhancing and is consistent with renal cancer. Benign lesions including angiomyolipomas will also enhance with gadolinium contrast. However, on T1-weighted images high signal fat content will be detected. Neither MRI nor CT imaging can differentiate an oncocytoma from renal cell carcinoma (Pretorius, 2000).

18. **b. aldosterone-producing adenoma.** Pheochromocytoma, adrenal cortical carcinoma, and metastatic lesions to the adrenal are usually of high signal intensity or bright on T2-weighted images (Korobkin, 1996). The benign adrenal myolipoma is easily demonstrated on T1-weighted images because fat contained within these lesions has a high signal or is bright compared with surrounding tissue.

19. **e. a T$_{1/2}$ of less than 10 minutes is consistent with a nonobstructed system.** A diuretic (usually furosemide 0.5 mg/kg) is administered when maximum collecting system activity is visualized. The T$_{1/2}$ is the time it takes for collecting system activity to decrease by 50% from that at the time of diuretic administration. This is highly technician dependent because the diuretic must be given when the collecting system is displaying maximum activity. Transit time thought the collecting system in less than 10 minutes is consistent with a normal, nonobstructed collecting system. T$_{1/2}$ of 10 to 20 minutes shows mild to moderate delay and may or may not be associated with a mechanical obstruction (Gambhir, 2004).

20. **a. has a higher diagnostic accuracy than CT for seminoma and nonseminoma testis cancer following chemotherapy.** There are some data on the use of PET/CT in testis cancer, where PET/CT was found to have a higher diagnostic accuracy than CT for staging and restaging in the assessment of a CT-visualized residual mass following chemotherapy for seminoma and nonseminomatous germ cell tumors (Albers, 1999; Hain, 2000).

Additional Study Points

1. Absorbed dose is measured in units called Gray (Gy). 1 rad = 0.01 Gy, or 1 centigray (cGy) = 1 rad.
2. The amount of energy absorbed by a tissue is referred to as the equivalent dose and is measured in Sieberts (Sb). Exposure of the eyes and gonads to radiation has a more significant biologic impact than exposure of other parts of the body. Exposure time during fluoroscopy should be minimized by using short bursts of fluoroscopy; positioning the image intensifier as close to the patient as feasible substantially reduces scatter radiation.
3. There are four basic types of iodinated contrast media: (1) ionic monomer, (2) nonionic monomer, (3) ionic dimer, (4) nonionic dimer.
4. Idiosyncratic anaphylactoid reactions are potentially fatal and are more common in patients with a prior history of adverse reactions to contrast media, asthmatics, diabetics, those with impaired renal and cardiac function, and those on β-adrenergic blockers.
5. It is common to have nausea, flushing, pruritus, urticaria, headache, and occasionally emesis after administration of contrast media.
6. Patients at high risk for adverse allergic reactions should be medicated with steroids, given 6 hours before the injection of contrast media, as well as antihistamines.
7. For retrograde pyelography it is useful to dilute contrast media by half with sterile saline, which facilitates identifying filling defects in the collecting system. There is a low risk of contrast reactions in patients in whom a retrograde or loopogram is performed.
8. One cycle per second is known as 1 Hertz (Hz). High-frequency ultrasonic transducers of 6 to 10 MHz are used to image structures near the surface. Deeper structures

require lower frequencies of 3.5 to 5 MHz. Axial resolution improves with increasing frequency, and depth of penetration decreases with increasing frequency.

9. Resistive index is the peek velocity minus the end-diastolic velocity over the peek systolic velocity. This is measured using the color flow Doppler with spectral display and is used to characterize renal artery stenosis, ureteral obstruction, and penile arterial insufficiency.

10. By convention, the liver is used as a benchmark for echogenicity. By convention, the cephalad aspect of the structure is to the left of the image.

11. Ultrasonography may produce injury due to mechanical effects caused by cavitation or by heat generation.

12. TcDTPA is primarily filtered by the glomerulus.

13. Because TcDMSA is both filtered by the glomerulus and secreted by the proximal tubule, it localizes in the renal cortex.

14. TcMAG3 is cleared mainly by tubular secretion.

15. A T one-half less than 10 minutes suggests an unobstructed system. A T one-half greater than 20 minutes is consistent with renal obstruction.

16. 18F fluorodeoxyglucose (FDG) is used as an imaging agent in PET scanning and takes advantage of the fact that tumors have increased glycolysis and decreased dephosphorylation.

17. Hounsfield units scale assigns a value of −1000 Hounsfield units for air. Dense bone is assigned a value of a +1000 Hounsfield units, and water is assigned 0 Hounsfield units.

18. With the exception of some indinavir stones, all renal and ureteral calculi may be detected by helical CT.

19. The advantage of MRI is high-contrast resolution of soft tissue on T1-weighted images. Fluid has a low signal and appears dark on T1-weighted images; on T2-weighted images, fluid has a high signal and appears bright. Gadolinium increases the brightness of T1-weighted images. Hemorrhage within a cyst results in a high signal on T1-weighted images.

chapter 5

Outcomes Research

Mark S. Litwin, MD, MPH

QUESTIONS

1. Barriers to health care access may include which of the following?
   a. Lack of health insurance
   b. Lack of transportation
   c. Beliefs about the health care system
   d. Culture
   e. All of the above

2. Costs of hospital care are best approximated by measuring:
   a. charges.
   b. collections.
   c. resources used.
   d. severity of illness.
   e. all of the above.

3. A true assessment of health care costs must include the amount of money spent on:
   a. facilities.
   b. disposable supplies.
   c. personnel.
   d. equipment.
   e. all of the above.

4. The introduction of diagnosis-related groups (DRGs) in the 1980s led to:
   a. longer hospital stays for most patients.
   b. shorter hospital stays for most patients.
   c. higher reimbursements for hospitals.
   d. higher reimbursements for physicians.
   e. increased costs.

5. Quality-adjusted life years (QALYs) are a metric used in:
   a. basic quality-of-life analysis in individual patients.
   b. cost-effectiveness analysis for populations of patients.
   c. patient satisfaction analysis for individual patients.
   d. cost-benefit analysis for individual patients.
   e. determining the number of years an individual is free of the condition.

6. Case mix is a metric that may be used in the study of medical outcomes to adjust for:
   a. comorbidity of a population cared for by a given provider.
   b. severity of illness in a population cared for by a given provider.

c. both.
d. neither.

7. In the Donabedian model of quality of care, measures of structure include:
   a. interpersonal skill with which a physician interacts with patients.
   b. perioperative mortality rates.
   c. patient satisfaction.
   d. board certification of physicians in a provider group.
   e. complication rates.

8. In the Donabedian model of quality of care, measures of outcome include:
   a. patient satisfaction.
   b. health-related quality of life.
   c. survival.
   d. all of the above.

9. Health-related quality of life is best assessed by:
   a. patients themselves.
   b. spouses or immediate family members of patients.
   c. primary care physicians caring for patients.
   d. specialists caring for patients.
   e. specially trained examiners.

10. Dysfunction and its related distress (also called "bother") are generally:
    a. perfectly correlated.
    b. completely independent.
    c. related but imperfectly correlated.
    d. measures of the same phenomenon.
    e. meaningful when the correlation coefficient is 0.1.

11. Disease-specific health-related quality of life domains in patients with urologic cancer include:
    a. physical function.
    b. emotional well-being.
    c. social function.
    d. sexual dysfunction.
    e. cardiac function.

12. In psychometric terms, reliability refers to how free an instrument is of:
    a. missing data.
    b. measurement error.
    c. grammatical or typographic errors.

d. invalid data.

e. selection bias.

13. When a scale has a coefficient alpha of 0.90, the scale has a high degree of:

a. alternate form reliability.

b. test-retest reliability.

c. internal consistency reliability.

d. concurrent validity.

e. construct validity.

ANSWERS

1. **d. All of the above.** Barriers to access may be financial or nonfinancial and include any factor that decreases the likelihood that an individual in need will receive medical services.

2. **c. resources used.** Charges are notoriously poor proxies for actual medical costs because of the way in which hospital budgets are calculated; actual collections do not account for deductibles, copayments, and opportunity costs.

3. **d. all of the above.** Each of the factors mentioned contributes to the total cost of health care.

4. **b. shorter hospital stays for most patients.** DRGs allow for the calculation of prospective payments to hospitals and as such have led to shorter lengths of stay; they have also led to decreased reimbursements to hospitals.

5. **b. cost-effectiveness analysis for populations of patients.** QALYs are used in population analysis and not for individual patients.

6. **c. both.** Measuring case mix allows for outcomes to be controlled for both the underlying medical diseases and the severity of the disease of interest among groups of patients under the care of a provider.

7. **d. board certification of physicians in a provider group.** Structural attributes of health care include clinician characteristics, such as board certification but not measures of process such as interpersonal style or outcome measures such as mortality and patient satisfaction.

8. **d. all of the above.** Each of these factors may be considered a valid measure of medical outcomes.

9. **a. patients themselves.** It is axiomatic that health-related quality-of-life outcomes be reported by patients themselves, as they perceive them.

10. **c. related but imperfectly correlated.** In the various domains of disease-specific health-related quality of life, function and bother are loosely associated with each other but measure discrete phenomena.

11. **d. sexual dysfunction.** Disease-specific, health-related, quality-of-life instruments focus on domains that are directly relevant to the specific disease or treatment.

12. **b. measurement error.** Reliability refers to what proportion of a test score is true and what proportion is due to chance variation (or measurement error).

13. **c. internal consistency reliability.** Cronbach's coefficient alpha is a well-established measure of internal consistency reliability.

Additional Study Points

1. Costs—what the provider spends to supply the service.
2. Charges—what the provider bills for the service, not necessarily what the provider collects for the service.
3. Resource utilization—takes into account the duration, frequency, and intensity of the service.
4. Length of stay—may be used to quantify resource utilization.
5. Cost-effectiveness is calculated by developing a probability model of possible medical outcomes for different interventions. The different interventions may then be compared taking into account costs.
6. Life years—the number of years lived for a population, not an individual patient.
7. Quality-adjusted life years—adjustment of the life years to account for the impact of various treatments on the health status of an individual.
8. Cost-benefit analysis—takes into account not only cost but other factors that may not have a monetary value such as extra years of life.
9. Case mix—refers to the severity of illness and the degree of comorbidity in a group of patients.

Basics of Urologic Surgery

Core Principles of Perioperative Care

Manish A. Vira, MD ● Louis R. Kavoussi, MD, MBA

QUESTIONS

1. A 64-year-old male is found to have an 8-cm left renal mass and presents to the office for evaluation regarding laparoscopic radical nephrectomy. He has a personal history of hypertension, non–insulin-dependent diabetes, and 30-pack-year tobacco use (quit 10 years ago). He has a strong family history of heart disease in that his father died at the age of 55 from a myocardial infarction. Further questioning reveals that he does not regularly exercise but is able to walk up three flights of stairs without shortness of breath. Before surgery, to minimize the risk of complication, the patient should:

   a. undergo routine preoperative testing with complete blood count, basic metabolic panel, electrocardiogram, and chest radiograph.

   b. be referred to cardiology consultation to determine if further testing is necessary.

   c. undergo noninvasive cardiac stress testing.

   d. undergo pulmonary function testing to determine the need for preoperative bronchodilators.

   e. be started on a perioperative β blocker to reduce the risk of perioperative myocardial ischemia.

2. With regard to unique patient populations, which of the following statements is true?

   a. Although elderly patients have an increased perioperative risk, recent larger trials have not found age as an independent risk factor for perioperative morbidity and mortality.

   b. Morbidly obese patients should undergo open rather than laparoscopic surgery because of increased risk of pulmonary complications.

   c. In a pregnant patient presenting with urolithiasis, if possible, operative intervention should be delayed until the second trimester.

   d. A patient who presents with a 30-pound weight loss over the previous 3 months should be started on parenteral feedings immediately postoperatively after elective surgery.

   e. In patients with liver disease, the primary determinant of postoperative risk is degree of liver function enzyme abnormality.

3. A 74-year-old male with muscle invasive bladder cancer is scheduled for radical cystectomy and ileal conduit urinary diversion. Preoperative urine culture shows no growth at 72 hours. The most important factor in prevention of surgical site infection in this patient is:

   a. preoperative bowel preparation with oral antibiotics (Nichols prep) and sodium phosphate solution (Fleet).

   b. administration of 2 g cefoxitin 1 hour before incision.

   c. continuation of perioperative antibiotics for 48 hours following surgery.

   d. preoperative hair removal with mechanical clippers and proper sterile preparation of the operative field.

   e. optimization of comorbid illness and nutritional status.

4. According to current guidelines in the prevention of thromboembolic complications, a 78-year-old male with a recent history of colon cancer, medical history of hypertension, coronary artery disease (postoperative angioplasty with two coronary stents), and chronic renal insufficiency (creatinine 2.9 mg/dL) undergoing laparoscopic transabdominal surgery should have pneumatic compression stockings and

   a. early ambulation.

   b. aspirin and early ambulation.

   c. low-molecular-weight heparin.

   d. low-molecular-weight heparin and aspirin.

   e. unfractionated heparin and aspirin.

5. A 72-year-old female with a history of asthma, mild congestive heart failure, and breast cancer is to undergo cystoscopy and placement of a midurethral sling. Of the following agents, the best choice for anesthesia induction would be:

   a. inhaled halothane.

   b. intravenous thiopental.

   c. inhaled desflurane.

   d. inhaled sevoflurane.

   e. intravenous succinylcholine.

6. The most appropriate indication for blood product transfusion is:

   a. packed red blood cells for an 82-year-old male with coronary artery disease and hematocrit of 31%.

b. fresh frozen plasma for a 69-year-old patient with an international normalized ratio (INR) of 1.6 scheduled to undergo laparotomy for a small bowel obstruction.

c. platelet transfusion for a 78-year-old male with chronic renal insufficiency who was scheduled to undergo partial nephrectomy and found to have a platelet count of 55,000 on preoperative testing.

d. packed red blood cells for a healthy 22-year-old male with a stable large retroperitoneal hematoma after motor vehicle accident and hematocrit of 21%.

e. Fresh frozen plasma for a 64-year-old female during resection of a large renal mass with inferior vena cava thrombus who experiences significant blood loss requiring 8 units of packed red blood cell transfusion.

7. In order to reduce the risk of iatrogenic injury to a patient in the operating room, the patient should:

a. be maintained with core body temperature between 36° C and 38° C throughout the perioperative period.

b. be instructed to bathe with an antiseptic solution the night before surgery.

c. be secured to the operating room table with fixed shoulder braces for procedures in steep Trendelenburg.

d. be positioned in the lithotomy position one leg at a time to ensure safe flexion of the hips.

e. be positioned and draped by the operating room staff before arrival of the surgeon.

8. In a patient undergoing an exploratory laparotomy for pelvic abscess following radical cystectomy, the best method of abdominal fascial closure is with:

a. polyglycolic acid (Dexon) suture with continuous closure.

b. silk suture with continuous closure.

c. polypropylene (Prolene) suture with interrupted closure.

d. polyglactin (Vicryl) suture with interrupted closure.

e. polydioxanone suture (PDS) with continuous closure.

ANSWERS

1. **e. be started on preoperative β blocker to reduce the risk of myocardial ischemia during the perioperative period.** This choice is best given the patient's multiple risk factors. Although cardiac stress testing may be considered, the patient's ability to climb three flights of stairs indicates a capacity of greater than 4 METS and therefore low risk of significant coronary artery disease. Although routine preoperative testing is performed widely, there is no evidence that routine testing reduces the risk of perioperative complications.

2. **c. In a pregnant patient presenting with urolithiasis, if possible, operative intervention should be delayed until the second trimester.** The second trimester represents the least anesthetic risk to the mother and fetus with regard to spontaneous abortion and teratogenicity. Although controversy exists as to the exact etiology, several recent trials have found age as an independent predictor of morbidity on multivariate analyses. Laparoscopic surgery is the preferred approach in morbidly obese patients secondary to the reduced risk of pulmonary and wound complications. Literature suggests that severely malnourished patients (>20 pounds weight loss in 3 months)

significantly benefit from 7 to 10 days of enteral (not parenteral) feedings *before* elective surgery. The primary determinants of the degree of severity in patients with cirrhosis are hepatic function and severity of clinical manitestations.

3. **b. administration of 2 g cefoxitin 1 hour before incision.** Administration of appropriate antibiotics within 60 minutes of incision has been shown to significantly decrease the incidence of surgical site infections. Recent meta-analyses from the colorectal literature indicate that mechanical bowel preparation does not decrease the risk of postoperative infections. Unless in the presence of active infection, perioperative antibiotics should be stopped after 24 hours of incision to decrease the risk of *Clostridium difficile* colitis. Although preoperative hair removal and optimization of nutritional status and comorbid illness improve surgical outcomes, there is no specific evidence that this reduces surgical site infections.

4. **e. unfractionated heparin and aspirin.** The clinical scenario describes a patient with high to highest risk of venous thromboembolism risk. As such, the patient would require both mechanical and pharmacologic prophylaxis. In a patient with renal insufficiency, unfractioned heparin is a better choice over low-molecular-weight heparin. There is no evidence that aspirin is effective in the prevention of venous thromboembolism, but in a patient with coronary stents, aspirin is important in the prevention of stent thrombosis in the perioperative period.

5. **d. inhaled sevoflurane.** This is an excellent choice for rapid induction in this patient secondary to its odorless and bronchodilation properties. Halothane can adversely affect left ventricular function and should be used with caution in patients with congestive heart failure. Desflurane has a pungent odor and is more suitable for maintenance of anesthesia during prolonged procedures. Intravenous thiopental can increase airway reactivity and is not appropriate in patients with asthma. Succinylcholine is appropriate for neuromuscular blockade and not commonly used for induction.

6. **c. platelet transfusion for a 78-year-old male with chronic renal insufficiency who was scheduled to undergo partial nephrectomy and found to have a platelet count of 55,000 on preoperative testing.** This patient has moderate thrombocytopenia with likely platelet dysfunction secondary to uremia undergoing a high bleeding risk procedure; therefore platelet transfusion is indicated. Current indications for packed red blood cell transfusion are maintenance of hematocrit of greater than 30% in patients with high risk of myocardial ischemia or in patients with hematocrit 21% to 30% with signs of inadequate oxygen carrying capacity. Fresh frozen plasma transfusion is indicated only in the presence of active bleeding rather than isolated INR elevation or large-volume transfusion.

7. **a. be maintained with core body temperature between 36° C and 38° C throughout the perioperative period.** Hypothermia by 1° C has been shown to increase surgical site infection and postoperative complications. There is no evidence that showering with an antiseptic solution the night before surgery decreases the incidence of wound infection. Fixed shoulder braces have been associated with an increased risk of brachial plexus injury and should not be used in the operating room. Both legs should be positioned simultaneously when placing

patients in the dorsal lithotomy position. Everyone in the operating room is responsible for patient safety, and therefore the surgeon should always be present for patient positioning.

8. **e. polydioxanone suture with continuous closure.** Continuous closure with PDS (slowly absorbable) suture has been shown to have the lowest wound failure rates. In the presence of infection, braided sutures (silk and Vicryl) should be avoided to prevent secondary wound infection and failure. Although nonabsorbable sutures may be used, these have been associated with increased postoperative patient discomfort. Fast-absorbing sutures (such as Dexon) should not be used in continuous fascial closure secondary to increased wound failure risks.

Additional Study Points

1. One must always determine whether a woman in the child-bearing years is pregnant before a surgical procedure. A urine pregnancy test is a simple method to do this.

2. The American Society of Anesthesiologists' classification is a significant predictor of operative mortality.

3. Preoperative cardiac evaluation is meant to identify serious coronary artery disease, heart failure, symptomatic arrhythmias, and the presence of a pacemaker or defibrillator. Major clinical predictors of cardiovascular risk are a recent myocardial infarction (within 1 month), unstable angina, evidence of an ischemic burden, decompensated heart failure, significant arrhythmias, and severe valvular disease.

4. Patients with an FEV1 of less than 30% predicted are at high risk for complications.

5. Perioperative β blockade is associated with a reduced risk of death among high-risk patients undergoing major non-cardiac surgical procedures. However, more recent data brings this into question.

6. Patients who have a depressed hypothalamic pituitary adrenal axis due to exogenous steroids should receive 50 to 100 mg of intravenous hydrocortisone before the induction of anesthesia and 25 to 50 mg every 8 hours thereafter until the patient's medication is resumed.

7. In the elderly, delirium can be the first clinical sign of hypoxia, metabolic, or infectious complications.

8. In the pregnant patient, postoperative pain is best managed with narcotic analgesics.

9. It is important to remember that for prophylaxis of venous thromboembolic disease and the use of antibiotic and mechanical bowel preps before intestinal surgery, the studies are often based on data obtained from nonurologic patients. The urologist must consider this when the procedure being performed is significantly different from the standard general surgical operation on which the data are based.

10. The half-life of warfarin is 36 to 42 hours, and it is recommended that warfarin be stopped 5 days before the surgical event.

11. For moderate to high-risk groups on anticoagulation therapy, a therapeutic bridge is performed using low-molecular-weight heparin. This may be stopped 12 hours before the procedure and instituted shortly after its completion.

12. The indications for fresh frozen plasma are immediate reversal of warfarin and replacement of specific clotting factors.

13. The most common cause of transfusion-related fatality is transfusion-related acute lung injury.

14. Hypothermia results in increased blood loss and an increase incidence of wound infection.

15. If hair is to be removed, it should preferably be removed immediately before the surgical event with clippers.

16. The surgical scar regains 3% of strength at 1 week, 20% at 3 weeks, and 80% at 3 months.

17. Rapidly absorbable sutures used for continuous fascia closure are associated with an increased incidence of incisional hernias.

Fundamentals of Instrumentation and Urinary Tract Drainage

Carlos E. Méndez Probst, MD ● Hassan Razvi, MD, FRCSC ●
John D. Denstedt, MD, FRCSC, FACS

QUESTIONS

1. What catheter type would be the most appropriate to drain a thick/viscous urine?
   a. 20-Fr two-way Foley catheter
   b. 20-Fr Nélaton catheter
   c. 20-Fr Malecot catheter
   d. 20-Fr Coudé catheter
   e. 16-Fr two-way Foley catheter

2. The French (Fr) number of a urethral catheter refers to the size of:
   a. total length.
   b. internal diameter.
   c. external circumference.
   d. internal circumference.
   e. volume of the retaining balloon.

3. The most import risk factor for developing a hospital-acquired urinary tract infection is:
   a. patient immunosuppression.
   b. history of previous urinary tract infection.
   c. type of catheter coating.
   d. use of an indwelling urethral catheter.
   e. failure to use a nonrefluxing urine collection bag.

4. The most important measure to prevent catheter-related urinary tract infections is the use of:
   a. sterile gloves at insertion.
   b. a closed drainage system.
   c. drainage system irrigation with antiseptic solution.
   d. antiseptic lubricant at insertion.
   e. perimeatal antibiotic ointment.

5. What is the most frequent complication of ureteral stents?
   a. Ureteral perforation
   b. Lower urinary tract symptoms
   c. Urinary tract infection
   d. Encrustation
   e. Pyelonephritis

6. Which is the most important risk factor for ureteral stent encrustation?
   a. Amount of conditioning film adherence to the catheter
   b. Hyperuricemia
   c. Hypercalciuria
   d. Stent indwelling time
   e. Shock wave lithotripsy therapy

7. What is the most biocompatible material for urinary biomaterial applications?
   a. Silicone
   b. Polyurethane
   c. Percuflex
   d. Nitinol
   e. Latex

8. The treatment most likely to be successful in eliminating a biomaterial related biofilm is:
   a. a 15-day course of gentamicin/cephalosporin antibiotic (Cextriaxone).
   b. oral nitrofurantoin until catheter removal.
   c. oral quinolone until catheter removal.
   d. urinary tract instillation with chemolysis/antibiotic solution.
   e. removal of the catheter.

ANSWERS

1. **c. 20-Fr Malecot catheter.** Because the goal is to drain thick fluids, this type of catheter has the largest available lumen size by size—it lacks a balloon inflation channel, which reduces the luminal surface area of other catheters.

2. **c. the external circumference.** The French size is a measure of the external, not internal, circumference of a catheter.

3. **d. use of an indwelling catheter.** As a foreign object inside a sterile cavity, it is responsible for more than 80% of the hospital-acquired urinary tract infections.

4. **b. a closed drainage system.** It is so far the only intervention supported by strong scientific evidence.
5. **b. Lower urinary tract symptoms.** Up to 90% of the stented patients have lower urinary tract symptoms, with more than half reporting an important negative impact in their quality of life.
6. **d. Stent indwelling time.** The rate of stone encrustation is 9.2% before 6 weeks, 47.5% in 6 to 12 weeks, and 76.3% after 12 weeks in polyurethane stents.

7. **a. Silicone.** This material has been found to be the most biocompatible; however, its handling characteristics have limited its clinical use.
8. **e. removal of the catheter.** Once a biofilm has established itself in the surface of a biomaterial, there is practically no way to remove or sterilize it.

Additional Study Points

1. One French or Ch is equal to 0.33 mm and refers to the total circumference of the outside of the catheter.
2. The use of feeding tubes as urethral catheters is to be discouraged.
3. The use of silicone catheters is associated with a lower incidence of urinary tract infections when compared with those made with latex.
4. Topical anesthesia requires a minimum of 10 minutes of exposure. Many studies have shown that it is not helpful in reducing pain in routine catheterization.
5. Routine use of catheter coatings is currently not supported by the available literature.
6. For selected patients, a suprapubic catheter results in less discomfort than a urethral catheter.
7. More than 80% of patients experience stent-related pain affecting daily activities, 32% report sexual dysfunction, and 58% report reduced work capacity.
8. The use of an α_1-adrenergic blocker has been demonstrated to be beneficial in reducing stent symptoms and pain.
9. Indwelling stent time should be limited to 4 months; after that it should be changed or removed. For pregnant patients, the time limit is 6 to 8 weeks.
10. A biofilm is the microorganism's attempt to control its immediate environment by limiting exposure to harmful factors while enhancing exposure to tropic factors. It usually consists of three layers: (1) innermost or linking film that is attached to the surface, (2) a base film that contains the microorganisms, and (3) an outer layer, which is the point of egress or access for organisms.

Principles of Endoscopy

Branden Duffey, DO ● Manoj Monga, MD, FACS

QUESTIONS

1. A catheter with an outer diameter of 1 mm is approximately how many French?
   a. 1
   b. 2
   c. 3
   d. 4.5
   e. 5

2. When selecting an endoscope for a particular procedure:
   a. the largest endoscope the urethra can accept should be used.
   b. the endoscope that provides the best irrigation should be used.
   c. flexible endoscopes should be used in most cases to prevent urethral trauma.
   d. rigid endoscopes should be used unless there is a specific indication or need for flexible instruments.
   e. the smallest scope that permits performance of the anticipated procedure should be used.

3. When comparing the advantages of flexible versus rigid cystoscopes, which of the following is FALSE?
   a. The rod-lens systems in rigid cystoscopes offer superior imaging quality compared with fiberoptic flexible cystoscopes.
   b. The larger internal lumen of a rigid cystoscope provides improved irrigant flow and thus visualization compared with flexible cystoscopes.
   c. There are more patient positioning options when performing flexible cystoscopy compared with rigid cystoscopy.
   d. Endoscope passage over an elevated bladder neck/median lobe may be easier with a flexible cystoscope compared with a rigid cystoscope.
   e. Flexible cystoscopes generally have a larger working channel compared with rigid cystoscopes, allowing passage of a wider variety of instruments.

4. Which of the following statements regarding patient preparation for cystourethroscopy is FALSE?
   a. Preoperative antimicrobial prophylaxis is not indicated before simple cystourethroscopy unless specific patient risk factors are present.
   b. When antimicrobial prophylaxis is indicated, the antimicrobials of choice are the fluoroquinolones and trimethoprim-sulfamethoxazole.

c. Preoperative intraurethral injection of a water-soluble lubricant-anesthetic has been shown in most randomized studies to improve patient comfort during flexible cystoscopy.
   d. Informed consent should be obtained, explaining the risks and benefits of the procedure.
   e. It is important to ensure the patient does not have a urinary tract infection before the procedure because mechanical manipulation and bladder distention may exacerbate the infection.

5. All of the following statements regarding endoscopic evaluation of a continent urinary diversion are correct EXCEPT:
   a. Detailed understanding of the diversion type and construction may facilitate successful cystoscopy.
   b. The Mitrofanoff and tapered/imbricated ileal continence mechanisms are quite sturdy and will permit aggressive manipulation.
   c. Simple filling and diagnostic procedures may be performed via the catheterizable channel, but percutaneous access should be performed if ancillary procedures are indicated.
   d. Visualization may be impaired by mucus, debris, bowel peristalsis, and tortuous afferent limbs.
   e. Afferent limbs are best evaluated with flexible endoscopes because they are well suited to navigate limb folding, kinking, and tortuosity.

6. Which of the following is TRUE regarding semirigid ureteroscopes?
   a. The optical system in most currently available semirigid ureteroscopes is the rod-lens system.
   b. Compared with flexible ureteroscopes they have smaller irrigation channels, reduced irrigant flow and visualization, and a smaller field of vision.
   c. The proximal ureter is routinely accessed with the semirigid ureteroscope in male patients.
   d. Semirigid ureteroscopy is typically utilized for diagnosis and treatment of a pathologic process below the iliac vessels.
   e. In males a longer urethra, relatively fixed prostate, and larger psoas muscles rarely prevent semirigid ureteroscopy above the iliac vessels.

7. Which of the following is TRUE regarding ureteral dilation to facilitate ureteroscopy?
   a. Ureteral dilation is most commonly required at the ureteropelvic junction.

b. Ureteral dilation is most commonly required in the mid ureter.

c. Ureteral dilation is least commonly required at the ureterovesical junction.

d. Ureterovesical junction dilation is indicated before routine ureteroscopy.

e. Ureteral dilation should be performed only when ureteroscope passage is impaired.

8. Which of the following statements regarding ureteral access sheaths (UASs) is FALSE?

a. UASs significantly reduce renal pressures during ureteroscopy.

b. UASs reduce operative time and cost when utilized during ureteroscopy.

c. UASs reduce ureteroscope damage and increase the time between instrument servicing.

d. UASs increase the risk of ureteral strictures.

e. UASs facilitate ureteroscope insertion, simple reentry, and calculi retrieval.

9. Which of the following statements regarding intracorporeal lithotriptors utilized during ureteroscopy is TRUE?

a. Ballistic lithotripsy utilizes electrical energy to generate a spark that leads to the formation of cavitation bubbles.

b. Holmium laser lithotripsy occurs primarily through a photothermal mechanism resulting in calculus vaporization.

c. Electrohydraulic lithotripsy (EHL) utilizes pneumatic or electrokinetic energy to drive a projectile body against a probe tip, creating a "jackhammer" effect.

d. The primary disadvantage of ballistic lithotripsy is the low safety margin relating to heat generated at the probe tip.

e. The primary disadvantage of EHL lithotripsy is poor probe flexibility that limits access to the lower pole.

10. Which of the following statements is TRUE regarding intracorporeal holmium:YAG laser lithotripsy?

a. The holmium:YAG laser effectively fragments all stone types except cystine stones.

b. Fragments produced by holmium:YAG laser lithotripsy are slightly larger compared with other intracorporeal lithotriptors.

c. Maintaining a pulse energy ≥1.0 J and varying pulse frequency facilitates efficient lithotripsy.

d. Energy from the holmium:YAG laser propagates 0.5 to 1.0 cm, providing a high margin of safety.

e. Holmium:YAG laser lithotripsy causes less calculus retropulsion compared with other lithotriptors.

11. Which of the following statements is FALSE regarding patient preparation for ureteroscopy?

a. Anesthetic options include local anesthesia with or without intravenous sedation, regional anesthesia, and general anesthesia.

b. Preoperative antimicrobial prophylaxis is not recommended before diagnostic ureteroscopy.

c. When indicated, the prophylactic antimicrobials of choice are the fluoroquinolones and trimethoprim-sulfamethoxazole.

d. Ureteroscopy may be performed in the supine, flank, or prone positions.

e. Both Trendelenburg and reverse-Trendelenburg positioning may facilitate laser lithotripsy.

12. Which of the following maneuvers should NOT be performed when difficulty is encountered passing a ureteroscope through the ureterovesical junction?

a. Rotate the beak of the ureteroscope while providing adequate irrigation.

b. Pass a guidewire through the working channel of the ureteroscope and advance the scope between the two "railroad" wires.

c. Dilate the distal ureter with a 10-mm radially expanding balloon dilator.

d. Dilate the distal ureter with a 6/10-Fr coaxial dilator over a guidewire.

e. Place an indwelling ureteral stent and allow passive dilation for 2 weeks.

ANSWERS

1. **c. 3.** Measurements in the French system refer to the outer diameter of an instrument or catheter in mm. The diameter of a circle is expressed by the formula $2\pi r$ where r = radius, or $d\pi$ where d = diameter. Thus, the French measurement of a catheter with an outer diameter of 1 mm is approximately 3.

2. **e. the smallest scope that permits performance of the anticipated procedure should be used.** Retrograde instrumentation of urinary tract can cause mucosal/urothelial trauma, leading to stricture formation. To minimize this risk, the smallest diameter endoscope that will accomplish the goals of the procedure should be selected.

3. **e. Flexible cystoscopes generally have a larger working channel compared with rigid cystoscopes, allowing passage of a wider variety of instruments.** In general, rigid cystoscopes have a larger working channel compared with flexible cystoscopes. The other answers are true statements regarding the pros of flexible or rigid cystoscopes.

4. **c. Preoperative intraurethral injection of a water-soluble lubricant-anesthetic has been shown in most randomized studies to improve patient comfort during flexible cystoscopy.** Most of the randomized prospective placebo-controlled studies have failed to demonstrate superiority of intraurethral lubricant-anesthetic over a standard lubricant. The other answer options are correct statements.

5. **b. The Mitrofanoff and tapered/imbricated ileal continence mechanisms are quite sturdy and will permit aggressive manipulation.** The Mitrofanoff and tapered/imbricated continent catheterizable channels tend to be fragile reconstructions. Aggressive instrumentation and manipulation can lead to stomal stenosis or loss of urinary continence.

6. **d. Semirigid ureteroscopy is typically utilized for diagnosis and treatment of a pathologic process below the iliac vessels.** Most semirigid ureteroscopes are based on fiberoptic systems; however, digital systems are also available. Semirigid ureteroscopes offer larger irrigation channels and improved irrigation, visualization, and field of

vision compared with flexible ureteroscopes. Frequently the proximal ureter may be safely accessed in female patients, but this is less common in males.

7. **e. Ureteral dilation should be performed only when ureteroscope passage is impaired.** Technologic advancements have permitted the miniaturization of ureteroscopes, eliminating the need for routine ureteral dilation. Ureteral dilation should only be performed when ureteroscope passage is impaired. Ureteral dilation is most commonly required at the ureterovesical junction, the narrowest portion of the ureter.

8. **d. UASs increase the risk of ureteral strictures.** Concerns regarding UAS-induced ureteral ischemia, necrosis, and stricture have largely been disregarded because the incidence of stricture after ureteroscopy with UAS has been demonstrated to be the same as with ureteroscopy alone (1.4%). The other answer choices illustrate the benefits of UAS use during ureteroscopy.

9. **b. Holmium laser lithotripsy occurs primarily through a photothermal mechanism resulting in calculus vaporization.** Ballistic lithotripsy harnesses pneumatic or electrokinetic energy sources to create a "jackhammer" effect with the ability to fragment all stone types. Because little heat is generated at the probe tip it has a high safety margin. EHL probes use electrical energy to create a cavitation bubble that collapses, causing shockwaves and microjets. Although EHL probes are quite flexible and inexpensive, the primary disadvantage of EHL lithotripsy is the propensity to damage ureteral mucosa and cause ureteral perforation.

10. **e. Holmium:YAG laser lithotripsy causes less calculus retropulsion compared with other lithotriptors.** Benefits of holmium:YAG laser lithotripsy are (1) the ability to fragment all stone types; (2) production of smaller fragments than other lithotriptors; (3) less stone retropulsion during lithotripsy; (4) stone free rates ≥90% in several case series; and (5) wide margin of safety. Efficient lithotripsy is facilitated by limiting the laser pulse energy to ≤1.0 J and varying the pulse frequency as needed. Energy generated by the holmium:YAG laser propagates no farther than 0.5 to 1.0 mm, providing a high margin of safety.

11. **b. Preoperative antimicrobial prophylaxis is not recommended before diagnostic ureteroscopy.** The best practice statement regarding antimicrobial prophylaxis released by the American Urological Association states that all patients undergoing ureteroscopy should receive preoperative antimicrobial prophylaxis and the duration of therapy should be ≤24 hours.

12. **c. Dilate the distal ureter with a 10-mm radially expanding balloon dilator.** All of the other options listed are accepted maneuvers when trouble is encountered while passing a ureteroscope past the ureterovesical junction. Balloon dilation is a valid option; however, a 4-mm balloon should be utilized to minimize ureteral trauma.

Additional Study Points

1. Simple endoscopy does not require prophylactic antibiotics unless there are risk factors.
2. If electrocautery is used, an electrolyte-free solution should be employed.
3. Narrow band imaging filters light into two separate bands that are absorbed by hemoglobin, aiding in identifying hypervascular lesions.
4. Five-aminolevulinic acid instilled in the bladder accumulates in neoplastic and inflammatory cells and fluoresces red when illuminated with blue light.
5. For ureteroscopy, the irrigants are typically physiologic solutions, such as normal saline. However, with a ureteral access sheath in place low osmolarity irrigant fluids may be utilized.
6. Complications of basketing include ureteral avulsion, intussusception, abrasion, perforation, postoperative stricture formation, and basket entrapment and retention.

chapter 9

Fundamentals of Laparoscopic and Robotic Urologic Surgery

Louis Eichel, MD ● Elspeth M. McDougall, MD, FRCSC, MHPE
● Ralph V. Clayman, MD

QUESTIONS

1. Absolute contraindications to laparoscopic surgery include all of the following EXCEPT:
   a. uncorrectable coagulopathy.
   b. hemodynamic instability.
   c. significant abdominal wall infection.
   d. suspected malignant ascites.
   e. extensive prior abdominal or pelvic surgery.

2. Of the following, which is considered a relative contraindication to laparoscopic surgery?
   a. Generalized peritonitis
   b. Massive hemoperitoneum
   c. Intestinal obstruction with intention to treat
   d. Extensive prior abdominal or pelvic surgery
   e. Abdominal wall infection

3. The best method of preoperative preparation for patients undergoing laparoscopic renal surgery is:
   a. a 3-day mechanical bowel preparation if an extraperitoneal or retroperitoneoscopic approach is anticipated.
   b. a mechanical bowel preparation and antibiotic preparation with Neomycin and metronidazole.
   c. for most uncomplicated patients, a clear liquid diet and a light mechanical bowel preparation the day before surgery.
   d. both an antibiotic and 3-day mechanical bowel preparation in patients who have had previous abdominal surgery if one anticipates encountering dense intra-abdominal adhesions.
   e. intravenous antibiotics 1 hour before surgery.

4. Which of the statements regarding pneumoperitoneum is TRUE?
   a. CO_2 as an insufflant can be dangerous because it can support combustion.
   b. CO_2 is most commonly used because it is insoluble in the blood.
   c. In patients with chronic respiratory disease, CO_2 is advantageous because it does not accumulate in the bloodstream.
   d. Argon gas would be an ideal insufflant owing to its low cost and poor solubility in blood.
   e. Nitrous oxide has previously been used for insufflation; however, it is no longer routinely used because of the potential for intra-abdominal explosion.

5. Studies have shown that during insufflation of the abdomen, 94% of the maximal intraperitoneal volume is achieved at an insufflation pressure of:
   a. 5 mm Hg.
   b. 10 mm Hg.
   c. 15 mm Hg.
   d. 20 mm Hg.
   e. 25 mm Hg.

6. Which of the following access techniques has the potential for less injury when obtaining a pneumoperitoneum and access to the abdomen for laparoscopy?
   a. Closed technique with Veress needle
   b. Closed technique with blind trocar insertion
   c. Open access technique
   d. Hand-port access
   e. Gasless technique

7. Which of the following hemostatic devices would be considered appropriate for control of a 6-mm vessel?
   a. Monopolar hook electrode
   b. Bipolar scissors
   c. Harmonic shears
   d. LigaSure device
   e. TissueLink device

8. Which of the following can be used to secure the renal vein?
   a. Titanium clips
   b. Hem-o-Lok plastic clips
   c. Endo GIA with 2.5-mm staples
   d. Endo GIA with 4.8-mm staples
   e. 5-mm LigaSure

9. For morcellation purposes, if the specimen is entrapped in a nylon impermeable sac (e.g., LapSac, Cook Urological, Spencer, IN) what is the recommended safest way to proceed?

a. Use of a high-speed morcellator

b. Ring forceps

c. Scissor morcellation

d. Kelly clamp

e. Ultrasonic tissuetripsy

10. Which of the following port sites most often requires formal closure with a fascial and peritoneal suture?

a. 5-mm nonbladed ports

b. 5-mm bladed ports

c. 10- to 12-mm nonbladed ports placed on the midline

d. 10- to 12-mm nonbladed ports placed on the midclavicular line

e. 10- to 12-mm nonbladed ports placed on the anterior axillary line

11. Which of the following pneumoperitoneum pressures is associated with the least perturbation in cardiac parameters, that is, change in stroke volume?

a. 12 mm Hg

b. 15 mm Hg

c. 18 mm Hg

d. 21 mm Hg

e. 24 mm Hg

12. Which of the following physiologic effects has been noted with establishment of pneumoperitoneum?

a. Increase in diaphragmatic motion

b. Increase in disturbances of gastrointestinal motility

c. Alkalosis

d. Decrease in urinary output

e. Increase in mesenteric vessel blood flow

13. Which of the following combinations best assesses the morbidity and mortality related to laparoscopic urology?

a. 2% morbidity, 0.8% mortality

b. 13% morbidity, 0.2% mortality

c. 20% morbidity, 0.5% mortality

d. 20% morbidity, 0.8% mortality

e. 25% morbidity, 0.8% mortality

14. What is the most common intra-abdominal site of injury associated with laparoscopic surgery?

a. Bowel injury

b. Vascular injury

c. Liver injury

d. Splenic laceration

e. Bladder injury

15. What is a characteristic of a blunt trocar, as compared with a bladed trocar?

a. The blunt trocar requires formal closure of the port site regardless of its size.

b. The blunt trocar takes less force to insert than the bladed trocar.

c. The blunt trocar decreases the chance of injury to the epigastric vessels.

d. The blunt trocar should only be placed in the midline.

e. The blunt trocar eliminates possible trocar injury to the bowel.

16. All of the following options for treatment of a gas embolism during laparoscopy are true EXCEPT:

a. hyperventilate the patient with 100% oxygen.

b. immediately cease insufflation.

c. place the patient in a head-down position.

d. advance a central venous line into the right side of the heart.

e. place the patient in a right lateral decubitus position with the left side up.

17. Pneumomediastinum, pneumothorax, and pneumopericardium associated with laparoscopy are a result of:

a. gas leaking along major blood vessels through congenital defects in the diaphragm.

b. gas passing through secondary enlargement of openings in the diaphragm.

c. diffusion of gas across the peritoneum and diaphragm.

d. a and b.

e. a and c.

18. If during insufflation of the abdomen the Veress needle is determined to have been placed into the iliac artery, which of the following is the best course of action?

a. Remove the Veress needle and proceed to open the abdomen

b. Remove the Veress needle and then proceed with insufflating at a different location

c. Leave the Veress needle in place and open the abdomen

d. Leave the Veress needle in place and proceed with insufflation of the abdomen at a different location

e. Call for a vascular surgery consult

19. What is the best management option if trocar injury to the iliac artery should occur during the placement of the first trocar?

a. Remove the trocar and open the abdomen immediately

b. Remove the trocar immediately and proceed with re-insufflation of the abdomen and placement of the trocar at an alternate site

c. Leave the trocar in place, consult a vascular surgeon, and convert to open laparotomy

d. Leave the trocar in place and proceed with insufflation of the abdomen and placement of another port at an alternate site

e. Remove the obturator and immediately flush the port with fibrin glue

20. Which of the following clinical presentations is commonly seen with a postoperative bowel injury after laparoscopy?

a. Abdominal distention and leukocytosis

b. Clinical signs of peritonitis and a high fever

c. Leukopenia, low-grade fever, and pain at one port site

d. High fever, abdominal distention, and leukocytosis

e. Low-grade fever, clinical findings of peritonitis, and abdominal distention

21. When a bladder injury is diagnosed postoperatively after a laparoscopic procedure, what is the best treatment?

a. Transurethral indwelling Foley catheter if it is an intraperitoneal injury of the bladder

b. Open repair if it is an extraperitoneal injury of the bladder

c. Laparoscopic or open repair if it is an intraperitoneal injury to the bladder

d. Laparoscopic repair if it is an extraperitoneal injury to the bladder

e. Transurethral injection of fibrin glue into the bladder injury site if it is an extraperitoneal injury to the bladder

22. During retroperitoneal renal laparoscopy, balloon dilatation should be performed in which of the following compartments?

a. Anterior pararenal space

b. Posterior pararenal space

c. Lateral pararenal space

d. Medial pararenal space

e. All of the above

23. Hypercarbia during laparoscopy may be related to all of the following EXCEPT which one?

a. Severe chronic respiratory disease

b. Subcutaneous emphysema

c. Increased insufflation pressures

d. Prolonged operative time

e. Radical nephrectomy

24. Possible advantages of retroperitoneal laparoscopy include all of the following EXCEPT:

a. less need for lysis of adhesions.

b. decreased risk of paralytic ileus.

c. decreased risk of port-site hernias.

d. direct rapid access to the renal hilum.

e. technically easier to learn.

25. After extraperitoneal pelvic lymph node dissection, the incidence of which one of the following is higher than with transperitoneal pelvic node dissection?

a. Urinoma

b. Lymphocele

c. Bowel injury

d. Laparoscopic repair if it is an extraperitoneal injury to the bladder

e. Shoulder/hip pain

26. All of the following instruments might be part of a hemorrhage control tray EXCEPT:

a. laparoscopic needle drivers.

b. laparoscopic Satinsky clamp and accompanying trocar.

c. Lapra-Ty clip applier and 6-inch length of 3-0 absorbable suture.

d. hemostatic agents (fibrin glue, gelatin matrix thrombin, etc.) plus laparoscopic applicators.

e. laparoscopic renal biopsy forceps.

27. Which of the following hemostatic agents requires a 20-minute set up time before use?

a. Tisseel

b. FloSeal

c. CrossSeal

d. BioGlue

e. CoSeal

28. Which of the following trocar types requires formal closure of the abdominal wall fascia in an adult patient?

a. An EndoTip trocar

b. A 12-mm fascial dilating trocar

c. A 5-mm bladed trocar

d. A 12-mm step trocar

e. A 12-mm bladed trocar

29. Which of the following relationships is true for port placement for laparoscopic suturing?

a. The angle produced by the horizontal plane and the instruments should be greater than 55 degrees and the angle between the needle drivers should be less than 25 degrees.

b. The angle produced by the horizontal plane and the instruments should be less than 55 degrees and the angle between the needle drivers should be between 25 and 45 degrees.

c. The angle produced by the horizontal plane and the instruments should be greater than 55 degrees and the angle between the needle drivers should be greater than 45 degrees.

d. The angle produced by the horizontal plane and the instruments should be less than 55 degrees and the angle between the needle drivers should be less than 25 degrees.

e. The angle produced by the horizontal plane and the instruments should be greater than 55 degrees and the angle between the needle drivers should be between 25 and 45 degrees.

30. During a procedure using the Da Vinci Robotic System the robot malfunctions and one of the grasping forceps is closed on a vital structure. The system is completely unresponsive. The appropriate action to safely disengage the instrument from the vital structure is to:

a. use the surgeon's console to override the system and robotically disengage the grasper.

b. remove the robotic instrument from the robotic arm.

c. use the sterile Allen wrench provided by the company to manually disengage the instrument and then remove it from the robotic arm.

d. use a hand-held laparoscopic instrument to pry open the jaws of the robotic instrument.

e. unplug the surgeon's console and robotic tower, plug them back in, and re-start the system.

ANSWERS

1. **e. extensive prior abdominal or pelvic surgery.** Absolute contraindications for laparoscopic surgery include uncorrectable coagulopathy, intestinal obstruction, abdominal wall infection, massive hemoperitoneum or hemoretroperitoneum, generalized peritonitis or retroperitoneal abscess, and suspected malignant ascites.

2. **d. Extensive prior abdominal or pelvic surgery.** When extensive intra-abdominal or pelvic adhesions are

suspected, close attention must be given to access into the abdomen whether this is by Veress needle or some open access technique. Alternatively, in these patients, a retroperitoneal approach may be preferable to a transperitoneal approach, but this is only a relative contraindication to performing laparoscopic surgery. All of the other options listed are absolute contraindications to laparoscopic surgery.

3. **c. for most uncomplicated patients, a clear liquid diet and a light mechanical bowel preparation the day before surgery.** For extraperitoneoscopy or retroperitoneoscopy, no bowel preparation is needed. For transperitoneal laparoscopic procedures, a light mechanical bowel preparation can be given in an effort to decompress the bowel. This usually consists of a clear liquid diet and a Dulcolax suppository or half bottle of magnesium citrate the day before the procedure.

4. **e. Nitrous oxide has previously been used for insufflation; however, it is no longer routinely used because of the potential for intra-abdominal explosion.** Most commonly, CO_2 is used as the insufflant because it does not support combustion and is very soluble in blood. However, in patients with chronic respiratory disease CO_2 may accumulate in the bloodstream to dangerous levels. In these patients, helium may be used for insufflation once the initial pneumoperitoneum has been established with CO_2. The drawback of helium is that, like air, it is much less soluble in the blood than CO_2. However, its use averts problems with hypercarbia. Other gases that were once used for insufflation, including room air, oxygen, and nitrous oxide, are no longer routinely used because of their potential side effects, such as air embolus or intra-abdominal explosion and potential to support combustion.

5. **c. 15 mm Hg.** During prospectively performed pressure-volume analysis in patients undergoing transperitoneal laparoscopic procedures, it was found that 94% of maximal intraperitoneal volume is achieved with an insufflation pressure of 15 mm Hg. Additional pressure did not significantly increase the volume. Furthermore, in a porcine study, elevation of the pneumoperitoneum pressure above 15 mm Hg did not significantly ease bladed trocar insertion.

6. **c. Open access technique.** A pneumoperitoneum can be more easily and, in one's early experience, more safely established using an open technique. However, its use involves making a larger incision and increases the chances of port-site gas leakage during the procedure. Studies in general surgery have shown the open technique to be as efficient as a closed approach.

7. **d. LigaSure device.** The LigaSure vessel-sealing system (Valleylab, Boulder, CO) consists of a 5- or 10-mm grasper/dissector connected to a bipolar radiofrequency generator. When the vascular structure is grasped by the instrument, the tissue is evaluated by feedback response system that subsequently delivers the optimal energy required to seal it more effectively. Therefore up to and including 7-mm veins and 5-mm arteries can be effectively secured with this device.

8. **c. Endo GIA with 2.5-mm staples.** The Universal 12-mm stapler (Covidien Ltd., Mansfield, MA) can be loaded with a variety of 30-, 45-, or 60-mm loads. Each staple load cartridge is color coded depending on the size of the staples: 2.0-mm staples (gray) or 2.5-mm staples (white) are preferred for vascular (renal vein) stapling, whereas 3.8-mm (blue) and 4.8-mm (green) staples are used in thicker tissues (ureter, bowel, bladder). The other choices are not appropriate for control of the renal vein.

9. **b. Ring forceps.** The LapSac (Cook Urological, Spencer, IN), which is made of nylon with a polyurethane inner coating and a polypropylene drawstring, is the least susceptible to tearing or leakage of cells. However, deployment of the LapSac and subsequent organ entrapment remain challenging endeavors. To aid in the opening of the LapSac the neck of the sack can be modified using a nitinol guidewire such that both ends of the guidewire exit the sack similar to the drawstring. The sack is loaded onto a nondisposable, two-tine LapSac introducer, introduced into the abdomen, and then unrolled, allowing the Nitinol guidewire to open the neck of the sack. The ring forceps is less likely to disrupt the sac.

10. **c. 10- to 12-mm nonbladed ports placed on the midline.** Currently, the shift from bladed to nonbladed trocars has resulted in a reduced need for port closure for even the 12-mm ports. The 12-mm ports that are not located on the midline do not require fascial closure. However, those on the midline are still considered to be at some risk for possible herniation; therefore most surgeons will close 10- to 12-mm nonbladed ports on the midline. All bladed port sites that are greater than 5 mm should be formally closed. Indeed, postoperative hernia rates with bladed trocars are reported at a frequency of 1.8% versus only 0.19% for the nonbladed trocars.

11. **a. 12 mm Hg.** Recent studies support a pneumoperitoneum pressure of 12 mm Hg, because this results in no perturbation in cardiac parameters, that is, no change in stroke volume, versus a pressure of 15 mm Hg. Working at lower pneumoperitoneum pressures has also been found to reduce postoperative pain. Also, a marked reduction in oliguria has been associated with working at 10 mm Hg pressure.

12. **d. Decrease in urinary output.** Because of increased intra-abdominal pressure from the pneumoperitoneum, diaphragmatic motion is limited. Laparoscopic surgery causes less significant disturbances of the gastrointestinal motility pattern compared with open surgery. Insufflation with CO_2 results in variable amounts of gas absorption, thereby raising the P_{CO_2} in the blood and creating an acidosis. Increased intra-abdominal pressure was found to be associated with a significant decrease in urinary output secondary to decreased blood flow to the renal cortex with an associated decrease in renal vein blood flow of up to 90% at 15 mm Hg.

13. **b. 13% morbidity, 0.2% mortality.** Historically, in large series, the overall incidence of laparoscopic complications in urology was in the range of 4%. Mortality was distinctly unusual, with a rate of 0.03% to 0.08%. However, a recent update from Johns Hopkins Hospital reported a 0.2% mortality rate and a 12% overall complication rate.

14. **b. Vascular injury.** The most common site of injury during laparoscopic surgery, in reports in the literature, is vascular in origin, occurring in 2.8% of patients, followed by bowel injury at 1.1%. The most often injured intra-abdominal organ was bowel at an incidence of 1.2%.

15. **c. The blunt trocar decreases the chance of injury to the epigastric vessels.** The use of only blunt trocars

decreases the chance of injury to the epigastric vessels by fivefold.

16. **e. place the patient in a right lateral decubitus position with the left side up.** The treatment for a suspected gas embolism is immediate cessation of insufflation and prompt desufflation of the peritoneal cavity. The patient is turned into a left lateral decubitus head-down position (i.e., right side up) to minimize right ventricular outflow problems. The patient is hyperventilated with 100% oxygen. Advancement of a central venous line into the right side of the heart with subsequent attempts to aspirate the gas may rarely be helpful. Use of hyperbaric oxygen and of cardiopulmonary bypass have also been reported.

17. **d. a and b.** Gas leaking along major blood vessels through congenital defects or secondary enlargement of openings in the diaphragm may lead to pneumomediastinum, pneumopericardium, and pneumothorax.

18. **d. Leave the Veress needle in place and proceed with insufflation of the abdomen at a different location.** If vascular injury should occur with the Veress needle, the needle should be left in place to identify the area of injury and insufflation of the abdomen can be re-performed at an alternate site and then the laparoscope inserted to identify the area of injury and to observe this as the Veress needle is removed to control any hemorrhage that may occur from the site.

19. **c. Leave the trocar in place, consult a vascular surgeon, and convert to open laparotomy.** A trocar injury to a major arterial vessel is a potentially life-threatening complication. The trocar should remain in place to tamponade the bleeding and also identify the area of injury once the abdomen is opened. The patient's blood should be typed and crossmatched, and immediate laparotomy should be performed and the site of vascular injury identified. A vascular surgery consult may be needed.

20. **c. Leukopenia, low-grade fever, and pain at one port site.** Postoperative bowel injury should be suspected in any patient who complains of increasing abdominal discomfort particularly at one port site and low-grade fever associated not uncommonly with leukopenia, although there usually will be a left shift in the differential white blood cell count. If this injury is unrecognized by these subtle clinical findings, the patient may succumb in 1 to 2 days. The diagnosis is made with a CT scan of the abdomen after oral administration of a contrast agent; it is recommended to obtain a delayed CT scan 4 to 6 hours later to best identify any small bowel leakage.

21. **c. Laparoscopic or open repair if it is an intraperitoneal injury to the bladder.** When bladder injury is diagnosed postoperatively the surgeon must determine whether the perforation is extraperitoneal or intraperitoneal. Extraperitoneal injury, without any complicating additional problems, may be treated by simple placement of a transurethral indwelling Foley catheter. Intraperitoneal injury is an indication for subsequent laparoscopic or open repair.

22. **b. Posterior pararenal space.** The space dorsolateral to the Gerota fascia is the posterior pararenal space. This is the space dilated during retroperitoneoscopy.

23. **e. Radical nephrectomy.** The potential for developing hypercarbia exists during both transperitoneal and preperitoneal laparoscopic procedures. Conceivably, this assumes greater importance in patients with preexisting airway and cardiovascular compliance. Vigilant perioperative anesthetic management is essential to prevent the development of potential complications related to CO_2 buildup. A rise in end-tidal CO_2 should prompt the anesthesiologist to adjust the respiratory rate and tidal volume to enhance CO_2 elimination. Simultaneously, the insufflation pressure of CO_2 should be decreased by the surgeon or, if need be, the operation should be halted and the abdomen desufflated until the end-tidal CO_2 returns to an acceptable level.

24. **e. technically easier to learn.** Retroperitoneoscopy is associated with unique anatomic orientation and a relatively restricted initial working area compared with transperitoneal laparoscopy. This results in a steeper learning curve.

25. **b. Lymphocele.** Absence of the peritoneal absorptive surface after extraperitoneoscopic lymphadenectomy may increase the risk of development of postoperative lymphocele.

26. **e. laparoscopic renal biopsy forceps.** The contents of a hemorrhage tray for laparoscopic surgery include the following:
Laparoscopic Satinsky clamp
10-mm suction/irrigation tip
Endo Stitch device with a 4-0 absorbable suture
Lapra-Ty clip applier and a packet of Lapra-Ty clips
6-inch length of 4-0 vascular suture on an SH needle with a
   Lapra-Ty clip preplaced on the end
2 laparoscopic needle drivers
Topical hemostatic agent of choice

27. **a. Tisseel.** Tisseel (Baxter, Glendale, CA) is a form of fibrin glue containing fibrinogen, calcium chloride, aprotinin, and thrombin. It is useful as a topical hemostatic agent as well as a tissue glue, but it has a 20-minute setup time and thus must be prepared well in advance of potential use.

28. **e. A 12-mm bladed trocar.** Of the choices listed, only a 12-mm bladed trocar site requires formal closure. Step trocars, EndoTip trocars, and fascial dilating trocars do not require closure. In adults, 5-mm trocars do not require closure.

29. **b. The angle produced by the horizontal plane and the instruments should be less than 55 degrees and the angle between the needle drivers should be between 25 and 45 degrees.** Frede and colleagues performed an in-vitro experiment performing laparoscopic suturing while varying trocar relationship to the horizontal plane and the distance between the two instrument trocars. They found that suturing was easiest when the angle between the horizontal plane and the instruments was less than 55 degrees and the angle between the two instruments was between 25 and 45 degrees (Frede et al, 1999).*

30. **c. Use the sterile Allen wrench provided by the company to manually disengage the instrument and then remove it from the robotic arm.** In the event of a system failure of the Da Vinci Robotic System (Intuitive Surgical, Sunnyvale, CA) during which the robotic arms are rendered nonfunctional, instrument jaws can be manually opened using a sterile Allen wrench provided by the company for this purpose.

---

*Sources referenced can be found in *Campbell-Walsh Urology, 10th Edition,* on the Expert Consult website.

Additional Study Points

1. Patients with massive ascites have an increased incidence of bowel injury when trocars are placed owing to the closer proximity of the bowel loops to the anterior abdominal wall.

2. The Veress needle is commonly placed at the superior boarder of the umbilicus; there is a potential risk of injury to the left common iliac vessels, aorta, and vena cava.

3. For transperitoneal trocar placement the trocars should be placed in a four-point diamond pattern such that the site of operation is encircled by the diamond.

4. When using a stapler, the tissue must be properly situated between the markers before the cartridge is fired. Otherwise, a portion of the tissue will not be encompassed by the stapler. A stapler should not be fired across any previously placed clips.

5. Before port removal is initiated the operative site and the intra-abdominal entry sites of each cannula should be carefully inspected for bleeding with the intra-abdominal pressure lowered to 5 mm Hg.

6. Patients with chronic obstructive pulmonary disease (COPD) may not be able to compensate for the absorbed CO_2 by increased ventilation and are at increased risk for hypercarbia up to 2 to 3 hours after the procedure.

7. Nitrous oxide insufflation reduces cardiac output and increases mean arterial pressure, heart rate, and central venous pressure. It also supports combustion.

8. In patients with severe COPD, one should consider using helium as an alternative for insufflation.

9. A drawback of using helium for insufflation is that it is much less soluble in blood than CO_2. Helium may be associated with a higher risk of gas embolism because of its lower blood solubility and thus the initial pneumoperitoneum should be established with CO_2 and then the insufflation should be maintained with helium.

10. Intra-abdominal pressures during laparoscopy should not be allowed to exceed 20 mm Hg over extended periods of time, and a working pressure of 10 to 12 mm Hg is recommended.

11. Increased intra-abdominal pressures may artificially elevate central venous pressure readings; and thus if it is critical to know right atrial filling pressures, a Swan-Ganz catheter should be placed.

12. During laparoscopy, diaphragmatic motion is limited and functional reserve capacity is decreased. There is a significant decrease in urinary output and decreased blood flow to mesenteric vessels as well as other abdominal organs, including liver, pancreas, stomach, spleen, and small and large bowel.

13. Excessive intra-abdominal pressure usually presents as an increase in ventilation pressure noted by the anesthesiologist.

14. Injury owing to capacitive coupling occurs when a charge is allowed to build up and not allowed to disperse via the abdominal wall. This condition may develop when a metal trocar is anchored to the skin with a nonconductive plastic grip. This type of trocar should not be used when using a current during the procedure.

Infections and Inflammation

chapter

10

Infections of the Urinary Tract

Anthony J. Schaeffer, MD ● Edward M. Schaeffer, MD, PhD

QUESTIONS

1. Acute pyelonephritis is the most likely diagnosis in a patient with:
   a. chills, fever, and flank pain.
   b. bacteria and pyuria.
   c. focal scar in renal cortex.
   d. delayed renal function.
   e. vesicoureteral reflux.

2. Bacteriuria without pyuria is indicative of:
   a. infection.
   b. colonization.
   c. tuberculosis.
   d. contamination.
   e. stones.

3. Nosocomial urinary tract infections (UTIs):
   a. occur in patients who are hospitalized or institutionalized.
   b. are caused by common bowel bacteria.
   c. can be suppressed by low-dose antimicrobial therapy.
   d. are due to reinfection.
   e. are due to bacterial persistence.

4. Most recurrent infections in female patients are:
   a. complicated.
   b. reinfections.
   c. due to bacterial resistance.
   d. due to hereditary susceptibility factors.
   e. composed of multiple organisms.

5. Rates of reinfection (i.e., time to recurrence) are influenced by:
   a. bladder dysfunction.
   b. renal scarring.
   c. vesicoureteral reflux.
   d. antimicrobial treatment.
   e. age.

6. The long-term effect of uncomplicated recurrent UTIs is:
   a. renal scarring.
   b. hypertension.
   c. azotemia.
   d. ureteral vesical reflux.
   e. minimal.

7. The ascending route of infection is least enhanced by:
   a. catheterization.
   b. spermicidal agents.
   c. indwelling catheter.
   d. fecal soilage of perineum.
   e. frequent voiding.

8. Approximately 10% of symptomatic lower UTIs in young, sexually active female patients are caused by:
   a. *Escherichia coli.*
   b. *Staphylococcus saprophyticus.*
   c. *Pseudomonas.*
   d. *Proteus mirabilis.*
   e. *Staphylococcus epidermidis.*

9. The virulence factor that is most important for adherence is:
   a. hemolysin.
   b. K antigen.
   c. pili.
   d. colicin production.
   e. O serogroup.

10. Phase variation of bacterial pili:
    a. occurs only in vitro.
    b. affects bacterial virulence.
    c. is characteristic of pyelonephritic *E. coli.*
    d. is irreversible.
    e. refers to change in pili length.

11. The finding that first suggested a biologic difference in women susceptible to UTIs is:
    a. increased adherence of bacteria to vaginal cells.
    b. decreased estrogen concentration in vaginal cells.
    c. elevated vaginal pH.
    d. nonsecretor status.
    e. postmenopausal status.

12. Increased bacterial adherence resulting in increased susceptibility of women to recurrent UTIs has not been demonstrated in:
    a. introital mucosa.
    b. urethral mucosa.
    c. buccal mucosa.
    d. vaginal fluid.
    e. bladder mucosa.

46

13. The primary bladder defense is:
    a. low urine pH.
    b. low urine osmolarity.
    c. voiding.
    d. Tamm-Horsfall protein (uromucoid).
    e. vaginal mucus.

14. The most significant sequela of renal papillary necrosis is renal:
    a. failure.
    b. abscess.
    c. obstruction.
    d. stone.
    e. cancer.

15. Severity and morbidity of bacteriuria is most morbid in patients with:
    a. spinal cord injuries.
    b. pregnancy.
    c. reflux.
    d. diabetes mellitus.
    e. HIV infection.

16. The most reliable urine specimen is obtained by:
    a. urethral catheterization.
    b. catheter aspiration.
    c. midstream voiding.
    d. suprapubic aspiration.
    e. antiseptic periurethral preparation.

17. The validity of a midstream urine specimen should be questioned if microscopy reveals:
    a. squamous epithelial cells.
    b. red blood cells.
    c. bacteria.
    d. white blood cells.
    e. casts.

18. Rapid screening methods for detecting UTIs should be used primarily for:
    a. low-risk asymptomatic patients.
    b. pregnant women.
    c. children.
    d. catheterized patients.
    e. elderly patients.

19. The most accurate test for evaluation of infection in the kidney is:
    a. the Fairley bladder washout test.
    b. ureteral catheterization.
    c. gallium scanning.
    d. CT.
    e. the antibody-coated bacteria test.

20. Urinary tract imaging is NOT usually indicated for recurrent UTIs in:
    a. women.
    b. girls.
    c. men.
    d. boys.
    e. spinal cord–injured patients.

21. The most sensitive imaging modality for diagnosing renal abscess is:
    a. ultrasonography.
    b. indium scanning.
    c. gallium scanning.
    d. excretory urography.
    e. CT.

22. Cure of UTIs depends most on an antimicrobial agent's:
    a. serum half-life.
    b. serum level.
    c. urine level.
    d. duration of therapy.
    e. frequency of therapy.

23. During the past 5 years, the least development of antimicrobial resistance has been observed for:
    a. ampicillin.
    b. cephalosporins.
    c. nitrofurantoin.
    d. fluoroquinolones.
    e. trimethoprim-sulfamethoxazole (TMP-SMX).

24. The ideal class of drugs for empirical treatment of uncomplicated UTIs is:
    a. aminopenicillins.
    b. aminoglycosides.
    c. fluoroquinolones.
    d. cephalosporins.
    e. nitrofurantoins.

25. Antimicrobial prophylaxis is characterized as:
    a. administration of an antimicrobial agent within 4 to 6 hours of the procedure.
    b. administration of an antimicrobial agent for a period of time covering the first 48 hours after the procedure.
    c. administration of an antimicrobial agent within 30 minutes of the initiation of a procedure and for a period of time covering the first 48 hours after the procedure.
    d. administration of an antimicrobial agent within 30 minutes of the initiation of a procedure and for a period of time that covers the duration of the procedure.
    e. administration of an antimicrobial agent the night before the initiation of a procedure and for a period of time that covers the duration of the procedure.

26. Antimicrobial prophylaxis for transurethral resection of the prostate is not indicated for patients with:
    a. valvular heart disease.
    b. prosthetic valves.
    c. unknown urine culture.
    d. sterile urine.
    e. indwelling catheter.

27. Prophylaxis for endocarditis should not be administered in patients with:
    a. a history of childhood heart murmurs.
    b. heart valves inserted more than 5 years ago.
    c. calcified heart valves associated with a murmur.
    d. all synthetic heart valves.
    e. cadaveric heart valves.

28. The host factor least likely to be associated with an increased risk of infection is:
    a. advanced age.
    b. a history of previous infection in the site/organ of interest.
    c. residence in a chronic care facility.
    d. indwelling orthopedic pins.
    e. coexistent infection.

29. Urine culture is not routinely recommended for the clinical diagnosis of acute cystitis in:
    a. young women.
    b. elderly women.
    c. children.
    d. men.
    e. patients with hematuria.

30. The drug of choice for uncomplicated cystitis in most young women is:
    a. TMP-SMX.
    b. fluoroquinolone.
    c. penicillin.
    d. cephalosporin.
    e. nitrofurantoin.

31. The optimal duration of antimicrobial therapy for symptomatic acute uncomplicated cystitis in women is:
    a. 1 day.
    b. 3 days.
    c. 7 days.
    d. 14 days.
    e. 21 days.

32. Treatment of asymptomatic bacteriuria is most indicated in patients who are:
    a. elderly.
    b. catheterized.
    c. pregnant.
    d. confused.
    e. incontinent.

33. Screening for bacteriuria is beneficial in:
    a. pregnant women.
    b. elderly patients.
    c. men.
    d. children.
    e. spinal cord–injured patients.

34. The most common cause of unresolved bacteriuria during antimicrobial therapy is:
    a. development of bacterial resistance.
    b. rapid reinfections.

c. azotemia.
    d. staghorn calculi.
    e. initial bacterial resistance.

35. Nitrofurantoin prophylaxis is effective because of the concentration of the drug in the:
    a. urine.
    b. vaginal mucus.
    c. bowel.
    d. serum.
    e. bladder.

36. The ideal antimicrobial agent for self-start therapy for a UTI is:
    a. a fluoroquinolone.
    b. a cephalosporin.
    c. nitrofurantoin.
    d. TMP-SMX.
    e. tetracycline.

37. The most common cause of acute pyelonephritis in young women is:
    a. vesicoureteral reflux.
    b. P-piliated bacteria.
    c. type 1 piliated bacteria.
    d. recurrent UTIs.
    e. bacterial endotoxin.

38. The optimal antimicrobial agent for treatment of acute uncomplicated pyelonephritis in women is:
    a. TMP-SMX.
    b. a cephalosporin.
    c. an aminoglycoside.
    d. a fluoroquinolone.
    e. nitrofurantoin.

39. A patient with acute pyelonephritis, persistent fever, and flank pain for 24 hours warrants:
    a. observation.
    b. CT.
    c. change in antimicrobial therapy.
    d. ultrasonography.
    e. blood cultures.

40. The overall mortality rate in emphysematous pyelonephritis is approximately:
    a. 5%.
    b. 10%.
    c. 20%.
    d. 40%.
    e. 60%.

41. In chronic renal abscess the predominant urographic abnormality is:
    a. calyceal distortion.
    b. renal mass.
    c. calculi.
    d. hydronephrosis.
    e. calyceal amputation.

42. The high mortality rate associated with perinephric abscess is primarily attributed to:
    a. bacterial hemolysis.
    b. diabetes mellitus.
    c. delay in diagnosis.
    d. inappropriate antimicrobial therapy.
    e. inadequate drainage.

43. The primary treatment for a small perirenal abscess in a functioning kidney is:
    a. nephrectomy.
    b. partial nephrectomy.
    c. open surgical drainage.
    d. percutaneous drainage.
    e. retrograde ureteral drainage.

44. Most patients with chronic pyelonephritis present with:
    a. hypertension.
    b. renal failure.
    c. chronic infection.
    d. flank pain.
    e. no symptoms.

45. The most common bacterial cause of xanthogranulomatous pyelonephritis is:
    a. *Escherichia coli.*
    b. *Pseudomonas.*
    c. *Klebsiella.*
    d. *Proteus mirabilis.*
    e. *Staphylococcus.*

46. It is hypothesized that the nidus for the Michaelis-Gutmann body is:
    a. renal papillae.
    b. bacterial fragments.
    c. calcium crystals.
    d. macrophages.
    e. uric acid stones.

47. Echinococcosis is rare in/among:
    a. the former Soviet Union.
    b. Eskimos.
    c. Native Americans.
    d. the United States.
    e. Eastern Europe.

48. The most reliable early clinical indicator of septicemia is:
    a. chills.
    b. fever.
    c. hyperventilation.
    d. lethargy.
    e. change in mental status.

49. Compared with nonpregnant women, pregnant women have a higher prevalence of:
    a. asymptomatic bacteriuria.
    b. acute cystitis.
    c. acute pyelonephritis.
    d. recurrent cystitis.
    e. bacterial persistence.

50. Clinical pyelonephritis during pregnancy is most commonly linked to:
    a. maternal sepsis.
    b. maternal anemia.
    c. maternal hypertension.
    d. eclampsia.
    e. congenital malformations.

51. The drug thought to be safe in any phase of pregnancy is:
    a. a fluoroquinolone.
    b. nitrofurantoin.
    c. a sulfonamide.
    d. penicillin.
    e. tetracycline.

52. The majority of elderly patients with bacteriuria are:
    a. asymptomatic.
    b. febrile.
    c. incontinent.
    d. confused.
    e. dysuric.

53. In the absence of obstruction, treatment of asymptomatic bacteriuria in the elderly:
    a. is cost effective.
    b. prevents renal failure.
    c. reduces mortality.
    d. reduces morbidity.
    e. is unnecessary.

54. The most common predisposing factor for hospital-acquired UTIs is:
    a. surgery.
    b. antimicrobial therapy.
    c. age.
    d. catheterization.
    e. diabetes mellitus.

55. The most effective measure for reducing catheter-associated UTI is:
    a. closed drainage.
    b. antimicrobial prophylaxis.
    c. catheter irrigation.
    d. intermittent catheterization.
    e. daily meatal care.

56. In spinal cord–injured patients the bladder drainage technique with the lowest complication rate is:
    a. clean intermittent catheterization (CIC).
    b. suprapubic drainage.
    c. indwelling catheter.
    d. condom catheter.
    e. suprapubic pressure.

57. Fournier gangrene in the early stage is least likely to be associated with scrotal:

    a. pain.

    b. discharge.

    c. crepitation.

    d. erythema.

    e. swelling.

Pathology

1. See Figure 10–1.

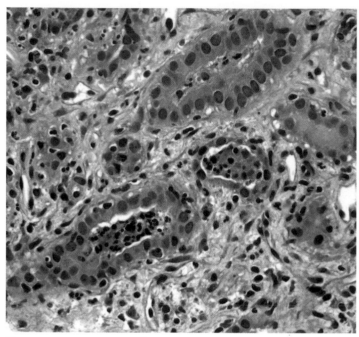

Figure 10–1.   (From Bostwick DG, Qian J, Hossain D. Non-neoplastic diseases of the prostate. In: Bostwick DG, Cheng L, editors. Urologic surgical pathology. 2nd ed. Edinburgh: Mosby; 2008.)

A 16-year-old girl has the acute onset of right flank pain and an enlarged kidney on imaging. A needle biopsy of the kidney is shown. The diagnosis is:

a. tuberculosis.

b. acute pyelonephritis.

c. malakoplakia.

d. nephroblastomatosis.

e. xanthogranulomatous pyelonephritis.

2. See Figure 10–2.

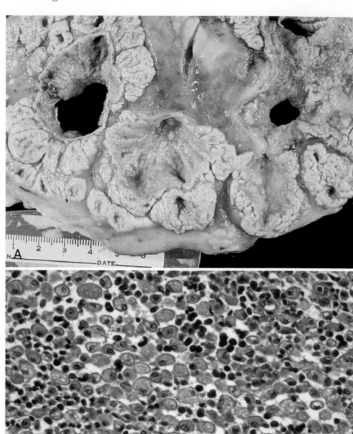

Figure 10–2.   (From Bostwick DG, Cheng L, editors. Urologic surgical pathology. 2nd ed. Edinburgh: Mosby; 2008.)

A 65-year-old man has a solid mass in his right kidney evident on imaging. A nephrectomy is done. The gross specimen is depicted in Figure 10–2A, and a photomicrograph is shown in Figure 10-2B. The diagnosis is:

a. renal abscess.

b. renal cell carcinoma, sarcomatoid variant.

c. renal cell carcinoma, clear cell variant.

d. xanthogranulomatous pyelonephritis.

e. malakoplakia.

3. See Figure 10–3.

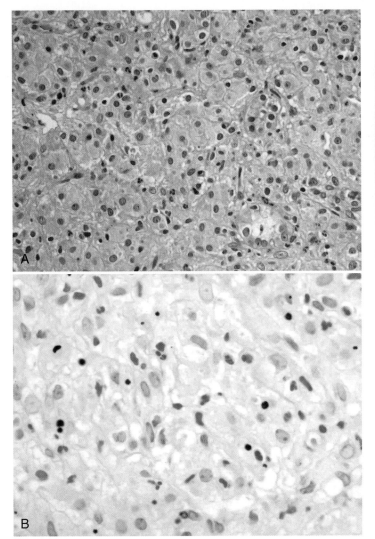

Figure 10–3.   (From Bostwick DG, Cheng L, editors. Urologic surgical pathology. 2nd ed. Edinburgh: Mosby; 2008.)

A 45-year-old woman is found to have a raised bladder lesion on cystoscopy. The microscopic findings from the biopsy specimen are shown. The diagnosis is:

a. herpesvirus infection.

b. malakoplakia.

c. adenocarcinoma.

d. endometriosis of the bladder.

e. inflammation.

Imaging

1. A 72-year-old man presents with right flank pain and fever. A contrast-enhanced CT scan is shown in Figure 10–4.

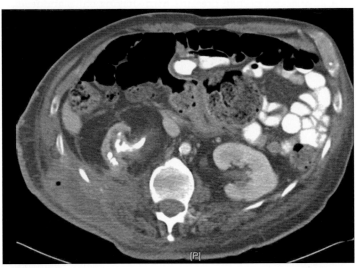

Figure 10–4.

The most likely diagnosis is:

a. acute right renal obstruction.

b. delayed excretion in left kidney.

c. cellulitis in right flank.

d. right perinephric abscess.

e. xanthogranulomatous pyelonephritis.

2. A 40-year-old woman presents with pelvic pain and fever. A contrast-enhanced CT scan is shown in Figure 10–5.

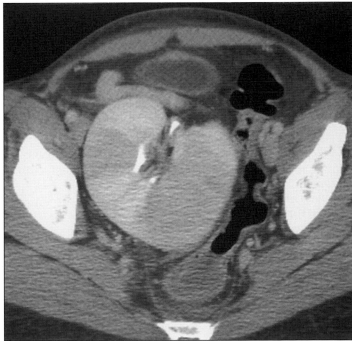

Figure 10–5.

The most likely diagnosis is:

a. renal infarct.

b. renal artery occlusion.

c. chronic pyelonephritis.

d. acute urinary obstruction.

e. acute pyelonephritis.

3. A 22-year-old woman presents with shaking chills and fever. An enhanced CT image is shown in Figure 10–6.

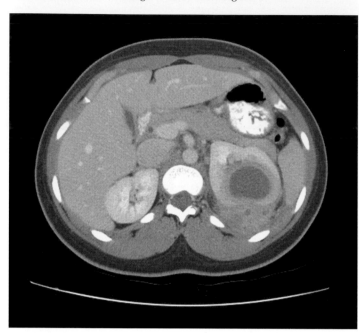

Figure 10–6.

The next step in management is:

a. percutaneous drainage.

b. nephrectomy.

c. partial nephrectomy.

d. open surgical drainage.

e. cystoscopy and retrograde urography.

ANSWERS

1. **a. chills, fever, and flank pain.** Acute pyelonephritis is a clinical syndrome of chills, fever, and flank pain that is accompanied by bacteriuria and pyuria, a combination that is reasonably specific for an acute bacterial infection of the kidney.

2. **b. colonization.** Bacteriuria without pyuria is generally indicative of bacterial colonization without infection of the urinary tract.

3. **a. occur in patients who are hospitalized or institutionalized.** Nosocomial or health care–associated UTIs occur in patients who are hospitalized or institutionalized and may be caused by *Pseudomonas* and other more antimicrobial-resistant strains.

4. **b. reinfections.** Of these recurrent infections, 71% to 73% are caused by reinfection with different organisms, rather than recurrence with the same organism.

5. **d. antimicrobial treatment.** Whether a patient receives no treatment or short-term, long-term, or prophylactic antimicrobial treatment, the risk of recurrent bacteriuria remains the same; antimicrobial treatment appears to alter only the time until recurrence.

6. **e. minimal.** The long-term effects of uncomplicated recurrent UTIs are not completely known, but, so far, no association between recurrent infections and renal scarring, hypertension, or progressive renal azotemia has been established.

7. **e. frequent voiding.** This route is further enhanced in individuals with significant soilage of the perineum with feces, women using spermicidal agents, and patients with intermittent or indwelling catheters.

8. **b. *Staphylococcus saprophyticus*.** *S. saprophyticus* is now recognized as causing approximately 10% of symptomatic lower UTIs in young, sexually active females, whereas it rarely causes infection in males and elderly individuals.

9. **c. pili.** Studies have demonstrated that interactions between FimH and receptors expressed on the luminal surface of the bladder epithelium are critical to the ability of many uropathogenic *E. coli* strains to colonize the bladder and cause disease.

10. **b. affects bacterial virulence.** This process is called phase variation and has obvious biologic and clinical implications. For example, the presence of type 1 pili may be advantageous to the bacteria for adhering to and colonizing the bladder mucosa but disadvantageous because the pili enhance phagocytosis and killing by neutrophils.

11. **a. increased adherence of bacteria to vaginal cells.** These studies established increased adherence of pathogenic bacteria to vaginal epithelial cells as the first demonstrable biologic difference that could be shown in women susceptible to UTI.

12. **e. bladder mucosa.** These studies individually and collectively support the concept that there is an increased epithelial receptivity for *E. coli* on the introital, urethral, and buccal mucosa that is characteristic of women susceptible to recurrent UTIs and may be a genotypic trait. Thus the vaginal fluid appears to influence adherence to cells and presumably vaginal mucosal colonization.

13. **c. voiding.** Bacteria presumably make their way into the bladder fairly often. Whether small inocula of bacteria persist, multiply, and infect the host depends in part on the ability of the bladder to empty.

14. **c. obstruction.** A patient who suffers from an acute ureteral obstruction caused by a sloughed papilla and who has a concomitant UTI should have the condition treated as a urologic emergency.

15. **a. spinal cord injuries.** Of all patients with bacteriuria, no group compares in severity and morbidity with those who have spinal cord injury.

16. **d. suprapubic aspiration.** A single aspirated specimen reveals the bacteriologic status of the bladder urine without introducing urethral bacteria, which can start a new infection.

17. **a. squamous epithelial cells.** The validation of the midstream urine specimen can be questioned if numerous squamous epithelial cells (indicative of preputial, vaginal, or urethral contaminants) are present.

18. **a. low-risk asymptomatic patients.** The main role of rapid screening methods for UTIs is in screening asymptomatic patients.

19. **b. ureteral catheterization.** Ureteral catheterization allows not only separation of bacterial persistence into upper and lower urinary tracts but also separation of the infection between one kidney and the other.

20. **a. women.** Several reports of women patients with recurrent UTIs show that excretory urograms are unnecessary for routine evaluation in women. Those who have special risk factors are excluded.

21. **e. CT.** CT and MRI are more sensitive than excretory urography or ultrasonography in the diagnosis of acute focal bacterial nephritis, renal and perirenal abscesses, and radiolucent calculi.

22. **c. urine level.** Efficacy of the antimicrobial therapy is critically dependent on the antimicrobial levels in the urine and the duration that this level remains above the minimum inhibitory concentration of the infecting organism. Thus resolution of infection is closely associated with the susceptibility of the bacteria to the concentration of the antimicrobial agent achieved in the urine.

23. **c. nitrofurantoin.** Over a 5-year period the prevalence of resistance to trimethoprim-sulfamethoxazole, ampicillin, and cephalothin increased significantly whereas resistance to nitrofurantoin and ciprofloxacin remained uncommon.

24. **c. fluoroquinolones.** The fluoroquinolones have a broad spectrum of activity that makes them ideal for the empirical treatment of UTIs.

25. **d. administration of an antimicrobial agent within 30 minutes of the initiation of a procedure and for a period of time that covers the duration of the procedure.** Surgical antimicrobial prophylaxis entails treatment with an antimicrobial agent before and for a limited time after a procedure to prevent local or systemic postprocedural infections.

26. **d. sterile urine.** Prolonged use of an indwelling urethral catheter is common in hospitalized patients and is associated with an increased risk of bacterial colonization with a 3% to 10% incidence of bacteriuria per catheter day in one study and 100% incidence of bacteriuria with long-term catheterization (>30 days). Prophylactic antimicrobial therapy during catheterization is not generally recommended because bacterial resistance can develop rapidly. Chronically catheterized patients have bacteriuria and should be treated therapeutically not with prophylaxis.

27. **a. a history of childhood heart murmurs.** The American Heart Association's recommendations on the prevention of bacterial endocarditis are based on the patient's risk of developing endocarditis and the likelihood that a procedure will cause bacteremia with an organism that can cause endocarditis. Prophylaxis is recommended for both high- and moderate-risk patients. High-risk patients include individuals with prosthetic heart valves, previous bacterial endocarditis, cyanotic congenital heart disease, and systemic-pulmonary shunts or conduits. Moderate-risk patients include other congenital malformations (excluding isolated secundum atrial septal defects, surgically repaired atrial septal defect, ventricular septal defects, or patent ductus arteriosus), acquired valvular dysfunction, hypertrophic cardiomyopathy, and mitral valve prolapse with valvular regurgitation and/or thickened leaflets. Antimicrobial prophylaxis is not recommended for patients with congenital malformations including isolated secundum atrial septal defects, surgically repaired atrial septal defect, ventricular septal defects, or patent ductus arteriosus; previous coronary artery bypass graft surgery; benign heart murmurs; previous Kawasaki disease or rheumatic fever without valvular dysfunction; or implanted pacemakers or defibrillators.

28. **d. indwelling orthopedic pins.** Bacterial seeding of implanted orthopedic hardware is a rare but morbid event. A joint commission of the American Urological Association, the American Academy of Orthopaedic Surgeons, and infectious disease specialists convened in 2003 and released an advisory statement on antibiotic prophylaxis for urologic patients with total joint replacement. In general, antimicrobial prophylaxis for urologic patients with total joint replacements, pins, plates, or screws is not indicated. Prophylaxis is advised for individuals at higher risk of seeding a prosthetic joint and include those with recently inserted implants (within 2 years).

29. **a. young women.** In women with recent onset of symptoms and signs suggesting acute cystitis and in whom factors associated with upper tract or complicated infection are absent a urinalysis that is positive for pyuria, hematuria, or bacteriuria or a combination should provide sufficient documentation of UTI and a urine culture may be omitted.

30. **a. TMP-SMX.** TMP and TMP-SMX are recommended in areas where the prevalence of resistance to these drugs among *E. coli* strains causing cystitis is less than 20%.

31. **b. 3 days.** Three-day therapy is the preferred regimen for uncomplicated cystitis in women.

32. **c. pregnant.** In populations other than those for whom treatment has been documented to be beneficial (e.g., pregnant women and patients undergoing urologic interventions), screening for or treatment of asymptomatic bacteriuria is not appropriate and should be discouraged.

33. **a. pregnant women.** In populations other than those for whom treatment has been documented to be beneficial (e.g., pregnant women and patients undergoing urologic interventions), screening for or treatment of asymptomatic bacteriuria is not appropriate and should be discouraged.

34. **e. initial bacterial resistance.** Most commonly, the bacteria are resistant to the antimicrobial agent selected to treat the infection.

35. **a. urine.** Nitrofurantoin, which does not alter the bowel flora, is present for brief periods at high concentrations in the urine and leads to repeated elimination of bacteria from the urine, presumably by interfering with bacterial initiation of infection.

36. **a. a fluoroquinolone.** Fluoroquinolones are ideal for self-start therapy because they have a spectrum of activity broader than that of any of the other oral agents and are superior to many parenteral antimicrobial agents, including aminoglycosides.

37. **b. P-piliated bacteria.** If vesicourethral reflux is absent, a patient bearing the P blood group phenotype may have special susceptibility to recurrent pyelonephritis caused by *E. coli* that have P pili and bind to the P blood group antigen receptors.

38. **d. a fluoroquinolone.** For patients who will be managed as outpatients, single-drug oral therapy with a fluoroquinolone is more effective than TMP-SMX for patients with domiciliary infections.

39. **a. observation.** Even though the urine usually becomes sterile within a few hours of starting antimicrobial therapy, patients with acute uncomplicated pyelonephritis may continue to have fever, chills, and flank pain for several more days after initiation of successful antimicrobial therapy. They should be observed.

40. **d. 40%.** Emphysematous pyelonephritis should be considered a complication of severe pyelonephritis rather than a distinct entity. The overall mortality rate is 43%.

41. **b. renal mass.** In a more chronic abscess, the predominant urographic abnormalities are those of a renal mass lesion.

42. **c. delay in diagnosis.** Although 71% of all the patients had eventual surgical treatment of their perinephric abscesses, the diagnostic delay of those patients admitted to medical services postponed definitive treatment and consequently caused higher mortality.

43. **d. percutaneous drainage.** Although surgical drainage, or nephrectomy if the kidney is nonfunctioning or severely infected, is the classic treatment for perinephric abscesses, renal ultrasonography and CT make percutaneous aspiration and drainage of small perirenal collections possible.

44. **e. no symptoms.** There are no symptoms of chronic pyelonephritis until it produces renal insufficiency, and then the symptoms are similar to those of any other form of chronic renal failure.

45. **d. *Proteus mirabilis*.** Although review of the literature shows *Proteus* to be the most common organism involved with xanthogranulomatous pyelonephritis, *E. coli* is also common.

46. **b. bacterial fragments.** It is hypothesized that bacteria or bacterial fragments form the nidus for the calcium phosphate crystals that laminate the Michaelis-Gutmann bodies.

47. **d. the United States.** In the United States the disease is rare, but it is found in immigrants from Eastern Europe or other foreign endemic areas or as an indigenous infection among Native Americans in the Southwest United States and in Eskimos.

48. **c. hyperventilation.** Even before temperature extremes and the onset of chills, bacteremic patients often begin to hyperventilate. Thus the earliest metabolic change in septicemia is a resultant respiratory alkalosis.

49. **c. acute pyelonephritis.** Pyelonephritis develops in 1% to 4% of all pregnant women and in 20% to 40% of pregnant women with untreated bacteriuria.

50. **a. maternal sepsis.** Women with asymptomatic bacteriuria are at higher risk for developing a symptomatic UTI that results in adverse fetal sequelae, complications associated with bacteriuria during pregnancy, and pyelonephritis and its possible sequelae, such as sepsis in the mother. Therefore all women with asymptomatic bacteriuria should be treated.

51. **d. penicillin.** The aminopenicillins and cephalosporins are considered safe and generally effective throughout pregnancy. In patients with penicillin allergy, nitrofurantoin is a reasonable alternative.

52. **a. asymptomatic.** Most elderly patients with bacteriuria are asymptomatic; estimates among women living in nursing homes range from 17% to 55%, as compared with 15% to 31% for their male cohorts.

53. **e. is unnecessary.** Prospective randomized comparative trials of antimicrobial or no therapy in elderly male and female nursing home residents with asymptomatic bacteriuria consistently document no benefit of antimicrobial therapy. There was no decrease in symptomatic episodes and no improvement in survival. In fact, treatment with antimicrobial therapy increases the occurrence of adverse drug effects and reinfection with resistant organisms and increases the cost of treatment. Therefore, asymptomatic bacteriuria in elderly residents of long-term care facilities should not be treated with antimicrobial agents.

54. **d. catheterization.** Catheter-associated bacteriuria is the most common hospital-acquired infection, accounting for up to 40% of such infections.

55. **a. closed drainage.** Careful aseptic insertion of the catheter and maintenance of a closed dependent drainage system are essential to minimize development of bacteriuria.

56. **a. clean intermittent catheterization.** Although never rigorously compared with indwelling urethral catheterization, CIC has been shown to decrease lower urinary tract complications by maintaining low intravesical pressure and reducing the incidence of stones.

57. **b. discharge.** Early on, the involved area is swollen, erythematous, and tender as the infection begins to involve the deep subcutaneous tissue. Pain is prominent, and fever and systemic toxicity are marked. The swelling and crepitus of the scrotum quickly increase, and dark purple areas develop and progress to extensive gangrene.

Pathology

1. **b. acute pyelonephritis.** There are numerous neutrophils within the interstitium and the renal tubules. The neutrophils in the tubules become white blood cell casts.

2. **d. xanthogranulomatous pyelonephritis.** The gross specimen shows xanthomatous nodules. The photomicrograph shows the characteristic foamy macrophages with neutrophils and cellular debris in the center of the nodule.

3. **b. malakoplakia.** Figure 10–3A shows von Hansemann histiocytes and Figure 10–3B demonstrates the Michaelis-Gutmann bodies, both of which are characteristic of this lesion.

Imaging

1. **d. right perinephric abscess.** The CT scan is obtained in the late arterial to nephrographic phase of the examination (the aorta is still opacified with contrast agent), before the excretion of the contrast agent. Thus option b is incorrect. There are multiple calculi in the right kidney, which is small and atrophic, indicating a chronic process (thus option a is incorrect). There is thickening of the perinephric fascia, and gas bubbles are seen in the posterior paranephric space, extending to the right flank. In addition, there are fluid collections in the posterior paranephric space and in the soft tissues of the right flank, making option d the most likely diagnosis. Xanthogranulomatous pyelonephritis is a chronic inflammatory condition associated with staghorn calculi. The affected kidney is usually enlarged rather than shrunken, as is the case here (making option e unlikely).

2. **e. acute pyelonephritis.** The image demonstrates a pelvic kidney with wedge-shaped area of decreased enhancement, characteristic of acute pyelonephritis. Renal infarcts cause areas of poor perfusion that are more sharply defined and more poorly enhancing than in the present case (making option a unlikely). The clinical history of fever also supports an infection. With renal artery occlusion (option b) the kidney would demonstrate no enhancement. Chronic pyelonephritis causes scarring in the kidney, and the nephrogram is usually normal. The renal contour in the present case is smooth, making option c unlikely. Acute urinary obstruction (option d) is ruled out because the visualized collecting system does not appear dilated.

3. **a. percutaneous drainage.** The image demonstrates a low-attenuation area in the posterior interpolar region of the left kidney, with perinephric fascial thickening, consistent with a renal abscess. Intravenous antimicrobial therapy with percutaneous drainage of renal abscesses is highly effective and is the treatment of choice. Antimicrobial therapy alone is unlikely to be effective given the size of the abscess. Nephrectomy, partial nephrectomy, and surgical drainage are rarely indicated in young patients with normally functioning kidneys. Cystoscopy is not warranted.

Additional Study Points

1. UTIs cause significant morbidity; they do not cause progressive renal failure unless significant comorbidities are present.
2. Increased receptors for uropathogenic *E. coli* on vaginal epithelial cells and buccal mucosal cells in women with recurrent UTIs imply a genetic etiology; moreover, hormonal changes may alter adherence of bacteria to the receptors in the vaginal epithelial cells explaining the cyclic nature of UTIs in women.
3. If appropriate antimicrobial therapy fails to eradicate bacteria and there is a rapid recurrence, imaging is indicated to determine abnormalities that may cause persistence.
4. In sepsis, low-dose dopamine has not been found to be efficacious, corticosteroids are controversial, granulocyte-stimulating factor has shown some promise, and protein-C is in clinical trial.

chapter
11

Prostatitis and Related Conditions, Orchitis, and Epididymitis

J. Curtis Nickel, MD, FRCSC

QUESTIONS

1. The prevalence of chronic prostatitis (diagnoses/symptoms) in population-based studies is approximately:
   a. <1%.
   b. 2% to 10%.
   c. >20%.
   d. 50%.
   e. unknown.

2. Which of the following etiologic agents or mechanisms has been unequivocally confirmed to be associated with prostatic inflammation?
   a. Intraprostatic ductal reflux
   b. Enterobacteriaceae species
   c. *Chlamydia* species
   d. *Ureaplasma* species
   e. *Corynebacterium* species

3. The most likely candidate for cryptic infection in category III prostatitis is:
   a. *Chlamydia*.
   b. *Ureaplasma*.
   c. nanobacteria.
   d. *Corynebacterium*.
   e. unknown.

4. The presence of white blood cells (WBCs) in the expressed prostatic secretion (EPS) of patients with category III chronic prostatitis/chronic pelvic pain syndrome (CP/CPPS):
   a. confirms significant prostatic inflammation.
   b. correlates with severity of symptoms.
   c. differentiates CP/CPPS patients from control patients.
   d. differentiates CP/CPPS IIIA patients from CP/CPPS IIIB patients.
   e. differentiates CP/CPPS II patients from CP/CPPS III patients.

5. What is the National Institutes of Health (NIH) Chronic Prostatitis Symptom Index?
   a. A 20-item validated questionnaire
   b. A research tool that is useful in clinical practice
   c. A symptom index for pain assessment
   d. An index that has been validated only in English
   e. A questionnaire that evaluates two domains of symptoms

6. An obese 26-year-old man has an 8-hour history of severe dysuria, stranguria, and suprapubic and perineal pain with fever. On examination, he has suprapubic tenderness and his prostate is enlarged, boggy, and exquisitely tender. Urinalysis shows pyuria. He continues to complain of symptoms despite insertion of a Foley catheter and has persistent fever after 30 hours of intravenous therapy with gentamicin and ampicillin. Culture grew *Escherichia coli*. The next best step in management is:
   a. change antibiotic to a third-generation cephalosporin.
   b. perform a transrectal ultrasonographic examination.
   c. perform a cystoscopic examination.
   d. perform a ultrasonography of the bladder.
   e. perform an intravenous pyelography.

7. A 36-year-old man has a 4-month history of dull perineal and suprapubic discomfort, postejaculatory pain, and moderate obstructive voiding symptoms. A pre-prostatic massage urine sample was sterile, and microscopic evaluation of the sediment showed 2 WBCs/high-powered field (hpf). No EPS was obtained during an uncomfortable digital rectal examination. A post-prostatic massage urine sample grew 10^2 *Staphylococcus epidermidis* organisms per milliliter, and microscopy of the sediment showed 10 to 12 WBCs/hpf. What is the NIH chronic prostatitis classification?
   a. Category I
   b. Category II
   c. Category IIIA
   d. Category IIIB
   e. Category IV

8. A 24-year-old man has an 8-month history of obstructive voiding symptoms and perineal and ejaculatory discomfort. A pre-prostatic massage urine sample was sterile, and microscopic evaluation of sediment showed 1 WBC/hpf. Microscopy of a minute amount of EPS showed 3 WBCs/

hpf. A post-prostatic massage urine sample was sterile, and microscopy of the sediment showed 2 WBCs/hpf. What is the NIH CP/CPPS classification?

a. Category I
b. Category II
c. Category IIIA
d. Category IIIB
e. Category IV

9. A 42-year-old man was treated for cystitis but continued to have dysuria, ejaculatory pain, and perineal/testicular discomfort after 7 days of antibiotics. The prostate examination was unremarkable. A midstream urine sample was sterile, but culture of a drop of EPS produced moderate growth of *Enterococcus faecalis*. A post-prostatic massage urine sample grew 10^2 *E. faecalis* organisms, and microscopic examination of the sediment showed 12 WBCs/hpf. What is the NIH classification?

a. Category I
b. Category II
c. Category IIIA
d. Category IIIB
e. Category IV

10. A 32-year-old man had been successfully treated for an *E. coli* cystitis with trimethoprim-sulfamethoxazole (7-day course) 4 months previously. A recurrence of similar symptoms was again successfully treated with ciprofloxacin (3 days), but no culture was done at this time. The patient presents 3 days after antibiotics were discontinued with continued perineal discomfort, ejaculatory pain, and mild dysuria. Pre- and post-prostatic massage urine and EPS samples were sterile. Evaluation of the EPS showed 20 WBCs/hpf. The prostate felt normal. What is the next best step?

a. Treat with anti-inflammatory agents
b. Do a standard Meares-Stamey four-glass test
c. Wait for 3 days and do a standard Meares-Stamey four-glass test
d. Restart trimethoprim-sulfamethoxazole
e. Restart fluoroquinolone antibiotics

11. A 47-year-old man has a 5-year history of perineal and suprapubic pain/discomfort and obstructive voiding symptoms that have not responded to multiple courses of antibiotics, α-adrenergic blockers, anti-inflammatory agents, repetitive prostatic massage, or phytotherapy. The prostate is tender, and the post-prostatic massage urine sample was sterile and showed 20 WBCs/hpf. The prostate-specific antigen (PSA) value was 1.2 mg/mL. The next best step is:

a. incision of bladder neck.
b. flow rate and bladder scan for residual urine.
c. video-urodynamics.
d. CT of pelvis.
e. cystoscopy and transrectal ultrasonography.

12. A 28-year-old man has been successfully treated for three episodes of cystitis (cultures not performed). He now presents with a 3-day history of frequency, urgency, dysuria, and suprapubic discomfort. The prostate feels normal

and is nontender. Results of an abdominal and pelvic ultrasonographic study were normal. A midstream culture done 24 hours earlier grew 10^5 *E. coli* organisms per milliliter. The next best step is:

a. a lower urinary tract localization test (two- or four-glass test).
b. several days of nitrofurantoin therapy followed by lower urinary tract localization test.
c. 4 weeks of fluoroquinolone therapy.
d. cystoscopy.
e. transrectal ultrasonography.

13. A 37-year-old man has a 3-month history of urinary frequency and urgency and discomfort localized to the perineum, suprapubic area, testes, and penis. A sterile post-prostatic massage urine sample showed 15 WBCs/hpf on microscopy. A year earlier the patient had been successfully treated for moderately severe symptoms with an unspecified antibiotic. He is allergic to many medications, including ciprofloxacin. The symptoms are now a significant bother and affecting his quality of life. The best initial treatment is a trial of:

a. an anti-inflammatory agent.
b. tetracycline.
c. trimethoprim-sulfamethoxazole.
d. trimethoprim.
e. carbenicillin.

14. A 58-year-old man with a 2-year history of symptomatic recurrent urinary tract infections with *Pseudomonas* (six to eight per year) is asymptomatic between treated episodes. *Pseudomonas aeruginosa* is localized to the EPS and post-prostatic massage (voided bladder 3, VB3) samples (but not the midstream urine sample, or VB2) during a period when he was asymptomatic. The EPS shows severe pyuria with WBC plugs or aggregates on microscopy. Transrectal ultrasonography shows extensive prostatic calcifications. Cystoscopy results are normal, residual urine is negligible, and the PSA value is 1.0 mg/mL. What is the best treatment?

a. Low-dose prophylactic antibiotics
b. Intraprostatic antibiotic injection
c. Radical transurethral resection of the prostate
d. Radical prostatectomy
e. Transurethral microwave thermotherapy

15. A 24-year-old man with a 6-year history of severe perineal pain with irritative and obstructive voiding symptoms has no significant benefits with 4 weeks of therapy with trimethoprim-sulfamethoxazole, anti-inflammatory agents, α-adrenergic blockers, or phytotherapy, respectively. Prostate-specific specimens were sterile and no WBCs were noted on microscopy. The physical examination had normal findings except for anal sphincter spasm and a tender but normal-feeling prostate gland. Video-urodynamics showed adequate funneling of the bladder neck with poor opening of the striated sphincter area and abnormal striated sphincter electromyographic activity during the emptying phase of micturition. The next step is:

a. 4 weeks of fluoroquinolone therapy.

b. muscle relaxant therapy.

c. bladder neck incision.

d. biofeedback.

e. transurethral microwave thermotherapy.

16. A 52-year-old man continues to have a high, spiking fever despite suprapubic catheterization and 36 hours of treatment with broad-spectrum intravenous antibiotics. Transrectal ultrasonography confirms a large prostatic abscess. The next best step is:

a. transperineal drainage.

b. transrectal aspiration.

c. transurethral drainage.

d. open drainage.

e. suprapubic aspiration.

17. α-Adrenergic blocker therapy for CP/CPPS:

a. is of proven value for CP/CPPS I.

b. is of proven value for CP/CPPS II.

c. is of proven value for CP/CPPS III.

d. is of proven value for CP/CPPS II and III.

e. May have value in some patients with CP/CPPS III.

18. Which of the following is the only non–organ-centric pharmacologic therapy that has been subjected to randomized placebo-controlled trials in CP/CPPS?

a. 5α-Reductase inhibitors

b. α-Adrenergic blockers

c. Antibiotics

d. Pharmacologic neuromodulators

e. Anti-inflammatory agents

19. An asymptomatic 65-year-old man undergoes a prostate biopsy because of an indistinct prostate asymmetry on digital rectal examination. The PSA value is 2.2 ng/mL. Pathologic examination reveals extensive glandular and periglandular infiltration with acute and chronic inflammatory cells. The next best step is:

a. observation.

b. 4 weeks of antibiotics and then reassessment.

c. 4 weeks of antibiotics and anti-inflammatory agents and then reassessment.

d. α-Adrenergic blocker therapy.

e. cystoscopy.

20. Which of the following invasive procedures has been shown to have efficacy compared with placebo-sham therapy in CP/CPPS?

a. Radical transurethral resection of the prostate

b. Transurethral balloon dilatation of prostate/bladder neck

c. Transurethral incision of the bladder neck

d. Microwave heat therapy

e. Transurethral needle ablation

Pathology

1. See Figure 11–1.

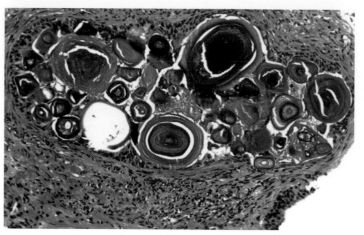

Figure 11–1.   (From Bostwick DG, Cheng L. Urologic surgical pathology. 2nd ed. Edinburgh: Mosby; 2008.)

A 65-year-old man undergoes transurethral resection of the prostate. The pathologic process depicted in the figure is most consistent with:

a. benign prostatic hyperplasia.

b. prostate cancer.

c. estrogen therapy.

d. stones at the surgical capsule.

e. endometrioid cancer of the utricle.

2. See Figure 11–2.

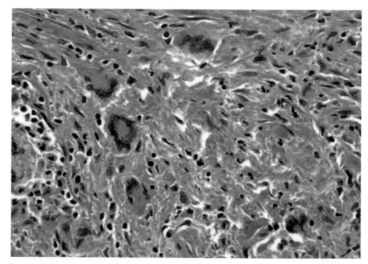

Figure 11–2.   (From Bostwick DG, Cheng L. Urologic surgical pathology. 2nd ed. Edinburgh: Mosby; 2008.)

A 70-year-old man had a transurethral resection of the prostate 10 years earlier. A repeat procedure is done. The patient most likely has:

a. tuberculosis.

b. BCG effect.

c. granulomatous prostatitis.

d. choriocarcinoma.

e. rheumatoid arthritis.

Imaging

1. A 40-year-old man with right scrotal pain is seen in the emergency department. Scrotal ultrasonography is performed (Fig. 11–3).

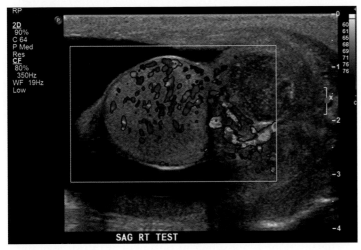

Figure 11–3.

The most likely diagnosis is:

a. adenomatoid tumor of epididymis.

b. testicular torsion.

c. primary testicular neoplasm.

d. epididymo-orchitis.

e. orchitis.

2. A 60-year-old man presents with pelvic and perineal discomfort, fever, and chills. A CT image is shown in Figure 11–4.

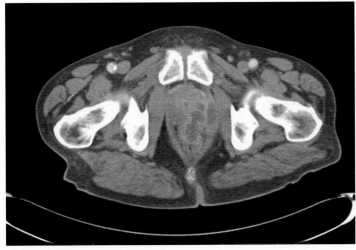

Figure 11–4.

The next step in management is:

a. MRI for staging.

b. antimicrobial therapy.

c. drainage.

d. retrograde urethrography.

e. transrectal prostate biopsy.

ANSWERS

1. **b. 2% to 10%.** Population-based studies employing the validated National Institutes of Health Chronic Prostatitis Symptom Index (NIH-CPSI) showed that the prevalence of prostatitis-like symptoms in the general population of men was between 2% and 10% (8.0% in Malaysia, 6.6% in Canada, 2.7% in Singapore, and approximately 2.2% in older men in Olmsted County, Minnesota).

2. **b. Enterobacteriaceae species.** The most common cause of bacterial prostatitis is the Enterobacteriaceae family of gram-negative bacteria.

3. **e. unknown.** A careful review of the evidence for and against the role of microorganisms—culturable, fastidious, or nonculturable—in type III prostatitis is equivocal, and etiologic mechanisms other than microorganisms must be considered.

4. **d. differentiates CP/CPPS IIIA patients from CP/CPPS IIIB patients.** The differentiation of the two subtypes of category III CPPS is dependent on cytologic examination of the urine and/or EPS: many white blood cells denote type IIIA; few to no white blood cells denote type IIIB.

5. **b. A research tool that is useful in clinical practice.** The National Institutes of Health Chronic Prostatitis Collaborative Research Network developed a reproducible and valid instrument to measure the symptoms and quality of life/impact of chronic prostatitis for use in research protocols as well as in clinical practice. The symptom index has also proved its usefulness in the evaluation and follow-up of patients in general clinical urologic practice.

6. **b. perform a transrectal ultrasonographic examination.** Development of a prostate abscess is best detected with transrectal ultrasonography. Patients with acute bacterial prostatitis are easily diagnosed and successfully treated with appropriate antibiotic therapy, as long as the clinician keeps a high index of suspicion for prostate abscess in patients who fail to respond quickly to the antibiotics.

7. **c. Category IIIA.** Diagnosis of CP/CPPS category IIIA, or inflammatory CPPS, is based on the presence of excessive leukocytes in EPS, a post-prostatic massage urine sample, or semen. 10^2 *Staphylococcus epidermidis* is a contaminant.

8. **d. Category IIIB.** Diagnosis of category IIIB CP/CPPS, or noninflammatory CPPS, rests on no significant leukocytes being found in similar specimens.

9. **b. Category II.** Category I is identical to the acute bacterial prostatitis category of the traditional classification system. Category II is identical to the traditional chronic bacterial prostatitis classification.

10. **e. Restart fluoroquinolone antibiotics.** The most important clue in the diagnosis of category II, chronic bacterial prostatitis, is a history of documented recurrent urinary tract infections. The fluoroquinolone should be continued for a minimum of 4 weeks.

11. **c. video-urodynamics.** A wide constellation of irritative and obstructive voiding symptoms is associated with CP/CPPS. Proposed causes to account for the persistent irritative and obstructive voiding symptoms include detrusor vesical neck or external sphincter dyssynergia, proximal or distal urethral obstruction, and fibrosis or hypertrophy of the vesical neck. Although flow rate and bladder scan can be done to further delineate these conditions, these

abnormalities can be clarified and diagnosed best by urodynamics, particularly video-urodynamics.

12. **b. several days of nitrofurantoin therapy followed by a lower urinary tract localization test.** In a patient who has acute cystitis the localization of bacteria in the EPS or VB3 specimen (post-prostatic massage sample) is impossible; and, in this case, the patient can be treated with a short course (1 to 3 days) of an antibiotic such as nitrofurantoin, which penetrates the prostate poorly but eradicates the bladder bacteriuria. Subsequent localization of bacteria in the post-prostatic massage urine sample or EPS sample is then diagnostic of category II prostatitis.

13. **d. trimethoprim.** Studies of animals with and without infection showed that trimethoprim concentrated in prostatic secretion and prostatic interstitial fluid (exceeding plasma levels) whereas sulfamethoxazole and ampicillin did not. It would be appropriate therefore to not prescribe the combination trimethoprim-sulfamethoxazole in a patient with multiple allergies.

14. **a. low-dose prophylactic antibiotics.** Prolonged therapy with low-dose prophylactic or suppressive antimicrobial agents can be considered for recurrent or refractory prostatitis, respectively.

15. **d. biofeedback.** On the basis of the possibility that the voiding and pain symptoms associated with CPPS may be secondary to some form of pseudodyssynergia during voiding or repetitive perineal muscle spasm, biofeedback has the potential to improve this process. Bladder neck incision in a young man should be avoided until after he has his family because of the possibility of retrograde ejaculation.

16. **c. transurethral drainage.** In patients who fail to respond quickly to antibiotics, a prostatic abscess is optimally drained by the transurethral incision route, although ultrasound-guided percutaneous aspiration (via any route) could be attempted first.

17. **e. may have value in some patients with CP/CPPS III.** Four randomized placebo-controlled trials have shown efficacy for terazosin, alfuzosin, and tamsulosin in patients with CPPS. However, two recent NIH-sponsored large randomized placebo controlled trials have not confirmed its efficacy in heavily pretreated chronic patients or in recently diagnosed α-adrenergic blocker–naive patients.

18. **d. Pharmacologic neuromodulators.** Neuromodulators (pregabalin) treat neuropathic pain and cannot be considered prostate-centric drugs, whereas all the other drugs that are listed and have been subjected to evaluation in randomized controlled trials could be considered organ centric.

19. **a. observation.** Asymptomatic inflammatory prostatitis (CP/CPPS IV) by definition does not require symptomatic therapy.

20. **d. Microwave heat therapy.** Although many uncontrolled trials employing heat therapy have shown benefit, three published studies have used sham controls.

Pathology

1. **a. benign prostatic hyperplasia.** Corpora amylacea fill benign prostatic acini. They are most often found in benign glands; however, on rare occasion they may be seen in association with carcinoma.

2. **c. granulomatous prostatitis.** Granulomatous prostatitis after transurethral resection of the prostate is characterized by aggregates of multinucleated giant cells. This condition is often found after chronic irritation.

Imaging

1. **d. epididymo-orchitis.** The image demonstrates skin thickening in the scrotum, hydrocele, and a complex hypoechoic mass in the enlarged epididymis that has no flow; color flow Doppler images demonstrate increased flow in the testis and in the remainder of the epididymis, consistent with epididymo-orchitis complicated by an epididymal abscess. These composite findings make the other listed possibilities less likely.

2. **c. drainage.** The CT image demonstrates low-attenuation areas in the prostate, primarily the left posterolateral aspect, with extension into the left periprostatic region. The appearance is most compatible with an abscess. This could be confirmed with transrectal ultrasonography. These findings on CT along with the clinical history and a rectal examination, which would reveal extreme tenderness, are sufficient to suggest a prostate abscess. Urgent drainage is prudent in such patients. Although urethral strictures and upper tract abnormalities may be the cause of recurrent urinary tract infections in a male, neither study is required urgently in a patient with a prostatic abscess. Antimicrobial therapy alone is not sufficient treatment at this stage of the infection. MRI may help in delineating the extent of involvement in equivocal cases but is unlikely to add more useful information when the results of CT and the physical examination are flagrantly abnormal. The appearance of the prostate on the CT image is not consistent with prostate cancer.

Additional Study Points

1. See Table 11–1 in *Campbell-Walsh Urology, 10th Edition* for a classification system for the prostatitis syndromes.

2. The most common cause of acute bacterial prostatitis is *Escherichia coli*.

3. Bacteria reside deep in the ducts of the prostate gland and form aggregates called biofilms that allow the bacteria to persist in the presence of antibiotics.

4. Factors that increase the risk of bacterial colonization of the prostate include (1) intraprostatic ductal reflux, (2) phimosis, (3) specific blood groups, (4) unprotected anal intercourse, (5) urinary tract infections, (6) acute epididymidis, (7) indwelling urethral catheters, and (8) condom catheter drainage.

5. Prostate-specific antigen levels can be markedly elevated during an episode of prostatitis.

6. Cytokines appear to play an important role in the development of prostatitis.

7. There is no validated level of WBCs in prostatic fluid that differentiates noninflammatory from inflammatory conditions; however, a finding of 5 to 10 WBCs/hpf is considered by many to be the upper limit of normal for prostatic fluid.

8. Patients with prostatitis-like symptoms who have no evidence of infection and complain of irritative voiding symptoms should have urine cytology performed.

9. Orchitis is rare and usually viral in origin; most cases of bacterial orchitis are secondary to local spread from the epididymidis.

10. Epididymitis usually results from spread of infection from bladder, urethra, or prostate via the vas deferens.

Bladder Pain Syndrome (Interstitial Cystitis) and Related Disorders

Philip M. Hanno, MD, MPH

QUESTIONS

1. Essential for the diagnosis of bladder pain syndrome/interstitial cystitis (BPS/IC) is the presence of:
   a. urinary urgency.
   b. pain or discomfort related to the bladder.
   c. glomerulations on cystoscopy.
   d. a Hunner ulcer.
   e. urinary frequency.

2. The definition of interstitial cystitis proposed by the National Institute of Arthritis, Diabetes, Digestive and Kidney Diseases (NIDDK) is best considered a:
   a. de facto definition of the disease.
   b. diagnostic pathway.
   c. definition applicable mainly to clinical research studies.
   d. historic document of no current value.
   e. purely symptom-based description of BPS/IC.

3. The best clinical evidence for a urine abnormality in BPS comes from:
   a. the absence of pain when a Foley catheter is left indwelling.
   b. relief of symptoms as a result of using narcotic analgesics.
   c. failure of conduit diversion to relieve symptoms.
   d. late occurrence of pain and bowel segment contraction after substitution cystoplasty and continent diversion.
   e. symptom relief associated with urinary alkalinization.

4. BPS/IC symptom and problem indices have been validated to:
   a. monitor disease progression or regression with or without treatment.
   b. correctly choose who should undergo cystectomy and diversion.
   c. determine on whom to perform diagnostic testing.
   d. accurately diagnose BPS/IC.
   e. determine appropriate candidates for clinical research.

5. Which of the following statements best categorizes the natural history of BPS/IC?
   a. The onset is generally insidious, occurring gradually over many years.
   b. Major deterioration in symptom severity is the rule.
   c. Symptoms follow a culture-documented urinary tract infection.
   d. Symptom resolution occurs regardless of treatment after 1 to 2 years.
   e. Onset is subacute with full development of the symptom complex over a relatively short time span.

6. Which statement best describes the relationship of BPS/IC to bladder cancer?
   a. BPS/IC is a premalignant lesion.
   b. BPS/IC is often associated with bladder cancer.
   c. A positive urine cytology can safely be ignored in patients with BPS/IC.
   d. No reports have documented an association of BPS/IC with subsequent development of bladder cancer.
   e. Dysplasia is a typical pathologic finding on bladder biopsy in BPS/IC patients.

7. The only animal with a known syndrome that appears to mimic BPS/IC is the:
   a. cat.
   b. rabbit.
   c. dog.
   d. goat.
   e. rat.

8. The antibiotic of choice for diagnosed BPS/IC is:
   a. doxycycline.
   b. none.
   c. gentamicin.
   d. ciprofloxacin.
   e. amoxicillin.

9. The cell most likely to play a central role in the pathogenesis of BPS is the:
   a. granulocyte.
   b. lymphocyte.
   c. mast cell.
   d. platelet.
   e. eosinophil.

10. Which statement best categorizes the potassium chloride test?
    a. It is soothing and calming to the painful bladder.
    b. It has high sensitivity and specificity for diagnosing BPS/IC.

c. It is an important element in choosing effective therapy.

d. It provides proof of abnormal mucosal permeability.

e. None of the above.

11. Bladder ulceration:

    a. is required to make a diagnosis of BPS/IC.

    b. is generally found in less than 10% of BPS patients.

    c. was not considered a part of the syndrome when it was initially described by Hunner.

    d. is synonymous with glomerulation.

    e. is pathognomonic of BPS/IC even in the absence of symptoms.

12. Exclusive use of the NIDDK criteria to diagnose BPS/IC would result in:

    a. an accurate depiction of the true prevalence of the condition.

    b. an improved treatment algorithm.

    c. increased diagnostic specificity.

    d. increased diagnostic sensitivity.

    e. a minimum of diagnostic testing and significant cost savings.

13. All but which ONE of the following disorders have a much higher prevalence in the BPS population than in the general population?

    a. Irritable bowel syndrome

    b. Diabetes

    c. Fibromyalgia

    d. Allergy

    e. Chronic fatigue syndrome

14. Where is the antiproliferative factor (APF) produced?

    a. Bladder urothelial cells

    b. Glomeruli

    c. Transitional urothelial cells in the upper tracts

    d. Mast cells

    e. Neutrophils

15. The postulated direct effect of antiproliferative factor is to:

    a. increase afferent neuron sensitivity.

    b. increase potassium efflux into urothelial cells.

    c. protect the surface glycosaminoglycan layer.

    d. elevate leukotriene levels.

    e. regulate growth factor production by bladder cells.

16. The central role of histopathology in BPS is to:

    a. determine whether the patient has ulcerative or nonulcerative disease (Hunner lesion).

    b. help determine the most efficacious treatment modality.

    c. predict prognosis.

    d. rule out other disorders that might be responsible for the symptoms.

    e. confirm the diagnosis with pathologic criteria.

17. Which of the following has the least in common with BPS?

    a. Vulvodynia

    b. Chronic bacterial prostatitis

    c. Orchialgia

    d. Penile pain

    e. Perineal and scrotal pain

18. Urodynamic findings typical of BPS include:

    a. uninhibited detrusor contractions.

    b. obstructed flow patterns.

    c. abnormal bladder compliance.

    d. decreased capacity and hypersensitivity.

    e. increased volume at first urge to void.

19. The finding of glomerulations:

    a. is significant only when cystoscopy is performed with the patient under anesthesia.

    b. is of no consequence in an asymptomatic patient.

    c. indicates a likelihood of response to laser fulguration of the bladder.

    d. is present only in patients with BPS.

    e. is sufficient to make a diagnosis of BPS.

20. The incidence of short-term spontaneous remission in BPS approaches:

    a. 50%.

    b. 100%.

    c. 30%.

    d. 10%.

    e. 75%.

21. Which test is potentially helpful for diagnosis, prognosis, and therapy?

    a. Potassium chloride test

    b. Intravesical heparin trial

    c. Bladder hydrodistention

    d. Bladder biopsy

    e. Urodynamics

22. Which of the following treatments is targeted to the glycosaminoglycan layer of the bladder?

    a. Sodium pentosan polysulfate

    b. Amitriptyline

    c. Hydroxyzine

    d. L-Arginine

    e. None of the above

23. Which of the following intravesical treatments has shown proven efficacy for BPS in pivotal U.S. Food and Drug Administration trials?

    a. BCG (bacille Calmette-Guérin)

    b. Hyaluronic acid

    c. Botulinum toxin

    d. Heparin

    e. None of the above

24. Which of the following statements is TRUE of narcotic analgesics?

    a. They have no place in the treatment of a chronic, nonmalignant condition such as BPS.

    b. They make patients physically dependent on them.

    c. They generally result in drug addiction when used for chronic pain.

d. They tend to cause diarrhea and sleeplessness.

e. All of the above

25. Which of the following is a reasonable surgical procedure to relieve the pain of BPS?

a. Transurethral fulguration of a Hunner lesion

b. Reduction cystoplasty

c. Sympathectomy and intraspinal alcohol injections

d. Cystolysis

e. Transvesical infiltration of the pelvic plexuses with phenol

26. The most important early step in the management of BPS is:

a. beginning intravesical treatment.

b. patient education.

c. initiating pentosan polysulfate therapy.

d. physical therapy.

e. strict adherence to "IC" diet.

27. A finding of detrusor overactivity on urodynamics in a patient with bladder pain in the absence of urinary urgency indicates:

a. the patient needs treatment with antimuscarinic medication.

b. the patient does not have BPS.

c. a urinary tract infection is likely.

d. neuromodulation would be the most effective treatment.

e. none of the above.

28. Men with irritative voiding symptoms and pelvic pain should be evaluated for:

a. chronic pelvic pain syndrome.

b. bacterial prostatitis.

c. bladder pain syndrome.

d. bladder carcinoma in situ.

e. all of the above.

29. The NIDDK Multidisciplinary Approach to the Study of Pelvic Pain (MAPP) is a 5-year multicenter program designed to:

a. test new treatments for BPS.

b. compile a long-term national database registration to follow BPS patients into the future.

c. gather data to justify officially changing the designation of "interstitial cystitis" to "bladder pain syndrome."

d. develop a rational treatment algorithm for BPS.

e. examine the chronic pelvic pain syndrome in men and BPS along with associated syndromes to better characterize the relationship among these disorders and enhance future diagnosis and treatment efforts.

30. Emotional, sexual, or physical abuse can be categorized as:

a. risk factors for BPS.

b. behaviors often attributed to patients with BPS.

c. unequivocally unrelated to BPS.

d. rare adverse events caused by medications used to treat BPS.

e. conditions for which there are no data to allow any tentative conclusions with regard to the relationship to BPS.

ANSWERS

1. **b. pain or discomfort related to the bladder.** Urgency, frequency, and the presence of glomerulations or a Hunner ulcer on endoscopy are often associated with BPS, but the presence of pain or discomfort is the primary component. IC may form a subgroup of the painful bladder group, but the criteria are not clear, and at this point the terms can be used interchangeably.

2. **c. definition applicable mainly to clinical research studies.** The definition of IC proposed by the NIDDK is best considered a definition applicable for use in research studies. It was never meant to define the disease but rather was developed to ensure that patients included in basic and clinical research studies were homogeneous enough that experts could agree on the diagnosis.

3. **d. late occurrence of pain and bowel segment contraction after substitution cystoplasty and continent diversion.** Substitution cystoplasty and continent diversion both fail in some BPS patients because of the development of pain in the bowel segment used or contraction of the bowel segment. Some studies have shown histologic changes in bowel segments used in BPS patients similar to those that occur in the IC bladder. Both of these findings provide circumstantial clinical evidence that the urine of BPS patients may have toxicity associated with the symptomatic expression of the disorder. However, data with regard to antiproliferative factor make this evidence suspect.

4. **a. monitor disease progression or regression with or without treatment.** Symptom and problem indices like the one developed by O'Leary and Sant are not intended to diagnose BPS/IC. Like the American Urologic Association Symptom Score for benign prostatic hypertrophy, these indices are designed to evaluate the severity of symptoms and to monitor disease progression or regression and response to treatment.

5. **e. Onset is subacute with full development of the symptom complex over a relatively short time span.** Several epidemiologic studies have concluded that the onset of BPS is commonly subacute rather than insidious. It presents more like one would expect an infectious disorder to present, rather than like a chronic disease process. Full development of the classic symptom complex takes place over a relatively short period of time. In the majority of cases it does not progress continuously but reaches its final stage rapidly and then continues without significant change in overall symptoms.

6. **d. No reports have documented an association of BPS/IC with subsequent development of bladder cancer.** In the 1970s, the Mayo Clinic documented bladder cancer in 12 of 53 men who had been treated for IC but the association was the result of incorrect diagnosis rather than progression. Peters and Kalinowski (2007)* and others have noted that patients with bladder cancer can be misdiagnosed as having BPS/IC.

7. **a. cat.** The feline urologic syndrome may represent the animal equivalent of BPS/IC. Approximately two thirds of cats with lower urinary tract disease have sterile urine and no evidence of other urinary tract disorders. A portion of these cats experience frequency and urgency of urination,

*Sources referenced can be found in *Campbell-Walsh Urology, 10th Edition,* on the Expert Consult website.

pain, and bladder inflammation. Glomerulations have been found in some of these cat bladders. Other findings similar to IC include bladder mastocytosis, increased histamine excretion, and increased bladder permeability.

8. **b. none.** Antibiotics are not indicated for the treatment of BPS/IC, nor have they been implicated as a causative factor. An empirical trial of doxycycline is reasonable in patients who have never had an antibiotic trial to treat the symptoms. Numerous studies have concluded that it is unlikely that active infection is involved in the ongoing pathologic process or that antibiotics have a role to play in treatment.

9. **c. mast cell.** Mast cells are strategically localized in the urinary bladder close to blood vessels, lymphatics, nerves, and detrusor smooth muscle. BPS appears to be a syndrome with neural, immune, and endocrine components in which activated mast cells play a central, although not primary, role in many patients.

10. **e. None of the above.** Up to 25% of patients meeting the NIDDK criteria for BPS/IC will have a negative KCl test. It is positive in the majority of patients with radiation cystitis, urinary tract infection, and nonbacterial prostatitis and in women with pelvic pain. It is neither sensitive nor specific for BPS/IC, is uncomfortable for the patients, and does not help to guide therapeutic decisions.

11. **b. is generally found in less than 10% of BPS patients.** Bladder ulceration (so-called Hunner ulcer) is more appropriately referred to as Hunner lesion and is found in a minority of patients with symptoms of BPS/IC. It is not a true ulcer but a "vulnus" or weakness or vulnerable area of the mucosa. A circumscribed red patch that cracks and bleeds with distention is best appreciated with the patient under anesthesia.

12. **c. increased diagnostic specificity.** Exclusive use of the NIDDK criteria to diagnose BPS would result in increased specificity and decreased sensitivity. Ninety percent of expert clinicians in the NIDDK database study agreed that patients diagnosed with IC by those criteria had IC. However, 60% of patients diagnosed by these clinicians as having BPS/IC did not fulfill the NIDDK criteria. Using the criteria as a basis for diagnosis would probably exclude the majority of patients with this symptom complex from the correct diagnosis.

13. **b. Diabetes.** Fibromyalgia, irritable bowel syndrome, chronic fatigue syndrome, and atopic allergic reactions are overrepresented in the BPS population. Studies are ongoing to find out the reason for such relationships in the NIDDK MAPP (Multidisciplinary Approach to the Study of Chronic Pelvic Pain) 5-year study. Diabetes has never been associated with an increased prevalence in patients with BPS.

14. **a. Bladder urothelial cells.** APF can be obtained from cultured uroepithelial cells and is not present in renal pelvic urine. It is associated with decreased production of heparin-binding epidermal growth factor–like growth factor.

15. **e. regulate growth factor production by bladder cells.** APF regulates growth factor production by bladder epithelial cells. It has been postulated that any of a variety of injuries to the bladder (infection, trauma, overdistention) in a susceptible individual may result in BPS if APF is present and suppresses production of heparin-binding epidermal growth factor–like growth factor.

16. **d. rule out other disorders that might be responsible for the symptoms.** The primary value of histopathology in BPS is to rule out other diseases that may account for the symptoms. The differentiation between ulcerative and nonulcerative disease is based on endoscopic features. There is no pathognomonic histologic finding for the disorder, nor can histology predict prognosis. Even a severely abnormal microscopic picture does not necessarily indicate a poor prognosis. At this time no data suggest that the treatment algorithm can be rationally predicated on the basis of the histologic findings alone.

17. **b. Chronic bacterial prostatitis.** BPS can be considered one of the pain syndromes of the urogenital and rectal area, all of which are well described but poorly understood. These include vulvodynia, orchialgia, perineal pain, penile pain, and rectal pain. Bacterial prostatitis is a well-understood entity with a known etiology and generally responds to treatment directed at the offending organism. NIH type 1 includes acute bacterial prostatitis and NIH type 2 denotes chronic bacterial prostatitis. Unlike NIH type 3 chronic pelvic pain syndrome/nonbacterial prostatitis, types 1 and 2 have no relationship to BPS.

18. **d. decreased capacity and hypersensitivity.** Cystometry in conscious BPS patients generally demonstrates normal function, the exception being decreased bladder capacity and hypersensitivity, perhaps exaggerated by the use of carbon dioxide as a medium. Pain on bladder filling, which reproduces the patient's symptoms, is very suggestive of IC. Bladder compliance in patients with IC is normal, because hypersensitivity would prevent the bladder from filling to the point of noncompliance.

19. **b. is of no consequence in an asymptomatic patient.** Glomerulations are not specific for BPS, and only when seen in conjunction with the clinical criteria of pain and frequency can the presence of glomerulations be viewed as potentially significant. Glomerulations can be seen after radiation therapy, in patients with bladder carcinoma, after exposure to toxic chemicals or chemotherapeutic agents, and in patients undergoing dialysis or after urinary diversion when the bladder has not filled for extended periods. They have also been reported in the majority of men with prostate pain syndromes. In the United States and Europe they are no longer viewed as important for diagnosis or management.

20. **a. 50%.** There is a 50% incidence of temporary remission unrelated to therapy, with a mean duration of 8 months. The clinical course of BPS is extremely variable, and it can be difficult to differentiate the effects of treatment from the natural history of the disease.

21. **c. Bladder hydrodistention.** Bladder hydrodistention with the patient under anesthesia is a common therapeutic modality employed for BPS, frequently as part of the diagnostic evaluation. Its primary value is in diagnosis of a Hunner lesion. Between 30% and 50% of patients experience some short-term relief in symptoms after the procedure. If a Hunner lesion is present, therapeutic response to resection or fulguration is excellent in many patients. About 30% of patients will note a brief exacerbation in their symptoms after hydrodistention. A bladder capacity under anesthesia of less than 200 mL indicates a poor prognosis.

22. **a. Sodium pentosan polysulfate.** The target of sodium pentosan polysulfate therapy is the glycosaminoglycan layer of the urothelium. This agent is an oral analogue of heparin. About 6% of an ingested dose is excreted in the urine. The

proposed mechanism of action is the correction of a glycosaminoglycan dysfunction, thus presumably reversing the abnormal epithelial permeability. It is marginally effective in about 30% of patients in placebo-controlled trials.

23. **e. None of the above.** None of these treatments has been proven efficacious for PBS/IC in double-blind placebo-controlled trials. Hyaluronic acid in both high and low concentrations and BCG have recently failed to show significant efficacy in large, multicenter American trials.

24. **b. They make patients physically dependent on them.** Narcotic analgesics can be very useful in a subset of BPS patients with severe disease. Unlike other classes of analgesics they have no therapeutic ceiling, dosing being limited by tolerance of side effects. They tend to cause constipation and can cause some sedation. Physical dependence is unavoidable, but physical addiction, a chronic disorder characterized by the compulsive use of a substance resulting in physical, psychological, or social harm to the user and the continued use despite that harm, is rare.

25. **a. Transurethral fulguration of a Hunner lesion.** Transurethral fulguration or laser irradiation of a Hunner lesion can provide symptomatic relief. None of the other procedures listed has any place in the treatment of BPS.

26. **b. patient education.** Patient education is the most important step in the initial treatment of BPS. This condition is chronic; the symptoms wax and wane, and remissions are not uncommon. It lends itself to practitioner abuse, and the uninformed, desperate patient is easy prey. Treatment is symptom driven, and an informed patient makes the best decisions.

27. **e. none of the above.** Clinically insignificant detrusor overactivity may be seen in 14% of patients with BPS, a rate of involuntary contractions that has been reported in normal subjects undergoing ambulatory urodynamics. The finding does not rule out the diagnosis of BPS, and treatment of this finding would be unlikely to result in improvement of the patient's bladder pain.

28. **e. all of the above.** BPS should be considered in the differential diagnosis of voiding disorders in men accompanied by irritative symptoms and pelvic pain. A rigorous BPS evaluation can be useful in differentiating BPS from bladder carcinoma in situ, functional or anatomic bladder outlet obstruction, and bacterial prostatitis. Many men with BPS have undergone what has proved to be unnecessary and ill-founded bladder neck surgery.

29. **e. examine the chronic pelvic pain syndrome in men and BPS along with associated syndromes to better characterize the relationship among these disorders and enhance future diagnosis and treatment efforts.** The question as to whether chronic pelvic pain syndrome in men (CPPS III), previously referred to as "nonbacterial prostatitis" and BPS are two different disorders or manifestations of one pathologic process forms part of the goal of the MAPP. Other goals are to outline the relationship of the urologic chronic pelvic pain syndromes with other chronic pain syndromes and learn why such syndromes tend to be associated clinically in the same patients.

30. **a. risk factors for BPS.** Emotional, sexual, and physical abuse have been shown to be risk factors in BPS, and this has been borne out in other studies. A Michigan study compared a control group of 464 women with 215 BPS/IC patients and found 22% of the control group having experienced abuse versus 37% of the patient group. Those with a history of sexual abuse may present with more pain and fewer voiding symptoms. How reliable these data are is not clear, and it would be wrong to jump to any conclusions about abuse in an individual patient. However, practitioners need to have sensitivity for the possibility of an abusive relationship history in all pain patients and in BPS patients in particular. When patients are found to have multiple diagnoses, the rate of previous abuse also increases; and these patients may need referral for further counseling at a traumatic stress center.

Additional Study Points

1. Bladder pain syndrome/interstitial cystitis (BPS/IC) is a condition that is diagnosed on a clinical basis and consists of chronic pelvic pain often exacerbated by bladder filling and associated with urinary frequency. This is a diagnosis of exclusion because there is no specific test or marker that is diagnostic. Interstitial cystitis may be a subgroup of this population that has typical histologic and cystoscopic features; however, those specific features are still subject to debate.

2. Patients with bladder pain syndrome have a 10-fold higher incidence of childhood voiding problems than do patients without the syndrome.

3. The female to male ratio is 5:1.

4. Antiproliferative factor (APF) is secreted by bladder epithelial cells, inhibits bladder epithelial cell proliferation, and is used as a marker of the disease. It may be the primary cause of syndrome in some patients. Urine antiproliferative factor appears to have the highest sensitivity and specificity of the markers studied for this disease.

5. Numerous studies indicate a role for increased sympathetic activity in interstitial cystitis. Whether this is a cause or effect is unknown.

6. Cross-sensitization among pelvic structures may contribute to chronic pain syndromes because this may result in alteration in function of adjacent pelvic organs.

7. Bladder compliance in patients with interstitial cystitis is normal.

8. Many patients find their symptoms adversely affected by certain food groups.

9. Amitriptyline, a tricyclic antidepressant, is the staple of oral treatment. Histamine-2 blockers such as cimetidine have shown some efficacy.

10. Intravesical agents such as silver nitrate, oxychlorosene (Clorpactin), dimethyl sulfoxide (DMSO), and sodium pentosan polysulfate (repairs the glycosaminoglycan layer) have all been used with limited success.

11. Long-term appropriate use of pain medication is an integral part of treatment of this disease.

12. Surgical treatment of this disease other than fulguration of a Hunner ulcer or hydrodistention should be an absolute last resort. Removal of the bladder or portions of the bladder has met with extremely limited success and is only rarely appropriate in highly selected circumstances.

13. Patient education, dietary manipulation, nonprescription analgesics, and pelvic floor relaxation sensation techniques constitute the initial treatment of BPS.

Sexually Transmitted Infections

Tara Lee Frenkl, MD, MPH ● Jeannette M. Potts, MD

QUESTIONS

1. The lifetime prevalence of human papillomavirus (HPV) infection among sexually active women is:
   a. 90%.
   b. 60% to 80%.
   c. 50%.
   d. 20% to 40%.
   e. less than 10%.

2. A very uncomfortable 36-year-old businessman returning from Thailand presents to his urologist with a 4-day history of worsening testicular swelling and pain. He has also noted dysuria but no penile discharge. The best empirical therapy is:
   a. ciprofloxacin, 500 mg PO, plus doxycycline, twice daily, for 7 days.
   b. ciprofloxacin, 500 mg PO, plus azithromycin, 1 g PO.
   c. ceftriaxone, 125 mg IM.
   d. tetracycline, 2 g PO.
   e. ceftriaxone, 125 mg IM, plus azithromycin, 1 g PO.

3. Trichomoniasis:
   a. can be treated with metronidazole in pregnant women during the second trimester.
   b. responds to a single dose of 500 mg of metronidazole.
   c. like many sexually transmitted diseases is more likely to be asymptomatic in women than in men.
   d. can be treated twice daily with metronidazole for 7 days but with greater gastrointestinal side effects than the single-dose therapy.
   e. can be harbored in the mouth and rectum.

4. A 62-year-old widower presents to his urologist concerned about a large painless, exfoliating lesion on his glans. He has no inguinal lymphadenopathy. He has been sexually active with one partner for the past 4 months. He has chronic bacterial prostatitis, and his urologist had recently initiated daily suppressive therapy with trimethoprim-sulfamethoxazole. The most likely diagnosis is:
   a. chancroid.
   b. amebiasis.
   c. lichen planus.
   d. drug reaction.
   e. primary syphilis.

5. A 32-year-old married man seeks counsel because his wife has been recently diagnosed with HPV infection after her annual cervical Papanicolaou smear. The couple has been married 8 years. The patient consumes alcohol in moderation and smokes half a pack of cigarettes per day. His history reveals no lower urinary tract symptoms, and his genital examination is normal. A microscopic urinalysis is acellular. He should be advised to:
   a. undergo androscopy.
   b. use condoms indefinitely.
   c. apply one course of 5-fluorouracil empirically.
   d. quit smoking.
   e. seek marriage counseling.

6. HIV testing should always be a consideration in any patient with possible STI exposure; however, which one of the following scenarios is least worrisome for HIV exposure or transmission?
   a. A patient suspected of having syphilis
   b. A patient with several umbilicated papules consistent with molluscum contagiosum virus in the groin and lower abdomen
   c. A woman with recurrent vaginal yeast infections
   d. A man who has a small papillomatous lesion on his shaft
   e. A person who had polymerase chain reaction (PCR)–proven chancroid, treated 5 years ago

7. Which one of the following statements about women and STIs is TRUE?
   a. Chancroid affects more women than it does men.
   b. Women with herpes simplex virus (HSV) infection are usually easily identified by the presence of vesicular eruptions in the perivaginal area.
   c. Cervical cancer may be considered an AIDS-defining illness.
   d. Women tend to seek prompt medical attention due to the high probability of symptomatology attributed to STIs.

e. Urologists can easily differentiate women with urinary tract infections from those with vaginal infections by taking a thorough history of their lower urinary tract symptoms.

8. Of the antibiotics listed below, the only group that is safe during pregnancy is:

a. erythromycin, azithromycin, ceftriaxone.

b. erythromycin, penicillin, tetracycline.

c. metronidazole, tetracycline, amoxicillin.

d. doxycycline, azithromycin, trimethoprim-sulfamethoxazole.

e. ciprofloxacin, cefixime, erythromycin.

9. A patient diagnosed with a primary infection due to HSV-2:

a. has probably had HSV-1 in the past.

b. can expect to have fewer recurrences than patients with HSV-1.

c. can expect to engage in intercourse safely without risk of transmission as soon as the lesions heal.

d. may have buccal lesions as well as genital ulcers.

e. should immediately begin suppression therapy.

10. In a patient who presents with a history or signs suggestive of syphilis, all of the following would be considered for the diagnosis EXCEPT:

a. sensitivity for rapid plasma reagin (RPR) and Venereal Disease Research Laboratory (VDRL) combined is 100% in secondary syphilis.

b. RPR and VDRL decrease and normalize with successful therapy.

c. positive HIV status may lead to higher false-negative serologic studies.

d. RPR and VDRL have a high rate of false-positive results.

e. fluorescent treponemal antibody (FTA) should be the initial screening test.

11. A 24-year-old female graduate student who "always" uses condoms presents with her first ever vesicular eruption on her labia, which appeared 2 days ago. Bilateral inguinal adenopathy is appreciated on examination, and the area is somewhat tender. The most important confirmatory test for this patient at this time is:

a. darkfield microscopy of the specimen scraped from the wound.

b. vaginal swabs for *Chlamydia* L1, L2, L3.

c. viral cultures for HSV.

d. PCR assay for *Haemophilus ducreyi*.

e. serum RPR or VDRL.

12. A 29-year-old homosexual male notices mild dysuria with a mucopurulent discharge within 2 weeks of his most recent sexual encounter. After obtaining cultures, empirical therapy is best given using a single dose of:

a. azithromycin, 1 g PO.

b. ciprofloxacin, 500 mg PO.

c. ciprofloxacin, 1000 mg PO.

d. ceftriaxone, 125 mg IM.

e. levofloxacin, 250 mg PO.

13. A patient is concerned about the sudden appearance of a single 1.5-cm ulcer with irregular borders. It is located on the distal part of his shaft and part of the proximal portion of his glands. All of the following are true EXCEPT:

a. genital ulcers can also result from noninfectious causes.

b. sensitivity for identification based on appearance alone is 31% to 35%.

c. coinfection of STIs occurs in approximately 10% of patients.

d. diagnosis can be reliably made by combining the appearance of the ulcer with the characteristic of inguinal adenopathy.

e. confirmatory cultures and serologic studies should be performed whenever possible.

Pathology

1. See Figure 13–1.

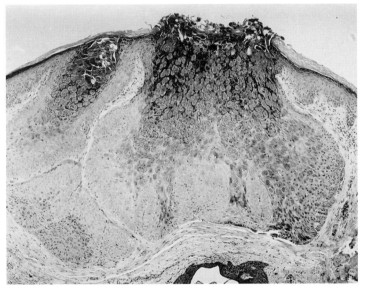

Figure 13–1.   (From Bostwick DG, Cheng L. Urologic surgical pathology. 2nd ed. Edinburgh: Mosby; 2008.)

A 23-year-old sexually active male noted the appearance of multiple 3-mm papules on the shaft of his penis. The papules are raised, are dome shaped, and have a central umbilication. The lesion is biopsied and depicted in Figure 13–1. The diagnosis is:

a. syphilis.

b. chancroid.

c. HPV infection.

d. molluscum contagiosum.

e. HSV infection.

2. See Figure 13–2.

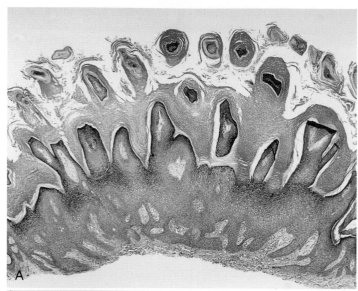

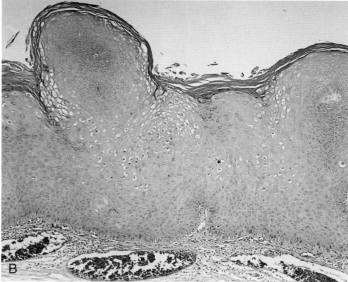

Figure 13–2.   (From Bostwick DG, Cheng L. Urologic surgical pathology. 2nd ed. Edinburgh: Mosby; 2008.)

A 23-year-old woman notices a cauliflower-like lesion on her vulva. She is sexually active. The lesion is sampled (see Fig. 13–2). The diagnosis is:

a. syphilis.

b. chancroid.

c. condyloma acuminatum or HPV infection.

d. molluscum contagiosum.

e. HSV infection.

ANSWERS

1. **b. 60% to 80%.** Epidemiologic studies indicate that this virus is extremely prevalent among sexually active women.

2. **e. ceftriaxone, 125 mg IM, plus azithromycin, 1 g PO.** Although ciprofloxacin is highly effective for the treatment of gonococcus, a quinolone-resistant strain has emerged in eastern Asia and the South Pacific. Either doxycycline or azithromycin would be appropriate to treat possible coinfection with *Chlamydia*.

3. **a. can be treated using metronidazole in pregnant women during the second trimester.** Metronidazole is safe during the second trimester of pregnancy and as a single 2-g dose or a better-tolerated regimen of 500 mg twice daily for 7 days can be administered to nonpregnant patients as well.

4. **d. drug reaction.** Although it would not be incorrect to suspect and test for an STI, a fixed drug reaction is the most probable condition in this setting.

5. **d. quit smoking.** An abnormal Papanicolaou smear does not imply infidelity given the long and variable latency of HPV. The only meaningful and practical suggestion is to recommend smoking cessation, because smoking in either partner is associated with higher rates of progression and malignancy.

6. **d. A man who has a small papillomatous lesion on his shaft.** Because of the ubiquitous nature of papillomatous lesions, it would be inappropriate to screen such patients for HIV, in the absence of any other risk factors.

7. **c. Cervical cancer may be considered an AIDS-defining illness.** Women are likely to contract STIs and suffer more from the consequences due to late diagnosis and prolonged asymptomatic periods. Because a woman's immune status can influence the behavior of HPV, cervical cancer is considered an AIDS-defining illness in patients who are HIV positive, similar to the way in which AIDS is defined in HIV-positive patients who are newly diagnosed with *Pneumocystis jiroveci*.

8. **a. erythromycin, azithromycin, ceftriaxone.**

9. **d. may have buccal lesions as well as genital ulcers.** Patients diagnosed with primary infection due to HSV-2 may expect more recurrences than in HSV-1 infection, can have buccal lesions, and will have asymptomatic shedding for up to 3 months after the first outbreak.

10. **e. fluorescent treponemal antibody (FTA) should be the initial screening test.** Because of decreased sensitivity in the setting of primary syphilis, FTA should not be part of initial screening. However, the physician must be aware of false-positive VDRL and RPR results, as well as the better sensitivity.

11. **c. viral cultures for HSV.** The most likely diagnosis is herpes simplex virus, given the latency period and tender, bilateral inguinal adenopathy and patient demographics. The most important point about this question, however, is the fact that condoms are not effective in preventing all infections.

12. **d. ceftriaxone, 125 mg IM.** Not only have quinolone-resistant strains of gonococcus affected Asia, but they have also become more frequently detected in homosexual males in the United States. Therefore, ceftriaxone would remain the most appropriate first choice for treatment.

13. **d. diagnosis can be reliably made by combining the appearance of the ulcer with the characteristic of inguinal adenopathy.**

Pathology

1. **d. molluscum contagiosum.** The pathology depicts the cytoplasmic inclusions known as molluscum bodies

or Henderson-Patterson bodies. These inclusions contain viral particles that initially stain eosinophilic but ultimately acquire a basophilic appearance. Gross lesions are small and dome shaped with a central umbilication.

2. **c. condylomata acuminatum or HPV infection.**
Notice the marked proliferation of squamous epithelium with papillomatous architecture and the lack of mitotic figures and a rather orderly noninvasive nature of the hypertrophied squamous epithelium.

Additional Study Points

1. When exposed to STIs women are more likely to become infected and less likely to be symptomatic.
2. There has been an increase in quinolone-resistant *Neisseria gonorrhoeae.*
3. Herpes simplex virus type 2 accounts for 90% of cases. Herpes simplex virus type 1 accounts for the remainder and is the common cause of cold sores; silent infection is common in this disease. The diagnosis is made by viral culture and subtyping.
4. Chancroid is caused by *Haemophilus ducreyi* and results in a painful, nonindurated ulcer covered by an exudate. Inguinal adenopathy occurs and may become suppurative.
5. Chancre of syphilis is single, painless, indurated, and clean. It is associated with nontender inguinal lymphadenopathy.
6. Latent syphilis is seropositive with no evidence of disease. Early latent syphilis occurs in less than 1 year. Late latent syphilis occurs beyond 1 year.
7. Primary syphilis is the acute infection. Secondary syphilis is manifested by mucocutaneous and constitutional signs and symptoms that are often associated with a maculopapular rash. Tertiary syphilis is a systemic disease involving the cardiovascular, skeletal, and central nervous system.
8. Serologic tests for syphilis should be confirmed with *Treponema* testing using either *T. pallidum* particle agglutination (TP-PA) or fluorescent treponemal antibody absorption (FTA-ABS) testing. RPR and VDRL correlate with disease activity. They usually become negative after treatment.
9. The Jarisch-Herxheimer reaction occurs when patients with syphilis are treated with penicillin, resulting in the release of toxic products when the treponemes are killed. The symptoms include headache, myalgia, fever, tachycardia, and increased respiratory rate.
10. Lymphogranuloma venereum presents as a single painless ulcer and painful inguinal adenopathy.
11. PCR assays are used for diagnosing chlamydial infection.
12. A strawberry rash on the vulva or strawberry cervix is seen in trichomoniasis.
13. Human papilloma virus (HPV) types 6 and 11 increase the risk for developing carcinoma of the external genitalia. More than 99% of cervical cancers and 84% of anal cancers are associated with HPV 16 or 18. The most common serotype associated with squamous cell carcinoma of the penis is HPV 16.
14. Biopsies of genital warts are not routinely indicated but should be performed when the wart is atypical, pigmented, indurated, or fixed and ulcerated.

Urologic Aspects of AIDS and HIV Infection

Thomas J. Walsh, MD, MS ● John N. Krieger, MD

QUESTIONS

1. Life expectancy in the countries most affected by HIV infection was:
   a. reduced by 15 years by the year 2000.
   b. reduced by 5 years by the year 2003.
   c. unchanged.
   d. reduced by 10 years by the year 2004.
   e. reduced by 5 years by the end of 2004.

2. With the availability of highly active antiretroviral therapy (HAART), blood screening, and treatment of sexually transmitted infections, the number of new HIV infections in the United States has:
   a. decreased to 20,000 per year.
   b. decreased to less than 10,000 per year.
   c. remained at a plateau of 40,000 infections per year.
   d. increased, but at a slower rate of 100,000 per year.
   e. increased to 75,000 per year.

3. Factors that influence sexual transmission of HIV include all of the following EXCEPT:
   a. sexually transmitted infections.
   b. antiretroviral therapy.
   c. circumcision status.
   d. anti-inflammatory therapy.
   e. gynecologic factors.

4. The typical course of untreated HIV infection includes all of the following EXCEPT:
   a. it takes 8 to 12 years from infection to death in the absence of treatment.
   b. it has three distinct phases.
   c. it occurs in 60% to 70% of patients.
   d. it takes more than15 years from infection to death in the absence of treatment.
   e. it is determined largely during the initial phase of infection.

5. The virologic set point indicates:
   a. the response to antiretroviral therapy.
   b. the risk for disease progression.
   c. prospects for HIV eradication.

d. effect of HAART on the viral reservoirs in lymphoid tissue.
   e. time from infection.

6. With complete and sustained suppression of HIV replication by antiretroviral therapy, it is estimated that HIV could be eliminated from an infected person in what time period?
   a. 3 to 6 months.
   b. 1 to 2 years.
   c. 3 to 4 years.
   d. 5 to 6 years.
   e. 10 years or more.

7. Herpetic lesions in an HIV-infected patient are not responding well to oral acyclovir. The following should be done:
   a. Obtain genital herpes culture and sensitivity testing.
   b. Determine the patient's HIV viral load and CD4 count.
   c. Change to an alternative oral drug.
   d. Change to IV acyclovir.
   e. Add photodynamic therapy.

8. The optimal approach to suspected voiding dysfunction in an HIV-infected patient begins with:
   a. urodynamic testing.
   b. standard pharmacologic measures.
   c. antiviral therapy.
   d. checking viral load.
   e. clean intermittent catheterization.

9. Most patients with presumed indinavir-containing urinary calculi require:
   a. extracorporeal shockwave lithotripsy.
   b. ureteroscopy.
   c. noncontrast CT for diagnosis.
   d. hydration, analgesics, and temporary cessation of indinavir.
   e. changing to an alternative protease inhibitor.

10. Which statement about HIV-associated nephropathy is incorrect?
    a. It is more common in black patients.
    b. It seldom presents as renal insufficiency.

c. It may present as proteinuria.

d. It often responds to HAART.

e. Echogenic kidneys with preserved size are shown on ultrasonography.

11. Kaposi sarcoma (KS):

   a. usually presents as renal disease.

   b. has an incidence that has changed little since the advent of HAART.

   c. is related to coinfection with both HIV and a herpesvirus.

   d. is related to activation of epithelial cells.

   e. is most common in patients who use intravenously administered drugs.

ANSWERS

1. **a. reduced by 15 years by the year 2000.** Life expectancy in the most affected sub-Saharan countries was reduced as much as 15 years by the year 2000, compared with projections in areas without HIV.

2. **c. remained at a plateau of 40,000 infections per year.** Despite antiretroviral therapy, blood screening, and treatment of sexually transmitted infections, the number of infections has remained at a plateau of 40,000 new HIV infections/year in the United States over the past decade.

3. **d. anti-inflammatory therapy.** Anti-inflammatory therapy is the only factor that has NOT been implicated as an epidemiologic risk factor for sexual transmission of HIV. Sexually transmitted diseases, antiretroviral therapy, circumcision status, and gynecologic factors have all been shown to influence the risk for sexual transmission of HIV.

4. **d. it takes more than 15 years from infection to death in the absence of treatment.** This is the only statement that is NOT supported by current data.

5. **b. the risk for disease progression.** During the transition from primary to chronic infection, HIV plasma RNA levels reach a virologic set point that predicts the rate of disease progression (Mellors et al, 1996).* The virologic set point varies among HIV-infected individuals and tends to remain stable in the same person during the chronic phase. The virologic set point that a person attains is determined by both the mechanisms involved in the establishment of chronic infection and by host factors that can modulate the course of HIV disease.

6. **e. 10 years or more.** Current estimates are that it may take 5 to 10 years or more to eliminate HIV, considering a half-life of 4 months for the long-lived infected CD4+ cells and provided that effective and durable suppression of viral replication is achieved by HAART.

7. **a. Obtain genital herpes culture and sensitivity testing.** Herpes simplex virus resistance should be suspected if lesions persist or recur despite antiviral therapy. Viral culture and resistance testing should be obtained, if possible.

8. **b. standard pharmacologic measures.** Standard pharmacologic measures are preferred for patients with mild dysfunction, and routine urodynamic investigation has proven to be of low yield.

9. **d. hydration, analgesics, and temporary cessation of indinavir.** Our experience is consistent with recommendations for conservative treatment in most cases, which include hydration, analgesics, and temporary cessation of indinavir.

10. **b. It seldom presents as renal insufficiency.** HIV-associated nephropathy typically presents as proteinuria in the nephrotic range (and often massive) and renal insufficiency.

11. **c. is related to coinfection with both HIV and a herpesvirus.** Coinfection with HIV and KS-associated herpesvirus increases the risk of developing KS 10,000-fold compared with KS-associated herpesvirus infection alone. The probability of developing KS after coinfection with both KS-associated herpesvirus and HIV approaches 50% over 10 years.

*Sources referenced can be found in *Campbell-Walsh Urology, 10th Edition,* on the Expert Consult website.

Additional Study Points

1. There are three main modes of HIV transmission: unprotected intercourse, contact with blood, and transmission from mother to child.

2. The presence of sexually transmitted infections increases the risk for concurrent HIV.

3. Ulcerative sexually transmitted infections including herpes, syphilis, and chancroid enhance the susceptibility to HIV per sexual contact.

4. Antiviral therapy for HIV does not necessarily make the patient noninfectious.

5. Men who are circumcised are at lower risk for HIV infection.

6. There are two types of HIV viruses: HIV-1 and HIV-2. There are very few cases of HIV-2 in the developed world, and it is less easily transmitted and less virulent than HIV-1.

7. HIV initially attaches to the CD4+ T-cell receptor.

8. Antiretroviral combination therapy delays the rate of progression of the disease and prolongs survival.

9. Overt AIDS is marked by a low CD4+ T-cell count.

10. Plasma HIV RNA load is the most accurate predictor of disease progression.

11. The diagnosis of HIV is made by screening for anti–HIV-1 and anti–HIV-2 antibodies using an enzyme-linked immunosorbent assay. If this is positive, confirmation is made using Western blot analysis. If the Western blot test is negative, then the enzyme-linked immunosorbent assay is falsely positive or the patient has an acute infection.

12. After treatment, the nadir of plasma HIV RNA predicts long-term outcome.

13. HIV testing is recommended for anyone diagnosed with a sexually transmitted infection or at risk for sexually transmitted infections.

14. Herpes simplex virus increases HIV replication in persons infected with both viruses.

15. Human papillomavirus infection increases the risk for carcinoma especially in HIV-infected hosts.

16. The most common intrascrotal pathologic process in AIDS patients is testicular atrophy.

17. Voiding dysfunction is common in patients with advanced HIV infection.

18. Urinary calculi have been associated with, most notably, protease inhibitors such as indinavir. These stones are soluble at an acidic pH.

19. HIV-associated nephropathy is a glomerular disease that often presents as proteinuria.

20. Patients with HIV are at particular increased risk for Kaposi sarcoma and non-Hodgkin lymphoma. Kaposi sarcoma presents as a raised, firm, indurated purplish plaque, reflecting the presence of abundant blood vessels, extravasated erythrocytes, and siderophages.

21. Human herpesvirus 8 is essential for all forms of Kaposi sarcoma.

22. HIV protease inhibitors are also potent antiangiogenic molecules and are useful in treating Kaposi sarcoma. However, localized lesions may be treated by irradiation, laser, cryotherapy, or intralesional injections of antineoplastic drugs. Corticosteroids should not be used to treat the lesions.

23. There may be an increased incidence of seminoma in patients with HIV infection.

Cutaneous Diseases of the External Genitalia

Richard Edward Link, MD, PhD

QUESTIONS

1. Which of the following is classified as a secondary skin lesion?
   a. Macule
   b. Papule
   c. Ulcer
   d. Vesicle
   e. Nodule

2. The periodic–acid Schiff stain is used to identify what organism in scraped or touched skin preparations?
   a. *Pseudomonas* sp.
   b. *Candida*
   c. *Corynebacterium minutissimum*
   d. Herpes simplex
   e. *Molluscum contagiosum*

3. Oral glucocorticosteroids are often used to treat dermatologic conditions and have a duration-of-effect lasting:
   a. 2 to 3 weeks.
   b. 30 to 90 minutes.
   c. 1 to 5 hours.
   d. 8 to 48 hours.
   e. 5 to 7 days.

4. The preferred dosage schedule for a short course of oral glucocorticosteroids used to treat a cutaneous disorder is:
   a. a single morning dose.
   b. a single evening dose.
   c. doses in the morning and evening.
   d. a dose every other day in the morning.
   e. re-dosing every 8 hours.

5. A 12-year-old boy has a long-standing history of asthma and occasional outbreaks of erythematous, pruritic papules on his scrotum and lower extremities. Which of the following options represents a rational approach to treating this condition?
   a. Long-term suppressive topical corticosteroids
   b. Frequent soaking in warm water to prevent the development of lesions
   c. Low-dose systemic corticosteroids
   d. The frequent application of emollients
   e. Application of a topical calcineurin inhibitor

6. Patch testing is a useful diagnostic test to identify:
   a. psoriasis.
   b. contact dermatitis.
   c. erythema gangrenosum.
   d. atopic dermatitis.
   e. Behçet disease.

7. The North American Contact Dermatitis Group identified a series of common allergens that were associated with contact dermatitis. Which allergen was the most common offending agent in contact dermatitis cases?
   a. Silver
   b. Textile dyes
   c. Ragweed
   d. Nickel sulfate
   e. Pet dander

8. A 35-year-old textile worker spills a small amount of green dye onto her left thigh. By the end of the workday, she is complaining of pain and burning over a 5-cm irregular patch of skin on her left thigh. What is the most likely diagnosis?
   a. Erysipelas
   b. Allergic contact dermatitis
   c. Hailey-Hailey disease
   d. Irritant contact dermatitis
   e. Koebner phenomenon

9. Following a recent exacerbation of genital herpes, a 22-year-old man notes the development of erythematous papules and targetoid lesions on his thighs, scrotum, and oral mucosa. The best next course of action is:
   a. oral antihistamines.
   b. systemic corticosteroids.
   c. observation.
   d. oral acyclovir.
   e. topical corticosteroids.

10. A 19-year-old woman is 2 days into a course of sulfonamides for an *Escherichia coli* urinary tract infection. She develops painful labial erosions that progress to a generalized rash with the formation of blisters. The most likely diagnosis is:
    a. erythema multiforme minor.
    b. Reiter syndrome.
    c. Stevens-Johnson syndrome.

d. pyoderma gangrenosum.

e. Sézary syndrome.

11. A 42-year-old circumcised man has a history of widely distributed erythematous plaques—most severe on his knees, elbows, inguinal folds, and glans penis. The condition has waxed and waned since he was in his early twenties. What is an appropriate therapy during an exacerbation?

a. Topical 3% liquor carbonis detergens in 1% hydrocortisone cream

b. Oral psoralen combined with ultraviolet radiation (PUVA)

c. Systemic corticosteroids

d. Topical 5-fluorouracil cream

e. Oral azathioprine

12. A 21-year-old man presents with dysuria, blurred vision, oral ulcers, and erythematous plaques in his genitalia. He has mild soreness in his knees and ankles. He is HIV negative and has had no prior history of sexually transmitted disease. What is a likely risk factor for development of this disorder?

a. Genital herpes simplex

b. The HLA-B27 haplotype

c. A history of atopic dermatitis

d. Exposure to benzene-containing chemicals

e. Family history of psoriasis

13. Which of the following statements is true about the treatment of symptomatic genital lichen planus?

a. Systemic corticosteroids can prevent the development of lesions.

b. In clinical trials, the most effective agent for treating lichen planus is systemic acitretin.

c. Systemic corticosteroids can shorten the time to clearance of existing lesions from 29 to 18 weeks.

d. Phytotherapy is the therapeutic modality of choice for treating lichen planus.

e. Metronidazole is an effective and well-established, first-line agent in the treatment of lichen planus.

14. The late stage of lichen sclerosus involving the glans penis is termed:

a. keratinizing balanoposthitis.

b. pseudoepitheliomatous, keratotic, and micaceous balanitis.

c. bowenoid papulosis.

d. balanitis xerotica obliterans.

e. Hailey-Hailey disease.

15. Which of the following cutaneous conditions has been associated with an increased risk of squamous cell carcinoma?

a. Lichen sclerosus et atrophicus

b. Lichen planus

c. Psoriasis

d. Bullous pemphigoid

e. Lichen nitidus

16. An 18-year-old man has a history of seizures following an automobile accident 2 weeks ago. He was sexually active prior to the accident. Today, he presents with a solitary, painful erosion on the penis. What course of action is appropriate at this time?

a. Do urethra swab for gonorrhea and chlamydia.

b. Consult with neurology to alter his antiseizure medication regimen.

c. Start oral acyclovir.

d. Do punch biopsy of the lesion.

e. Start oral doxycycline.

17. A 35-year-old, previously healthy woman has noted the rapid development of sharply demarcated, pruritic, red-brown plaques over a large extent of her skin surface. The plaques are particularly dense in her nasolabial folds and perianal area, and the nails are spared. What is the next step?

a. Systemic corticosteroids

b. HIV test

c. Skin culture for *Malassezia furfur*

d. Examination of the lesions under ultraviolet (UV) light

e. Biopsy of the lesions

18. In patients with pemphigus vulgaris, the characteristic clinical sign showing loss of epidermal cohesion is:

a. the dimple sign.

b. the Asboe-Hansen sign.

c. the Leser-Trélat sign.

d. the dimple sign.

e. the bullous blanching sign.

19. Which of the following statements is FALSE concerning pemphigus vulgaris?

a. The majority of pemphigus patients have painful oral mucosal erosions.

b. Pemphigus appears to have an autoimmune pathogenesis.

c. Blisters appear to form due to loss of keratinocyte cell–cell adhesion.

d. Treatment of pemphigus relies on systemic corticosteroids.

e. Given enough time, even advanced cases of pemphigus generally resolve spontaneously without sequelae.

20. Which of the following dermatoses has an association with celiac disease?

a. Dermatitis herpetiformis

b. Hailey-Hailey disease

c. Behçet disease

d. Bullous pemphigoid

e. Psoriasis

21. Which of the following is not a vesicobullous dermatosis?

a. Hailey-Hailey disease

b. Pyoderma gangrenosum

c. Pemphigus vulgaris

d. Zoon balanitis

e. Linear IgA bullous dermatoses

22. Which agent has been shown to be effective in treating linear IgA bullous dermatoses?

a. Azathioprine

b. Cyclosporine

c. Dapsone

d. Metronidazole

e. Sulfonylurea

23. A 45-year-old woman has pruritic, foul-smelling blistering in the inframammary folds and groin. The skin findings are confluent areas of vesicles with fragile blisters. Which of the following statements is FALSE concerning this condition?

   a. The condition is usually worse during the summer months.

   b. Intralesional corticosteroids may be effective for treatment.

   c. Involvement of the vulva is common in women.

   d. Wide local excision may be necessary in refractory cases.

   e. Laser vaporization has been applied successfully to this condition.

24. A 35-year-old man presents with painful ulcerations in his mouth and on his penis, as well as blurred vision and a history of recurrent epididymitis. What is the likely diagnosis?

   a. Behçet disease

   b. Oculocutaneous aphthous ulcer syndrome

   c. Epidermolysis bullosa

   d. Fabry disease

   e. Pyoderma gangrenosum

25. Which of the following statements is FALSE concerning pyoderma gangrenosum?

   a. Pyoderma gangrenosum most likely has an autoimmune mechanism of pathogenesis.

   b. There is an association with collagen vascular disease.

   c. Corticosteroids may play a role in management.

   d. The presence of vacuolated keratinocytes in an inflammatory background is pathognomonic for this condition.

26. Which of the following cutaneous conditions has an association with borderline personality disorder?

   a. Factitial dermatitis

   b. "Innocent" traumatic dermatitis

   c. Sézary syndrome

   d. Munchausen syndrome by proxy

   e. Behçet disease

27. The most common organisms causing erysipelas are:

   a. dermatophytes.

   b. *Staphylococcus aureus.*

   c. *Streptococcus pyogenes.*

   d. *Escherichia coli.*

   e. *Pseudomonas* sp.

28. Which of the following statements is FALSE concerning Fournier gangrene?

   a. The mortality rate even with modern treatment may be greater than 15%.

   b. Most of the cases of Fournier gangrene are caused by *Streptococcus pyogenes.*

   c. Alcoholism is a significant risk factor for development of Fournier gangrene.

d. In severe cases, debridement may need to extend into the chest wall.

e. Fournier gangrene can be caused by either a cutaneous, urethral, or perirectal source of infection.

29. An 18-year-old woman develops a pruritic rash over her thighs and buttocks after using a whirlpool spa. Her face and upper extremities are spared. What is the likely diagnosis?

   a. Candidal intertrigo

   b. Pseudomonal folliculitis

   c. Contact dermatitis

   d. Scabies infestation

   e. Herpes simplex

30. Which of the following conditions has an association with hyperhidrosis?

   a. Atopic dermatitis

   b. Trichomycosis axillaris

   c. Hidradenitis suppurativa

   d. Psoriasis

   e. Genital lichen planus

31. A patient being treated for tinea cruris has significant scrotal involvement. What alternative diagnosis does this suggest?

   a. Seborrheic dermatitis

   b. Erythrasma

   c. Cutaneous candidiasis

   d. Hidradenitis suppurativa

   e. Contact dermatitis

32. Which of the following is a treatment for scabies that is contraindicated in pediatric patients?

   a. Lindane

   b. Dapsone

   c. Permethrin

   d. Ivermectin

   e. Doxycycline

33. Which of the following statements concerning Bowen disease is incorrect?

   a. Bowen disease and squamous cell carcinoma in situ are the same condition.

   b. Bowen disease involving the glans penis is termed erythroplasia of Queyrat.

   c. Bowen disease may be treated with topical imiquimod.

   d. Bowen disease is associated with human papillomavirus (HPV) type 6 and 11.

   e. Mohs microsurgery may play a role when tissue preservation is critical.

34. Which of the following statements concerning verrucous carcinoma is correct?

   a. Verrucous carcinoma has a high propensity to metastasize.

   b. Verrucous carcinoma should not be treated with primary radiotherapy due to the risk of anaplastic transformation.

   c. Verrucous carcinoma is an exceedingly rare malignancy of the genitalia.

d. Verrucous carcinoma is associated with HPV type 16 and 18.

e. Verrucous carcinoma may grow very rapidly and destroy local tissue.

35. What is the most common site of presentation for Kaposi sarcoma in immunocompetent individuals?

   a. Chest
   b. Face
   c. Lower extremities
   d. Genitalia
   e. Palms

36. The following malignancy has been found concurrently in lesions of pseudoepitheliomatous, keratotic, and micaceous balanitis:

   a. basal cell carcinoma.
   b. cutaneous T-cell lymphoma.
   c. squamous cell carcinoma.
   d. verrucous carcinoma.
   e. Kaposi sarcoma.

37. Which of the following statements about extramammary Paget disease (EPD) is FALSE?

   a. EPD is an adenocarcinoma.
   b. EPD is associated with another underlying malignancy in more than 60% of cases.
   c. EPD has been associated with malignancies of the urethra and bladder.
   d. EPD lesions show vacuolated Paget cells on histopathologic exam.
   e. The vulva is the most common genital site involved in women.

38. Patients with cutaneous T-cell lymphoma who develop hematologic involvement are given the diagnosis of:

   a. lymphoid papulosis.
   b. mycosis fungoides.
   c. pagetoid reticulosis.
   d. Sézary syndrome.
   e. Fabry disease.

39. Which of the following conditions has the most in common histologically with pearly penile papules?

   a. Psoriasis
   b. Tuberous sclerosis
   c. Molluscum contagiosum
   d. Herpes simplex

40. The most effective treatment for Zoon balanitis is:

   a. topical 5-fluorouracil.
   b. topical corticosteroids.
   c. circumcision.
   d. laser therapy.
   e. topical calcineurin inhibitors.

41. Skin tags are also termed:

   a. fibrofolliculomas.
   b. angiokeratomas.
   c. hamartomas.
   d. acrochordons.
   e. dermatofibromas.

42. The Leser-Trélat syndrome refers to:

   a. the rapid progression of lichen planus associated with the HLA-B27 haplotype.
   b. an abrupt increase in the size and number of seborrheic keratoses, suggesting internal malignancy.
   c. the combination of hand, foot, and genital psoriasis.
   d. the development of brown macules on the genitalia, unrelated to sun exposure.
   e. the combination of oral and genital ulcers often seen in Behçet disease.

ANSWERS

1. **c. Ulcer.** Secondary skin lesions develop as the skin condition evolves or are caused by scratching or superinfection. A secondary skin lesion is classified morphologically as a scale, crust, erosion, ulcer, atrophy, or scar.

2. **b. *Candida*.** To identify cutaneous fungi, such as dermatophytes and *Candida* species, periodic acid–Schiff (PAS) staining may be applied to scraped or touched skin specimens.

3. **d. 8 to 48 hours.** Oral glucocorticosteroids (GCS) are absorbed in the jejunum with peak plasma concentrations occurring in 30 to 90 minutes. Despite short plasma half-lives of 1 to 5 hours, the duration-of-effect of GCS lasts between 8 and 48 hours, depending on the agent.

4. **a. a single morning dose.** For short-term (≤3 weeks) treatment of dermatologic conditions such as allergic contact dermatitis, a single morning dose of oral glucocorticosteroids is given to minimize suppression of the hypothalamic-pituitary-adrenal axis.

5. **d. The frequent application of emollients.** The condition described is atopic dermatitis (AD or eczema), which is associated with susceptibility to irritants and proteins, as well as the tendency to develop asthma and allergic rhinitis. Intense pruritus is the hallmark of AD, and controlling the patient's urge to scratch is critical for successful treatment. Removal of various "trigger factors" from the environment (such as chemicals, detergents, and household dust mites) may be beneficial in some cases. The mainstay of treatment for AD includes gentle cleaning with nonalkali soaps and the frequent use of emollients.

6. **b. contact dermatitis.** Patch testing is a simple technique of exposing an area of skin to a variety of potential allergens in a grid template. Generally performed by dermatologists, patch testing can help to confirm the diagnosis of allergic contact dermatitis and the allergen involved.

7. **d. Nickel sulfate.** In 2003, the North American Contact Dermatitis Group (NACDG) reported a long list of common allergens implicated in allergic contact dermatitis based on patch testing results. The most common sensitizing allergen identified was nickel sulfate, which is a common component of costume jewelry and belt buckles.

8. **d. Irritant contact dermatitis.** Irritant contact dermatitis results from a direct cytotoxic effect of an irritant chemical touching the skin and is responsible for approximately 80% of contact dermatitis cases. Occupational exposure is also common. Examples of

offending agents include soaps, metal salts, acid- or alkali-containing compounds, and industrial solvents.

9. **c. Observation.** Erythema multiforme (EM) minor is an acute, self-limited skin disease characterized by the abrupt onset of symmetrical fixed red papules that may evolve into target lesions. The majority of cases are precipitated by herpesvirus type I and II, with herpetic lesions usually preceding the development of target lesions by 10 to 14 days. Although continuous suppressive acyclovir may prevent EM episodes in patients with herpes infection, administration of the drug after development of target lesions is of no benefit. With observation alone, the natural history of EM minor is spontaneous resolution after several weeks without sequelae, although recurrences are common.

10. **c. Stevens-Johnson syndrome.** Stevens-Johnson syndrome (SJS) is a life-threatening severe allergic reaction with features similar to extensive skin burns. A vast array of inciting factors has been implicated in the development of SJS, with drug exposures being the most commonly identified. Nonsteroidal anti-inflammatory agents are the most frequent offending agents followed by sulfonamides, tetracycline, penicillin, doxycycline, and anticonvulsants.

11. **a. Topical 3% liquor carbonis detergens in 1% hydrocortisone cream.** Psoriasis is a papulosquamous disorder affecting up to 2% of the population with a relapsing and remitting course. For genital psoriasis, the mainstay of therapy is the use of low-potency topical corticosteroid creams for short courses. Photochemotherapy combining an ingested psoralen with ultraviolet radiation (PUVA) has been used extensively to treat psoriasis. However, a dose-dependent increase in the risk of genital squamous cell carcinoma has been associated with high-dose PUVA therapy for psoriasis elsewhere on the body. Genital shielding during PUVA therapy is strongly recommended; therefore this modality is contraindicated for treating psoriatic lesions localized to genital skin.

12. **b. The HLA-B27 haplotype.** Reiter syndrome is a syndrome composed of urethritis, arthritis, ocular findings, oral ulcers and skin lesions. It is generally preceded by an episode of either urethritis (*Chlamydia, Gonococcus*) or gastrointestinal infection (*Yersinia, Salmonella, Shigella, Campylobacter, Neisseria,* or *Ureaplasma* species) and is more common in HIV- positive patients. There is a strong genetic association with the HLA-B27 haplotype.

13. **c. Systemic corticosteroids can shorten the time to clearance of existing lesions from 29 to 18 weeks.** Although bothersome pruritus is common with lichen planus (LP), asymptomatic lesions on the genitalia do not require treatment. The primary modality of treatment for symptomatic lesions is topical corticosteroids, although for severe cases, systemic corticosteroids have been shown to shorten the time course to clearance of LP lesions from 29 to 18 weeks.

14. **d. balanitis xerotica obliterans.** Lichen sclerosis (LS) is a scarring disorder, with a predilection for the external genitalia of both sexes, characterized by tissue pallor, loss of architecture, and hyperkeratosis. The late stage of this disease is called balanitis xerotica obliterans, which can involve the penile urethra and result in troublesome urethral stricture disease.

15. **a. Lichen sclerosus et atrophicus.** Despite the similarities in name, lichen sclerosis (LS) shares little in common with lichen planus and lichen nitidus other than

pruritus and a predilection for the genital region. Another critical distinction is that LS has been associated with squamous cell carcinoma of the penis, particularly those variants not associated with human papillomavirus, and may represent a premalignant condition. Biopsy is worthwhile both to confirm the diagnosis and exclude malignant change.

16. **b. Consultation with neurology to alter his antiseizure medication regimen.** The association of epileptic seizures and a solitary painful genital lesion is suspicious for a diagnosis of Behçet disease (BD). Other causes for genital ulceration, however, including aphthous ulcers, syphilis, herpes simplex, and chancroid, must be considered before a diagnosis of BD is made. In this case, the patient's neurologic issues should take priority over treatment for his genital ulcer.

17. **b. HIV test.** Seborrheic dermatitis (SD) is a common skin disease characterized by the presence of sharply demarcated, pink-yellow to red-brown plaques with a flaky scale. Particularly in immunosuppressed individuals, SD may involve a significant proportion of the body surface area. Extensive and/or severe SD should raise concerns for possible underlying HIV infection.

18. **b. The Asboe-Hansen sign.** The loss of epidermal cohesion seen in pemphigus vulgaris leads to the characteristic Asboe-Hansen sign: spreading of fluid under the adjacent normal-appearing skin away from the direction of pressure on a blister.

19. **e. Given enough time, even advanced cases of pemphigus generally resolve spontaneously without sequelae.** Severe cases of pemphigus vulgaris without appropriate treatment may be fatal due to the loss of the epidermal barrier function of large areas of affected skin. Treatment usually depends on systemic corticosteroids, although minimization of steroid dose is an important goal to limit side effects. The addition of immunosuppressive agents, such as azathioprine and cyclophosphamide, may be beneficial due to their corticosteroid-sparing effect.

20. **a. Dermatitis herpetiformis.** Dermatitis herpetiformis (DH) is a cutaneous manifestation of celiac disease and is generally associated with gluten sensitivity. Diagnosis can be confirmed by biopsy and direct immunofluorescence, which shows a granular pattern of IgA deposition at the basement membrane. Treatment includes the use of dapsone and a strict gluten-restricted diet.

21. **b. Pyoderma gangrenosum.** Pyoderma gangrenosum (PG) is an ulcerative skin disease associated with systemic illnesses, including inflammatory bowel disease, arthritis, collagen vascular disease, and myeloproliferative disorders. The classic morphologic presentation of PG is painful cutaneous and mucous membrane ulceration, often with extensive loss of tissue and a purulent base.

22. **c. Dapsone.** Characteristic clinical features of linear IgA bullous dermatosis (LABD) include vesicles and bullae arranged in a combination of circumferential and linear orientations. Treatment with either sulfapyridine or dapsone is usually effective in controlling LABD and long-term spontaneous remission rates of 30% to 60% have been described.

23. **c. Involvement of the vulva is common in women.** Hailey-Hailey disease (HH) is an autosomal dominant blistering dermatosis that has a predilection for the intertriginous areas including the groin and perianal region.

Symptoms include an unfortunate combination of pruritus, pain, and a foul odor. Because heat and sweating exacerbate the condition, HH tends to worsen during the summer months. In women, disease in the inframammary folds is common, although vulvar disease is unusual. For disease resistant to medical therapy, wide excision and skin grafting have been effective, as have local ablative techniques such as dermabrasion and laser vaporization.

24. **a. Behçet disease.** When oral and genital aphthous ulcers are coexistent, the clinician should consider the diagnosis of Behçet disease (BD). BD is a generalized relapsing and remitting ulcerative mucocutaneous disease that likely involves a genetic predisposition and an autoimmune mode of pathogenesis. Affected individuals may also suffer from epididymitis, thrombophlebitis, aneurysms, and gastrointestinal, neurologic, and arthritic problems.

25. **d. The presence of vacuolated keratinocytes in an inflammatory background is pathognomonic for this condition.** Pyoderma gangrenosum (PG) is an ulcerative skin disease associated with systemic illnesses, including inflammatory bowel disease, arthritis, collagen vascular disease, and myeloproliferative disorders. It most commonly affects women between the 2nd and 5th decade of life and likely has an autoimmune pathogenesis given its association with other autoimmune diseases. As was the case in Behçet disease, no specific diagnostic laboratory test or histopathologic feature is pathognomonic for PG, although a history of underlying systemic disease may raise suspicion.

26. **a. Factitial dermatitis.** Factitial dermatitis is a psychocutaneous disorder in which the individual self-inflicts cutaneous lesions, usually for an unconscious motive. An association between factitial dermatitis and borderline personality disorder appears to exist.

27. **c. *Streptococcus pyogenes*.** Erysipelas is a superficial bacterial skin infection limited to the dermis with lymphatic involvement. In contrast to the cutaneous lesion of cellulitis, erysipelas generally has a raised and distinct border at the interface with normal skin. The causative organism is usually *Streptococcus pyogenes*.

28. **b. Most of the cases of Fournier gangrene are caused by *Streptococcus pyogenes*.** Fournier gangrene (FG) is a potentially life-threatening progressive infection of the perineum and genitalia. In the genital region, most cases of FG are caused by mixed bacterial flora, which include gram-positive, gram-negative, and anaerobic bacteria.

29. **b. Pseudomonal folliculitis.** Folliculitis is a common disorder characterized by perifollicular pustules on an erythematous base. It occurs most frequently in heavily hair-bearing areas such as the scalp, beard, axilla, groin, and buttocks and can be exacerbated by local trauma from shaving, rubbing, or clothing irritation. Folliculitis has also been associated with the use of contaminated hot tubs and swimming pools, with the offending organism usually *Pseudomonas aeruginosa*.

30. **b. Trichomycosis axillaris.** Trichomycosis axillaris (TA) is a superficial bacterial infection of axillary and pubic hair caused by *Corynebacterium*, which is associated with hyperhidrosis. Shaving can provide immediate improvement, and antibacterial soaps may prevent further infection. For pubic TA, clindamycin gel, bacitracin, and oral erythromycin have also proven effective.

31. **c. Cutaneous candidiasis.** Tinea cruris is the term given to dermatophyte infection of the groin and genital area and is commonly known as "jock itch." The inner thighs and inguinal region are the most commonly affected areas, and the scrotum and penis are usually spared in men. Significant scrotal involvement should raise suspicion for cutaneous candidiasis as an alternative diagnosis.

32. **a. Lindane.** As in the case of pediculosis pubis, the treatment of choice for scabies is 5% permethrin cream applied to the entire body overnight, with a second application one week later. An alternative scabicide, lindane, is not favored due to both central nervous system (CNS) toxicity in children and a rising rate of resistance among mites.

33. **d. Bowen disease is associated with human papilloma virus type 6 and 11.** Bowen disease occurring on the mucosal surfaces of the male genitalia is referred to as erythroplasia of Queyrat. In that location, coinfection with human papilloma virus type 8, 16, 39, and 51 has been identified. In contrast, the variant of squamous cell carcinoma termed "verrucous carcinoma" has been associated with human papilloma virus type 6 and 11 infection but not with the more classically oncogenic type 16 and 18.

34. **b. Verrucous carcinoma should not be treated with primary radiotherapy due to the risk of anaplastic transformation.** Verrucous carcinoma (VC) is a slow-growing, locally aggressive, exophytic, low-grade variant of squamous cell carcinoma that has little metastatic potential. It most commonly occurs in uncircumcised men on the glans or prepuce, although similar lesions can be found on the vulva, vagina cervix, or anus. Treatment is preferably by local excision. Primary radiotherapy is relatively contraindicated due to the potential for anaplastic transformation with a subsequent increase in metastatic potential.

35. **c. Lower extremities.** Kaposi sarcoma (KS) in immunocompetent individuals presents as slowly growing, blue-red pigmented macules on the lower extremities. Although oral and gastrointestinal lesions may occur, the genitalia are seldom involved. This is in contrast to the case with AIDS, in which a solitary genital lesion may be the first manifestation of KS. The clinical features of KS in AIDS patients are diverse, ranging from a single lesion to disseminated cutaneous and visceral disease.

36. **d. verrucous carcinoma.** Pseudoepitheliomatous, keratotic, and micaceous balanitis (PEKMB) is a rare entity characterized by the development of a thick, hyperkeratotic plaque on the glans penis of older men. There remains controversy as to whether PEKMB is a premalignant condition. PEKMB was originally thought to be a purely benign process, although several case reports have documented the presence of concurrent verrucous carcinoma associated with this lesion.

37. **b. EPD is associated with another underlying malignancy in more than 60% of cases**. Extramammary Paget disease (EPD) is an uncommon intraepithelial adenocarcinoma of sites bearing apocrine glands. There is an important association between EPD and another underlying malignancy in 10% to 30% of cases. In the male, associations between urethral, bladder, rectal, and apocrine malignancies with EPD have been described.

38. **d. Sézary syndrome.** Cutaneous T-cell lymphoma (CTCL) represents a group of related neoplasms derived from T cells

that home to the skin. CTCL generally presents with pruritus, which must be differentiated from a variety of benign dermatoses, including psoriasis, eczema, superficial fungal infections, and drug reactions. Patients may subsequently develop hematologic involvement (termed "Sézary syndrome") and cutaneous plaques, erosions, ulcers, or frank skin tumors.

39. **b. Tuberous sclerosis.** Pearly penile papules (PPP) are white, dome-shaped, closely spaced, small papules located on the glans penis. Histologically, these lesions are angiofibromas similar to the lesions seen on the face in tuberous sclerosis.

40. **c. circumcision.** Zoon balanitis, also called plasma cell balanitis, occurs in uncircumcised men from the 3rd decade onward. Squamous cell carcinoma and extramammary Paget disease should be excluded, often by biopsy. Circumcision appears to be proof against development of the disease and can be performed to cure the majority of cases. For patients averse to circumcision, topical corticosteroids may provide symptomatic relief, and laser therapy may also have a role.

41. **d. Acrochordons.** Skin tags (acrochordons, fibroepithelial polyps) are soft, skin-colored, pedunculated lesions that can be present anywhere on the body. It is important to distinguish these lesions from the hamartomatous skin lesions (multiple fibrofolliculomas) associated with Birt-Hogg-Dube syndrome, which are histologically distinct from common skin tags.

42. **b. an abrupt increase in the size and number of seborrheic keratoses, suggesting internal malignancy.** The presence of brown macules unrelated to sun exposure suggests a diagnosis of seborrheic keratoses (SK). This condition may commonly involve the genitalia but generally spares the mucous membranes, palms, and soles of the feet. An abrupt increase in the size and number of multiple seborrheic keratoses (SK) has been termed Leser-Trélat syndrome and has been implicated as a cutaneous marker of internal malignancy. The HLA-B27 haplotype is associated with Reiter syndrome, not rapidly progressive lichen planus.

Additional Study Points

1. Topical application of steroids may result in systemic absorption resulting in significant side effects.
2. The majority of cases of erythema multiforme are precipitated by herpesvirus type I and II, with the herpetic lesions usually preceding the development of the target lesions by two weeks.
3. The major form of erythema multiforme is called Stevens-Johnson syndrome, which has a protracted course of 4 to 6 weeks and may have a mortality approaching 30%. Nonsteroidal anti-inflammatory agents, sulfonamides, tetracyclines, penicillin, doxycycline, and anticonvulsants are the most common offending agents.
4. Reiter syndrome comprises urethritis, arthritis, ocular findings (conjunctivitis), oral ulcers, and skin lesions. It is generally preceded by an episode of urethritis or a gastrointestinal infection. It is more common in HIV-positive patients.
5. The triad of clinical features in Behçet syndrome consists of mucocutaneous lesions of the oral cavity, genitalia, and uveitis. The ulcers are painful.
6. Hidradenitis suppurativa is an epithelial disorder of hair follicles that occurs in the apocrine gland–bearing skin, which results in a marked inflammatory response with formation of abscesses and sinus tracks.
7. Ecthyma gangrenosum is a result of pseudomonal septicemia and may result in gangrenous ulcers.
8. Dermatophytes are fungi of three genera: *Trichophyton*, *Microsporum*, and *Epidermophyton*. Tinea cruris, an infection of the groin and genital skin, may be caused by one of these fungi. Postinflammatory hyperpigmentation occurs with this disease and may not indicate an active infection.
9. Bowenoid papulosis consists of multiple small erythematous papules and is associated with human papillomavirus (HPV) type 16.
10. Angiokeratomas of Fordyce are vascular ectasias of dermal blood vessels. They are 1 to 2 mm, red or purple papules and may be the source of troublesome scrotal bleeding.

16

Tuberculosis and Other Opportunistic Infections of the Genitourinary System

Islam A. Ghoneim, MD, PhD • John C. Rabets, MD • Steven D. Mawhorter, MD, DTM&H

QUESTIONS

1. Which of the following statements about the epidemiology of tuberculosis is TRUE?
   a. Tuberculosis (TB) incidence has increased in the United States since the 1990s.
   b. Tuberculosis incidence among Asian immigrants is comparable to that for persons born in the United States.
   c. Tuberculosis incidence is decreasing worldwide.
   d. Tuberculosis occurs predominantly in patients with acquired immunodeficiency syndrome (AIDS) late in the course of their disease (CD4+ T-cell count of <200 cells/mm^3).
   e. Globally, tuberculosis is the most common opportunistic infection in AIDS patients.

2. The spread of *Mycobacterium tuberculosis* is least dependent on which of the following?
   a. Size of the bacillary inoculum inhaled
   b. Infectivity of the mycobacterial strain
   c. Duration of exposure to the source case
   d. Immune status of the source case
   e. Immune status of the exposed individual

3. Which of the following statements regarding tuberculosis is correct?
   a. Humans are not the only reservoir for *M. tuberculosis*.
   b. Renal tuberculosis is usually the result of activation of prior blood-borne metastatic renal infection.
   c. Epididymitis is a rare presenting symptom of genitourinary tuberculosis.
   d. Transmission of genitourinary tuberculosis from male to female is common.
   e. Renal tuberculosis is most common in children younger than 5 years of age.

4. Which one of the following conditions is most likely to reactivate a dormant *M. tuberculosis* infection?
   a. Human immunodeficiency virus (HIV) infection
   b. Pulmonary hypertension
   c. Emphysema
   d. Allergic asthma
   e. Osteoarthritis

5. The Centers for Disease Control and Prevention (CDC) has recommended defining a tuberculin reaction of 5 mm of induration as positive for which of the following?
   a. Infants
   b. Intravenous drug abusers
   c. Homeless individuals
   d. Diabetics
   e. HIV-positive individuals

6. The radiologic test that is most useful for evaluating the anatomic manifestations of genitourinary tuberculosis is:
   a. ultrasonography.
   b. intravenous pyelography.
   c. computed tomography.
   d. magnetic resonance imaging.
   e. retrograde pyelography.

7. All of the following features of genitourinary tuberculosis can be seen on an intravenous urogram EXCEPT:
   a. infundibular stenosis.
   b. renal calcifications.
   c. ureteral stricture.
   d. "thimble" bladder.
   e. vesicoureteral reflux.

8. Which of the following antituberculous drugs can cause visual changes?
   a. Isoniazid
   b. Streptomycin
   c. Rifampicin
   d. Pyrazinamide
   e. Ethambutol

9. Which form of tuberculosis is usually treated for more than 6 months?
   a. Pulmonary
   b. Genitourinary

c. Osteomyelitis

d. Nodal

e. Concomitant pulmonary and genitourinary

10. Hepatic toxicity from isoniazid (INH) is:

a. preventable with vitamin B6.

b. irreversible.

c. evident almost immediately after initiation of therapy.

d. manifested as hyperbilirubinemia.

e. often normalizes after several months of continued therapy.

11. Which of the following statements regarding surgery for genitourinary tuberculosis is correct?

a. Patients should have at least 4 to 6 weeks of extensive chemotherapy before surgery.

b. Lack of renal calcification is not a contraindication to partial nephrectomy.

c. Open surgical drainage of an abscess is usually required.

d. There is no indication for an epididymectomy in the modern era of chemotherapy.

e. Strictures at the ureteropelvic junction are common and frequently require endopyelotomy.

12. Which of the following statements regarding intravesical bacillus Calmette-Guérin (BCG) treatment is FALSE?

a. Quinolones should be avoided during BCG treatment.

b. BCG should be administered immediately after a transurethral resection.

c. Serious side effects are uncommon.

d. BCG sepsis treatment begins with isoniazid.

e. BCG is commonly used to reduce recurrence rates of superficial urothelial carcinoma.

13. Which of the following statements about *Schistosoma haematobium* and its life cycle is TRUE?

a. Worm pairs are principally located in the hepatic vasculature in humans.

b. It is common in South America.

c. Human infection is acquired by exposure to fresh water that harbors infected snails.

d. Worm pairs have life spans estimated between 3 and 6 months.

e. Sexual reproductive phase occurs in snails.

14. When one evaluates a patient for *S. haematobium* infection, which one of the following statements is TRUE?

a. An active infection can be diagnosed by the presence of laterally spined eggs in the urine.

b. An active infection has the full complement of egg stages present.

c. A history of living or traveling in Africa means that the patient has been to endemic areas.

d. The intensity of infection is inversely related to the egg burden found in tissues or body fluids.

e. Calculating the number of eggs per 10 mL of urine is not an indication of the intensity of the infection.

15. The human host response to *S. haematobium* is characterized by which one of the following?

a. T-cell–dependent host responses modulate granuloma formation.

b. Granulomatous host response to the schistosome eggs does not cause the pathologic tissue changes.

c. Eosinophil-mediated killing is effective against adult worms.

d. HIV-positive patients with lower CD4+ T-cell counts have higher egg burdens than patients with normal CD4+ T-cell counts.

e. A "sandy patch" is a granulomatous ulcer.

16. Which one of the following is the most common clinical presenting symptom presentation of acute *S. haematobium* infection?

a. Katayama fever

b. Swimmer's itch

c. Renal failure

d. Calcified bladder

e. Hematuria

17. Bilharzial bladder cancer occurring in patients with *S. haematobium* infection:

a. Is often manifested at 20 to 30 years of age.

b. Squamous cell carcinoma accounts for 30% to 40% of the cancers.

c. Nitrates, nitrite, N-nitroso compounds, and tryptophan metabolites have been identified in elevated amounts in the urine of patients with schistosomiasis-associated bilharzial bladder cancer.

d. More than 40% of the squamous cell carcinomas are well differentiated.

e. Patients can frequently be treated with partial cystectomy.

18. A 43-year-old woman from Madagascar has schistosomal obstructive uropathy (SOU). Which of the following statements is true?

a. The SOU usually obstructs the ureters symmetrically.

b. The obstruction would likely be at the ureteropelvic junction (UPJ).

c. If treated while the disease is active, hydronephrosis may resolve.

d. There is no change in ureteral function until radiologically demonstrable disease is noted.

19. A 24-year-old man who had recently come from Syria had been previously diagnosed with urinary schistosomiasis. He had not received any treatment. His medical records from Syria noted that he had an *S. haematobium* infection, and an intravenous pyelogram had demonstrated severe hydroureter on the left with a segmental distal ureteral lesion and delayed excretion. He has a normal creatinine level. Initial management should include:

a. cystoscopy with ureteral stent placement.

b. cystoscopy with ureteral stent placement and intravesical medical therapy.

c. medical management with oral praziquantel.

d. percutaneous nephrostomy tube placement followed by medical therapy.

e. distal ureterectomy and primary reimplantation into the bladder.

20. Filarial disease is characterized by all of the following EXCEPT:

    a. Elephantiasis of the limbs, chyluria, fever, localized lymphangitis, and hydrocele formation are seen.

    b. Biopsy and removal of involved lymph nodes are often necessary.

    c. Obstructive lymphatic disease occurs in patients who are repeatedly infected.

    d. The female mosquito (*Culex pipiens*) is the vector.

    e. After inoculation, larvae travel through the lungs through the blood before settling in their ultimate destination, large lymphatic vessels.

21. A 34-year-old shepherd from Spain has dull bilateral flank pain and intermittent microscopic hematuria. If a parasite is responsible for the patient's complaints, which of the following statements is correct?

    a. Hanging groin, or scrotal elephantiasis, may ultimately develop.

    b. Ivermectin is a first-line treatment option.

    c. Needle aspiration of any lesion is indicated before initiating therapy.

    d. Thick-walled fluid-filled cysts with calcified walls are diagnostic.

    e. Metronidazole is a first-line treatment option.

22. A 70-year-old retired career soldier develops pulmonary infiltrates and *Escherichia coli* bacteremia after receiving high-dose steroid therapy as part of lymphoma treatment. Motile structures are seen on urinalysis. The presence of which organism can explain his constellation of findings?

    a. *Trichomonas vaginalis*

    b. *Entamoeba histolytica*

    c. *Escherichia coli*

    d. *Cryptococcus neoformans*

    e. *Strongyloides stercoralis*

23. Which fungus is the most common cause of systemic fungal infection in severely immunocompromised patients?

    a. *Aspergillus*

    b. *Cryptococcus neoformans*

    c. *Blastomyces*

    d. *Histoplasma*

    e. *Mucor*

24. What is the most prevalent underlying disease associated with a single episode of candiduria?

    a. Malignancy

    b. Diabetes

    c. Collagen disease

    d. Neurogenic bladder

    e. Concomitant antibiotic administration

25. The recommended treatment for vulvovaginal candidiasis is:

    a. vinegar douches.

    b. intravaginal amphotericin lavage.

    c. one week of oral therapy with fluconazole.

    d. a single oral dose of fluconazole.

    e. saline vaginal irrigations.

26. Which of the following statements is FALSE regarding genitourinary candidiasis?

    a. The bladder may have a "snow effect" appearance on cystoscopy.

    b. The patient rarely develops urinary obstruction.

    c. The patient with candiduria is usually asymptomatic.

    d. Foley catheters in the postsurgical patient increase the risk for acquiring candiduria.

    e. The patient may need the placement of various drains to clear infections.

27. All of the following are major predisposing factors for renal candidal infection in pediatric patients EXCEPT:

    a. indwelling intravascular catheters.

    b. maternal diabetes mellitus.

    c. low birth weight.

    d. prematurity.

    e. broad-spectrum antibiotics.

28. When treating candiduria which of the following apply?

    a. Foley catheters or intravenous lines are not risk factors.

    b. Treat with topical agents.

    c. Not all patients with candiduria need treatment.

    d. Fungal balls resolve with medical therapy.

    e. Patients undergoing urologic procedures may be observed.

29. Aspergillosis outbreaks can be seen in:

    a. shepherds.

    b. aviaries.

    c. the central United States.

    d. dialysis centers.

    e. the western United States.

30. In AIDS patients, which genitourinary organ becomes the "reservoir" for *Cryptococcus* after treatment of cryptococcal meningitis?

    a. Kidney

    b. Bladder

    c. Epididymis

    d. Kidney

    e. Prostate

31. Radiographic findings may be similar to those of tuberculosis in which genitourinary fungal infection?

    a. Candidiasis

    b. Hydatid disease

    c. Schistosomiasis

    d. Coccidioidomycosis

    e. Phycomycosis

32. *Candida krusei* and *C. glabrata* are resistant to which drug?

    a. Amphotericin B

    b. Fluconazole

    c. Itraconazole

    d. Flucytosine

    e. Ketoconazole

ANSWERS

1. **e. Globally, tuberculosis is the most common opportunistic infection in AIDS patients.**
2. **d. Immune status of the source case.** The probability that a person will become infected depends on the duration of exposure to the source case, the size of the bacillary inoculum inhaled, and the infectivity of the mycobacterial strain. Virtually all AIDS patients with a positive purified protein derivative (PPD) test develop active TB during their lifetime unless antituberculous prophylaxis is offered.
3. **b. Renal tuberculosis is usually the result of activation of prior blood-borne metastatic renal infection.** Genitourinary TB is caused by metastatic spread of the organism through the bloodstream during the initial infection. The kidney is usually the primary organ infected in urinary disease, and other parts of the urinary tract become involved by direct extension.
4. **a. Human immunodeficiency virus (HIV) infection.** Most persons control the initial infection and develop no clinical illness. They have dormant bacilli, which may begin to produce disease years later after debilitating disease, trauma, corticosteroids, immunosuppressive therapy, diabetes, or AIDS.
5. **e. HIV-positive individuals.**
6. **c. computed tomography.** CT has become more widely available and has arguably replaced intravenous urography (IVU) as the imaging modality of choice for the diagnosis and evaluation of genitourinary TB. The latest CT software allows the creation of three-dimensional reconstructed images, adding another dimension to the images that a CT scan can produce. It is at least the equal of IVU in identifying caliceal abnormalities, hydronephrosis or hydroureter, autonephrectomy, amputated infundibulum, urinary tract calcifications, and renal parenchymal cavities.
7. **e. vesicoureteral reflux.** Renal lesions can be visualized on IVU. They may appear as a distortion of a calyx, as a calyx that is fibrosed and completely occluded (lost calyx from infundibular stenosis), as multiple small calyceal deformities, or as severe calyceal and parenchymal destruction. Other manifestations of genitourinary TB that can be visualized on IVU include ureteral dilatation above an ureterovesical junction (UVJ) stricture or a rigid fibrotic ureter with multiple strictures. The cystographic phase of the IVU can give valuable information about the condition of the bladder, which may be small and contracted (thimble bladder) or irregular, with filling defects and bladder asymmetry.
8. **e. Ethambutol.** Ethambutol rarely causes retrobulbar neuritis and should be discontinued if ocular changes occur. Changes in visual acuity and red-green color perception are early findings, and these parameters should be tested at baseline and every 4 to 6 weeks.
9. **c. Osteomyelitis.** Six-month regimens are effective for most forms of TB, including genitourinary TB, with the exception of disseminated TB, TB osteomyelitis, and TB meningitis.
10. **e. often normalizes after several months of continued therapy.** INH is associated with hepatic "toxicity" in 10% to 20% of patients, usually in the form of asymptomatic elevations in transaminase levels. This occurs after 6 to 8 weeks of therapy and may normalize with continued INH treatment. Close follow-up is appropriate to monitor for concerning progression of toxicity.
11. **a. Patients should have at least 4 to 6 weeks of extensive chemotherapy before surgery.**
12. **b. BCG should be administered immediately after a transurethral resection.** To avoid systemic absorption and therefore reduce the risk of major adverse reactions, one should wait 3 weeks after transurethral resection before starting BCG treatment.
13. **c. Human infection is acquired by exposure to fresh water that harbors infected snails.** On deposition into fresh water (not salt), the miracidia emerge as short-lived, ciliated larvae that swim and seek hosts.
14. **c. A history of living or traveling in Africa means that the patient has been to endemic areas.** Transmission of *S. haematobium* occurs in 53 countries in the Middle East and in most of the African continent. In Southwest Asia, it is found in Southern Yemen, Yemen, Saudi Arabia, Lebanon, Syria, Turkey, Iraq, and Iran (World Health Organization, 2009).*
15. **a. T-cell–dependent host responses modulate granuloma formation.** The host responds to egg antigens by forming granulomas around the egg, which is a T–cell-dependent host response. This immune response also facilitates egg transit across mucosa. Hence, larger egg counts are found in more immune-competent individuals.
16. **e. Hematuria.**
17. **d. More than 40% of the squamous cell carcinomas are well differentiated.**
18. **c. If treated while the disease is active, hydronephrosis may resolve.** If diagnosis is delayed and the schistosomiasis becomes chronic or inactive, then obstructive uropathy becomes the most common chronic condition requiring surgery.
19. **c. medical management with oral praziquantel.** In general, surgery is reserved for complications that have not responded to adequate medical treatment within a reasonable follow-up time (e.g., obstructive uropathy) or for those mandating immediate intervention, such as intractable bladder hemorrhage.
20. **b. Biopsy and removal of involved lymph nodes is often necessary.** This may result in additional complications if attempted.
21. **d. Thick-walled fluid-filled cysts with calcified walls are diagnostic.** Diagnosis can be made by plain film radiography, ultrasonography, or CT, which shows a thick-walled, fluid-filled spherical cyst, often with a calcific cyst wall. Praziquantel or albendazole given for 7 to 10 days before a procedure may minimize or prevent secondary seeding by daughter cysts, if the primary cyst accidentally ruptures after needle aspiration or surgical intervention.
22. **e. *Strongyloides stercoralis*.** This parasite can be asymptomatically maintained by autoreinfection for decades after acquisition worldwide. The career soldier may have been infected in WWII or Viet Nam. Immunosuppression, (especially with corticosteroids) can lead to *Strongyloides* hyperinfection, that is, dissemination of larvae to extra-intestinal organs with mortality rates as high as 85%. The migrating worms carry gram-negative bacteria on their coat,

---

*Sources referenced can be found in *Campbell-Walsh Urology*, 10th Edition, on the Expert Consult website.

which may result in bacteremia or infection of the genitourinary system.

23. **a. *Aspergillus*.** Disseminated *Aspergillus* is a major opportunistic fungus in patients compromised by malignancy, diabetes mellitus, AIDS, immunosuppressive agents, and organ transplantation.

24. **b. Diabetes.** In a documented single episode of candiduria, the major associated illnesses included diabetes mellitus (39%), urinary tract disease (37.7%), malignancy (22.2%), and malnutrition (17%).

25. **d. a single oral dose of fluconazole.** Treatment with oral fluconazole (a single 150-mg dose) is as effective as topical intravaginal therapy in the treatment of vulvovaginal candidiasis.

26. **b. The patient rarely develops urinary obstruction.**

27. **b. maternal diabetes mellitus.**

28. **c. Not all patients with candiduria need treatment.** It should be emphasized that *Candida* species in the urine may represent contamination of the specimen during collection or colonization, without true infection. However, the persistence of candiduria requires evaluation and consideration of treatment.

29. **d. dialysis centers.** Outbreaks of disease have been attributed to contaminated air conditioning systems, surgical theaters, dialysis fluid, and construction dust.

30. **e. Prostate.**

31. **d. Coccidioidomycosis.**

32. **b. Fluconazole.**

Additional Study Points

1. Hematogenous spread of tuberculosis occurs to the kidney, epididymis, and fallopian tubes.
2. The likelihood of reactivation of dormant TB increases with diabetes and immunosuppression, such as with HIV infection and malignancies.
3. Healing tubercles result in extensive fibrosis, which may cause infundibular stenosis and ureteral pelvic junction stricture.
4. Tuberculosis usually affects the lower ureter. Tuberculosis of the bladder is secondary to infection from the kidney.
5. Lower urinary tract symptoms are the commonest presentation of genitourinary tuberculosis; up to 25% of patients will present with sterile pyuria.
6. When culturing for tuberculosis, the first morning void specimen is most appropriate.
7. Pipe-stem ureter and bladder contracture may be sequelae of tuberculosis.
8. Surgical treatment is reserved for a nonfunctional kidney and to correct obstructive effects of fibrosis rather than to remove infected tissues.
9. First-line drugs for treating tuberculosis are rifampicin, INH, pyrazinamide, and ethambutol.
10. Pyridoxine must be given with INH to prevent a peripheral neuropathy.
11. Patients must have a minimum of 3 to 6 weeks of medical treatment before surgical therapy is undertaken in those with active infection.
12. Strictures of the ureter usually occur in the distal third.
13. *Schistosoma haematobium* has a terminal spine and dwells principally in the perivesical venous plexuses.
14. Schistosomiasis may cause inflammatory polyps of the bladder, sandy spots in the bladder (which represent submucosal egg deposition), calcification of the entire outline of the bladder, and strictures of the ureter with hydronephrosis. It may be associated with bladder cancer.
15. Squamous cell carcinoma of the bladder is the most common histologic variant occurring as a result of schistosomiasis. These cancers are usually well differentiated or verrucous and therefore carry an overall good prognosis.
16. *Wuchereria bancrofti* accounts for 90% of human lymphatic filariasis.
17. Obstructive lymphatic disease typically occurs in people who have multiple reinfections.
18. *Wuchereria bancrofti* results in chyluria and filarial hydrocele, and occasional extensive scrotal and penile lymphedema.
19. *Trichomonas vaginalis* is a flagellate protozoan organism and causes vaginitis in women and urethritis, epididymitis, prostatitis, and occasional infertility in men.

Molecular and Cellular Biology

Basic Principles of Immunology in Urology

Stuart M. Flechner, MD, FACS ● James H. Finke, PhD ● Robert L. Fairchild, PhD

QUESTIONS

1. Antigen presentation involves both uptake of foreign proteins and processing to form peptide/MHC complexes. Each of the following immune responsive cell types can carry out this function EXCEPT:
   a. granulocytes.
   b. vascular endothelial cells.
   c. monocytes.
   d. macrophages.
   e. dendritic cells.

2. Transplants between two siblings who are histocompatibility leukocyte antigen (HLA) identical (perfect class I and II match) can be rejected. This is primarily a consequence of:
   a. direct antigen presentation.
   b. differences in complement proteins.
   c. indirect antigen presentation.
   d. differences in childhood antimicrobial vaccination.
   e. differences in numbers of circulating platelets.

3. Lymphocyte activation depends on complex interactions between many intracellular enzymes, transcription factors, and electrolytes. The influx of which electrolyte is most important for T-cell activation?
   a. Sodium
   b. Magnesium
   c. Potassium
   d. Phosphorus
   e. Calcium

4. Anergy describes a state of immune nonresponsiveness to antigenic stimulation. The most effective way to induce a state of anergy is by:
   a. splenic irradiation.
   b. delivery of signal 1 and signal 2.
   c. depletion of complement proteins.
   d. delivery of signal 1 without signal 2.
   e. depletion of helper CD4+ T cells.

5. Each of the following characteristics describes the utility and adaptability of the immune system EXCEPT:
   a. memory.
   b. rapid amplification.
   c. identification of self.
   d. antigen restriction.
   e. nonspecific defense mechanisms.

6. Innate immune responses are nonspecific and include all of the following EXCEPT:
   a. natural killer cells.
   b. antibody-dependent cell-mediated cellular cytotoxicity.
   c. complement.
   d. acute-phase proteins.
   e. physical and mucosal barriers.

7. Which cell surface glycoprotein is commonly referred to as the "pan–T-cell marker" due to its presence on all T lymphocytes?
   a. CD3
   b. CD4
   c. CD8
   d. CD28
   e. CD45

8. The part of an IgG antibody molecule that interacts with cell surface receptors on other immune reactive cells such as natural killer (NK) cells is the:
   a. hypervariable region.
   b. disulfide bonds.
   c. amino-terminal end of the antibody.
   d. Fc fragment.
   e. Fab fragment.

9. The family of transcription factors termed nuclear factor of activated T cells (NFAT) are essential for T-cell activation and clonal expansion through the expression of the gene for:
   a. interferon-γ (IF-γ).
   b. transferrin.
   c. tumor necrosis factor.
   d. interleukin-2 (IL-2).
   e. IL-10.

10. The receptor on B cells that recognizes antigen and transmits signals to the nucleus for gene expression is:
    a. the T-cell receptor.
    b. the surface IgD molecule.
    c. the surface IgM molecule.
    d. CD40.
    e. CD28.

11. The JAK/STAT signaling pathways are critical in regulating cytokine expression. Inborn deficiencies in these pathways may lead to diseases such as:
    a. Burkitt lymphoma.
    b. Wilms tumor.
    c. neuroblastoma.
    d. retinoblastoma.
    e. severe combined immunodeficiency.

12. The initial contact of host immunoresponsive cells with foreign antigen or transplanted donor tissue takes place in the:
    a. peripheral lymph nodes.
    b. thymus gland.
    c. spleen.
    d. bursa of Fabricius.
    e. bone marrow.

13. Programmed cell death, apoptosis, is a mechanism responsible for the elimination of aged, damaged, autoimmune, or redundant cells. Caspase proteins are responsible for executing the suicide program by:
    a. release of granzyme B.
    b. activating the alternative complement pathway.
    c. activating natural killer cells.
    d. mediating DNA fragmentation and condensation.
    e. release of perforin.

14. Tolerance describes the absence of lymphocyte reactivity to specific antigens that have been previously encountered by the immune system. Known mechanisms of tolerance include each of the following EXCEPT:
    a. deletion of reactive T cells.
    b. deletion of reactive B cells.
    c. blocking by antigen-antibody complexes.
    d. clonal anergy by delivery of signal 1 without costimulation.
    e. suppression of immune responses by regulatory cells.

15. Chemokines are chemoattractant cytokines that localize various cell populations to tissue sites of inflammation. Each of the following cell types respond to chemokines EXCEPT:
    a. erythrocytes.
    b. granulocytes.
    c. natural killer cells.
    d. dendritic cells.
    e. monocytes.

16. Although most human tumors are antigenic, the immune system is often not a significant barrier to tumor growth and metastasis. A major reason for the relative weakness of the immune system to eradicate tumors is:
    a. absence of costimulation by tumors leading to anergy.
    b. tumor-induced alterations of immune function.
    c. impaired function of tumor neovasculature.
    d. rapid tumor cell proliferation.
    e. lack of tumor cell Fc receptors.

17. Tumor cell destruction by the immune system often is weak due to tumor cell escape mechanisms, which include all of the following EXCEPT:
    a. tumor cell release of IL-2.
    b. reduced expression of major histocompatibility complex (MHC) class I and II molecules on tumor cells.
    c. tumor cell and local release of IL-10.
    d. ligation of tumor cell FAS by the FAS ligand (FASL) to induce apoptosis of host T cells.
    e. tumor cell and local release of transforming growth factor-β (TGF-β).

18. Immunotherapy for metastatic renal cell carcinoma in humans has included the use of cytokines such as IFN-γ and IL-2. The objective response rate (both complete and partial responses) has been demonstrated in what percentage of patients?
    a. 95%
    b. 75%
    c. 55%
    d. 35%
    e. 15%

19. Extracellular bacteria are susceptible to killing by phagocytosis and complement, but some have developed capsules to block these mechanisms. The most effective immune counter-measure for bacterial encapsulation is the:
    a. classical complement pathway.
    b. alternative complement pathway.
    c. opsonization of bacteria by circulating antibodies.
    d. increased secretion of TGF-β in tears.
    e. increased beating of bronchial cilia.

20. Clearance of intracellular bacteria is most dependent on which immune cell population?
    a. Macrophages
    b. Plasma cells
    c. Natural killer cells
    d. Dendritic cells
    e. Primed T lymphocytes

21. Passive immune therapy may be particularly useful for patients with immunodeficiency. Passive therapy is delivered by:
    a. attenuated viral organisms.
    b. lyophilized vaccines.
    c. heterologous serum.
    d. live viral organisms.
    e. cow's milk.

22. Toll-like receptors can be engaged by all of the following EXCEPT:
    a. bacterial flagellin.
    b. bacterial lipopolysaccharides.
    c. calcium.
    d. double-stranded viral RNA.
    e. paclitaxel.

23. Recognition of Toll-like receptors by microbial products can activate all of the following immune mechanisms EXCEPT:

    a. adaptive immunity.

    b. intracellular microbial killing.

    c. innate immunity.

    d. IgE antibody formation.

    e. expression of costimulatory molecules.

24. DNA microarrays depend on the ability of target nucleic acid sequences to:

    a. bind to the surface of activated lymphocytes.

    b. hybridize to complementary oligonucleotides or polymerase chain reaction (PCR) products.

    c. engage the T-cell receptor (TCR).

    d. bind to antibody fixed to a glass slide.

    e. fix complement.

25. Gene expression profiling using DNA microarrays can be used to distinguish the following characteristics of urologic cancers EXCEPT:

    a. pathologic stage of the malignancy.

    b. diagnosis and classification of the malignancy.

    c. monitoring the host response to the malignancy.

    d. discovery of targets for treatment of the malignancy.

    e. definition of the clinical prognosis of the malignancy.

26. Which of the following events do not play a role in the initiation of TCR signaling after engagement with antigen and MHC class II molecules?

    a. TCR interaction with CD4 coreceptor

    b. TCR interaction with CD8 coreceptor

    c. Phosphorylation of TCR and CD3 immunoreceptor tyrosine-based activation motifs (ITAMs) by LCK and FYN kinases

    d. Recruitment of ZAP-70 to TCR and its activation

    e. Activation of the adaptor molecule, linker of activation in T cells (LAT)

27. Which of the following is a FALSE statement regarding the JANUS family of kinases?

    a. The 4 JAK kinases are not constitutively associated with various cytokine receptors.

    b. The JAK kinases regulate different cytokine receptors.

    c. The cytokine-receptor binding causes dimerization of receptor chains resulting in JAK activation and phosphorylation of receptors.

    d. The STATs are recruited to receptors and phosphorylated by JAK kinases.

    e. Mutation in JAK3 results in severe combined immunodeficiency.

28. Which of the following statements is TRUE regarding programmed cell death (apoptosis)?

    a. It is a mechanism for the elimination of aged, damaged, and autoimmune cells or cells no longer needed for differentiation.

    b. It is a mechanism for inducing a primary immune response.

    c. The proteins responsible for executing apoptosis, caspases, are JAK kinases.

    d. Caspase-8 is the initiator caspase for apoptosis initiated by FAS and the T-cell receptor.

    e. BCL-2 and BCL-XL are antiapoptotic proteins that protect the nucleus from damage.

29. The development of an effective immune response to cancer cells is dependent on appropriate antigen presentation by dendritic cells and the subsequent activation of CD4+ and CD8+ T cells. Which of the statements listed below are TRUE?

    a. Many human tumors express antigenic epitopes that can be recognized by either CD4+ T cells or by CD8+ T cells.

    b. T cells can destroy tumor cells by several mechanisms, which include the elaboration of granules containing pore forming proteins, the upregulation of FASL that can bind FAS receptors, and the activation of macrophages.

    c. IFN-γ production by lymphocytes is necessary but not sufficient for promoting antitumor immune response.

    d. Tumors may evade T-cell detection because of a loss of MHC class I/II molecules or because of a decrease in expression of transporter proteins associated with antigen processing.

    e. T-reg cells, TGF-β, IL-10, gangliosides, and prostaglandin represent potential immune suppressive mechanisms within the tumor microenvironment.

ANSWERS

1. **a. granulocytes.** Macrophages, monocytes, some B cells, Langerhans cells of the skin, dendritic reticulum cells, and vascular endothelial cells can process and present antigen.

2. **c. indirect antigen presentation.** The evidence for an indirect recognition pathway for alloantigens comes from observations that rejection can take place even if donor and recipient share most, if not all, MHC antigens.

3. **e. Calcium.** This event also leads to the opening of the calcium channels in the plasma membrane, which further increases Ca^{2+} levels. Elevated intracellular Ca^{2+} results in the activation of the enzyme calcineurin, which is a cytosolic serine/threonine protein phosphatase that regulates the activation of a family of transcription factors termed nuclear factor of activated T cells (NFAT).

4. **d. delivery of signal 1 without signal 2.** In fact, stimulation by signal 1 alone leads to a state of anergy, whereby the T cell becomes unresponsive to further stimulation by antigen.

5. **d. antigen restriction.** Unique characteristics that help explain the utility and adaptability of the immune system against many different foreign invaders include (1) the ability to identify self from nonself, (2) specificity, (3) memory, and (4) rapid amplification.

6. **b. antibody-dependent cell-mediated cellular cytotoxicity.** Innate defense mechanisms represent nonspecific barriers to invaders, which rely primarily on physical barriers, phagocytic cells, natural killer cells, complement, acute phase proteins, lysozyme, and the interferons.

7. **a. CD3.** Each T-cell precursor retains the pan–T-cell CD3 marker, which is the signal-transducing complex closely linked to the T-cell receptor.

8. **d. Fc fragment.** The Fc fragment does not bind antibody but is responsible for fixation to complement and attachment of the molecule to the cell surface.

9. **d. interleukin-2.** NFAT along with other transcription factors plays a critical role in T-cell activation and clonal expansion through activation of the IL-2 gene.

10. **b. the surface IgD molecule.** The receptor on B cells that recognizes antigen and transmits signals to the nucleus for gene expression is composed of a cell surface immunoglobulin containing heavy and light chains with variable regions.

11. **e. severe combined immunodeficiency.** The biologic importance of different JAKs and STATs has been revealed by deficiencies of these proteins both in human and animal models. Mutations in JAK3 have resulted in patients having severe combined immunodeficiency (SCID) that is similar to X-linked SCID, which occurs because of a mutation in the common cytokine receptor γ chain.

12. **a. peripheral lymph nodes.** Activation of specific T cells and the generation of an immune response require transport of antigenic components to the lymphoid tissue. For the induction of most T-cell–mediated immune responses, the crucial antigen-presenting cell is the dendritic cell, which is interspersed throughout peripheral tissues.

13. **d. mediating DNA fragmentation and condensation.** The proteins responsible for executing the suicide program, the caspases, are essentially common to all the stimuli and pathways and mediate the nuclear and cytoplasmic alterations characteristic of apoptotic cell death. The specific roles of each member of the caspase cascade are gradually becoming defined, whereby caspases 3, 6, and 7 have been identified as the terminal effectors mediating DNA fragmentation and chromatin condensation.

14. **c. blocking by antigen-antibody complexes.** An important mechanism mediating tolerance to self-proteins is the deletion of self-reactive T cells and B cells during maturation. Clonal anergy of T cells is induced by T-cell receptor engagement of peptide/MHC complexes in the absence of costimulatory signals. An active mechanism of tolerance mediated by T cells with suppressive or downregulatory activities may also be induced to inhibit immune responses to self and exogenous antigens.

15. **a. erythrocytes.** Cytokines with chemoattractant properties, chemokines, are also crucial in mediating localization and trafficking of leukocytes to tissue sites during physiologic processes, including inflammation and homeostasis.

16. **b. tumor-induced alterations of immune function.** Tumor-induced alterations in the functional status of immune cells may be responsible for the poor development of antitumor immunity in many cancer patients.

17. **a. tumor cell release of IL-2.** Natural killer cells can recognize and destroy some tumors, particularly those of lymphoid origin, without any exogenous activation. Reduction in or loss of MHC class I and class II expression by tumors, including renal cell carcinoma, has been well documented. In some tumors, there is also decreased expression of transporter proteins associated with antigen processing (TAP proteins). Among the best studied immunosuppressive molecules overexpressed in the tumor microenvironment is the Th2 cytokine IL-10. TGF-β is also thought to contribute to the suppression of tumor immunity. Evidence suggests that the downregulation of antitumor immunity may be due in part to the induction of the FAS apoptotic pathway in T cells.

18. **e. 15%.** It is clear from these and other studies that a subset of individuals with metastatic renal cancer does respond favorably to cytokine therapy; however, they represent a minority of patients (<15% response rate).

19. **c. opsonization of bacteria by circulating antibodies.** Many of these bacterial mechanisms can be overridden by host antibodies, which are soluble or secreted on external mucosal surfaces. Circulating antibodies can directly bind to bacterial exotoxins and "neutralize" them. They can also bind to the encapsulated bacteria, which will permit ingestion by polymorphs and macrophages.

20. **e. Primed T lymphocytes.** Clearance of these intracellular microbes depends directly on T cells, which in turn must activate the infected macrophages. Specifically primed T cells react with processed antigen derived from the intracellular bacteria in association with MHC class II molecules on the macrophage surface.

21. **c. heterologous serum.** Protection against a specific infection can be passively transferred from one individual to another by serum containing preformed antibodies. This type of passive immunity is generally short-lived, because the half-life of immunoglobulins is 1 to 2 weeks. Patients with immunodeficiency diseases may actually be sustained by regular treatments with pooled nonspecific human immune globulin treatments.

22. **c. calcium.** Toll-like receptors are cell surface glycoproteins that need physical contact with other macromolecules such as bacterial flagellins, lipopolysaccharides, phytins, or nucleic acids. Minerals such as calcium are too small.

23. **d. IgE antibody formation.** Engagement of Toll-like receptors activates various cellular immune responses. IgE antibody on the surface of mast cells promotes degranulation and allergy. IgE antibody is constitutively expressed on basophils/mast cells.

24. **b. hybridize to complementary oligonucleotides or PCR products.** DNA microarrays or gene chips are tests performed in a laboratory. They depend on the natural ability of two complementary strands of nucleic acids to hybridize to each other. The others are in-vivo biologic processes.

25. **a. pathologic stage of the malignancy.** DNA microarrays can identify a unique molecular signature of a cancer, which represents the sum of genes upregulated or downregulated by the tumor. This can help classify the specific cancer, aid in identifying potential molecular targets for therapy, or possibly predict outcome of therapy. The pathologic stage of the cancer is a description of its extent in the host. It is usually defined clinically, often aided by radiologic and histologic evaluation.

26. **b. TCR interaction with CD8 coreceptor.** The interaction of the TCR and class II HLA antigens requires the stabilization of CD4 on T cells. Class I antigen would be required to engage the CD8 molecules. The initiation of further downstream intracellular events is dependent on the cell surface engagement of class II antigen and CD4.

27. **a. The 4 JAK kinases are not constitutively associated with various cytokine receptors.** The JANUS family of kinases are constitutively expressed and are associated with various cell surface cytokine receptors. Once these receptors are engaged the JAK kinases become activated and promote cytokine gene expression.

28. **a. It is a mechanism for the elimination of aged, damaged, and autoimmune cells or cells no longer**

needed for differentiation. The proteins responsible for executing the suicide program are the caspases, and they can be triggered by a number of mechanisms such as FAS and TNFR but not the T-cell receptor or JAK kinases.

29. **All of the statements are true.**
   a. Many human tumors express antigenic epitopes that can be recognized by either CD4+ T cells or by CD8+ T cells.
   b. T cells can destroy tumor cells by several mechanisms, which include the elaboration of granules containing pore-forming proteins, the upregulation of FASL that can bind FAS receptors, and the activation of macrophages.
   c. IFN-γ production by lymphocytes is necessary but not sufficient for promoting antitumor immune response.
   d. Tumors may evade T-cell detection because of a loss of MHC class I/II molecules or because of a decrease in expression of transporter proteins associated with antigen processing.
   e. T-reg cells, TGF-β, IL-10, gangliosides, and prostaglandin represent potential immune suppressive mechanisms within the tumor microenvironment.

Additional Study Points

1. The immune response is divided into innate immunity and adaptive immunity.
2. Innate immunity is nonspecific and involves polymorphonuclear leukocytes, macrophages, natural killer cells, compliment, acute-phase proteins, interferons, and lysosomes, among others.
3. Adaptive immunity is specific and involves lymphocytes, antibodies, and cytokines.
4. Natural killer cells do not require prior contact with the antigen and are not MHC restricted.
5. Immune responses may be either humoral or cellular. The humoral response involves antibodies, whereas the cellular response involves macrophages, T cells, dendritic cells, etc.
6. The thymus is responsible for the selection and education of T cells; the bone marrow is responsible for the education of B cells, which produce antibody.
7. Dendritic cells process antigen and present it to the T cells. T cells present antigen to B cells. B cells make antibody.
8. The MHC markers (HLA) are divided into class I and class II.
9. All nucleated cells express HLA class I antigens, whereas class II antigens are primarily found on B cells, monocytes, macrophages, and antigen presenting cells.
10. The major histocompatibility complex (MHC) is located on chromosome 6. Current tissue typing checks for three class I antigens—HLA-A, HLA-B, and HLA-C, and two class II antigens—HLA-DR and HLA-DQ. A six-antigen match refers to HLA-A, HLA-B, and HLA-DR.
11. The T-cell receptor, or TCR, is responsible for the initial step in T-cell activation upon encounter with an antigen. During antigen priming CD4+ T cells produce cytokines.
12. Chemokine production is primarily regulated by the cytokine environment. Chemokines attract leukocytes to the area in which they are located.
13. T lymphocytes are central to the generation of an effective tumor immune response.
14. Activation of CD8+ T cells that recognize tumor-associated antigens presented by MHC class I molecules and CD4+ T cells that respond to tumor-associated antigens presented by MHC class II molecules represents the most effective tumor immune response.
15. There are five classes of antibodies: IgA, IgG, IgM, IgD, and IgE. They are produced by plasma cells (B cells).

Molecular Genetics and Cancer Biology

Mark L. Gonzalgo, MD, PhD ● Alan Keith Meeker, PhD, MA

QUESTIONS

1. DNA is composed of all of the following elements EXCEPT:
   a. a base, either a purine or a pyrimidine.
   b. a sugar, called ribose.
   c. a phosphate.
   d. two complementary strands.
   e. hydrogen bonds.

2. The physical chemistry of DNA bases requires:
   a. uracil to form hydrogen bonds with guanine.
   b. purine to form hydrogen bonds with another purine.
   c. pyrimidine to form hydrogen bonds with a purine.
   d. adenine to form hydrogen bonds with cytosine.
   e. thymine to form hydrogen bonds with guanine.

3. Which of the following does DNA gene expression require?
   a. Linear DNA to be converted into linear RNA, a process called translation
   b. Conversion of linear RNA into a linear set of amino acids, a process called transcription
   c. Protein synthesis exclusively within the nucleus
   d. Mitosis
   e. A mechanism to bridge the gap between the genetic code and protein synthesis

4. Which of the following statements about transcriptional regulation is NOT true?
   a. Two general components involved in transcriptional regulation are specific sequences in the RNA and proteins that interact with those sequences.
   b. In addition to the genetic information carried within the nucleotide sequence of DNA, it provides specific docking sites for proteins that enhance the activity of the transcriptional machinery.
   c. Specific sequences within the promoter or enhancer region of a gene are called response elements.
   d. DNA sequences, often referred to as consensus sequences, are found in many genes and respond in a coordinated manner to a specific signal.
   e. It is an important mechanism to ensure coordinated gene expression.

5. What is alternative splicing?
   a. A form of protein modification occurring after a mature polypeptide is produced
   b. A modification to DNA during meiosis
   c. A process of including or excluding certain exons in an mRNA transcript
   d. A process in which novel RNA sequences are randomly inserted into a transcript
   e. A method of RNA degradation

6. Which of the following statements is TRUE regarding the nuclear matrix?
   a. It has the same protein composition in every tissue type.
   b. It is the site of mRNA transcription.
   c. It has the same protein composition whether a cell is proliferating or undergoing differentiation.
   d. It provides a mechanism to trace the cell type of origin for a cancer, because the nuclear matrix is identical within tissue types.
   e. It is a form of DNA.

7. What happens in the process of translation?
   a. The RNA message of four parts (the nucleotides A, U, C, and G) is converted into 20 amino acids by using a functional group of three adjacent nucleotides called a codon.
   b. Each amino acid is encoded by only one codon.
   c. Shifts in the reading frame are of no consequence in the production of the polypeptide chain, because of the fidelity of template DNA.
   d. Single-base substitutions always encode for the identical amino acid, known as a polymorphism.
   e. Transfer of genetic information from the DNA to the RNA occurs.

8. Which of the following statements about ubiquitination is NOT true?
   a. Ubiquitination is an important regulatory mechanism of a cell, used in the efficient disposal of proteins.
   b. A small protein called ubiquitin is linked to a protein, tagging it for destruction.
   c. The proteosome is the site of protein-ubiquitin complex degradation.

d. The proteosome has a cylindrical shape.

e. The targeted inhibition of proteosome function appears to enhance cancer progression.

9. Which of the following statements about oncogenes is TRUE?

a. They are mutated forms of abnormal genes, known as proto-oncogenes.

b. They can be produced by an inactivating mutation of a proto-oncogene, resulting in the silencing of the gene.

c. They can be produced by gene amplification, resulting in many copies of the gene, or by chromosomal rearrangement.

d. They are always due to retroviruses, capable of inducing malignant transformation of normal cells.

e. They are endogenous cancer-fighting genes.

10. Which of the following statements about hypermethylation is TRUE?

a. It is a direct change to the DNA sequence, similar to a mutation that alters the normal base-pairing.

b. It occurs exclusively on cytosine nucleotides in the dinucleotide sequence CG.

c. Somatic methylation of CpG dinucleotides in the regulatory regions of genes is very often associated with increased transcriptional activity, leading to increased expression of that gene.

d. In cancer, hypermethylation is associated with enhanced activity of oncogenes, and demethylation may be an effective strategy for the treatment of cancer.

e. It marks cells for ubiquitination.

11. Von Hippel–Lindau (VHL) disease predisposes patients to:

a. epididymal carcinoma.

b. clear cell renal carcinoma.

c. papillary renal cell carcinoma.

d. adrenocortical carcinoma.

e. all of the above.

12. Hereditary prostate carcinoma is estimated to account for what percentage of total patients diagnosed with prostate cancer before 55 years of age?

a. 0% to 10%

b. 11% to 20%

c. 21% to 30%

d. 31% to 40%

e. 41% to 50%

13. Hereditary prostate cancer genes that have been proven to cause prostate carcinoma include:

a. ELAC2.

b. MSR1.

c. RNASEL.

d. none of the above.

e. all of the above.

14. Which of the following hereditary tumor syndromes are associated with genitourinary tumors?

a. Von Hippel–Lindau syndrome

b. Birt-Hogg-Dube syndrome

c. Beckwith-Wiedemann syndrome

d. None of the above

e. All of the above

15. Which of the following cancer-associated chromosomal abnormalities would be most likely to be associated with inactivation of a tumor suppressor gene?

a. Inversion

b. Tetraploidy

c. Amplification

d. Deletion

e. Double minutes

16. Polymorphisms:

a. are sporadic mutations.

b. usually have functional significance.

c. can alter expression of genes.

d. occur rarely in normal population.

e. all of the above.

17. The two main points of control in the cell cycle are:

a. S and G_0.

b. S and the G_2M boundary.

c. M and the G_1S boundary.

d. G_1S and G_2M boundaries.

e. G_2 and M.

18. The *TP53* tumor suppressor gene plays a critical role in which of the following processes?

a. Apoptosis

b. Angiogenesis

c. DNA replication

d. Signal transduction

e. All of the above

19. Which of the following is an alternative splice variant of $TP16^{INK4a}$?

a. $TP27^{kip1}$

b. $TP57^{kip2}$

c. $TP15^{INK4b}$

d. $TP14^{ARF}$

e. $TP21^{cip1}$

20. INK4 family members inhibit the activity of:

a. cyclin D/CDK4.

b. cyclin E/CDK2.

c. cyclin A/CDK2.

d. cyclin B/CDC2.

e. all of the above.

21. Cyclin-CDK complexes primarily function at the G_1S boundary by:

a. dephosphorylation of RB.

b. phosphorylation of MDM2.

c. dephosphorylation of E2F.

d. phosphorylation of E2F.

e. phosphorylation of RB.

22. The regulatory proteins at the G_2M checkpoint primarily respond to:

a. hypoxia.

b. nutrient-poor environment.

c. DNA damage.

d. cytokines.

e. all of the above.

23. Nucleotide excision repair primarily protects the cell from DNA damage caused by:

a. reactive oxygen species.

b. DNA polymerase errors.

c. double-stranded breaks.

d. ultraviolet light.

e. all of the above.

24. Which of the following repair pathways is responsible for repairing double-stranded DNA breaks?

a. MSH2/MSH6

b. Homologous recombination

c. Nucleotide excision repair

d. Mismatch repair

e. None of the above

25. Which of the following genes has been linked to double-stranded break repair?

a. *TP53*

b. *VHL*

c. *BRCA1*

d. *RB*

e. *PTEN*

26. Procaspases are activated by which of the following?

a. Phosphorylation

b. Ubiquitination

c. Dimerization

d. Mitochondrial import

e. Proteolytic cleavage

27. Ligand-dependent apoptosis is an attractive therapeutic target because activation is:

a. independent of *TP53*.

b. dependent on *TP53*.

c. independent of caspases.

d. dependent on caspases.

e. dependent on RB.

28. The *TP53*-induced apoptosis is mediated through:

a. APAF-1/caspase 9.

b. CD95 receptor.

c. TRAIL.

d. BCL-2.

e. TP21^{cip}.

29. Pro-apoptotic BCL-2 family members function by:

a. digesting the mitochondria.

b. increasing the cellular membrane permeability.

c. increasing the mitochondrial membrane permeability.

d. directly activating executioner caspases.

e. increasing nuclear membrane permeability.

30. The enzyme telomerase immortalizes cells by:

a. protecting the cells from DNA damage.

b. stabilizing *TP53*.

c. allowing the cell to grow in a nutrient-poor environment.

d. inhibiting apoptosis.

e. maintaining chromosomal length.

31. Telomere loss can lead to all of the following EXCEPT:

a. irreversible cell cycle exit, termed senescence.

b. apoptosis.

c. DNA hypomethylation.

d. chromosomal instability.

e. increased tumor initiation.

32. Which of the following chromosomal rearrangements is NOT typically associated with a genitourinary malignancy?

a. Fusion of BCR to ABL by chromosome translocation

b. Fusion of TMPRSS2 to ERG by intrachromosomal deletion

c. Fusion of MITF/TFE gene family members by chromosome translocation

d. Isochromosome 8q

e. Loss of chromosome 9

33. An isochromosome of 12p has been identified in which genitourinary carcinoma?

a. Testis

b. Prostate

c. Renal

d. Bladder

e. Penile

ANSWERS

1. **b. a sugar, called ribose.** Ribose is an element of RNA, not DNA. In a rudimentary form, DNA is the fusion of three different elements: a base (either a pyrimidine or a purine), a sugar (in the case of DNA, called 2-deoxyribose; for RNA, called ribose), and a phosphate (that links individual nucleotides together). The repeating connections between the phosphates and the sugars provide the backbone from which the information-carrying bases protrude. In its "resting" or nonreplicating form, this chain of elements forms a helix of two complementary strands; this double helix is held together by hydrogen bonds.

2. **c. a pyrimidine to form hydrogen bonds with a purine.** The double helix is held together by the formation of hydrogen bonds between the pyrimidine on one strand and the purine base on the other. Uracil is in RNA not DNA. Purines do not form bases with purines. The purine adenine (A) always forms 2 hydrogen bonds with the pyrimidine thymine (T), and the purine guanine (G) always forms 3 hydrogen bonds with the pyrimidine cytosine (C), one consequence being that A-T bonding is weaker than G-C bonding.

3. **e. A mechanism to bridge the gap between the genetic code and protein synthesis.** The physical locations of DNA and its genetic code, and protein synthesis and the manifestation of that code are separate: DNA is in the nucleus, and protein synthesis is cytoplasmic. The DNA message must be converted into mRNA by a process called transcription in the nucleus. The mRNA is transferred into the cytoplasm, where the mRNA is converted into a protein by a process called translation.

4. **a. Two general components involved in transcriptional regulation are specific sequences in**

the RNA and proteins that interact with those sequences. Specific sequences in the DNA, called response elements, bind to the nuclear proteins that control transcription. Importantly, this provides a mechanism to coordinate gene expression by providing similar docking sites for genes that need to be expressed at specific time points. Whereas mRNA transcription, stability, transport, and translation are all highly regulated, they are not controlled by the transcriptional machinery binding to specific mRNA sequences.

5. **c. A process of including or excluding certain exons in an mRNA transcript.** A specific gene may have multiple similar (not identical) forms (isoforms). This is accomplished by having specific exons included or excluded from the final mRNA transcript. This allows one DNA sequence to produce several protein products that have different functions. It is not a random process but is very tightly regulated to ensure that the correct mRNA transcript is produced in the correct cell at the correct point in time.

6. **b. It is the site of mRNA transcription.**

7. **a. The RNA message of four parts (the nucleotides A, U, C, and G) is converted into 20 amino acids by using a functional group of three adjacent nucleotides called a codon.** There is significant redundancy, with several codons encoding for each amino acid. As a result, the RNA sequence between individuals can be different and yet still encode the same amino acid sequence (a polymorphism). However, some polymorphisms do result in amino acid changes. Shifts in reading frame are the most deleterious mutations because they result in a change in all the codons after the insertion/deletion, and thus a dramatic change in the amino acid sequence occurs.

8. **e. The targeted inhibition of proteosome function appears to enhance cancer progression.** Degradation of proteins in the cell is an active, not passive, process. Ubiquitination is the process by which proteins are tagged for transport to the proteosome for destruction. Perturbation of this process is often found in cancer, and therefore inhibition of ubiquitination is a promising therapy for cancer.

9. **c. They can be produced by gene amplification, resulting in many copies of the gene, or by chromosomal rearrangement.** There are at least three ways a proto-oncogene can be converted into an oncogene. First, a mutation can occur within the coding sequence, producing a permanently activated form of the gene. A second mechanism converting a proto-oncogene into an oncogene is through gene amplification. A third mechanism of oncogene formation is through chromosomal rearrangement.

10. **b. It occurs exclusively on cytosine nucleotides in the dinucleotide sequence CG.** Hypermethylation is a normal process by which DNA is modified by the addition of a methyl group to a cytosine nucleotide in a CpG DNA sequence. There is no change in the DNA sequence. Methylation results in gene silencing, that is, decreased expression of the gene. As a result, hypermethylation in cancer is associated with decreased transcription and, therefore, reduces expression of tumor suppressor genes. Ubiquitination decreases levels of proteins but does so by increasing the degradation of the protein. Whereas alterations in ubiquitination occur in cancer, they are not directly related to methylation.

11. **b. clear cell renal carcinoma.** VHL is a hereditary tumor syndrome that predisposes patients to clear cell renal carcinoma, retinal angiomas, pheochromocytomas, hemangiomas of the CNS, epididymal cystadenomas, and pancreatic islet cell tumors. It is not associated with epididymal, papillary renal cell, or adrenocortical carcinomas.

12. **e. 41% to 50%.** Although the inherited form of prostate cancer is estimated to be responsible for only 9% of all prostate cancer, it is implicated in 43% of cases of disease diagnosed before 55 years of age.

13. **d. none of the above.** All of the genes above have been linked to prostate cancer by both linkage studies examining families with a strong predisposition to prostate cancer and in some cases by case control studies examining polymorphisms within these genes. However, no data have conclusively demonstrated that these genes cause prostate cancer.

14. **e. All of the above.** Each of these syndromes includes increased risk of specific genitourinary malignancies among the spectra of pathologies.

15. **d. Deletion.** A common mechanism of tumor supressor gene inactivation is through deletion of the gene or a chromosomal region containing the gene. The other abnormalities listed produce either no net loss of genetic material or lead to a gain of genetic material, a finding often associated with increase oncogene activity due to increased copy number of the oncogene.

16. **c. can alter expression of genes.** With the cloning of the human genome, it has become apparent that genetic anomalies are not limited to high-risk individuals; over 10 million common genetic variants exist. These are not mutations but are normal differences in the human genome. Although the majority have no functional significance, variants within the reading frame of the gene can change the amino acid sequence, variants within the promoter can alter transcription of a gene, and variants in close proximity to intron–exon boundaries can alter splicing.

17. **d. G_1S and G_2M boundaries.**

18. **a. Apoptosis.** Active *TP53* binds to the promoter region of *TP53*-responsive genes and stimulates the transcription of genes responsible for cell cycle arrest, repair of DNA damage, and apoptosis. *TP53* responds to DNA damage by inducing cell cycle arrest through *TP21^{cip1}* and then transcriptionally activating DNA repair enzymes. If the cell cannot arrest growth and/or repair the DNA, *TP53* induces apoptosis. Whereas angiogenesis, DNA replication, and signal transduction are all critical cellular processes, *TP53* does not directly influence any of them.

19. **d. TP14^{ARF}.** TP14^{ARF} was originally identified as an alternative splice variant of the CDK inhibitor TP16^{INK4a}. It has been demonstrated that TP14^{ARF} functions not by acting as a CDK inhibitor but by degrading MDM2. The acronym "ARF" refers to the fact that an alternate reading frame was used in this splice variant.

20. **a. cyclin D/CDK4.** The INK4 family of CDK inhibitors directly inhibits the assembly of cyclin D with CDK4 and CDK6 by blocking the phosphorylation of the cyclin D–CDK4/6 complex. This phosphorylation is necessary for activation of the complex.

21. **e. phosphorylation of RB.** Phosphorylation is the attachment of a phosphate to a protein. It alters the conformation of the protein and therefore is an excellent

method of regulating gene function. Cyclin-CDK complexes phosphorylate RB or its family members, TP107 and TP130. Phosphorylated RB can no longer bind to members of the E2F family of transcription factors. Free E2F heterodimerizes with DP1 or DP2 and transcriptionally activates genes important in DNA replication, such as DNA polymerase-A, and in the cell cycle, such as E2F-1. Dephosphorylation of RB has the opposite effect. E2F regulation does not occur directly though phosphorylation or dephosphorylation. MDM2 regulates TP53 and is not directly affected by cyclin-CDK complexes.

22. **c. DNA damage.** Hypoxia, nutrient-poor environment, and cytokines are all signals to the cell that it is not in an environment that is conducive to cellular division. These signals influence the cell BEFORE it invests its energy in replicating the DNA, that is, it is a G_1S checkpoint. If DNA damage occurs, it is critical the errors are repaired before cellular division. Therefore DNA damage can lead to cell cycle arrest at both the G_1S and G_2M checkpoints.

23. **d. ultraviolet light.** Nucleotide excision repair (NER) is a major defense against DNA damage caused by ultraviolet radiation and chemical exposure. NER acts on a wide range of alterations that result in large local distortions in DNA by recognizing distortions in the DNA helix, excising the damaged DNA, and replacing it with the correct sequence. Base excision repair is the primary mechanism for repairing damage caused by reactive oxygen species. Mismatch repair is the primary mechanism for polymerase errors. Double-stranded break repair is the primary mechanism for repairing double-stranded breaks.

24. **b. Homologous recombination.** Homologous recombination (HR) is one of two mechanisms for repairing DNA double-stranded breaks, the other being nonhomologous end joining (NHEJ). In homologous recombination, the normal undamaged sister chromatid is used as a template to repair the damaged segment of DNA.

25. **c. BRCA1.** BRCA1 is associated with familial breast and ovarian cancer. It is believed that the breast cancer susceptibility gene BRCA1 (as well as BRCA2) play an important role in homologous recombination as well as sensing DNA damage. Both BRCA1 and BRCA2 are part of an enzymatic complex with RAD51- and BRCA1-associated RING domain 1 (BARD1). This complex is recruited by proliferating cell nuclear antigen (PCNA) to regions that have undergone DNA damage to repair DNA breaks.

26. **e. Proteolytic cleavage.** Procaspases are the larger, inactive precursor forms of the caspase proteins. Specific proteolytic cleavage is required for their activation. The caspases themselves are proteases and once activated proceed to cleave and activate other caspases, thus

facilitating a proteolytic cascade that serves to amplify the initial apoptotic signal.

27. **a. independent of TP53.** The identification of ligand-dependent apoptosis receptors may have a profound impact on therapy. Most cancer therapies (e.g., chemotherapy and external beam radiotherapy) depend on TP53 to induce apoptosis in the cancer cell. Because TP53 is mutated in more than half of malignancies, TP53-independent pathways for apoptosis are of great clinical interest. Because ligand-dependent apoptosis is independent of TP53, these receptors and ligands are attractive and novel treatment targets.

28. **a. APAF-1/caspase 9.** The TP53-induced apoptosis is dependent on the APAF-1/caspase 9 activation pathway.

29. **c. increasing the mitochondrial membrane permeability.** Although each proapoptotic BCL-2 family member responds to different stimuli, the principal mechanism by which these family members induce cell death is by increasing mitochondrial membrane permeability.

30. **e. maintaining chromosomal length.** Telomerase immortalizes cells by maintaining the ends of the chromosomes, or telomeres, which normally shorten with each cell division.

31. **c. DNA hypomethylation.** Normal cells closely monitor their telomere lengths and, should they fall below a critical threshold length, will initiate either cell senescence or apoptosis. If key players in these responses (e.g., TP53) are mutated then chromosomal instability may result contributing to cancer initiation. To date, there is not a strong connection known for telomere loss and loss of DNA methylation.

32. **a. Fusion of BCR to ABL by chromosome translocation.** This particular chromosomal abnormality is typically found in chronic myelogenous leukemia patients, not in solid tumors. TMPRSS2-ERG gene fusions are found in ≈50% of prostate cancer cases; MITF/TFE gene family translocations have been associated with a subset of renal cell carcinomas; isochromosome 8q is found in a subset of prostate cancers and is often associated with the loss of 8p; loss of chromosome 9 is observed in a subset of urothelial cancers, and enumeration of this chromosome by fluorescence in-situ hybridization (FISH) is one of the components of a molecular test used for detecting bladder cancer.

33. **a. Testis.** The urologic malignancy most closely linked to a karyotypic abnormality is a testis tumor. A 12p isochromosome was first identified in a testis tumor in the 1980s, and experimentally this cytogenetic hallmark of testicular tumors has diagnostic and prognostic value.

Additional Study Points

1. Cancer cells have (1) genetic instability, (2) autonomous growth, (3) insensitivity to external antiproliferative signals, (4) resistance to apoptosis, (5) unlimited cell division, (6) angiogenesis, (7) invasive behavior, and (8) ability to evade the immune system.
2. RNA contains coding sequences (exons) and noncoding sequences (introns).
3. Loss of function of both alleles of a tumor suppressor gene is typically required for carcinogenesis.
4. Tumor suppressor genes regulate and control cellular growth. Oncogenes promote cell growth.
5. Certain tumor suppressor genes do not follow the two-hit hypothesis and may be inhibited by one alteration.
6. Cyclin-dependent kinases (CDK) are involved in synthetic activities of the cell cycle.
7. The regulatory portion of the CDK protein is called the cyclin and may also assist in substrate specificity.

8. The key point in the late G_1–cell phase at which the cell cycle becomes insensitive to extra cellular signals is termed the restriction point.

9. If the cell cannot arrest growth or repair DNA damage, *TP53* often induces apoptosis.

10. Hypermethylation of CpG islands results in transcriptional downregulation, while hypomethylation of these regions increases the potential for gene activity.

11. More than 70% of prostate cancers are thought to harbor some form of a recurrent gene fusion.

12. Family history is one of the strongest predictors of prostate cancer risk.

13. The VHL gene is found to be mutated in over half of sporadic renal cell carcinoma cases.

14. High-density, single nucleotide polymorphism (SNP) microarrays have been used in genome-wide association studies to identify DNA sequence variants associated with cancer risk.

15. Telomeres are structures composed of specialized repetitive DNA complexed with telomere-specific binding proteins located at the ends of every human chromosome and serve to stabilize and protect the end.

16. Progressive telomere shortening acts as a mitotic clock-signaling cell cycle exit (death), once telomeres reach a shortened threshold length.

17. Apoptosis is an orderly process in which the contents of dying cells are degraded, packaged, and then engulfed by neighboring macrophages. This activity does not produce an inflammatory response.

18. Defects in the apoptotic cascade can profoundly influence tumor response to chemotherapy and radiotherapy.

19. Effective chemotherapy and radiation therapy in large part are dependent on apoptosis.

20. Apoptosis is mediated by the caspases.

Regenerative Medicine in Urology: Stem Cells, Tissue Engineering, and Cloning

Anthony Atala, MD

QUESTIONS

1. Currently, possible tissue replacements for reconstruction include which of the following?
   a. Native nonurologic tissues
   b. Homologous tissues
   c. Heterologous tissues
   d. Artificial biomaterials
   e. All of the above

2. The most common types of synthetic prostheses for urologic use are made of:
   a. latex.
   b. silicone.
   c. urethane.
   d. biodegradable polymers.
   e. polyvinyl.

3. What does tissue engineering involve?
   a. The principles of cell transplantation
   b. The principles of materials science
   c. The use of matrices alone
   d. The use of matrices with cells
   e. All of the above

4. In tissue engineering, when autologous cells are used:
   a. donor tissue is dissociated into individual cells.
   b. cells are either implanted directly into the host or expanded in culture.
   c. cells are attached to a support matrix.
   d. the cells and matrix are implanted in vivo.
   e. all of the above are relevant.

5. Which of the following statements is true regarding biomaterials?
   a. They facilitate the localization and delivery of cells.
   b. They facilitate the localization and delivery of bioactive factors.
   c. They define a three-dimensional space for the formation of new tissues.

   d. They guide the development of new tissues with appropriate function.
   e. All of the above are true.

6. Types of biomaterials that have been used for engineering genitourinary tissues include which of the following?
   a. Naturally derived materials
   b. Acellular tissue matrices
   c. Synthetic polymers
   d. All of the above
   e. None of the above

7. Procedures and techniques that allow for the exclusion of nonurologic tissues during augmentation cystoplasty include which of the following?
   a. Autoaugmentation
   b. Ureterocystoplasty
   c. Tissue expansion
   d. Tissue engineering
   e. All of the above

8. In demucosalized intestinal segments for urinary reconstruction, removal of the mucosa and submucosa may lead to:
   a. contraction of the intestinal patch.
   b. mucosal regrowth.
   c. tissue necrosis.
   d. decreased vascularity.
   e. angiogenesis.

9. Permanent synthetic materials, when used in continuity with the urinary tract, have been associated with:
   a. mechanical failure.
   b. emboli.
   c. calculus formation.
   d. a and c.
   e. none of the above.

10. Urothelium is associated with:
    a. a high reparative capacity.
    b. an inherent capacity for artificial extracellular matrix attachment.

c. frequent malignant differentiation.

d. poor growth parameters.

e. none of the above.

11. Major limitations in phallic reconstructive surgery include which of the following?

a. The availability of adequate growth factors

b. The availability of sufficient autologous tissue

c. The availability of adequate surgical techniques

d. All of the above

e. None of the above

12. What is the most prevalent form of renal replacement therapy?

a. Organ transplantation

b. Dialysis

c. Bioartificial hemofilters

d. Bioartificial renal tubules

e. Engineered functional renal structures

13. The ideal bulking substance for the endoscopic treatment of reflux and incontinence should have what characteristic?

a. Easily injectable

b. Nonantigenic

c. Nonmigratory

d. Volume stable

e. All of the above

14. Which of the following statements regarding microencapsulated cells is true?

a. They have a semipermeable barrier.

b. They are protected from the host's immune system.

c. They allow for physiologic release of substances.

d. They provide a long-term delivery system of byproducts.

e. All of the above.

15. What are the most common cell sources for tissue engineering today?

a. Embryonic stem cells

b. Induced pluripotent stem cells

c. Autologous primary cells

d. Stem cells derived from nuclear transfer techniques

e. None of the above

ANSWERS

1. **e. All of the above.** Whenever there is a lack of native urologic tissue, reconstruction may be performed with native nonurologic tissues (skin, gastrointestinal segments, or mucosa from multiple body sites), homologous tissues (cadaver fascia, cadaver, or donor kidney), heterologous tissues (bovine collagen), or artificial materials (silicone, polyurethane, Teflon).

2. **b. silicone.** The most common type of synthetic prostheses for urologic use is made of silicone.

3. **e. All of the above.** Tissue engineering follows the principles of cell transplantation, materials science, and engineering toward the development of biologic

substitutes that would restore and maintain normal function. Tissue engineering may involve matrices alone, wherein the body's natural ability to regenerate is used to orient or direct new tissue growth, or the use of matrices with cells.

4. **e. all of the above are relevant.** When cells are used for tissue engineering, donor tissue is dissociated into individual cells. They may be implanted directly into the host or expanded in culture, attached to a support matrix, and reimplanted after expansion. The implanted tissue can be heterologous, allogeneic, or autologous.

5. **e. All of the above are true.** Biomaterials facilitate the localization and delivery of cells and/or bioactive factors (e.g., cell adhesion peptides and growth factors) to desired sites in the body, define a three-dimensional space for the formation of new tissues with appropriate structure, and guide the development of new tissues with appropriate function.

6. **d. All of the above.** Generally, three classes of biomaterials have been used for engineering genitourinary tissues: naturally derived materials (e.g., collagen and alginate), acellular tissue matrices (e.g., bladder submucosa and small intestinal submucosa), and synthetic polymers (e.g., polyglycolic acid [PGA], polylactic acid [PLA], and poly[lactic-coglycolic acid] [PLGA]).

7. **e. All of the above.** Because of the problems encountered with the use of gastrointestinal segments, numerous investigators have attempted alternative methods, materials, and tissues for bladder replacement or repair. These include autoaugmentation, ureterocystoplasty, methods for tissue expansion, seromuscular grafts, matrices for tissue regeneration, and tissue engineering using cell transplantation.

8. **a. contraction of the intestinal patch.** It has been noted that removal of only the mucosa may lead to mucosal regrowth, whereas removal of the mucosa and submucosa may lead to retraction of the intestinal patch.

9. **d. a and c.** Usually, permanent synthetic materials used for bladder reconstruction succumb to mechanical failure and urinary stone formation, and degradable materials lead to fibroblast deposition, scarring, graft contracture, and a reduced reservoir volume over time.

10. **a. a high reparative capacity.** It has been well established for decades that the bladder is able to regenerate generously over free grafts. Urothelium is associated with a high reparative capacity. Bladder muscle tissue is less likely to regenerate in a normal manner.

11. **b. The availability of sufficient autologous tissue.** One of the major limitations of phallic reconstructive surgery is the availability of sufficient autologous tissue.

12. **b. Dialysis.** Although dialysis therapy is currently the most prevalent form of renal replacement therapy, the relatively high morbidity and mortality rates have prompted investigators to seek alternative solutions involving ex-vivo systems.

13. **e. All of the above.** The ideal substance for the endoscopic treatment of reflux and incontinence should be injectable, nonantigenic, nonmigratory, volume stable, and safe for human use.

14. **e. All of the above.** Microencapsulated Leydig cells offer several advantages, such as serving as a semipermeable

barrier between the transplanted cells and the host's immune system, as well as allowing for the long-term physiologic release of testosterone.

15. **c. Autologous primary cells.** Most current strategies for engineering urologic tissues involve harvesting of autologous cells from the host diseased organ. However, in situations in which extensive end-stage organ failure is present, a tissue biopsy may not yield enough normal cells for expansion. Under these circumstances, the availability of pluripotent stem cells may be beneficial.

Additional Study Points

1. Stem cells may be either embryonic or adult. Embryonic stem cells may be harvested from (1) a blastocyst, (2) amniotic fluid, or (3) the placenta. Adult stem cells are usually isolated from a specific organ or bone marrow.

2. Stem cells have the ability to self renew, to differentiate into a number of cell types and to form clonal populations.

3. Altered nuclear transfer is a technique in which a genetically modified nucleus from a somatic cell is transferred into a human oocyte. The resulting embryo develops into a blastocyst but cannot implant into a uterus. The ethical advantage is that a fully developed organism is not created.

4. Adult stem cells have been discovered in many organs in the body and may serve as primary mechanisms of repair for injuries of these organs.

5. The ideal biomaterial provides regulation of cell behavior in order to promote development of functional new tissue. The cell behavior regulated includes but is not limited to cell adhesion, proliferation, migration, and differentiation. There are three types of biomaterials that are used: (1) naturally derived materials such as collagen or alginate (a polysaccharide isolated from seaweed), (2) acellular tissue matrices such as bladder submucosal or small intestine submucosal, and (3) synthetic polymers such as polyglycolic acid.

6. Formation of new blood vessels and capillaries occur by two mechanisms: vasculogenesis, in which new capillaries are formed from undifferentiated cells, and angiogenesis, in which new capillaries form by sprouting from preexisting capillaries.

7. In normal wound healing, epithelial cell in growth is initiated from the wound edges. This type of healing for a distance of more than a few millimeters results in fibrosis and scar formation. Matrices or matrices implanted with cells on the open wound allow greater wound coverage with the hope of less fibrosis.

8. Most free grafts for bladder replacement show an adequate urothelial layer, but the muscular layer is not fully developed.

Reproductive and Sexual Function

Male Reproductive Physiology

Paul J. Turek, MD, FACS, FRSM

QUESTIONS

1. Embryologically, the vas deferens and body of the epididymis are derived from what developmental structure?
   a. Müllerian ducts
   b. Wolffian ducts
   c. Urogenital ridge
   d. Gubernaculum testis
   e. Metanephros

2. The proportion of testicular volume comprised of seminiferous tubules in the human testis is:
   a. 5%.
   b. 10% to 20%.
   c. 50% to 60%.
   d. 70% to 80%.
   e. 90% to 95%.

3. Which hormones play a central role in regulation of Sertoli cell function?
   a. LH, FSH
   b. FSH, estradiol
   c. Prolactin, LH
   d. FSH, testosterone
   e. ABP, testosterone

4. The majority of the fluid in the male ejaculate is derived from:
   a. the epididymides.
   b. the ejaculatory ducts.
   c. the seminal vesicles.
   d. the testes.
   e. the prostate.

5. Blood supply for the testes is derived from all of the following sources EXCEPT:
   a. the internal spermatic artery.
   b. the deferential artery.
   c. the external spermatic artery.
   d. the cremasteric artery.
   e. the pudendal artery.

6. A 25-year-old bodybuilder eschews the merits of "natural" bodybuilding and cycles and stacks injectable anabolic steroids regularly to maximize muscle bulk. His fertility potential would be expected to be:
   a. normal, because exogenous testosterone does not impair production of endogenous testosterone.

   b. low, because exogenous testosterone stimulates pituitary production of follicle-stimulating hormone (FSH) and luteinizing hormone (LH).
   c. low, because exogenous testosterone inhibits pituitary production of FSH and LH.
   d. low, because exogenous testosterone is not as potent as endogenous testosterone at nurturing spermatogenesis.
   e. normal, because intratestis testosterone concentrations are 50 times higher than serum levels, whether or not the blood contains exogenous testosterone.

7. Structural elements of the blood–testis barrier are observed in:
   a. Sertoli–Sertoli cell junctions.
   b. Leydig cells.
   c. basement membranes.
   d. desmosomes between spermatocytes.
   e. spermatids.

8. How do elevated levels of prolactin influence testosterone production?
   a. Inhibit gonadotrophin-releasing hormone (GnRH) and LH
   b. Indirectly inhibit Sertoli cells
   c. Directly inhibit Leydig cells
   d. Upregulate inhibin
   e. Downregulate activin

9. What is the normal developmental pattern of spermatogenic cells?
   a. Sertoli, spermatogonia, spermatocyte
   b. Spermatocyte, spermatogonia, spermatid
   c. Spermatid, Sertoli, spermatocyte
   d. Spermatogonia, spermatid, spermatocyte
   e. Spermatogonia, spermatocyte, spermatid

10. Which testis hormone is the major feedback inhibitor of LH secretion?
    a. Testosterone
    b. Inhibin
    c. Activin
    d. Prolactin
    e. Sertolin

11. What is the normal volume for adult human testes?
    a. 5 mL
    b. 10 mL
    c. 20 mL

d. 30 mL

e. 40 mL

12. Major components of the epididymis include:

a. caput, corpus, and cauda.

b. globus minor, ductus deferens, and cauda.

c. rete testis, efferent ductules, and caput.

d. efferent ductules, caput, and cauda.

e. septa, efferent ductules, and corpus.

13. Which of the following is characteristic of meiosis?

a. Cellular DNA content doubles during the first (meiotic) cell division.

b. Chromosome number is maintained.

c. Homologous chromosomes (nonsister) pair during the second cell division.

d. Crossing over is present.

e. Centromeres do not divide.

14. When does a testosterone peak occur during a human male's life?

a. 2 months

b. 6 to 9 months

c. 30 to 40 years

d. 50 to 60 years

e. >70 years

15. With chronic obstruction, optimal sperm quality is found in what region of the epididymis?

a. Rete testis

b. Efferent ducts

c. Proximal epididymis

d. Midepididymis

e. Distal epididymis

16. Which of the following occurs during spermiogenesis?

a. Division of type B spermatogonia to form primary spermatocytes

b. Cellular remodeling within the basal compartment of the seminiferous tubule

c. DNA replication

d. Nuclear compaction

e. Cytokinesis

17. Changes to sperm during epididymal transit include:

a. increased positive charge.

b. sulfhydryl reduction.

c. decreased phospholipid content.

d. reduced membrane rigidity.

e. increased capacity for glycolysis.

18. Which of the following germ cell types is considered a true stem cell?

a. Elongating spermatids

b. Primary spermatocytes

c. Round spermatids

d. Secondary spermatocytes

e. Type A spermatogonia

19. During their development within the male reproductive tract prior to ejaculation, sperm spend the majority of time in which organ?

a. Epididymis

b. Ejaculatory ducts

c. Seminal vesicle

d. Testis

e. Vas deferens

20. The sperm region containing mitochondria is the:

a. tail.

b. head.

c. acrosome.

d. midpiece.

e. axoneme.

21. Which of the following statements about testosterone is most accurate?

a. It is produced by the exocrine testis.

b. It exists mainly in the unbound or "free" form in the circulation.

c. It is regulated by follicle-stimulating hormone.

d. Its production is increased by excess prolactin.

e. Its metabolite is dihydrotestosterone (DHT).

22. Spermiogenesis includes all of the following processes EXCEPT:

a. loss of cytoplasm.

b. formation of the acrosome.

c. flagellar formation.

d. migration of cytoplasmic organelles.

e. cell division.

23. After ejaculation the contents of the vas deferens are:

a. returned to the seminal vesicles.

b. maintained in the ampulla.

c. released into the ejaculatory ducts.

d. propelled back into the epididymis.

e. released into the bladder.

ANSWERS

1. **b. Wolffian ducts.** Mullerian ducts regress in the male. The indifferent gonad migrates to the urogenital ridge to become the testis. The gubernaculum testis is associated with the testis.

2. **d. 70% to 80%.** In humans, interstitial tissue takes up 20% to 30% of the total testicular volume.

3. **d. FSH, testosterone.** FSH and testosterone play the most important role in the regulation of Sertoli cell function, including androgen binding protein (ABP) production.

4. **c. the seminal vesicles.** At least 65% to 70% of ejaculate volume is derived from the seminal vesicles, with the remainder from the vas deferens (with sperm) and prostatic secretions. Periurethral glands may also contribute a small amount of fluid to the normal ejaculate.

5. **e. the pudendal artery.** The arterial supply to the human testis and epididymis is derived from three sources: the internal spermatic artery, the deferential artery, and the external spermatic or cremasteric artery.

6. **c. low, because exogenous testosterone inhibits pituitary production of FSH and LH.** Because of negative feedback inhibition that maintains homeostatic balance in the pituitary-gonadal axis, excess testosterone of any type will cause anterior pituitary production of LH and FSH to fall. This results in azoospermia in most men on anabolic steroids, but the effect will vary based on the dose, frequency, and duration of the cycles and stacking regimen.

7. **a. Sertoli–Sertoli cell junctions.** Sertoli–Sertoli tight junctions prevent the deep penetration of electron-opaque tracers into the seminiferous epithelium from the testicular interstitium. The tight junctions between Sertoli cells segregate premeiotic germ cells (spermatogonia) from meiotic and postmeiotic germ cells.

8. **a. Inhibit GnRH and LH.**

9. **e. Spermatogonia, spermatocyte, spermatid.** Proceeding from the least to the most differentiated, they are named dark type A spermatogonia (Ad); pale type A spermatogonia (Ap); type B spermatogonia (B); preleptotene primary spermatocytes (R); leptotene primary spermatocytes (L); zygotene primary spermatocytes (z); pachytene primary spermatocytes (p); secondary spermatocytes (II); and Sa, Sb1, Sb2, Sc, Sd1, and Sd2 spermatids.

10. **a. Testosterone.** Inhibin and activin regulate FSH secretion by feedback inhibition. Prolactin, in excess, can downregulate LH secretion.

11. **c. 20 mL.** Although ethnic and racial differences do exist, 20 mL is considered the normal testis volume.

12. **a. caput, corpus, and cauda.** Anatomically, the epididymis is divided into three regions: the caput, the corpus, and the cauda epididymis. On the basis of histologic criteria, each of these regions can be subdivided into distinct zones separated by transition segments.

13. **d. Crossing over is present.** Crossing over of sister chromatids and exchange of genetic material is the hallmark of chromosomal recombination during meiosis. This does not occur in mitosis. Other unique characteristics of meiosis are that homologous chromosomes pair during meiosis I (the first cell division) and that chromosome numbers are half (haploid) that of mitotic cells.

14. **a. 2 months.** A testosterone peak occurs at approximately 2 months of age. A peak occurs earlier during the first trimester of gestation, and a third occurs later at puberty.

15. **c. Proximal epididymis.** Studies in men with congenital absence of the vas deferens or epididymal obstruction from vasectomy frequently report poor motility in sperm aspirated from the distal epididymis, with optimal sperm quality and motility in the proximal epididymis.

16. **d. Nuclear compaction.** In spermiogenesis, cell division, or cytokinesis, does not occur. In addition, the adluminal compartment, and not the basal compartment, is involved. Spermatids, and not spermatogonia, are the cell types undergoing metamorphosis.

17. **e. increased capacity for glycolysis.** Sperm undergo numerous metabolic changes during epididymal transit. Animal studies describe the acquisition of an increased capacity for glycolysis, changes in intracellular pH and calcium content, modification of adenylate cyclase activity, and alterations in cellular phospholipid and phospholipid-like fatty acid content.

18. **e. Type A spermatogonia.** Type A spermatogonia are the only true stem cell in the testis because they can both self renew or differentiate down the spermatogenic pathway.

19. **d. Testis.** Sperm spend 45 to 60 days developing in the testis and 2 to 12 days in the epididymis.

20. **d. midpiece.** The middle segment of the sperm is a highly organized, consisting of helically arranged mitochondria surrounding a set of outer dense fibers and the characteristic 9 + 2 microtubular structure of the axoneme.

21. **e. Its metabolite is dihydrotestosterone (DHT).** Testosterone is converted to DHT in target tissue by 5-α reductase. Testosterone is produced by the endocrine testes, exists mainly in bound forms in plasma and is mainly regulated by LH, not FSH. Excess prolactin decreases testosterone production.

22. **e. cell division.** During spermiogenesis, the products of meiosis, the round Sa spermatids, metamorphose into mature spermatids. During this process, extensive changes occur in both the spermatid cytoplasm and the nucleus, but cell division is not required. These changes include loss of cytoplasm, formation of the acrosome, formation of the flagellum, and migration of cytoplasmic organelles to positions characteristic of the mature sperm.

23. **d. propelled back into the epididymis.** Studies have shown that after sexual stimulation or ejaculation, the contents of the vas deferens are propelled back toward the cauda epididymis, because the distal portion of the vas deferens contracts with greater amplitude, frequency, and duration than does the proximal portion.

Additional Study Points

1. Testosterone, dihydrotestosterone, and estradiol are translocated to nuclear DNA recognition sites and regulate the transcription of target genes.
2. The hypothalamus is anatomically linked to the pituitary gland by both a portal vascular system and neuronal pathway. The hypothalamic hormone GnRH (sometimes called LHRH) stimulates the secretion of luteinizing hormone and follicle-stimulating hormone.
3. GnRH output exhibits three types of rhythmicity: (1) seasonal—peaking in the spring, (2) circadian—peaking in the early morning, and (3) pulsatile—periodic peaks per 24 hours. The importance of pulsatile GnRH secretory pattern is demonstrated when a GnRH agonist is given; this eliminates the pulsatile activity and therefore suppresses GnRH output.
4. Both androgens and estrogens regulate LH secretion through negative feedback.
5. Increased levels of prolactin abolish gonadotropin pulsatility by interfering with the episodic GnRH release, thus causing a reduction in LH and FSH.
6. Testosterone is metabolized to dihydrotestosterone and estradiol.
7. Sertoli cells produce inhibin, which inhibits FSH and activin, which then stimulates FSH and accounts for the

relatively secondary independence of FSH from GnRH secretion.

8. Negative feedback for testosterone occurs at the hypothalamus; for estrogens, it occurs at the pituitary.

9. The SRY (sex-determining region Y gene) on the short arm of the Y chromosome is a critical gene for sex determination.

10. Dihydrotestosterone masculinizes the external genitalia; müllerian inhibiting substance prevents müllerian duct development, i.e., uterus, and fallopian tubes and proximal third of the vagina.

11. A progressive decline in testosterone and sperm production occurs with age.

12. Androgen production during the early male neonate's life is thought to hormonally imprint the hypothalamus, liver, and prostate.

13. The blood–testes barrier is more appropriately termed blood seminferous tubule barrier; this allows sperm development to occur in an immunologically privileged site.

14. An insult to the testes, such as biopsy, torsion, or trauma, will not induce antisperm antibodies if it occurs before puberty.

15. Embryonic-like cells obtained from adult testis biopsies exhibits pluripotency and can form all three germ layers.

16. The azoospermic factor region (AZF) is located on the long arm of the Y chromosome. Deletions in this region are found in some patients with abnormal spermatogenesis.

17. With paternal age, there are increases in structural chromosomal abnormalities in sperm and autosomal-dominant mutations leading to sentinel phenotypes in offspring.

18. See Table 20–3 in *Campbell-Walsh Urology, 10th Edition.*

19. Lymph from the caput and corpus epididymis travels the same route as that for the testes. Lymph from the cauda epididymis joins the vas deferens and terminates in the external iliac nodes. There is a blood–epididymis barrier that extends from caput to cauda epididymis.

20. The epididymis serves to transport sperm, store it, increase fertility, and promote motility maturation. Epididymal function is temperature and androgen dependent.

21. A component of the semen coagulation, semenogelin, is a component of semen coagulation produced in the seminal vesicle. Seminal vesicle secretions have an alkaline pH and contain antioxidant enzymes, fructose, vitamin C, flavins, and prostaglandins.

Male Infertility

Edmund Sabanegh, Jr., MD • Ashok Agarwal, PhD

QUESTIONS

1. Infertility is defined as failure to conceive after:
   a. 3 months of regular, unprotected intercourse.
   b. 6 months of regular, unprotected intercourse.
   c. 9 months of regular, unprotected intercourse.
   d. 1 year of regular, unprotected intercourse.
   e. 2 years of regular, unprotected intercourse.

2. What percent of infertility is at least partially attributed to a male cause?
   a. 10%
   b. 20%
   c. 25%
   d. 50%
   e. 75%

3. All of the following are indications for a male infertility evaluation EXCEPT:
   a. patients with risk factors for male infertility.
   b. failure to conceive after 1 year of regular, unprotected intercourse.
   c. presence of female infertility risk factors.
   d. history of mumps orchitis before puberty.
   e. any couple questioning male fertility potential.

4. Which of the following is true regarding infertility?
   a. Primary infertility is defined as infertility that is primarily due to a male factor.
   b. Secondary infertility indicates prior conception with the current or previous partner.
   c. Optimal sexual frequency for couples attempting to conceive is every third day.
   d. Ovulation kits measure midcycle follicle-stimulating hormone (FSH) levels to help time intercourse around ovulation.
   e. Baseline pregnancy rates for normal couples are 50% per cycle.

5. All of the following lubricants are recommended for patients attempting to conceive EXCEPT:
   a. KY jelly.
   b. vegetable oil.
   c. raw egg white.
   d. preseed.
   e. none of the above.

6. Antibiotics known to be directly spermatotoxic include all of the following EXCEPT:
   a. nitrofurantoin.
   b. gentamycin.
   c. erythromycin.
   d. ciprofloxacin.
   e. tetracycline.

7. Which of the following is correct regarding medication and its association with impaired spermatogenesis?
   a. Sulfalazine is associated with irreversible reduction in sperm count and morphology.
   b. Tamsulosin causes an increase in antegrade ejaculation.
   c. Finasteride results in dose-dependent reduction in sperm motility.
   d. Cimetidine inhibits androgen production.
   e. Marijuana increases serum testosterone levels.

8. When performing a physical examination of the infertile male, which statement is TRUE?
   a. Assessment of the presence or absence of vas deferens is ideally performed with ultrasound.
   b. The normal adult testis volume is 20 mL.
   c. A grade 2 varicocele is one that is visible through the scrotal skin.
   d. A rectal examination assessing for the presence of a midline cyst is important in the evaluation of a man with unilateral absence of the vas deferens.
   e. A right-sided vericocele is of no consequence.

9. All the following are true statements regarding semen analysis EXCEPT:
   a. Abstinence of 2 to 7 days before a semen analysis is optimal.
   b. Two separate samples at least 7 days apart should be analyzed.
   c. Coitus interruptus is an accurate and reliable method of obtaining semen.
   d. Only 50% of men will have a recognizable cause of infertility on the basis of the standard semen analysis.
   e. The most common cause of low-volume ejaculate is incomplete collection.

10. Which statement about semen analysis is TRUE?
    a. Any degree of sperm agglutination is considered abnormal.

b. Normal sperm count is reported as greater than 40 million sperm per milliliter.

c. Antisperm antibodies usually manifest themselves through abnormal morphology.

d. The acrosome compromises 20% of the sperm head.

e. The Endtz test is used to differentiate nonsperm round cells in semen between white blood cells and immature germ cells.

11. All the following statements are true regarding a postcoital (PCT) test EXCEPT:

a. Indications for a postcoital test include hyperviscous sperm, unexplained infertility, and low-volume sperm with unexplained infertility.

b. The cervical mucus must be examined 2 to 8 hours after normal intercourse 1 day before ovulation.

c. A normal result is 5 progressively motile sperm per high-power field (HPF) in the cervical mucus.

d. The most common cause of an abnormal PCT is improper timing of the test.

e. Men with hypospadias may have an abnormal PCT.

12. Which of the following is TRUE regarding sperm function tests?

a. Enzymes important in the acrosome reaction include acrosin and trypsin.

b. The acrosome reaction test and sperm penetration assay (SPA) are clinically important and relevant tests.

c. An acrosome reaction test may be useful in patients with severe teratospermia and round-headed sperm.

d. In a PCT, good-quality mucus with shaking sperm indicate abnormal sperm penetration.

e. In the SPA, successful penetration is indicated by absent sperm heads within the oocyte cytoplasm.

13. All the following statements are true regarding anti-sperm antibodies (ASA) EXCEPT:

a. Direct ASA testing detects antibodies bound to sperm.

b. Indirect ASA testing is done only in females.

c. Tight junctions between Sertoli cells regulate the blood-testis barrier.

d. Vasectomy is the most common cause of the development of ASA.

e. Other conditions such as torsion, infection, and testicular trauma all may result in the breakdown of the blood-testis barrier and development of ASA.

14. Types of ASA include all of the following EXCEPT:

a. sperm agglutinating types of antibodies that cause the agglutination of sperm and reduced motility.

b. sperm immobilizing types of antibodies that result in shaking of sperm.

c. spermatotoxic antibodies that result in a complement-dependent destruction of sperm.

d. acceptable normal values of ASA by World Health Organization (WHO) standards are less than 40%.

e. in a patient with ASA and inability to bind in a zona pellucida test, intracytoplasmic sperm injection (ICSI) is the treatment of choice.

15. Which of the following is TRUE regarding reactive oxygen species (ROS) testing in semen?

a. ROS testing usually does not result in sperm damage or abnormal sperm parameters.

b. High levels of ROS are an independent marker of male factor infertility.

c. The chemiluminescence assay is not an accurate means to determine the presence of ROS.

d. ROS levels for healthy donors are 2.5×10^4 cpm/20 million.

e. The evidence does not suggest use of antioxidants in male infertility patients with elevated ROS.

16. DNA fragmentation is associated with all of the following EXCEPT:

a. smoking.

b. chemotherapy.

c. leukocytospermia.

d. oxidative stress.

e. vaginal lubricants.

17. Which of the following is TRUE regarding the effects of sperm DNA damage?

a. DNA damage is correlated positively with poor semen parameters, especially low sperm concentration and low sperm motility, leukocytospermia, and oxidative stress.

b. Elevated DNA fragmentation index (DFI) is associated with poorer results in conventional IVF.

c. DFI is usually lower in ejaculated sperm compared with sperm obtained from testicular tissue.

d. Elevated DNA fragmentation is not associated with lower in-vivo pregnancy rates.

e. DFI has been shown to be the etiology of idiopathic infertility.

18. All of the following warrant an endocrine evaluation in a male infertility patient EXCEPT:

a. oligospermia with counts less than 10 mil/mL.

b. erectile dysfunction.

c. decreased libido.

d. gynecomastia.

e. premature ejaculation.

19. Initial hormone evaluation in an infertile man with severe oligospermia includes:

a. testosterone and FSH.

b. FSH and LH.

c. FSH, LH, and prolactin.

d. FSH and inhibin B.

e. LH, prolactin, and free testosterone.

20. Which of the following is TRUE regarding genetic testing in male infertility patients?

a. 25% of all infertile males will have structural and numerical chromosomal abnormalities.

b. Genetic testing with karyotype and Y-chromosome microdeletion is indicated for all patients with azoospermia or severe oligospermia.

c. Y-chromosome microdeletion exists in 50% of patients with azoospermia.

d. CFTR mutations are identified in only 10% of patients with congenital bilateral absence of vas deferens (CBAVD).

e. None are true.

21. Which of the following is TRUE regarding ejaculatory duct obstruction (EJDO)?

a. Normal volume azoospermia is a common presentation for EJDO.

b. EJDO will often present with low-volume azoospermia.

c. Seminal vesicle width greater than 12 to 15 mm is suggestive of obstruction.

d. In a patient with suspected EJDO, seminal pH will usually be around 8.

e. If any sperm is found in seminal vesicle aspiration at the time of transrectal ultrasonography (TRUS), the diagnosis of EJDO is confirmed.

22. All of the following statements are true regarding radiologic examination of the male infertile patient EXCEPT:

a. Scrotal ultrasound is recommended for the diagnosis and potential treatment of subclinical varicoceles.

b. Testicular microlithiasis are noted in 3% of subfertile men but are not thought to be a precursor for testicular cancer.

c. Testicular germ cell tumors are more common in men with infertility, and a screening ultrasound is recommended when there is any concern on physical examination.

d. Abdominal ultrasonography is indicated in men with unilateral absence of the vas deferens or CBAVD that is not associated with CFTR mutation due to an increased incidence of upper tract anomalies.

e. Venography is the gold standard for the diagnosis of varicocele and is usually performed at the time of venous embolization.

23. Late maturation arrest (MA) is characterized by:

a. the presence of only Sertoli cells and Leydig cells in the biopsy tissue.

b. elevated FSH and LH levels.

c. presence of elongated spermatids in the seminiferous tubules.

d. patients with normal sperm counts.

e. small testis size.

24. All of the following statements are true regarding azoospermia EXCEPT:

a. Pretesticular etiologies of azoospermia are usually endocrine in nature.

b. Testicular cause of azoospermia is also known as primary testis failure.

c. Secondary testis failure is characterized by high serum gonadotropin levels and small testis size.

d. Post-testicular causes constitute 40% of cases of azoospermia.

e. Low-volume azoospermia with normal testis size and palpable vas is a common presentation for testicular failure.

25. All of the following statements are true regarding semen abnormalities in infertility EXCEPT:

a. Endocrinopathies are rarely observed in oligospermic males with sperm counts greater than 10 mil/mL.

b. Only 25% of males presenting for an infertility evaluation will have normal bulk semen parameters.

c. Teratospermia is a common finding and of minimal clinical significance in the absence of bizarre morphology.

d. Asthenospermia is often iatrogenic from delayed processing in the andrology laboratory.

26. The mechanism of varicocele-induced impaired spermatogenesis is thought to be:

a. heat injury from excess pooling of blood in dilated spermatic veins.

b. excess turbulent flow through dilated veins that causes a pressure injury to the testicle.

c. reflux of splenic metabolites, which is directly gonadotoxic.

d. higher testosterone levels in the peritesticular vasculature, which inhibit spermatogenesis.

e. a lower degree of oxidative stress due to excessive venous pooling.

27. Indications for varicocelectomy include all of the following EXCEPT:

a. a clinical varicocele in a male with known infertility.

b. adolescent males with ipsilateral testis size reduction of 20% compared with the contralateral testis.

c. dull ipsilateral scrotal pain.

d. a subclinical varicocele in a patient with abnormal semen parameters.

e. a clinical varicocele in an infertility patient with an elevated DNA fragmentation index.

28. Which of the following is TRUE regarding outcomes for varicocele ligation?

a. An average increase in motility by 20%

b. Improved semen parameters in about two thirds of patients

c. Improvement in semen parameters in men with genetic infertility (e.g., Y-chromosome microdeletion)

d. Spontaneous fertilization rates of 75%

e. No improvement in semen parameters in azoospermic patients

29. Which of the following is TRUE regarding the effect of cryptorchidism in male infertility?

a. The literature does not support improved fertility with early orchiopexy.

b. Mechanisms for cryptorchid-induced testis failure include testicular dysgenesis, impaired endocrine axis, immunologic damage, and obstruction.

c. These patients often have low FSH levels and small testes.

d. Both unilateral and bilateral cryptorchidism have equivalent effects on male fertility.

e. The level of the cryptorchid testis is not predictive of spermatogenic impairment.

30. An azoospermic male presents for evaluation of infertility. He has small testes bilaterally and gynecomastia. Of note, he tells you that he works at a pet store cleaning the dog kennel because he does not notice the smell. The best treatment for his infertility is:

    a. testosterone replacement.

    b. clomiphene.

    c. bromocriptine.

    d. gonadotropins.

    e. pseudoephedrine hydrochloride.

31. A 21-year-old male comes into your clinic for advice regarding his fertility potential. He states that in his childhood, he was always the tallest in his class. However, he stopped growing halfway through middle school. On physical examination, he is noted to have a large penis. Which of the following is the correct statement regarding his fertility potential?

    a. He may recover spermatogenesis if he starts treatment with gonadotropins.

    b. He is likely to cause a pregnancy with or without treatment with corticosteroids.

    c. He needs an MRI of the head to accurately diagnose the pituitary lesion.

    d. Exogenous testosterone should be given to the patient to support spermatogenesis.

    e. He will need to be catheterized after an ejaculation and have that sperm used for intrauterine insemination.

32. A 32-year-old male presents to your clinic with new-onset erectile dysfunction. As part of your detailed history he informed you that he has been having some difficulty with his vision for the past 6 months and does not feel safe driving anymore. Optimal treatment for this patient is:

    a. cabergoline.

    b. testosterone.

    c. gonadotropins.

    d. pseudoephedrine hydrochloride.

    e. bromocriptine.

33. A 21-year-old male presents to your office for an infertility evaluation after his wife's reproductive endocrinologist ordered a semen analysis that demonstrated azoospermia. His past medical history is unremarkable except that the onset of puberty was at the age of 16. On physical examination, the patient is a tall and slender male with 4 mL testes bilaterally. Which of the following statements is TRUE?

    a. Most of these patients have a mosaic genetic pattern.

    b. This patient's condition is a rare genetic cause of nonobstructive azoospermia.

    c. He is at higher risk for breast and testicular cancer.

    d. Successful sperm retrieval is impossible in these patients.

    e. Advanced paternal age is a risk factor for this condition.

34. Which of the following is TRUE regarding Y-linked microdeletion?

    a. The AZF region is located on the Yq portion of the Y-chromosome.

    b. AZFa deletions are common in patients with nonobstructive azoospermia.

    c. Isolated microdeletions of regions of the AZFb region are the norm.

    d. Patients with AZFc microdeletions may have sperm in the ejaculate.

    e. MicroTESE is often successful in patients with AZFa microdeletion.

35. A 38-year-old male presents to your clinic for evaluation of primary infertility and azoospermia. The patient was adopted and does not know his family history. When questioning his sexual history, he states that when he ejaculates, it is usually a small amount, but he thought that was normal for him. He has normal-sized testes, and a rectal examination demonstrates a normal prostate with no midline cyst. On TRUS, small atretic seminal vesicles are seen. His FSH and testosterone levels are normal. Which of the following is TRUE regarding his infertility?

    a. A scrotal ultrasound is necessary for the diagnosis.

    b. A testicular biopsy will usually demonstrate maturation arrest.

    c. Eighty percent of these patients have a mutation on the CFTR gene on chromosome 9.

    d. Genetic counseling is usually not necessary in these patients.

    e. Optimal management of these patients involves sperm harvesting and ICSI.

36. All of the following statements are true regarding ejaculatory dysfunction in patients with spinal cord injuries EXCEPT:

    a. Blood pressure monitoring and preparation with sublingual nifedipine are important in patients prone to autonomic dysreflexia.

    b. Penile vibratory stimulation (PVS) is a reliable means of sperm retrieval in patients with incomplete spinal cord lesions above T12.

    c. Electroejaculation (EEJ) is usually reserved for patients who fail a trial of PVS.

    d. Sigmoidoscopy is performed both before and after EEJ to check for preexisting rectal injuries or injuries related to the procedure itself.

    e. Catheterization and instillation of a sperm-friendly media into the bladder are often performed to improve sperm survival in the bladder.

37. Which of the following is TRUE regarding empiric therapy of male infertility?

    a. Aromatase inhibitor therapy will decrease testosterone-to-estradiol ratios after 3 months of treatment.

    b. Treatment of idiopathic infertility with gonadotropins has been shown to increase pregnancy rates by 50%.

    c. Clomiphene therapy is superior to tamoxifen at improving sperm counts in patients with idiopathic infertility.

    d. Empiric treatment with antioxidants in men with elevated DNA fragmentation index will improve fragmentation rates and ICSI-derived pregnancy.

    e. All patients with idiopathic infertility should be treated with a 6-month course of letrozole.

ANSWERS

1. **d. 1 year of regular, unprotected intercourse.** The American Society of Reproductive Medicine classically defines infertility as the absence of conception after 12 months of regular, unprotected intercourse.

2. **b. 20%.** Another 30% involves both a male and a female factor. This underlies the importance of a male evaluation in couples with infertility.

3. **d. history of mumps orchitis before puberty.** Prepubertal mumps orchitis has minimal effects on fertility and would thus not be considered a significant male risk factor for infertility. All of the other choices represent appropriate indications for a male infertility evaluation.

4. **b. Secondary infertility indicates prior conception with the current or previous partner.** Primary infertility, on the other hand, is defined as infertility without any history of conception. Optimal sexual frequency is every other day near the time of ovulation, maximizing the opportunity of viable sperm to encounter the oocyte; more frequent intercourse does not allow replenishment of adequate numbers of spermatozoa within the epididymis. Ovulation kits are able to predict ovulation by measuring midcycle LH surge. Baseline pregnancy rates for fertile couples are between 20% and 25% per month.

5. **a. KY jelly.** KY jelly and many other commonly used vaginal lubricants adversely affect sperm motility, and some may be spermicidal. Couples attempting to conceive should avoid using vaginal lubricants or use the minimal amount possible. Natural lubricants such as those listed have a less potent effect on sperm motility.

6. **d. ciprofloxacin.** Of the listed antibiotics, all are known to be directly spermatotoxic with the exception of ciprofloxacin.

7. **d. Cimetidine inhibits androgen production.** Androgen production is inhibited by spironolactone, ketoconazole, and cimetidine. Sulfalazine is known to cause a reversible reduction in sperm concentration and motility. α Blockers in general (and tamsulosin in particular) are known to cause retrograde ejaculation. 5-α reductase inhibitors cause a reduction in semen volume, as well as erectile and ejaculatory dysfunction. Finally, marijuana is known to cause a reduction in testosterone levels and decreased sperm count with seminal leukocytes.

8. **b. The normal adult testis volume is 20 mL.** Diagnosis of CBAVD is made by physical examination alone. A grade 2 varicocele is one that is palpable in the standing position without valsalva. Midline cysts on rectal exam may be a cause of ejaculatory duct obstruction.

9. **c. Coitus interruptus is an accurate and reliable method of obtaining semen.** Often the initial drops of ejaculate that are lost contain the largest concentration of spermatozoa.

10. **e. The Endtz test is used to differentiate nonsperm round cells in semen between white blood cells and immature germ cells.** It is a useful assay to indicate the presence and degree of leukocytospermia and potent source of oxidative stress in seminal plasma. A small degree of sperm agglutination is normal according to WHO criteria. Normal sperm count is considered greater than 20 million sperm per milliliter. Antisperm abnormalities usually manifest themselves as abnormal sperm agglutination. The acrosome usually compromises 40% to 70% of the head area.

11. **c. A normal result is 5 progressively motile sperm per HPF in the cervical mucus.** A normal result for a postcoital test is greater than 10 to 20 progressively motile sperm/HPF in the cervical mucus. Most men with glanular or distal hypospadias will have a normal PCT; however, some men with midshaft or more proximal hypospadias may have an abnormal result.

12. **c. An acrosome reaction test may be useful in patients with severe teratospermia and round-headed sperm.** The test checks for the presence and activity of the acrosome. The acrosome makes up the majority of the volume of the sperm head. Two important enzymes in acrosome function include acrosin and hyaluronidase. But the acrosome reaction test and the SPA have minimal clinical significance. Shaking sperm in a PCT classically indicates antisperm antibodies. Successful penetration in a SPA is tested by swollen sperm heads within the oocyte cytoplasm.

13. **b. Indirect ASA testing is only done in females.** Indirect ASA testing detects antibodies in the serum and may be clinically relevant in females (such as in the case of shaking sperm on a PCT) or as a test for the detection of antibodies in males.

14. **d. acceptable normal values of ASA by WHO standards are less than 40%.** Acceptable normal values by 1992 WHO standards include less than 10% by IgG (mixed antiglobulin reaction) and 20% by immunobead test.

15. **b. High levels of ROS are an independent marker of male factor infertility.** ROS has been shown to be an independent marker for male infertility in leukocytospermic samples. ROS is associated with DNA damage and may demonstrate as morphologic abnormalities in routine semen analysis.

16. **e. vaginal lubricants.** All the other choices are associated with elevated DNA fragmentation index.

17. **a. DNA damage is correlated positively with poor semen parameters, especially low sperm concentration and low sperm motility, leukocytospermia, and oxidative stress.** DFI is correlated with oligoasthenospermia and elevated ROS. A cutoff of 30% in in-vivo DFI is associated with a decrease in in-vivo fertilization rates. DFI is actually lower in testicular sperm compared with ejaculated sperm; thus the use of intratesticular sperm in patients with elevated DFI is recommended for ICSI. DFI has not been definitively shown to be causative for idiopathic infertility.

18. **e. premature ejaculation.** Whereas previously all men presenting with male infertility underwent an endocrine evaluation, these are now usually performed in men with a specific indication. With the exception of premature ejaculation, all of the other choices are an indication to perform an endocrine evaluation in a patient with male infertility.

19. **a. testosterone and FSH.** Although not universally agreed on, a reasonable progression of hormone analysis would be a morning testosterone and FSH, and if these were abnormal, one should repeat morning testosterone, LH, and prolactin (especially in low testosterone).

20. **b. Genetic testing with karyotype and Y-chromosome microdeletion is indicated for all patients with azoospermia or severe oligospermia.** Genetic abnormalities are rare in men with infertility; however, 10% to 15% of azoospermic men will have a karyotype abnormality. In addition, 10% to 15% of men with azoospermia or severe oligospermia may have microdeletions of the Y-chromosome in addition. CFTR mutations are found in 80% of men with CBAVD.

21. **b. EJDO will often present with low-volume azoospermia,** with an acidic pH usually reflecting only prostatic secretions. Occasional sperm may be present in seminal vesicles on men without EJDO, but findings of 3 or more sperm/HPF in the seminal vesicle usually indicate EJDO.

22. **a. Scrotal ultrasound is recommended for the diagnosis and potential treatment of subclinical varicoceles.** Treatment of subclinical varicoceles currently has no role in the management of male infertility. The other statements are correct regarding imaging and male infertility.

23. **c. presence of elongated spermatids in the seminiferous tubules.** Patients with maturation arrest usually have severe oligospermia or azoospermia and classically have gonadotropin levels within the normal range and normal testes size. Early versus late maturation arrest is usually distinguished by the presence of elongated spermatids.

24. **e. Low-volume azoospermia with normal testis size and palpable vas is a common presentation for testicular failure.** Patients with testis failure typically have normal-volume azoospermia and small testis size. The other statements are all true.

25. **b. Only 25% of males presenting for an infertility evaluation will have normal bulk semen parameters.** Over 50% of males presenting for a male infertility evaluation will have normal bulk semen parameters, underlying the importance of an accurate history to detect any other occult female factors or other issues that may be responsible for the lack of conception.

26. **a. heat injury from excess pooling of blood in dilated spermatic veins.** Although there is considerable debate on the issue, varicocele-induced spermatotoxicity is thought to be due to elevated intrascrotal temperature, although the true etiology is likely multifactorial.

27. **d. a subclinical varicocele in a patient with abnormal semen parameters.** Repair of subclinical varicoceles has no role currently in the management of male infertility.

28. **b. Improved semen parameters in about two thirds of patients**. Although varicocele repair may return sperm to the ejaculate in azoospermia, there is no benefit in males with genetic azoospermia. Improvements are reported to be around 10 mil/mL in sperm concentration, 10% motility improvement, and WHO morphology increases of 3%.

29. **b. Mechanisms for cryptorchid-induced testis failure include testicular dysgenesis, impaired endocrine axis, immunologic damage, and obstruction.** The literature does suggest some modest improvement in fertility with early orchiopexy before the age of 4. Men with unilateral orchiopexy have minimal effects on fertility with paternity rates similar to age-matched controls. The level of the cryptorchid testis is usually associated with the degree of spermatogenic impairment.

30. **d. gonadotropins.** This is a classic presentation of Kallman syndrome, associated with hypogonadotropic hypogonadism and midline facial defects, as well as anosmia. Appropriate treatment is gonadotropin replacement.

31. **b. He is likely to cause a pregnancy with or without treatment with corticosteroids.** The clinical presentation of congenital adrenal hyperplasia is variable, the most severe of which presents neonatally with excessive virilization and salt-wasting. Milder forms may present later in adolescence with early puberty, advanced skeletal maturation, and excessive phallic enlargement. In a small series of these patients, 60% of men were able to cause pregnancies with or without treatment with corticosteroids.

32. **a. cabergoline.** Although bromocriptine is an appropriate therapy for hyperprolactinemia, cabergoline has a longer half-life allowing for more infrequent dosing and improved side effect profile without compromising therapeutic efficacy.

33. **e. Advanced paternal age is a risk factor for this condition.** Klinefelter syndrome is the most common cause of genetic nonobstructive azoospermia. Advancing paternal age is associated with higher rates of XY sperm and higher probability of KS offspring. These men are at higher risk for breast cancer, extragonadal mediastinal germ cell tumors, and non-Hodgkin lymphoma. With advanced microTESE techniques, sperm retrieval is possible in 69% of these patients.

34. **d. Patients with AZFc microdeletions may have sperm in the ejaculate.** Men with AZFc microdeletion may have severe oligospermia. Thus all men with severe oligospermia should get genetic testing including screening for Y-chromosome microdeletions. AZFa deletions are rare, and AZFb deletions usually occur along with microdeletions of the AZFc segment as well. MicroTESE is not recommended in males with AZFa microdeletions because the success of sperm retrieval is extremely small.

35. **e. Optimal management of these patients involves sperm harvesting and ICSI.** This patient has CBAVD. Eighty percent of patients with CBAVD have mutations on the *CFTR* gene on chromosome 7. Genetic counseling is necessary for these patients. Spermatogenesis is maintained as a rule, and sperm harvest with IVF is usually the appropriate treatment for these patients.

36. **b. Penile vibratory stimulation (PVS) is a reliable means of sperm retrieval in patients with incomplete spinal cord lesions above T12.** PVS is usually a reliable means of sperm retrieval in patients with complete spinal cord lesions above T10. The rest of the statements are true regarding neurogenic ejaculatory dysfunction.

37. **d. Empiric treatment with antioxidants in men with elevated DNA fragmentation index will improve fragmentation rates and ICSI-derived pregnancy.** Empiric medical treatment of male infertility in men with idiopathic infertility is a controversial subject with few randomized data demonstrating benefit. However, antioxidant therapy has been shown to improve DNA fragmentation index and is recommended in men attempting to conceive.

Additional Study Points

1. Sixty to seventy-five percent of couples will conceive within 6 months of unprotected intercourse. Ninety percent will conceive by 1 year.
2. Human spermatogenesis requires 64 days to complete with an additional 5 to 10 days of epididymal transit time.
3. Sperm will survive between 2 and 5 days in favorable cervical mucus. Therefore the frequency of intercourse during the time of ovulation should be every 2 days.
4. Mesh hernia repairs can induce a dense fibroblastic reaction and may cause vas occlusion.
5. Varicoceles are present in 15% of normal males and in 19% to 41% of males presenting with primary infertility.
6. Varicoceles on the right side that do not decompress in the supine position require studies to rule out retroperitoneal pathology.
7. Because secretions of the seminal vesicles are alkaline and have a high fructose content, an acidic pH and the absence of fructose in semen indicate absence of the vas or seminal vesicles in an azoospermic individual.
8. Sperm motility is recognized as the most important predictor of the functional aspect of spermatozoa.
9. The ENDTZ test is used to identify leukocytes.
10. α-Glucosidase is a specific marker for epididymal function.
11. Large quantities of sperm are not normally present in the seminal vesicles.
12. Testicular microlithiasis is common and does not represent an increased risk for germ cell tumor development, nor does it necessitate continued surveillance.
13. Germinal cell aplasia is found in 20% to 40% of inguinal testes and 90% of intra-abdominal testes.

Surgical Management of Male Infertility

Marc Goldstein, MD, DSc (Hon)

QUESTIONS

1. Which of the following venous structures are intentionally preserved during varicocelectomy?
   a. External spermatic veins
   b. Internal spermatic veins
   c. Gubernacular veins
   d. Deferential (vasal) veins
   e. Cremasteric veins

2. In the evaluation for vasectomy reversal, which clinical finding is suggestive of epididymal obstruction?
   a. Varicocele
   b. Hydrocele
   c. Sperm granuloma
   d. Normal serum follicle-stimulating hormone (FSH) level
   e. Vasal gap larger than 2 cm

3. Which of the following is NOT an indication for crossed vasovasostomy?
   a. Right: inguinal vas obstruction and normal testis
      Left: patent vas and atrophic testis
   b. Right: epididymal obstruction, patent vas, and normal testis
      Left: ejaculatory duct obstruction and normal testis
   c. Right: inguinal vas obstruction and normal testis
      Left: epididymal obstruction, patent vas, and normal testis
   d. Right: epididymal obstruction and patent vas above vasectomy site
      Left: sperm in testicular end of vas and vasectomy site in convoluted vas
   e. Right: congenital absence of epididymis and normal patent vas
      Left: normal testis and partial absence of vas ending retroperitoneally

4. Compared with the other surgical options for varicocelectomy, the advantages of performing a subinguinal microsurgical varicocelectomy include all of the following EXCEPT:
   a. lower rate of arterial injury.
   b. lower rate of postoperative hydrocele.
   c. lower rate of varicocele recurrence.
   d. fewer number of veins ligated.
   e. lower overall complication rate.

5. Which maneuvers should be avoided when bridging a large vasal gap during vasovasostomy?
   a. Mobilization of the vas deferens toward the external inguinal ring
   b. Dissection of the sheath of the convoluted vas deferens off the epididymis and allowing the testis to drop upside down
   c. Separation of the cauda and corpus epididymis from the testis
   d. Mobilization of the vas deferens toward the internal inguinal ring
   e. Unraveling of the convoluted vas deferens

6. In which of the following scenarios is a testis biopsy least helpful?
   a. Failure to retrieve motile sperm from the epididymis
   b. Sperm retrieval for nonobstructive azoospermia
   c. Diagnostic evaluation of men with congenital absence of vas and normal FSH levels
   d. Diagnostic evaluation in azoospermic men with normal findings on scrotal examination and normal serum testosterone and FSH levels
   e. Sperm retrieval for men diagnosed with Sertoli cell–only pattern in the testes

7. Which of the following scenarios has the lowest rate for sperm return to ejaculate after vasectomy reversal?
   a. Motile sperm in the vas and vasovasostomy
   b. Nonmotile sperm in the vas and vasovasostomy
   c. Motile sperm in the vas and unilateral crossed vasovasostomy
   d. Thick, white vasal fluid devoid of sperm and vasovasostomy
   e. Copious clear vasal fluid but no sperm and vasovasostomy

8. In the evaluation for azoospermia, all of the following tests should be considered to confirm a diagnosis of obstructive azoospermia EXCEPT:
   a. transrectal ultrasonography.
   b. testicular biopsy.
   c. serum antisperm antibody assay.
   d. epididymal biopsy.
   e. serum testosterone and FSH assay.

9. Which of the following is TRUE regarding varicocele?

   a. Treatment in infertile men rarely results in improved semen parameters.

   b. Severity of testicular insult is related to the size of the varicoceles.

   c. Severity of testicular insult from varicocele is duration independent.

   d. Because of the severity of testicular insult, repair of large varicoceles is not warranted.

   e. Surgical treatment of subclinical varicoceles results in greater improvement in semen quality than treatment of large varicoceles.

10. After a bilateral vasoepididymostomy, a patient remained azoospermic in two semen analyses until 6 months postoperative, when the analysis revealed 8 million sperm/mL with 60% motility. What is the next management step?

    a. A plan for intrauterine insemination with ejaculated sperm

    b. A plan for assisted reproduction with intracytoplasmic sperm injection (ICSI) and ejaculated sperm

    c. Cryopreservation of semen

    d. No follow-up necessary

    e. Scrotal ultrasound

11. Which of the following is a disadvantage of the intussusception vasoepididymostomy?

    a. Inability to assess epididymal fluid for sperm before setting up for anastomosis

    b. Lower patency rate than end-to-side techniques

    c. Difficult hemostasis

    d. Placement of sutures into a collapsed epididymal tubule

    e. Transection of the epididymis required before anastomosis

12. All of the following situations are appropriate for assisted reproduction with ICSI as a first line of treatment EXCEPT:

    a. obstruction with multiple failures of reconstruction.

    b. mild oligoasthenospermia with varicoceles and a female partner of 29 years of age.

    c. Klinefelter syndrome.

    d. only a few viable sperm found in the ejaculate.

    e. postchemotherapy azoospermia.

13. In which of the following settings are vasovasostomy and vasoepididymostomy contraindicated?

    a. Previous vasectomy more than 20 years ago

    b. Concomitant scrotal pain

    c. Concomitant hydrocele

    d. Concomitant varicoceles

    e. Nonobstructive azoospermia

14. In the presence of epididymal obstruction, which of the following statements is FALSE?

    a. The quality of sperm is better in caput than caudal tubules.

    b. Vasoepididymostomy to the caudal tubules has a better patency rate than to the caput tubules.

    c. Vasovasostomy can yield a satisfactory patency rate.

   d. A scrotal sonogram may demonstrate epididymal fullness and hydrocele.

   e. Intraoperative sperm cryopreservation is possible.

15. Which of the following statements is FALSE regarding microsurgical testicular sperm extraction?

    a. Sertoli cell–only pattern is a contraindication for the procedure.

    b. Large seminiferous tubules typically give a higher sperm yield.

    c. It is best performed percutaneously.

    d. It can better preserve the blood supply to testis parenchyma than a nonmicrosurgical wound.

    e. It should be used in men with nonobstructive azoospermia.

16. All of the following are expected outcomes of varicocele repair EXCEPT:

    a. improved sperm motility.

    b. increased risk of multiple gestation.

    c. improved sperm counts.

    d. elevated serum testosterone levels.

    e. return of sperm to the ejaculate in azoospermic men.

17. A 30-year-old man presenting with primary infertility was found to be azoospermic on two semen analyses. For which of the following findings is a diagnostic biopsy indicated?

    a. Ejaculate volume below 2 mL with negative fructose

    b. Semen pH less than 7.2

    c. Palpable vasa, normal serum FSH, normal testis volume, and negative antisperm antibodies

    d. Serum FSH of 25 IU/L and 12-mL soft testis

    e. Absence of vasa deferentia and normal serum FSH level

18. In which of the following scenarios is a vasogram indicated?

    a. Azoospermia, Sertoli cell only on testis biopsy

    b. Azoospermia, testicular volume of 10 mL, FSH value 25 IU/L

    c. Azoospermia, normal testicular volume, biopsy revealing active spermatogenesis

    d. Azoospermia, no palpable vasa deferential

    e. Sperm count 5 mil/mL, 5% motility, grade 2 varicoceles bilaterally

19. All of the following diagnoses can be made from a radiocontrast vasogram EXCEPT:

    a. inguinal vasal obstruction.

    b. ejaculatory duct obstruction.

    c. seminal vesicle agenesis.

    d. spermatogenic failure.

    e. partial agenesis of vasa deferentia.

20. All of the following are potential complications of transurethral resection of the ejaculatory ducts EXCEPT:

    a. urinary incontinence.

    b. retrograde ejaculation.

    c. recurrent epididymitis.

    d. testicular atrophy.

    e. contamination of semen with urine.

21. What is the pathogenesis of postvaricocelectomy hydrocele?
    a. Increased testicular venous pressure
    b. Lymphatic obstruction
    c. Soft tissue fibrosis
    d. Arterial injury
    e. Catch-up growth of testes

22. Which of the following is TRUE regarding the ejaculatory duct?
    a. It is a single midline duct formed by the confluence of the seminal vesicle ducts.
    b. It enters into the middle of the verumontanum.
    c. It joins with the prostatic ducts.
    d. It is a paired duct formed by the confluence of each seminal vesicle duct and vasa deferentia.
    e. It enters directly into the vesicle trigone.

23. All of the following are potential complications of vasography EXCEPT:
    a. vasal obstruction at the site of vasography.
    b. perivasal hematoma.
    c. sperm granuloma at the site of vasography.
    d. injury to the vasal artery.
    e. retrograde ejaculation.

24. What is the estimated percentage of men who develop antisperm antibodies after vasectomy?
    a. 0% to 20%
    b. 20% to 40%
    c. 40% to 60%
    d. 60% to 80%
    e. 80% to 100%

25. Intraoperatively during a vasectomy reversal, a sperm granuloma is found on the left side. What does this indicate?
    a. Concomitant epididymal obstruction that requires a vasoepididymostomy
    b. Infection requiring postoperative antibiotics
    c. The need for genetic counseling
    d. That sperm will be found at the testicular end of the vas
    e. That the procedure should be abandoned and the patient should undergo re-exploration in 3 months

26. When is the best time to perform vasography?
    a. At the time of diagnostic testis biopsy
    b. At the time of reconstruction if a prior testis biopsy result was normal
    c. At the time of scrotal ultrasonography with color flow Doppler
    d. At the time of transrectal ultrasonography revealing normal seminal vesicles
    e. At the time of electroejaculation

27. Twelve years after vasectomy, a man was found on routine examination to have asymptomatic sperm granulomas bilaterally. All of the following scenarios are true EXCEPT:
    a. Microrecanalization is possible with the appearance of rare sperm in the ejaculate.

    b. If vasectomy reversal is performed, only bilateral vasovasostomy is likely to be necessary.
    c. The epididymides are unlikely to be indurated.
    d. The epididymides are likely to be obstructed.
    e. No treatment is necessary for asymptomatic sperm granuloma.

28. A midline cyst compressing the ejaculatory duct is found on a transrectal ultrasonographic scan. What does the presence of sperm in the cyst aspirate suggest?
    a. Congenital absence of vas on at least one side
    b. Nonobstructive azoospermia
    c. Bilateral epididymal obstruction
    d. The possibility of XXY karyotype
    e. Patency of a vas deferens and epididymis on at least one side

29. After transurethral resection of the ejaculatory ducts, the patient develops retrograde ejaculation. What is the next step of management?
    a. Watchful waiting
    b. Intrauterine insemination
    c. ICSI
    d. A trial of pseudoephedrine
    e. Electroejaculation

30. One year after vasovasostomy, a progressive decline in sperm motility and sperm counts is noted. What does this indicate?
    a. Progressive spermatogenic failure
    b. Infection
    c. Arterial injury to the testis and epididymis
    d. Ejaculatory duct obstruction
    e. Stricture of the vasovasostomy

31. In which of the following scenarios would a diagnostic testicular biopsy provide valuable clinical information?
    a. Men with azoospermia, atrophic testes, and an FSH level of 25 IU/L
    b. Men with a 47 XXY karyotype
    c. Men with a fecundity history who seek vasectomy reversal
    d. Men with primary infertility, azoospermia, normal physical examination findings, and a normal serum FSH level
    e. Men with anejaculation caused by high spinal cord injury

32. Which of the following is TRUE regarding retractile testes in adults?
    a. As in the pediatric population, surgical repair is never indicated.
    b. A dartos pouch operation is the treatment of choice.
    c. Simple three-stitch orchiopexy of the tunica albuginea to the dartos, as for torsion prophylaxis, is effective in preventing retraction.
    d. Bilateral orchiopexy is necessary for unilateral retractile testis.
    e. Torsion of the testis is a common complication.

33. Which of the following is TRUE regarding vasoepididymostomy?
    a. End-to-side anastomosis currently has the highest patency rate.
    b. Microsurgical technique does not significantly improve the surgical outcome.
    c. Assisted reproduction with ICSI is a more cost-effective option.
    d. It should be reserved for azoospermia patients with spermatogenic arrest.
    e. It should be performed only to an epididymal tubule containing sperm.

34. When a vasoepididymostomy is performed for fertility reasons, which of the following should be routinely done in the same setting?
    a. Intraoperative epididymal sperm aspiration for sperm cryopreservation
    b. Testicular biopsy for sperm cryopreservation
    c. A touch preparation of testicular tissue
    d. A squash preparation of testicular tissue
    e. A radiocontrast vasogram

35. Which of the following is the most important factor in ensuring a high patency rate after a vasovasostomy?
    a. Age of the patient
    b. Time since vasectomy
    c. Surgeon's technique and experience
    d. Presence of motile sperm in the vasal fluid
    e. Presence of a sperm granuloma at the vasectomy site

36. Which of the following surgical sperm retrieval techniques is inappropriate for the clinical situation indicated?
    a. PESA for congenital absence of vas
    b. Percutaneous testicular sperm aspiration (TESA) after failed vasoepididymostomy
    c. Electroejaculation in a man with postretroperitoneal lymph node dissection for left testicular embryonal carcinoma
    d. Microsurgical epididymal sperm aspiration (MESA) for spermatogenic maturation arrest
    e. Testicular sperm extraction (TESE) in a man with azoospermia from chemotherapy

ANSWERS

1. **d. Deferential (vasal) veins.** All veins within the cord, with the exception of the vasal veins, are doubly ligated. Scrotal or gubernacular collateral veins have been demonstrated radiographically to be the cause of 10% of recurrent varicoceles. All external spermatic veins are identified and doubly ligated with hemoclips and divided. The gubernaculum is inspected for the presence of veins exiting from the tunica vaginalis. These are either cauterized or doubly ligated.

2. **b. Hydrocele.** The presence of a hydrocele in the presence of excurrent ductal system obstruction is often associated with secondary epididymal obstruction. Surgeons attempting reconstruction should be aware of the possibility of the need for a vasoepididymostomy.

3. **d. Right: epididymal obstruction, patent vas above vasectomy site, and normal testis; Left: sperm in testicular end vas and vasectomy site in convoluted vas.** Crossover is indicated in the following circumstances: (1) unilateral inguinal obstruction of the vas deferens associated with an atrophic testis on the contralateral side. A crossover vasovasostomy should be performed to connect a healthy testicle to the contralateral unobstructed vas. (2) Obstruction or aplasia of the inguinal vas or ejaculatory duct on one side and epididymal obstruction on the contralateral side. It is preferable to perform one anastomosis with a high probability of success (vasovasostomy) than two operations with a much lower chance of success such as unilateral vasoepididymostomy and contralateral transurethral resection of the ejaculatory ducts.

4. **d. fewer number of veins ligated.** At the subinguinal level, significantly more veins are encountered, the artery is more often surrounded by a network of tiny veins that must be ligated, and the testicular artery has often divided into two or three branches, making arterial identification and preservation more difficult without using a microscope for the procedure.

5. **e. Unraveling of the convoluted vas deferens.** When large vasal gaps are present, a gauze-wrapped index finger is used to bluntly separate the cord structures from the vas. Blunt finger dissection through the external ring will free the vas to the internal ring if additional abdominal side length is necessary. These maneuvers will leave all the vasal vessels intact. When the vasal gap is extremely large, additional length can be achieved by dissecting the entire convoluted vas free of its attachments to the epididymal tunica, allowing the testis to drop upside down. If the amount of the vas removed is so large that even these measures fail to allow a tension-free anastomosis, the incision can be extended to the internal inguinal ring, the floor of the inguinal canal cut, and the vas rerouted under the floor, as in a difficult orchiopexy. An additional 4 to 6 cm of length can be obtained by dissecting the epididymis off of the testis from the vasoepididymal junction to the caput epididymis. The superior epididymal vessels are left intact and provide adequate blood supply to the testicular end of the vas. With this combination of maneuvers, gaps up to 10 cm wide can be bridged. The convoluted vas should not be unraveled. This disturbs the blood supply at the anastomotic line.

6. **c. Diagnostic evaluation of men with congenital absence of vas and normal FSH levels.** Testis biopsy is indicated in azoospermic men with testes of normal size and consistency, palpable vasa deferentia, and normal serum FSH levels. Under these circumstances, biopsy will distinguish obstructive azoospermia from primary seminiferous tubular failure. In the testes of men with congenital absence of vasa, biopsy always reveals normal or at least some spermatogenesis and biopsy is not necessary before definitive sperm aspiration and in-vitro fertilization (IVF) with ICSI.

7. **d. Thick, white vasal fluid devoid of sperm and vasovasostomy.** If the fluid expressed from the vas is found to be thick, white, water insoluble, and like toothpaste in quality, microscopic examination rarely reveals sperm. Under these circumstances, the tunica

vaginalis is opened and the epididymis inspected. If clear evidence of obstruction is found (e.g., an epididymal sperm granuloma with dilated tubules above and collapsed tubules below), vasoepididymostomy is performed. When the surgeon is in doubt or is not experienced with vasoepididymostomy, vasovasostomy should be performed. However, only 15% of men with bilateral absence of sperm in the vasal fluid after barbotage and intensive search will have sperm return to the ejaculate after vasovasostomy.

8. **d. epididymal biopsy.** Before attempted surgical reconstruction of the reproductive tract, spermatogenesis in the patient should be evident. A testicular biopsy may be indicated to confirm the presence of spermatogenesis. Men with a low semen volume should have a transrectal ultrasonographic scan to alert one to the possibility of an additional ejaculatory duct obstruction. For serum and antisperm antibody studies, the presence of serum antisperm antibodies corroborates the diagnosis of obstruction and the presence of active spermatogenesis. At present, this test is of unknown prognostic value and is optional. For serum FSH assay, men with small, soft testes should have serum FSH measured. An elevated FSH level suggests impaired spermatogenesis and potentially a poorer prognosis.

9. **b. Severity of testicular insult is related to the size of the varicoceles.** Larger varicoceles appear to cause more damage than small varicoceles; large varicoceles are associated with greater preoperative impairment in semen quality than are small varicoceles.

10. **c. Cryopreservation of semen.** With the older end-to-end or end-to-side vasoepididymostomy method, at 14 months after surgery 25% of initially patent anastomoses have shut down. For this reason, we recommend banking sperm both intraoperatively and as soon as sperm appear in the ejaculate postoperatively.

11. **a. Inability to assess epididymal fluid for sperm before setting up for anastomosis.** This method, also known as the *triangulation technique,* was introduced by Berger. There are several advantages of this method over previous techniques (see Table 22–3 in *Campbell-Walsh Urology, 10ᵗʰ Edition*): Two or three sutures placed in the epididymal tubule provide four and six points of fixation, and the anastomosis is virtually bloodless. However, one cannot assess tubular fluid for sperm before the anastomosis setup.

12. **b. mild oligoasthenospermia with varicoceles and a female partner of 29 years of age.** Assisted reproduction can be offered to men with surgically unreconstructable obstruction such as congenital absence of the vas deferens; men with few viable sperm in the ejaculate; azoospermic men with varicoceles (half of these men will respond to varicocelectomy with return of enough sperm to ejaculate to achieve pregnancy using IVF with ICSI); and men with nonobstructive azoospermia.

13. **e. Nonobstructive azoospermia.** Before attempted surgical reconstruction of the reproductive tract, spermatogenesis in the patient should be evident. A prior history of natural fertility prevasectomy is usually adequate. In other cases, a testicular biopsy may be indicated to confirm the presence of spermatogenesis.

14. **c. Vasovasostomy can yield a satisfactory patency rate.** If clear evidence of obstruction is found, vasoepididymostomy is performed. When there is doubt or

the physician is not experienced with vasoepididymostomy, vasovasostomy should be performed. However, only 15% of men with bilateral absence of sperm in the vasal fluid after barbotage and an intensive search will have sperm return to the ejaculate after vasovasostomy.

15. **c. It is best performed percutaneously.** The use of an operating microscope for standard open diagnostic testes biopsy allows identification of an area in the tunica albuginea free of blood vessel, minimizing the risk of injury to the testicular blood supply and allowing a relatively blood-free biopsy specimen.

16. **b. increased risk of multiple gestation.** Varicocelectomy results in significant improvement in the findings of semen analysis in 60% to 80% of men. Reported pregnancy rates after varicocelectomy vary from 20% to 60%. A randomized controlled trial of surgery versus no surgery in infertile men with varicoceles revealed a pregnancy rate of 44% at 1 year in the surgery group versus 10% in the control group. In our series of 1500 microsurgical operations, 43% of couples were pregnant at 1 year and 69% at 2 years when couples with female factors were excluded. Microsurgical varicocelectomy results in return of sperm to the ejaculate in 50% of azoospermic men with palpable varicoceles. Repair of large varicoceles results in a significantly greater improvement in semen quality than repair of small varicoceles. In addition, large varicoceles are associated with greater preoperative impairment in semen quality than are small varicoceles, and consequently overall pregnancy rates are similar regardless of varicocele size. Some evidence suggests that the younger the patient is at the time of varicocele repair, the greater the improvement after repair and the more likely the testis is to recover from varicocele-induced injury. Varicocele recurrence, testicular artery ligation, and postvaricocelectomy hydrocele formation are often associated with poor postoperative results. In infertile men with low serum testosterone levels, microsurgical varicocelectomy alone results in substantial improvement in serum testosterone levels.

17. **c. Palpable vasa, normal serum FSH, and normal testis volume and negative antisperm antibodies.** Men with a positive antisperm antibody assay are always obstructed, and a biopsy is not necessary. Men with elevated FSH levels and small, soft testes always have nonobstructive azoospermia.

18. **c. Azoospermia, normal testicular volume, biopsy revealing active spermatogenesis.** The absolute indications for vasography are azoospermia, plus complete spermatogenesis with many mature spermatids on testis biopsy and at least one palpable vas. Relative indications for vasography are severe oligospermia with normal testis biopsy, a high level of sperm-bound antibodies that may be due to obstruction, low semen volume, and poor sperm motility (partial ejaculatory duct obstruction).

19. **d. spermatogenic failure.** Vasography should answer the questions: Are there sperm in the vasal fluid? Is the vas obstructed? If the testis biopsy reveals many sperm, then the absence of sperm in vasal fluid indicates obstruction proximal to the vasal site examined, most likely an epididymal obstruction. Vasography is done in this case with saline or indigo carmine to confirm the patency of the

seminal vesicle end of the vas before vasoepididymostomy. Copious vasal fluid containing many sperm indicates vasal or ejaculatory duct obstruction, and formal contrast vasography is performed to document the exact location of the obstruction. Copious thick, white fluid without sperm in a dilated vas indicates secondary epididymal obstruction in addition to potential vasal or ejaculatory duct obstruction.

20. **d. testicular atrophy.** Reflux of urine into the ejaculatory ducts, vas, and seminal vesicles occurs after a majority of resections. This can be documented by voiding cystourethrography or by measuring semen creatinine levels. Reflux can lead to acute and chronic epididymitis. Recurrent epididymitis often results in epididymal obstruction. The incidence of epididymitis after transurethral resection is probably underestimated. Symptomatic chemical epididymitis may occur from refluxing urine. If epididymitis is chronic and recurrent, vasectomy or even epididymectomy may be necessary. Even when care has been taken to spare the bladder neck, retrograde ejaculation is common after transurethral resection. Transurethral instrumentation can increase the risk of urethral stricture.

21. **b. Lymphatic obstruction.** Analysis of the protein concentration of hydrocele fluid indicates that hydrocele formation after varicocelectomy is due to lymphatic obstruction.

22. **d. It is a paired duct formed by the confluence of each seminal vesicle duct and vasa deferentia.** The ejaculatory ducts course between the bladder neck and the verumontanum and exit at the level of and along the lateral aspect of the verumontanum.

23. **e. retrograde ejaculation.** Complications of vasography include stricture, injury to the vasal blood supply, hematoma, and sperm granuloma. Multiple attempts at percutaneous vasography using sharp needles can result in stricture or obstruction at the vasography site. Careless or crude closure of a vasotomy can also result in stricture and obstruction. Non-water-soluble contrast agents may also result in stricture and should not be employed for vasography. If the vasal blood supply is injured at the site of vasography, vasovasostomy proximal to the vasography site may result in ischemia, necrosis, and obstruction of the intervening segment of vas. A bipolar cautery should be used for meticulous hemostasis at the time of vasostomy to prevent hematoma in the perivasal sheath. Leaky closure of a vasography site may lead to the development of a sperm granuloma, which can result in structure or obstruction of the vas.

24. **d. 60% to 80%.** Systemic effects of vasectomy have been postulated. Vasectomy disrupts the blood-testis barrier, resulting in detectable levels of serum antisperm antibodies in 60% to 80% of men. Some studies suggest that the antibody titers diminish 2 or more years after vasectomy. Others suggest that these antibody titers persist. However, neither circulating immune complexes nor deposits are increased after vasectomy.

25. **d. The sperm will be found at the testicular end of the vas.** A sperm granuloma at the testicular end of the vas suggests that sperm have been leaking at the vasectomy site. This vents the high pressures away from the epididymis and is associated with a better prognosis for restored fertility regardless of the time interval since vasectomy.

26. **b. At the time of reconstruction, if a prior testis biopsy result was normal.** There is no need to perform vasography at the time of testis biopsy for azoospermia unless immediate reconstruction is planned and the touch or wet preparation biopsy reveals mature sperm with tails. If performed carelessly, vasography can cause stricture or even obstruction at the vasography site, which can complicate subsequent reconstruction.

27. **d. The epididymides are likely to be obstructed.** Sperm granulomas form when sperm leak from the testicular end of the vas. Sperm are highly antigenic, and an intense inflammatory reaction occurs when sperm escape outside the reproductive epithelium. Sperm granulomas are rarely symptomatic. The presence or absence of a sperm granuloma at the vasectomy site seems to be of importance in modulating the local effects of chronic obstruction on the male reproductive tract. The sperm granuloma's complex network of epithelialized channels provides an additional absorptive surface that helps vent the high intraluminal pressure in the obstructed excurrent ducts. Numerous animal studies have correlated the presence or absence of sperm granuloma at the vasectomy site with the degree of epididymal and testicular damage. Species that always develop granulomas after vasectomy have minimal damage to the seminiferous tubules. Some studies of men undergoing vasectomy reversal have revealed somewhat higher success rates in men who have a sperm granuloma at the vasectomy site, whereas another large study has not. Although sperm granulomas at the vasectomy site are present microscopically in 10% to 30% of men undergoing reversal, it is likely that, given enough time, virtually all men develop sperm granulomas at the vasectomy site, the epididymis, or the rete testis. When chronic postvasectomy pain is localized to the granuloma, excision and occlusion of the vasa with intraluminal cautery usually relieve the pain and prevent recurrence. Men with postvasectomy congestive epididymitis may be relieved of pain by open-ended vasectomy designed to purposefully produce pressure, relieving sperm granuloma.

28. **e. Patency of a vas deferens and epididymis on at least one side.** The fine-needle aspirate is examined for sperm. If sperm are present, it means at least one vas and epididymis are patent.

29. **d. A trial of pseudoephedrine.** Pseudoephedrine (Sudafed), 120 mg orally 90 minutes before ejaculation, may prevent retrograde ejaculation. If this is not successful, sperm can be retrieved from alkalinized urine and used for either intrauterine insemination or IVF with ICSI.

30. **e. Stricture of the vasovasostomy.** Late stricture and obstruction are disappointingly common. Progressive loss of sperm motility followed by decreasing counts indicates stricture.

31. **d. Men with primary infertility, azoospermia, normal physical examination findings, and a normal serum FSH level.** Testis biopsy is indicated in azoospermic men with testis of normal size and consistency, palpable vasa deferentia, and normal serum FSH levels.

32. **b. A dartos pouch operation is the treatment of choice.** When scrotal orchiopexy is performed for retractile testis, a dartos pouch operation should be performed. Simple suture orchiopexy of the tunica albuginea of the testis to the dartos, such as is performed sometimes to prevent torsion, will not prevent retraction of these testes into the groin. Creation of a dartos pouch will keep the testis well down into the scrotum and permanently prevent

retraction. This is also the most reliable and safest technique for the prevention of testicular torsion.

33. **e. It should be performed only to an epididymal tubule containing sperm.** Specific treatments for male factor infertility such as microsurgical reconstruction for obstructive azoospermia and varicocelectomy for impaired testes remain the safest and most cost-effective ways of managing infertile men. Microsurgical approaches allow accurate approximation of the vasal mucosa to that of a single epididymal tubule, resulting in marked improvement in the patency and pregnancy rates. If the level of obstruction is not clearly delineated, after the buttonhole opening is made in the tunica, a 70-μm diameter tapered needle from the 10-0 nylon microsuture is used to puncture the epididymal tubule, beginning as distal as possible, and fluid is sampled from the puncture site. When sperm are found, the puncture sites are sealed with microbipolar forceps, a new buttonhole is made in the epididymal tunica just proximally, and the tubule is prepared as described previously. Patency rates with the intussusception technique can exceed 80%. With the classic end-to-side or older end-to-end method, the patency rate is about 70% and 43% of men with sperm will impregnate their wives after a minimum follow-up of 2 years.

34. **a. Intraoperative epididymal sperm aspiration for sperm cryopreservation.** Once sperm are identified, they are aspirated into glass capillary tubes and flushed into media for cryopreservation.

35. **c. Surgeon's technique and experience.** The responsibilities assumed by the surgeon demand the utmost in judgment and skill. Many of the procedures described in this chapter are among the most technically demanding in all of urology. Acquisition of the skills required to perform them demands intensive laboratory training in microsurgery and a thorough knowledge of the anatomy and physiology of the male reproductive system.

36. **d. MESA for spermatogenic maturation arrest.** MESA is indicated for men with normal spermatogenesis and unreconstructable obstruction such as congenital bilateral absence of the vas deferens.

Additional Study Points

1. If the vas is transected at two different locations, the intervening segment will likely fibrose due to lack of blood supply.
2. In repairing a hydrocele, the epididymis is often splayed and one should leave a generous border around the epididymis to avoid injuring it.
3. When sperm are retrieved before any repair, it is prudent to cryo preserve some for future use, if necessary.
4. Following vaso epididymotomy, 50% to 85% of men will have sperm in the ejaculate; about half of these men will foster a pregnancy.
5. The indications for testicular sperm extraction are failure to find sperm in the epididymis and nonobstructive azoospermia.
6. During microsurgical testicular sperm extraction, larger tubules are more likely to yield sperm.
7. About 85% of patients following vaso vasostomy will have sperm in their ejaculate; a little more than half will foster a pregnancy.

Physiology of Penile Erection and Pathophysiology of Erectile Dysfunction

Tom F. Lue, MD, ScD (Hon), FACS

QUESTIONS

1. The tunica albuginea:
   a. consists of a single layer of strong fibrous tissue, enclosing both the corpora cavernosa and the corpus spongiosum.
   b. is a bilayered structure enclosing most of the corpora cavernosa but is single layered around the entire corpus spongiosum.
   c. is commonly called the Buck fascia of the penis.
   d. consists of collagen, smooth muscle, and elastic fibers.
   e. extends all the way to the glans penis to give the glans penis a strong covering.

2. The thickness of the tunica albuginea:
   a. is the same throughout the entire penis.
   b. is less in the pendulous portion of the penis.
   c. is less at the ventral groove of the penis.
   d. remains the same during both the flaccid and the erect phases of the penis.
   e. determines the girth of the penis.

3. The following statements about the accessory pudendal artery are true EXCEPT:
   a. It may arise from the obturator artery.
   b. It may travel anterior to the prostate.
   c. It may be damaged during radical prostatectomy.
   d. It may be the dominant blood supply to the corpus cavernosum.
   e. It is present in just 10% of men.

4. The arterial supply of the corpus cavernosum is usually from the:
   a. external pudendal artery.
   b. accessory pudendal artery.
   c. cavernous artery.
   d. the dorsal artery.
   e. inferior epigastric artery.

5. The venous channels draining the corpus cavernosum:
   a. originate in the center of the corpus cavernosum
   b. originate in the emissary veins.
   c. originate in the subtunical venules.

   d. drain exclusively via the dorsal vein of the penis.
   e. drain exclusively via the cavernous vein.

6. Reduced penile venous outflow during erection is due to:
   a. active constriction of the superficial and deep dorsal veins.
   b. opening of penile arterio-venous shunts.
   c. compression of the subtunical venules and emissary veins by the tunica albuginea.
   d. active constriction of emissary veins.
   e. relaxation of the ischiocavernous muscle.

7. Penile erection involves:
   a. arterial dilation and venous constriction.
   b. relaxation of the ischiocavernous muscle.
   c. arterial dilation, venous compression, and sinusoidal relaxation.
   d. contraction of the smooth muscles within the corpus cavernosum.
   e. filling and expansion of the sinusoidal spaces by nitric oxide.

8. The innervation of the penis comes from:
   a. S2-4 spinal segments.
   b. T10-12 and S2-4 spinal segments.
   c. the dorsal nerve.
   d. the cavernous nerve.
   e. all of the above.

9. The ischiocavernous and bulbocavernous muscles are:
   a. innervated by the pudendal nerve.
   b. responsible for the rigid phase of erection.
   c. important in the expulsion of semen during ejaculation.
   d. striated muscles.
   e. all of the above.

10. Stimulation of which area of the brain has been reported to induce penile erection?
    a. Paraventricular area of the hypothalamus
    b. Midbrain raphe
    c. Substantia nigra
    d. Nucleus paragigantocellularis
    e. A 5-catecholamine cell group and locus ceruleus

11. The principal neurotransmitter mediating penile erection is:
    a. prostaglandin E 1.
    b. nitric oxide.
    c. norepinephrine.
    d. acetylcholine.
    e. neuropeptide P.

12. Of the ion channels identified on the penile smooth muscle, which two have been shown to be involved in penile erection?
    a. Sodium and chloride channels
    b. Calcium and potassium channels
    c. Titanium sodium and potassium channels
    d. Chloride and calcium channel
    e. Calcium and phosphate channels

13. The action of nitric oxide within the penile smooth muscle cell involves:
    a. activation of adenylyl cyclase and elevation of cyclic AMP.
    b. activation of phosphodiesterase type 4.
    c. opening of calcium channels resulting in elevated cytosolic calcium levels.
    d. activation of guanylyl cyclase and elevation of cyclic GMP.
    e. closure of potassium channels.

14. Which of the following molecules is involved in detumescence of the penis?
    a. Nitric oxide
    b. Phosphodiesterase type 5
    c. Phosphodiesterase type 3
    d. Acetylcholine
    e. Neuropeptide P

15. Gap junctions:
    a. are a communication between the tunica albuginea and the sinusoid space.
    b. are a communication between the glans penis and the corpora cavernosa.
    c. are a communication between the corpus cavernosum and corpus spongiosum.
    d. are a communication between intracavernous muscle cells.
    e. have similar content of the connexin 43 protein in diabetic and healthy rats.

16. Neurotransmitters involved in modulating sexual function in the brain include:
    a. epinephrine, testosterone, and prolactin.
    b. dopamine, norepinephrine, serotonin, and oxytocin.
    c. endothelin and calcitonin gene-related peptide (CGRP).
    d. vasoactive intestinal polypeptide (VIP) and acetylcholine.
    e. all of the above.

17. Apomorphine:
    a. has a strong analgesic action but is not a narcotic.
    b. is a central-acting dopamine receptor agonist.
    c. produces penile erection when injected into the corpus cavernosum.
    d. is an inhibitor of phosphodiesterase type 5 similar to sildenafil.
    e. is often used as an antiemetic.

18. Central norepinephrine transmission seems to enhance sexual function as evidenced by:
    a. clonidine, an α_2-adrenergic agonist that enhances sexual function.
    b. yohimbine, an α_2-adrenergic antagonist that enhances sexual function.
    c. intracavernous injection of phenylephrine, which produces penile erection.
    d. oral phentolamine, which enhances penile erection.
    e. intracavernous injection of papaverine, which produces penile erection.

19. The Massachusetts Male Aging Study (MMAS):
    a. reported the prevalence of erectile dysfunction (ED) in the United States is about 50% at age 50, 60% at age 60, and 70% at age 70 (including mild, moderate, and severe ED).
    b. reported the prevalence rate of severe ED remains the same, but prevalence rate of mild ED increases with age,
    c. is an MMAS hospital–based, cross-sectional survey of sexual function in men and women in the United States.
    d. surveyed more than 1700 hospitalized patients between 1995 and 1997.
    e. estimated that the incidence rate of ED is about 20 million new cases per year in the United States.

20. A 58-year-old man complained of impotence after radical prostatectomy for cancer of the prostate. Impotence after radical prostatectomy is frequently a result of injury to which of the following?
    a. The dorsal nerve of the penis
    b. The cavernous nerves
    c. The genitofemoral nerve
    d. The sympathetic ganglion
    e. The ilioinguinal nerve

21. The function of testosterone includes each of the following EXCEPT:
    a. enhances sexual interest.
    b. increases frequency of sexual acts.
    c. increases the frequency of nocturnal erections but has little or no effect on fantasy or visually induced erections.
    d. maintains nitric oxide synthase (NOS) activity in the penis (in rats).
    e. prevents hair loss in men.

22. Cavernosal (Venogenic) ED is a disease of the:
    a. deep dorsal vein.
    b. emissary vein.
    c. preprostatic venous plexus.
    d. tunica albuginea or cavernous smooth muscle.
    e. internal pudendal vein.

23. Which of the following is NOT part of the normal aging process?
    a. Greater latency to erection and loss of forceful ejaculation

b. Decreased ejaculatory volume and a longer refractory period

c. Decreased frequency and duration of nocturnal erection

d. Decrease in penile tactile sensitivity

e. Complete ED

24. ED associated with diabetes can be a result of:

a. psychologic impact.

b. neurologic deficit.

c. arterial insufficiency.

d. endothelial cell dysfunction.

e. all of the above.

25. The following are proposed molecular mechanisms of diabetic ED EXCEPT:

a. impaired nitric oxide (NO) synthesis.

b. increased levels of oxygen free radicals.

c. elevated levels of advanced glycosylation end products, which quench NO.

d. selective degeneration of nitric oxide synthase–containing nerves.

e. decreased level of phosphodiesterase type 5.

26. The causes of ED in an animal model of hyperlipidemia and hypercholesterolemia include each of the following EXCEPT:

a. increased production of contractile thromboxane and prostaglandin.

b. increased production of oxytocin.

c. the contractile effect of oxidized low-density lipoprotein.

d. release of superoxide radicals.

e. increased production of NOS inhibitors.

27. Which brain area has been reported to control nocturnal penile erection?

a. Paraventricular area of the hypothalamus

b. Midbrain raphe

c. Substantia nigra

d. Nucleus paragigantocellularis

e. Lateral preoptic area

28. The following statements about endothelin are true EXCEPT:

a. It may induce relaxation or contraction dependent on receptor binding.

b. It is synthesized in the sinusoidal endothelium.

c. It is thought to play a role in maintaining the corporal smooth muscle in a semicontracted state at rest.

d. Inhibition of endothelin action by an inhibitor of the ETa receptor enhances penile erection in men with ED.

e. It works by activation of phospholipase C beta to induce IP3 production and increase intracellular calcium concentration.

29. All of the following are true about the metabolic syndrome in men EXCEPT that it:

a. has been associated with increased incidence of ED.

b. has been associated with hypogonadism.

c. occurs in association with increased peripheral adipose tissue.

d. consists of insulin resistance, obesity, hypertension, and dyslipidemia.

e. has been associated with hypoprolactinemia.

30. All of the following are branches of the common penile artery EXCEPT:

a. dorsal artery.

b. bulbourethral artery.

c. perineal artery.

d. helicine arteries.

e. cavernous artery.

ANSWERS

1. **b. is a bilayered structure enclosing most of the corpora cavernosa but is single layered around the entire corpus spongiosum.** Inner-layer bundles support and contain the cavernous tissue and are oriented circularly. Radiating from this inner layer are intracavernous pillars that act as struts to augment the septum and provide essential support to the erectile tissue. Outer-layer bundles are oriented longitudinally, extending from the glans penis to the proximal crura; they insert into the inferior pubic rami but are absent between the 5 and the 7 o'clock positions. In contrast, the corpus spongiosum lacks an outer layer or intracorporeal struts, ensuring a low-pressure structure during erection.

2. **c. is less at the ventral groove of the penis.** The strength and thickness of the tunica correlate in a statistically significant fashion with location. The most vulnerable area is located on the ventral groove (between the 5 and 7 o'clock positions), where the longitudinal outer layer is absent; most prostheses tend to extrude here, and this is where tears usually occur with fractures of the penis.

3. **e. It is present in just 10% of men.** In many instances, however, accessory arteries exist, arising from the external iliac, obturator, vesical and femoral arteries. In some men they may constitute the dominant or only arterial supply to the corpus cavernosum. In a study of 20 fresh human cadavers, Droupy and colleagues (1997)* reported three patterns of penile arterial supply: type I arising exclusively from internal pudendal arteries (3/20); type II arising from both accessory and internal pudendal arteries (14/20); and type III arising exclusively from accessory pudendal arteries (3/20). Nehra and colleagues (2008) studied 79 consecutive patients with a history of ED and noted that 35% had an accessory pudendal artery, typically arising from the obturator artery. In these men, the accessory pudendal artery was the dominant blood supply in 54% and the only corporal blood supply in 11%. The importance of accessory pudendal artery preservation during radical prostatectomy was demonstrated by Mulhall and colleagues (2008), who reported more rapid recovery of sexual function in men who underwent artery-sparing radical prostatectomy.

4. **c. cavernous artery.** The cavernous artery effects tumescence of the corpus cavernosum and enters it at the hilum of the penis, where the two crura merge. Along its course, it gives off many helicine arteries, which supply the trabecular erectile tissue and the sinusoids. These helicine

---

*Sources referenced can be found in *Campbell-Walsh Urology, 10th Edition,* on the Expert Consult website.

arteries are contracted and tortuous in the flaccid state and become dilated and straight during erection.

5. **c. originate in the subtunical venules.** The venous drainage from the three corpora originates in tiny venules leading from the peripheral sinusoids immediately beneath the tunica albuginea. These venules travel in the trabeculae between the tunica and the peripheral sinusoids to form the subtunical venous plexus before exiting as the emissary veins.

6. **c. compression of the subtunical venules and emissary veins by the tunica albuginea.** Reduced venous outflow from the corpora cavernosa involves (1) compression of the subtunical venous plexuses between the tunica albuginea and the expanded sinusoids, reducing venous outflow; (2) stretching of the tunica to its capacity, which occludes the emissary veins between the inner circular and outer longitudinal layers and further decreases venous outflow to a minimum.

7. **c. arterial dilation, venous compression, and sinusoidal relaxation.** Sexual stimulation triggers release of neurotransmitters from the cavernous nerve terminals. This results in relaxation of these smooth muscles and the following events: (1) dilation of the arterioles and arteries by increased blood flow in both the diastolic and systolic phases; (2) trapping of the incoming blood by the expanding sinusoids; (3) compression of the subtunical venous plexuses between the tunica albuginea and the peripheral sinusoids, reducing venous outflow.

8. **e. all of the above.** In humans, the T10 to T12 segments are most often the origin of the sympathetic fibers, and the chain ganglia cells projecting to the penis are located in the sacral and caudal ganglia. The parasympathetic pathway arises from neurons in the intermediolateral cell columns of the second, third, and fourth sacral spinal cord segments. The preganglionic fibers pass in the pelvic nerves to the pelvic plexus, where they are joined by the sympathetic nerves from the superior hypogastric plexus. The cavernous nerves are branches of the pelvic plexus that innervate the penis. The dorsal nerve of the penis joins other nerves to become the pudendal nerve. The latter enters the spinal cord via the S2-S4 roots to terminate on spinal neurons and interneurons in the central gray region of the lumbosacral segment. Activation of these sensory neurons sends messages of pain, temperature, and touch by means of spinothalamic and spinoreticular pathways to the thalamus and sensory cortex for sensory perception.

9. **e. all of the above.** The Onuf nucleus in the second to fourth sacral spinal segments is the center of somatomotor penile innervation. These nerves travel in the sacral nerves to the pudendal nerve to innervate the ischiocavernosus and bulbocavernosus muscles. Contraction of the ischiocavernosus muscles produces the rigid-erection phase. Rhythmic contraction of the bulbocavernosus muscle is necessary for ejaculation.

10. **a. Paraventricular area of the hypothalamus.** The erectile response induced by injection of apomorphine into the paraventricular area can be suppressed by blockers of both dopamine and oxytocin receptors. Injection of oxytocin into the paraventricular area also induces erection, but this cannot be blocked by dopamine receptor blockers. These findings suggest that dopaminergic neurons activate oxytocinergic neurons in the paraventricular area and that the release of oxytocin produces erection.

11. **b. nitric oxide.** Relaxation of the cavernous smooth muscle is the key to penile erection.
    Nitric oxide released by nNOS contained in the terminals of the cavernous nerve initiates the process.
    Upon entering the smooth muscle cells, NO stimulates the production of cyclic GMP.
    Cyclic GMP activates protein kinase G, which in turn opens the potassium channels and closes the calcium channels.
    Low cytosolic calcium favors smooth muscle relaxation.
    The smooth muscle regains its tone when cGMP is degraded by phosphodiesterase.

12. **b. Calcium and potassium channels.** The intracellular second messengers mediating smooth muscle relaxation, cAMP and cGMP, activate their specific protein kinases, which phosphorylate certain proteins to cause opening of potassium channels, closing of calcium channels, and sequestration of intracellular calcium by the endoplasmic reticulum. The resultant fall in intracellular calcium leads to smooth muscle relaxation.

13. **d. activation of guanylyl cyclase and elevation of cyclic GMP.** The most physiologically relevant receptor for NO is soluble guanylyl cyclase (sGC), and the NO-sGC-cGMP pathway is responsible for the vasorelaxing effect of many endothelium-dependent vasodilators including histamine, estrogens, insulin, corticotrophin-releasing hormone, nitrovasodilators, and acetylcholine. This pathway is also principally responsible for erection.

14. **b. Phosphodiesterase type 5.** With the exception of PDE6, which is specifically expressed in photoreceptor cells, all 10 PDEs have been identified in the corpus cavernosum. However, there is ample evidence that PDE5 is by far the principal PDE for the termination of cavernous cGMP signaling.

15. **d. are a communication between intracavernous muscle cells.** During erection and detumescence, communication should exist among cavernous smooth muscles to mediate synchronized relaxation and contraction. Several studies have demonstrated the presence of gap junctions in the membrane of adjacent muscle cells. These intercellular channels allow exchange of ions such as calcium and second-messenger molecules. The major component of gap junctions is connexin-43, a membrane-sparing protein of less than 0.25 μm that has been identified between smooth muscle cells of human corpus cavernosum. Cell-to-cell communication through these gap junctions most likely explains the synchronized erectile response, although their pathophysiologic impact is still unclear.

16. **b. dopamine, norepinephrine, serotonin, and oxytocin.** A variety of neurotransmitters (dopamine, norepinephrine, serotonin [5-HT]) and neural hormones (oxytocin, prolactin) have been implicated in regulation of sexual function. It is suggested that dopaminergic and adrenergic receptors may promote sexual function and 5-HT receptors inhibit it.

17. **b. is a central-acting dopamine receptor agonist.** Five different dopamine receptors have been cloned (D1 to D5), and several of these exist in multiple forms. In men, apomorphine, which stimulates both D1 and D2 receptors, induces erection that is unaccompanied by sexual arousal.

18. **b. yohimbine, an α₂-adrenergic antagonist that enhances sexual function.** Central norepinephrine transmission seems to have a positive effect on sexual

function. In both humans and rats, inhibition of norepinephrine release by clonidine, an α_2-adrenergic agonist, is associated with a decrease in sexual behavior, and yohimbine, an α_2-receptor antagonist, has been shown to increase sexual activity.

19. **a. reported the prevalence of ED in the United States is about 50% at age 50, 60% at age 60, and 70% at age 70 (including mild, moderate, and severe ED).** From the prevalence rates reported in the MMAS study, between the ages of 40 and 70 years, the probability of complete ED increased from 5.1% to 15%, moderate dysfunction increased from 17% to 34%, and mild dysfunction remained constant at about 17%.

20. **b. The cavernous nerves.** Because of the close relationship between the cavernous nerves and the pelvic organs, the incidence of iatrogenic impotence from pelvic surgical procedures is reportedly high: radical prostatectomy, 43% to 100%; abdominal perineal resection, 15% to 100%.

21. **e. prevents hair loss in men.** Mulligan and Schmitt (1993) concluded that testosterone (1) enhances sexual interest; (2) increases the frequency of sexual acts; and (3) increases the frequency of nocturnal erections but has little or no effect on fantasy-induced or visually stimulated erections.

22. **d. tunica albuginea or cavernous smooth muscle.** Veno-occlusive dysfunction may result from a variety of pathophysiologic processes: degenerative tunical changes; fibroelastic structural alterations; insufficient trabecular smooth muscle relaxation; and venous shunts. Degenerative changes (Peyronie disease, old age, and diabetes) or traumatic injury to the tunica albuginea (penile fracture) can impair the compression of the subtunical and emissary veins. In Peyronie disease, the inelastic tunica albuginea may prevent the emissary veins from closing.

23. **e. Complete ED.** A number of studies have indicated a progressive decline in sexual function in "healthy" aging men. Masters and Johnson (1977) noted a number of changes in older men including greater latency to erection, less turgidity, loss of forceful ejaculation and decreased volume, and a longer refractory period. Decreased frequency and duration of nocturnal erection with increasing age was reported in a group of men who had regular intercourse. Other research has also indicated a decrease in penile tactile sensitivity with age.

24. **e. all of the above.** Diabetes mellitus may cause ED by affecting one or a combination of the following: psychologic well-being, central nervous system function, androgen secretion, peripheral nerve activity, endothelial cell function, and smooth muscle contractility.

25. **e. decreased level of phosphodiesterase type 5.** In diabetic animal models, diabetes causes endothelial cell dysfunction, resulting in an increased prevalence of vascular disease. Other effects include decreased nNOS, reduced activity of eNOS, oxidative stress, increased advanced glycation end products (AGEs), decreased elastin, reduced vascular endothelial growth factor (VEGF), hypercontractility of cavernous erectile tissue, and decreased smooth muscle/collagen ratio leading to impairment of the veno-occlusive mechanism.

26. **b. increased production of oxytocin.** The effect of hypercholesterolemia on erectile function has been studied in different experimental models. In hypercholesterolemic rabbits, although the endothelial NO/cGMP pathway is impaired, neuronal vasodilation does not appear affected. The NO/cGMP pathway effect likely owes to increased superoxide production or endogenous NOS inhibitors such as NG-monomethyl-L-arginine monoacetate (L-NMMA) and asymmetrical dimethylarginine (ADMA). L-arginine supplementation reverses endothelium-dependent relaxation impairment. In a more severe ischemic experimental model, rabbits underwent balloon de-endothelization of the iliac arteries followed by a high-cholesterol diet. They developed both penile arterial insufficiency and veno-occlusive dysfunction owing to decreased expandability of the cavernous smooth muscle. As a result of the impaired NO activity, production of contractile thromboxane and prostaglandin increased, leading to potentiation of neurogenic contractions of the cavernous smooth muscle.

27. **e. Lateral preoptic area.** Nocturnal erection occurs mostly during rapid-eye-movement (REM) sleep. Positron emission tomography scanning of humans in REM sleep shows increased activity in the pontine area, the amygdala, and the anterior cingulate gyrus but decreased activity in the prefrontal and parietal cortex. The mechanism that triggers REM sleep is located in the pontine reticular formation; the cholinergic neurons in the lateral pontine tegmentum are activated, whereas the adrenergic neurons in the locus ceruleus and the serotonergic neurons in the midbrain raphe are silent. This differential activation may be responsible for these nocturnal erections. In rats, the area of the brain that appears to control nocturnal penile tumescence is the lateral preoptic area (LPOA).

28. **d. Inhibition of endothelin action by an inhibitor of the ETa receptor enhances penile erection in men with ED.** Endothelin, a potent vasoconstrictor produced by the endothelial cells, has also been suggested to be a mediator for detumescence. Endothelin-1 is a member of a family of three peptides and is a potent constrictor synthesized by the sinusoidal endothelium. Its presence in human cavernous tissue suggests the participation of this peptide in the regulation of trabecular smooth muscle. Endothelin also potentiates the constrictor effects of catecholamines on trabecular smooth muscle. Two receptors for endothelin, ETA and ETB, mediate the biologic effects of endothelin in vascular tissue: ETA receptors mediate contraction, whereas ETB receptors induce relaxation.

29. **e. has been associated with hypoprolactinemia.** The metabolic syndrome (MetS) includes glucose intolerance, insulin resistance, obesity, dyslipidemia, and hypertension. Higher prevalence of ED (26.7%) in men with MetS relative to controls (13%) has been reported. Furthermore, the prevalence of ED increases as the number of MetS components increases. In an analysis of the Baltimore Longitudinal Study of Aging in which men were followed for a mean of 5.8 years, the authors confirmed that the prevalence of MetS increases with age and that MetS is associated with lower androgen levels. They also found that lower total T levels, along with lower sex hormone binding globulin (SHBG) levels, predict a higher incidence of MetS. Men with MetS have an increased prevalence of ED, reduced endothelial function score, and higher circulating concentrations of C-reactive protein compared with men without metabolic disorders. Low levels of androgens in men with ED and obesity were also reported by Corona and colleagues (2008).

30. **c. perineal artery.** The internal pudendal artery becomes the common penile artery after giving off a branch to the perineum. The three branches of the penile artery are the dorsal, bulbourethral, and cavernous. Distally, they join to form a vascular ring near the glans. The dorsal artery is responsible for engorgement of the glans during erection. The bulbourethral artery supplies the bulb and corpus spongiosum. The cavernous artery effects tumescence of the corpus cavernosum and enters it at the hilum of the penis, where the two crura merge. Along its course, it gives off many helicine arteries, which supply the trabecular erectile tissue and the sinusoids. These helicine arteries are contracted and tortuous in the flaccid state and become dilated and straight during erection.

Additional Study Points

1. See Table 23–10 in *Campbell-Walsh Urology, 10th Edition* for the classification of male ED.
2. Sexual stimulation triggers release of neurotransmitters from the cavernous nerve terminals. This results in relaxation of the smooth muscles and (a) dilation of arteries; (b) trapping of incoming blood by the expanding sinusoids; (c) compression of the subtunical venous plexuses between the tunica albuginea and the peripheral sinusoids reducing venous outflow; (d) stretching of the tunica to capacity, which occludes the emissary veins; (e) an increase in PO2; and (f) further pressure increases with contraction of the ischio-cavernosus muscles.
3. The sympathetic system causes detumescence (norepinephrine is the neural transmitter).
4. Thiazide diuretics may be responsible for impotence.
5. Luteinizing hormone-releasing hormone agonists result in the reduction of sexual desire in 70% of patients.
6. Sexual dysfunction is a common event after the induction of antiretroviral therapy.
7. The prevalence of ED is three times higher in diabetic men, occurs at an earlier age, and increases with the duration of the disease.
8. The metabolic syndrome consisting of glucose intolerance, insulin resistance, obesity, dyslipidemia, and hypertension increases the risk of ED.
9. About half of the people with chronic renal failure have significant sexual dysfunction. Moreover, following transplantation about half continue to have ED.
10. Primary ED is a life-long inability to initiate or maintain an erection. In most cases it is psychogenic, but in a small number it is due to maldevelopment of the penis and/or blood and nerve supply.
11. Aging is the single most important contributing factory to ED.
12. Endothelial dysfunction is the final common pathway to ED in patients with hyperlipidemia, diabetes mellitus, hypertension, and chronic renal failure.

chapter
24

Evaluation and Management of Erectile Dysfunction

Arthur L. Burnett, MD, MBA, FACS

QUESTIONS

1. A predictor for the development of erectile dysfunction (ED) is:
   a. endocarditis.
   b. osteoarthritis.
   c. peptic ulcer disease.
   d. stroke.
   e. dementia.

2. Goal-directed management:
   a. reflects patient preferences for management.
   b. applies an understanding of therapeutic options.
   c. accepts the patient's derivation of satisfaction.
   d. requires the acceptance of sexual disorders by patients.
   e. omits a thorough discussion with the treating physician.

3. A patient with ED who has a low risk for cardiovascular events should:
   a. undergo cardiac stress testing.
   b. receive cardiologic referral.
   c. receive counseling for lifestyle modifications.
   d. initiate statin therapy.
   e. be reassured that there is no need for cardiovascular health intervention.

4. It is appropriate to categorize the etiology of ED because:
   a. organic ED indicates a role for risk reduction therapy.
   b. psychogenic ED implies normal ability to attain an erection.
   c. psychogenic ED demands psychiatric intervention.
   d. mixed ED demands specialist referral.
   e. mixed ED encompasses a sexual desire disorder.

5. Self-administered questionnaires for ED:
   a. are impractical for clinical practice.
   b. define cardiac risk.
   c. indicate depression causality.
   d. supplant objective diagnostic tests.
   e. monitor responsiveness to treatments.

6. Recommended serum laboratory testing for men with sexual problems typically include:
   a. a hemoglobin A1C level.
   b. a lipid profile.
   c. thyroid function tests.
   d. a prolactin level.
   e. a PSA measurement.

7. The diagnostic advantage of Duplex ultrasound of the penis relative to the combined intracavernous injection and stimulation (CIS) test is its:
   a. combination of a pharmacologic stimulus.
   b. inclusion of audiovisual stimulation.
   c. bypass of neurologic and hormonal influences affecting erection.
   d. application of independent assessor rating.
   e. quantification of penile vascular status.

8. Penile angiography aims to:
   a. provide anatomic information regarding the arterial and venous structures of the penis.
   b. distinguish congenital variations from acquired abnormalities of the penile vasculature.
   c. establish the functional significance of penile vascular abnormalities.
   d. depict functional abnormalities in combination with the administration of a vasodilatory agent.
   e. define penile anatomy suitable for surgical revascularization.

9. Penile tumescence and rigidity monitoring is useful in discerning the:
   a. role of central neurologic processes involved in erections.
   b. integrity of physiologic erection aggregately.
   c. quality of sexually relevant erections.
   d. erection responsiveness independent of anxiety disorders.
   e. psychogenic etiology for erectile disorders.

10. The best indicator of hypogonadism is:

    a. a screening questionnaire.

    b. a total serum testosterone measurement.

    c. a free serum testosterone measurement.

    d. a bioavailable serum testosterone measurement.

    e. an intratesticular testosterone measurement.

11. Efficacy of androgen replacement therapy for sexual dysfunction is best judged by:

    a. testosterone measurement increase above midnormal range.

    b. testosterone measurement increase at maximal normal range.

    c. patient-reported improvement in sexual function.

    d. testosterone measurement increase to normal range.

    e. clinical findings of anthropometric improvement.

12. Optimization of effect for PDE5 inhibitors is best achieved by:

    a. daily dosing.

    b. reducing the frequency of sexual intercourse attempts.

    c. increasing food intake with dosing.

    d. applying sexual stimulation.

    e. using twice-maximal dosages.

13. A small dose of medication is used when initiating intracavernosal injection therapy for the patient with ED associated with:

    a. performance anxiety.

    b. diabetes mellitus.

    c. hypogonadism.

    d. pelvic trauma.

    e. priapism.

14. Vacuum erection device therapy is particularly advantageous when the ED presentation is associated with:

    a. young age.

    b. Peyronie disease.

    c. hemophilia.

    d. glanular insufficiency.

    e. penile fibrosis.

15. The best indication for performing arterial revascularization in the treatment of ED is the clinical presentation of:

    a. aging.

    b. diabetes mellitus.

    c. cardiovascular disease.

    d. cigarette smoking.

    e. perineal trauma.

ANSWERS

1. **d. stroke.** Predictors for the development of ED include age, lower education, diabetes mellitus, cardiovascular disease (including hypertension and stroke), cigarette smoking (active and passive exposure), and obesity.

2. **c. accepts the patient's derivation of satisfaction.** Goal-directed management aims to allow the patient or couple to make an informed selection of the preferred therapy for sexual fulfillment on the basis of a sound understanding of all treatment options after completing a thorough discussion with the treating physician. The approach recognizes that patients vary in their acceptance of their sexual disorders, their interest to pursue management, and their manner of deriving satisfaction from treatment.

3. **c. receive counseling for lifestyle modifications.** According to current principles for ED management, even patients at low risk for cardiovascular events should receive the minimum recommendations for cardiovascular disease management, which include counseling for lifestyle modifications and regular health monitoring.

4. **a. organic ED indicates a role for risk-reduction therapy.** An attempt to ascertain the potential etiology of ED may facilitate therapeutic objectives. The suggestion of organic ED, possibly having a physical disease state correlation, may involve a modifiable condition such as cigarette smoking and physical inactivity.

5. **e. monitor responsiveness to treatments.** Self-report measures have served as brief and practical tools that document the presence, severity, and responsiveness to treatment of ED. They do not delineate an etiologic basis for ED.

6. **b. lipid profile.** Recommended tests typically include fasting glucose, complete blood count, lipid profile, and serum total testosterone. Other tests as listed are optional or may be done as needed.

7. **e. quantification of penile vascular status.** Duplex ultrasound of the penis offers all diagnostic components of the CIS test. In addition, it adds quantification of blood flow in the penis.

8. **e. define penile anatomy suitable for surgical revascularization.** Penile angiography depicts the anatomy of the arterial supply of the penis for consideration of surgical revascularization.

9. **b. integrity of physiologic erection aggregately.** The monitoring of penile tumescence and rigidity affords a basic evaluation of the functional integrity of physiologic penile erection. It does not define a psychogenic cause for ED.

10. **d. bioavailable serum testosterone measurement.** The best indicator of androgen status is the calculated bioavailable testosterone (free testosterone and albumin-bound testosterone).

11. **c. patient-reported improvement in sexual function.** The efficacy of testosterone supplementation is best judged by clinical response of improved sexual function subjectively rather than a precise testosterone determination.

12. **d. applying sexual stimulation.** Strategies to optimize response to PDE5 inhibitors include properly applying sexual stimulation, reducing food intake, escalating drug dosing to maximal recommended dosages as needed, and repeating attempts with the medications several times with sexual activity.

13. **a. performance anxiety.** It is generally recommended that a small dose of vasoactive medication should be used in this setting with patients having nonvasculogenic forms of ED.

14. **d. glanular insufficiency.** Vacuum therapy achieves engorgement of blood within the glans penis in addition to the corpora cavernosa, such that it is particularly

advantageous for patients experiencing glanular insufficiency.

15. **e. perineal trauma.** Arterial surgery should be performed selectively on patients younger than 55 years who are nonsmokers and nondiabetics, with the absence of venous leakage and confirmation radiographically of stenosis of the external pudendal artery, which is usually induced by trauma.

Additional Study Points

1. The prevalence of ED in the adult male is 20%.
2. Men with ED are 45% more likely than men without ED to experience a cardiac event within 5 years of diagnosis.
3. The IIEF questionnaire has five domains: erectile function, orgasmic function, sexual desire, intercourse satisfaction, and overall satisfaction.
4. Erections observed with nocturnal penile tumescence monitoring do not necessarily equate with erections sufficient for sexual performance.
5. Cavernous arterial insufficiency is suggested when peek systolic velocity is less than 25 cm/sec. A peek systolic velocity greater than 35 cm/sec defines normal cavernous arterial inflow.
6. Free testosterone and albumin-bound testosterone comprise the bioavailable testosterone.
7. Testosterone production is circadian with the peak occurring in the morning.

Priapism

Gregory A. Broderick, MD

QUESTIONS

1. Ischemic priapism is a persistent erection marked by each of the following clinical and pathophysiologic characteristics EXCEPT:
   a. rigidity of the corpora cavernosa.
   b. bright red corporal blood.
   c. hypoxic and acidotic corporal environment.
   d. painful rigidity.
   e. thrombus within the sinusoidal spaces.

2. Each of the following are etiologies typically associated with ischemic priapism EXCEPT:
   a. sickle cell disease.
   b. straddle injury.
   c. cocaine use.
   d. spider bite.
   e. pharmacologic erection therapy.

3. Sickle cell disease is a risk factor for ischemic priapism; the pathophysiologic mechanisms include each of the following EXCEPT:
   a. decreased content of HgbS in the plasma.
   b. HgbS polymerizes when deoxygenated.
   c. scavenging of nitric oxide.
   d. arginine catabolism removing substrate for NO synthesis.
   e. adhesive interactions among sickle cells, endothelial cells, and leukocytes.

4. Prolonged erection in males 40 years of age and older is usually attributed to:
   a. sickle cell disease.
   b. hematologic malignancy.
   c. erectile dysfunction pharmacotherapy.
   d. prostate cancer.
   e. testosterone supplementation.

5. Case reports have documented prolonged erections and rarely priapism in men using phosphodiesterase (PDE) type-5 inhibitor therapies. Associated risks for prolonged erection/priapism include each of the following EXCEPT:
   a. daily dosing.
   b. combination with intracavernous injection.
   c. history of penile trauma.

   d. psychotropic medications.
   e. narcotic use.

6. The associations and pathophysiology of high-flow priapism include each of the following EXCEPT:
   a. straddle injury.
   b. coital trauma.
   c. birth canal injury to the newborn male.
   d. cold-knife urethrotomy.
   e. hemodialysis.

7. The critical pathologic change occurring in the cavernosal tissue at 4 hours after the onset of ischemic priapism is:
   a. irreversible cavernous damage and erectile dysfunction.
   b. the beginning of glucopenia.
   c. the beginning of hypercoagulable thrombotic conditions.
   d. the deterioration of cavernous smooth muscle contractile responses.
   e. cavernous fibrosis.

8. The nitric oxide/cGMP signaling pathway is implicated in the pathogenesis of priapism on the basis of scientific work showing:
   a. guanylate cyclase activity upregulation.
   b. guanylate cyclase activity downregulation.
   c. nitric oxide synthase activity upregulation.
   d. PDE type-5 activity upregulation.
   e. PDE type-5 activity downregulation.

9. An adolescent with sickle cell disease presents with a 6-hour erection. Initial cavernous blood gas results show P_{O_2} 30 mm Hg, P_{CO_2} 60 mm Hg, and pH 7.25. The first therapeutic step should be:
   a. oral terbutaline.
   b. oral pseudoephedrine.
   c. intracavernous aspiration.
   d. exchange transfusion.
   e. distal surgical shunt.

10. The characteristic blood flow defect of ischemic priapism found on color Duplex ultrasonography is:
    a. normal cavernosal artery inflow.
    b. increased cavernosal artery inflow.
    c. decreased or absent cavernosal artery inflow.

d. arteriovenous blush.

e. sinusoidal fistula.

11. After initial intracavernous treatment for ischemic priapism, blood gas sampling produces an equivocal mixed-venous blood result. Priapism resolution is best confirmed by:

a. color Duplex ultrasonography.

b. penile scintigraphy.

c. corpus cavernosography.

d. penile arteriography.

e. pelvic CT scan.

12. After a second session of intracavernous treatment consisting of aspiration/irrigation with phenylephrine administration, the priapic penis remains turgid. Cavernosal blood gas results are Po_2 40 mm Hg, Pco_2 50 mm Hg, and pH 7.35. The next step should be:

a. observation.

b. oral sympathomimetic.

c. repeat intracavernous treatment.

d. distal surgical shunt.

e. proximal surgical shunt.

13. Phenylephrine is the preferred sympathomimetic used in the treatment of ischemic priapism because of its:

a. α_1-selective activity.

b. α_1 and α_2 activity.

c. β_1-selective activity.

d. β_2-selective activity.

e. combined α and β activities.

14. The best indication for arterial embolization in the management of high-flow priapism is:

a. unlikely spontaneous resolution.

b. failure of sympathomimetic therapy.

c. reduction of recurrent priapism risk.

d. reduction of subsequent erectile dysfunction risk.

e. patient preference to intervene.

15. Persistent penile rigidity after a technically successful proximal surgical shunt procedure in a patient with a 72-hour episode of ischemic priapism is an indication for:

a. observation.

b. gonadotropin-releasing hormone agonist therapy.

c. pudendal artery ligation.

d. distal surgical shunt.

e. penile prosthesis surgery.

16. The mother of a child with sickle cell disease complains that her son has recently been awakening with erections lasting 3 to 4 hours. She is concerned that similar occurrences have been a warning sign for a major priapism. All of the following are appropriate management options EXCEPT:

a. trial of nightly oral sympathomimetic drug.

b. trial of low-dosage, daily PDE type-5 inhibitor.

c. a gonadotropin-releasing hormone agonist or antiandrogen.

d. intracavernous injection of phenylephrine in the morning.

17. Evidence-based studies of priapism therapies and outcomes are rare. A recent investigation of adult sickle cell disease patients presenting with ischemic priapism subjected all men to a standard protocol of aspiration and phenylephrine injections. Long-term sexual health function outcomes revealed complete ED in men with duration of priapism:

a. less than 12 hours.

b. 12 to 24 hours.

c. longer than 36 hours.

d. longer than 48 hours.

e. longer than 72 hours.

18. An adult male presents with ischemic priapism of 8 hours' duration. He fails to respond to serial aspiration and intracavernous injection after 4 hours in the emergency department. The recommended intervention at this time should be:

a. hydration, nasal oxygen, and keeping the patient NPO for 8 hours to avoid risks of emergent intubation.

b. a percutaneous distal penile shunt.

c. an open distal shunt.

d. an open proximal shunt.

e. a saphenous vein shunt.

19. Radiographic imaging may be helpful in the diagnosis and management of priapism. Each of the following is correct EXCEPT:

a. color Doppler in the evaluation of a persistent erection following treatments for ischemic priapism.

b. penile arteriography to differentiate high-flow from ischemic priapism.

c. MRI to diagnose corporal thrombus in men with refractory priapism or when there has been a significant delay in presentation.

d. MRI in the differential diagnosis of corporal metastasis.

20. A 36-year-old male is referred for a diagnosis of priapism after he slipped while climbing aboard his yacht. He initially had a saddle bruise on his perineum and pain; the next morning he awoke with persistent erection. The patient has a board of directors meeting at the end of the week and wants immediate treatment. The correct management strategy is:

a. penile aspiration and α-adrenergic injection in the office or emergency department.

b. penile arteriography.

c. angio-embolization after a thorough discussion of chances for spontaneous resolution and risks of treatment-related erectile dysfunction.

d. color Doppler ultrasound–guided corporal exploration to ligate fistula.

e. distile penile shunt.

ANSWERS

1. **b. bright red corporal blood.** Ischemic priapism is a persistent erection marked by rigidity of the corpora cavernosa and little or no cavernous arterial inflow. In ischemic priapism there are time-dependent changes in the corporal metabolic environment with progressive hypoxia, hypercarbia, and acidosis. The patient typically complains of

penile pain after 6 to 8 hours, and examination reveals a rigid erection. After 48 hours thrombus can be found in the sinusoidal spaces and smooth muscle necrosis with fibroblast-like cell transformation is evident.

2. **b. straddle injury.** Nonischemic priapism is much rarer than ischemic priapism, and the etiology is largely attributed to trauma. Forces may be blunt or penetrating, resulting in laceration of the cavernous artery or one of its branches within the corpora. The etiology most commonly reported is a straddle injury to the crura.

3. **a. decreased content of HgbS in the plasma.** The clinical features are seen in homozygous SCD patients: chronic hemolysis, vascular occlusion, tissue ischemia, and end-organ damage. HbS polymerizes when deoxygenated, injuring the sickle erythrocyte, activating a cascade of hemolysis and vaso-occlusion. Membrane damage results in dense sickling of red cells, causing adhesive interactions among sickle cells, endothelial cells, and leukocytes. Hemolysis releases hemoglobin into the plasma. Free Hbg reacts with nitric oxide (NO) to produce methemoglobin and nitrate. This is a scavenging reaction; the vasodilator NO is oxidized to inert nitrate. Sickled erythrocytes release arginase-I into blood plasma, which converts l-arginine into ornithine, effectively removing substrate for NO synthesis. Oxidant radicals further reduce NO bioavailability. The combined effects of NO scavenging and arginine catabolism result in a state of NO resistance and insufficiency termed *hemolysis-associated endothelial dysfunction*. Therapeutic interventions include transfusion to decrease the relative concentrations of HgbS in the plasma.

4. **c. erectile dysfunction pharmacotherapy.** The introduction of intracavernous pharmacotherapy approximately 2 decades ago led to a pronounced increase in the incidence of prolonged erection and true priapism. Prolonged erection is more commonly reported than is priapism, following therapeutic or diagnostic injection of intracavernous vasoactive medications. In many communities patients receiving intracavernous medications for erectile dysfunction will outnumber patients with sickle cell disease. The majority of men requiring treatment for erectile dysfunction are middle aged to older men. In worldwide clinical trials of the Alprostadil Study Group, prolonged erection (defined as 4 to 6 hours) was 5%, and priapism (>6 hours) was described in 1% of subjects. In papaverine/phentolamine/alprostadil intracavernous injection programs, prolonged erections have been reported in 5% to 35% of patients.

5. **a. daily dosing.** Few cases reports have documented priapism following a PDE type-5 inhibitor therapy. These reports suggest that men with the following conditions were at increased risk for priapism: sickle cell disease, spinal cord injury, men who used a PDE type-5 inhibitor recreationally, men who used a PDE type-5 inhibitor in combination with intracavernous injection, men with a history of penile trauma, men on psychotropic medications, and men abusing narcotics. Tadalafil 5 mg daily dosing caused no priapism in a phase II clinical study of 281 men with history of lower urinary tract symptoms secondary to benign prostatic hyperplasia for 6 weeks, followed by dosage escalation to 20 mg once daily for 6 weeks.

6. **e. hemodialysis.** Nonischemic priapism is much rarer than ischemic priapism, and the etiology is largely attributed to trauma. Forces may be blunt or penetrating,

resulting in laceration of the cavernous artery or one of its branches within the corpora. The etiology most commonly reported is a straddle injury to the crura. Other mechanisms include coital trauma, kicks to the penis or perineum, pelvic fractures, birth canal trauma to the newborn male, needle lacerations, complications of penile diagnostics, and vascular erosions complicating metastatic infiltration of the corpora. Although accidental blunt trauma is the most common etiology, high-flow priapism has been described following iatrogenic injury: cold-knife urethrotomy, Nesbitt corporoplasty, and deep dorsal vein arterialization. Any mechanism that lacerates a cavernous artery or arteriole can produce unregulated pooling of blood in sinusoidal space with consequent erection.

7. **d. the deterioration of cavernous smooth muscle contractile responses.** In ischemic priapism there are time-dependent changes in the corporal metabolic environment with progressive hypoxia, hypercarbia, and acidosis. In-vitro studies have demonstrated that when corporal smooth muscle strips are exposed to a hypoxic condition, α-adrenergic stimulation fails to induce corporal smooth muscle contraction. Histologically, by 12 hours corporal specimens show interstitial edema, progressing to destruction of the sinusoidal endothelium, exposure of the basement membrane, and thrombocyte adherence at 24 hours.

8. **e. PDE type-5 activity downregulation.** Recent scientific advances have shown that priapism is associated with decreased PDE-5 functional regulation in the penis. The relative lack of this molecular factor needed for controlling chemical signaling of penile erection accounts for stuttering and ischemic priapism in sickle cell patients. Experimental models of corpus cavernosum smooth muscle cells suggest that cyclic nucleotide cGMP is produced in low steady-state amounts under the influence of priapism-related destruction of the vascular endothelium and thus reduced endothelial nitric oxide activity. This situation downregulates the set point of PDE type-5 function, secondary to altered cGMP-dependent feedback control mechanisms. When nitric oxide is neuronally produced in response to erectogenic stimulus or during sleep-related erectile activity, cGMP production surges in a manner that leads to excessive erectile tissue relaxation because of basally insufficient functional PDE type-5 to degrade the cyclic nucleotide.

9. **c. intracavernous aspiration.** The history and blood gases define an ischemic priapism event, which warrants immediate attempts at decompression/aspiration of the corpora cavernosa. In sickle cell disease, concurrent systemic treatments may be offered but relief of the penile ischemia should be pursued aggressively. Aspiration should be repeated until no more dark blood can be seen coming out of the corpora and bright red blood is obtained. This process decreases the intracavernous pressure, relieves pain, and resuscitates the corporal environment removing anoxic, acidotic, and hypercarbic blood.

10. **c. decreased or absent cavernosal artery inflow.** In presentations of ischemic priapism, minimal or absent blood flow in the cavernosal arteries is found using color Doppler ultrasonography. Color Doppler ultrasound is an adjunct to the corporal aspirate in differentiating ischemic from nonischemic priapism. Patients with ischemic priapism will have no blood flow in the cavernous arteries; the return of

cavernous artery waveform will accompany successful detumescence. Patients with nonischemic priapism have normal to high blood-flow velocities in the cavernous arteries; an effort should be made to localize the characteristic blush of color emanating from flow signal of the disrupted cavernous artery or arteriolar-sinusoidal fistula.

11. **a. color Duplex ultrasonography.** This tool is the most reliable and least invasive imaging technique to differentiate ischemic from nonischemic priapism. Color Doppler ultrasound should always be considered in the evaluation of a full or partial erection after treatments for ischemic priapism. The differential diagnosis includes resolved ischemia with persistent tenderness and penile edema, persistent ischemia, or conversion to a high-flow state.

12. **a. observation.** These blood gas results are consistent with normal mixed venous blood. The turgid penis may be due to tissue edema. Observation is appropriate at this time.

13. **a. α_1-selective activity.** According to American Urological Association Guidelines, aspiration followed by intracavernous injection of sympathomimetic drugs is the standard of care in the medical treatment of ischemic priapism. Sympathomimetic pharmacotherapies (phenylephrine, etilephrine, ephedrine, epinephrine, norepinephrine, metaraminol) cause smooth muscle contraction in the corpora. Phenylephrine is a selective α_1-adrenergic receptor agonist, with minimal β-mediated inotropic and chronotropic cardiac effects. There are no comparative trials of sympathomimetic injectables in the management of priapism.

14. **e. patient preference to intervene.** Nonischemic priapism should generally be managed by observation. Arterial priapism is not an emergency. Spontaneous resolution or response to conservative therapy has been reported in up to 62% of published series. Persistent partial erection from high-flow priapism may be from months to years. There are no comparative outcome studies of intervention versus conservative management, but there are sufficient case descriptions in children to recommend initial watchful waiting. Adult patients demanding immediate relief can be offered selective arterial embolization.

15. **e. penile prosthesis surgery.** Unfortunately, the natural history of untreated ischemic priapism or priapism refractory to interventions is severe fibrosis, penile length loss, and complete erectile dysfunction. The exact time point when penile prosthesis becomes a reasonable option is unclear, but most series describe complete ED in men who have had ischemic priapism for 36 to 72 hours. The advantages of early penile implantation in the acute management of ischemic priapism are preservation of penile length and a technically easier implantation; delayed implantation is technically challenging due to corporal fibrosis.

16. **c. a gonadotropin-releasing hormone agonist or antiandrogen.** The goals of managing stuttering ischemic priapism are prevention of future episodes, preservation of erectile function, and reducing the trauma to the patient from priapism management. A trial of daily oral sympathomimetic therapy, a trial of oral PDE type-5 inhibitor therapy, or intracavernous injection of phenylephrine should be considered in the management of children and adults with stuttering ischemic priapism associated with hemoglobinopathies. GnRH agonists or antiandrogens may be used in adults but should not be used in patients who have not achieved full sexual maturation and adult stature.

17. **c. longer than 36 hours.** In those patients where priapism was reversed, spontaneous erection (with or without sildenafil) was reported in 100% of men when priapism was reversed in less than 12 hours; 78% when reversed by 12 to 24 hours; and 44% when reversed by 24 to 36 hours. No patient reported spontaneous erection after priapism duration of more than 36 hours.

18. **b. a percutaneous distal penile shunt.** The objective of shunt surgery is reoxygenation of the corpus cavernosum. The shared principle of all shunting procedures is to reestablish corporal inflow by relieving venous outflow obstruction. A distal cavernoglanular shunt should be the first choice of shunting procedures because it is technically easier to perform than proximal shunting. Percutaneous distal shunting is less invasive than open distal shunting and can be attempted in the emergency department with local anesthetic. Anesthesiologists must be educated that ischemic priapism is an emergency and sexual function outcomes are time dependent; appropriate airway precautions should be taken for emergent intubation as needed in the surgical management of priapism.

19. **b. penile arteriography to differentiate high-flow from ischemic priapism.** Color Doppler ultrasound (CDU) is an adjunct to the corporal aspirate in differentiating ischemic from nonischemic priapism. CDU imaging should include corporal shaft and transperineal assessment of the crural bodies when there is a history of penile trauma or straddle injury. CDU should always be considered in the evaluation of a persistent or partial erection after treatments for ischemic priapism. Penile arteriography is too invasive as a diagnostic procedure to differentiate ischemic from nonischemic priapism. Penile arteriography should be reserved for the management of high-flow priapism, when embolization is planned. There are three possible roles for MRI: imaging of a well-established arteriolar-sinusoidal fistula; identifying corporal thrombus; and identifying corporal metastasis.

20. **c. angio-embolization after a thorough discussion of chances for spontaneous resolution and risks of treatment-related erectile dysfunction.** Arterial priapism is not an emergency and may be managed expectantly. Diagnosis of high-flow priapism is best made by penile/perineal color Doppler ultrasound. Penile aspiration and injection of α-adrenergic agents is not recommended for HFP. Angio-embolization should be preceded by a thorough discussion of chances for spontaneous resolution, risks of treatment-related erectile dysfunction, and lack of significant consequences expected from delaying interventions. Overall success rates with embolization are high, although a single treatment carries a recurrence rate of 30% to 40%. Where angio-embolization fails or is contraindicated, surgical ligation is reasonable. Formation of a pseudocapsule at the site of a sinusoidal fistula may take weeks to months following trauma. Color Doppler ultrasound guidance is recommended during exploration to locate fistula.

Additional Study Points

1. Ischemic priapism is the result of little or no cavernous arterial inflow.
2. Interventions 48 to 72 hours beyond the onset of ischemic priapism have little benefit in preserving potency.
3. Stuttering priapism is recurrent, unwanted, painful erections in men, usually with sickle cell disease.
4. Nonischemic or high-flow arterial priapism is usually the result of trauma, and the corpora are tumescent but not rigid.
5. The etiology of the majority of ischemic priapism is idiopathic; however, it may be associated with alcohol or drug abuse, perineal trauma, and sickle cell disease.
6. Priapism following a PDE-5 inhibitor usually occurs in men with other risk factors.
7. On rare occasion, following reversal of ischemic priapism, high-flow priapism may occur. Doppler ultrasound is useful in making this diagnosis.
8. Ischemic priapism and stuttering priapism are the result of NO imbalance.
9. In ischemic priapism, aspiration alone will be curative in a third of the patients.
10. Phenylephrine, 200 µg/mL given in 1-mL aloquats, not to exceed a total dose of 2 mg, is used to treat ischemic priapism.
11. Aspiration has no role in high-flow priapism other than for diagnosis; it plays no role in treatment.
12. PDE-5 inhibitor therapy has been used to treat stuttering priapism in men with sickle cell disease.
13. When surgical therapy is indicated, a cavernosal glanular shunt should be the first choice.
14. Spontaneous resolution of high-flow arterial priapism generally occurs in two thirds of patients.

Premature Ejaculation

John P. Mulhall, MD, MSc (Anat)

QUESTIONS

1. The neurotransmitter most involved in ejaculation is:
   a. oxytocin.
   b. nitric oxide.
   c. serotonin.
   d. acetylcholine.
   e. adrenaline.

2. The first portion of the ejaculate is secreted by the:
   a. prostate.
   b. seminal vesicle.
   c. vas deferens.
   d. bulbourethral glands.
   e. glands of Littre.

3. In the U.S. National Health and Social Life Survey (Laumann et al, 1999),* the prevalence of premature ejaculation (PE) was:
   a. 10%.
   b. 20%.
   c. 30%.
   d. 40%.
   e. 50%.

4. In the Global Study of Sexual Attitudes and Behaviors, the highest prevalence of PE was seen in:
   a. Europe.
   b. North America.
   c. South America.
   d. Asia.
   e. the Middle East.

5. The final common pathway in PE is (there may be more than one correct answer):
   a. hyposensitivity of 5-HT1A receptors.
   b. hypersensitivity of 5-HT1A receptors.
   c. hyposensitivity of 5-HT2C receptors.
   d. hypersensitivity of 5-HT2C receptors.
   e. hypersensitivity of dopamine receptors.

6. Polymorphisms in which gene have been implicated in PE?
   a. *SERT*
   b. Nitric oxide synthase gene
   c. *DAT1*
   d. *Ob*
   e. *RE-1*

7. The hormone most implicated in PE development is:
   a. testosterone.
   b. thyroxine.
   c. prolactin.
   d. cortisol.
   e. ACTH.

8. Evidence suggests that the most effective SSRI agent for PE is:
   a. citalopram.
   b. fluoxetine.
   c. fluvoxamine.
   d. paroxetine.
   e. sertraline.

9. SSRI agents for prolongation of intravaginal ejaculatory latency time achieve optimal therapeutic efficacy:
   a. within 2 days.
   b. at 1 week.
   c. at 2 weeks.
   d. at 4 weeks.
   e. at 3 months.

10. SSRI withdrawal syndrome occurs at what time point after stopping SSRI agents abruptly?
    a. Within 12 hours
    b. 24 hours
    c. 1 to 3 days
    d. 5 days
    e. 1 week

11. The serotonin syndrome in patients using SSRI agents is manifested by:
    a. diarrhea.
    b. myoclonus.
    c. polydipsia.
    d. urticaria.
    e. petechiae.

---

*Sources referenced can be found in *Campbell-Walsh Urology, 10th Edition,* on the Expert Consult website.

ANSWERS

1. **c. serotonin.** Serotonin is the primary neurotransmitter involved in ejaculation. Manipulation of its synaptic levels

results in alterations in ejaculatory latency time. Oxytocin plays some role in orgasm. Nitric oxide is the primary neurotransmitter for erection. Acetylcholine plays little role in erectile physiology other than to modulate adrenergic tone. Adrenaline is the primary detumescence neurotransmitter.

2. **d. bulbourethral glands.** In humans, the composition of the ejaculate is released from participating organs in a particular order. The first portion of the ejaculate is provided by the bulbourethral glands followed by some fluid from the prostate. Afterwards, the main fraction of the ejaculate including the bulk of the spermatozoa is contributed by the epididymis and vas deferens, along with prostatic and seminal vesicle contributions.

3. **c. 30%.** One of the first large-scale prospective studies to assess the prevalence of PE was the U.S. National Health and Social Life Survey conducted in the early 1990s (Laumann et al, 1999). One of the major aims of this study was the assessment of the variation of timing and sequence of individual sex activity in response to life course events and changes in social and cultural environment. This study was interview based, and one of the sexual issues assessed in the study was PE. This survey used an area probability sample of 3442 men aged 19 to 59 years. Subjects were questioned regarding "climaxing too early" over the course of the preceding 12 months. The prevalence of PE in the study was 29%.

4. **d. Asia.** In the Global Study of Sexual Attitudes and Behaviors (GSSAB), Laumann and colleagues conducted an international poll of 13,618 male subjects in 29 countries. Subjects were questioned in either face-to-face or telephone interviews and in certain countries by mailed questionnaires. The prevalence of PE, which in this analysis was defined using a single question regarding "achieving orgasm too quickly," ranged from 20% to 30% with significant geographic variation. In this analysis the lowest prevalence of PE was reported in the Middle East at 12.4%, while the highest prevalence occurred in Southeast Asia at 30.5%.

5. **Both b and c.** The combination of hypersensitivity of the proejaculation receptors (5-HT$_{1A}$) and hyposensitivity of the antiejaculation receptors (5-HT2C) is believed to result in premature ejaculation.

6. **a. SERT.** Recent evidence has demonstrated that polymorphisms in the *SERT* gene, the gene encoding for the serotonin transporter (5HTT), may predispose patients to shorter intravaginal ejaculatory latency times. The 5-HTT functioning is moderated by a polymorphism in the 5-HT key promoter region of the SERT gene (5-HTTLPR). 5-HTTLPR has a short and a long allele, with genotypes of L/L, S/L, and SS. The S allele reduces transcriptional efficiency of the 5-HTT gene promoter resulting in reduced 5-HTT expression and reduced serotonin uptake compared with the L allele. Notably the S allele has been associated with a nearly 50% reduction in the expression of the 5-HTTLPR protein, vulnerability for mood disorders, inadequate response to SSRI medications, and their side effects.

7. **b. thyroxine.** Some evidence supports the concepts that hyperthyroidism is associated with PE. Low levels of testosterone may be associated with delayed ejaculation. None of the other hormones are involved in ejaculatory physiology.

8. **d. paroxetine.** Using a daily treatment regimen, paroxetine has been shown to have the highest efficacy (IELT fold increase of 9), followed by sertraline (4) and fluoxetine (4). A meta-analysis on SSRI use in PE focused on eight randomized, double-blind studies of the SSRI and tricyclic antidepressant for treatment of PE including the stopwatch assessment of IELT. The rank order of efficacy of IELT increase was paroxetine, sertraline, clomipramine, fluoxetine, and placebo. There is little evidence that citalopram or fluvoxamine are of any significant benefit.

9. **d. at 4 weeks.** The function of SSRI agents is mediated through receptor modulation. Thus a period of exposure is required before the receptor function is altered to permit increased ejaculatory latency time. For most patients, most SSRI agents will require 3 to 4 weeks to maximize their effect.

10. **c. 1 to 3 days.** SSRI "discontinuation or withdrawal syndrome," a group of physical and psychological symptoms including nausea, vomiting, dizziness, headache, ataxia, drowsiness, excitement, anxiety, and insomnia begins 1 to 3 days after the drug cessation and may continue for more than a week in some patients. This syndrome is usually reversible by SSRI reintroduction. Thus it is recommended that SSRI should be gradually withdrawn over 2 to 4 weeks.

11. **b. myoclonus.** Drug-drug interactions (DDIs) with SSRI agents are common, leading potentially to the "serotonin syndrome," a group of serious, persistent symptoms including myoclonus, hyperreflexia, sweating, shivering, dyscoordination, and mental status changes.

Additional Study Points

1. Emission is controlled by the sympathetic nervous system.
2. The expulsion phase is controlled by the somatic nervous system via the pudendal nerve.
3. Cerebral serotonin (5-HT) plays an inhibitory role in ejaculation.
4. Selective serotonin reuptake inhibitor (SSRI)–induced elevated levels of serotonin in the synapse result in prolongation of ejaculation latency time.
5. A definitive link between circumcision status and sexual function has not been established.
6. The definition of premature ejaculation involves a rapid ejaculation combined with negative personal feelings.
7. Evidence supports a role for genetic factors, hyperthyroidism, and prostatitis in this disorder.
8. Pharmacologic agents used in treating the disorder include selective serotonin reuptake inhibitors and tricyclic antidepressants.

27

Prosthetic Surgery for Erectile Dysfunction

Drogo K. Montague, MD

QUESTIONS

1. The three treatments that have had the most impact on the history of erectile dysfunction management are:
   a. inflatable penile prostheses, penile arterial surgery, and PDE5 inhibitors.
   b. inflatable penile prostheses, penile venous ligation, and PDE5 inhibitors.
   c. inflatable penile prostheses, intracavernous injections, and PDE5 inhibitors.
   d. intracavernous injections, penile venous ligation, and PDE5 inhibitors.
   e. intracavernous injections, penile arterial surgery, and PDE5 inhibitors.

2. The most important difference between a prosthetic erection and a normal erection is that the prosthetic erection:
   a. is usually shorter.
   b. has less girth.
   c. has less sensitivity.
   d. has greater rigidity.
   e. is cooler.

3. The feature that differentiates the AMS 700 LGX prosthesis from others is:
   a. penile girth expansion.
   b. penile length expansion.
   c. that it has two pieces.
   d. that it is preconnected.
   e. that it is prefilled.

4. The three most commonly used surgical approaches for penile prosthesis implantation are:
   a. ventral penile, infrapubic, and inguinoscrotal.
   b. subcoronal, inguinoscrotal, and penoscrotal.
   c. ventral penile, infrapubic, and penoscrotal.
   d. inguinoscrotal, infrapubic, and penoscrotal.
   e. subcoronal, infrapubic, and penoscrotal.

5. Compared with the penoscrotal approach, the infrapubic approach has the following advantage:
   a. It avoids dorsal nerve injury.
   b. It allows scrotal pump anchoring.
   c. It provides better corporeal exposure.
   d. It allows reservoir placement under direct vision.
   e. There is less chance of infection.

6. The traditional method of sizing corpora for cylinders:
   a. sizes them correctly.
   b. undersizes them by 1 cm.
   c. undersizes them by 2 cm.
   d. oversizes them by 1 cm.
   e. oversizes them by 2 cm.

7. Cylinders that are too long for the corp ora result in:
   a. an S-shaped deformity and premature failure.
   b. an S-shaped deformity and poor rigidity.
   c. premature failure and poor rigidity.
   d. premature failure and pain.
   e. an S-shaped deformity and pain.

8. For most patients, the ideal inflatable penile prosthesis reservoir location is:
   a. the inguinal canal.
   b. the scrotum.
   c. the retropubic space.
   d. between the rectus muscle and the peritoneum.
   e. extraperitoneal, lateral to the rectus muscle.

9. Wearing the penis up on the lower abdomen (anatomic position) postoperatively helps to:
   a. prevent upward penile curvature.
   b. prevent downward penile curvature.
   c. minimize pain.
   d. avoid infection.
   e. avoid autoinflation.

10. Following penile prosthesis implantation, failure to reach orgasm is best avoided by:
    a. supplemental testosterone.
    b. using a water-soluble lubricant.
    c. not inflating the device to high cylinder pressures.
    d. having adequate foreplay.
    e. using a rear-entry position.

11. Infected penile prostheses are best treated by:
    a. removal of the single infected component.
    b. removal of all prosthetic components.

c. twelve weeks of broad spectrum antibiotics.

d. hyperbaric oxygen.

e. 12 weeks of broad-spectrum antibiotics + hyperbaric oxygen.

12. Five months following three-piece inflatable penile prosthesis implantation, the recipient complains of persistent scrotal pain. Physical examination is normal except for adherence of the scrotal skin to the pump. The most likely cause of this man's symptoms and physical findings is:

a. allergy to silicone.

b. mechanical irritation from too much pumping.

c. overly tight undergarments.

d. infection with gram-positive organisms.

e. infection with gram-negative organisms.

13. The following coatings for penile prosthesis are being used in attempts to lower the infection rates:

a. minocycline, rifampin, and polyvinylpyrrolidone.

b. gentamicin, vancomycin, and polyvinylpyrrolidone.

c. gentamicin, vancomycin, and rifampin.

d. gentamicin, rifampin, and povidone-iodine (Betadine).

e. minocycline, vancomycin, and povidone-iodine (Betadine).

14. Infection rates following penile prosthesis revision surgery have been shown to be equivalent to infection rates following first-time penile prosthesis implantation. This is most likely due to:

a. 6 weeks of postrevision, wide-spectrum, intravenous antibiotics.

b. irrigation with hydrogen peroxide, povidone-iodine (Betadine), and multiple antibiotic solutions.

c. hydrophilic-coated devices.

d. antibiotic-coated devices.

e. removal of all prosthetic components.

15. During three-piece inflatable penile prosthesis implantation while the right corpus cavernosum is being dilated, the 8-mm dilator comes out the urethral meatus. Which approach should be used to manage this intraoperative complication?

a. Repair the urethra, continue using the implant, and leave the urethral catheter as a stent for 3 weeks.

b. Repair the urethra, continue using the implant, and insert a suprapubic tube.

c. Abandon the implant, and leave the urethral catheter in for 10 days.

d. Abandon the implant, repair the urethra, and leave the urethral catheter as a stent for 3 weeks.

e. Abandon the implant, repair the urethra, and insert a suprapubic tube.

ANSWERS

1. **c. inflatable penile prostheses, intracavernous injections, and PDE5 inhibitors.** In the 1970s and 1980s there was considerable enthusiasm regarding penile arterial revascularization and penile venous ligation surgery.

However, long-term results with these two treatment modalities have generally been disappointing and consequently these procedures are no longer commonly performed.

2. **a. is usually shorter.** In our experience shortness of the prosthetic erection is the most common cause for patient dissatisfaction. The other difference between a prosthetic erection and a normal erection is the absence of glans tumescence.

3. **b. penile length expansion.** The middle fabric layer of the AMS 700 LGX cylinder provides both controlled girth and length expansion.

4. **e. subcoronal, infrapubic, and penoscrotal.** The subcoronal incision should only be used to implant malleable or positionable devices.

5. **d. It allows reservoir placement under direct vision.** This is the only advantage of the infrapubic surgical approach.

6. **e. oversizes them by 2 cm.** The correct cylinder size is one whose length is the same as the length of an imaginary line that runs lengthwise through the center of the corpus cavernosum. Traditional sizing techniques overestimate this length by approximately 2 cm.

7. **a. an S-shaped deformity and premature failure.** A malleable prosthesis that is too long may cause pain, but a cylinder that is too long does not. Rigidity is usually not affected.

8. **c. the retropubic space.** When the reservoir is in the retropubic space, autoinflation of the prosthesis is less likely.

9. **b. prevent downward penile curvature.** While healing is taking place, a pseudocapsule forms around the prosthesis. If the cylinders are held down by an undergarment as this capsule is forming, they may develop downward curvature.

10. **d. having adequate foreplay.** If a man inflates his prosthesis, he is able to have coitus. However, unless he is sexually aroused, he may be unable to reach orgasm.

11. **b. removal of all prosthetic components.** Although only the scrotal pump may appear clinically to be infected, all components of the prosthesis are joined by tubing and the entire device should be considered infected.

12. **d. infection with gram-positive organisms.** Organisms such as *Staphylococcus epidermidis* typically cause a low-grade infection manifested by these symptoms and clinical findings. Infections due to gram-negative organisms commonly occur earlier and are associated with erythema and often drainage of pus from the wound.

13. **a. minocycline, rifampin, and polyvinylpyrrolidone.** Coloplast's three-piece inflatable penile prosthesis is coated with polyvinylpyrrolidone. American Medical System's three-piece inflatable penile prostheses are coated with minocycline and rifampin.

14. **e. removal of all prosthetic components.** Infection rates following repeat penile prosthesis surgery approach the rates seen with first-time penile prosthesis implantation if the entire device is replaced.

15. **c. Abandon the implant, and leave the urethral catheter in for 10 days.** If the implant is not abandoned, the urethra is unlikely to heal and the entire device is at risk of infection.

Additional Study Points

1. There are three types of penile prostheses in common use: (1) semirigid, (2) two-piece inflatable, and (3) three-piece inflatable. Normal penile flaccidity and erection is best achieved with a three-piece prosthesis.

2. Device removal is required when there is infection or erosion through the skin.

3. Safe insertion of the reservoir in the retropubic space requires an empty bladder.

4. Infections occurring within the first few weeks following an implant are more likely to be associated with gram-negative bacteria as opposed to those occurring 6 months or later, which are associated with gram-positive bacteria.

5. Late prosthetic infections can occur due to hematogenous spread.

6. Early penile prosthesis reimplantation after removal of an infection penile prosthesis following eradication of infection minimizes loss of penile length.

7. When one of the cylinders fails, many patients can have successful coitus with only one functional cylinder.

8. In one study, 70% of patients with a penile prosthesis were still sexually active, whereas only 40% of patients who were using penile injections continued to be sexually active.

Peyronie Disease

Gerald H. Jordan, MD, FACS, FAAP (Hon), FRCS (Hon) ●
Kurt A. McCammon, MD, FACS

QUESTIONS

1. Which of the following statements regarding Peyronie disease is correct?
   a. Most patients with Peyronie disease understand the effects of their disease and thus require little counseling.
   b. The majority of patients with Peyronie disease will eventually require surgery.
   c. Surgery, when required, can be viewed as palliation for the effects of the Peyronie disease process.
   d. In many patients with Peyronie disease, medical therapy has proved curative.
   e. The vast majority of patients will require prosthetic placement.

2. All of the following are associated with the development of Peyronie disease EXCEPT:
   a. angiotensin-converting enzyme inhibitors.
   b. β-adrenergic blockers.
   c. Paget disease of the bone.
   d. diabetes mellitus.
   e. phenytoin use.

3. Which of the following statements regarding Peyronie disease is NOT correct?
   a. Smith, using an autopsy study, found the asymptomatic incidence of Peyronie disease to be 22%.
   b. The symptomatic incidence of Peyronie disease has risen and now is estimated to be approximately 16%.
   c. The average age at onset of Peyronie disease is in the middle 50s.
   d. The asymptomatic prevalence of Peyronie disease is established to be 0.4% to 1.0%.
   e. The vast majority of patients with signs of Peyronie disease will have spontaneous resolution of the effects of the disease.

4. With regard to Peyronie disease, select the correct statement:
   a. Phosphodiesterase-5 (PDE5) inhibitor medications and the approved intracavernosal injection agents are contraindicated for use in Peyronie patients.
   b. PDE5 inhibitors may directly lead to the development of Peyronie disease.
   c. Prolonged use of papaverine and phentolamine (Regitine) has been implicated as a cause of intracorporeal fibrosis.
   d. The vacuum erection device (VED) is contraindicated for use in the Peyronie disease patient.

   e. Constriction rings are directly proven to be associated with the development of Peyronie disease.

5. With regard to the anatomy of the penis pertinent to Peyronie disease the:
   a. linear longitudinal layer attenuates at the 12-o'clock position (dorsal midline).
   b. circular lamina of the tunica albuginea attenuates at the 6-o'clock position (ventral midline).
   c. septal fibers interweave with the circular fiber lamina of the tunica albuginea.
   d. longitudinal lamina of the tunica albuginea is thickest at the ventral midline.
   e. midline septal fibers interweave with the thickened periurethral outer lamina.

6. Current theory about the etiology of Peyronie disease includes all of the following EXCEPT:
   a. The inciting event leading to Peyronie disease seems to be buckling trauma during erection.
   b. Transforming growth factor-β1 (TGF-β1) has been implicated as a cause of the abnormal disordered healing.
   c. Recent investigations also implicate the downregulation of factors known to be antifibrotic.
   d. Accumulation of plaque has been associated with other disorders governed by increased cholesterol and lipid levels.
   e. There is a downregulation of antifibrotic factors in Peyronie disease.

7. The natural history of Peyronie disease results in:
   a. the majority of patients presenting with sudden onset of stable deformity.
   b. many patients requiring surgery to resolve their painful erections.
   c. all patients eventually developing a stable deformity.
   d. frequent total resolution of the Peyronie disease process.
   e. those who have curvature have painful erections.

8. All of the following statements are TRUE with regard to the relationship of erectile dysfunction and Peyronie disease EXCEPT:
   a. In many of the older published series, the stratification of erectile problems, functional versus organic, is not clear. Currently with better validated instruments, stratification is included in most series.

b. The highly emotional aspects of Peyronie disease are expressed in many men via disordered erectile function.

c. Many men tend to abandon their sexual activities in response to the emotional trauma of Peyronie disease.

d. Surgery to address cavernous veno-occlusive dysfunction is often effective in men with Peyronie disease.

e. Often, with corrective surgery, disorders of erectile function seen preoperatively resolve with the surgical process.

9. Which of the following statements is TRUE with regard to the presenting complaints of patients with Peyronie disease?

a. Distal flaccidity occurs because of vascular blockage due to involvement of the spongy erectile tissue of the corpora cavernosa by the plaque.

b. Migratory penile deformity is usually due to the development of additional plaque.

c. Pain with intercourse rarely disappears without surgical therapy.

d. Foreshortening of the penis is a frequent complaint of patients with Peyronie disease.

e. Indentation of the corpora cavernosa is usually of cosmetic concern only.

10. For the medical management of Peyronie disease:

a. vitamin E has been proven to be highly efficacious.

b. aminobenzoate potassium (Potaba) has not been proven definitively to be efficacious.

c. nonsteroidal anti-inflammatory agents have been proven to be efficacious.

d. colchicine is thought to be efficacious by virtue of effects on purine metabolism.

e. tamoxifen, by virtue of its action on tubulin, has proved to be highly efficacious.

11. All of the following statements are TRUE with regard to intralesional injection protocols for Peyronie disease EXCEPT:

a. Intralesional corticosteroids are not recommended.

b. Verapamil injection protocols are logistically laborious, but the injections are well tolerated.

c. Collagenase is believed to work by dissolving collagen, thus allowing for plaque expansion and reinitiation of remodeling.

d. Interferon injections are proposed to work by mechanisms similar to those of verapamil but are associated with postinjection systemic symptoms.

e. Both verapamil and interferon are believed to have action based on their property of blocking cell division and thus purging the system of TGF-β.

12. Surgery is absolutely indicated in patients with Peyronie disease for which of the following?

a. Persistent pain with erection

b. Severe foreshortening of the penis

c. Erectile dysfunction or curvature that precludes intercourse

d. Indentation of the penis not related to issues of penetration

e. All of the above

13. When surgery is planned for Peyronie disease, which statement is TRUE?

a. Algorithms are the best mechanisms to determine surgical candidacy.

b. Corporoplasty techniques are technically straightforward and thus are the best for the surgeon who does not operate frequently on Peyronie disease patients.

c. Corporoplasty techniques, in most series, have better results for preservation of erectile function and thus are clearly superior for all Peyronie disease patients who are surgical candidates.

d. Incision and grafting techniques using synthetic "graft" material (e.g., Gore-Tex, Silastic) have been proven, in large series, to be highly effective.

e. Incision and grafting techniques, in emerging well-stratified studies, have been shown to effectively straighten the penis and preserve erectile function in Peyronie disease patients.

ANSWERS

1. **c. Surgery, when required, can be viewed as palliation for the effects of the Peyronie disease process.** Fortunately, however, most patients only require counseling, education, and reassurance. Although medical therapy is used, few studies have shown medical therapy to have proven efficacy. A minority of patients will have deformity that precludes their having intercourse, which is one of the indications for surgery. In the patient who is adequately sexually active, performing corrective surgery, just to make things better, cannot be recommended. The vast majority of patients with Peyronie disease thus do not require surgery, and, in most, prosthetic implantation can be avoided.

2. **a. angiotensin-converting enzyme inhibitors.** Peyronie disease is associated with Dupuytren contracture. Thirty to 40 percent of Peyronie disease patients will also have findings compatible with Dupuytren contracture. Other associated conditions include plantar fascial contracture (Ledderhose disease) and tympanosclerosis. Peyronie disease is also reported to be associated with external trauma to the penis, diabetes mellitus, Paget disease of the bone, history of urethral instrumentation, β-adrenergic blocker use, and phenytoin use; and now more and more patients are being seen with the only identifiable other association being that of having had a radical prostatectomy.

3. **b. The symptomatic incidence of Peyronie disease has risen and now is estimated to be approximately 16%.** The symptomatic incidence of Peyronie disease has previously been estimated at 1%. However, with the advent of pharmacologic treatment for erectile dysfunction, the incidence is clearly rising and can be quite conservatively estimated to be 4% to 5% now. In white men the average age at onset of Peyronie disease is approximately 53 years of age. The asymptomatic prevalence was estimated at 0.4% to 1%. It is reasonable to suggest that the asymptomatic prevalence of Peyronie disease is also increasing. An autopsy study of 100 men without a known history of Peyronie disease found 22 of the 100 men to have lesions histologically compatible with Peyronie disease.

4. **c. Prolonged use of papaverine and phentolamine (Regitine) has been implicated as a cause of intracorporeal fibrosis.** The phosphodiesterase-5 (PDE5)

inhibitor medications and the approved intracavernosal injection agents are not approved for Peyronie disease patients. This is because these patients were excluded during the final phase studies reviewed for drug approval. There has never been any suggestion that PDE5 inhibitors are directly causally related to the development of Peyronie disease. There are emerging data that would suggest that certain endothelial integrity can be preserved with the initiation of PDE5 inhibitor therapy; and, in fact, recent data suggest that the use of PDE5 inhibitors may be therapeutic for Peyronie disease patients. Cyclic guanosine monophosphate (GMP), which is one of the mediators of penile erection, is produced by nitric oxide activation of guanylyl cyclase. Cyclic GMP is also antifibrotic in Peyronie disease plaques. Long-term administration of sildenafil, a PDE inhibitor, impedes cyclic GMP breakdown and has been shown to prevent Peyronie disease plaque formation in rat models. Intracavernosal injection therapy has not been directly implicated as causative in Peyronie disease. It has certainly been theorized that repeated trauma from insertion of the needle could stimulate a Peyronie disease–like process. The prolonged use of papaverine and phentolamine has been shown to create intracorporeal fibrosis. The vacuum erection device is not contraindicated for use in Peyronie disease patients; and, in fact, there are protocols that are examining the vacuum device as a possible treatment method for patients with Peyronie disease.

5. **c. septal fibers interweave with the circular fiber lamina of the tunica albuginea.** The tunica albuginea is bilaminar throughout most of its circumference. It is composed of an outer longitudinal layer and an inner circular layer. The tunica albuginea varies in thickness from 1.5 to 3 mm depending on the position on the circumference. The outer longitudinal layer attenuates in the ventral midline, and thus the tunica is monolaminar at that point. The outer longitudinal layer is thickest on the ventrum adjacent to the corpus spongiosum and on the dorsum and thinnest on the lateral aspect.

6. **d. Accumulation of plaque has been associated with other disorders governed by increased cholesterol and lipid levels.** Somers and Dawson (1997)* have shown that Peyronie disease most likely begins with buckling trauma causing injury to the septal insertion of the tunica albuginea. It has been proposed that the avascular nature of the tunica albuginea may impede clearance of many tissue growth factors, particularly transforming growth factor (TGF)-β1. TGF-β1 has been implicated in a number of cases of soft tissue fibrosis as well as with erectile dysfunction. The TGFs are also capable of autoinducement. Recent investigations have also implicated the failure of downregulation of matrix metalloproteinase (MMP) in the abnormal scarring process of Peyronie disease. Failure of downregulation of MMP also has been implicated in a number of disease processes. MMPs function as antifibrotic factors. α₁-Antitrypsin, which is a proteinase inhibitor, has also been implicated as a possible factor in the development of Peyronie disease. Recent investigation has not verified that implication; however, it was found that α₁-antitrypsin levels do vary with age.

7. **c. all patients eventually developing stable deformity.** In most cases of Peyronie disease there are two phases: an active phase that often can be associated with painful erections and migratory deformity of the penis and the quiescent phase, which is characterized by stabilization of the deformity and inevitably with disappearance of painful erections if they were present. Up to one third of patients, however, will present with what appears to be sudden development of painless and stable deformity. A review by Mulhall interestingly shows that in a large cohort of men with Peyronie disease one third presented with erectile dysfunction at the time that they presented with Peyronie disease and a significant percentage of them had erectile dysfunction that preceded their notice of the onset of Peyronie disease and its diagnosis. This confirms the work of other authors.

8. **e. Often, with corrective surgery, disorders of erectile function seen preoperatively resolve with the surgical process.** In publications concerning the natural history of disease, erectile dysfunction is prominently mentioned. In the older literature, patients were not stratified with regard to the functional issues versus the organic issues as they relate to erectile dysfunction. Jones, in 1977, dealt best with the counseling issues of men with sexual dysfunction and described the counseling of a man with Peyronie disease as being much the same as counseling a person who has suffered a death and is grieving. Recent data show that most men indicated that the impact of Peyronie disease on their life was severe. That data verify much of what Jones reported. The emotions expressed by many of the men who were interviewed ranged from anger to frustration to hopelessness. A major point made by Jones in dealing with Peyronie disease patients is to avoid or limit emotional factors. Patients and their partners need to hear the suggestion that they must "keep sexual expression alive." Recent data show that men with Peyronie disease, even though not in a steady relationship, do continue to have sex; however, it was usually "very different than it used to be," and most were very concerned that their condition would worsen to the point that they would be unable to have sexual intercourse in the future. Cavernous veno-occlusive disease (CVOD) is seen in patients with Peyronie disease, and the precise mechanism is not clear. What is clear is that surgery to address CVOD is virtually never effective in Peyronie disease patients.

9. **d. Foreshortening of the penis is a frequent complaint of patients with Peyronie disease.** The presenting symptoms of Peyronie disease include (1) in many cases penile pain with erection, (2) penile deformity, (3) shortening of the penis with and without an erection, (4) notice of a plaque or indurated area in the penis, and (5) in many patients erectile dysfunction. Some patients complain of being awakened in the morning with pain during their erection. Spontaneous improvement in pain with erection virtually always occurs as the inflammation resolves. However, this must not be confused with pain during intercourse. Pain during intercourse often does persist and is due to the mechanical forces of intercourse on the curved penis. Distal flaccidity is frequently noted, but it is believed to be due to the mechanical effects of the plaque, limiting stretching of the midline septal fibers and thus creating a hinge effect at that area. Studies have shown that proximally and distally to the plaque the pressures within the corpora cavernosa are the same.

10. **b. Aminobenzoate potassium (Potaba) has not been proven definitively to be efficacious.** Any discussion

*Sources referenced can be found in *Campbell-Walsh Urology, 10th Edition,* on the Expert Consult website.

on the medical management of Peyronie disease begins with the disclaimer that few medical management regimens have been subjected to double-blind drug testing. Vitamin E has not been subjected to blinded or controlled studies and thus has not been proven to be efficacious. The prolonged use of high-dose vitamin E is not recommended because of its anticoagulation effects. Aminobenzoate potassium has been looked at in a small blinded study that showed it to be efficacious, but subsequent studies have not verified those results. Additionally, at therapeutic doses, patients complain of gastrointestinal side effects when taking aminobenzoate potassium. Colchicine binds tubulin and causes it to depolymerize and thus inhibits mobility and adhesion of leukocytes but also inhibits mitosis by disrupting spindle cell fibers and thus functions as a very potent anti-inflammatory agent. Tubulin is also involved in the process of wound contracture. Colchicine also stimulates collagenases. Nonsteroidal anti-inflammatory drugs and corticosteroids have been used anecdotally; however, no studies support an indication for the use of these drugs. Tamoxifen is thought to facilitate the release of TGF-β from fibroblasts; however, recent studies have not shown the use of tamoxifen to be effective in Peyronie disease patients.

11. **e. Both Verapamil and interferon are believed to have action based on their property of blocking cell division and thus purging the system of TGF-β.** A number of intralesional injection protocols have been examined. It is the recommendation of the consensus committee on penile curvatures that the use of intralesional corticosteroids be eliminated or at least initiated with extreme caution because of the rather significant local side effects, the inconsistent pattern of improvement in well-established curvature, the lack of studies showing proven efficacy, and reports of patients who believed their condition deteriorated after the injections. A number of nonblinded studies have suggested efficacy with the use of intralesional verapamil, but no blinded studies suggest that the use of verapamil as an intralesional agent is efficacious. Collagenase has been subjected to two double-blind studies, but intralesional collagenase is currently available only on study protocol. The use of interferons as intralesional therapy for Peyronie disease was reported in 1991. The mechanism of action of interferon is very similar to that proposed for verapamil. Verapamil is well tolerated. Complications are associated only with the injection procedure per se and are minimal. However, almost all patients injected with interferon develop a "flulike" syndrome. Both verapamil and interferon interfere with the "manufacture" or exocytosis of collagen.

12. **c. Erectile dysfunction or curvature that precludes intercourse.** For a patient to be a surgical candidate the patient must have stable and mature disease. Indications for surgery include deformity that precludes intercourse and/or erectile dysfunction that precludes intercourse. Surgery for persistent pain or for foreshortening only rarely provides good results and thus is strongly not recommended.

13. **e. Incision and grafting techniques, in emerging well-stratified studies, have been shown to effectively straighten the penis and preserve erectile function in Peyronie disease patients.** For a patient to be a surgical candidate, the patient must have mature/quiescent disease. The patient likewise should be significantly disabled with regard to the performance of intercourse by either the curvature and/or the associated erectile dysfunction. A number of corporoplasty techniques have been proposed, and all have been shown to be relatively effective. Corporoplasty techniques are not necessarily straightforward techniques; in some cases achieving an adequately straight penis can be technically quite complex. In past series, corporoplasty techniques have been shown to have a better rate of preservation of preoperative erectile function, as compared with excision and grafting techniques. Well-stratified studies that have been recently performed have shown excellent rates of preservation of erectile function with incision and grafting techniques. Because foreshortening is a cardinal finding for most patients with Peyronie disease, surgery that further "foreshortens the penis" is often not well accepted by nor palatable to the patient. Thus, in determining candidacy for surgery, and in determining the recommended surgical technique, a number of factors must be taken into account: (1) the patient's current symptoms; (2) the patient's stratification with regard to erectile function; (3) the predominant direction of curvature and location of the plaque; and (4) the patient's goals, after a course of education and counseling. In general, there are no large series that show effective use of synthetic graft materials. Those materials can be useful in patients who are having concomitant insertion of a penile prosthesis. In my experience, however, the use of the synthetic graft materials as "stand alone grafts" usually does not provide adequate results.

SUMMARY

Peyronie disease is not the "terminal/no hope" diagnosis that many patients believe it is, and in some cases have been told that it is. With proper counseling and education, proper stratification, and proper tailoring of the approach to patients, most can be effectively managed.

Additional Study Points

1. Surgery for Peyronie disease is at best palliation.
2. TGF-β1 is thought to be involved in the formation of a Peyronie plaque.
3. Peyronie disease has two phases: (1) an active phase associated with painful erections and changing deformity and (2) a quiescent phase characterized by stabilization.
4. Complete spontaneous resolution of Peyronie disease is infrequent.
5. The simultaneous occurrence of erectile dysfunction with Peyronie disease is not an infrequent occurrence.
6. Spontaneous improvement of pain almost always occurs as the inflammation resolves.
7. To examine the penis for plaques it should be examined on stretch.
8. The deformities of Peyronie disease may be migratory before stabilizing.
9. One third of patients will develop dystrophic calcification in the plaque.
10. If a dermal graft is to be used, it should be 30% larger than the defect.
11. When penile prostheses are used in patients with Peyronie disease and when incisions in the plaques are required, the incisions should be closed with synthetic patch materials such as Gore-Tex.

Androgen Deficiency in the Aging Male

Alvaro Morales, MD, FACS, FRCS

QUESTIONS

1. The prevalence of symptomatic testosterone (T) deficiency in American men 30 to 70 years of age is:

   a. unknown.

   b. 2%.

   c. 6%.

   d. 10%.

   e. 14%

2. Which of the following statements regarding testosterone (T) production and metabolism is NOT correct?

   a. T is produced by the Leydig cells under the control of luteinizing hormone (LH) only.

   b. T is produced by brain cells, but this portion is not measurable in serum.

   c. T is produced by conversion from other androgens such as dehydroepiandrosterone (DHEA).

   d. T is produced in decreased amounts in the presence of hyperprolactinemia.

   e. T bound to sex hormone–binding globulin (SHBG) is active in the prostate.

3. Which of the following statements regarding the clinical diagnosis of androgen deficiency in aging is TRUE?

   a. Screening questionnaires (Androgen Deficiency in Aging Males [ADAM], Aging Male Survey [AMS]) have high (>75%) specificity.

   b. Serum T trigger level for symptoms ranges narrowly among individuals.

   c. Recurrence of symptoms is highly reproducible for each individual's serum T levels, with interruption of therapy.

   d. Signs and symptoms of hypogonadism are specific; biochemical support is desirable but not mandatory.

   e. Sarcopenia and osteopenia/osteoporosis are fundamental elements for the diagnosis of the condition.

4. Which of the following biochemical assays best reflects tissue-available testosterone?

   a. Total T

   b. Free T by direct radioimmunoassay using a T analog with low affinity for SHBG

   c. Free T by equilibrium dialysis

   d. Free androgen index

   e. Salivary T

5. Which of the following statements is TRUE?

   a. Intraindividual variations in serum T levels are insignificant; repeat measurements for diagnosis, therefore, are not necessary.

   b. Intraindividual variations in serum T levels are less apparent with assays for bioavailable T.

   c. In older men (>65 years) borderline levels of T with normal gonadotropins rule out the diagnosis of hypogonadism.

   d. Repeatedly finding borderline serum T levels in the presence of clinical manifestations of T deficiency justifies a trial of T supplementation.

   e. Repeatedly finding borderline serum total T levels in the presence of clinical manifestations of T deficiency is an indication for ordering a direct radioimmunoassay of free T using a T analog assay with low affinity for SHBG.

6. Alterations in other hormones, besides sex steroids, occur with aging. Which of the following is NOT true?

   a. Growth hormone decreases at a rate similar to T.

   b. Melatonin production by the pineal gland decreases with aging.

   c. Prolactin production is not affected by aging.

   d. Leptin increases with aging and more so in the presence of hypogonadism.

   e. SHBG decreases in healthy aging.

7. Which of the following is NOT a contraindication for T therapy in males?

   a. Breast cancer

   b. Gynecomastia

   c. Angina pectoris

   d. Heart failure

   e. Polycythemia

8. The safety and efficacy of T therapy are not conclusively established. Which of the following is NOT a recommendation by the Institute of Medicine (IOM) Committee on Testosterone and Aging?

   a. Focus on populations most likely to benefit.

   b. Use T for treatment, not for prevention, of disease.

   c. Focus on clinical outcomes with preliminary evidence of benefit.

d. Begin with short-term safety trials.

e. Conduct long-term studies only if short-term efficacy is established.

9. A 58-year-old, type 2 diabetic, hypertensive man presents with low libido, poor quality erections, and low energy but no depression. His medications include insulin, gemfibrozil, enalapril, and metoclopramide. Examination shows weak dorsalis pedis, moderate muscle wasting, and soft testes. Prostate and penis examinations were normal. Biochemistry includes HbA1c: 13% (normal, 4 to 6); prostate-specific antigen (PSA): 0.8 ng/L (normal, <4); total T: 210 ng/dL (normal, 300 to 800); and prolactin: 60 ng/mL (normal, <20). The next step is to:

a. measure free T by direct RIA.

b. repeat prolactin assessment.

c. order MRI of the pituitary.

d. initiate T replacement therapy.

e. initiate treatment with cabergoline or bromocriptine.

10. A 67-year-old man presents with a history of radical retropubic prostatectomy (RRP) for a Gleason sum 7 adenocarcinoma of the prostate 6 years previously. He complains of fatigue and markedly decreased sexual desire and quality of erections. PSA: <0.1; bioavailable T: 1.6 nmoL/L (normal, 2 to 9); LH: 6.7 (normal, <18). Repeat bioavailable T: 1.4 nmoL/L. The next step is to:

a. not consider him a candidate for supplemental T.

b. wait for 4 more years (10 since RRP) to consider supplemental T.

c. consider administration of a weak androgen such as DHEA.

d. inform him of the risks and, with his consent, administer T.

e. inform him of the risks and advise him against T therapy.

ANSWERS

1. **c. 6%.** The incidence is 500,000 new cases per year. Traditionally, the prevalence of hypogonadism in the aging man was inferred from population projections. The Massachusetts Male Aging Study reported a crude incidence of 12.3 per 1000 person-years, leading to a prevalence of 481,000 new cases per year. The same group estimated that 5.6% not only had hypogonadism but are symptomatic.

2. **a. T is produced by the Leydig cells under the control of luteinizing hormone (LH) only.** LH modulates most of the biosynthesis of T by the Leydig cells. However, neural influences from the paraventricular nucleus of the hypothalamus and ghrelin actively regulate Leydig cell activity. Small amounts of androgens are produced in the brain. In some tissues such as the prostate, T bound to SHBG can activate SHBG receptors and produce effects within the cell (see Fig. 29–1 in *Campbell-Walsh Urology, 10th Edition*).

3. **c. Recurrence of symptoms is highly reproducible for each individual's serum T levels, with interruption of therapy.** The sensitivity of the screening questionnaires is high (~80%), but their specificity is low (<50%). There is a wide interindividual variation for the T level, triggering specific symptoms of hypogonadism (probably depending on the number of CAG repeats in the androgen receptor). However, after an adequate response to treatment, discontinuation of T administration triggers symptoms at highly reproducible T levels in each individual. Manifestations of hypogonadism are not specific and are seen in other conditions (healthy aging, depression, hypothyroidism). Neither the clinical picture nor the biochemical assays individually are sufficient for diagnosis and management of late-onset hypogonadism (see Fig. 29–2 and Table 29–3 in *Campbell-Walsh Urology, 10th Edition*).

4. **c. Free T by equilibrium dialysis.** Total T is usually sufficient for the initial diagnosis. It may be misleading in conditions associated with an elevation in SHBG levels (healthy aging, hyperthyroidism, obesity). Radioimmunoassay for free T is imprecise and should never be ordered. The most accurate test in this situation is the free T value obtained by equilibrium dialysis or by centrifugal ultrafiltration. These tests are expensive and cumbersome. The free androgen index is also inadequate, and the value of salivary T has not been definitively established. Calculated free and bioavailable T tests are accurate and simpler alternatives (see Table 29–4 in *Campbell-Walsh Urology, 10th Edition*).

5. **d. Repeatedly finding borderline serum T levels in the presence of clinical manifestations of T deficiency justifies a trial of T supplementation.** Longitudinal studies have shown a significant variation in serum T levels over short periods, in the same individuals with any assays, and specifically with measurement of bioavailable T. A repeat measurement is, therefore, advisable. The hypothalamus and the pituitary age together with the gonads. The feedback mechanisms are usually blunted in the elderly, and a decrease in number and function of Leydig cells is infrequently associated with elevation of gonadotropins. In the presence of florid clinical manifestations of hypogonadism but a questionable biochemistry, a short (3 month) trial of T supplementation is justified. The assay that should not be used is a commonly available and frequently ordered one: direct radioimmunoassay of free T using a labeled T analog with low affinity for SHBG. It has poor accuracy and most closely reflects the measurement of total T (see Table 29–4 in *Campbell-Walsh Urology, 10th Edition*).

6. **e. SHBG decreases in healthy aging.** DHEA, growth hormone, melatonin, and thyroxine decrease with aging; and their deficiency shares many of the manifestations of hypogonadism. Prolactin is not particularly affected by the aging process, but hyperprolactinemia can be induced by medications. In addition to aging, SHBG might increase in several situations. Therefore, misdiagnosis of eugonadism may occur when only total T is measured. SHBG-bound T is largely inaccessible to tissues, although there are some notable exceptions, such as the prostate (see Table 29–5 in *Campbell-Walsh Urology, 10th Edition*).

7. **c. Angina pectoris.** Breast cancer growth is stimulated by estrogen (from peripheral conversion/aromatization of T). The same mechanism is considered responsible for the development of gynecomastia during androgen therapy. T has been shown to be a coronary and peripheral vasodilator (through nongenomic mechanisms). Although rare, fluid retention may occur in the elderly; therefore, the administration of T should be regarded with caution. Modest increases in red blood cell mass are common after T therapy. Occasionally, polycythemia may be significant, particularly in the elderly.

8. **d. Begin with short-term safety trials.** The IOM report includes an extensive review of the literature and a set of recommendations for future research in T therapy. The panel believed that efficacy of T treatment has not yet been demonstrated and recommended, therefore, that efficacy must be established first by clinical trials. Only if efficacy is demonstrated should long-term safety trials similar to the Women's Health Initiative be conducted (see Table 29–7 in *Campbell-Walsh Urology, 10th Edition*). Thus, short-term efficacy trials were recommended, not short-term safety trials.

9. **d. initiate T replacement therapy.** The combination of symptoms associated with small, soft testes and a marked decrease in total T levels constitutes a clear indication for T supplementation. There is increasing evidence that insulin resistance is associated with a decrease in Leydig cell T secretion. Initiation of treatment based on the clinical picture and clearly decreased T levels is justified, but prudence dictates that the initial result be confirmed. Although bioavailable T is a more accurate reflection of androgenicity than total T, in this particular case it is not necessary: bioavailable T testing is more expensive and cumbersome to perform. Assessment of the pituitary is generally recommended but, at this man's age, it would not be surprising to find normal LH levels despite profound hypogonadism. The moderate prolactin elevation is most likely drug induced (metoclopramide), and the drug should be discontinued (see Table 29–4 and Fig. 29–3 in *Campbell-Walsh Urology, 10th Edition*).

10. **d. inform him of the risks and, with his consent, administer T.** T administration is an absolute contraindication in the presence of prostate cancer, but there is no evidence that this patient is harboring it. Recommendations regarding T supplementation in this situation are based on limited and, mostly, anecdotal information. However, when there is severe testosterone deficiency syndrome (TDS) with significant interference in the quality of life, a trial of T treatment may be justified. Good clinical judgment plays an important role in a situation like this. If T treatment is initiated, the initial follow-up must be frequent and particularly careful. An elevation of the PSA is a clear indication that prostate cells are present and T administration should then be discontinued. Most likely this will lead to a return of the PSA value to the pretreatment levels. Familiarity with the Consensus Recommendations on the use of supplemental T is strongly advised.

Additional Study Points

1. With aging there is a change in the gonadal hypothalamic pituitary axis.

2. The number of Leydig cells decrease with aging and there is a reduction in the diurnal variation of T, suggesting desensitization of Leydig cells to LH with aging.

3. Circulating T is 98% bound to SHBG and albumin. T bound to albumin is more readily unbound than that bound to SHBG.

4. With aging, changes in enzyme receptor function and responsiveness of cells to the balance between T and dihydrotestosterone occur at different rates in individuals, which makes setting an absolute level of hormone deficiency difficult for a particular individual.

5. Metabolism of T takes place mainly in the liver, prostate, and skin; and the catabolic products are excreted in the urine.

6. The CAG repeat sequence on the androgen receptor is maximal in man (about 22 triplets) and is less in other species. There is an increased androgen response of the receptor in men with shorter CAG repeats. The androgen receptor may be activated not only by T but also by protein kinase C and other factors.

7. Hypogonadal men have increased levels of leptin and insulin. They are more likely to be obese. Hypogonadism correlates with elevated serum glucose and triglyceride levels. There is an increase in total body fat mass and fasting insulin resistant index.

8. Administration of T in older men is associated with decreased visceral fat, decreased glucose concentration, and increased sensitivity to insulin.

9. The diagnosis of TDS cannot be based on absolute levels of serum T or symptoms and requires a matter of judgment. However, among the most prominent symptoms of this syndrome are tiredness, decreased sexual desire, and dysphoria (mood of general dissatisfaction, depression).

10. It appears that bioavailable free T is better correlated with symptoms of TDS than is total T. Measurement of T should be restricted to the morning hours because that is the peak point of secretion. In younger men there is a normal circadian rhythm that is blunted as men age.

11. As men age, growth hormone decreases, which may result in changes in lean muscle mass, bone density, hair distribution, and the pattern of obesity. In addition, there is a reduction in DHEA, melatonin, and thyroxine. Serum leptin levels increase.

12. Hypogonadism is associated with increased mortality in males.

13. Serum T increases bone mineral density. Higher levels of circulating T correlate with a lower cardiovascular risk. Lower levels correlate with hypoactive sexual desire.

14. The presence of prostate or breast cancer is an absolute contraindication for T treatment. There is little evidence to indicate that in the normal male without prostate cancer supplementation with T for periods of up to 3 years increases prostate growth.

15. Serum PSA thresholds for normal values are less in hypogonadal men.

16. T increases red cell mass.

Female Sexual Function and Dysfunction

Courtenay Kathryn Moore, MD

QUESTIONS

1. What is the normal vaginal pH for premenopausal women?
   a. 2.0 to 3.0
   b. 3.5 to 4.5
   c. 5.5 to 6.5
   d. 6.5 to 7.5
   e. >7.5

2. A patient presents with complaints of an abnormal vaginal discharge. A wet mount of the secretions show clue cells. How should the patient be treated?
   a. No treatment is required. Clue cells are normal vaginal flora.
   b. The patient should be treated with ciprofloxacin.
   c. The patient and her partner should be treated with ciprofloxacin.
   d. The patient should be treated with metronidazole (Flagyl).
   e. The patient and her partner should be treated with metronidazole (Flagyl).

3. When is a vascular workup not indicated in a woman with sexual complaints?
   a. In a woman with sexual arousal problems with a history of a pelvic fracture
   b. In a postmenopausal woman complaining of dyspareunia
   c. In an obese, diabetic, hypertensive woman with sexual arousal disorder
   d. In a woman with sexual arousal disorders unresponsive to other therapies
   e. In a woman with sexual arousal disorders after radical pelvic surgery

4. What is the most common type of female sexual disorder?
   a. Dyspareunia
   b. Vaginismus
   c. Hypoactive sexual desire disorder
   d. Orgasmic disorder
   e. Sexual arousal disorder

5. Which is not a contraindication to testosterone therapy?
   a. Androgenic alopecia
   b. Obesity
   c. Hirsutism
   d. Polycystic ovary syndrome
   e. Liver dysfunction

6. Which medications have known sexual side effects?
   a. Cocaine
   b. Selective serotonin reuptake inhibitors
   c. Histamine-2 blockers
   d. β-Adrenergic blockers
   e. All of the above

7. A 27-year-old woman presents with complaints of dyspareunia, dysuria, vaginal discharge, and some dribbling of urine. On physical examination there is fullness of the anterior vaginal wall. On palpation the patient reports tenderness, and drainage per urethra is noted. What is the most likely diagnosis and what imaging modality would best confirm the diagnosis?
   a. Cystocele/Dynamic MRI of the pelvis
   b. Bartholin gland cyst/No imaging required
   c. Vaginal candidiasis/No imaging required
   d. Urethral diverticulum/MRI of the pelvis
   e. Urethral carcinoma/CT of the pelvis

8. What conditions cause low free testosterone levels in women?
   a. Oral contraceptives
   b. Prolactinoma
   c. Cushing disease
   d. Aging
   e. All of the above

9. Which of the following statements is FALSE?
   a. Studies have found no significant difference in the estrogen levels of women with and without clinically diagnosed hypoactive sexual desire disorders.
   b. The administration of exogenous estrogens in patients with hypoactive sexual desire disorder has been shown to improve sexual desire.
   c. Treatment with progesterone alone has not been shown to improve sexual desire in either premenopausal or menopausal women.
   d. In studies of both naturally and surgically menopausal women, the administration of testosterone alone, without estrogen replacement therapy, has been shown to improve desire, arousal, and sexual fantasies.

e. New data suggest that testosterone therapy is beneficial in premenopausal women with hypoactive sexual desire disorder who have low circulating testosterone levels.

10. Which of the following structures are not embryologically homologous?

   a. Bartholin glands and Cowper glands
   b. Skene glands and the prostate
   c. Penis and clitoris
   d. Scrotum and labia minora
   e. None of the above

11. The dorsal nerve of the clitoris is the terminal branch of what nerve?

   a. Inferior hemorrhoidal nerve
   b. Superficial perineal nerve
   c. Deep perineal nerve
   d. Genitofemoral nerve
   e. Ilioinguinal nerve

12. Complications of testosterone therapy in women include all of the following EXCEPT:

   a. virilization.
   b. hyperpigmentation.
   c. acne.
   d. hirsutism.
   e. hyperlipidemia.

ANSWERS

1. **b. 3.5 to 4.5.** Normal vaginal pH in premenopausal women is 3.5 to 4.5. After menopause the vaginal pH becomes more basic secondary to a drop in estrogen levels.

2. **d. The patient should be treated with metronidazole (Flagyl).** The patient has bacterial vaginosis given the clue cells on her wet mount. The patient but not her partner should be treated with metronidazole.

3. **b. In a postmenopausal woman complaining of dyspareunia.** The most likely cause of dyspareunia in a postmenopausal woman is atrophic vaginitis, which should be treated with topical estrogen therapy. Indications for vascular testing include (1) women with sexual arousal disorders who have exposure to multiple vascular risk factors, (2) women who have suffered pelvic fractures, and (3) women with sexual arousal disorders unresponsive to other therapies.

4. **c. Hypoactive sexual desire disorder.** Hypoactive sexual desire disorder (HSDD) is the most common female sexual disorder.

5. **b. Obesity.** Contraindications to testosterone therapy include androgenic alopecia, hirsutism, seborrhea or acne, polycystic ovary syndrome, liver dysfunction, and estrogen depletion.

6. **e. All of the above.** See Table 30–3 in *Campbell-Walsh Urology, 10th Edition* for discussion of medications with known sexual side effects.

7. **d. Urethral diverticulum/MRI of the pelvis.** The patient has a symptomatic urethral diverticulum as characterized by the three Ds: dyspareunia, dysuria, postvoid dribbling. MRI is the imaging modality of choice.

8. **e. All of the above.** Hyperprolactinemia, Cushing disease, aging, and oral contraceptives all cause decreases in circulating free testosterone in women. Hyperprolactinemia from a prolactinoma and Cushing disease cause adrenal suppression and androgen insufficiency. Free testosterone levels also decrease with aging and increases of sex hormone–binding globulin from oral contraceptives binds free testosterone, decreasing levels of free testosterone.

9. **b. The administration of exogenous estrogens in patients with hypoactive sexual desire disorder has been shown to improve sexual desire.** Numerous studies have also shown no change in sexual desire with the administration of exogenous estrogen therapy alone in women. However, administration of both estrogen and androgen in natural and surgically menopausal woman has been shown to restore normal levels of sexual desire.

10. **d. Scrotum and labia minora.** In males the scrotum is homologous to the female labia majora. The penile urethra is homologous to the labia minora.

11. **c. Deep perineal nerve.** The pudendal nerve branches into three nerves: the inferior hemorrhoidal nerve, superficial perineal nerve, and the deep perineal nerve. The dorsal nerve of the clitoris is the terminal branch of the deep perineal nerve.

12. **b. hyperpigmentation.** Virilization, acne, hirsutism, hyperlipidemia, menstrual irregularities, liver dysfunction, seborrhea, and male pattern baldness are all possible complications of exogenous testosterone therapy in women.

Additional Study Points

1. Studies suggest that 43% of women and 31% of men experience sexual dysfunction.
2. Testosterone production in women comes directly from the ovaries and adrenal glands and, unlike estrogen and progesterone levels that fall abruptly with menopause, testosterone levels diminish gradually throughout life.
3. Sexual neutrality or being receptive to rather than initiating sexual activity is considered a normal variation of female sexual functioning.
4. Women with incontinence are up to three times more likely to experience decreased arousal and infrequent orgasms and increased dyspareunia.
5. Lack of estrogen may not directly impair female arousal and desire, but it impairs sexual function by resulting in a decreased vasocongestion and lubrication and increased vaginal epithelial atrophy.
6. Progesterones have an indirect effect on sexual function by increasing depressive moods.
7. Optimal female sexual health requires physical, emotional, and mental well-being.

Male Genitalia

31

Neoplasms of the Testis

Andrew J. Stephenson, MD, FACS, FRCSC ● Timothy D. Gilligan, MD, MS

QUESTIONS

1. The following adult male germ cell tumor (GCT) subtypes arise from intratubular germ cell neoplasia (ITGCN) EXCEPT:
   a. embryonal tumor.
   b. choriocarcinoma.
   c. classic seminoma.
   d. spermatocytic seminoma.
   e. teratoma.

2. Which of the following statements is TRUE regarding spermatocytic seminoma?
   a. Cryptorchidism is a risk factor.
   b. It may occur as a mixed GCT with other histologic GCT subtypes.
   c. It may contain i(12p) mutations.
   d. Bilateral testicular involvement may occur in 2% to 3% of cases.
   e. Metastatic spermatocytic seminoma is rare.

3. Which of the following GCT subtypes is most likely to spread hematogenously?
   a. Choriocarcinoma
   b. Embryonal carcinoma
   c. Immature teratoma
   d. Teratoma with malignant transformation
   e. Seminoma

4. A 24-year-old man presents with a solid, painless, right intratesticular mass confirmed by scrotal ultrasonography. His left testis is normal. Serum tumor markers show a human chorionic gonadotropin (hCG) value of 96 mU/mL (upper limit: <5 mU/mL) and an α-fetoprotein (AFP) value of 58 ng/mL (upper limit: <11 ng/mL). The most likely histologic finding in the right testis is:
   a. pure teratoma.
   b. pure seminoma.
   c. pure embryonal carcinoma.
   d. pure yolk sac tumor.
   e. choriocarcinoma.

5. Which of the following is an acceptable indication for testis-sparing surgery?
   a. 1.3-cm solid intratesticular mass with a normal contralateral testis
   b. Suspected benign testicular lesion
   c. 2.4-cm solid mass in a solitary testis
   d. Hypogonadal male with 1.2-cm solid intratesticular mass in a solitary testis

   e. Small (<1 cm) hyperechoic lesion suggestive of a "burned out" primary tumor in a patient with disseminated nonseminomatous GCT (NSGCT) with serum-elevated AFP and hCG

6. A 37-year-old man presents with a 5-cm left testicular mass. CT reveals a 6-cm para-aortic mass but no evidence of distant metastases. Serum tumor markers show an AFP level of 1100 ng/mL (upper limit: <11 ng/mL) and an hCG level of 80 mU/mL (upper limit: <5 mU/mL). Left inguinal orchiectomy reveals a mixed GCT with 60% embryonal carcinoma, 30% yolk sac tumor, 5% seminoma, and 5% teratoma. The next best management step is:
   a. retroperitoneal lymph node dissection (RPLND).
   b. induction chemotherapy with three cycles of bleomycin-etoposide-cisplatin.
   c. induction chemotherapy with four cycles of bleomycin-etoposide-cisplatin.
   d. to obtain repeat serum tumor marker levels in 7 days.
   e. CT-guided biopsy of the para-aortic mass.

7. All of the following patients would be classified as "poor-risk" by International Germ Cell Cancer Collaborative Group (IGCCCG) classification criteria EXCEPT those with:
   a. testicular seminoma with brain metastases.
   b. primary mediastinal NSGCT.
   c. testicular NSGCT with rising postorchiectomy AFP of 15,000 ng/mL (upper limit: <11 ng/mL).
   d. primary retroperitoneal NSGCT with liver metastases.
   e. testicular NSGCT with rising postorchiectomy hCG of 93,000 mU/mL (upper limit: <5 mU/mL).

8. A 34-year-old African-American man with a left testicular mass undergoes inguinal orchiectomy that reveals a 1.2-cm pure seminoma that is confined to the testis with no evidence of lymphovascular invasion or rete testis invasion. His postorchiectomy serum tumor markers are within the normal range. CT of the chest-abdomen-pelvis reveals no evidence of retroperitoneal lymphadenopathy and no evidence of pulmonary metastases. However, on the chest images, there is evidence of bulky hilar adenopathy bilaterally. The next best management step is:
   a. induction chemotherapy with four cycles of bleomycin-etoposide-cisplatin.
   b. induction chemotherapy with four cycles of etoposide-cisplatin.
   c. mediastinoscopy and biopsy.
   d. close observation..
   e. bilateral thoracotomy and resection.

9. A 43-year-old man with clinical stage IIA left seminoma receives dog-leg radiation therapy to the retroperitoneum and ipsilateral pelvis with a boost to his solitary 2-cm para-aortic mass. Six months after completing treatment, surveillance CT reveals a persistent para-aortic mass that has now grown to 2.8 cm. The remainder of his metastatic evaluation is negative, and his serum tumor marker levels are all within normal limits. The next best management step is:

   a. RPLND.

   b. CT-guided biopsy of the retroperitoneal mass.

   c. close observation until the mass regresses or the patient develops distant metastases.

   d. induction chemotherapy with three cycles of bleomycin-etoposide-cisplatin.

   e. salvage chemotherapy with four cycles of paclitaxel-ifosfamide-cisplatin.

10. A 41-year-old man has ITGCN discovered on biopsy of an atrophic right testis during investigations for infertility due to azoospermia. He has a prior history left inguinal hernia repair. His left testis is normal in size and consistency, and there is evidence of normal spermatogenesis on testicular biopsy. His serum luteinizing hormone (LH), follicle-stimulating hormone (FSH), and testosterone levels are within the normal range. The most appropriate treatment for the ITGCN in the right testis at this time is:

   a. inguinal orchiectomy.

   b. low-dose radiation therapy.

   c. carboplatin.

   d. observation.

   e. transscrotal orchiectomy.

11. Which of the following factors is NOT associated with the presence of occult metastases in clinical stage I NSGCT?

   a. Lymphovascular invasion

   b. Absence of yolk sac tumor in the primary tumor

   c. Percentage of embryonal carcinoma in the primary tumor

   d. Elevated preorchiectomy AFP level

   e. Advanced primary tumor stage

12. A 27-year-old convict at a correctional facility presents for management of clinical stage I left NSGCT. He has a history of enlarging left testicular mass for 12 months that was discovered incidentally during a routine physical examination by the prison physician. Pathologic examination of the orchiectomy specimen revealed a 1.2-cm mixed GCT (40% seminoma, 40% embryonal carcinoma, 20% yolk sac tumor) confined to the testis without evidence of lymphovascular invasion. His postorchiectomy serum tumor markers are within normal limits. He has a history of multiple incarcerations in the past, and his viral serology is positive for hepatitis C. The most appropriate treatment is:

   a. adjuvant radiation therapy to the retroperitoneum and ipsilateral pelvis.

   b. surveillance.

   c. chemotherapy with two cycles of bleomycin-etoposide-cisplatin.

   d. chemotherapy with two cycles of carboplatin.

   e. RPLND.

13. Which of the following factors is NOT associated with the presence of necrosis/fibrosis in residual masses after first-line chemotherapy?

   a. Absence of teratoma in the primary tumor

   b. Residual mass size

   c. Percentage shrinkage of mass after chemotherapy

   d. Prechemotherapy mass size

   e. Lymphovascular invasion

14. A 37-year-old man presents for treatment of a 1.2-cm left testicular mixed GCT (40% teratoma, 40% seminoma, 15% embryonal carcinoma, 5% yolk sac tumor) confined to the testis without evidence of lymphovascular invasion. His postorchiectomy serum tumor marker levels are within normal limits. Chest CT shows no evidence of metastatic disease. Abdominopelvic CT shows a 7-mm nodule in the paracaval location just inferior to the right renal hilum. The remainder of the CT study is unremarkable. His past medical history is also unremarkable. The most appropriate management is:

   a. CT-guided biopsy of the paracaval lesion.

   b. RPLND.

   c. two cycles of chemotherapy with bleomycin-etoposide-cisplatin.

   d. observation.

   e. three cycles of chemotherapy with bleomycin-etoposide-cisplatin.

15. The following factors are associated with the presence of occult distant metastases in patients with clinical stage IIA-B NSGCT EXCEPT:

   a. elevated postorchiectomy hCG.

   b. lymphovascular invasion.

   c. retroperitoneal mass size.

   d. large primary tumor with involvement of the scrotal skin.

   e. retroperitoneal lymphadenopathy outside the primary landing zone.

16. The following are independent risk factors for relapse after postchemotherapy RPLND EXCEPT:

   a. evidence of viable malignancy in resected specimens.

   b. incomplete resection.

   c. rising pre-RPLND serum tumor markers.

   d. poor-risk disease at diagnosis by IGCCCG criteria.

   e. prior RPLND.

17. A 34-year-old man with right clinical stage III NSGCT (100% embryonal carcinoma) with good-risk features by IGCCCG criteria receives induction chemotherapy with three cycles of bleomycin-etoposide-cisplatin. At completion of chemotherapy his serum tumor markers are within normal limits. On postchemotherapy CT studies he has a 1.7-cm mass (4.8 cm at diagnosis) in the interaortocaval region and a 0.8-cm mass in the para-aortic region (2.3 cm at diagnosis). He also has bilateral pulmonary nodules in the right lower lobe (0.6 cm; 1.4 cm at diagnosis) and left upper lobe (0.8 cm; 1.6 cm at diagnosis). The most appropriate management is:

   a. four cycles of vinblastine-ifosfamide-cisplatin second-line chemotherapy.

b. resection of the interaortocaval mass.

c. bilateral postchemotherapy RPLND.

d. bilateral thoracotomy and resection of residual pulmonary masses.

e. CT-guided biopsy of the pulmonary mass(es).

18. Which of the following statements is FALSE concerning late relapse of NSGCT?

a. Surgical resection is the primary treatment modality.

b. Yolk sac tumor is the most common malignant histology.

c. The incidence is increasing.

d. The retroperitoneum is the most common site.

e. The outcome is poor relative to those with early NSGCT relapse.

19. A 35-year-old man with clinical stage IIC left mixed GCT (50% embryonal, 40% teratoma, 10% yolk sac) with good-risk features by IGCCCG criteria receives three cycles of bleomycin-etoposide-cisplatin chemotherapy. At the start of chemotherapy his AFP was 380 ng/mL (upper limit: <11 ng/mL), and this has normalized at the end of chemotherapy. Restaging CT shows the solid para-aortic mass has increased from 5.3 cm to 8.9 cm with displacement of the aorta and left kidney as well as new lymphadenopathy in the left common iliac and left obturator region. The patient complains of recent onset of left-sided back pain. The most appropriate management is:

a. RPLND and pelvic lymph node dissection.

b. CT-guided biopsy of the para-aortic mass.

c. four cycles of paclitaxel-ifosfamide-cisplatin as second-line chemotherapy.

d. two cycles of bleomycin-etoposide-cisplatin followed by carboplatin-etoposide high-dose chemotherapy and autologous stem cell rescue.

e. bleomycin-etoposide-cisplatin plus radiation therapy.

20. The rationale for single-agent carboplatin as treatment for clinical stage I seminoma is based on the following factors EXCEPT:

a. absence of teratoma.

b. less neurotoxicity compared with cisplatin.

c. less nephrotoxicity compared with cisplatin.

d. less ototoxicity compared with cisplatin.

e. similar efficacy to cisplatin.

21. Late complications of infradiaphragmatic dog-leg radiotherapy include the following EXCEPT:

a. peptic ulcer disease.

b. coronary artery disease.

c. secondary malignancy.

d. ejaculatory dysfunction.

e. impaired spermatogenesis.

22. The rationale for surveillance in clinical stage I seminoma is based on the following factors EXCEPT:

a. utility of serum tumor markers to identify relapse at an early and curable stage.

b. relapses are cured in virtually all cases by deferred dog-leg radiotherapy.

c. lack of validated histopathologic prognostic factors to identify a high-risk subset.

d. improved short- and long-term toxicity compared with primary radiotherapy and carboplatin.

e. 15% to 20% of patients are cured by orchiectomy.

23. A 44-year-old man with clinical stage III left testicular seminoma with IGCCCG good-risk features has a discrete 2.4-cm residual para-aortic mass (3.8 cm at diagnosis) after receiving three cycles of bleomycin-etoposide-cisplatin chemotherapy. His pulmonary nodules have regressed completely. His serum tumor markers are within the normal range. The most appropriate management is:

a. postchemotherapy radiation therapy to the residual mass.

b. fluorodeoxyglucose-labeled positron emission tomography (FDG-PET) at least 4 weeks after completing chemotherapy.

c. observation.

d. postchemotherapy surgical resection of the residual mass.

e. four cycles of paclitaxel-ifosfamide-cisplatin as second-line chemotherapy.

24. A 42-year-old asymptomatic man presents for management of right NSGCT (80% embryonal carcinoma, 10% teratoma, 10% choriocarcinoma). His preorchiectomy hCG value was 15,000 mU/mL (upper limit: <5 mU/mL), and this has risen to 50,800 mU/mL after orchiectomy. Chest CT shows numerous pulmonary nodules. There is evidence of multiple masses in the interaortocaval region (largest 4.8 cm) and masses in the para-aortic region (largest 2.6 cm). The most appropriate management is:

a. three cycles of bleomycin-etoposide-cisplatin chemotherapy.

b. RPLND.

c. four cycles of bleomycin-etoposide-cisplatin chemotherapy.

d. CT of the head.

e. two cycles of bleomycin-etoposide-cisplatin followed by carboplatin-etoposide high-dose chemotherapy and autologous stem cell rescue.

25. Which of the following statements is FALSE regarding treatment-related toxicity?

a. Two cycles of platin-based chemotherapy does not increase one's risk of developing cardiovascular disease or secondary malignant neoplasm (SMN).

b. Frequent CT body imaging may increase the risk of SMN.

c. The risk of cardiovascular disease is highest among patients receiving mediastinal radiotherapy.

d. Exposure to cisplatin-based chemotherapy and history of cigarette smoking are associated with similar risks of cardiovascular disease and SMN.

e. Suprahilar dissection, vascular reconstruction, and hepatic resection are risk factors for chylous ascites after RPLND.

26. Which of the following are NOT similarities between Leydig cell tumors and GCT?

i. Both are associated with a history of cryptorchidism.

ii. Radical inguinal orchiectomy is the initial treatment of choice.

iii. Bilateral tumors occur in 2% to 3% of cases.

iv. Both may be associated with gynecomastia.

v. The retroperitoneum is the most common site of metastatic disease.

   a. i, ii, and iii

   b. i and iii

   c. i, ii, iii, and iv

   d. v only

   e. All the above

27. A 54-year-old man presents with an enlarging right inguinal mass. On examination, a palpable mass is noted in the right inguinal region that extends into the right hemiscrotum. The testis cannot be distinguished from this mass. Staging CT reveals a heterogeneous, infiltrative, area of low intensity mass (–20 Hounsfield units), 6 × 9 cm, involving the right spermatic cord and extending from the inguinal canal into the scrotum with displacement of the right testis. There is no evidence of retroperitoneal lymphadenopathy or distant metastases. The most appropriate management is:

   a. inguinal orchiectomy followed by adjuvant radiotherapy.

   b. inguinal orchiectomy alone.

   c. transscrotal orchiectomy.

   d. inguinal orchiectomy followed by ifosfamide-based adjuvant chemotherapy.

   e. inguinal orchiectomy followed by RPLND.

Pathology

1. A 26-year-old man has a right radical orchiectomy for an embryonal carcinoma of the testis. At the time of surgery a contralateral biopsy is performed (Fig. 31–1).

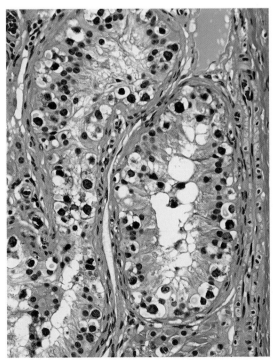

Figure 31–1.   (From Bostwick DG, Cheng L. Urologic surgical pathology. 2nd ed. Edinburgh: Mosby; 2008.)

The patient should be advised that:

   a. he has an embryonal cancer of low volume in the contralateral testis.

   b. he probably will be infertile.

   c. he has a Leydig cell tumor.

   d. he has a Sertoli cell tumor.

   e. he has an increased likelihood of having a GCT in the remaining testis.

2. A 35-year-old man has an asymptomatic right scrotal mass. Testicular ultrasonography reveals a 3-cm heterogeneous intratesticular mass. A right radical orchiectomy is performed and the histology is depicted in Figure 31–2.

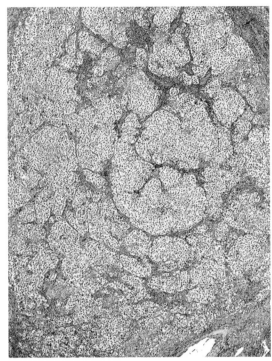

Figure 31–2.   (From Bostwick DG, Cheng L. Urologic surgical pathology. 2nd ed. Edinburgh: Mosby; 2008.)

The patient has:

   a. seminoma.

   b. embryonal carcinoma.

   c. yolk sac cancer.

   d. choriocarcinoma.

   e. teratoma.

3. A 32-year-old man has a right radical orchiectomy for a testicular mass. Preoperatively his AFP value was normal and his hCG level was elevated at 5000 units. The histology is depicted in Figure 31–3.

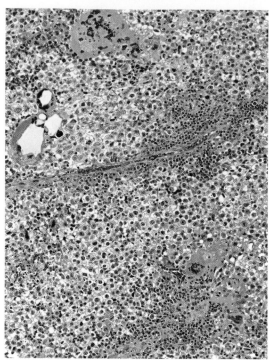

Figure 31–3.   (From Bostwick DG, Cheng L. Urologic surgical pathology. 2nd ed. Edinburgh: Mosby; 2008.)

A CT of the retroperitoneum and lungs reveals no evidence of metastatic disease. The next step in management should be:

a. induction chemotherapy.

b. head CT for possible brain metastases.

c. RPLND.

d. repeat serum markers.

e. FDG-PET.

4. A 50-year-old man has a right radical orchiectomy for a testicular mass. The histology is depicted in Figure 31–4.

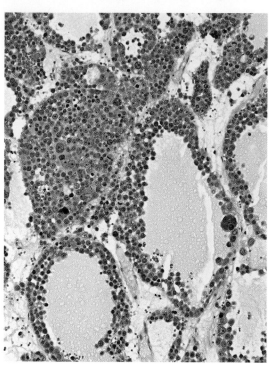

Figure 31–4.   (From Bostwick DG, Cheng L. Urologic surgical pathology. 2nd ed. Edinburgh: Mosby; 2008.)

The patient should:

a. have chemotherapy for lymphoma.

b. have chemotherapy for embryonal cancer.

c. have radiation therapy for seminoma.

d. have a biopsy of the contralateral testis.

e. be told that the excision is curative and there is a low likelihood that he will ever develop metastases.

5. A 20-year-old man has a right radical orchiectomy. The pathology is depicted in Figure 31–5.

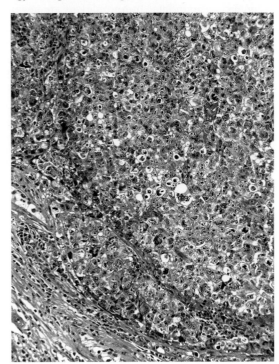

Figure 31–5.   (From Bostwick DG, Cheng L. Urologic surgical pathology. 2nd ed. Edinburgh: Mosby; 2008.)

His hCG and AFP values are elevated and a CT reveals no evidence of metastatic disease. Three weeks later repeat AFP and hCG testing show no change in either marker. The patient should be advised to:

a. have induction chemotherapy.

b. have an RPLND.

c. undergo observation.

d. receive radiotherapy below the diaphragm.

e. repeat the hCG and AFP tests in another month.

6. A 25-year-old man has a right radical orchiectomy and the histology is depicted in Figure 31–6.

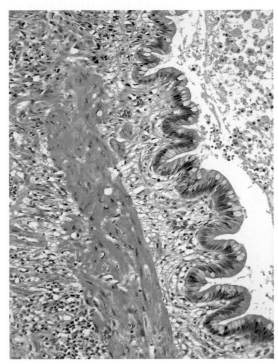

Figure 31–6.   (From Bostwick DG, Cheng L. Urologic surgical pathology. 2nd ed. Edinburgh: Mosby; 2008.)

The patient's markers are negative; however, there is a 3-cm mass in the retroperitoneum. He is given chemotherapy, and the mass shrinks to 2.8 cm. The patient should be advised to

a. have a retroperitoneal lymphadenectomy.

b. have salvage chemotherapy.

c. get a FDG-PET scan.

d. receive radiation therapy.

e. be observed.

Imaging

1. A 36-year-old man noted a firm left scrotal mass. He was hit in the groin 1 month earlier with a tennis ball. Currently he has no pain, fever, or chills. The testicular ultrasound image is depicted in Figure 31–7.

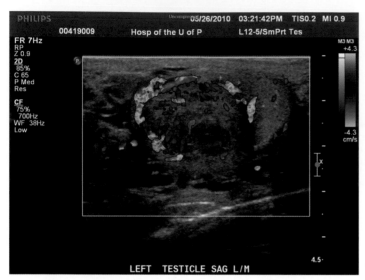

Figure 31–7.

The most likely diagnosis is:

a. ruptured testis with peritesticular hematoma.

b. testicular neoplasm.

c. epidermoid cyst.

d. dilated rete testis.

e. testicular abscess.

2. A 32-year-old man had a left radical orchiectomy. Pathologic evaluation reveals a mixed GCT containing seminoma and embryonal cell carcinoma. Tumor markers are negative. The CT image depicted in Figure 31–8 was obtained 1 day post operation. Chest CT is negative.

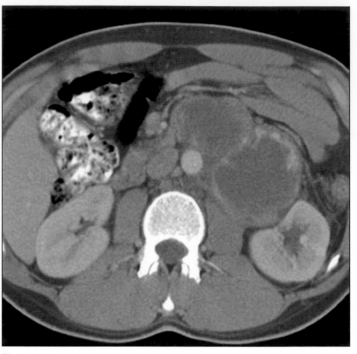

Figure 31–8.

The next step in management is:

a. biopsy.

b. radiation therapy.

c. chemotherapy.

d. RPLND.

e. repeat CT in 1 week to confirm a postsurgical inflammatory response.

ANSWERS

1. **d. spematocytic seminoma.** ITGCN is the common precursor lesion for all types of adult male GCT with the exception of spermatocytic seminoma. Pediatric GCTs do not typically arise from ITGCN.

2. **e. Metastatic spermatocytic seminoma is rare.** Spermatocytic seminoma differs from other GCT subtypes in that it does not arise from ITGCN, cryptorchidism is not a risk factor, bilaterality has not been reported, it does not express i(12p) or placental alkaline phosphatase, and it does not occur as a mixed GCT with other GCT subtypes. Only one documented case of metastasis has been reported, and these lesions are almost always cured by orchiectomy.

3. **a. Choriocarcinoma.** With the exception of choriocarcinoma, the most common route of disease dissemination is via lymphatic channels from the primary tumor to the retroperitoneal lymph nodes and subsequently to distant sites. Choriocarcinoma has a propensity for hematogenous dissemination. Yolk sac tumors in children are thought to spread hematogenously as well.

4. **c. pure embryonal carcinoma.** Pure embryonal carcinoma may produce both AFP and hCG. Pure seminoma is associated with elevated serum hCG levels in 15% of cases

but does not produce AFP. Pure teratoma typically is not associated with elevated serum tumor markers, although slightly elevated AFP levels may be observed. Choriocarcinoma is uniformly associated with elevated hCG levels but does not produce AFP. The vast majority of yolk sac tumors produce AFP but they do not produce hCG.

5. **b. Suspected benign testicular lesion.** Testis-sparing surgery should be considered only in patients with suspected GCT who have normal testicular androgen production and who have a small (<2 cm) tumor either in a solitary testis or in the setting of bilateral synchronous testicular GCT. Testis-sparing surgery should not be performed in patients with suspected GCT who have a normal contralateral testis. Testis-sparing surgery may also be considered in patients with suspected benign testicular lesions such as an epidermoid cyst or adenomatoid tumor arising from the tunica albuginea.

6. **d. to obtain repeat serum tumor marker levels in 7 days.** Patients with elevated serum tumor markers before orchiectomy should have these levels measured after orchiectomy to assess whether the levels are declining, stable, or rising. Management decisions should not be made based on serum tumor marker levels before orchiectomy. Patients with rising postorchiectomy serum tumor marker levels should receive chemotherapy. The IGCCCG classification of metastatic NSGCT is based on the postorchiectomy serum tumor marker levels.

7. **a. testicular seminoma with brain metastases.** According to IGCCCG classification criteria there is no "poor risk" category for metastatic seminoma. Patients with metastatic seminoma who have nonpulmonary visceral metastases (e.g., liver, bone, brain) are classified as at intermediate risk. Metastatic NSGCT patients with mediastinal primary tumor *or* nonpulmonary visceral metastases *or* postochiectomy AFP > 10,000 ng/mL, *or* postorchiectomy hCG of 50,000 mU/mL are classified as at poor risk.

8. **c. mediastinoscopy and biopsy.** The presence of distant metastasis in the absence of retroperitoneal disease or elevated serum levels of tumor markers is uncommon, particularly for patients with testicular seminoma. As such these patients should undergo biopsy and histologic confirmation of the suspected lesion before management decisions are made.

9. **b. CT-guided biopsy of the retroperitoneal mass.** The risk of teratoma at metastatic sites is less of a consideration for metastatic seminoma than NSGCT. Although rare, seminoma may transform into NSGCT elements, and this should be considered in patients with metastatic seminoma who fail to respond to conventional therapy. These patients should undergo biopsy and histologic confirmation of the suspected lesion before management decisions are made. Either an open or a laparoscopic biopsy of the para-aortic mass is an acceptable approach if the CT-guided biopsy is not feasible or the result is nondiagnostic. However, an RPLND should not be performed without histologic confirmation of NSGCT pathology.

10. **a. inguinal orchiectomy.** Inguinal orchiectomy and low-dose radiation therapy are associated with the highest rates of local control of ITGCN. In a patient with a normal contralateral testis (particularly if future paternity is desired), inguinal orchiectomy is the preferred choice owing to the deleterious effects of radiation therapy on spermatogenesis within the contralateral testis.

11. **d. Elevated pre-orchiectomy AFP level.** Preorchiectomy serum tumor marker levels are not associated with the presence of occult metastases in clinical stage I NSGCT. The presence of postorchiectomy serum tumor marker levels in clinical stage I NSGCT indicates the presence of occult systemic disease.

12. **c. chemotherapy with two cycles of bleomycin-etoposide-cisplatin.** Chemotherapy is associated with the lowest risk of recurrence and is thus preferred over surveillance for patients who are anticipated to be noncompliant with surveillance imaging and testing (even for patients at low risk for occult metastases). Chemotherapy and RPLND are associated with similar rates of long-term cure, but the former may be preferable in patients with transmissible diseases. Adjuvant radiation therapy and carboplatin are standard treatment approaches for clinical stage I seminoma.

13. **e. Lymphovascular invasion.** Absence of teratoma in the primary tumor, prechemotherapy and postchemotherapy mass size, and percentage shrinkage of mass with chemotherapy are all associated with the presence of necrosis/fibrosis in residual masses after first-line chemotherapy. However, none of these factors (alone or together) is sufficiently accurate to exclude the presence of residual teratoma or viable malignancy in patients with residual masses greater than 1 cm. Lymphovascular invasion is associated with the presence of occult metastases in patients with clinical stage I NSGCT and has no impact on the histology of residual masses after chemotherapy.

14. **d. observation.** Patients at low-risk for metastatic disease with indeterminate CT findings should be closely observed because small (<1 cm) retroperitoneal lesions may represent false-positive findings, particularly if they are located outside the primary landing zone. A CT-guided biopsy would be technically difficult to perform given the lesion size and its proximity to the renal vessels.

15. **b. lymphovascular invasion.** Lymphovascular invasion is associated with the presence of occult metastases in patients with clinical stage I NSGCT, but it has not been associated with an increased risk of distant metastases in patients with clinical or pathologic stage II disease. Elevated postorchiectomy serum tumor markers, bulky (>3 cm) retroperitoneal masses, or retroperitoneal lymphadenopathy outside the primary landing zone are associated with an increased risk of systemic relapse after RPLND. Thus clinical stage IIA-B patients with these features are recommended to receive induction chemotherapy. Scrotal invasion by the primary tumor is associated with an increased risk of metastasis to the inguinal lymph nodes, which are considered nonregional lymph nodes.

16. **d. poor-risk disease at diagnosis by International Germ Cell Cancer Collaborative Group (IGCCCG) criteria.** Although patients with poor-risk GCT have diminished survival and are more likely to have viable malignancy or incomplete resection at postchemotherapy RPLND, IGCCCG risk category is not a predictor of relapse independent of the histology of resected masses or completeness of resection. "Desperation" postchemotherapy RPLND in the setting of rising serum tumor markers after second- or third-line chemotherapy and reoperative RPLND

are other conditions associated with an increased risk of relapse.

17. **c. bilateral postchemotherapy RPLND.** Approximately one third of patients will have residual masses at multiple anatomic sites, and these patients should undergo resection of all sites of measurable residual disease because discordant histology between anatomic sites is reported in 22% to 46% of cases. However, the presence of necrosis in postchemotherapy RPLND specimens is highly predictive of necrosis at other sites. Thus, postchemotherapy RPLND should be performed before resection of residual masses at other sites. Observation of small residual masses at other sites is a reasonable option if the histology of the RPLND specimen is necrosis. Patients with viable malignancy discovered at postchemotherapy resection should have all residual masses resected and are usually treated with an additional two cycles of chemotherapy. A full course of second-line chemotherapy is reserved for patients with either serologic or radiographic progression during or after first-line chemotherapy.

18. **e. The outcome is poor relative to those with early NSGCT relapse.** Until recently, late relapse has been associated with a worse prognosis than early relapse, although more recent data suggest these patient groups have a similar probability of cure. Disease-free rates of 50% to 60% are reported after treatment of early and late relapse.

19. **b. CT-guided biopsy of the para-aortic mass.** Patients with good-risk metastatic NSGCT who have dramatic progression of their disease with first-line chemotherapy despite normalization of serum tumor marker levels should be considered to have either growing teratoma syndrome or teratoma with malignant transformation. The presence of an enlarging solid mass and new sites of disease suggest a malignant process. An enlarging mass only with cystic appearance is more suggestive of growing teratoma syndrome. A CT-guided biopsy to identify the presence of malignant transformation is indicated because this finding may influence the choice of chemotherapy.

20. **e. similar efficacy to cisplatin.** All of the randomized trials in advanced GCT in which a cisplatin-based regimen has been compared with a carboplatin-based regimen have reported superior outcomes with cisplatin. The rationale for single-agent carboplatin is based on reduced toxicity compared with cisplatin and 65% to 90% response rates reported in studies of carboplatin in advanced seminoma.

21. **d. ejaculatory dysfunction.** Dog-leg radiotherapy for clinical stage I seminoma is associated with infertility due to the direct effects of radiation on the germinal epithelium with resultant impaired spermatogenesis. Infertility related to ejaculatory dysfunction is not association with radiation therapy and is most commonly associated with RPLND.

22. **a. utility of serum tumor markers to identify relapse at an early and curable stage.** Only 15% of seminomas produce elevations in serum hCG, and serum tumor marker levels are uncommonly elevated in the vast majority of patients with clinical stage I seminoma at diagnosis or at the time of relapse. This is in contrast to clinical stage I NGSCT in which serum tumor markers are commonly the first (and only) manifestation of disease relapse.

23. **c. observation.** In contrast to advanced NSGCT, only 10% of residual masses in advanced seminoma after first-line chemotherapy contain viable malignancy (90% contain fibrosis/necrosis only) and residual teratoma is less of a consideration. Spontaneous resolution of these masses will occur in the majority of cases. Approximately 30% of discrete residual masses greater than 3 cm will contain viable malignancy. FDG-PET is a useful adjunct to postchemotherapy staging CT to determine the need for postchemotherapy surgical resection. Residual masses larger than 3 cm that are PET negative and those less than 3 cm can be safely observed because of the high probability of necrosis/fibrosis. FDG-PET has no role in the characterization of residual masses less than 3 cm.

24. **d. CT of the head.** Choriocarcinoma spreads hematogenously and widely. Brain metastases should be suspected in any patient with a very high hCG level. Thus, patients with high hCG levels at diagnosis should have staging CT or MRI studies of the brain. Choriocarcinomas are highly vascular and tend to hemorrhage during chemotherapy, which may have catastrophic consequences in those patients with brain metastases. Brain metastases are also associated with a poor prognosis, and these patients should receive four cycles of bleomycin-etoposide-cisplatin as first-line chemotherapy, as should any patient with an hCG level over 5000 mU/mL at the time chemotherapy is initiated.

25. **a. Two cycles of platin-based chemotherapy does not increase one's risk of developing cardiovascular disease or SMN.** Although the risk of late complications of chemotherapy is dose dependent there appears to be no safe lower limit. Thus even patients receiving one to two cycles of platin-based chemotherapy may have an increased risk of late toxicity.

26. **b. i and iii.** Unlike GCT, Leydig cell tumors are not associated with a history of cryptorchidism and bilateral tumors have not been reported.

27. **a. inguinal orchiectomy followed by adjuvant radiotherapy.** A large, infiltrative mass involving the spermatic cord in an adult man is a sarcoma until proven otherwise. The low-intensity signal on CT and patient age make liposarcoma the most common histology. Paratesticular liposarcoma rarely metastasize but tend to recur locally. Thus, adjuvant radiotherapy may be used to decrease the risk of local recurrence.

Pathology

1. **e. he has an increased likelihood of having a GCT in the remaining testis.** The patient has intratubular germ cell neoplasia as evidenced by enlarged hyperchromatic nuclei and a lack of a spermatogenesis. This carries an increased risk for developing a GCT.

2. **a. seminoma.** Notice the sheathlike pattern of small cells interspersed with fibrous septa that contain lymphocytes, the hallmarks of seminoma.

3. **d. repeat serum markers.** The patient has seminoma with syncytiotrophoblasts. Approximately 15% of patients with seminoma have elevated hCG and will demonstrate syncytiotrophoblasts.

4. **e. be told that the excision is curative and there is a low likelihood that he will ever develop metastases.** This is a spermatocytic seminoma with a very low malignant potential. Notice the small basophilic cells and the multinucleated tumor giant cell, which are characteristic for spermatocytic seminoma.

5. **a. have induction chemotherapy.** This patient has an embryonal carcinoma: notice the primitive, anaplastic epithelial cells. With persistently elevated serum markers the patient should undergo induction chemotherapy.

6. **a. have RPLND.** The tumor depicted is a teratoma: notice the mature enteric epithelium. Because the specimen is in the primary tumor there is a high likelihood that there is residual teratoma in the retroperitoneal mass. This tumor is chemoinsensitive and should be resected.

Imaging

1. **b. testicular neoplasm.** The ultrasound image shows an irregular, vascular mass in the left testis that also has microlithiasis. This is most consistent with a testicular neoplasm. It is not unusual for patients to have a history of groin trauma before presentation.

2. **c. chemotherapy.** The CT image shows a large (>5 cm) para-aortic mass that represents metastatic adenopathy. Because this represents bulky retroperitoneal disease (stage IIC), chemotherapy is the best option.

Additional Study Points

1. Germ cell tumors (GCTs) occur bilaterally approximately 2% of the time. The risk factors for developing GCTs include cryptorchidism, a family history of testicular cancer, a previous history of testicular cancer, and intratubular germ cell neoplasia (ITGCN).

2. In men with a history of GCTs, the finding of testicular microlithiasis on ultrasonography in the contralateral testis is associated with an increased risk of intratubular germ cell neoplasia; the significance of microlithiasis in the general population, however, is unclear.

3. One to 5 percent of GCTs are extragonadal; they are generally less sensitive to chemotherapy and are more likely to contain yolk sac tumor elements than tumors arising in the testis.

4. On rare occasion teratomas may transform into somatic malignancies such as rhabdomyosarcoma, adenocarcinoma, and neuroendocrine tumors.

5. Two thirds of patients with GCTs have diminished fertility.

6. Choriocarcinomas and seminomas do not produce AFP.

7. The half-life of AFP is 5 to 7 days; that of hCG is 24 to 36 hours.

8. The primary landing zone in the retroperitoneum for right testicular tumors is the interaortocaval lymph nodes; for left testicular tumors it is the periaortic lymph nodes; the pattern of lymph drainage in the retroperitoneum is from right to left.

9. Patients with persistently elevated AFP and hCG after orchiectomy are given induction chemotherapy.

10. In clinical stage I disease approximately 25% of patients will have metastases.

11. Lymphovascular invasion and a prominent component of embryonal carcinoma are risk factors for metastases in NSGCTs.

12. In seminomas, risk factors for metastases are rete testis involvement and tumor size greater than 4 cm.

13. Patients with bulky retroperitoneal lymph node disease greater than 3 cm should receive induction chemotherapy.

14. After initial treatment, patients with enlargement of a retroperitoneal mass or an increase in markers should undergo salvage chemotherapy. Consideration may be given to a CT-guided biopsy under selected circumstances.

15. Patients with an NSGCT, undetectable markers, and a residual mass greater than 1 cm after chemotherapy should undergo surgical resection.

16. Approximately half of those patients who have surgical resection of a retroperitoneal mass following chemotherapy will harbor teratoma or a viable malignancy. The remainder will have fibrosis.

17. Patients with viable malignancy in residual masses after salvage chemotherapy have a poor prognosis.

18. In patients with seminomas who are treated with chemotherapy, the size of the residual mass is highly predictive of viable tumor. Masses less than 3 cm rarely have viable tumor in them, whereas about a third of residual masses greater than 3 cm contain viable malignancy.

19. Late toxicity of chemotherapy includes peripheral neuropathy, Raynaud phenomenon, hearing loss, hypogonadism and infertility, secondary malignant neoplasms, and cardiovascular disease.

20. Ninety percent of Leydig cell tumors and Sertoli cell tumors are benign and 10% are malignant.

21. The most common testicular neoplasm in men older than 50 is lymphoma.

22. Cystadenoma of the epididymis is associated with von Hippel-Lindau syndrome; adenomatoid tumor of the epididymis is benign.

23. Liposarcoma is the most common paratesticular tumor in the adult. Rhabdomyosarcoma is the most common paratesticular tumor in the child.

Surgery of Testicular Tumors

Joel Sheinfeld, MD ● George J. Bosl, MD

QUESTIONS

1. A 23-year-old man undergoes a right orchiectomy for seminoma followed by chemotherapy for a 10-cm retroperitoneal mass. His tumor markers are normal both before and after treatment. After treatment his mass is 5 cm. Which of the following statements is TRUE?

   a. Residual retroperitoneal disease can usually be resected completely.

   b. The probability of viable disease in the retroperitoneum is approximately 25%.

   c. Postchemotherapy retroperitoneal lymph node dissection (RPLND) is associated with low morbidity.

   d. Postchemotherapy radiation therapy is warranted.

   e. Percutaneous biopsy is accurate.

2. Which of the following is TRUE regarding testicular anatomy?

   a. The right testicular vein drains to the right renal vein.

   b. The left testicular artery arises from the left renal artery.

   c. The left testicular lymphatic drainage is to the interaortocaval and paracaval nodes.

   d. The right testicular lymphatic drainage is to paracaval, interaortocaval, and para-aortic nodes.

   e. The right testicular artery arises from the right renal artery.

3. A 19-year-old man presents with a 5-cm para-aortic mass. Needle biopsy of the mass reveals a nonseminomatous germ cell tumor (NSGCT). He is given four cycles of etoposide-cisplatin chemotherapy. The left testes, which had a 2-cm mass before treatment, is now without any abnormality on ultrasound or physical examination and his tumor markers have normalized. Which of the following is appropriate treatment of his testes?

   a. Observation

   b. Radiation therapy

   c. Radical left inguinal orchiectomy

   d. Testicular biopsy and orchiectomy if viable disease remains

   e. Bilateral orchiectomy

4. Which of the following is the most common site for late recurrence of NSGCT?

   a. Retroperitoneum

   b. Lung

   c. Liver

   d. Brain

   e. Mediastinum

5. Which of the following associations is correct when describing the events of ejaculation?

   a. Lumbar sympathetics and bulbourethral muscle contraction

   b. Bladder neck contraction and pudendal somatic nerves

   c. Sympathetic fibers and bladder neck contraction

   d. Pelvic parasympathetics and emission

   e. Lumbar sympathetics and erection

6. During postchemotherapy RPLND each of the following structures can be ligated without attendant morbidity EXCEPT the:

   a. inferior mesenteric vein.

   b. inferior mesenteric artery.

   c. right and left testicular arteries.

   d. right renal vein.

   e. lumbar arteries.

7. Which of the following is NOT correct regarding laparoscopic RPLND?

   a. It is feasible when performed by experienced laparoscopists.

   b. Therapeutic efficacy is well established.

   c. It is associated with shorter recovery times than open RPLND.

   d. There are fewer postoperative analgesic requirements than with open RPLND.

   e. There is low morbidity in postchemotherapy RPLND.

8. A 23-year-old man undergoes right orchiectomy for a mixed NSGCT without vascular invasion. Results of physical examination and CT of the chest, abdomen, and pelvis are normal, and the patient's preoperative human chorionic gonadotropin (hCG) value is elevated and remains elevated after orchiectomy. Which of the following is the most appropriate treatment?

   a. Surveillance

   b. Two cycles of platinum-based chemotherapy

   c. Four cycles of etoposide-cisplatin or three cycles of bleomycin-etoposide-cisplatin

   d. RPLND

   e. Radiation to retroperitoneum

9. A 33-year-old man undergoes left orchiectomy for NSGCT and his serum tumor markers normalize. Imaging reveals a 2-cm mass in the para-aortic region, and he undergoes primary RPLND. During the operation excessive bleeding leads to an incomplete resection. Pathology reveals four positive lymph nodes, the largest of which measures 3.5 cm with extranodal extension. Which of the following is the most appropriate therapy?
   a. Observation
   b. Redo RPLND
   c. Two cycles of platinum-based chemotherapy
   d. Four cycles of etoposide-cisplatin or three cycles of bleomycin-etoposide-cisplatin
   e. Salvage chemotherapy

10. Abnormal fertility in testicular cancer patients is associated with all of the following EXCEPT:
   a. chemotherapy.
   b. primary germ cell defect.
   c. nerve-sparing RPLND.
   d. circulating levels of hCG.
   e. radiation to scrotum.

11. Which of the following is the strongest risk factor for postoperative pulmonary complications in bleomycin-treated patients?
   a. Preoperative pulmonary function test results
   b. Concentration of inspired oxygen during operation
   c. Fluid administered in the perioperative period
   d. History of acute bleomycin toxicity
   e. Age

12. A 25-year-old man undergoes four cycles of etoposide-cisplatin for stage IIB NSGCT. Postchemotherapy CT of the chest, abdomen, and pelvis is normal. There was no teratoma in the primary tumor. What is the probability of residual teratoma or viable cancer in the retroperitoneum?
   a. 0%
   b. 5%
   c. 20%
   d. 45%
   e. 100%

13. Which of the following is the most common adjunctive procedure performed during postchemotherapy RPLND?
   a. Splenectomy
   b. Left nephrectomy
   c. Right nephrectomy
   d. Vena caval resection
   e. Bowel resection

14. Which of the following is TRUE regarding resection of residual thoracic disease after chemotherapy for NSGCT?
   a. It is unsafe to perform in conjunction with RPLND.
   b. It is unnecessary if retroperitoneal specimens reveals fibrosis.
   c. It is more likely to reveal fibrosis in the setting of a solitary pulmonary mass and fibrosis in the retroperitoneum.

   d. It is not necessary to remove a right lung nodule if a left lung nodule reveals fibrosis.
   e. It can be safely performed via the same incision as RPLND.

15. A 21-year-old man undergoes four cycles of etoposide-cisplatin after right-sided orchiectomy for mixed NSGCT. During postchemotherapy RPLND the para-aortic lymph nodes above the inferior mesenteric artery reveal viable GCT on frozen section. The remainder of the dissection should include:
   a. paracaval and interaortocaval tissue.
   b. interaortocaval tissue.
   c. paracaval, interaortocaval, and para-aortic tissue below the inferior mesenteric artery.
   d. no further dissection.
   e. right suprahilar tissue.

16. Malignant transformation, that is, into non–germ cell elements, is a feature associated with:
   a. seminoma.
   b. yolk sac tumors.
   c. embryonal carcinoma.
   d. teratoma.
   e. choriocarcinoma.

17. A 24-year-old patient with stage IIC NSGCT completes induction chemotherapy with complete resolution of a 6-cm para-aortic mass. His α-fetoprotein (AFP) level has normalized; the hCG is markedly elevated. Appropriate therapy at this point is:
   a. radiation therapy to the retroperitoneum.
   b. salvage chemotherapy.
   c. full RPLND.
   d. exploratory laparotomy.
   e. modified RPLND.

18. The most common site of relapse for patients with clinical stage I NSGCT on surveillance is the:
   a. brain.
   b. liver.
   c. chest.
   d. retroperitoneum.
   e. supraclavicular nodes.

19. The most common site for retroperitoneal recurrence after RPLND is the:
   a. interaortocaval region.
   b. paracaval region.
   c. para-aortic region.
   d. interiliac region.
   e. precaval region.

20. After meticulous bilateral primary RPLND with negative lymph nodes, the most likely pattern of relapse includes:
   a. brain metastasis.
   b. liver metastasis.
   c. lung metastasis.
   d. elevated serum tumor markers.
   e. both c and d.

21. Arguments against primary chemotherapy for clinical stage I NSGCT include all of the following EXCEPT:
    a. possible nephrotoxicity, ototoxicity, neurotoxicity, cardiovascular toxicity.
    b. potential late relapse secondary to chemorefractory elements, particularly teratoma.
    c. myelosuppression.
    d. risk of acute leukemia.
    e. retrograde ejaculation.

22. Incidence of teratoma in the retroperitoneum in patients with pathologic stage II NSGCT after primary RPLND is:
    a. 0% to 5%.
    b. 6% to 10%.
    c. 11% to 20%.
    d. 21% to 30%.
    e. >50%.

23. Late relapse of GCT is characterized by:
    a. poor clinical outcome.
    b. the retroperitoneum being the most common site.
    c. an elevated AFP level.
    d. chemoresistance.
    e. all of the above.

ANSWERS

1. **b. The probability of viable disease in the retroperitoneum is approximately 25%.** Postchemotherapy residual masses in the setting of pure seminoma are a difficult problem to manage. The morbidity of complete RPLND is great owing to the severe desmoplastic reaction surrounding the tumor. The ability to perform a complete RPLND is rare. Residual masses greater than 3 cm are associated with a 27% chance of harboring viable malignancy in a study from Memorial Sloan-Kettering Cancer Center.

2. **d. The right testicular lymphatic drainage is to paracaval, interaortocaval, and para-aortic nodes.** Lymphatic drainage is critical to the understanding of metastatic spread of testicular tumor. The left testis drains mainly to the para-aortic nodes. However, the right testis drains into the interaortocaval, precaval, preaortic lymph nodes. The right testicular vein drains directly into the vena cava, and the left testicular vein drains into the left renal vein. Both testicular arteries arise from the aorta between the renal and inferior mesenteric arteries.

3. **c. Radical left inguinal orchiectomy.** Delayed orchiectomy after chemotherapy is indicated because the testes represents a privileged site and is often refractory to chemotherapy. Up to 50% of testes removed in this setting will contain either viable GCT or teratoma (Simmonds, 1995).*

4. **a. Retroperitoneum.** The most common site of late recurrence for both teratoma and viable NSGCT is the retroperitoneum and when associated with viable GCT is associated with a mortality rate of 75%.

5. **c. Sympathetic fibers and bladder neck contraction.** Lumbar sympathetic fibers control the act of emission innervating the seminal vesicles, vas deferens, and prostate. Bladder neck contraction is also controlled via sympathetic nerves and is necessary for antegrade ejaculation. Pudendal somatic nerves control the rhythmic contractions of the perineal muscles and bulbourethral muscle.

6. **d. right renal vein.** The inferior mesenteric artery can be ligated in younger patients without ischemic injury to the colon providing the marginal arterial supply is intact. Lumbar arteries are routinely divided to expose the tissue behind the great vessels. The right renal vein has limited anastomotic flow, and ligation will lead to proteinuria and loss of kidney function.

7. **b. Therapeutic efficacy is well established.** Although no randomized trial has been conducted, multiple studies describing the feasibility of laparoscopic RPLND have been reported. In general the postoperative pain and recovery times are shorter than with open RPLND. However, owing to the short median follow-up and the frequent use of adjuvant chemotherapy, no statement can yet be made regarding therapeutic efficacy.

8. **c. Four cycles of etoposide-cisplatin or three cycles of bleomycin-etoposide-cisplatin.** This patient has stage I-S disease, and RPLND alone in this setting is associated with a high incidence of postoperative persistently elevated tumor markers. Full induction chemotherapy is warranted with four cycles of etoposide-cisplatin or three cycles of bleomycin-etoposide-cisplatin.

9. **d. Four cycles of etoposide-cisplatin or three cycles of bleomycin-etoposide-cisplatin.** Due to the findings of viable disease, extranodal extension, and nodes greater than 2 cm this patient is not a good candidate for observation. The operation described is incomplete and no interaortocaval dissection was performed; therefore it cannot be assumed that this patient is without evidence of disease and adjuvant chemotherapy with two cycles is not standard. Reoperation in this setting is not warranted unless there is a persistent mass after full induction chemotherapy.

10. **c. nerve-sparing RPLND.** Patients undergoing primary prospective nerve-sparing RPLND have similar paternity rates to testicular cancer patients on surveillance. The other choices are all either reversible or permanent causes of subnormal fertility in testicular cancer patients.

11. **c. Fluid administered in the perioperative period.** The single most important risk factor for postoperative pulmonary complications in patients previously treated with bleomycin is the overall fluid and blood transfusion requirements.

12. **c. 20%.** The interpretation of postchemotherapy CT scans as normal or abnormal is subject to variability. However in the three large series of RPLND in the setting of a "normal" CT scan the findings of teratoma or viable GCT ranged from 20% to 30%.

13. **b. Left nephrectomy.** The left kidney is the most common organ removed in most series of postchemotherapy RPLND. Twenty percent of patients in the series of Nash and associates required nephrectomy, and these patients usually presented with hilar or suprahilar left-sided residual masses (Nash et al, 1998).

14. **c. It is more likely to reveal fibrosis in the setting of a solitary pulmonary mass and fibrosis in the**

---

*Sources referenced can be found in *Campbell-Walsh Urology*, 10th Edition, on the Expert Consult website.

retroperitoneum. The predictors of fibrosis in thoracic specimens include fibrosis in the retroperitoneum, solitary mass, and pretreatment tumor markers. In the setting of fibrosis in the retroperitoneum there is a 30% chance of finding discordant histologic findings in the chest. Even in the presence of a benign pathologic process in one lung there can still be teratoma or viable GCT in the contralateral lung.

15. **c. paracaval, interaortocaval, and para-aortic tissue below the inferior mesenteric artery.** The presence of left-sided viable disease makes full bilateral dissection mandatory. Prospective nerve-sparing techniques can be employed in this setting in select candidates to preserve antegrade ejaculation.

16. **d. teratoma.** Teratoma may undergo malignant transformation. At present there are no reliable factors to predict this event.

17. **b. Salvage chemotherapy.** Surgical cures with a rising serum tumor marker after induction chemotherapy are very rare, and patients should receive second-line chemotherapy.

18. **d. retroperitoneum.** Sixty to 70 percent of patients with stage I NSGCT who experience relapse on surveillance will have retroperitoneal metastasis (± elevated serum tumor markers). Approximately 90% of relapses occur the first year and almost 98% within the first 2 years.

19. **c. para-aortic region.** The most common site for retroperitoneal relapse after RPLND for both right and left primary tumors is the para-aortic region. There are two reasons for this: (1) this region is excluded in some published modified right-sided templates and (2) obtaining adequate exposure in this area is more technically demanding.

20. **e. both c and d.** Brain and liver metastases are rare after a primary RPLND. If a thorough bilateral resection has been performed, retroperitoneal relapses are rare as well. Pulmonary and/or serologic recurrences are the most common in this setting.

21. **e. retrograde ejaculation.** Retrograde ejaculation may result from RPLND but not chemotherapy.

22. **d. 21% to 30%.** The two largest series from Indiana University and Memorial Sloan-Kettering Cancer Center show a 21% to 30% incidence of teratoma in positive retroperitoneal nodes. The incidence increases with clinical stage and the presence of teratoma in the primary tumor.

23. **e. All of the above.** Late relapse of GCT is characterized by 5-year survival rates less than 50%. This setting is further characterized by chemoresistance, an elevated AFP, and the fact that 50% to 80% of the patients will have retroperitoneal disease.

Additional Study Points

1. The proper performance of a radical inguinal orchiectomy includes mobilizing the cord 1 to 2 cm proximal to the internal inguinal ring and individually ligating the vas deferens and cord vessels with silk sutures so that the stump may be identified if an RPLND is performed.

2. When an orchiectomy has been performed through the scrotum, in patients who have a low-stage seminoma, the radiation portals should be extended to include the ipsilateral groin and scrotum; for those with low-stage NSGCT the scrotal scar should be excised along with the spermatic cord remnant; and for those who have received a full cycle of platinum-based chemotherapy, only the cord stump need be removed at the time of RPLND.

3. The right testicular lymphatics drain to the interaortocaval lymph nodes followed by precaval and pericaval nodes. The left testicular lymphatics drain to the periaortic and preaortic lymph nodes.

4. Contralateral lymphatic flow is more commonly seen in right-sided tumors than left-sided tumors.

5. There is a 20% to 30% incidence of positive nodes in clinical stage I disease and approximately a 25% relapse rate in such patients who are placed on a surveillance protocol.

6. Suprahilar metastases are rare in low-stage NSGCT. Three to 23 percent of patients with positive nodes at RPLND will have extra-template disease. The most common site of residual suprahilar disease is in the retrocrural space.

7. It is extremely important to secure all lymphatic vessels with either clips or ties, particularly in the region of the right renal artery and diaphragmatic crus, when performing a primary RPLND to minimize injury to the cisterna chyli, which could result in chylous ascites.

8. In the presence of documented or suspected metastatic disease a full bilateral dissection should be performed. In selected cases, preservation of individual nerve fibers may be performed.

9. The anterior split over the vena cava is not likely to damage nerve fibers; however, the anterior split over the aorta risks injury to these fibers.

10. The most important nerves to preserve antigrade ejaculation are those arising from the L3-4 ganglia. To preserve nerve fibers, a dissection on the aorta should only be performed after the nerve fibers have been identified and isolated.

11. There is a sevenfold increase in cardiovascular complications in men treated with platinum-based chemotherapy.

12. All patients should be given the opportunity to bank sperm before RPLND.

13. Lymphovascular invasion, higher T stage, tumor involvement of the cord, capsule, or scrotum, and a high percentage of embryonal carcinoma are associated with an increased incidence of retroperitoneal relapse. Most relapses occur within the first 2 years and are rare after 5 years. The absence of teratoma in the primary tumor does not preclude its presence in the retroperitoneum.

14. Elevated tumor marker levels after orchiectomy require systemic chemotherapy as the next step not RPLND.

15. Patients best suited for RPLND are those with clinical stage IIA and low-volume, less than 3-cm ipsilateral disease (stage IIB).

16. Sixty percent of patients with testicular cancer have subnormal pretreatment semen analyses. Sixty-five percent of men on surveillance can impregnate their partner after orchiectomy.

17. Bilateral RPLND is the standard template for patients with pathologic stage II NSGCT.

18. Bleomycin causes restrictive pulmonary fibrosis with increased collagen deposition and makes the patient highly susceptible to fluid overload.

19. Increased serum concentration of AFP and hCG after primary platinum-based chemotherapy is usually characterized by unresectable viable tumor, and salvage chemotherapy rather than excision of the mass is recommended.

20. After chemotherapy, retroperitoneal masses are composed of necrosis/fibrosis in 50%, teratoma in 40%, and viable GCT in 10%. A residual mass after salvage chemotherapy is composed of viable GCT in 50%, teratoma in 40%, and fibrosis in 10%. If viable GCT is present in the RPLND specimen and the tumor has been completely resected, the addition of two cycles of platinum-based chemotherapy provides a survival benefit.

21. The clinical behavior of a teratoma is unpredictable, and complete resection is required.

22. After chemotherapy, RPLND is indicated for NSGCT primary tumors in which the residual mass is larger than 1 cm. RPLND may be eliminated after chemotherapy if there was no evidence of the disease in the retroperitoneum before chemotherapy.

23. Late relapses occur in 2% to 4% of patients, and more than half of late relapses occur beyond 10 years, emphasizing the need for prolonged follow-up.

24. If the aortic wall is stripped of its adventitia, it should be replaced with a synthetic graft because delayed rupture may occur.

25. Tumor involvement of the superior mesenteric artery, celiac axis, or porta hepatis usually precludes resection. After chemotherapy, resection of residual masses should be accompanied by a complete RPLND. The standard bilateral dissection is the prudent approach.

26. Incidental appendectomy during RPLND increases the risk of infection and should not be performed.

27. After chemotherapy for seminoma, residual masses very rarely contain teratoma and are extremely difficult technically to remove. Thus a residual mass less than 3 cm should be observed, patients with masses larger than 3 cm should have positron emission tomography, and if a viable seminoma is noted then additional chemotherapy is indicated.

28. After chemotherapy, spermatogenesis may take 3 years to return to normal.

Laparoscopic Retroperitoneal Lymphadenectomy for Testicular Tumors

Mohamad E. Allaf, MD ● Louis R. Kavoussi, MD, MBA

QUESTIONS

1. A 23-year old man presented after undergoing transscrotal orchiectomy for presumed hydrocele. Pathologic examination reveals embryonal carcinoma with vascular invasion. Serum levels of tumor markers and results of physical examination and CT of the chest, abdomen, and pelvis are normal. Which of the following approaches is appropriate?
   a. Observation
   b. Retroperitoneal lymph node dissection (RPLND)
   c. RPLND plus excision of scrotal scar
   d. RPLND plus scrotectomy and inguinal lymph node dissection
   e. RPLND plus scrotal and inguinal radiation

2. Late relapse is a feature most commonly associated with:
   a. seminoma.
   b. yolk sac tumor.
   c. embryonal carcinoma.
   d. choriocarcinoma.
   e. teratoma.

3. A 25-year-old man with a stage IIC nonseminomatous germ cell tumor (NSGCT) has completed primary platinum-based chemotherapy. Tumor marker levels have normalized according to appropriate half-life, and he underwent bilateral postchemotherapy RPLND. Final pathologic analysis revealed a focus of yolk sac tumor. Appropriate therapy at this point is:
   a. careful observation.
   b. radiation therapy.
   c. two additional cycles of platinum-based chemotherapy.
   d. four additional cycles of platinum-based chemotherapy.
   e. re-exploration in 6 weeks.

4. A 20-year-old man with clinical stage I NSGCT undergoes laparoscopic RPLND. During surgery a 2-cm lymph node is encountered. Which of the following is the next step?
   a. Abort the procedure and administer chemotherapy
   b. Convert to an open procedure
   c. Perform a unilateral template dissection and administer chemotherapy
   d. Continue the procedure and perform a full bilateral dissection
   e. None of the above

5. The most common cause of open conversion during laparoscopic RPLND is:
   a. intraoperative discovery of bulky lymphadenopathy.
   b. failure to progress.
   c. bowel injury.
   d. hypercapnia.
   e. bleeding.

6. Two weeks after laparoscopic RPLND a patient complains of abdominal distention and emesis. CT reveals ascites. Diagnostic paracentesis confirms the diagnosis of chylous ascites. The next best step is:
   a. reassurance and discharge.
   b. reoperation to identify and treat the source of lymphatic leak.
   c. placement of peritoneal drain and initiation of a low-fat diet.
   d. initiation of somatostatin.
   e. hydration and initiation of a low-fat diet.

7. A 20-year-old man undergoes laparoscopic RPLND after right radical orchiectomy for an NSGCT. All of the following regions should be dissected clear of all lymphatic tissue EXCEPT:
   a. right spermatic cord.
   b. paracaval region.
   c. interaortocaval region.
   d. retrocrural region.
   e. precaval region.

8. Potential advantages to laparoscopic compared with open RPLND include all of the following EXCEPT:
   a. improved cosmesis.
   b. shorter convalescence.
   c. improved disease-free survival.
   d. shorter interval to chemotherapy when necessary.
   e. faster return to normal activities.

ANSWERS

1. **c. RPLND plus excision of scrotal scar.** In the setting of scrotal contamination and clinical stage I disease the patient is best managed with RPLND and wide excision of the scrotal scar. The remainder of the cord also should be removed. Observation is not optimal, owing to the presence of vascular invasion and scrotal contamination.

2. **e. teratoma.** Late relapse of germ cell tumor after definitive therapy is defined as recurrence more than 2 years after completion of therapy and being without evidence of disease. Teratoma is the most common histologic subtype involved in cases of late relapse. This is likely due to its combination of prolonged doubling time and chemotherapy resistance.

3. **c. two additional cycles of platinum-based chemotherapy.** The patient's prognosis is related to serum tumor marker level at the time of RPLND, prior treatment burden, and the pathologic findings for the resected specimen. If viable GCT is present at any site but all disease is completely resected, two additional cycles provide survival benefit in this subset of patients. Einhorn reported only 2 long-term survivors of 22 patients (9%) with completely resected viable germ cell tumor after cisplatin, bleomycin, and vinblastine chemotherapy if additional postoperative chemotherapy was not given. Fox and colleagues reported that 70% of patients with completely resected viable GCT after primary chemotherapy followed by two cycles of postoperative chemotherapy remained disease free compared with none of seven patients without additional chemotherapy.

4. **d. Continue the procedure and perform a full bilateral dissection.** Whenever a suspicious lymph node is identified a full bilateral dissection should be performed.

Chemotherapy will not compensate for an inadequate retroperitoneal dissection.

5. **e. bleeding.** The most common reason for conversion to an open procedure is uncontrollable bleeding, and vascular injury is cited as the most common intraoperative complication. This occurs less than 5% of the time in experienced hands.

6. **e. hydration and initiation of a low-fat diet.** Chylous ascites is a devastating complication that occurs less than 2% of the time after primary laparoscopic (and open) RPLND. Initiation of a low-fat diet, hydration, and drainage of the fluid is usually the first step in the management. Reoperation is considered only when all other options have been exhausted.

7. **d. retrocrural region.** The superior boundary of dissection templates does not include lymph nodes superior to the renal hilum.

8. **c. improved disease-free survival.** No study has demonstrated any difference in disease-free survival comparing open or laparoscopic approaches to node dissection.

Additional Study Points

1. Patients who have small volume retroperitoneal disease (pN1) are cured 70% of the time by a radical RPLND.
2. RPLND is the treatment of choice for patients with stage I NSGCTs with teratoma.
3. All patients undergoing RPLND should be offered preoperative sperm banking.
4. In nerve-sparing techniques for RPLND, great care should be taken around the lumbar veins because these are adjacent to the sympathetic chain.

Tumors of the Penis

Curtis A. Pettaway, MD ● Raymond S. Lance, MD ● John W. Davis, MD

QUESTIONS

1. Which of the following penile lesions does NOT have malignant potential?
   a. Balanitis xerotica obliterans
   b. Condylomata acuminata
   c. Coronal papillae
   d. Bowen disease
   e. Leukoplakia

2. Which of the following infections is associated with cervical dysplasia?
   a. HIV infection
   b. Herpesvirus infection
   c. Gonorrhea
   d. Human papillomavirus (HPV) infection
   e. Lymphogranuloma venereum

3. What is the major difference between Bowen disease and erythroplasia of Queyrat?
   a. Loss of rete pegs
   b. Keratin staining
   c. Viral etiologic agents
   d. Location
   e. Treatment options

4. Kaposi sarcoma of the AIDS-related (epidemic) type is associated with which of the following etiologic agents?
   a. HPV type 16
   b. Human herpesvirus (HHV) type 8
   c. HPV type 32
   d. *Haemophilus ducreyi* (chancroid [soft chancre])
   e. Coxsackievirus type 23

5. Where do penile cancers most commonly arise?
   a. Glans
   b. Shaft
   c. Frenulum
   d. Coronal sulcus
   e. Scrotum

6. Which of the following is not considered a risk factor for the development of squamous cell carcinoma of the penis?
   a. Cigarette smoke
   b. HPV infection
   c. Phimosis
   d. Gonorrhea
   e. Chewing tobacco

7. All of the following are preventive strategies to decrease the incidence of penile cancer EXCEPT:
   a. Circumcision after 21 years of age
   b. Avoiding sexual promiscuity
   c. Daily genital hygiene
   d. Avoiding cigarette smoke
   e. Circumcision before puberty

8. Which of the following statements regarding penile cancer is FALSE?
   a. Cancer may develop anywhere on the penis.
   b. Because of the associated discomfort, patients usually present to physicians within the first month of noting the lesion.
   c. Phimosis may obscure the nature of the lesion.
   d. Penetration of the Buck fascia and the tunica albuginea by the tumor permits invasion of the vascular corpora.
   e. Cancer cells reach the contralateral inguinal region because of lymphatic cross-communications at the base of the penis.

9. Before a treatment plan for penile cancer is initiated, which of the following is TRUE?
   a. Adequate biopsies to determine stage are unimportant because all patients should be treated with amputation.
   b. Radiologic studies play no role in decision making.
   c. DNA flow cytometry should be performed on virtually all specimens because it provides crucial information.
   d. Tumor stage grade and vascular invasion status all provide prognostically important information.
   e. No disfiguring therapy is indicated, because spontaneous remissions have been noted in approximately 10% of cases.

10. Which of the following statements is TRUE regarding the natural history of penile cancer?
    a. Metastases from the primary tumor often involve lung, liver, or bone as initial sites.
    b. Lymphatic drainage from the primary tumor is ipsilateral alone in most cases.
    c. Metastasis often initially involves spread from the corpora cavernosa to the pelvic lymph nodes.

d. Metastasis initially involves inguinal lymph nodes beneath the fascia lata.

e. Metastasis initially involves inguinal lymph nodes above the fascia lata.

11. Which of the following statements concerning hypercalcemia in patients with penile cancer is TRUE?

a. It is more commonly due to massive bone metastases than bulky soft tissue metastases.

b. It is often related to uremia due to ureteral obstruction.

c. It may be due to the action of parathyroid hormone–like substances released from the tumor.

d. It is related to the action of osteoblasts on bone formation.

e. It is managed with aggressive diuretic administration as first-line therapy.

12. The following statements are true regarding imaging tests in patients with penile cancer EXCEPT:

a. Both ultrasonography and MRI lack sensitivity for the detection of corpus cavernosum involvement.

b. CT is not an appropriate test for determining primary tumor stage.

c. CT may be beneficial in detecting enlarged inguinal nodes in obese patients or those who have had prior inguinal therapy.

d. Lymphangiography can detect abnormal architecture in normal-sized lymph nodes.

e. Inguinal palpation is preferred to CT and lymphangiography for determining inguinal nodal status.

13. According to the 2006 version of the International Union Against Cancer/TNM staging system for penile cancer, which of the following statements is TRUE?

a. Primary tumor stage is based on the size of the primary lesion.

b. Lymph node stage is based on the resectability of involved nodes.

c. Stage T2 tumors are based on biopsy and involve corpora cavernosa only.

d. Large verrucous carcinomas are considered stage Ta.

e. Stage T1 tumors may involve the urethra at the meatus.

14. What is the strongest prognostic factor for survival in penile cancer?

a. The presence of lymph node metastasis

b. The grade of the primary tumor

c. The stage of the primary tumor

d. Vascular invasion presence in the primary tumor

e. The extent of lymph node metastasis

15. Criteria for curative surgical resection (>70% 5-year survival) in patients treated for lymph node metastasis include all of the following EXCEPT:

a. No more than two positive inguinal lymph nodes

b. No positive pelvic lymph nodes

c. Absence of extranodal extension of cancer

d. Unilateral metastasis

e. A single metastasis of only 6 cm

16. Surgical staging of the inguinal region is strongly considered under all of the following conditions EXCEPT:

a. palpable adenopathy.

b. stage T2 or greater primary tumor.

c. presence of vascular invasion in primary tumor.

d. presence of predominantly high-grade cancer in primary tumor.

e. stage Ta tumors.

17. A watchful waiting strategy toward the management of the inguinal region in patients with no palpable adenopathy is recommended for all of the following situations EXCEPT:

a. primary tumor stage Tis.

b. primary tumor stage Ta.

c. primary tumor stage T1, grade I.

d. primary tumor stage T1, grade II.

e. noncompliant patients.

18. Strategies to minimize the morbidity of inguinal staging in patients with no palpable adenopathy include all the following EXCEPT:

a. superficial inguinal lymph node dissection.

b. modified complete inguinal dissection.

c. standard ilioinguinal dissection.

d. sentinel lymph node biopsy.

e. dynamic sentinel node biopsy.

19. Which of the following inguinal staging procedures is considered the "gold standard" for detecting microscopic metastases while limiting both morbidity and false-negative findings?

a. Inguinal node biopsy

b. Superficial inguinal dissection

c. Sentinel lymph node dissection

d. Fine-needle aspiration cytology

e. Sentinel lymph node biopsy

20. For patients with proven unilateral metastasis at presentation, all of the following surgical considerations are true EXCEPT:

a. Ipsilateral ilioinguinal lymphadenectomy should be performed.

b. A contralateral staging procedure is not indicated.

c. A contralateral staging procedure is indicated.

d. Both a superficial dissection and a deep ipsilateral dissection are performed.

e. Ipsilateral pelvic dissection provides useful prognostic information.

21. Adjuvant or neoadjuvant chemotherapy should be considered in addition to surgery for all of the following EXCEPT:

a. single pelvic nodal metastasis.

b. extranodal extension of cancer.

c. fixed inguinal masses.

d. two unilateral inguinal nodes with focal metastases.

e. single 6-cm inguinal lymph node.

22. The majority of penile cancers are histologically:

a. melanoma.

b. bowenoid papulosis.

c. squamous cell carcinoma.

d. epidemic Kaposi sarcoma.

e. verrucous carcinoma.

23. Which of the following chemotherapeutic agents used in combination therapy for penile cancer has been associated with significant pulmonary toxicity?

 a. Bleomycin

 b. Methotrexate

 c. Cisplatin

 d. 5-Fluorouracil (5-FU)

 e. Paclitaxel

24. Indications for radiation therapy as primary treatment for penile cancer include which of the following?

 a. Young, sexually active patient with a small lesion

 b. Patient refuses surgery

 c. Patient with inoperable tumor who needs local treatment but desires to retain the penis

 d. None of the above

 e. a, b, and c

25. Primary penile melanoma is thought to be rare for what reason?

 a. Penile skin is protected from exposure to the sun.

 b. Keratin content in penile skin is decreased.

 c. Penile blood supply precludes such tumor development.

 d. Effective topical chemotherapy exists.

 e. None of the above

26. Lymphomatous infiltration of the penis is most likely secondary to which condition?

 a. Autoimmune disorder

 b. Diffuse disease

 c. Metastasis from a distant primary tumor

 d. Chronic infection

 e. Previous venereal infection

27. What is the most frequently encountered sign of metastatic involvement of the penis?

 a. Pain

 b. Urethral discharge

 c. Ecchymoses

 d. Priapism

 e. Preputial swelling

28. Which of the following features of Buschke-Löwenstein tumor characterizes it as different from condyloma acuminatum?

 a. Propensity for early distant metastasis

 b. Disruption of the rete pegs

 c. Loss of pigmentation

 d. Autoamputation

 e. Invasion and destruction of adjacent tissue by compression

29. Which of the following statements about how verrucous carcinoma of the penis differs from classic Buschke-Löwenstein tumor is TRUE?

 a. The terms describe the same disease.

b. Verrucous carcinoma sometimes exhibits spontaneous regression.

c. Proportion of melanin pigment in verrucous carcinoma is higher than in Buschke-Löwenstein tumor.

d. Simultaneous bilateral inguinal metastases occur commonly with Buschke-Löwenstein tumor.

e. Circumcision is not protective for verrucous carcinoma.

30. Small lesions of erythroplasia of Queyrat may be successfully treated with which of the following?

 a. Topical 5% 5-FU

 b. Neodymium:yttrium-aluminum-garnet (Nd:YAG) laser

 c. Local excision

 d. External-beam radiation therapy

 e. All of the above

ANSWERS

1. **c. Coronal papillae.** Coronal papillae present as linear, curved, or irregular rows of conical or globular excrescences, varying from white to yellow to red, arranged along the coronal sulcus. They are considered acral angiofibromas. These lesions have not been associated with malignancy.

2. **d. Human papillomavirus (HPV) infection.** HPV is recognized as the principal etiologic agent in cervical dysplasia and cervical cancer.

3. **d. Location.** Carcinoma in situ of the penis is referred to by urologists and dermatologists as erythroplasia of Queyrat if it involves the glans penis or prepuce and as Bowen disease if it involves the remainder of the penile shaft skin, genitalia, or perineal region.

4. **b. Human herpesvirus (HHV) type 8.** HHV type 8—also known as Kaposi sarcoma-associated herpesvirus—is strongly suspected to be the etiologic agent of epidemic (AIDS-related) Kaposi sarcoma.

5. **a. Glans.** Penile tumors may present anywhere on the penis but occur most commonly on the glans (48%) and prepuce (21%).

6. **d. Gonorrhea.** No convincing evidence has been found linking penile cancer to other factors such as occupation, other venereal diseases (gonorrhea, syphilis, herpes), marijuana use, or alcohol intake.

7. **a. Circumcision after 21 years of age.** Adult circumcision appears to offer little or no protection from subsequent development of the disease. These data suggest that the crucial period of exposure to certain etiologic agents may have already occurred at puberty and certainly by adult age, rendering later circumcision relatively ineffective as a prophylactic tool for penile cancer.

8. **b. Because of the associated discomfort, patients usually present to physicians within the first month of noting the lesion.** Patients with cancer of the penis, more than patients with other types of cancer, seem to delay seeking medical attention. In large series, from 15% to 50% of patients have been noted to delay medical care for more than a year.

9. **d. Tumor stage, grade, and vascular invasion status all provide prognostically important information.** Confirmation of the diagnosis of carcinoma of the penis, an assessment of the depth of invasion and tumor grade by the combination of an adequate biopsy, and complete clinical assessment are beneficial before the initiation of definitive

therapy. Biopsy can be performed as a frozen section immediately before definitive therapy in some cases.

10. **e. Metastasis initially involves inguinal lymph nodes above the fascia lata.** The lymphatics of the prepuce form a connecting network that joins with the lymphatics from the skin of the shaft. These tributaries drain into the superficial inguinal nodes (the nodes external to the fascia lata).

11. **c. It may be due to the action of parathyroid hormone–like substances released from the tumor.** Parathyroid hormone and related substances may be produced by both tumor and metastases that activate osteoclastic bone resorption.

12. **a. Both ultrasonography and MRI lack sensitivity for the detection of corpus cavernosum involvement.** The sensitivity of ultrasonography for detecting cavernosum invasion was 100% in one study. This study confirmed the value of ultrasonography in assessing the primary tumor also reported by other investigators. For lesions suspected of invading the corpus cavernosum, both ultrasonography and contrast-enhanced MRI may provide unique information, especially when organ-sparing surgery is considered.

13. **d. Large verrucous carcinomas are considered stage Ta.** According to this staging system, designations for primary tumors are as follows: Tx indicates that the primary tumor cannot be assessed; T0 indicates no evidence of tumor; Tis indicates carcinoma in situ; Ta indicates noninvasive verrucous carcinoma; T1 indicates tumor invading subepithelial connective tissue; T2 indicates tumor invading corpus spongiosum or cavernosum; T3 indicates tumor invading urethra or prostate; and T4 indicates tumor invading other adjacent structures.

14. **e. The extent of lymph node metastasis.** The presence and extent of metastasis to the inguinal region are the most important prognostic factors for survival in patients with squamous penile cancer.

15. **e. A single metastasis of only 6 cm.** Pathologic criteria associated with long-term survival after attempted curative surgical resection of inguinal metastases (i.e., 80% 5-year survival) include (1) minimal nodal disease (up to two involved nodes in most series), (2) unilateral involvement, (3) no evidence of extranodal extension of cancer, and (4) the absence of pelvic nodal metastases. A lymph node larger than 4 cm is often associated with extranodal extension of cancer.

16. **e. stage Ta tumors.** Tumor histologic type associated with little or no risk for metastasis includes those patients with primary tumors exhibiting (1) carcinoma in situ or (2) verrucous carcinoma.

17. **e. noncompliant patients.** Noncompliant patients with any degree of invasion in the primary tumor specimen should have an inguinal staging procedure recommended.

18. **c. standard ilioinguinal dissection.** In patients with no evidence of palpable adenopathy who are selected to undergo inguinal procedures by virtue of adverse prognostic factors within the primary tumor, the goal is to define whether metastases exist with minimal morbidity for the patient. A variety of treatment options for this purpose have been reported and include (1) fine-needle aspiration cytology, (2) node biopsy, (3) sentinel lymph node biopsy, (4) extended sentinel lymph node dissection, (5) dynamic

sentinel node biopsy, (6) superficial dissection, and (7) modified complete dissection.

19. **b. Superficial inguinal dissection.** One series found that the sensitivity of fine-needle aspiration cytology was approximately 71% in 18 patients with clinically negative lymph nodes. This finding and the technical difficulty with lymphangiography make aspiration less practical as a staging technique for patients with no palpable lymph nodes. Biopsies directed to a specific anatomic area can be unreliable in identifying microscopic metastasis and are no longer recommended.

20. **b. A contralateral staging procedure is not indicated.** Support for a bilateral procedure is based on the finding of bilateral lymphatic drainage from the primary site in the majority of cases and contralateral metastases in more than 50% of patients so treated in some series even if the contralateral nodal region was negative to palpation.

21. **d. two unilateral inguinal nodes with focal metastases.** For patients requiring ilioinguinal lymphadenectomy because of the presence of metastases, adjuvant chemotherapy should be considered for those exhibiting more than two positive lymph nodes, extranodal extension of cancer, or pelvic nodal metastasis. Reports from one center further confirmed the value of adjuvant chemotherapy. Of 25 node-positive patients treated with adjuvant combination vincristine-bleomycin-methotrexate chemotherapy, 82% survived 5 years, compared with 37% of 31 patients treated with surgery alone.

22. **c. squamous cell carcinoma.** The majority of tumors of the penis are squamous cell carcinomas demonstrating keratinization, epithelial pearl formation, and various degrees of mitotic activity.

23. **a. Bleomycin.** Response rates of bleomycin whether as a single agent or in combination with other agents has not been shown to be superior to cisplatin alone but has been associated with significant pulmonary toxicity and death in several series of patients treated for metastatic penile cancer.

24. **e. a, b, and c.** Radiation therapy may be considered in a select group of patients: (1) young individuals presenting with small (2 to 4 cm), superficial, exophytic, noninvasive lesions on the glans or coronal sulcus; (2) patients refusing surgery as an initial form of treatment; and (3) patients with inoperable tumor or distant metastases who require local therapy to the primary tumor but who express a desire to retain the penis.

25. **a. Penile skin is protected from exposure to the sun.** Melanoma and basal cell carcinoma rarely occur on the penis, presumably because the organ's skin is protected from exposure to the sun.

26. **b. Diffuse disease.** When lymphomatous infiltration of the penis is diagnosed, a thorough search for systemic disease is necessary.

27. **d. Priapism.** The most frequent sign of penile metastasis is priapism; penile swelling, nodularity, and ulceration have also been reported.

28. **e. Invasion and destruction of adjacent tissues by compression.** The Buschke-Löwenstein tumor differs from condyloma acuminatum in that condylomata, regardless of size, always remain superficial and never invade adjacent tissue. Buschke-Löwenstein tumor displaces, invades, and destroys adjacent structures by compression. Aside from this unrestrained local growth, it demonstrates no signs of

malignant change on histologic examination and does not metastasize.

29. **a. The terms describe the same disease.** Buschke-Löwenstein tumor is synonymous with verrucous carcinoma and giant condyloma acuminatum.

30. **e. All of the above.** When lesions are small and noninvasive, local excision, which spares penile anatomy and function, is satisfactory. Circumcision will adequately treat preputial lesions. Fulguration may be successful but often results in recurrences. Radiation therapy has successfully eradicated these tumors, and well-planned, appropriately delivered radiation results in minimal morbidity. Topical 5-FU as the 5% base causes denudation of malignant and premalignant areas while preserving normal skin. There are also reports of successful treatment with Nd:YAG laser.

Additional Study Points

1. Pearly penile papules or papillomas are normal and generally found on the glans penis or corona.

2. Zoon balanitis presents as an erythematous plaque that pathologically reveals a plasma cell infiltrate and is cured by circumcision. Grossly, it is difficult to distinguish from carcinoma in situ.

3. Lesions associated with the development of penile cancer include cutaneous horn, balanitis xerotica obliterans, and pseudoepitheliomatous micaceous and keratotic balanitis.

4. Bowenoid papulosis meets all the histologic criteria for carcinoma in situ; however, the course is invariably benign.

5. Kaposi sarcoma is classified as (1) not associated with immunodeficiency and with an indolent and rarely fatal course, (2) associated with immunosuppressive treatment that is often reversed by modification of the immunosuppressive medications, (3) African Kaposi sarcoma, and (4) HIV-related Kaposi sarcoma. If surgical treatment is required, localized excision is often successful.

6. Carcinoma in situ of the glans is called erythroplasia of Queyrat; if carcinoma in situ is on the shaft of the penis it is called Bowen disease.

7. On the penis there are multiple cross connections of lymphatics so that drainage can occur to either inguinal region.

8. The overwhelming majority of penile squamous cell carcinomas occur on the glans, the prepuce, or corona.

9. Vascular invasion and perineural invasions are strong predictors of lymph node metastases. Distant metastases occur late in the course of the disease and are rare without recognized significant inguinal and pelvic lymphadenopathy.

10. Tis, TA, T1, grade 1 and grade 2 tumors are at low risk for metastases.

11. T2 or greater and grade 3 tumors have a greater than 50% incidence of metastases.

12. The criteria associated with long-term survival after inguinal lymphadenectomy include (1) minimal nodal disease, (2) unilateral involvement, (3) no evidence of extranodal extension, and (4) absence of pelvic node metastases.

13. Inguinal lymphadenectomy should be bilateral when performed on patients at initial presentation. If, on the other hand, the patient presents with unilateral adenopathy at a prolonged time after the initial presentation and treatment of the primary lesion, a unilateral inguinal node dissection may be considered.

Surgery of Penile and Urethral Carcinoma

David S. Sharp, MD ● Kenneth W. Angermeier, MD

QUESTIONS

1. The following statements regarding biopsy of a penile lesion are true EXCEPT:
   a. Biopsy provides confirmation of the histologic diagnosis.
   b. Dorsal slit may be required to expose the glans penis or inner preputial skin.
   c. If possible, adjacent normal tissue should be included to help assess depth of invasion.
   d. Biopsy findings provide prognostic information.
   e. If the lesion involves the urethral meatus, urethroscopy should be performed to evaluate the distal urethra.

2. Laser therapy may provide effective treatment for all of the following lesions EXCEPT:
   a. invasive stage T2 lesions.
   b. carcinoma in situ.
   c. bowenoid papulosis.
   d. superficial stage Ta penile cancers.
   e. dysplastic penile lesions.

3. Techniques that may allow improved delineation of the extent of superficial penile cancer during laser therapy include all of the following EXCEPT:
   a. photodynamic diagnosis and autofluorescence.
   b. preparation of the treatment area with 5% acetic acid.
   c. application of iced saline to the treatment area.
   d. frozen-section biopsies.
   e. c and d.

4. Mohs micrographic surgery provides for:
   a. compromise of long-term local control.
   b. effective therapy for invasive tumors (stage T2 or greater).
   c. retention of function and anatomic integrity of the penis.
   d. effective therapy for large lesions.
   e. a technically simple procedure for excision of penile carcinoma.

5. All of the following statements regarding conservative surgical excision for penile carcinoma are true EXCEPT:
   a. Careful long-term surveillance following surgery is necessary.
   b. Frozen-section biopsies are usually not needed during these procedures.
   c. Glans defects after tumor excision that are not amenable to primary closure may be covered with a split-thickness skin graft or a flap of outer preputial skin.
   d. Glansectomy and circumcision remove the entire contents of the preputial cavity.
   e. Conservative excision provides tissue for tumor grading and assessment of margins.

6. Successful local control by partial penectomy depends on which of the following?
   a. Division of the penis at least 2 cm proximal to the gross tumor
   b. Cleanliness of the patient
   c. Use of adjuvant chemotherapy
   d. Status of inguinal nodes
   e. History of smoking

7. Partial penectomy:
   a. requires creation of a perineal urethrostomy.
   b. provides for normal sexual function in greater than 70% of men.
   c. is required less often than total penectomy.
   d. results in local recurrence rates of less than 10%.
   e. is intended to result in the need for the patient to sit to void.

8. Efforts designed to improve the accuracy of dynamic sentinel lymph node biopsy include all of the following EXCEPT:
   a. using an ultrasensitive gamma ray detection probe.
   b. routine inguinal exploration in the absence of radiotracer visualization.
   c. extended pathologic analysis of excised lymph nodes.

d. intraoperative palpation of the wound for abnormal nodes.

e. preoperative inguinal ultrasonography with fine-needle aspiration of any abnormal-appearing nodes.

9. When compared with the standard groin dissection, the modified groin dissection has all of the following features EXCEPT:

a. The node dissection excludes regions lateral to the femoral artery and caudad to the fossa ovalis.

b. The saphenous vein is preserved.

c. The transposition of the sartorius muscle is eliminated.

d. The required incision is longer.

e. Decreased morbidity.

10. Which of the following statements regarding radical ilioinguinal lymphadenectomy is TRUE?

a. The fascia lata remains intact.

b. The saphenous vein may be preserved in the setting of low-volume disease.

c. Rotation of the gracilis muscle is performed to cover the exposed femoral vessels.

d. The femoral nerve is visualized superior to the iliacus fascia.

e. A laparoscopic approach has not been reported.

11. A pelvic node dissection for male penile cancer should include all of the following areas EXCEPT:

a. Distal common iliac nodes.

b. Para-aortic and paracaval node dissection.

c. External iliac nodes.

d. Obturator group of nodes.

e. a and b.

12. Which of the following measures may help prevent lymphedema after a radical ilioinguinal node dissection?

a. Preservation of Colles fascia in the flap dissection

b. Low-dose heparin in the perioperative period

c. A 6-week delay between treatment of the primary tumor and the node dissection

d. Postoperative bed rest and elastic stockings

e. Obliteration of dead space during wound closure

13. What is the most frequent site of both stricture disease and urethral cancer in the male?

a. Pendulous urethra

b. Fossa navicularis

c. Bulbomembranous urethra

d. Prostatic urethra

e. Urethral meatus

14. Which of the following is TRUE concerning distal urethral carcinoma in the male?

a. Prognosis depends on histologic cell type.

b. Penectomy is usually indicated for tumors infiltrating the corpus spongiosum.

c. Prognosis is worse than for bulbomembranous urethral cancer.

d. Conservative surgical therapy is not effective.

e. Biopsy most commonly demonstrates transitional cell carcinoma.

15. When a delayed urethrectomy is performed in a male patient after radical cystectomy, which of the following is necessary to ensure a complete dissection and decrease the risk of a local recurrence?

a. Removal of the fossa naviculesis and urethral meatus

b. Bilateral groin dissections

c. Total penectomy

d. Intraoperative ultrasound imaging

e. Cauterization of the urethral bed

16. Which of the following statements regarding urethral tumor recurrence after cystectomy and orthotopic urinary diversion is FALSE?

a. It seems to occur more frequently than after cutaneous diversion.

b. Some patients with carcinoma in situ may be successfully treated with urethral infusion of bacillus Calmette-Guérin (BCG).

c. Urethrectomy and cutaneous diversion can often be done using bowel tissue from the existing neobladder.

d. Surveillance consists of urine cytology and symptom assessment.

e. Urethrectomy with conversion to a continent cutaneous diversion may be possible in some patients.

17. Possible causes for female urethral carcinoma include all of the following EXCEPT:

a. childhood urinary tract infections.

b. leukoplakia.

c. chronic irritation or urinary tract infections.

d. proliferative lesions such as caruncles.

e. human papillomavirus infection.

18. What is the most common histologic type of proximal urethral cancer in women?

a. Adenocarcinoma

b. Squamous cell carcinoma

c. Melanoma

d. Transitional cell carcinoma

e. Lymphoma

19. What is the most significant prognostic factor for local control and survival in female urethral cancer?

a. Anatomic location and extent of the tumor

b. Age at presentation

c. Histologic type of the tumor

d. Hematuria

e. Urinary retention

20. Radiation therapy for female urethral carcinoma is most successful:

a. as a single modality for proximal invasive tumors.

b. when used in conjunction with chemotherapy for low-stage distal urethral tumors.

c. at controlling distant metastatic disease.

d. at controlling small lesions in the distal urethra.

e. as neoadjuvant therapy prior to excision of locally advanced proximal urethral cancer.

Pathology

1. See Figure 35–1.

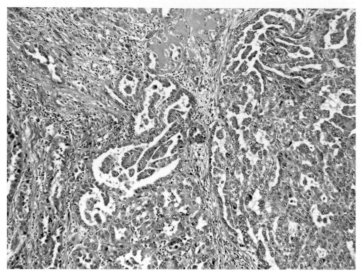

Figure 35–1.

A 64-year-old female has had urethral pain for the past 6 months. A 1-cm mass is palpable in the miduretheral area. A biopsy of the mass is depicted in the figure below. The diagnosis is:

a. squamous cell carcinoma.

b. adenocarcinoma.

c. transitional cell carcinoma.

d. normal urethral epithelium

e. inverted papilloma.

2. See Figure 35–2.

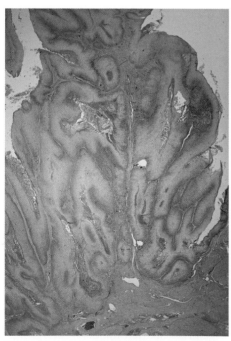

Figure 35–2.

A 65-year-old man has a cauliflower-type lesion on his foreskin, he is sexually active. The lesion is biopsied and depicted below. It is:

a. Kaposi sarcoma.

b. verrucous vulgaris.

c. chancroid.

d. verrucous carcinoma.

e. lymphogranuloma venereum.

3. See Figure 35–3.

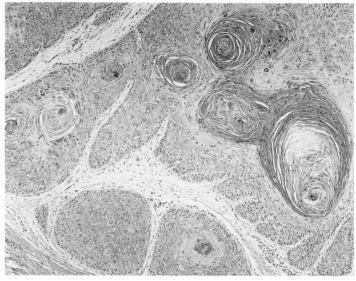

Figure 35–3.

A 75-year-old man has a red raised lesion on his glands that has been present for the past 6 months. The lesion is biopsied and depicted below. The diagnosis is:

a. squamous cell carcinoma.

b. adenocarcinoma.

c. Kaposi sarcoma.

d. transitional cell carcinoma.

e. epithelium inclusion body.

ANSWERS

1. **d. Biopsy findings provide prognostic information.** Before the administration of therapy, a biopsy is required to provide histologic confirmation of the diagnosis of penile cancer and staging information by assessing the depth of microscopic invasion. Adjacent normal tissue should be included to evaluate invasion, a crucial differential point with regard to planning definitive surgery. A dorsal slit may be necessary to expose a lesion within the preputial cavity, and, if the urethral meatus is involved, urethroscopy should be performed to assess the distal urethra.

2. **a. Invasive stage T2 lesions.** Laser therapy has gained popularity in recent years for the treatment of premalignant lesions and carcinoma in situ (Bowen disease, erythroplasia of Queyrat, bowenoid papulosis), and some stage Ta and small T1 penile cancers.

3. **c. application of iced saline to the treatment area.** Photodynamic visualization and autofluorescence have been described as aids to guiding frozen-section biopsies during laser therapy of superficial penile cancer, whereas coating the treatment area with 5% acetic acid often results in acetowhite staining of occult areas of squamous cell carcinoma.

4. **c. Retention of function and anatomic integrity of the penis.** Mohs micrographic surgery allows for retention of function and anatomic integrity of the penis without compromising local control rates in small (<1 to 2 cm) superficial noninvasive and small T1 tumors. It is contraindicated for larger or more invasive lesions.

5. **b. Frozen-section biopsies are usually not needed during these procedures.** Frozen-section biopsies are an essential component of conservative excision for penile carcinoma to ensure complete tumor eradication.

6. **a. Division of the penis at least 2 cm proximal to the gross tumor.** Successful local control by partial penectomy depends on division of the penis at least 2 cm proximal to the gross tumor extent.

7. **d. results in local recurrence rates of less than 10%.** Partial penectomy results in a local recurrence rate of 0% to 8%. It is performed more often than total penectomy, does not generally require creation of a perineal urethrostomy, and provides adequate sexual function in a relatively small percentage of men.

8. **a. using an ultrasensitive gamma ray detection probe.** Techniques reported to increase the accuracy of dynamic sentinel lymph node biopsy include preoperative inguinal ultrasonography with needle biopsy of any suspicious nodes, routine inguinal exploration even in the absence of radiotracer visualization, intraoperative palpation of the wound for abnormal nodes, and extended pathologic analysis of any excised lymph nodes.

9. **d. The required incision is longer.** The modified groin dissection differs from the standard dissection in that (1) the skin incision is shorter; (2) the node dissection is limited, excluding regions lateral to the femoral artery and caudad to the fossa ovalis; (3) the saphenous veins are preserved; and (4) the transposition of the sartorius muscles is eliminated.

10. **b. The saphenous vein may be preserved in the setting of low-volume disease.** In a radical inguinal lymphadenectomy, the fascia lata is divided longitudinally, and the sartorius muscle is rotated to cover the femoral vessels. The femoral nerve is usually not seen because it lies beneath the iliacus fascia lateral to the femoral artery. In the setting of low-volume nodal disease, it is acceptable to spare the saphenous vein, if feasible, to attempt decreasing the risk of lower-extremity complications.

11. **b. Para-aortic and paracaval node dissection.** The pelvic lymphadenectomy includes the distal common iliac, external iliac, and obturator groups of nodes. No further therapeutic benefit is gained from proximal iliac or para-aortic node dissection.

12. **d. Postoperative bed rest and elastic stockings.** Efforts to minimize lymphedema during the initial postoperative period include applying thigh-high elastic wraps or stockings and elevating the foot of the bed.

13. **c. Bulbomembranous urethra.** The incidence of urethral stricture in men later developing a carcinoma of the urethra ranges from 24% to 76% and most frequently involves the bulbomembranous urethra, which is also the portion of the urethra most commonly involved by tumor.

14. **b. Penectomy is usually indicated for tumors infiltrating the corpus spongiosum.** In general, anterior urethral carcinoma is more amenable to surgical control, and the patient's prognosis is better than that for posterior urethral carcinoma, which is often associated with extensive local invasion and distant metastasis.

15. **a. Removal of the fossa navicularis and urethral meatus.** It is important that the fossa navicularis and meatus are also taken in the dissection, because of the high incidence of involvement of the squamous epithelium.

16. **a. It seems to occur more frequently than after cutaneous diversion.** Studies to date suggest that urethral tumor recurrence after orthotopic urinary diversion is less common than after cutaneous diversion. In the presence of an orthotopic neobladder, urethral surveillance consists of urine cytology and symptom assessment. Success has been reported in selected patients treated with urethral infusion of BCG for urethral carcinoma in situ after orthotopic diversion. After urethrectomy, cutaneous diversion can often be done using bowel tissue from the existing neobladder, eliminating the need to take additional small bowel tissue out of the circuit.

17. **a. childhood urinary tract infections.** Causes associated with subsequent development of malignancy include chronic irritation or urinary tract infections; proliferative lesions such as caruncles, papillomas, adenomas, and polyps; leukoplakia of the urethra; parturition; human papillomavirus infection.

18. **b. Squamous cell carcinoma.** Carcinomas of the proximal or entire urethra tend to be high grade and locally advanced, with squamous cell carcinoma accounting for 60%; transitional cell carcinoma 20%; adenocarcinoma 10%; undifferentiated tumor and sarcomas 8%; and melanoma 2%.

19. **a. Anatomic location and extent of the tumor.** The most significant prognostic factor for local control and survival is the anatomic location and extent of the tumor, with low-stage distal urethral tumors having a better prognosis than high-stage proximal urethral tumors.

20. **d. at controlling small lesions in the distal urethra.** Radiation therapy alone, as with surgical excision, is often sufficient to control small lesions in the distal urethra.

Pathology

1. **b. adenocarcinoma.** The patient has a midurethral diverticulum in which adenocarcinoma has developed. This is the most common type of cancer found in a female urethral diverticulum and the second most common type of urethral cancer in the female.

2. **d. verrucous carcinoma.** Note invasion at the base. This lesion is locally invasive but normally does not metastasize.

3. **a. squamous cell carcinoma.** Note infiltrative nature of lesion and the formation of keratin pearls.

Additional Study Points

1. If the patient is uncircumcised, circumcision is recommended at the time of laser therapy.

2. The Nd:YAG laser has a penetration depth of 3 to 6 mm and is the preferred laser for treatment of penile carcinoma. Laser treatment has a recurrence rate of approximately 20%. It is best used for patients with carcinoma in situ or small-volume T1 disease.

3. In addition to cancer control, the goals of penile surgery for carcinoma include the ability to stand to void and preservation of sexual function.

4. Increased penile stump length may be accomplished by releasing the suspensory ligaments.

5. Penile cancer is not a unilateral disease and may metastasize to either groin regardless of location of the primary lesion.

6. Immediate resection of clinically occult lymph node metastases in patients with penile cancer results in improved survival when compared to waiting until metastatic lymph nodes become palpable before performing a groin dissection.

7. A radical groin dissection may be therapeutic and on occasion is used for palliation.

8. Penile cancer does not metastasize to the pelvic nodes without involvement of the inguinal nodes.

9. In the male, squamous cell carcinoma constitutes 80% of the histology, transitional cell 15%, adenocarcinoma and others 5%. In the female, squamous cell carcinoma accounts for 50% to 70%, adenocarcinoma 25%, and transitional cell carcinoma 10%.

10. In the male the anterior urethra lymphatics drain to the inguinal nodes, the posterior urethra lymphatics drain to the pelvic nodes.

11. In the female, the anterior urethra (distal third) lymphatics drain to the inguinal nodes. The posterior urethra lymphatics (proximal two thirds) drain to the external and internal iliac and obturator lymph nodes.

12. Transitional cell carcinoma, which involves the prostatic urethral stoma, significantly increases the probability of urethral recurrence.

13. Adenocarcinoma is the most common type of tumor to occur in a urethral diverticulum.

14. Distal urethral cancers in both men and women have a more favorable prognosis than proximal urethral cancers.

Surgery of the Penis and Urethra

Gerald H. Jordan, MD, FACS, FAAP (Hon), FRCS (Hon) ● Kurt A. McCammon, MD, FACS

QUESTIONS

1. With regard to the physical characteristics of tissue, which of the following statements is TRUE?
   a. They are a function of the collagen-elastin architecture because it is suspended in a mucopolysaccharide matrix.
   b. Only select tissues have inherent tissue tension.
   c. Extensibility can be used synonymously with compliance.
   d. Physical properties of grafts are a function of the superficial dermal or laminar area.
   e. Physical characteristics of flaps vary by the thickness of the underlying fat.

2. In tissue transfer terms, which of the following statements concerning grafts is TRUE?
   a. The process of take can be accelerated by increasing graft mass.
   b. A graft is tissue excised from a donor site that reestablishes its blood supply by revascularization.
   c. During inosculation, the first phase of take, the graft exists at below core body temperature.
   d. Conditions of take are a reflection of only the graft host bed (e.g., scarring, infection).
   e. During imbibition true "connection" of the microvasculature occurs.

3. With regard to the microanatomy of the grafts using skin as a model, which of the following statements is TRUE?
   a. The intradermal plexus is at the interface of the superficial dermis and the deep dermis.
   b. The subdermal plexus is carried at the juncture of the deep dermis and the underlying tissue.
   c. The lymphatics are most richly distributed in the adventitial dermis.
   d. The adventitial dermis, because of its collagen content, accounts for the majority of the physical characteristics.
   e. The subdermal plexus has a rich distribution of small vessels.

4. Grafts of all kinds can be termed split thickness or full thickness. Choose the best answer below with regard to these.
   a. A split-thickness skin graft exposes the vessels of the subdermal plexus.
   b. Exposing the subdermal plexus conveys less fastidious vascular characteristics.
   c. Mesh grafts are created by cutting slits in the epidermis or epithelium.
   d. A full-thickness skin graft is fastidious because of the nature of the subdermal plexus, among other variables.
   e. A split-thickness graft is for the most part composed of epithelium and reticular dermis.

5. With regard to the grafts used most commonly in genitourinary reconstructive surgery, which of the following statements is TRUE?
   a. Thin full-thickness skin is an optimal replacement for the tunica albuginea of the corpora cavernosa.
   b. Bladder epithelial graft is fastidious, because of the nature of the superficial lamina.
   c. Oral mucosal grafts are thought to have a panlaminar plexus.
   d. Tunica vaginalis graft has proved to be a very reliable one for single-stage urethral reconstruction.
   e. Dermal grafts have been used with good success for urethral reconstruction.

6. If a flap is classified according to elevation technique, which of the following statements is TRUE?
   a. All peninsula flaps would by definition be a random flap.
   b. Some peninsula flaps maintain the tissue continuity but divide the vascular continuity.
   c. A true island flap could also be called a paddle.
   d. The microvascular free transfer flap relies on the principle of flap delay.
   e. An island flap would by definition be an axial flap.

7. With regard to the anatomy of the penile shaft, which of the following statements is TRUE?
   a. Throughout most of the length of the penis, the septum is a true competent septum.
   b. The erectile tissues of the normal corpora cavernosa are separated from the tunica by the space of Smith.
   c. The dorsal arteries of the penis are carried in envelope fashion in the dartos fascia.
   d. The Buck fascia is loosely areolar and lies immediately beneath the skin.
   e. The Buck fascia attenuates on the venarum, lateral to the corpus spongiosum.

8. According to consensus, the urethra should be divided into six entities. Which of the following statements is most accurate?
   a. The fossa navicularis is that portion of the urethra that is most dorsally displaced with regard to the surrounding spongy erectile tissue.

b. The bulbous urethral portion is invested by the thickest portion of the corpus spongiosum.

c. The bulbous urethra at its proximal extent is part of the posterior urethra.

d. The membranous urethra is invested by the most proximal aspect of the corpus spongiosum.

e. The membranous urethra, throughout its length is surrounded by the external rhabdosphincter.

9. With regard to the arterial vascularization of the deep structures of the penis, which of the following statements is TRUE?

a. The circumflex cavernosal arteries are uniform in number and distribution.

b. The arteries to the bulb arborize into the spongy erectile tissue of the glans.

c. The common penile artery represents the end continuation of the superficial external pudendal artery.

d. The common penile artery divides to become the cavernosal artery and the dorsal arteries, after branching off the circumflex cavernosal arteries.

e. The blood supply of the deep structures of the penis is derived from the common penile artery, which is the continuation of the internal pudendal artery after it branches off its perineal branch and the posterior scrotal arteries.

10. With regard to the innervation to the penis, which of the following statements is TRUE?

a. The cavernosal nerves are purely parasympathetic and are the extensions of the nervi erigentes.

b. The pudendal nerves accompany the dorsal artery of the penis and the dorsal vein of the penis as they run through the obturator foramen.

c. The dorsal nerve arises in the Alcock canal as a branch of the pudendal nerve.

d. The dorsal nerves throughout their course are prominent, large nerve bundles.

e. The skin of the shaft of the penis is innervated by a branch of the femoral nerve.

11. With regard to the Colles fascia, which of the following statements is TRUE?

a. The Colles fascia is the perineal component of the Camper fascia.

b. The Colles fascia attaches at its posterior margin to the midline fusion of the ischial cavernosus muscle.

c. The Colles fascia joins with the dartos fascia (tunica dartos) of the scrotum.

d. The Colles fascia becomes contiguous with the Buck fascia in the posterior triangle of the perineum.

e. The Colles fascia inserts laterally on the thigh to the quadriceps fascia.

12. With regard to the anterior triangle of the perineum, which of the following statements is TRUE?

a. The ischiocavernosus muscles laterally attach to the inner surface of the ischium and insert in the midline into the Buck fascia.

b. The bulbous spongiosum muscles (midline fusion of the ischial cavernosus muscles) insert posteriorly to the anal sphincter.

c. The perineal body represents a confluence of fascial structures.

d. The perineal body has a prominent neurovascular pedicle within it that provides autonomic innervation to the pelvic diagram.

e. The superficial anal sphincter is contiguous with the dorsal aspect of the bulbospongiosus musculature.

13. Select the correct statement from below.

a. When one encounters the endoscopic findings consistent with urethral hemangioma, one must be alert to exclude the diagnosis of urethral carcinoma.

b. Laser therapy has been very successfully used for the management of large urethral hemangiomas.

c. Reiter syndrome includes the triad of stomatitis, arthritis, and urethritis.

d. In Reiter syndrome, the urethritis is usually mild and self-limiting.

e. Urethral hemangioma does not commonly involve the corpus spongiosum.

14. Select the correct statement from below.

a. Lichen sclerosus/balanitis xerotica obliterans (LS/BXO) is the genital manifestation of psoriasis.

b. Lichen sclerosus/balanitis xerotica obliterans (LS/BXO) is a disease of middle-aged adults and is virtually never seen in younger adults or adolescents.

c. Amyloidosis is a rare disease involving the urethra. It presents as a urethral mass, and patients may experience hematuria, dysuria, or urethral obstruction.

d. In most cases in patients presenting with amyloidosis, aggressive excision is often required.

e. Lichen sclerosus virtually never involves the urethra proximal to the fossa navicularis.

15. Which of the following statements concerning urethral fistula associated with hypospadias repair is TRUE?

a. Fistula closure, in the majority of cases, requires tissue transfer.

b. In acute fistulas, resuturing and reinstitution of diversion should be considered.

c. Fistulas associated with inflammatory strictures usually resolve with aggressive antibiotic therapy.

d. Fistulas associated with hypospadias repair can respond to fulguration and closure with tissue glue.

e. Fistulas often recur, not because of a problem at the fistula site but because of stenosis or obstruction distal to the fistula site.

16. With regard to urethral meatal stenosis in childhood, which of the following statements is TRUE?

a. Meatal stenosis is a frequent complication of phimosis.

b. Meatal stenosis is frequently associated with upper tract changes, and all patients should be evaluated with ultrasonography and voiding cystourethrography.

c. When ammoniacal meatitis is noted, often a short course of meatal dilation and steroid cream application will resolve the problem.

d. When meatal stenosis is present, usually a dorsally based YV advancement flap repair is preferred.

e. Meatal stenosis in childhood is frequently associated with concomitant lichen sclerosus.

17. When treating a patient with penile amputation, which of the following statements is TRUE?

a. Replantation is not a consideration in self-inflicted injury, because most of these patients are chronically psychotic and will eventually try to amputate the penis again.

b. If the distal part of the penis is not available, even if the amputation involves mostly skin with much of the shaft preserved, it is recommended that the remaining shaft be buried in the scrotum.

c. In the case of amputation associated with avulsion, debridement to undivided tissue must precede penile replantation.

d. The classic technique for replantation involves coaptation of the dorsal nerve, the deep dorsal vein, and the cavernosal arteries.

e. The McRoberts technique of macroreplantation is not the preferred method of management for these patients, but when the situation warrants it, it is very successful.

18. With regard to the management of external trauma, which of the following statements is TRUE?

a. Because of the nature of the genital tissues, aggressive initial debridement must be undertaken.

b. The eventual effect of a genital burn may be to unacceptably tether and/or incarcerate the penis.

c. The gracilis flap is ideally suited for coverage of large perineal or groin wounds.

d. Complications of direct irradiation to the penis can usually be resolved with split-thickness skin grafts.

e. Thermal burns frequently involve the deep tissues of the genitalia.

19. Concerning genital lymphedema, which of the following statements is TRUE?

a. Reconstruction for lymphedema that is the consequence of the indirect effects of radiation is best accomplished with excision of the tissues and coverage with split-thickness skin grafts (STSGs).

b. In reconstruction for lymphedema, it is essential to maintain the parietal tunica vaginalis of the testes intact with grafting over that location.

c. When considering reconstruction for lymphedema, full-thickness skin grafts (FTSGs) are preferable because of the distribution of the lymphatics in the superficial (adventitial) dermis.

d. In the case of genital lymphedema, it is not unusual for the immune response of the tissues to be altered and for patients to have significant involvement with genital papillomas.

e. Not unusually, in cases where the genital lymphedema is localized, the midline of the scrotum can be preserved for reconstruction.

20. Which of the following statements is most accurate concerning anterior urethral stricture disease?

a. It causes limitation of the urethral lumen because of the bulk of the scar.

b. It most often is limited to the urethral epithelium.

c. It implies a scarring process, usually involving both the epithelium and the underlying spongy erectile tissue of the corpora cavernosa.

d. It causes limitation of the urethral lumen because of contraction and noncompliance of the scar.

e. It is metaplastic process of the urethral epithelium.

21. Which of the following statements concerning pelvic fracture urethral distraction defects is TRUE?

a. It involves the tissues of the epithelium as well as the underlying erectile tissues of the corpora cavernosa.

b. It involves the tissues of the epithelium as well as the underlying erectile tissue of the corpus spongiosum.

c. It is not a true stricture but rather fibrosis that results from distraction of the urethra.

d. The stricture process can often be occult because of the unpredictable involvement of the urethral tissues.

e. The defect is usually predictably proximal to the external sphincter at the junction of the prostatic urethra with the membranous urethra.

22. Which of the following statements regarding strictures resulting from LS/BXO is true?

a. They are usually associated with the scarring extending deeply into the corpus spongiosum.

b. They usually begin as meatal stenosis associated with ammoniacal balanitis/meatitis.

c. They often resolve with the use of antibiotics.

d. The process has been definitively shown to be the result of infectious inflammation of the urethral tissues caused by *Borrelia burgdorferi*.

e. They are most successfully reconstructed with penile skin islands carried on the dartos fascia.

23. When one is treating a patient in retention or a patient experiencing difficult catheter placement, which of the following statements is TRUE?

a. Endoscopy defines the nature of the difficulty.

b. The patient can usually be effectively treated with filiform follower dilation.

c. Optimal management may mean placement of a suprapubic catheter.

d. Imaging results are usually not informative.

e. Once the retention has been dealt with, patients rarely need further evaluation.

24. In determining the anatomy of the stricture, all of the following provide useful information EXCEPT:

a. MRI.

b. high-resolution ultrasonography.

c. contrast studies.

d. urethroscopy.

e. calibration with Bougie à boule.

25. With regard to the modalities for evaluation of the urethra, which of the following statements is TRUE?

    a. Extravasation of contrast material during retrograde urethrography inevitably implies poor technique.

    b. Distention of the urethra during sonourethrogram often confuses findings.

    c. Contrast material suitable for intravenous injection should be used for all retrograde urethrogram studies.

    d. Contrast material thickened with lubricating gels better define the stricture length.

    e. Because retrograde urethrogram is not informative in the posterior urethra, visualization of the anterior urethra usually suffices.

26. With regard to planning of reconstruction for urethral stricture, which of the following statements is TRUE?

    a. Even if a patient does not have retention, placement of a suprapubic tube may help define strictured areas.

    b. Tightly stenotic areas should be dilated to pass endoscopes proximally.

    c. The effects of hydrodilation are manifested most immediately distal to the area of narrowest stenosis.

    d. Calibration of strictured areas to 16 Fr or greater reliably predicts the potential for segments to contract.

    e. Sonourethrogram by itself accurately predicts depth of spongiofibrosis.

27. With regard to direct visual internal urethrotomy, which of the following statements is TRUE?

    a. Strictures are best incised at the 12-o'clock position.

    b. Deep incision of the corpus spongiosum has been shown to optimize long-term results.

    c. In optimally selected patients, long-term success of internal urethrotomy is approximately 90%.

    d. Internal urethrotomy should be the first procedure considered for any stricture of the anterior urethra.

    e. It can be associated with erectile dysfunction.

28. Concerning permanently implanted urethral stents, which of the following statements is TRUE?

    a. Long-term follow-up (10- and 11-year data) shows that if a permanently implanted stent is patent at 4.0 to 4.5 years, then long-term patency can be expected.

    b. Permanently implantable stents are indicated for short strictures of the bulbous urethra and, when so employed, are associated with short-term success in the range of approximately 84%.

    c. They are rarely complicated by persistent perineal pain.

    d. They are useful for short strictures of the pendulous urethra.

    e. They are useful in cases of failed skin patch urethroplasty.

29. All of the following are either absolute or strong relative contraindications to the use of the Urolume stent EXCEPT:

    a. distraction injuries of the membranous urethra.

    b. patients who have strictures associated with urethral fistula.

    c. patients with short strictures of the bulbous urethra not associated with significant spongiofibrosis.

    d. patients who are younger than 50 years old who are reasonable candidates for urethral reconstruction.

    e. children with bulbous urethral stricture disease.

30. Concerning anterior urethral reconstruction, which of the following statements is TRUE?

    a. Excision and primary anastomosis reconstruction is severely limited and useful only for very proximal strictures 1 to 2 cm in length.

    b. Performance of the excision and primary anastomosis technique is facilitated by dissection of the corpus spongiosum to the level of the glans penis.

    c. Success requires total excision of the fibrosis with a widely spatulated anastomosis.

    d. Reconstruction is facilitated by development of the intracrural space with infrapubectomy.

    e. In cases of longer strictures, excision with partial anastomosis allowing one wall to granulate offers acceptable results.

31. With regard to techniques of urethral reconstruction, which of the following statements is TRUE?

    a. The Monseur technique employed the use of mesh split-thickness skin.

    b. Excision with strip anastomosis and onlay (augmented anastomosis) is an excellent form of reconstruction for strictures too long to be dealt with only by excision and primary anastomosis.

    c. The Barbagli operation combines the use of excision with staged augmented anastomosis.

    d. The use of the spongioplasty maneuver requires the total excision of all spongiofibrosis.

    e. Vessel-sparing excision with primary anastomosis is not useful for distal bulbous urethral strictures.

32. With regard to genital skin flap operations for anterior urethral reconstruction, which of the following statements is TRUE?

    a. Flap operations are best applied as individual techniques and require the surgeon to become intimately familiar with the individual steps of each technique.

    b. The operation can conceptually become one operation with multidimensional application.

    c. The operations are all based on mobilization of the extended Buck fascia.

    d. The operations require a comfortable understanding of the extended circumflex iliac superficial vascular pattern.

    e. They are of limited value in patients who have been previously circumcised.

33. With regard to flap procedures for anterior urethral reconstruction, which of the following statements is TRUE?

    a. The scrotal skin island is a problematic flap and should be avoided at all cost.

    b. The circular skin islands, mechanically, are facilitated by dividing the dartos fascial flaps ventrally.

    c. The "tubed flaps" in general are optimal for cases of short- to moderate-length strictures.

    d. The length of tubed segments can be limited by the aggressive mobilization of the corpus spongiosum.

e. Combined tissue transfer, the combination of graft patch and flap patch, has been shown to be superior to tubed reconstruction.

34. With regard to strictures associated with LS/BXO, which of the following statements is TRUE?
   a. The Urolume stent has proved to be an excellent option.
   b. Staged skin graft procedures have yielded excellent durable results.
   c. Because LS/BXO is a generalized skin condition, oral mucosa has been considered for reconstruction, with initial encouraging results.
   d. Patch flap techniques have provided excellent long-term success rates.
   e. In most cases, because the lumen is severely stenotic, urethral resection with tubed flap reconstructive is preferable.

35. Which of the following statements concerning urethral distraction injuries is TRUE?
   a. They are usually associated with full-thickness spongiofibrosis.
   b. Although they can involve any part of the membranous urethra, they most frequently occur at the juncture of the membranous urethra with the bulbous urethra.
   c. They can be partial, and this difference is easily defined by contrast studies.
   d. They are best managed with an aligning catheter placed to traction.
   e. Inevitably are associated with injury to the pudendal nerves.

36. Pelvic fracture urethral distraction injuries are:
   a. optimally first evaluated with contrast studies.
   b. often evaluated with an endoscope in the anterior urethra and a cystogram with the patient straining to void.
   c. always defined with simultaneous cystogram and retrograde urethrogram.
   d. always complicated by postoperative incontinence when contrast material is seen in the posterior urethra.
   e. never be evaluated with endoscopy in the acute-injury phase.

37. With regard to continence after reconstruction for pelvic fracture urethral distraction injuries, which of the following statements is TRUE?
   a. Location of the injury along the course of the membranous urethra is not associated with continence postoperatively.
   b. Continence can be accurately predicted by contrast studies.
   c. Continence is best predicted by the appearance of the bladder neck on endoscopy.
   d. Continence is best addressed after a procedure to reestablish urethral continuity is performed.
   e. Continence is best in patients with partial distraction injuries.

38. All of the following maneuvers facilitate reconstruction of pelvic fracture urethral distraction injuries without creating chordee or foreshortening of the penis EXCEPT:
   a. development of the intracavernosal (intracrural) space.
   b. infrapubectomy.
   c. mobilization of the proximal corpus spongiosum.
   d. division of the attachment of the bulbospongiosum to the perineal body.
   e. dissection of the scarred Buck fascia from the corpus spongiosum.

39. With regard to failures of reconstruction of posterior urethral distraction primary anastomotic technique, which of the following statements is TRUE?
   a. Most failures are due to technical anastomotic issues.
   b. Long-segment failures are readily amenable to direct-vision internal urethrotomy with Urolume stent placement.
   c. Patients with one intact pudendal artery are at risk for ischemic stenosis of the corpus spongiosum.
   d. Patients with reconstitution of an injured pudendal vessel, even if reconstitution was a unilateral phenomenon, are excellent candidates for posterior urethral reconstruction.
   e. Inevitably, redo reconstruction requires a procedure using tissue transfer.

40. In dealing with the entity of chordee without hypospadias, which of the following statements is TRUE?
   a. Correction of curvature is often achieved with mobilization of the corpus spongiosum alone.
   b. It often can be corrected with maneuvers that lengthen the foreshortened ventral skin.
   c. Is best straightened by an incision and grafting operation.
   d. Division of the urethra/corpus spongiosum is virtually always indicated.
   e. It is usually present with either ventral curvature or ventral curvature associated with torsion.

41. With regard to congenital curvature of the penis, which of the following statements is TRUE?
   a. If length is an issue, the patient probably is more correctly characterized as having chordee without hypospadias.
   b. It is optimally managed with incision and grafting to avoid foreshortening of the penis.
   c. In most cases, despite dissection and incision of tissues that appear inelastic, most patients require incision with grafting.
   d. Correction is facilitated by tourniquet occlusion during artificial erections.
   e. Curvature is usually dorsal.

42. With regard to acquired curvatures of the penis that are not Peyronie disease, which of the following statements is TRUE?
   a. Most are characterized by prominent dorsal scars.
   b. In most cases, global cavernosal veno-occlusive dysfunction (CVOD) is not a complicating factor.

c. They are virtually never associated with "minimal" buckling trauma.

d. Patients often have significant penile foreshortening.

e. There is usually an association with either hypospadias or epispadias.

ANSWERS

1. **a. They are a function of the collagen-elastin architecture because it is suspended in a mucopolysaccharide matrix.** All tissue has inherent physical characteristics, and those are extensibility, inherent tissue tension, and the vesicoelastic properties of stress relaxation and creep. The physical characteristics of a transferred unit are primarily a function of the helical arrangement of collagen along with the elastin cross linkages. The collagen-elastin architecture is suspended in a mucopolysaccharide matrix that influences the vesicoelastic properties. The physical properties of skin and the other grafts appropriate for urethral reconstruction are mainly a function of the deep laminar or dermal layer. It is that layer that has the most extensive collagen-elastin architecture.

2. **b. A graft is tissue excised from a donor site that reestablishes its blood supply by revascularization.** Tissue can be transferred as a graft (see Fig. 36–1 in *Campbell-Walsh Urology, 10th Edition*). The term graft implies that tissue has been excised and transferred to a graft host bed, where a new blood supply develops by a process that has been termed take. Take requires approximately 96 hours and occurs in two phases. The initial phase, termed imbibition, takes about 48 hours, and during that phase the graft survives by "drinking" nutrients from the adjacent graft host bed. During that phase, the graft temperature is less than core body temperature. The second phase, termed inosculation, also requires about 48 hours and is the phase during which true microcirculation is reestablished in the graft. During that phase, the temperature of the graft rises to core body temperature. Processes that interfere with the vascularity of the graft host bed thus interfere with graft take. The process of take is also influenced by the nature of the grafted tissue. Thus a split-thickness unit in most cases is much less fastidious from a vascular standpoint and also much less fastidious from the standpoint of total mass of the grafted tissue. However the trade-off with split-thickness tissue is that it does not generally carry "the physical characteristics" and is thus prone to contraction. All of these conditions must be recognized and included in the planning process when one elects a form of reconstruction (i.e., primary versus staged).

3. **b. The subdermal plexus is carried at the juncture of the deep dermis and the underlying tissue.** The superficial plexus or intradermal plexus is carried at approximately the interface of the epithelium and the superficial dermis. The subdermal plexus exists at the interface of the deep dermis and the subcutaneous tissues. That skin is termed the reticular dermis. The superficial dermis and skin is termed the adventitial dermis and is equivalent to the superficial lamina. The majority of the lymphatics are in the deep dermal layer or reticular dermal layer, and this can be compared with the deep laminar layer. The collagen content of that layer is much greater than in the superficial layer. Thus that layer is believed to account for the physical characteristics of the tissue. The intradermal

or superficial plexus in most tissues is generally composed of many small vessels. The subdermal layer or deep plexus consists of much more sparsely distributed vessels, which are larger. In the case of the bladder epithelial graft, the perforators connecting the deep plexus to the superficial plexus are much more frequently distributed than in skin. In buccal mucosa, the layered arrangement is lost and the microvasculature consists of a panlaminar plexus.

4. **d. A full-thickness skin graft is fastidious because of the nature of the subdermal plexus, among other variables.** If a graft is carried as a full-thickness unit (FTG), it carries the covering. It carries the superficial dermis or lamina with all of the characteristics attributable to that layer. In most cases, the plexus (subdermal plexus) is composed of larger vessels that are more sparsely distributed. The graft is thus fastidious in its vascular characteristics. A split- thickness skin graft thus carries the epithelium and the underlying superficial dermis.

5. **c. Oral mucosal grafts are thought to have a panlaminar plexus.** In the case of the oral mucosal graft, there is a panlaminar plexus. In the case of the bladder epithelial graft, there is a superficial and a deep plexus; however, the plexuses are connected by many more perforators. The dermal graft for years has been used to augment the tunica albuginea. Mature vein grafts show evidence of take to the vas vasorum. Other grafts that have been utilized for single-stage urethral reconstruction include rectal mucosa grafts, dermal grafts, and tunica vaginalis graft. The results using dermal grafts and tunica vaginalis grafts are not acceptable, and these grafts are not considered to be good grafts for urethral reconstruction. There are only a small series that have reported the use of rectal mucosal grafts. The precise process of take, to our knowledge, has not been well defined. In recent years, acellular collagen matrix has been proposed as an alternative to the grafts mentioned earlier. The precise mechanism of action of these "grafts" is not well defined. It may well be that these grafts serve as a biologic dressing only and then become replaced by lateral ingrowths from the adjacent epithelial layer. The future probably lies in the use of cultured tissues for grafts.

6. **e. An island flap would by definition be an axial flap.** A peninsula flap is a flap in which the vascular and cutaneous continuities of the flap base are left intact. Peninsula flaps can be elevated on either random vasculature or axial vasculature, depending on the location of the donor site (see Figs. 36–2 and 36–3 in *Campbell-Walsh Urology, 10th Edition*). An island flap is a flap in which the vascular continuity is maintained; however, the cuticular continuity is divided (see Fig. 36–3B in *Campbell-Walsh Urology, 10th Edition*). The microvascular free transfer flap (free flap) (see Fig. 36–3C in *Campbell-Walsh Urology, 10th Edition*) has both the vascular continuity and the cuticular continuity interrupted. The vascular continuity is then reestablished at the recipient site. A true island flap is elevated on dangling vessels. The terminology thus should not be confused with what is most commonly used for urethral reconstruction, fascial flaps carrying skin islands or skin paddles.

7. **b. The erectile tissues of the normal corpora cavernosa are separated from the tunica by the space of Smith.** The corpora cavernosa are not separate structures but constitute a single space with free communication through an incompetent midline septum,

composed of multiple strands of elastic tissue similar to that making up the tunica albuginea. The erectile tissue is separated from the tunica albuginea by a thin layer of areolar connective tissue that was described by Smith. The Buck fascia is directly abutted to the tunica albuginea of the corpora cavernosa. The Buck fascia surrounds the adventitia of the corpora spongiosum in envelope fashion, and the dorsal neurovascular structures are contained in envelope fashion between the superficial and deep laminar of the Buck fascia on the dorsum. The Buck fascia is thus "devoted" to the deep structures (see Fig. 36–5 in *Campbell-Walsh Urology, 10ᵗʰ Edition*). The dartos fascia is loosely areolar and lies immediately beneath the skin. It is in that fascial layer that the arborizations of the superficial external pudendal vessels and the posterior scrotal vessels are carried.

8. **b. The bulbous urethral portion is invested by the thickest portion of the corpus spongiosum.** The fossa navicularis is contained within the spongy erectile tissue of the glans penis and terminates at the junction of the urethral epithelium with the skin of the glans. The bulbous urethra is covered by the midline fusion of the ischiocavernosus musculature and is invested by the bulbospongiosum of the proximal corpus spongiosum. It becomes larger and lies closer to the dorsal aspect of the corpus spongiosum, exiting from its dorsal surface prior to the posterior attachment of the bulbospongiosum to the perineal body. The membranous urethra is the portion that traverses the perineal pouch and is partially surrounded by the external urethral sphincter. This segment of the urethra is unattached to fixed structures, has the distinction of being the only portion of the male urethra that is not invested by another structure, and is lined with a delicate transitional epithelium (see Fig. 36-7 in *Campbell-Walsh Urology, 10ᵗʰ Edition*).

9. **e. The blood supply to the deep structures of the penis is derived from the common penile artery, which is the continuation of the internal pudendal artery after it branches off its perineal branch and the posterior scrotal arteries.** From that point onward, it is termed the common penile artery. As it nears the urethral bulb, the artery divides into its three terminal branches as follows: (1) the bulbourethral arteries, which enter the proximal corpus spongiosum; (2) the dorsal artery, which travels along the dorsum of the penis contained in envelope fashion between the superficial and deep lamina of the Buck fascia; and (3) the cavernosal arteries, usually a single artery, which arise and penetrate the corpora cavernosa at the hilum and run the length of the penile shaft. The circumflex cavernosal arteries are given off at varying locations along the dorsal artery, but their distribution is neither uniform nor dependable (see Fig. 36–12 in *Campbell-Walsh Urology, 10ᵗʰ Edition*).

10. **c. The dorsal nerve arises in the Alcock canal as a branch of the pudendal nerve.** The cavernosal nerves are a combination of the parasympathetic and visceral afferent fibers that constitute the autonomic nerves of the penis. These provide the nerve supply to the erectile apparatus. The pudendal nerves enter the perineum with the internal pudendal vessels through the lesser sciatic notch at the posterior border of the ischiorectal fossa. They run in the fibrofascial pudendal canal of Alcock to the edge of the urogenital diaphragm. Each dorsal nerve of the penis arises in the Alcock canal as the first branch of the pudendal nerve. On the shaft, their fascicles fan out to supply proprioceptive and sensory nerve terminals in the tunica of the corpora cavernosa and sensory terminals in the skin. The skin of the penis is innervated by branches of the genitofemoral nerve.

11. **c. The Colles fascia joins with the dartos fascia (tunica dartos) of the scrotum.** The Colles fascia joins with the dartos fascia (tunica dartos) of the scrotum, and a fold of this fascia projects backward beneath the fibers of the bulbospongiosus muscle. Anteriorly, the Colles fascia fuses and becomes continuous with the membranous layer of the subcutaneous connective tissue of the anterior abdominal wall (the Scarpa fascia). The Colles fascia extends laterally over the highest insertion at the fascia.

12. **a. The ischiocavernosus muscles laterally attach to the inner surface of the ischium and insert in the midline into the Buck fascia.** The ischiocutaneous muscles cover the crura of the corpora cavernosa. They attach to the inner surfaces of the ischium and ischial tuberosities on each side and insert at the midline into the Buck fascia, surrounding the crura at their junction below the arcuate ligament of the penis. The bulbospongiosus muscles are located in the midline of the perineum. They are attached to the perineal body posteriorly and to each other in the midline, as they encompass the bulbospongiosum and crura of the corpora cavernosa at the base of the penis. These muscles are confluent with the ischiocavernosus muscles laterally, and at their insertion into the Buck fascia. The anal sphincters are in the posterior perineal triangle.

13. **d. In Reiter syndrome, the urethritis is usually mild and self-limiting.** Because all reported cases of urethral hemangioma have been benign, management is dependent on the size and location of the lesion. Most are relatively localized, but extensive involvement is occasionally seen. For smaller lesions, laser treatment has been successful and produces less scarring. The preferred treatment for larger lesions is open excision and urethral reconstruction. Reiter syndrome is characterized by a classic triad of arthritis, conjunctivitis, and urethritis. Urethral involvement is usually mild, self-limiting, and a minor portion of the disease.

14. **c. Amyloidosis is a rare disease involving the urethra. It presents as a urethral mass, and patients may present with hematuria, dysuria, or urethral obstruction.** BXO has in the past been the term used to describe the genital presentation of lichen sclerosus. By the recent Consensus Conference, the term BXO has become synonymous with lichen sclerosus, and lichen sclerosus is the favored terminology. It is the most common cause of meatal stenosis. Lichen sclerosus appears as a whitish plaque that may involve the prepuce, glans penis, urethral meatus, and fossa navicularis. Several reports have suggested the association with chronic infection with the spirochete *Borrelia burgdorferi*. Although previously thought to be rare, lichen sclerosus (BXO) is commonly found at the time of circumcisions performed beyond the neonatal period. Long-term antibiotic therapy may also be helpful to improve the inflammation as secondary infection of the inflamed tissue may occur. We have typically used tetracycline, but a trial of long-term penicillin (or

advanced-generation erythromycin) may be warranted. Amyloidosis, a rare disease, should be considered in the evaluation of any patient with a urethral mass. The differential diagnosis includes urethral neoplasm. Cystoscopy and transurethral biopsy is indicated. Patients may present with hematuria, dysuria, or urethral obstruction. Most patients can be followed expectantly. Urethral strictures associated with LS can involve long segments of the anterior urethra.

15. **e. Fistulas often recur, not because of a problem at the fistula site but because of stenosis or obstruction distal to the fistula site.** Treatment of a urethral fistula must be directed not only toward the defect but also toward the underlying process leading to its development. In cases of urethral reconstruction, especially reconstruction for hypospadias, fistula often occurs or recurs because of distal obstruction and high-pressure voiding. After urethral surgery, fistulas can develop immediately or as delayed complications. Repair of the fistula may be delayed at a minimum of 6 months to allow for complete resolution of the inflammation. Fistulas associated with inflammatory strictures occur as periurethral tracts and develop secondary to high-pressure voiding of infected urine. Repair requires suprapubic drainage, and treatment of the infection requires incision and drainage of any abscesses present. One must be very cautious in treating the patient with urethral fistulas but without a chronic history of obstructive voiding symptoms. In many cases, fistula or periurethral abscess may be the hallmark symptom of urethral carcinoma. Fistulas associated with failed hypospadias repair often are relatively large and can require substantial urethral reconstruction in order to address them.

16. **c. When ammoniacal meatitis is noted, often a short course of meatal dilation and steroid cream application will resolve the problem.** Meatal stenosis in the male child appears to be a consequence of circumcision, which allows for ammoniacal meatitis. In children seen with ammoniacal meatitis, we usually start them with meatal dilation using steroid cream. Within a week, the process seems to settle down. Anecdotally, the fusion of the ventral meatus skin, which causes meatal stenosis, seems to be avoided. Because childhood meatal stenosis truly represents a fusion of the ventral urethral meatus, dividing the thin membrane of fusion is preferred. This leaves the child with a slit-shaped meatus; the use of a dorsal YV maneuver can be required in special circumstances, but for most cases it can be avoided and should be because of the cosmetic deformity of the glans that it leaves.

17. **e. The McRoberts technique of macroreplantation is not the preferred method of management for these patients, but when the situation warrants it, it is very successful.** Often the amputation is self-inflicted, usually during an acute psychotic break. This should not preclude replantation unless the patient adamantly refuses such treatment. Even then, with a court order and the agreement of two or more surgeons, replantation may be undertaken. If possible, microreplantation should be carried out. This technique consists of an anatomic approximation of the tunica albuginea of the corporeal bodies, a spatulated two-layer anastomosis of the urethra. The dorsal nerves are coapted using an epineural technique unless the injury is distal, at

which point a vesicular coaptation may be required. The dorsal vein is anastomosed, and the dorsal arteries are anastomosed. Anastomosis of the cavernosal arteries is not possible and should not be attempted (see Fig. 36–15 in *Campbell-Walsh Urology, 10th Edition*). If the situation is such that microreplantation cannot be undertaken, then the technique described by McRoberts can be carried out. His series and other series show that a high degree of success can be expected after replantation without microvascular reanastomosis. In most of the patients, however, they will have numbness distal to the replant site. With microreplantation, it is not at all unusual for patients to have excellent sensation distal to the area of injury and to have resumption of normal erectile function.

If the patient presents with the distal part having been disposed of or otherwise unavailable, then the wound should be closed. Often the penis will have been stretched during the amputation and an excess of skin will have been removed, leaving a good length intact with denuded penile shaft structures. In that case, the corporeal bodies would be closed, the urethral meatus must be spatulated, and the penis can be immediately covered with a split-thickness skin graft. If the injury occurs because of avulsion, replantation is not an option as the stretch injury to the spermatic vessels or vessels of the penis causes unpredictable damage to the endothelium.

18. **b. The eventual effect of a genital burn may be to unacceptably tether and/or incarcerate the penis.** The physiologic functions of genital tissues cannot be accurately duplicated. The unique vascularity of genital tissue allows for less aggressive rather than more aggressive debridement. In many patients, the penis will have become incarcerated in contracted scar tissue after healing of the acute injury. Successful transposition of a gracilis musculocutaneous flap introduces compliant vascular tissue and skin into the area, allowing release of the penile shaft. The gracilis musculocutaneous flap is not particularly well suited for the coverage of large perineal or groin defects; however, the posterior thigh flap offers excellent bulky sensate tissues. Therapeutic radiation can produce chronic suppurative gangrene. These lesions are not amenable to reconstruction. Chemical burns to the genitalia usually cause damage to the superficial structures. In the case of chemical burn, vigorous irrigation must be accomplished because chemical burns can cause long-term issues with scarring and tethering; involvement of the deep structures usually does not occur.

19. **a. Reconstruction for lymphedema that is the consequence of the indirect effects of radiation is best accomplished with excision of the tissues and coverage with split-thickness skin grafts (STSGs).** Patients with lymphedema can readily undergo reconstruction. When the lymphedematous tissue has been excised, the testes will be free and, as in a degloving injury, they must be fixed in the midline in an anatomically correct position. The shaft of the penis should be covered with an STSG. If the scrotum cannot be closed, a meshed STSG is used to cover the testes, as described. Not uncommonly, these patients have hydroceles, the parietal tunica vaginalis must be excised, and grafting can be done directly onto the visceral tunica vaginalis of the testicles. Unlike the full-thickness skin flap (FTSF), split-thickness skin carries little of

the reticular dermis and hence few of the lymphatic channels. Reaccumulation of lymphedema will occur within an FTSG and can recur in a thick STSG. In many cases of lymphedema limited to the genitalia, the posterior scrotal skin and the lateral scrotal skin are spared from the lymphedematous process. Thus, in some cases, primary closure after excision can be accomplished using these tissues. If grafting is required, using these tissues to blend the grafts into the groin and perineum technically is much easier. The lymphedematous process involves recurrent cellulitis, lymphedema, and the development of lymphangiectasia. Lymphangiectasia can look like genital papilloma; however, it is a very different process. If there is any question, biopsy can clarify the issue.

20. **d. It causes limitation of the urethral lumen because of contraction and noncompliance of the scar.** The term urethral stricture refers to anterior urethral disease. By virtue of the Consensus Conference, obliterative processes of the membranous urethra, such as those associated with pelvic fracture, would be referred to as pelvic fracture urethral distraction defects and other narrowing processes of the posterior urethra are correctly referred to as either contractures or stenoses. Thus the term urethral stricture describes a process that involves the urethral epithelium along with the spongy erectile tissue of the corpus spongiosum, and this is referred to as spongiofibrosis. In some cases, the scarring process can extend through the tissues of the corpus spongiosum and into the adjacent tissues. It is contraction of the scar that reduces the urethral lumen. Squamous metaplasia is often seen involving the urothelium of the urethra proximal to a narrow caliber urethral stricture.

21. **c. It is not a true stricture but rather fibrosis that results from distraction of the urethra.** By virtue of the Consensus Conference, narrowing of the posterior urethra is not referred to as a stricture. Those obliterative processes associated with pelvic fracture are termed pelvic fracture urethral distraction defects (PFUDD). PFUDD is an obliterative process of the posterior urethra that has resulted in fibrosis and is the defect of distraction of the urethra in that area. Although the distraction defect can be lengthy in some cases, the actual process involving the tissues of the urethra is usually confined.

22. **a. They are usually associated with the scarring extending deeply into the corpus spongiosum.** Some evidence suggests that the progression of the stricture to eventually involve the entire anterior urethra may be due to high-pressure voiding that causes intravasation of urine into the glands of Littre, inflammation of these glands, and, perhaps, microabscesses and deep spongiofibrosis. Whether the urethral changes and eventual fibrosis are also related to bacterial injury, to our knowledge, has not been well defined. Literature does not show resolution of the stricture process with the use of antibiotics. Whereas the spirochete *Borrelia burgdorferi* has been implicated in lichen sclerosus elsewhere, there is no literature that absolutely implicates it in the process that is seen on the genitalia referred to as lichen sclerosus/BXO. Currently, because LS is a skin disease, it is recommended that tissue other than skin be used for reconstruction.

23. **c. Optimal management may mean placement of a suprapubic catheter.** When a patient cannot void, an attempt is made to pass a urethral catheter. If the catheter does not pass, the nature of the obstruction is determined by dynamic retrograde urethrography. Thus most cases are managed with acute dilation, and clearly there are many instances in which this is not the best course for the patient. When there is doubt, we determine the nature of the stricture if possible, and not uncommonly, we place a suprapubic cystostomy catheter to treat the acute situation and allow time for a more appropriate treatment plan to be devised. Although detailed imaging is not always available, flexible endoscopy is very useful in allowing a glide wire to be passed through the area of stenosis; however, the anatomy of this stricture process cannot be determined just by endoscopy.

24. **a. MRI.** To devise an appropriate treatment plan, it is important to determine the location, length, depth, and density of the stricture (spongiofibrosis). The length and location of the stricture can be determined using radiographs, urethroscopy, and ultrasonography. The depth and density of the scar in the spongy tissue can be deduced from the physical examination, the appearance of the urethra in contrast studies, the amount of elasticity noted on urethroscopy, and the depth and density of fibrosis as evidenced by ultrasonographic evaluation of the urethra, although the absolute length of spongiofibrosis may not be evident on ultrasonographic evaluation. MRI has been suggested as useful in patients with pelvic fracture urethral distraction, particularly in cases in which the anatomy of the pelvis has become significantly distorted. With regard to anterior urethral stricture, however, MRI has not been useful, with the exception of those cases in which there is urethral carcinoma. In those cases, MRI can provide invaluable information concerning the spread of the tumor. Bougie à boule calibration can be very helpful.

25. **c. Contrast material suitable for intravenous injection should be used for all retrograde urethral studies.** Extravasation during retrograde urethrography is possible in patients in whom the urethra is markedly inflamed. For this reason, contrast studies should be carried out with contrast material that is suitable for intravenous injection. Contrast materials that have been thickened with lubricating jelly can be a source of problems and offer little benefit. Real-time ultrasonographic evaluation of the urethra after it has been filled with a lubricating jelly or saline has been described by McAninch. If the patient is not in a steep lateral oblique position for the retrograde urethrogram, the length of the stricture will be underestimated. For a retrograde urethrogram to be valid, entire visualization of the urethra, from meatus to bladder neck is imperative.

26. **a. Even if a patient does not have retention, placement of a suprapubic tube may help define strictured areas.** In selected patients, we have found it useful to place a suprapubic tube to defunctionalize the urethra. After 6 to 8 weeks, if there will be a constriction of an area that was hydrodilated with voiding, the tendency for that constriction to occur should become apparent. It is imperative, however, to completely evaluate the urethra proximal and distal to the stricture with endoscopy and bougienage during surgery, to ensure that all of the involved urethra is included in the reconstruction. Whereas hydraulic pressure generated by voiding may keep segments proximal to the stricture patent, unless these segments are included in the repair, they are at risk for contraction after obstruction of the narrow-caliber segment is relieved with

reconstruction. For this reason, any abnormal areas of the urethra that are proximal to a narrow-caliber segment of the stricture must be treated with suspicion. If the lumen does not appear to demonstrate evidence of diminished compliance, then we presume that area to be uninvolved in active stricture disease. However, coning down of the urethra suggests its involvement in the scar. Use of a sonourethrogram is felt by some to accurately establish length of stricture but not the extent of spongiofibrosis.

27. **e. It can be associated with erectile dysfunction.** Many surgeons have learned to perform internal urethrotomy by making a single incision at the 12-o'clock position. This location might be questioned, however, based on the location of the urethra within the corpus spongiosum. Distally, although the anterior aspect of the corpus spongiosum is thicker, a deep incision in the more distal aspects of the anterior urethra will certainly enter the corpora cavernosa, and these incisions have been associated with the creation of erectile dysfunction. The most common complication of internal urethrotomy is recurrence of stricture. Less commonly noted complications of internal urethrotomy include bleeding and extravasation of irrigation fluid into the perispongiosal tissues. One report using actuarial technique showed the curative success rate of internal urethrotomy to be 29% to 30% for all patients. Other evaluations have confirmed this success rate. However, there are a number of studies that do show which strictures best respond to internal urethrotomy. These are strictures of the bulbous urethra that are less than 1.5 cm in length and are not associated with dense or deep spongiofibrosis (i.e., straddle injuries). In those particular cases, long-term success has been shown to be 75% to 78%. For strictures outside the bulbous urethra, most studies do not show internal urethrotomy to have long-term success.

28. **b. Permanently implantable stents are indicated for short strictures of the bulbous urethra and, when so employed, are associated with short-term success in the range of approximately 84%.** Removable urethral stents are designed to prevent the process of epithelialization from incorporating the stent into the urethral wall and are left in place for as long as 6 months to a year before being removed. The greatest experience with these removable stents comes from Israel, and centers there report good success in small numbers of patients. Removable urethral stents are currently only available in the United States as part of clinical trials. Permanently implantable stents have been approved for use in the United States for a number of years. Milroy's study shows a success rate of approximately 84% at 4.5 years using the permanently implantable Urolume endourethral stent. That success rate is almost identical to the initial data from a North American study. However, 11-year follow-up from the North American study does not show durability, and overall the success rate is less than 30%. Likewise, long-term data from the Netherlands would indicate that the initial enthusiasm for the use of these stents has waned because of lack of durability. Young patients, in particular, complain of perineal pain, often associated with vigorous activity even when the stent is properly implanted in the bulbous urethra. Placement of the stents in the pendulous portion of the urethra is contraindicated. The use of permanently implanted stents is being questioned, in general, with the development of a number of temporary/removable urethral stents.

29. **c. patients with short strictures of the bulbous urethra not associated with significant spongiofibrosis.** Patients who have had pelvic fracture urethral distraction injuries are not candidates for the use of the Urolume endoprosthesis. The use of the Urolume endoprosthesis in these patients is specifically contraindicated. Patients who have undergone prior substitution urethral reconstruction, particularly when skin has been incorporated into the urethra, have been shown to be very poor candidates for implantation with the Urolume endoprosthesis. These patients are a strong relative contraindication. Patients who have had significant urethral straddle trauma have strictures that are associated with deep spongiofibrosis, and these patients are likewise not good candidates for implantation. There are many centers in Europe and South America, where the Urolume endoprosthesis has been employed for 15 to 16 years, that are now advocating the use of the Urolume endoprosthesis only in patients who are older than 50 years of age and/or who have other significant medical problems that would make the option of open urethral reconstruction less appealing. The use of the Urolume endoprosthesis in pediatric or adolescent patients has never been advocated.

30. **c. Success requires total excision of the fibrosis with a widely spatulated anastomosis.** It has now been demonstrated with certainty that the most dependable technique of anterior urethral reconstruction is the complete excision of the area of fibrosis, with a primary reanastomosis of the normal ends of the anterior urethra. The best results are achieved when the following technical points are observed: (1) the area of the fibrosis is totally excised; (2) the urethral anastomosis is widely spatulated, creating a large ovoid anastomosis; (3) the anastomosis is tension free; and (4) epithelial apposition is achieved. With vigorous mobilization, development of the intercrural space, and detachment of the bulbospongiosum from the perineal body, significant lengths of stricture can be excised and reanastomosed. For very proximal bulbous strictures, tension-free anastomosis can be facilitated by the dissection of the membranous urethra. As a rule, the closer the stricture is to the membranous urethra, the longer it can be and still be reconstructed by anastomotic techniques. The tenet that excision and primary anastomosis should be the goal for all bulbous strictures is one that is being further reinforced by current series published. While guideline lengths of 1 to 2 cm are valuable for planning, most would agree that if excision and primary anastomosis is possible it should be done, and, with aggressive dissection and the maneuvers described earlier, often strictures much longer than the "guideline lengths" can be so reconstructed.

31. **b. Excision with strip anastomosis and onlay (augmented anastomosis) is an excellent form of reconstruction for strictures too long to be dealt with only by excision and primary anastomosis.** A number of grafts have been used for reconstruction as follows: (1) full-thickness skin graft, (2) split-thickness skin graft for staged techniques, (3) the bladder epithelial graft, (4) the buccal mucosal grafts, and (5) in small series, the rectal mucosal graft. The place of the acellular matrixes, as well as cultured tissues, is being studied at a number of

institutions. Early reports are quite favorable, but long-term follow-up is lacking, and series size at this point is small.

Monseur described a technique in which the urethra was opened on the dorsum and was then sewn open. Barbagli modified that operation by adding a graft to the opened stricturotomy. The place for spongioplasty has been debated. Spongioplasty is really only appropriate in the bulbous urethra, and certainly spongioplasty cannot be used if there is extensive spongiofibrosis involving the bulbospongiosum. Vessel-sparing excision with primary anastomosis has been proposed for short-length, very proximal, anterior urethral stricture or membranous urethral stenosis.

32. **b. The operation can conceptually become one operation with multidimensional application.** A number of applications of genital skin islands, mobilized on either the dartos fascia of the penis or the tunica dartos of the scrotum, have been proposed for repair of urethral stricture disease. In the past, these flap operations were considered to be separate procedures. We suggest that all of these procedures are really different applications of a single concept, proposed by the microinjection studies of Quartey. Skin islands, as mentioned, can be viewed as passengers on fascial flaps, and the design of flaps for urethral reconstruction can be done parallel to the design of flaps for reconstruction in general. These procedures using skin islands oriented on the penile dartos fascia have been also useful for reconstruction of the fossa navicularis. There are three important considerations for the use of flaps in urethral reconstruction: (1) the nature of the flap tissue, (2) the vasculature of the flap, and (3) the mechanics of flap transfer. The skin must be nonhirsute for urethral reconstruction. In addition, for donor site consideration, it is most convenient to use the areas of redundant nonhirsute genital skin. These skin islands can be reliably elevated even in patients who have been circumcised.

33. **d. The length of tubed segments can be limited by the aggressive mobilization of the corpus spongiosum.** The literature has made it clear that onlay procedures (graft or flap) are attended with a higher success rate than are tubularized skin islands. Tubularized grafts and skin islands should therefore be avoided, if possible. When tubularized segments cannot be avoided, the length of these segments can be limited by combining aggressive mobilization and excision. Tubularized flaps, without question, provide better results than tubularized grafts. There are now few small series that seek to avoid tubed-flap reconstruction by using the combination of a graft spread-fixed to "reestablish the urethral plate" combined with flap onlay. At this point, there is only short follow-up, but that short follow-up has not proven an advantage.

34. **c. Because lichen sclerosus/BXO is a generalized skin condition, oral mucosa has been considered for reconstruction, with initial encouraging results.** Special mention must be made regarding reconstruction for strictures associated with LS/BXO. With the advent of flap techniques, many centers embraced these techniques for these strictures. However, analysis of results of these patients from several large centers has shown a very high recurrence rate. Because of that, these centers adjusted by applying staged graft techniques. Interestingly, staged graft techniques using skin grafts again had a very high recurrence rate on a number of analyses. It is theorized that because LS/BXO is a skin condition, the use of skin as a flap, a single-stage graft,

or a staged graft does not preclude involvement of the skin with the LS/BXO inflammatory process. At the time of this writing, this center has completed a cursory assessment of our series of patients with LS/BXO-associated strictures who underwent reconstruction with flap-skin island techniques and skin graft. Preliminary results at our center are not as dismal as from other centers, but the success rate is clearly less (approximately 60%) than for non–LS/BXO-associated strictures. At present, a number of centers now believe that, for reconstruction of stricture associated with LS/BXO, staged oral graft techniques should be employed. Short follow-up suggests better success with this approach.

35. **b. Although they can involve any part of the membranous urethra, they most frequently occur at the juncture of the membranous urethra with the bulbous urethra.** Urethral distraction injuries are the result of blunt pelvic trauma and accompany about 10% of pelvic fracture injuries. Although it is possible to totally disrupt the urethra with a straddle injury, these injuries most commonly involve only the bulbous urethra. Distraction injuries of the membranous urethra have been compared to plucking an apple (prostate) off its stem (the membranous urethra). This analogy implies that the injury most frequently occurs at the apex of the prostate. Experience shows that this is not the case, however, and the most frequent point of distraction is at the departure of the membranous urethra from the bulbospongiosum. In the postpubescent male, the injury seldom involves the prostatic urethra. In the prepubescent male, in whom the prostatic urethra is more fragile, the injury can extend into that area. Many injuries appear not to totally distract the entire circumference of the urethra. Instead, a strip of epithelium is left intact. In these patients, the placement of an aligning catheter may allow the urethra to heal virtually unscarred or with an easily managed stricture. Because of flexible endoscopy equipment, placement of an aligning catheter is relatively straightforward. Because of the ready availability of flexible cystoscopes, some centers are now evaluating, acutely, these injuries only with endoscopy. Aligning catheters are just what the name implies, a guide, not a mechanism for placing traction on the bladder and prostate. The incidence of vascular injury at the level of the deep internal pudendal arteries has been significantly underestimated in the PFUDD population.

36. **a. optimally first evaluated with contrast studies.** Although location of the distraction injury has been demonstrated to be an important factor in continence after reconstruction, this information should be a factor only in patient counseling before the reconstruction and not in the treatment approach. The length of the defect is an important consideration and must be determined as precisely as possible. Lack of contrast material in the posterior urethra gives some information, albeit inconclusive, about the integrity of the bladder neck. When the patient is successfully relaxing to void and the cystogram outlines the posterior urethra, a simultaneous retrograde urethrogram nicely outlines the length of the distraction defect. However, this situation is the exception rather than the rule, and retrograde urethrograms are most useful for determining whether the anterior urethra is normal. If the anterior urethra is normal, it has been our experience, as well as that of others, that a successful anastomotic repair is ensured. In fact, a primary anastomosis

has been shown to be possible even with some involvement of the anterior urethra. Thus primary anastomosis is unquestionably the goal in all of these patients until it is proved impossible to do. When the proximal urethra is not visualized on simultaneous cystogram with urethrogram, endoscopy through the suprapubic tract in combination with retrograde urethrogram can be used to outline the defect.

37. **d. Continence is best addressed after a procedure to reestablish urethral continuity is performed.** We have found, and others have reported, that the competence of the bladder neck is difficult to accurately assess before the reestablishment of urethral continuity. Even in cases in which an obvious scar is noted to involve the bladder neck, follow-up of these patients after the urethral reconstruction establishes continuity of the urethra has found many patients with more than adequate continence. Still other patients are believed to have incontinence due to scar incarceration of the bladder neck. In our experience, however, this is an infrequent occurrence, and the appearance of the bladder neck by any modality available is not predictive of continence. It is currently our practice to reestablish the continuity of the urethra, and in cases in which there are concerns about continence, to forewarn the patient before the urethral reconstruction. Colopinto and others have not shown an association of ultimate continence as related to the location of the distraction injury.

38. **d. division of the attachment of the bulbospongiosum to the perineal body.** Development of the intracrural space, mobilization of the corpus spongiosum, infrapubectomy, and, if needed, rerouting of the corpus spongiosum all shorten the course that the corpus spongiosum must traverse and allow reconstruction without attendant chordee. Division of the attachments of the bulbospongiosum to the perineal body is, in fact, the maneuver that facilitates anterior urethral reconstruction. Whereas some centers prefer to divide the corpus spongiosum very proximally during the mobilization of the corpus spongiosum, the most favored mechanism mobilizes the entire bulbospongiosum, divides the proximal blood supply if it has not been disrupted by the trauma itself, and divides then through the area of the distraction fibrosis (see Figs. 36–35 to 36–38 in *Campbell-Walsh Urology, 10th Edition*). Dissection of the scarred Buck fascia greatly increases the elasticity of the mobilized corpus spongiosum.

39. **d. Patients with reconstitution of an injured pudendal vessel, even if reconstitution was a unilateral phenomenon, are excellent candidates for posterior urethral reconstruction.** With the techniques discussed, or similar techniques, curative rates for reconstruction of posterior urethral distraction injuries are in the high 90% range according to the work of the authors. Failures are not, in large centers, due to technical problems (i.e., anastomotic restenosis). In general, failures are indicative of ischemia of the proximal corpus spongiosum with ensuring stenosis of the mobilized corpus spongiosum. We found that many patients had evidence of either unilateral or bilateral pudendal artery lesions but that most had evidence of vascular reconstruction. We found that patients with an intact pudendal artery on one side often were potent and were reliably cured with reconstruction. We found that patients with only reconstituted vessels, either

unilateral or bilateral, never were potent but were reliably reconstructed. Shenfeld, along with others, has reported a reasonably large series of patients undergoing redo posterior urethral reconstruction using a primary anastomotic technique.

40. **e. It is usually present with either ventral curvature or ventral curvature associated with torsion.** In many cases, there are abnormalities of the ventral penile skin. In patients who have chordee without hypospadias, the photograph will reveal an erect penis commensurate with the size of the detumescent penis, whereas in the congenital curvature patient the erect penis will be noticeably large. Many of our patients are also evaluated preoperatively by our sex therapy colleague. Because of their congenital anomaly, these patients often become relatively reclusive and have poor self and genital images. Even in patients with obvious abnormalities of the corpus spongiosum (i.e., poor ventral fusion or frank bifid corpus spongiosum), wide mobilization usually reveals that it is not the corpus spongiosum that remains as the ventral limiting factor. In most patients, the penis will remain curved due to the inelasticity of the ventral aspect of the corpora cavernosa. If the epithelial tube has served as an adequate urethra (i.e., it is not stenotic), the morbidity of the urethral division and subsequent need for urethral reconstruction must be considered before undertaking such a procedure. In children, after mobilization and excision of the dysgenetic tissues, the residual chordee can usually be corrected by making a longitudinal incision with a sharp blade. If this maneuver is not sufficient, the dorsal neurovascular structures can be mobilized in concert with the Buck fascia and a small ellipse or ellipses of dorsal tunica albuginea excised and closed with watertight plicating sutures.

41. **a. If length is an issue, the patient probably is more correctly characterized as having chordee without hypospadias.** Patients with congenital curvature of the penis can have ventral, lateral (which is most often to the left), and/or unusually dorsal curvature. Patients usually present as otherwise healthy young men between the ages of 18 and 30. Many of these patients will have noticed curvature before puberty but will have presumed it to be normal. With puberty, however, they discover that the curvature is not normal. We do not routinely recommend a tourniquet device, because constricting devices can conceal the proximal limits of the curvature. This is of most significance in cases of ventral curvatures that frequently extend proximally. In patients with ventral curvature, there may be some illusion of thickening of the dartos fascia and the Buck fascia, and in those patients, the fibrous tissue is mobilized and completely excised. After these issues are excised, the artificial erection is repeated, and an occasional patient will have a completely straightened curvature. Most patients, however, suffer from a differential elasticity between the dorsal and ventral aspects of the corporeal bodies, and although the curvature may have been lessened, it will persist, unless further procedures are done to straighten the penis. Because the size of the erect penis is usually not a problem in these cases of congenital curvature, we have chosen the second option. If the patient falls into the category of chordee without hypospadias, if shortness of the penis is an issue, we do not hesitate to use incisions with grafts to correct the curvature.

42. **b. In most cases, global cavernosal veno-occlusive dysfunction (CVOD) is not a complicating factor.**
When a young man presents with an acquired curvature of the penis, one must always allow the possibility of Peyronie disease. Occasionally, however, a patient or his initial-care physician will ignore the stigmata of the trauma (often described as "minimal" by patients), and the patient will present with a noticeable lateral scar that causes both indentation of the lateral aspect of the penis and, in some cases, curvature. Patients who had preexisting lateral curvature may actually notice that their penis has been straightened by the trauma, but they are disturbed by the concavity caused by the scar. The pathology of a subclinical fracture of the penis is believed to be due to either the disruption of the outer longitudinal layer of the tunica albuginea during the buckling trauma only or the disruption of both layers of the tunica albuginea during buckling trauma but with preservation of the Buck fascia. These patients usually have normal erectile function, and there is no association with concomitant global CVOD. However, the association of CVOD and trauma of the penis continues to be seen, and some patients, after fracture-type injuries of the penis, will have significant problems with erectile dysfunction. These injuries are not associated with shortening of the penis. It is the lack of erectile dysfunction and penile shortening that help distinguish these patients from those with Peyronie disease. Although foreshortening of the penis is not a characteristic of either the injury itself or the resulting scar in either of these injuries, these patients are not thought to be best treated by approaching the opposite aspect of the scar and excising an ellipse of the tunica. This would result in bilateral scars, which will cause bilateral indentation of the penis, and although the penis will have been straightened by the correction, most patients are upset by the cosmetic and functional result of a near-circumferential indentation of the penis. Curvatures associated with hypospadias or epispadias are not acquired curvatures.

Additional Study Points

1. A meshed split-thickness graft that is applied to the genitalia should not be expanded but rather placed on the recipient site without expansion to allow collections from beneath the graft to escape.
2. Split-thickness grafts do not contain lymphatics; however, full-thickness grafts do.
3. Split-thickness grafts do not develop sensation; however, sensation may be present due to its presence in the deep structures beneath the graft.
4. Tunica vaginalis grafts result in aneurysmal dilatation when they are used for large defects.
5. The superficial dorsal penile vein usually drains to the left saphenous vein; the deep dorsal and circumflex veins lying beneath the Buck fascia drain to the periprostatic plexus.
6. The Buck fascia is adjacent to the deep structures of the penis; the dartos fascia is next to the skin.
7. Lichen sclerosus is a disease of the skin and may involve large portions of the genital skin; therefore using the genital skin for reconstruction may result in recurrence of the disease.
8. Lichen sclerosus may be a premalignant lesion and often results in meatal stenosis.
9. A spontaneous urethral fistula or unexplained periurethral abscess may be the harbinger of a urethral carcinoma.
10. Circumcision provides protection for men in areas of endemic HIV.
11. Cellulitis may be a problem in patients who have genital lymphedema.
12. As a general rule in the urethra, flaps are best suited for distal reconstruction, grafts for proximal reconstruction.
13. In the repair of a urethral stricture, a small soft silastic catheter is used to stent the anastomosis, and often a suprapubic tube is placed to divert the urine.
14. For urethral distraction injuries (posterior urethral disruptions), an aligning catheter, at the very worst, facilitates subsequent reconstruction and, at best, may leave the patient with an endoscopically manageable urethra.

37

Surgery of the Scrotum and Seminal Vesicles

Parviz K. Kavoussi, MD ● Raymond A. Costabile, MD

QUESTIONS

1. Which of the following vessels has the least direct contribution to the arterial supply of the vas deferens?
   a. Deferential artery
   b. Internal spermatic artery
   c. Superior vesicle artery
   d. Inferior epigastric artery
   e. Inferior epididymal artery

2. The best reason for using the no-scalpel vasectomy technique is:
   a. it has a higher sterilization rate than standard vasectomy with incision.
   b. patients are rendered sterile in less time.
   c. it is easier to learn than the standard technique.
   d. it results in a lower rate of complications, including hematoma and infection.
   e. it results in a higher rate of reversibility.

3. The no-scalpel technique for vasectomy reduces the rate of:
   a. hematoma.
   b. vasectomy failures.
   c. recanalization.
   d. injury to testicular artery.
   e. chronic orchalgia.

4. Vasectomy failure rate when both the abdominal and testicular ends of the divided vas deferens are occluded with hemoclips is:
   a. less than 1%.
   b. 5% to 10%.
   c. 10% to 20%.
   d. 20% to 30%.
   e. 50% to 60%.

5. The technical aspect shown to decrease vasectomy failure rates the most is:
   a. no-scalpel technique.
   b. conventional technique.
   c. fascial interposition of dartos fascia between the divided ends of the vas deferens.
   d. occluding both ends of the divided vas deferens with hemoclips.

   e. occluding both ends of the divided vas deferens thermally with the use of intraluminal cautery.

6. The technical aspect when performing vasectomy to make vasectomy reversal easier in the future is:
   a. no-scalpel technique.
   b. not excising a long segment of vas deferens.
   c. dividing the vas deferens as close to the epididymis as possible.
   d. occluding both ends of the divided vas deferens with hemoclips.
   e. occluding both ends of the divided vas deferens thermally with the use of intraluminal cautery.

7. Vasectomy has been established to be associated with:
   a. prostate cancer.
   b. dementia.
   c. cardiovascular disease.
   d. atherosclerosis.
   e. a 10% incidence of chronic scrotal pain.

8. What is the estimated percentage of men who develop antisperm antibodies after vasectomy?
   a. 0% to 20%
   b. 20% to 40%
   c. 40% to 60%
   d. 60% to 80%
   e. >80%

9. Which of the following is an indication for repeat vasectomy?
   a. Painless sperm granuloma
   b. Motile sperm found in semen analysis 3 months after vasectomy
   c. Nonmotile sperm found in semen analysis 3 months after vasectomy
   d. Persistent testicular pain 3 months after vasectomy
   e. All of the above

10. Pressure-induced injury following vasectomy occurs in:
    a. the testis.
    b. the ejaculatory duct.
    c. the epididymis.
    d. the vas deferens.
    e. the seminal vesicles.

11. In the management of chronic orchialgia, which of the following statements is TRUE?
    a. Imaging studies are not indicated.
    b. Varicocele is not a significant contributor of chronic scrotal pain.
    c. Orchiectomy usually relieves the pain.
    d. Denervation of the cord may offer relief in selected cases.
    e. Diagnostic epididymal puncture should be performed to rule out chronic bacterial epididymitis.

12. Which of the following is TRUE regarding hydrocelectomy?
    a. Hematoma is the least frequent complication.
    b. The Jaboulay bottleneck operation is associated with a high recurrence rate.
    c. The Lord plication is an ideal operation for long-standing postinfectious hydroceles.
    d. Sclerotherapy is often the treatment of choice for young men of reproductive age.
    e. The Jaboulay bottleneck operation is associated with a low recurrence rate.

13. A nontransilluminating, nontender mass is noted in the epididymis on physical examination and confirmed to be solid by sonography. What is the most likely diagnosis?
    a. Epididymal cyst
    b. Adenomatoid tumor
    c. Spermatocele
    d. Testicular tumor
    e. Hydrocele

14. Men who were treated with epididymectomy for chronic epididymitis responded the most favorably if:
    a. there was a palpable epididymal abnormality.
    b. there was no palpable abnormality, but there were sonographic changes of the epididymis.
    c. there were no palpable abnormalities and no sonographic changes of the epididymis.
    d. they had improvement of pain with spermatic cord block.
    e. none of the above apply.

15. Which of the following is TRUE regarding retractile testes in adults?
    a. As in children, surgical repair is never indicated.
    b. A dartos pouch orchidopexy is the treatment of choice.
    c. Simple three-stitch orchiopexy of the tunica albuginea to the dartos, as for torsion prophylaxis, is effective in preventing retraction.
    d. Bilateral orchiopexy is necessary for a unilateral retractile testis.
    e. Coexisting varicocele is common.

16. The most appropriate approach to a long-standing, thick-walled, loculated hydrocele is:
    a. excision of the hydrocele sac.
    b. the Jaboulay bottleneck technique.
    c. the Lord plication technique.
    d. the inguinal approach.
    e. sclerotherapy.

17. In men with chronic orchitis without an identifiable bacterial pathogen, antibiotics:
    a. decrease the length of symptoms.
    b. improve the severity of symptoms.
    c. decrease the length of time to full activity.
    d. are steadily being prescribed more frequently empirically.
    e. none of the above apply.

18. When a clinically palpable varicocele is encountered in a patient with orchalgia, varicocelectomy will resolve the pain:
    a. 10% of the time.
    b. 25% of the time.
    c. 50% of the time.
    d. 75% of the time.
    e. 90% of the time.

19. What is the embryologic origin of the seminal vesicles?
    a. Müllerian duct
    b. Ectodermal ridge
    c. Distal mesonephric duct
    d. Swelling of the distal paramesonephric duct
    e. Neural crest cells

20. What percentage of the ejaculate volume is made up of seminal vesicle secretions?
    a. 5% to 10%
    b. 20% to 30%
    c. 60% to 80%
    d. 90%
    e. The seminal vesicle does not contribute to the seminal plasma volume.

21. What artery is the major blood supply to the seminal vesicle?
    a. Hypogastric
    b. Vesiculodeferential artery
    c. Inferior vesicle
    d. Internal iliac
    e. Deep dorsal penile

22. Decreased T1 signal intensity on MRI, along with increased T2 intensity of seminal vesicles, is indicative of which process?
    a. Inflammation of the seminal vesicles
    b. Hemorrhage within the seminal vesicles
    c. Seminal vesicle tumors
    d. Seminal vesicle cysts
    e. Normal seminal vesicles

23. Agenesis of the seminal vesicle is associated with significant ipsilateral renal anomalies. What is the embryologic reason for this?
    a. A genetic defect links seminal vesicle agenesis to renal agenesis.
    b. A mutation occurs in the cystic fibrosis transmembrane regulator gene.
    c. There was an insult to the mesonephric duct at approximately 12 weeks' gestation.

d. There was an embryologic insult to the mesonephric duct earlier than 7 weeks' gestation.

e. There is no association between agenesis of the seminal vesicle and ipsilateral renal anomalies.

24. What disorder is frequently associated with bilateral agenesis of the seminal vesicles?
    a. Cystic fibrosis
    b. Kartagener syndrome
    c. Young syndrome
    d. Kallmann syndrome
    e. Klinefelter syndrome

25. What causes the majority of seminal vesicle cysts?
    a. Ejaculatory duct stone
    b. Obstruction of the ejaculatory duct
    c. Inflammation
    d. Renal agenesis
    e. Trisomy 21

26. What is the most common type of malignant neoplasm found in seminal vesicles?
    a. Primary adenocarcinoma
    b. Sarcoma
    c. Cystosarcoma phyllodes
    d. Metastatic tumors
    e. Amyloidosis

27. What is the best initial test for a suspected seminal vesicle abnormality?
    a. CT
    b. Transrectal ultrasonography
    c. MRI
    d. Fine-needle biopsy
    e. Vasography

28. What is the best method to differentiate a benign from malignant seminal vesicle mass?
    a. Biopsy of the lesion
    b. Contrast medium–enhanced CT
    c. Gadolinium–enhanced MRI
    d. Transrectal ultrasonography
    e. Rectal examination

29. What is the best surgical approach to a congenital lesion of the seminal vesicle?
    a. The perineal route because this has the quickest recovery
    b. The transcoccygeal route because these are usually large lesions
    c. The laparoscopic route so that the ipsilateral kidney can be dealt with concomitantly and recovery may be shorter
    d. The paravesical route because this has a lower incidence of postoperative erectile dysfunction
    e. The transvesical route because rectal injury is much less likely

30. What is the best indication for the transcoccygeal approach to the seminal vesicle?
    a. Need for exploration of the ipsilateral kidney
    b. Patient with previous suprapubic and/or perineal surgery

c. Patient wishing to maintain potency
d. Patient with bilateral large seminal vesicle lesions
e. Patient with metastatic tumor to the seminal vesicle

31. In a patient with a seminal vesicle abscess, the treatment of choice is:
    a. laparoscopic unroofing.
    b. transvesical excision of the seminal vesicle.
    c. aspiration and antibiotic instillation.
    d. endoscopic unroofing by deep transurethral resection.
    e. retropubic approach to unroof the abscess.

ANSWERS

1. **c. Superior vesicle artery.** The superior vesicle artery does not supply the vas deferens, whereas all of the other arteries listed may have a branch to the vas deferens.

2. **d. it results in a lower rate of complications, including hematoma and infection.** This method eliminates the scalpel incision, results in fewer hematomas and infections, and leaves a much smaller wound than conventional methods of accessing the vas deferens for vasectomy.

3. **a. hematoma.** The no-scalpel technique significantly decreases the rate of hematomas, infections, and pain during the procedure.

4. **a. less than 1%.** Vasectomy failure rate when both the abdominal and tesicular ends of the divided vas deferens are occluded with hemoclips is less than 1%.

5. **c. fascial interposition of dartos fascia between the divided ends of the vas deferens.** Interposition of dartos fascia between the divided ends of the vas deferens is a technique for occlusion that has been reported to reduce the recanalization rate to nearly zero.

6. **b. not excising a long segment of vas deferens.** The technical aspects when performing vasectomy to make vasectomy reversal easier in the future include not excising a long segment of vas deferens, dividing the vas deferens approximately 3 cm cephalad to the cauda of the epididymis in the straight portion of the vas deferens, and simply transecting the vas deferens followed by low-voltage cautery occlusion and then by fascial interposition.

7. **e. a 10% incidence of chronic scrotal pain.** Vasectomy has not been established to be associated with prostate cancer, dementia, cardiovascular disease, or atherosclerosis, although it has been associated with a 10% incidence of chronic scrotal pain.

8. **d. 60% to 80%.** Vasectomy disrupts the blood-testis barrier, resulting in detectable levels of serum antisperm antibodies in 60% to 80% of men.

9. **b. Motile sperm found in semen analysis 3 months after vasectomy.** If any motile sperm are found in the ejaculate 3 months after vasectomy, consideration should be given to repeating the procedure.

10. **c. the epididymis.** The brunt of pressure-induced damage after vasectomy falls on the epididymis and efferent ductules.

11. **d. Denervation of the cord may offer relief in selected cases.** Microsurgical total denervation of the spermatic cord is a procedure used with reported success in several small series.

12. **e. The Jaboulay bottleneck operation is associated with a low recurrence rate.** The Jaboulay bottleneck

operation, in which the sac edges are sewn together behind the cord, reduces the chance of recurrence caused by reapposition of the edges of the hydrocele sac.

13. **b. Adenomatoid tumor.** Most nontransilluminable solid epididymal masses are benign adenomatoid tumors.

14. **a. there was a palpable epididymal abnormality.** A retrospective review of men who underwent epididymectomy for chronic epididymitis showed that outcomes were best when the patient had a palpable epididymal abnormality on physical examination. Men in this study without a palpable abnormality, but with sonographic changes, had slightly worse outcomes, and those with neither a palpable abnormality nor a demonstrable ultrasonographic abnormality did not improve with epididymectomy.

15. **b. A dartos pouch orchidopexy is the treatment of choice.** Creation of a dartos pouch will keep the testis well down into the scrotum and permanently prevent retraction.

16. **a. excision of the hydrocele sac.** Excising the hydrocele is recommended for long-standing, thick-walled, loculated hydroceles.

17. **d. are steadily being prescribed more frequently empirically.** Despite evidence that up to 75% of patients with epididymitis/orchitis do not have an identifiable bacterial urinary tract infection concomitantly with their clinical epididymitis, antibiotics are routinely given. Empirical antibiotic administration in the absence of positive urine cultures has been steadily increasing, from 75% to 95% between the years of 1965 and 2005 and is not indicated.

18. **c. 50% of the time.** When a clinically palpable varicocele is encountered in a patient with orchalgia, varicocelectomy will resolve the pain 50% of the time.

19. **c. Distal mesonephric duct.** The seminal vesicle develops as a dorsolateral bulbous swelling of the distal mesonephric duct at approximately 12 fetal weeks.

20. **c. 60% to 80%.** The secretions from the seminal vesicle contribute 60% to 80% of the ejaculate volume.

21. **b. Vesiculodeferential artery.** The blood supply to the seminal vesicle is from the vesiculodeferential artery, a branch of the superior vesical artery.

22. **a. Inflammation of the seminal vesicles.** Seminal vesiculitis shows decreased signal intensity on the T1-weighted image, whereas the T2-weighted image intensity is higher than that of both fat and the normal seminal vesicle.

23. **d. There was an embryologic insult to the mesonephric duct earlier than at 7 weeks' gestation.** Unilateral agenesis of the seminal vesicles has an incidence of 0.6% to 1% and may be associated with unilateral absence of the vas deferens, as well as ipsilateral renal anomalies.

24. **a. Cystic fibrosis.** Seventy to 80 percent of men with bilateral absence of the vas deferens or seminal vesicles are carriers of the genetic mutation associated with cystic fibrosis. Conversely, 80% to 95% of men with cystic fibrosis have bilateral absence of the vas deferens or seminal vesicles.

25. **b. Obstruction of the ejaculatory duct.** Cysts of the seminal vesicles may be either congenital or acquired and are thought to be due to obstruction of the ejaculatory duct.

26. **d. Metastatic tumors.** Very few primary tumors of the seminal vesicles have been reported. It is more common for carcinoma of the bladder, prostate, or rectum, or lymphoma to secondarily involve the seminal vesicles.

27. **b. Transrectal ultrasonography.** Transrectal ultrasonography is the preferred initial test for seminal vesicle abnormality, owing to its low invasiveness, ease of performance, and ability to perform concomitant transrectal biopsies.

28. **a. Biopsy of the lesion.** Transrectal ultrasonography and biopsy of the seminal vesicle mass is accurate and easily accomplished.

29. **c. The laparoscopic route so that the ipsilateral kidney can be dealt with concomitantly and recovery may be shorter.** Although data are limited for laparoscopic excision of benign seminal vesicle disease alone, this approach appears to afford superb visualization with minimal postoperative morbidity and shorter hospitalization, compared with the open surgical alternatives.

30. **b. Patient with previous suprapubic and/or perineal surgery.** In individuals for whom the perineal or supine position may be difficult to maintain, or for those who have had multiple suprapubic or perineal surgeries, the transcoccygeal approach may be useful.

31. **d. endoscopic unroofing by deep transurethral resection.** If the abscess is in the portion of the seminal vesicle adjacent to the prostate, a deep transurethral resection into the prostatic substance, just distal to the bladder neck at the 5-o'clock or 7-o'clock position, may be effective in relieving the problem. However, a CT-guided aspiration and drain placement is becoming the preferred least-traumatic option.

Additional Study Points

1. Since scrotal cases are considered clean rather than sterile, prophylactic antibiotics are recommended preoperatively. Hair removal should occur immediately before the procedure.

2. Fournier gangrene is a necrotizing fasciitis that involves the skin and subcutaneous tissue and requires broad-spectrum antibiotics, including a third-generation cephalosporin, an aminoglycoside, and metronidazole. These patients require fluid resuscitation, and when hemodynamically stable, debridement. Daily debridement in the operating room until all nonviable tissue is removed should be subsequently performed.

3. Ninety-seven percent of patients undergoing open-ended vasectomy develop sperm granulomas.

4. Division of the vas deferens during vasectomy should occur at least 3 cm from the epididymitis. There is no vasectomy technique that is 100% effective; over 80% of the patients achieve azoospermia at 3 months following vasectomy.

5. When the testis is removed for orchalgia, pain relief is better achieved if the orchiectomy is performed

through an inguinal incision rather than a transscrotal incision.

6. There is no association between vasectomy and prostate cancer, cardiovascular disease, atherosclerosis, or dementia.

7. Any surgical manipulation of the epididymis results in azoospermia on that side.

8. Leaving a scrotal drain after scrotal procedures does not lessen the complication rate or the development of postoperative hematomas.

9. When repairing large hydroceles the epididymis and spermatic vessels may be splayed by the hydrocele, and care must be taken to identify them to avoid injury.

10. Microsurgical denervation of the spermatic cord has been employed for the treatment of orchalgia with reported success rates as high as two thirds achieving pain relief. It should only be considered if a cord block is successful.

11. Seminal vesicle cysts are associated with ipsilateral renal agenesis or dysplasia in two thirds of patients and have been associated with polycystic kidney disease.

Renal Physiology and Pathophysiology

chapter 38

Renal Physiology and Pathophysiology

Daniel A. Shoskes, MD, MSc, FRCSC • Alan W. McMahon, MD

QUESTIONS

1. The AT1 receptor:
   a. has a more pronounced vasoconstriction on the afferent rather than the efferent arteriole.
   b. is the receptor for angiotensin I.
   c. protects against ischemia-reperfusion injury by intrarenal dilation.
   d. mediates increased release of aldosterone.
   e. is not expressed in the kidney.

2. Which of the following statements about endothelin is FALSE?
   a. Stimulation of endothelin-1 (ET-1) decreases sodium excretion.
   b. Endothelin is the most potent vasoconstrictor yet identified.
   c. ET-1 release is inhibited by nitric oxide.
   d. ET-1 release stimulates aldosterone secretion.
   e. ET-1 release reduces renal blood flow.

3. Which of the following is a vasodilator of the renal artery?
   a. Endothelin
   b. Carbon monoxide
   c. Atrial natriuretic peptide
   d. Norepinephrine
   e. Angiotensin II

4. Which of the following is FALSE regarding carbon monoxide and the enzyme hemoxygenase?
   a. Hemoxygenase-2 (HO-2) is a constitutive enzyme.
   b. HO-1 is an inducible enzyme.
   c. Increased carbon monoxide (CO) increases ischemia-reperfusion injury in the kidney.
   d. HO-1 expression helps to maintain renal medullary blood flow.
   e. HO-1 produces CO through the catabolism of heme.

5. Which of the following regarding erythropoiesis is FALSE?
   a. Reduced erythropoiesis and anemia are common in chronic renal disease.
   b. Erythropoiesis is inhibited by low circulating oxygen tension.
   c. During chronic inflammation, erythropoiesis is decreased.
   d. The kidney makes most of the erythropoietin in the body.
   e. There are erythropoietin receptors in many organs of the body.

6. Which of the following is TRUE about sodium and the kidney?
   a. By definition, hypernatremia is always associated with elevated total body sodium content.
   b. Normal compensation for hyponatremia is decreased antidiuretic hormone (ADH) secretion and thirst suppression.
   c. Abnormal elevation of serum lipids can lead to a false, elevated measurement of serum sodium.
   d. If asymptomatic hyponatremia does not improve within 24 hours, intravenous hypertonic saline should be started.
   e. In therapy for symptomatic hyponatremia, the goal should be a normal serum sodium value of 135 mEq/L within 48 hours.

7. The syndrome of inappropriate antidiuretic hormone secretion (SIADH):
   a. is associated with decreased aquaporin expression in the kidney.
   b. is always seen in patients with hypervolemia.
   c. is associated with high total body sodium.
   d. is triggered by low circulating volume.
   e. may be treated with lithium or demeclocycline.

8. Which of the following regarding therapy for hyponatremia is FALSE?
   a. Fluid overload as a result of hypertonic saline infusion should be treated with a loop diuretic such as furosemide.
   b. Too rapid correction can lead to a cerebral demyelination syndrome.
   c. Aggressive therapy should be discontinued when the serum sodium concentration is raised 10% or symptoms subside.
   d. Intranasal desmopressin is a useful adjuvant therapy.
   e. For acute severe hyponatremia with symptoms, a typical infusion rate of hypertonic saline would be 1 mL/kg/hr.

9. Diabetes insipidus:
   a. may be classified as nephrogenic or urogenic.
   b. is associated with inappropriately concentrated urine.
   c. is associated with hypervolemia.
   d. is associated with mutations of the genes producing aldosterone.
   e. results in impairment of maximum concentrating ability of the kidney due to loss of the medullary osmotic gradient.

10. Which of the following regarding potassium is FALSE?
    a. Angiotensin-converting enzyme (ACE) inhibitors may be a cause of hypokalemia.
    b. Potassium is primarily an intracellular ion.
    c. Acidosis drives potassium out of the cell into the circulation.
    d. High-sodium load in the distal tubule promotes potassium excretion.
    e. Upper limit for safe intravenous potassium infusion is 40 mEq/hr.

11. Which of the following regarding hyperkalemia is FALSE?
    a. Hemolysis of the blood sample may falsely elevate the measured potassium.
    b. Hyperkalemia can cause peaked T waves on the electrocardiogram (ECG).
    c. All patients with a serum potassium value greater than 5.5 mEq/L require immediate therapy.
    d. Nebulized albuterol can reduce serum potassium by promoting an intracellular shift of potassium.
    e. Intravenous calcium does not lower serum potassium but is given to protect the heart from the effects of hyperkalemia.

12. Which of the following is TRUE about acid handling?
    a. Normal pH in the blood is 7.56 to 7.60.
    b. Normal body metabolism produces less than 1000 mmol of acid per day.
    c. All acids produced by metabolism can be excreted by the lungs.
    d. Immediate response to an acid load is through buffers in the blood.
    e. Ammonia (NH_4) is the most important buffer in the blood.

13. Which of the following regarding renal handling of acid is FALSE?
    a. Most bicarbonate is reabsorbed in the distal collecting tubule.
    b. Lungs can excrete volatile acid, but the kidneys must excrete fixed acid.
    c. Carbonic anhydrase catalyzes the production of H^+ and HCO_3^- from H_2O and CO_2.
    d. Chronic respiratory acidosis should lead to increased H^+ in the kidney.
    e. Ammonium ion (NH_4^+) is produced from glutamine, primarily by proximal tubular cells.

14. A patient who has a blood pH of 7.2 has:
    a. pure metabolic acidosis.
    b. pure respiratory acidosis.
    c. acidemia.
    d. a blood buffer system that is not working.
    e. a mixed acid-base disturbance.

15. In a patient with acidosis:
    a. increasing the blood HCO_3^- level increases the anion gap.
    b. direct bicarbonate loss from the kidney would lead to metabolic acidosis and a normal anion gap.
    c. lactic acidosis usually presents as a nonanion gap metabolic acidosis.
    d. appropriate respiratory compensation for a metabolic acidosis is decreased respiration with an increased P_{CO_2}.
    e. It is not possible to have both a respiratory and metabolic acidosis at the same time.

16. Which of the following regarding renal tubular acidosis (RTA) is FALSE?
    a. The hallmark of RTA type I is a hyperchloremic metabolic acidosis with a high urinary pH (>5.5) in the presence of persistently low serum HCO_3^-.
    b. Type I RTA is also called distal RTA.
    c. Type II RTA is more common in children.
    d. The hallmark of type IV RTA is hypokalemia.
    e. The form of RTA most commonly associated with renal calculi is type I.

17. Which of the following regarding metabolic alkalosis is FALSE?
    a. Paradoxical aciduria may occur due to distal tubule injury.
    b. Excessive nasogastric fluid loss can lead to metabolic alkalosis that is chloride responsive.
    c. Appropriate respiratory compensation is decreased respiration and increased P_{CO_2}.
    d. Hyperaldosteronism can lead to chloride-resistant metabolic alkalosis.
    e. Therapy for chloride-responsive metabolic alkalosis requires replacement of chloride AND fluid volume.

18. Which of the following is NOT a function of ADH?
    a. Increased aquaporin-2 insertion into the luminal membrane of the collecting duct
    b. Increased urea transporter insertion into the luminal membrane of the collecting duct
    c. Increased systemic vascular resistance
    d. Increased sodium reabsorption
    e. Increased free water excretion in response to hypernatremia

19. Which of the following is TRUE about vitamin D metabolism?
    a. Vitamin D deficiency is uncommon in chronic renal failure.
    b. Dermally synthesized cholecalciferol is the most potent form of vitamin D.
    c. Dermally synthesized cholecalciferol must be hydroxylated by both the liver and kidney for maximal potency.

d. Vitamin D activity is mediated through membrane-bound vitamin D receptors.

e. Vitamin D increases renal excretion of calcium.

20. Which of the following regarding parathyroid hormone (PTH) is FALSE?

a. PTH secretion is increased by hypocalcemia.

b. PTH secretion is increased by hyperphosphatemia.

c. PTH receptors are found mainly in bone and kidney.

d. PTH increases calcium and phosphorus reabsorption in the distal tubule.

e. PTH helps regulate 1,25(OH)-vitamin D levels by increasing 1α-hydroxylase activity.

21. Renal blood flow (RBF):

a. is equal in all parts of the kidney.

b. accounts for 5% to 10% of cardiac output.

c. courses through the glomerulus through the afferent arteriole and exits through the efferent venule.

d. is similar in men and women.

e. is one of the determinants of the glomerular filtration rate.

22. All of the following can increase total glomerular flow rate (GFR) EXCEPT increased:

a. RBF.

b. intraglomerular (hydraulic) pressure.

c. glomerular permeability.

d. efferent arteriolar resistance.

e. functioning nephron number.

23. All of the following are important in GFR regulation EXCEPT:

a. afferent arteriolar tone.

b. distal tubule chloride concentrations.

c. angiotensin II.

d. nitric oxide.

e. serum osmolality.

24. All of the following statements regarding GFR assessment are true EXCEPT:

a. Plasma creatinine is an accurate marker of early reductions in GFR.

b. Inulin clearance is an accurate but impractical measurement of GFR.

c. Twenty-four–hour creatinine clearance overestimates GFR by 10% to 20%.

d. Use of the four-variable modification of diet in renal disease (MDRD) formula improves the accuracy of the plasma creatinine.

e. Plasma urea is an unreliable estimate of GFR.

25. Which of the following regarding glucose handling in the kidney is FALSE?

a. Glucose is freely filtered across the glomerulus.

b. Glucose reabsorption is facilitated by specific glucose transporters in the proximal convoluted tubule (PCT).

c. Glucose reabsorption is linked to bicarbonate reabsorption in the PCT.

d. Glucose reabsorption is 100% up to plasma glucose levels of 400 mg/dL.

e. Glucose reabsorption is a passive process.

26. Which of the following about the proximal convoluted tubule is FALSE?

a. It functions as a bulk transporter, rather than a fine-tuner of ultrafiltrate.

b. It is able to increase or decrease reabsorption rates in response to changes in GFR.

c. It has a minor role in sodium reabsorption.

d. It reabsorbs 80% of filtered water, mainly through aquaporin-1 water channels.

e. It is the major site of bicarbonate reabsorption.

27. All of the following are true regarding the loop of Henle EXCEPT:

a. It is responsible for the generation of a hypertonic medullary interstitium, which is necessary for urinary concentration.

b. It is able to increase or decrease reabsorption rates in response to changes in GFR.

c. The descending limb is highly water permeable.

d. The thin ascending limb actively reabsorbs sodium, chloride, and urea.

e. The thick ascending limb is impermeable to water.

28. Which of the following about the thick ascending limb of the loop of Henle is FALSE?

a. Twenty-five percent of filtered sodium is actively reabsorbed by the furosemide-sensitive NKCC2 cotransporter.

b. Calcium and magnesium reabsorption is inhibited by furosemide.

c. Potassium is reabsorbed and returned to the systemic circulation by renal outer medullary potassium (ROMK) channels.

d. It is the site of uromodulin secretion.

e. Ten to 20 percent of filtered bicarbonate is reabsorbed in the thick ascending limb of the Henle loop (TALH).

29. Regarding the distal convoluted tubule, all the following statements are true EXCEPT:

a. The DCT reabsorbs 10% of filtered sodium by the thiazide-sensitive NCC cotransporter.

b. Sodium reabsorption is dependent solely on luminal sodium concentrations.

c. Calcium reabsorption is paracellular and influenced by sodium reabsorption.

d. Magnesium reabsorption is transcellular by luminal magnesium channels.

e. Loop diuretics increase sodium reabsorption in the DCT.

30. All of the following statements are TRUE about the collecting tubule EXCEPT:

a. The collecting tubule is designed for fine tuning, rather than bulk transport, of ultrafiltrate.

b. Sodium reabsorption is regulated by aldosterone and occurs passively through luminal sodium channels.

c. Potassium reabsorption is dependent on both aldosterone and luminal flow rates.

d. The collecting tubule is impermeable to water at all times.

e. Intercalated cells are largely responsible for acid-base regulation in the collecting tubule.

Pathology

1. See Figure 38–1.

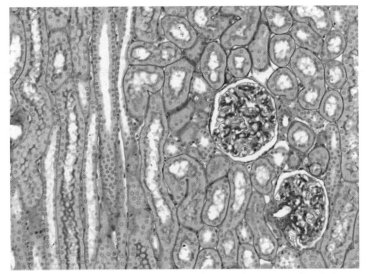

Figure 38–1. (From Bostwick DG, Cheng L. Urologic surgical pathology. 2nd ed. Edinburgh: Mosby; 2008.)

A 26-year-old diabetic has a percutaneous renal biopsy. The microscopic diagnosis is:

a. glomerulosclerosis.

b. interstitial nephritis.

c. normal medulla.

d. normal cortex.

e. acute tubular necrosis.

ANSWERS

1. **d. mediates increased release of aldosterone.** AT1, the receptor for angiotensin II, mediates the release of aldosterone. Intrarenal dilatation is mediated through AT2.

2. **a. Stimulation of the endothelin-1 (ET-1) decreases sodium excretion.** Despite reduction in renal blood flow, stimulation of ET-1 by endothelin increases net sodium excretion.

3. **b. Carbon monoxide.** The others are vasoconstrictors.

4. **c. Increased carbon monoxide (CO) increases ischemia-reperfusion injury in the kidney.** CO is protective against renal ischemia-reperfusion injury.

5. **b. Erythropoiesis is inhibited by low circulating oxygen tension.** Erythropoiesis is increased by low circulating oxygen tension.

6. **b. Normal compensation for hyponatremia is decreased antidiuretic hormone (ADH) secretion and thirst suppression.**

7. **e. may be treated with lithium or demeclocycline.** Lithium or demeclocycline may be used to treat SIADH.

8. **d. Intranasal desmopressin is a useful adjuvant therapy.** Desmopressin is useful to treat hypernatremia caused by diabetes insipidus.

9. **e. results in impairment of maximum concentrating ability of the kidney due to loss of the medullary osmotic gradient.** In both nephrogenic and neurogenic diabetes insipidus, maximum concentrating ability of the kidney is impaired owing to loss of the medullary osmotic gradient.

10. **a. Angiotensin-converting enzyme (ACE) inhibitors may be a cause of hypokalemia.**

11. **c. All patients with a serum potassium value greater than 5.5 mEq/L require immediate therapy.** Patients with mild elevation of potassium, especially when chronic and not associated with ECG changes, do not require emergent therapy.

12. **d. Immediate response to an acid load is through buffers in the blood.**

13. **a. Most bicarbonate is reabsorbed in the distal collecting tubule.** Most bicarbonate reabsorption in the kidney occurs in the proximal tubule.

14. **c. acidemia.** The only thing that is certain with a low pH is that there is acidemia. This may be caused by metabolic, respiratory, or mixed disorders.

15. **b. Direct bicarbonate loss from the kidney would lead to metabolic acidosis and a normal anion gap.** Direct bicarbonate loss is "measured" in the anion gap and therefore leads to metabolic acidosis with a normal anion gap.

16. **d. The hallmark of type IV RTA is hypokalemia.** RTA type IV is most commonly associated with hyperkalemia. Aldosterone deficiency or resistance leads to decreased secretion of potassium in the distal tubule.

17. **a. Paradoxical aciduria may occur due to distal tubule injury.** Metabolic alkalosis is often associated with hypovolemia and elevated aldosterone. In an attempt to conserve sodium and water, H+ may be exchanged with sodium, leading to aciduria, despite the presence of systemic alkalosis.

18. **e. Increased free water excretion in response to hypernatremia.** ADH decreases free water excretion in response to hypernatremia in an attempt to return plasma osmolality back to normal.

19. **c. Dermally synthesized cholecalciferol must be hydroxylated by both the liver and kidney for maximal potency.** Cholecalciferol is minimally active, but potency increases 100 times after it is hydroxylated at the 1- and 25-position to form calcitriol.

20. **d. PTH increases calcium and phosphorus reabsorption in the distal tubule.** PTH increases phosphorus excretion in the kidney.

21. **e. is one of the determinants of the glomerular filtration rate.**

22. **c. glomerular permeability.** Glomerular permeability is already maximal under normal conditions for water and small solutes, so GFR will not increase significantly with increased glomerular permeability. Rather, one sees increased filtration of larger substances such as albumin.

23. **e. serum osmolality.** GFR is not affected significantly by serum osmolality.

24. **a. Plasma creatinine is an accurate marker of early reductions in GFR.** Plasma creatinine is a very insensitive marker of early reductions in GFR, because

increases in tubular secretion of creatinine keep plasma levels from rising until there has been a significant reduction in GFR.

25. **d. Glucose reabsorption is 100% up to plasma glucose levels of 400 mg/dL.** The reabsorptive threshold for glucose is about 200 mg/dL. Plasma levels above this result in urinary glucose wasting.

26. **c. It has a minor role in sodium reabsorption.** The PCT accounts for 65% of sodium reabsorption, the most of any tubular segment.

27. **d. The thin ascending limb actively reabsorbs sodium, chloride, and urea.** Reabsorption of sodium, chloride, and urea occurs passively in the thin ascending limb.

28. **c. Potassium is reabsorbed and returned to the systemic circulation by renal outer medullary potassium (ROMK) channels.** Potassium is recycled in the thick ascending limb of the Henle loop (TALH) rather than reclaimed so that luminal potassium concentrations change very little.

29. **c. Calcium reabsorption is paracellular and influenced by sodium reabsorption.** Calcium reabsorption is transcellular through ECaC1 channels, and paracellular calcium movement is inhibited by claudin 8.

30. **d. The collecting tubule is impermeable to water at all times.** Water permeability is low in the basal state but increases markedly under the influence of ADH.

Pathology

1. **a. normal kidney cortex.** Notice the fine-tufted glomeruli with the vessel entering. Also notice the minimal amount of interstitial tissue. The tubules with the smaller lumen and larger cells are proximal tubules; the tubules with the thinner cells and wider lumens are distal tubule cells. Glomeruli, proximal, and distal tubules are located in the cortex, not in the medulla.

Additional Study Points

1. The determinants of GFR are hydraulic pressure (intra-arterial pressure), which promotes filtration; oncotic pressure, which opposes filtration; permeability of the glomerular basement membrane, which is normally maximal for water and small molecules; and pressure in Bowman space, which opposes filtration.

2. GFR is regulated through two mechanisms: autoregulation, which is an intrinsic property of arterial smooth muscle, and tubular glomerular feedback, which involves the renin angiotensin system.

3. The ideal substance to measure GFR is freely filtered and not metabolized, secreted, or reabsorbed by the kidney. Because creatinine is secreted by the renal tubule it is not ideal; however, due to the ease of measurement, it is practical. When bowel is placed in the urinary tract, electrolytes, water, and substances used to measure GFR are reabsorbed by the bowel, thus rendering them less than ideal agents for determining GFR in this circumstance.

4. The Cockcroft-Gault and the MDRD formulae calculate GFR from serum creatinine and thus do not require a urine collection. They take into account the patient's age, sex, and race. They are generally good approximations of GFR, and in selected circumstances, one may be preferred over the other.

5. For each doubling of plasma creatinine there is an approximately 50% reduction in GFR.

6. Renal blood flow is 20% of cardiac output. Cortical blood flow is approximately 5 times as great as medullary blood flow.

7. Sixty to 65% of filtrate is reabsorbed in the proximal tubule.

8. The bulk of bicarbonate is reclaimed in the proximal tubule.

9. The thick ascending limb of Henle reabsorbs sodium in excess of water and is important for maintaining the medullary osmotic gradient. It is here that loop diuretics have their action.

10. The kidney secretes protons to maintain acid-base balance in the cortical collecting duct. When a proton is secreted as ammonium, its effect on urinary pH is minimal, and therefore it does not generate a significant hydrogen ion gradient; whereas, when protons are secreted and coupled with sulfate and/or phosphate (titratable acid), the urine pH is lowered, thus increasing the hydrogen ion gradient and limiting the ability of the kidney to secrete additional protons by this mechanism.

11. Tamm-Horsfall protein is the matrix of renal tubule casts.

12. Atrial natriuretic peptide (ANP) is produced in the atrium, and promotes natriuresis. It is useful in monitoring myocardial function.

13. Vasopressin, in addition to increasing water reabsorption, increases sodium reabsorption, promotes potassium secretion, increases adrenocorticotropic hormone (ACTH) production, and releases factor VIII and von Willebrand factor.

14. Vitamin D becomes biologically active in the kidney and (a) increases intestinal absorption of calcium, (b) regulates osteoblastic activity, (c) increases reabsorption of calcium in the kidney and, (d) suppresses parathyroid (PTH) release.

15. Parathyroid hormone increases bone reabsorption, increases renal reabsorption of calcium and promotes phosphate secretion, and stimulates production of calcitriol, the active form of vitamin D.

chapter 39

Renovascular Hypertension and Ischemic Nephropathy

Amr Fergany, MD, PhD ● Andrew C. Novick, MD

QUESTIONS

1. The rate-limiting step in the renin-angiotensin-aldosterone cascade is:
   a. secretion of angiotensinogen by the liver.
   b. conversion of angiotensinogen to angiotensin I.
   c. conversion of angiotensin I to angiotensin II.
   d. secretion of aldosterone from the adrenal cortex.
   e. secretion of adrenocorticotropic hormone from the anterior pituitary.

2. The major site of synthesis of systemic renin is:
   a. the liver.
   b. the lung.
   c. the brain.
   d. the kidney.
   e. the adrenal gland.

3. Renin secretion is mediated by all of the following EXCEPT:
   a. diminished potassium delivery to the distal tubule.
   b. diminished chloride delivery to the distal tubule.
   c. diminished stretch of the afferent arteriole.
   d. β-adrenergic stimulation of the kidney.
   e. exogenous prostaglandins.

4. Angiotensin-converting enzyme (ACE):
   a. is a specific enzyme that converts angiotensin I to angiotensin II.
   b. is a nonspecific enzyme that has several functions in vivo.
   c. forms angiotensin I from angiotensinogen.
   d. is the only enzyme in the formation of angiotensin II that cannot be pharmacologically modulated.
   e. is the major enzyme for degradation of angiotensin II.

5. Angiotensin II stimulates all the following actions EXCEPT:
   a. cardiac muscle hypertrophy.
   b. thirst.
   c. vasoconstriction.
   d. secretion of aldosterone.
   e. secretion of epinephrine.

6. Under conditions of decreased renal perfusion, angiotensin II regulates glomerular filtration through:
   a. afferent arteriolar vasodilatation.
   b. afferent arteriolar vasoconstriction.
   c. efferent arteriolar vasodilatation.
   d. efferent arteriolar vasoconstriction.
   e. main renal artery vasoconstriction.

7. Experimental models of renovascular hypertension are characterized by:
   a. a close resemblance to human clinical renovascular hypertension.
   b. the early volume-dependent phase of hypertension.
   c. the late renin-dependent phase of hypertension.
   d. constant sensitivity to ACE inhibition.
   e. dynamic change through different pathophysiologic phases.

8. Atheroembolism (cholesterol embolism):
   a. frequently contributes to deterioration of renal function in patients with atherosclerotic renal artery stenosis.
   b. occurs mainly in young patients with fibrous renal artery disease.
   c. is usually managed by exploration and immediate surgical repair.
   d. is usually managed by percutaneous transluminal angioplasty.
   e. is a benign phenomenon, usually limited to the lower extremities, that rarely involves the kidney.

9. The presence of anatomic renal artery stenosis:
   a. indicates that surgical or endovascular repair is necessary.
   b. should be excluded in every patient with high blood pressure.
   c. is only significant if stenosis is more than 70%.
   d. is only significant if associated with other vascular (e.g., aortic) disease.
   e. is exclusively the result of renal artery atherosclerosis.

10. The diagnosis of renal artery stenosis:
    a. is usually confirmed through laboratory testing.
    b. is based on wide radiologic screening of asymptomatic patients.
    c. is based on radiologic confirmation of clinically suspicious cases.
    d. is generally not pursued in azotemic patients.
    e. can be confirmed by clinical examination alone.

11. Definitive diagnosis of renal artery stenosis is currently provided through:
    a. duplex ultrasonography.
    b. rapid sequence intravenous urography.
    c. intraoperative digital subtraction angiography.
    d. magnetic resonance angiography.
    e. intra-arterial angiography.

12. Duplex ultrasonography as a tool to diagnose renal artery stenosis:
    a. has the advantage of providing excellent anatomic detail.
    b. is limited by the need to transport patients to an imaging facility.
    c. can provide all the necessary information for treatment of patients with ischemic nephropathy.
    d. is not useful as a screening test for patients where renal artery stenosis is suspected.
    e. has the advantage of mobility, widespread availability, noninvasiveness, and no effect on renal function.

13. Carbon dioxide digital subtraction angiography:
    a. is an invasive diagnostic modality that is especially useful in patients with renal insufficiency.
    b. is a noninvasive diagnostic technique that minimizes the risk associated with iodinated contrast angiography.
    c. is associated with a higher incidence of arterial wall trauma than is standard angiography.
    d. cannot be used if angioplasty is contemplated.
    e. is associated with a high incidence of allergic complications and gas embolism.

14. Medical management for patients with renal artery stenosis:
    a. rarely succeeds in controlling hypertension.
    b. is the best chance for maintaining renal function.
    c. is appropriate therapy for young patients with ischemic nephropathy.
    d. is generally preferred for children.
    e. is appropriate therapy for older patients with mild hypertension.

15. Nephrectomy as a treatment option for renal artery stenosis:
    a. is indicated for hypertension caused by a unilateral, small, poorly functioning kidney.
    b. is indicated for bilateral renal artery stenosis, provided that total renal function is normal.
    c. is usually indicated in cases of ischemic nephropathy rather than renovascular hypertension.
    d. should be performed exclusively using open surgical technique and not laparoscopically.
    e. rarely provides long-term therapeutic benefit even in properly selected cases.

16. Revascularization of ischemic kidneys:
    a. should be performed only in patients with ischemic nephropathy.
    b. should be performed only in patients with renovascular hypertension.
    c. provides inferior long-term benefit compared with medical management.
    d. leads to stabilization, but not improvement, of renal function.
    e. may be performed surgically or percutaneously.

17. Percutaneous transluminal angioplasty of the renal arteries:
    a. can be performed under ultrasonographic guidance.
    b. is currently performed using coaxial dilators placed through the femoral artery.
    c. currently employs a dilatation balloon passed through the femoral or axillary artery.
    d. is useful only for cases of atherosclerotic renal artery disease.
    e. is the preferred modality for treating branch renal artery disease.

18. The best therapeutic results after percutaneous angioplasty can be expected with the following arterial lesions:
    a. renal artery aneurysm.
    b. ostial renal artery atherosclerotic stenosis.
    c. branch renal artery atherosclerotic stenosis.
    d. main renal artery fibrous stenosis.
    e. branch renal artery fibrous stenosis.

19. Complications of percutaneous angioplasty:
    a. should never be managed surgically.
    b. include contrast allergy, as well as femoral and renal artery trauma.
    c. occur in 30% to 50% of cases.
    d. are not related to operator experience.
    e. should always be managed by immediate surgery.

20. Technical success for percutaneous angioplasty in cases of fibrous dysplasia can be expected to be:
    a. less than 50%.
    b. 50% to 60%.
    c. 65% to 75%.
    d. 75% to 85%.
    e. 90% or more.

21. Results of percutaneous angioplasty in cases of atherosclerotic renal artery stenosis are worse than in cases of fibrous disease because:
    a. atherosclerotic plaque is more difficult to dilate using angiographic balloons.
    b. atherosclerotic lesions are tighter and do not allow passage of the guidewire.
    c. femoral artery atherosclerosis usually precludes arterial access.
    d. renal artery atherosclerotic lesions are usually ostial and part of aortic wall plaque.
    e. renal artery atherosclerosis usually involves arterial branches and responds poorly to dilatation.

22. The use of endovascular stents as treatment for renal artery stenosis:
   a. has increased the rate of emergency surgery because of complications of angioplasty.
   b. has increased the rate of immediate postangioplasty success.
   c. is reserved mainly for cases of fibrous renal artery stenosis.
   d. is the preferred technique for angioplasty in children.
   e. necessitates arterial access through the axillary artery.

23. Continued deterioration of renal function after renal artery stent placement may be due to all of the following EXCEPT:
   a. acute thrombosis of the renal artery.
   b. cholesterol embolism.
   c. a slightly larger stent than the renal artery diameter.
   d. restenosis of the renal artery.
   e. progressive glomerulosclerosis.

24. Which of the following statements regarding atherosclerotic renal artery disease is incorrect?
   a. It is the most common type of renal artery disease.
   b. It is more common in men than in women.
   c. It is usually not associated with manifestations of generalized atherosclerosis.
   d. It is more common in patients older than 50 years of age.
   e. It usually involves the proximal 2 cm of the main renal artery.

25. The most useful clinical marker or markers of progressive atherosclerotic renal artery obstruction are:
   a. poorly controlled hypertension.
   b. poorly controlled hypertension and a decrease in kidney size.
   c. poorly controlled hypertension and an increase in serum creatinine level.
   d. a decrease in kidney size and an increase in serum creatinine level.
   e. all of the above.

26. All of the following represent clinical clues to the presence of atherosclerotic renal artery disease EXCEPT:
   a. evidence of generalized atherosclerosis.
   b. patient age younger than 50 years.
   c. unilateral small kidney.
   d. mild azotemia.
   e. severe hypertension.

27. The most common cause of unilateral renal atrophy in patients older than 50 years of age is:
   a. congenital hypoplasia.
   b. chronic pyelonephritis.
   c. atherosclerotic renal artery disease.
   d. fibrous renal artery disease.
   e. chronic glomerulonephritis.

28. Clinical clues suggesting renal salvageability with complete arterial occlusion include all of the following EXCEPT:
   a. kidney size greater than 9 cm.
   b. angiographic evidence of collateral vascular supply.

   c. nondiseased glomeruli as seen on a renal biopsy specimen.
   d. function of the involved kidney as revealed by isotope renography.
   e. absence of contralateral compensatory renal hypertrophy.

29. The percentage of end-stage renal disease cases that are currently thought to be caused by ischemic nephropathy is:
   a. 0% to 5%.
   b. 6% to 10%.
   c. 15% to 20%.
   d. 50% to 60%.
   e. 80% to 90%.

30. The natural history of renal artery atherosclerosis is best characterized as being:
   a. unpredictable and varying in each case.
   b. gradually improving.
   c. progressive and unremitting.
   d. not a threat to renal function.
   e. associated with remissions and exacerbation.

31. Renal artery stenosis causing ischemic nephropathy is:
   a. most commonly due to atherosclerosis of the renal arteries.
   b. easy to diagnose because of characteristic symptoms.
   c. usually occurs in younger, healthier patients.
   d. results in mild renal impairment of no clinical significance.
   e. usually diagnosed as focal disease affecting the renal arteries.

32. The class of antihypertensive drugs having a specific deleterious effect on renal function in cases of renal artery stenosis is:
   a. vasodilators.
   b. calcium channel blockers.
   c. ACE inhibitors.
   d. β-adrenergic blockers.
   e. ganglion blockers.

33. Which of the following investigations is best suited as an initial screening test for renal artery stenosis in a 65-year-old woman with generalized atherosclerosis, diabetes mellitus, and a serum creatinine value of 2.5 mg/dL?
   a. CT angiography
   b. Intra-arterial digital subtraction angiography
   c. Captopril test
   d. Duplex ultrasonography of the renal arteries
   e. Determination of differential renal vein renin

34. Which of the following best describes the outcome of patients with ischemic nephropathy who undergo dialysis?
   a. They have the poorest survival of all patients.
   b. They have the best survival of all patients.
   c. Infection is the major cause of mortality.
   d. Long-term survival is a realistic goal.
   e. Complications with vascular access make peritoneal dialysis a better choice.

35. Patients with end-stage renal failure from ischemic nephropathy:
    a. are always beyond the point of regaining renal function with revascularization.
    b. are the best candidates for revascularization.
    c. may be suitable candidates for revascularization if renal salvage criteria are met.
    d. tolerate permanent dialysis exceptionally well.
    e. should undergo only angioplasty for revascularization.

36. Which of the following is the most common type of renal arterial aneurysm?
    a. Fusiform
    b. Saccular
    c. Dissecting
    d. Post-traumatic
    e. Intrarenal

37. A 30-year-old healthy woman is evaluated for hypertension and noted to have a 4-cm noncalcified renal artery aneurysm. Factors that affect treatment include all the following EXCEPT:
    a. the absence of calcification.
    b. the patient's age.
    c. the absence of hematuria.
    d. the size of the aneurysm.
    e. hypertension.

38. Arteriovenous fistulas resulting from needle biopsy of the kidney:
    a. generally heal spontaneously within 2 weeks.
    b. are not amenable to transcatheter angiographic occlusion.
    c. usually require total or partial nephrectomy for treatment.
    d. generally heal spontaneously within 18 months.
    e. are an uncommon cause of acquired renal arteriovenous fistulas.

39. In which of the following clinical settings is surgical excision of a renal arterial aneurysm clearly NOT indicated?
    a. Dissecting aneurysm
    b. Calcified aneurysm 1.5 cm in diameter
    c. Aneurysm causing hypertension
    d. Noncalcified aneurysm 3.0 cm in diameter
    e. Aneurysm increasing in size on sequential angiograms

40. Renal arterial aneurysms may cause hypertension through all of the following mechanisms EXCEPT:
    a. extrinsic compression of renal arterial branches.
    b. turbulent blood flow within an aneurysm.
    c. associated arteriolar nephrosclerosis.
    d. associated renal artery stenosis.
    e. peripheral renal embolism.

41. The most common cause of an acquired renal arteriovenous fistula is:
    a. blunt renal trauma.
    b. renal carcinoma.
    c. renal surgery.

    d. penetrating renal trauma.
    e. closed renal biopsy.

42. The most common method of surgical treatment of symptomatic congenital arteriovenous fistulas has been:
    a. aortorenal bypass with saphenous vein.
    b. total or partial nephrectomy.
    c. bench surgery and autotransplantation.
    d. individual ligation of interconnecting arteriovenous channels.
    e. aortorenal bypass with hypogastric artery.

43. The most appropriate method of management for a patient with unilateral renal arterial embolism secondary to a myocardial ventricular aneurysm is:
    a. systemic anticoagulation.
    b. observation.
    c. aortorenal bypass.
    d. surgical renal artery embolectomy.
    e. segmental renal arterial resection and reanastomosis.

44. Which of the following statements regarding acute renal arterial thrombosis is FALSE?
    a. It commonly occurs in the proximal two thirds of the main renal artery.
    b. It may be due to trauma.
    c. It more commonly involves the right renal artery.
    d. It may be due to atherosclerosis.
    e. It may be managed with percutaneous intra-arterial infusion of streptokinase.

45. Combined repair of aortic and renal artery atherosclerosis:
    a. is recommended to decrease patient morbidity from multiple procedures.
    b. has a low morbidity in cases of bilateral renal artery repair.
    c. can be performed with a combination of open and endovascular repair.
    d. should not be performed using a combination of open and endovascular repair.
    e. cannot be performed as a staged procedure.

46. Regarding selection of patients for endovascular treatment (stenting) of atherosclerotic renal artery stenosis:
    a. Any patient with renal artery stenosis should be offered this procedure.
    b. Procedure-related morbidity is so low that most patients are good candidates.
    c. Most unselected patients have good results with acceptable morbidity.
    d. Selection criteria should be as strict as surgical selection to minimize patient morbidity.
    e. Higher morbidity than open surgery results in fewer number of suitable patients.

47. Which of the following is correct regarding treatment of renal artery aneurysms?
    a. Conservative management by observation is the most appropriate strategy.
    b. If surgery is required, nephrectomy is the best option.

c. Endovascular stents have no role in managing this condition.

d. Ex-vivo repair with autotransplantation is sometimes required.

e. Rupture of the aneurysm is the only indication for treatment.

48. In patients with significant renal artery stenosis to a solitary kidney:

a. volume expansion with decreasing renin secretion occurs.

b. the acute phase of renovascular hypertension is severe and prolonged.

c. there is minimal risk of ischemic nephropathy.

d. medical management with ACE inhibitors is optimal.

e. medical management with antihypertensive medication is usually easy to achieve.

49. An 18-year-old man is found to be hypertensive (BP 190/110 mm Hg). Subsequent evaluation includes renal angiography, which reveals a unilateral tight (90%) renal artery stenosis that is smooth and associated with an intimal dissection and prominent collateral vessels. The next step in management should be:

a. Medical treatment is the long-term treatment of choice.

b. Emergency open surgical repair should be undertaken.

c. This lesion will not progress; observation is the best option.

d. Percutaneous angioplasty should be undertaken after institution of medical treatment.

e. A threat to renal function may necessitate dialysis.

50. An 82-year-old man is being evaluated angiographically for aortic atherosclerotic disease. An acute deterioration of renal function occurs over the following 2 days. All of the following statements are true EXCEPT:

a. Repeat angiography to exclude renal artery thrombosis and possible emergency revascularization is needed.

b. Atheroembolism may be the reason for deterioration of renal function.

c. Nephrotoxicity from radiographic contrast agent may be responsible for renal function deterioration.

d. Duplex ultrasonography of the renal artery is a reasonable study to exclude renal artery thrombosis.

e. Supportive care, as needed, is the best option in this situation.

ANSWERS

1. **b. conversion of angiotensinogen to angiotensin I.** The basic cascade of the renin-angiotensin-aldosterone system (RAAS) involves conversion of angiotensinogen to angiotensin I through the action of renin. This is the rate-limiting step for the entire system, and, accordingly, control of renin release regulates the activity of the whole system.

2. **d. kidney.** Renin is a single–polypeptide chain aspartyl protease that is secreted from the juxtaglomerular cells of the afferent arteriole. The kidney is the major site of renin production, although renin mRNA is found in several other tissues where the local renin-angiotensin system functions.

3. **a. diminished potassium delivery to the distal tubule.** Reduction of distal tubule salt delivery stimulates renin secretion and vice versa. Although sodium was initially thought to be responsible for this action, it now appears that the signal for macula densa–controlled renin release is the alteration of tubular chloride concentration.

4. **b. is a nonspecific enzyme that has several functions in vivo.** ACE is expressed in several tissues where the local RAAS functions. Renal ACE is localized to the glomerular endothelial cells and the proximal tubule brush border, where it might play a role in cleaving filtered protein for reabsorption. Within the central nervous system (CNS), ACE is found in several locations, where it functions in the local RAAS. This local CNS RAAS is thought to have dipsogenic and hypertensive effects, as well as to stimulate vasopressin secretion. Adrenal ACE is found predominantly in the medulla, where it is thought to stimulate catecholamine secretion. ACE is found abundantly in the testes and prostate, in the Leydig cells, and in cytoplasmic droplets in sperm. In the female reproductive tract, ACE is found in follicular and fallopian tube oocytes. The precise role of ACE in the reproductive system has not been elucidated.

5. **e. secretion of epinephrine.** Angiotensin II acts directly on the adrenal glomerulosa cells to stimulate aldosterone secretion, which is accomplished through increased desmolase activity and increased conversion of corticosterone to aldosterone. This serves to augment the salt reabsorptive actions of angiotensin II to conserve sodium. Vasoconstriction and release of aldosterone occur immediately and are of short duration, supporting the role of angiotensin II in maintaining tissue perfusion in hypovolemia. Other actions, such as vascular growth and ventricular hypertrophy, are slower in onset and longer in duration, lasting for several days or weeks.

6. **d. efferent arteriolar vasoconstriction.** One of the most important actions of angiotensin II is the autoregulation of glomerular filtration rate (GFR) in response to changes in renal perfusion. This action is effected through changes in vascular resistance, as well as mesangial cell tone. Angiotensin II causes a marked increase in efferent arteriolar resistance in cases of renal hypoperfusion but does not affect afferent arteriolar resistance unless there is an increase in renal perfusion pressure. The result of this disproportionate increase in efferent over afferent resistance is an increase in capillary hydraulic pressure, and subsequently in filtration pressure, maintaining GFR in the face of decreased renal perfusion.

7. **e. dynamic change through different pathophysiologic phases.** Renovascular hypertension has been demonstrated in two models of experimental Goldblatt hypertension: the two-kidney, one-clip model (2K,1C), in which one renal artery is clipped and the contralateral kidney is in place and normal; and the one-kidney, one-clip model (1K,1C), in which one renal artery is clipped and the contralateral kidney is removed. Neither of the models remains static but rather passes through an acute phase, a transition phase, and then a final chronic phase. In cases of 2K,1C hypertension, a chronic phase is eventually reached after several days or weeks, when unclipping of the stenotic kidney fails to normalize blood pressure. In this chronic phase, the elevated perfusion pressure as well as high levels of angiotensin II, have resulted in widespread arteriolar damage to the contralateral kidney. Excretory function (natriuresis) of the contralateral kidney declines, resulting in

extracellular volume expansion, decrease of circulating angiotensin II levels, and gradual development of a "volume-dependent" type of hypertension.

8. **a. frequently contributes to deterioration of renal function in patients with atherosclerotic renal artery stenosis.** The organs most commonly affected by atheroembolism are the kidney, spleen, pancreas, and gastrointestinal tract. Renal effects take the form of deteriorating renal function, usually after a precipitating event. The decline in renal function can vary in severity from slowly progressive to rapid acute renal failure. Gradual improvement of renal function occurs after the event, but recurrent episodes lead to progressive loss of renal function with time.

9. **c. is only significant if stenosis is more than 70%.** Renal artery stenosis becomes hemodynamically significant when the stenosis exceeds 70% of the lumen. Most patients with hypertension suffer from essential hypertension, and thus it is not indicated to investigate them for renal arterial disease. Renal artery stenosis can be the result of atherosclerosis, fibromuscular dysplasia, as well as other less common diseases.

10. **c. is based on radiologic confirmation of clinically suspicious cases.** The clinical clues serve in the selection of patients who should be studied for the possible presence of renal artery stenosis. For patients with suspected renovascular hypertension, a number of tests are available for functional diagnosis of renovascular hypertension. These tests (plasma renin activity, captopril test, captopril renography, and renal vein renin assays) diagnose hyperactivity of the RAAS but provide no anatomic information regarding the offending arterial lesion. Anatomic delineation of the arterial lesion guides the treatment decisions and is obtained by intra-arterial angiography, which remains the most definitive study and the "gold standard" against which other diagnostic techniques are compared.

11. **e. intra-arterial angiography.** Intra-arterial angiography remains the gold standard for diagnosing renal artery disease, and it is the test to which other tests are compared. However, angiography is not suitable for use as a preliminary screening tool for all patients suspected of having renal artery stenosis.

12. **e. has the advantage of mobility, widespread availability, noninvasiveness, and no effect on renal function.** Duplex ultrasonography of the renal arteries is a noninvasive anatomic study that has shown excellent ability for screening and diagnosis of renal artery stenosis. The equipment is mobile and can be moved to critically ill patients. It is also widespread, relatively easy to use, and does not depend on kidney function nor affect kidney function. It does not provide anatomic detail, because it depends on measuring blood flow velocity in the renal artery and comparing that to the blood flow velocity in the aorta.

13. **a. is an invasive diagnostic modality that is especially useful in patients with renal insufficiency.** Carbon dioxide has been introduced as a contrast agent for intra-arterial injection in an effort to reduce contrast nephrotoxicity from iodinated contrast material. Carbon dioxide has no effect on renal function, making it an ideal agent for use in patients with renal insufficiency.

14. **e. is appropriate therapy for older patients with mild hypertension.** In patients with atherosclerotic renal vascular hypertension, more vigorous attempts at medical management are warranted, because these patients are older and often have extrarenal vascular disease. Therefore multiple-drug regimens that control blood pressure are often the preferred approach.

15. **a. is indicated for hypertension caused by a unilateral, small, poorly functioning kidney.** Advances in both surgical renal vascular reconstruction and medical antihypertensive therapy have limited the role of total or partial nephrectomy in the management of patients with renal artery disease. These operations are only occasionally indicated in patients with severe arteriolar nephrosclerosis, severe renal atrophy, noncorrectable renal vascular lesions, and renal infarction.

16. **e. may be performed surgically or percutaneously.** Intervention with surgery or endovascular therapy is best reserved for patients whose hypertension cannot be adequately controlled or when renal function is threatened by advanced vascular disease.

17. **c. currently employs a dilatation balloon passed through the femoral or axillary artery.** The original Gruntzig coaxial technique uses an 8- or 9-Fr renal guiding catheter through which a 4.3- or 4.5-Fr balloon catheter is passed over a guidewire traversing the stenotic segment through a femoral arterial puncture. Modification of the original technique and balloon catheters have allowed the use of a 5-Fr femoral artery puncture through which a 5-Fr diagnostic catheter is passed to the renal artery using the Seldinger technique. An axillary approach may be used to perform renal percutaneous transluminal angioplasty, when the renal arteries originate at an acute angle from the abdominal aorta, as well as in cases with severe pelvic atherosclerosis, occlusion, or the presence of bypass grafts in the pelvic or abdominal areas.

18. **d. main renal artery fibrous stenosis.** The results of angioplasty for fibrous dysplasia of the main renal artery have been excellent and equal to those obtained with surgical revascularization; therefore angioplasty is the initial treatment of choice in such cases.

19. **b. include contrast allergy, as well as femoral and renal artery trauma.** The complications of percutaneous transluminal angioplasty include those of standard angiography (complications related to arterial puncture and to the use of iodinated contrast material), as well as specific complications related to manipulation of the renal arteries. Transient deterioration of renal function is the most frequent complication and is related to the contrast load delivered during the procedure. Technical mishaps during percutaneous transluminal angioplasty may lead to an intimal dissection or even thrombosis of the renal artery.

20. **e. 90% or more.** Percutaneous transluminal angioplasty is usually performed in cases of fibrous dysplasia without stent placement and has become the primary modality of treatment for these lesions. With the use of modern equipment and increasing experience with the technique, technical success has been more than 90%. A beneficial blood pressure response—that is, cure of hypertension or improvement in blood pressure control—can be expected in more than 80% and up to 100% of cases.

21. **d. renal artery atherosclerotic lesions are usually ostial and part of aortic wall plaque.** Renal artery

stenosis in cases of arteriosclerosis obliterans is usually bilateral and ostial or very proximal in the main renal artery. In most ostial cases, this represents encroachment of the atherosclerotic plaque in the abdominal aorta upon the origin of the renal artery rather than primary renal artery disease. The patients affected by atherosclerotic renal artery stenosis are also different from patients with fibrous dysplasia of the renal arteries in that they are generally older and have a number of comorbid medical conditions, as well as generalized atherosclerosis affecting the coronary and carotid arteries or the peripheral vascular tree. Associated essential hypertension and nephrosclerosis are usually present. All of the previously mentioned factors, as well as the propensity for atheroembolism in patients with generalized arteriosclerosis obliterans, make percutaneous transluminal angioplasty in cases of arteriosclerosis obliterans renal artery stenosis less successful and associated with higher morbidity (and some mortality) than in cases of fibrous dysplasia.

22. **b. has increased the rate of immediate postangioplasty success.** In the only prospective study comparing percutaneous transluminal angioplasty alone versus the procedure with stenting in ostial atherosclerosis, 85 patients were randomized to receive either treatment. Technical success was higher in the group receiving stents (88% vs. 57%), and patency at 6 months was 75% for patients in the group receiving stents versus 29% for the patients undergoing the procedure alone. In patients with successful primary procedures, restenosis occurred in 14% of the patients with stents and in 48% of patients undergoing percutaneous transluminal angioplasty alone. Stenting for immediate or late failure of the procedure was required in 12 (of 42) patients in the group undergoing percutaneous transluminal angioplasty alone. This study reflects the overall higher success of percutaneous transluminal angioplasty with stenting in treating ostial atherosclerosis when compared with the procedure alone and probably also justifies the increasing trend to perform primary stenting in these cases to avoid exposing patients to a secondary procedure.

23. **c. a slightly larger stent than the renal artery diameter.** Complications of percutaneous transluminal angioplasty with stenting were not found to be significantly different from those of percutaneous transluminal angioplasty alone in a prospective study comparing both procedures. Specifically, rates in both groups for bleeding-related complications were 19% and 10% for cholesterol embolism; the rate for access site pseudoaneurysm and renal artery injury was slightly higher with stent placement (7% vs. 5%). Transient deterioration of renal function secondary to contrast nephrotoxicity was noted in 24% of patients undergoing the procedure alone and in 21% of patients undergoing the procedure with stent placement.

24. **c. It is usually not associated with manifestations of generalized atherosclerosis.** Recent epidemiologic studies indicate that atherosclerotic renal artery disease is quite common in patients with generalized atherosclerosis obliterans, regardless of whether renovascular hypertension is present.

25. **d. a decrease in kidney size and an increase in the serum creatinine level.** Clinical follow-up of patients in our study also revealed that significantly more patients with progressive disease developed deterioration of overall renal function (a decrease in kidney size or an increase in the serum creatinine level) compared with patients with stable disease. Interestingly, serial blood pressure control was equivalent in these two groups, indicating that it is not a useful clinical marker for progressive atherosclerotic renal artery stenosis.

26. **b. patient age younger than 50 years.** Studies indicate that clinical screening for atherosclerotic renal artery disease is appropriate in older patients with most or all of the following features: (1) evidence of generalized atherosclerosis; (2) a decrease in the size of one or both kidneys; (3) renal insufficiency, even of a mild extent, particularly in patients with no obvious underlying cause; (4) the development of progressive azotemia after restoration of normotension with medical antihypertensive therapy; (5) coronary artery disease; (6) a history of congestive heart failure; and (7) peripheral vascular disease.

27. **c. atherosclerotic renal artery disease.** The screening of patients for atherosclerotic renal artery disease is based in part on an early (1965) study by Gifford and colleagues.* These investigators found that in 53 of 75 older patients (71%) with unilateral renal atrophy, the renal atrophy was caused by stenosing atherosclerotic renal artery disease. Of equal importance was the finding that 22 of these 53 patients (42%) also had unsuspected atherosclerotic renal artery disease involving the opposite normal-sized kidney. Subsequently, Lawrie and colleagues reviewed 40 patients with renal atrophy caused by total arterial occlusion and noted contralateral atherosclerotic renal artery stenosis in 31 patients (78%). These observations underscore the high incidence of renal artery disease, often bilateral, in patients with generalized atherosclerosis and diminished renal size.

28. **e. absence of contralateral compensatory renal hypertrophy.** Complete occlusion of the renal artery most often ends in irreversible ischemic damage of the involved kidney. In some patients with gradual arterial occlusion, however, the viability of the kidney can be maintained through the development of collateral arterial supply. Helpful clinical clues suggesting renal salvageability in such cases include the following: (1) angiographic demonstration of retrograde filling of the distal renal arterial tree, by collateral vessels on the side of the total arterial occlusion; (2) a renal biopsy showing well-preserved glomeruli; (3) kidney size greater than 9 cm; and (4) function of the involved kidney as revealed by isotope renography or intravenous pyelography. When such criteria are present, restoration of normal renal arterial flow can lead to recovery of renal function.

29. **b. 6% to 10%.** The exact incidence of end-stage renal disease caused by atherosclerotic renal artery disease in the United States is not known. In a report from England, Scoble and colleagues prospectively performed renal arteriography in all new patients with end-stage renal disease during an 18-month period. Atherosclerotic renal artery disease was the cause of end-stage renal disease in 6% of all patients and in 14% of patients older than 50 years of age. Approximately 300,000 patients in the United States are currently being maintained by chronic dialysis. Their median age is greater than 60 years, and a majority of

---

*Sources referenced can be found in *Campbell-Walsh Urology, 10th Edition,* on the Expert Consult website.

patients have evidence of generalized atherosclerosis obliterans. Although the exact number of patients with end-stage renal disease caused by atherosclerotic renal artery disease is not known, these data suggest that there are several thousand patients in this category.

30. **c. progressive and unremitting.** Natural history data clearly show that atherosclerotic renal artery disease progresses in many patients and that loss of functioning renal parenchyma is a common sequela of such progression.

31. **a. most commonly due to atherosclerosis of the renal arteries.** Atherosclerosis of the renal arteries, usually as part of generalized atherosclerosis, is the most common cause of ischemic nephropathy. This is a silent disease that requires clinical suspicion for diagnosis. The condition usually occurs in older patients with generalized atherosclerosis and can progress to significant renal impairment and the need for renal replacement therapy.

32. **c. ACE inhibitors.** Another important clinical clue to the presence of significant atherosclerotic renal artery stenosis is the development of progressive azotemia after medical control of blood pressure in patients with significant hypertension. ACE inhibitor agents can lead to deterioration of renal function through loss of efferent arteriolar vasoconstrictor tone in the kidney.

33. **d. Duplex ultrasonography of the renal arteries.** Duplex ultrasonography offers significant advantages as a diagnostic tool for renal artery stenosis. It is noninvasive, uses portable equipment that is relatively inexpensive and widely available, does not use iodinated contrast material, and has no effect on renal function. Azotemia does not affect the results of the study, and no discontinuation of antihypertensive medications is required.

34. **a. They have the poorest survival of all patients.** Patients with renal vascular disease as the cause of end-stage renal disease had the poorest survival of all patients who have had dialysis, with a 27-month median survival time and a 12% 5-year survival rate.

35. **c. may be suitable candidates for revascularization if renal salvage criteria are met.** Occasional patients with end-stage renal disease from ischemic nephropathy have been encountered; renal function in these patients has been salvageable with revascularization. The basis for this has been the presence of chronic bilateral total renal arterial occlusion when, fortuitously, the viability of one or both kidneys has been maintained through collateral vascular supply. In such cases, revascularization can yield dramatic recovery of renal function.

36. **b. Saccular.** Saccular aneurysms are the most common type and account for about 75% of renal artery aneurysms. They generally occur at the bifurcation of the renal artery, perhaps because of an inherent weakness in the wall of the artery at this point.

37. **c. the absence of hematuria.** Factors that appear to predispose to aneurysmal rupture include absent or incomplete calcification, aneurysmal diameter greater than 2.0 cm, coexisting hypertension, and pregnancy (females of childbearing age).

38. **d. generally heal spontaneously within 18 months.** Approximately 70% of fistulas occurring after needle biopsy of the kidney close spontaneously within 18 months.

39. **b. Calcified aneurysm 1.5 cm in diameter.** A small (<2.0 cm) well-calcified renal arterial aneurysm in an asymptomatic normotensive patient does not require operative intervention. These aneurysms can be followed with serial plain abdominal radiographs to detect any change in size.

40. **c. associated arteriolar nephrosclerosis.** The majority of renal arterial aneurysms are small and asymptomatic. Renovascular hypertension is reported to occur in 15% to 75% of patients and may be due to turbulent flow within an aneurysm, associated arterial stenosis, dissection, arteriovenous fistula formation, thromboembolism, or compression of adjacent arterial branches by a large aneurysm.

41. **e. closed renal biopsy.** Acquired fistulas are the most common type of fistula, accounting for 70% to 75% of all renal arteriovenous fistulas. On angiography, they appear as solitary communications between an artery and a vein. By far the most common cause is iatrogenic trauma resulting from needle biopsy of the kidney.

42. **b. total or partial nephrectomy.** Various operations have been used in the surgical treatment of renal arteriovenous fistulas. Most congenital or cirsoid fistulas have been managed with total or partial nephrectomy, because of the difficulty of completely excising the many small communicating vessels.

43. **a. systemic anticoagulation.** Patients with unilateral renal arterial embolic occlusion generally have serious underlying extrarenal disease and are best managed nonoperatively with systemic anticoagulation.

44. **c. It more commonly involves the right renal artery.** Renal arterial thrombosis commonly involves the proximal or middle third of the main renal artery, whereas renal arterial embolization generally involves peripheral arterial branches. Acute arterial occlusion is more common on the left side, because of the more acute angle between the left renal artery and the aorta.

45. **c. can be performed with a combination of open and endovascular repair.** The morbidity of a combined repair, especially when both renal arteries are involved, is especially high, and this justifies a staging technique, where the renal arteries are repaired separate from the aorta, or a combined open/endovascular approach.

46. **d. Selection criteria should be as strict as surgical selection to minimize patient morbidity.** Procedure-related morbidity from renal artery stenting is substantial with possible mortality. This requires attention to patient comorbidities before recommending the procedure. At the same time, the chance of a beneficial outcome should be carefully evaluated regarding the renal function, the size of the kidneys, as well as the anatomic distribution of disease.

47. **d. Ex-vivo repair with autotransplantation is sometimes required.** A variety of treatment methods are available for treatment of renal artery aneurysms. Surgical repair commonly requires ex-vivo reconstruction and autotransplantation due to involvement of the branches of the renal artery. Endovascular stents have recently been used to exclude the aneurysm from the main renal artery and effectively treat it. Nephrectomy should be the last resort in complicated cases. Such treatment modalities should be instituted before complications, especially rupture of the aneurysm, occur.

48. **a. volume expansion with decreasing renin secretion occurs.** In patients with stenosis to the artery of a solitary kidney, the situation is similar to a one-kidney,

one-clip experimental model of renovascular hypertension. The acute renin-dependent phase of hypertension is short, rapidly passing into the chronic phase, characterized by volume expansion and gradually decreasing renin secretion. In the clinical situation, medical management is usually difficult, and the patients face the risk of developing ischemic nephropathy and deterioration of renal function. Acute deterioration of renal function can be precipitated by the use of ACE inhibitors in this situation.

49. **d. Percutaneous angioplasty should be undertaken after institution of medical treatment.** This appearance is typical of an intimal fibroplasia. These lesions are usually progressive and can result in intimal dissection with occlusion of the main renal artery or its branches. Renal function is not usually threatened in unilateral lesions. Long-term medical treatment is not a good option

in younger patients to avoid the complications of long-term treatment, which does not stop disease progression. Initial control of blood pressure should be undertaken medically followed by an attempt at endovascular repair, which is usually successful. Surgical revascularization should be reserved for failure of percutaneous angioplasty.

50. **a. Repeat angiography to exclude renal artery thrombosis and possible emergency revascularization is needed.** This scenario is most commonly explained by atheroembolism to the kidneys after manipulation of an atherosclerotic aorta. Less common causes may be contrast nephrotoxicity or thrombosis of the renal arteries. The best option is to provide supportive care to the patient, as needed, and avoid further manipulation of the aorta. Duplex ultrasonography is a good noninvasive test to assess patency of the main renal artery, if occlusion or thrombosis is suspected.

Additional Study Points

1. There is an extremely high morbidity and mortality in patients who require dialysis due to end-stage renal disease resulting from atherosclerotic renal artery occlusion.

2. There are two major pathologic causes of renal artery disease: (1) atherosclerosis and (2) fibrous dysplasia.

3. In unilateral renal artery stenosis with a normal contralateral kidney, hypertension is due to angiotensin-induced vasoconstriction.

4. In bilateral renal artery stenosis or in renal artery stenosis in a solitary kidney, hypertension is due to volume overload.

5. CT angiography and magnetic resonance angiography do not visualize the distal renal arterial tree well.

6. Except in rare circumstances, functional testing for renal vascular hypertension has been largely replaced by anatomic imaging of the renal artery lesions.

7. Causes of renal vascular hypertension in children include fibromuscular dysplasia, vasculitis, neurofibromatosis, and neuroblastoma.

8. Widespread glomerular hyalinization indicates irreversible ischemic renal injury and suggests that there would be little benefit from relief of renal artery obstruction.

9. Extensive atherosclerotic disease precludes renal revascularization.

10. When the aorta is severely diseased, renal revascularization on the left may be accomplished with a splenorenal bypass, and on the right with a hepatorenal bypass or a supraceliac lower thoracic aorta renal bypass.

11. A transient deterioration of renal function is not infrequently seen following a contrast load in patients with significant renal artery stenosis and limited renal function.

12. A Page kidney results from compression of the renal parenchyma, usually due to a hematoma. It produces renin-dependent hypertension.

13. Minimally invasive treatment by balloon angioplasty with or without arterial stenting is the preferred method of treatment in patients with severe hypertension or ischemic nephropathy due to atherosclerosis.

Upper Urinary Tract Obstruction and Trauma

chapter 40

Pathophysiology of Urinary Tract Obstruction

Iqbal Singh, MCh (Urology), DNB (Genitourinary Surgery), MS, DNB ● Jack W. Strandhoy, PhD ● Dean G. Assimos, MD

QUESTIONS

1. In unilateral ureteral obstruction, which of the following is responsible for contralateral compensatory renal growth?
   a. Augmented extracellular matrix synthesis and growth of mesangial cells
   b. Increased mitochondrial respiration
   c. Increased proliferation of the residual nephrons
   d. Deposition and growth of fibroblasts in the renal interstitial tissues
   e. None of the above

2. Which of the following histopathological findings predicts the recovery of renal function at the time of pyeloplasty?
   a. Increased collagen in the renal parenchyma
   b. Increased elastin in renal parenchyma
   c. Increased collagen and elastin in renal parenchyma
   d. Increased fibroblasts, renal mesangial cells, and nephrons
   e. Increased renal insulin-like growth factor binding protein-3 (IGFBP-3), matrix metalloproteinase-9 (MMP-9), interleukin-10 (IL-10), and transforming growth factor-β (TGF-β)

3. When comparing contrast-enhanced color Doppler imaging (CECDI), magnetic resonance angiography (MRA), and computed tomographic angiography (CTA) for detecting crossing vessels associated with ureteropelvic junction obstruction:
   a. MRA is the most sensitive.
   b. CTA is the most sensitive.
   c. CECDI has the highest specificity.
   d. the comparative accuracy of all the three modalities ranges from 93% to 100%.
   e. all the above are incorrect.

4. Which of the following correctly defines the ability of magnetic resonance urography (MRU) to assess renal function?
   a. MRU with gadopentetate dimeglumine contrast accurately estimates global renal function.
   b. MRU with gadopentetate dimeglumine contrast accurately estimates differential renal function.
   c. MRU with contrast is not indicated to assess renal function in patients with renal insufficiency.
   d. MRU correlates well with renal scintigraphy.
   e. All of the above.

5. There is a low risk for development of nephrogenic systemic fibrosis after contrast MRI in patients with:
   a. obstructive uropathy.
   b. normal renal function.
   c. diabetic nephropathy.
   d. ischemic nephropathy.
   e. none of the above.

6. Internalized ureteral stent failure is more common in patients with:
   a. advanced cancer.
   b. normal renal function.
   c. solitary kidneys.
   d. horseshoe kidneys.
   e. duplicated collecting systems.

7. In pelvic lipomatosis:
   a. lower urinary tract symptoms are uncommon.
   b. constipation is uncommon.
   c. pain is rare.
   d. hypertension occurs in up to one third of patients.
   e. patients often present in retention.

8. Which of the following is a sign of pelvic lipomatosis?
   a. Radiolucent areas in pelvis on plain abdominal radiography
   b. Bilateral hydronephrosis
   c. Medial location of the lower ureters
   d. Extrinsic compression of the rectum
   e. All of the above

9. Endometriosis of the urinary tract:
   a. most commonly involves the ureter.
   b. most commonly involves the urethra.
   c. is associated with cystitis glandularis.
   d. involves the ureter in 15% to 20% of the cases.
   e. more commonly involves the right ureter than the left.

10. Circumcaval ureter:
    a. is more common in females.
    b. only involves the right ureter.
    c. is only treated in the presence of ureteral obstruction.
    d. does not occur in situs inversus.
    e. is best diagnosed with ultrasonography.

11. If a pulsatile mass is palpated on rectal examination, which of the following is suspected?
    a. Ovarian vein thrombophlebitis
    b. Aortic aneurysm
    c. Rectal tumor
    d. Internal iliac artery aneurysm
    e. Internal hemorrhoid

12. Retroperitoneal fibrosis can be caused by:
    a. tuberculosis.
    b. histoplasmosis.
    c. actinomycosis.
    d. pelvic surgery.
    e. all of the above.

13. Which of these predict poor functional recovery after relief of ureteral obstruction?
    a. Absence of pyelolymphatic backflow
    b. Good compliance of the collecting system
    c. Presence of minimal obstruction
    d. Normal renal cortical thickness
    e. Absence of infection

14. Ureteral stenting is preferred over percutaneous nephrostomy in patients with:
    a. advanced cervical cancer.
    b. uncorrected coagulopathy.
    c. ureteral stone with suspected sepsis.
    d. hydronephrosis of pregnancy.
    e. all of the above.

15. Endometriosis with ureteric obstruction is best treated by:
    a. nephrectomy.
    b. ureteral stenting and administration of danazol.
    c. ureteral stenting and administration of leuprolide acetate.
    d. hysterectomy, bilateral salpingo-oophorectomy, and ureterolysis.
    e. ureterolysis.

16. All of the following drugs are associated with the development of retroperitoneal fibrosis EXCEPT:
    a. methamphetamine.
    b. morphine.
    c. propranolol.
    d. LSD.
    e. haloperidol.

17. Postobstructive diuresis is:
    a. generally prolonged.
    b. usually self-limited.
    c. not associated with hypernatremia.
    d. common with unilateral obstruction in a patient with two kidneys.
    e. associated with concentrated urine initially.

18. The release of tumor necrosis factor-α (TNF-α) in obstructive uropathy is stimulated by:
    a. angiotensin II.
    b. cysteinyl aspartate–specific proteinases.
    c. cytochrome c.
    d. tissue inhibitors of metalloproteinases (TIMPs).
    e. all of the above.

19. Which of the following characterizes obstructive nephropathy when compared to hydronephrosis?
    a. Renal function impairment
    b. Bilateral ureteral dilation
    c. Unilateral ureteral dilation
    d. Calyceal blunting
    e. None of the above

20. Which of these urinary changes occur after relief of bilateral ureteral obstruction?
    a. Increased sodium excretion
    b. Decreased phosphate excretion
    c. Decreased potassium excretion
    d. Decreased magnesium excretion
    e. None of the above

21. Which of the following is thought to play a role in postobstructive diuresis after release of bilateral ureteral obstruction?
    a. Increased renal aquaporin-2 water channels
    b. Increased renal aquaporin-3 water channels
    c. Increased antidiuretic hormone (ADH)
    d. Increased atrial natriuretic peptide
    e. Increased aldosterone

22. After 5 hours of unilateral ureteral obstruction, which of the following occurs in the obstructed kidney?
    a. Increased renal plasma flow
    b. Increased glomerular filtration
    c. Shift of blood flow from the outer to the inner cortex
    d. Increased sodium delivery to the macula densa
    e. Decrease in renal vein renin levels

23. Atrial natriuretic peptide induces which of the following?
    a. Decrease in urinary sodium excretion
    b. Increase in afferent arteriolar dilation
    c. Increase in efferent arteriolar dilation
    d. Decrease in glomerulotubular feedback
    e. Increase in renin production

24. Which of the following occurs after bilateral ureteral obstruction?
    a. Shift of blood flow to the outer renal cortex
    b. Decrease in atrial natriuretic peptide
    c. Decrease in collecting system pressure during the first day
    d. Increase in renal plasma flow at 8 hours
    e. None of the above

25. Which of the following may promote tubular interstitial fibrosis in the obstructed kidney?
    a. Increase in renal metalloproteinase levels
    b. Increase in expression of transforming growth factor-β
    c. Administration of enalapril
    d. Administration of losartan
    e. Decrease in phosphorylation of SMAD proteins

26. A difference between unilateral (UUO) and bilateral ureteral obstruction (BUO) is that:
    a. fractional excretion of sodium after relief of obstruction is greater in BUO.
    b. atrial natriuretic peptide levels are higher in UUO.
    c. risk of postobstructive diuresis is less with BUO.
    d. urinary pH is higher in UUO.
    e. new-onset hypertension is more common with UUO.

27. Which of the following is true of compensatory renal growth?
    a. Glomerular number increases.
    b. Insulin-like growth factor-1 is inhibitory.
    c. It increases with age.
    d. Hypertrophic and hyperplastic growth occur.
    e. It is more common with partial obstruction.

28. The chance for renal recovery after ureteral obstruction is most influenced by:
    a. early relief of obstruction.
    b. presence of extrarenal pelvis.
    c. presence of a solitary kidney.
    d. uninfected urine.
    e. Normal blood pressure.

29. Which of the following is expected in a kidney that has been obstructed for 1 month?
    a. Increased renal pelvic pressure
    b. Reduced Na^+, K^+-ATPase activity
    c. Reduced urinary pH
    d. Reduced tubulointerstitial fibrosis
    e. Increased aquaporin-2 water channels

30. Reduced expression of sodium transporters in the obstructed kidney may be due to:
    a. reduced delivery of sodium to the nephron.
    b. renal ischemia.
    c. increased renal interstitial pressure.
    d. increased prostaglandin E_2 (PGE_2).
    e. all of the above.

31. A reduction in concentrating ability of the obstructed kidney is due to:
    a. decreased ADH expression.
    b. maintenance of a medullary hypertonicity and reduced glomerular flow rate (GFR).
    c. increased renal aquaproin-1 water channels.
    d. decreased renal aquaporin-2 water channels.
    e. urea backflux from the inner medullary collecting duct.

32. A persistent concentrating defect after relief of bilateral ureteral obstruction (BUO) is primarily due to:
    a. continued excessive secretion of atrial natriuretic peptide.
    b. decreased synthesis of aquaporins.
    c. decreased synthesis of cyclic AMP.
    d. persistent hypokalemia.
    e. decreased release of ADH from the posterior pituitary.

33. In studies of complete UUO for 24 hours, renal blood flow has been shown to:
    a. briefly cease with ureteral clamping and then gradually return toward control.
    b. gradually decline over the course of the constriction.
    c. increase by 25% and remain elevated during the obstruction.
    d. increase over an hour and then steadily decrease.
    e. remain unchanged during clamping and undergo reactive hyperemia upon release.

34. Ureteral and tubular pressure changes in experimental unilateral ureteral occlusion over 24 hours are characterized by:
    a. a continued increase due to urine secretion.
    b. an immediate decrease as flow ceases.
    c. an increase followed by a decrease.
    d. no change due to extravasation of tubule fluid.
    e. no change due to contralateral renal compensation.

35. Which of the following have been implicated in the initial rise in renal blood flow in UUO?
    a. Adenosine and bradykinin
    b. Atrial natriuretic peptide and platelet-activating factor
    c. Dopamine and acetylcholine
    d. Prostaglandin and nitric oxide
    e. Endothelin and angiotensin II

36. Experimental evidence has implicated which of the following vasoconstrictor lipids with the decreased renal blood flow in the third phase of UUO?
    a. Ergosterol
    b. Plasminogen activating inhibitor-1
    c. Prostaglandin E_2
    d. Leukotriene C_4
    e. Thromboxane A_2

37. Which of the following best explains the greater fractional excretion of sodium that follows the release of BUO compared with UUO?
    a. Better-preserved glomerular filtration rate with UUO than with BUO
    b. Greater expansion of extracellular volume with BUO than with UUO
    c. More contralateral compensation with BUO than with UUO
    d. Less renal vasoconstriction with BUO than with UUO
    e. More secretion of aldosterone with BUO than with UUO

38. Obstruction causes which of the following disturbances in the renal regulation of acid-base balance?
    a. Decreased bicarbonate reclamation in the proximal tubule
    b. Decreased H^+-ATPase expression in the collecting duct
    c. Greater buffering of acid loads by glutamine breakdown to NH_3
    d. Decreased proportion of H^+ buffered as titratable acid rather than as NH_4^+
    e. Urine pH above 7.4

39. Ureteral obstruction causes which of the following metabolic increases in the kidney?
    a. ATP synthesis
    b. Glycolytic capacity in the cortex
    c. Medullary consumption of oxygen
    d. Ratio of lactate to pyruvate in renal tissue
    e. Use of glucose metabolism by the proximal tubule

40. Which of the following contribute(s) to obstruction-induced tubulointerstitial fibrosis?
    a. Angiotensin II
    b. Metalloproteinase inhibitors
    c. Transforming growth factor-β
    d. Nuclear factor-κB
    e. All of the above

41. Obstruction induces apoptosis, or programmed cell death, of nephrons. Tumor necrosis factor-α causes inflammation in the kidney and stimulates which key family of enzymes involved in apoptosis?
    a. Aminopeptidases
    b. Caspases
    c. Metalloproteinases
    d. Phosphatases
    e. Reverse transcriptases

42. Which of the following studies best predicts whether renal functional recovery will occur after reconstruction of an obstructed kidney?
    a. Diuretic-mercaptoacetyltriglycine (MAG)-3 scan
    b. Diuretic–diethyltriaminepentaacetic acid (DTPA) scan
    c. Duplex ultrasonography of the kidneys
    d. Dimercaptosuccinic acid (DMSA) renogram
    e. Unenhanced magnetic resonance urogram

43. A 40-year-old man has anorexia, fatigue, and a serum creatinine value of 4.6 mg/dL. CT reveals severe bilateral hydronephrosis and a retroperitoneal soft tissue mass encasing the great vessels and ureters. The next step is:
    a. CT-guided biopsy of the mass.
    b. open surgical biopsy of the mass.
    c. placement of bilateral ureteral stents.
    d. corticosteroid therapy.
    e. ureterolysis.

44. Pelvic lipomatosis is associated with:
    a. cystitis glandularis.
    b. prostatic urethral elongation.
    c. bladder neck elevation.

d. extrinsic compression of the rectum.
e. all of the above.

45. Which of the following may cause either intrinsic or extrinsic obstruction of the ureter in women?
    a. Gravid uterus
    b. Endometriosis
    c. Tubo-ovarian abscess
    d. Ovarian remnant
    e. Fibroid uterus

46. A 69-year-old woman has bilateral ureteral obstruction secondary to locally invasive cervical cancer. What is the likelihood of stent failure within the first 3 months?
    a. 5%
    b. 15%
    c. 30%
    d. 50%
    e. 90%

47. A patient has asymptomatic unilateral, mild hydronephrosis 1 week after repair of an abdominal aortic aneurysm. Serum creatinine value is normal. The next step is:
    a. corticosteroid therapy.
    b. tamoxifen therapy.
    c. ureteral stent placement.
    d. exploratory laparotomy.
    e. observation with serial imaging.

48. In a patient with an obstructing ureteral stone, administration of nonsteroidal anti-inflammatory drugs will induce a reduction in all of the following EXCEPT:
    a. collecting system pressure.
    b. renal blood flow.
    c. renal aquaporin-2 water channels.
    d. diuresis.
    e. pain score.

49. A 55-year-old, otherwise healthy woman has a chronically obstructed left kidney and normal right kidney. Which differential renal function for the left kidney would best serve as a cutoff point below which nephrectomy should be performed and above which salvage should be considered?
    a. 5%
    b. 10%
    c. 25%
    d. 35%
    e. 45%

50. Angiotensin-converting enzyme (ACE) inhibitors or angiotensin receptor blockers attenuate the decrease in GFR caused by ureteral obstruction by reducing constriction at which level?
    a. Afferent arteriole
    b. Efferent arteriole
    c. Glomerular capillary
    d. Juxtaglomerular mesangial cell
    e. Renal artery

51. Postobstructive diuresis and natriuresis is seen more often following relief of BUO rather than UUO because:
    a. renal sodium transporters are decreased only during BUO.
    b. third-space sequestration of fluid is greater with UUO.
    c. atrial natriuretic peptide secretion decreases during UUO.
    d. contralateral increases in transporters attenuates natriuresis of UUO.
    e. greater increases in vasopressin (ADH) with BUO inhibit sodium transport.

ANSWERS

1. **a. Augmented extracellular matrix synthesis and growth of mesangial cells.** When the kidney enlarges in compensatory renal growth, there is augmented extracellular matrix synthesis and growth of mesangial cells (Kasinath et al, 2006; Sinuani et al, 2006).*

2. **c. Increased collagen and elastin in renal parenchyma.** Histopathologic findings may predict recovery of renal function. The presence of increased collagen and elastin in renal parenchyma at the time of pyeloplasty has been shown to have a negative impact on recovery of renal function (Kim et al, 2005; Kiratli et al, 2008).

3. **d. the comparative accuracy of all the three modalities ranges from 93% to 100%.**

4. **e. All the above** can be used to assess renal function. MRU has been demonstrated to have an excellent correlation with the renal isotope GFR in the adult (Abo El-Ghar-2 et al, 2008) and pediatric patients (Jones et al, 2008) with obstructed kidneys. The incorporation of intravenous administration of gadopentetate-DTPA has allowed a dynamic, functional assessment of the collecting system that correlates well with diuretic renal scintigraphy, yet provides far greater anatomic detail than nuclear studies. Differential GFR can be assessed with postimaging processing, and contrast washout can be measured to calculate renal clearance, differentiating dilated systems from obstructed systems (Rohrschneider et al, 2002; Chu et al, 2004).

5. **b. normal renal function.** The use of gadodiamide-based MRI in patients with renal insufficiency [GFR < 30 mL/min] has been seen to increase the risk of NSF. The risk of nephrogenic systemic fibrosis associated with the use of some gadolinium agents (especially gadodiamide) in patients with renal insufficiency [GFR < 30 mL/min] limit the utility of contrast MRI in such patients (Broome et al, 2007; Frokaier et al, 2007; Sadowski et al, 2007; Abo El-Ghar-2 et al, 2008).

6. **a. advanced cancer.** Ureteral stenting may not be as effective for treating patients with extrinsic ureteral obstruction. Docimo and Dewolf (1989) reported a mean 43% failure rate in ureteral stents placed for extrinsic ureteral obstruction, the majority related to malignancy. The association of stent failure and poor renal function has been reported by others (McCullough et al, 2008). The presence of extrinsic ureteral obstruction due to

bladder or prostatic pathology, especially advanced malignancies, is another risk factor for stent failure (Danilovic et al, 2005).

7. **d. hypertension occurs in up to one third of patients** (Klein et al, 1988; Heyns, 1991). Approximately one half of patients present with lower urinary tract symptoms and one quarter with bowel symptoms, typically constipation. Suprapubic, back, flank, or perineal discomfort can also be an initial clinical manifestation.

8. **e. All of the above.** There are various radiologic signs of pelvic lipomatosis. On plain film, increased pelvic lucency may be noted; proliferation of the mature unencapsulated pelvis fat may lead to severe bilateral hydroureteronephrosis. In contrast to retroperitoneal fibrosis, which usually affects the proximal and midureters, pelvic lipomatosis causes significant displacement of the distal ureters medially (Lin et al, 2007). CT may demonstrate pelvic fat and extrinsic compression of the rectum (Susmano and Dolin, 1979).

9. **d. involves the ureter in 15% to 20% of the cases.** The bladder is the most common organ involved when endometriosis afflicts the urinary tract.

10. **c. is only treated in the presence of ureteral obstruction.** The other options are incorrect.

11. **d. Internal iliac artery aneurysm.** An iliac artery aneurysm should be suspected, if a pulsatile mass is palpated on rectal examination (Marino et al, 1987). The diagnosis can be made with various imaging studies including ultrasonography, MRI, and CT.

12. **e. all of the above.** Unique infections can cause retroperitoneal fibrosis, such as tuberculosis, histoplasmosis, and actinomycosis. It can occur after abdominal or pelvic surgery as well as abdominal trauma. Radiation and systemic chemotherapy have also been reported to induce it (Fassina et al, 2006; Vaglio et al, 2006).

13. **a. Absence of pyelolymphatic flow.** Factors that have a positive influence on functional recovery include a smaller degree of obstruction, greater compliance of the collecting system, and presence of pyelolymphatic backflow (Shokeir et al, 2002). Conversely, older age and decreased renal cortical thickness are predictors of diminished recovery of renal function (Lutaif et al, 2003).

14. **b. uncorrected coagulopathy.** If the patient with obstructive uropathy has an uncorrectable coagulopathy or platelet abnormality, ureteral stenting is indicated. Compared with percutaneous nephrostomy placement, stent insertion may require greater x-ray exposure (Mokhmalji et al, 2001). This may be of concern in pregnant patients, particularly early in gestation when the fetus is most sensitive to radiation effects (McAleer and Loughlin, 2004). Percutaneous nephrostomy should be strongly considered if pyonephrosis is suspected.

15. **d. hysterectomy, bilateral salpingo-oophorectomy, and ureterolysis.**

16. **b. morphine.** Drugs suspected to cause retroperitoneal fibrosis include methysergide, hydralazine, reserpine, haloperidol, LSD, methyldopa, β blockers, ergotamine alkaloids, and amphetamines.

17. **b. usually self limited.** Postobstructive diuresis is generally self-limited and is generally associated with initial hyposthenuric urine. Release of obstruction can result in marked diuresis and natriuresis.

18. **a. angiotensin-II.** The release of TNF-α, a potent inflammatory cytokine, is stimulated by angiotensin,

---

*Sources referenced can be found in *Campbell-Walsh Urology, 10th Edition,* on the Expert Consult website.

especially in the first few hours of renal obstruction. It can upregulate its own expression as well as that of other inflammatory mediators, such as interleukin-1, platelet-activating factor, nitric oxide, eicosanoids, and cell adhesion molecules.

19. **a. Renal function impairment.** The term obstructive nephropathy should be reserved for the damage to the renal parenchyma that results from an obstruction to the flow of urine anywhere along the urinary tract. The term hydronephrosis implies dilatation of the renal pelvis and calyces and can occur without obstruction.

20. **a. Increased sodium excretion.** There is a profound increase in sodium excretion after relief of bilateral ureteral obstruction. This is due to ANP and perhaps reduced sodium transporters. The massive natriuresis enhances excretion of phosphate, potassium, and magnesium.

21. **d. Increased atrial natriuretic peptide (ANP).** The accumulation of extracellular volume stimulates the synthesis and release of ANP, which promotes increased GFR and sodium excretion. Decreases in the aquaporin water channels in the kidney further promote the diuresis.

22. **c. Shift of blood flow from the outer to the inner cortex.** There is a shift of blood flow from the outer to inner cortex with UUO that is opposite to that which is seen with BUO. At the 5-hour interval of UUO, there is a reduction in renal plasma flow and GFR that results in diminished sodium delivery to the macula densa.

23. **b. Increase in afferent arteriolar dilation.** By promoting dilation of the afferent arteriole and constriction of the efferent arteriole, ANP increases GFR. It also decreases the sensitivity of tubuloglomerular feedback, inhibits renin release, and increases the ultrafiltration coefficient.

24. **a. Shift of blood flow to the outer renal cortex.** There is a shift of blood flow to the outer renal cortex with BUO in contrast to the reversed pattern with UUO.

25. **b. Increase in expression of transforming growth factor-β.** There is increased expression of TGF-β with obstruction that contributes to an increase in the extracellular matrix of the kidney and promotes inflammation. TGF-β is activated by angiotensin II, and animal models have demonstrated that pharmacologic methods of inhibiting angiotensin II reduces the fibrosis occurring after obstruction.

26. **a. fractional excretion of sodium after relief of obstruction is greater in BUO.** The increased fractional excretion of sodium in BUO is due to volume expansion, resulting in increased levels of ANP and the overall increased solute load.

27. **d. Hypertrophic and hyperplastic growth occur.** Compensatory renal growth of the unaffected kidney has been demonstrated, and animal models indicate that both hyperplastic and hypertrophic growth can occur. These growth patterns may depend on the age of the subject. Insulin-like growth factor-1 is thought to stimulate this event. It is more prominent in the immature kidney. Animal models have demonstrated that glomerular number does not increase during this process.

28. **a. early relief of obstruction.** Although the other distractors influence recovery of renal function after release of obstruction, prompt eradication of obstruction provides the best approach for salvage.

29. **b. Reduced Na⁺, K⁺-ATPase.** Obstruction results in a reduction in sodium transporters, including Na^+, K^+-ATPase.

It also promotes tubulointerstitial fibrosis, reduction in aquaporin channels, and acidification defects. The collecting system pressure should not be increased at this point.

30. **e. all of the above.** All of the factors listed may contribute to a reduction in sodium transporters.

31. **d. decreased renal aquaporin-2 water channels.** The concentrating defect that occurs with obstruction is not due to inadequate levels of ADH. Choices b, c, and e result in enhanced concentrating ability, whereas a reduction in aquaporin-2 water channels does the opposite.

32. **b. decreased synthesis of aquaporins.** Li and coworkers (2001) showed that the polyuria after release of BUO correlated with a decreased expression of aquaporins 1, 2, and 3. Over a 30-day period, the expressions of AQP-2 and -3 gradually normalized, but the expression of AQP-1 remained decreased. The reduced rate of synthesis and mobilization of water channels into the nephron membranes accounts for a decreased response to exogenous vasopressin or cyclic AMP.

33. **d. increase over an hour and then steadily decrease.** Renal blood flow initially rises in the first phase, because of afferent arteriolar vasodilatation. In phase 2, efferent arteriolar constriction keeps ureteral pressure elevated, but in phase 3, both preglomerular and postglomerular vasoconstriction reduces renal blood flow and ureteral pressure.

34. **c. an increase followed by a decrease.** The first phase is characterized by a rise in both ureteral pressure and renal blood flow lasting 1 to 1.5 hours. This is followed by a decline in renal blood flow (RBF) and a continued increase in ureteral (tubular) pressure lasting until the 5th hour of occlusion. The final phase involves a further decline in RBF and a progressive decline in ureteral pressure.

35. **d. Prostaglandin and nitric oxide.** Studies during the early, vasodilatory phase of UUO have shown that the increase in RBF can be prevented by prostaglandin synthesis inhibitors, such as indomethacin or other nonsteroidal anti-inflammatory drugs (NSAIDs). Intravenous administration of indomethacin before ureteral ligation results in a decline in renal blood flow without the initial vasodilatation. In addition, administration of nitric oxide (NO) synthesis inhibitors, such as N-nitro-L-arginine methyl ester (L-NAME) or N-monomethyl-L-arginine (L-NMMA), attenuates the initial rise in RBF with occlusion in rats, and when L-NMMA was discontinued, the rise in RBF was restored in 10 minutes. These findings provide evidence for a role of prostaglandins and nitric oxide in reducing preglomerular afferent arteriolar vascular resistance in the early phase of UUO.

36. **e. Thromboxane A₂.** In the vasoconstrictive established phase of UUO, inhibitors of thromboxane synthesis have shown reduced vasoconstriction, reduced renal TxB_2 production, the stable metabolite of TxA_2, and an increase in the ratio of prostacyclin to thromboxane production. Administration of a thromboxane receptor blocker also improved renal function in rats after 24 hours of UUO.

37. **b. Greater expansion of extracellular volume with BUO than with UUO.** With bilateral obstruction, the contralateral renal unit does not have the opportunity for compensation as with UUO. Extracellular volume may be greatly expanded so that postobstructive diuresis is most commonly seen in this type of obstruction. After relief of BUO, the increased extracellular volume with attendant salt

and water buildup, urea and other osmolytes, and increased production of atrial natriuretic peptide and potentially other natriuretic substances all contribute to a profound natriuresis and a fractional excretion for sodium that is greater than after relief of UUO.

38. **b. Decreased H⁺-ATPase expression in the collecting duct.** The cumulative evidence shows a major acidification defect in the distal nephron. Release of obstruction does not result in bicarbonaturia, indicating that proximal reclamation remains intact. There is a defect in the proximal handling and breakdown of glutamine, which means that a higher proportion of protons are buffered as titratable acid. The best evidence indicates a defect in the expression of H⁺-ATPase in the collecting duct. Even so, because there is a deficit in filtered and excreted phosphate, fewer protons can be buffered by phosphate so that the pH of the urine may be lower in spite of a total net decrease in H⁺ secretion.

39. **d. Ratio of lactate to pyruvate in renal tissue.** Obstruction causes a shift from oxidative metabolism to anaerobic respiration. This results in a reduction of renal ATP levels and an increase in the renal lactate to pyruvate ratio. The proximal tubule has relatively little glycolytic capacity and uses ketone bodies, fatty acids, glutamine, and lactate for mitochondrial ATP synthesis. The proximal convoluted tubule cannot use glucose for oxidative metabolism.

40. **e. All of the above.** See Figure 37–3 in *Campbell-Walsh Urology, 9th Edition,* for an overview of the processes leading to inflammation and increased matrix synthesis and components of fibrosis. Tubule cells, macrophages, and fibroblasts all contribute to the fibrotic process. The mediators of angiotensin II, growth factors, and cytokines contribute to the process and offer opportunities for pharmacologic intervention.

41. **b. Caspases.** Cysteinyl aspartate–specific proteinases (caspases) are known to mediate apoptotic cell death in obstructed kidneys. This is a family of 12 enzymes, and caspase 3 and 8 are best correlated with renal cell apoptosis. Increases in TNF-α and binding of its two receptors initiate events along with stimulation of NF-κB. Growth factors modify the process and offer opportunities for therapeutic intervention.

42. **d. Dimercaptosuccinic acid (DMSA) renogram.** The DMSA renogram has been shown to be superior to DTPA or MAG-3 for the prediction of renal recovery (Thompson and Gough, 2001). Although some have successfully used these other radiotracers to predict functional recovery, the cortical phase of the renogram is the critical factor. Doppler ultrasonography and magnetic resonance urography (MRU) have not been demonstrated to predict renal recovery.

43. **c. placement of bilateral ureteral stents.** In the acutely ill patient, initial therapy should be directed at draining the obstructed kidneys. Biopsy should be undertaken after metabolic stabilization. An underlying malignancy may be present in 8% to 10% of cases of suspected retroperitoneal fibrosis. This is most commonly obtained percutaneously, but open surgical biopsy may be necessary. Definitive therapy of retroperitoneal fibrosis, whether medical or surgical, should be delayed until after adequate drainage has been obtained and malignancy has been excluded.

44. **e. all of the above.** Cystitis glandularis is present in 40% of patients with pelvic lipomatosis. Elongation of the prostatic urethra and elevation of the bladder neck are commonly encountered mechanical effects of the pelvic lipomatosis and may preclude rigid cystoscopy. Hence, the urologist should be aware of these and be prepared to perform flexible cystoscopy if needed. Extrinsic compression of the rectum has also been identified in these patients.

45. **b. Endometriosis.** In the female patient, the gravid uterus, endometrial implants, a tubo-ovarian abscess, an ovarian remnant, and fibroids all may cause extrinsic compression and obstruction of the ureter. The ureter is involved in 15% to 20% of endometriosis cases of the urinary tract. In addition to extrinsic obstruction, ureteral implants may involve the ureteral lumen and cause intrinsic obstruction.

46. **d. 50%.** Ureteral stenting is recognized to be less effective in the management of extrinsic ureteral obstruction, particularly when it is due to malignancy. In a prospective study, a 56% failure rate was noted at 3 months. A similar study noted that over 40% of those stents that ultimately failed had failed within 6 days of initial placement. If ureteral stenting is performed in patients with extrinsic obstruction due to malignancy, close follow-up is warranted.

47. **e. observation with serial imaging.** Hydronephrosis in the early postoperative period is common and resolves spontaneously in a majority of these patients. Intervention may be required, if symptoms arise or renal functional impairment is noted.

48. **c. renal aquaporin-2 water channels.** NSAIDs have been shown to significantly reduce pain in patients treated for acute ureteral obstruction. NSAIDs have also been demonstrated to reduce renal blood flow and collecting system pressure. This may contribute to the reduction in diuresis seen after relief of obstruction. An additional mechanism for the reduced collecting system pressure and reduced diuresis is an NSAID-mediated preservation of aquaporin-2 water channels, preventing the downregulation of aquaporin-2 channels otherwise seen in the obstructive setting.

49. **b. 10%.** The usual cutoff point for nephrectomy is 10% or less of total renal function being supplied by the affected kidney. This has not been prospectively studied but is based on common clinical practice, and, as such, this must be tempered by clinical insight into the overall status of the patient.

50. **a. Afferent arteriole.** Reduced preglomerular resistance increases glomerular capillary pressure and filtration rate.

51. **d. contralateral increases in transporters attenuates natriuresis of UUO.** Diuresis and natriuresis occurs primarily after release of BUO because volume expansion, release of ANP, and decreases in the tubular sodium transporters all occur. With UUO, transporter synthesis increases in the unobstructed kidney to help compensate and reduce excretory losses in the obstructed kidney.

Additional Study Points

1. With unilateral ureteral obstruction, renal blood flow increases during the first 1 to 2 hours. It begins to decrease at 3 to 4 hours and markedly declines after 5 hours of obstruction.

2. The increase in renal blood flow in unilateral ureteral obstruction is a result of relaxation of afferent arterials in which PGE_2 and nitrous oxide play a role.

3. Reduction in whole-kidney GFR after prolonged obstruction is due to afferent arteriolar vaso-constriction mediated by the renin-angiotensin system. Thus angiotensin II is an important mediator of reduced renal blood flow in the second and third phases of ureteral obstruction. Moreover, thromboxane A_2 may also contribute.

4. In bilateral ureteral obstruction, there is a modest increase in renal blood flow lasting approximately 2 hours, followed by a profound decline in renal blood flow.

5. In unilateral ureteral obstruction there is a shift of blood flow from the outer cortex to inner cortex. In bilateral ureteral obstruction, the shift is in the opposite direction toward the outer cortex.

6. With the release of bilateral obstruction, a postobstructive diuresis may occur that is much greater than in unilateral ureteral obstruction due to accumulated solutes and volume expansion.

7. Partial neonatal obstruction may impair nephrogenesis.

8. Following complete ureteral obstruction, urine is reabsorbed by (1) extravasation at the calyceal fornix, (2) pyelo-venous backflow, (3) pyelolymphatic backflow, and (4) tubular reabsorption.

9. Following obstruction, there is a disregulation of the aquaporin water channels in the proximal tubule, descending loop, and collecting duct, which may contribute to long-term polyuria.

10. The excretion of sodium following the relief of bilateral ureteral obstruction is greater than after unilateral ureteral obstruction, because in bilateral obstruction there is retention of sodium, water, urea, and other osmotic substances and an increase of atrial natriuretic factor, all of which stimulate a profound natriuresis.

11. Obstruction causes a defect in urinary acidification in the distal tubule involving a defect in ammonium production.

12. Compensatory renal growth decreases progressively with increasing age. While the kidney does enlarge, there is not an increase in nephrons or number of glomeruli after birth.

13. Functional recovery has been reported as long as 150 days following relief of unilateral ureteral obstruction.

14. Older age and decreased cortical thickness are predictors of diminished recovery following relief of obstruction.

15. Recovery of renal function following relief of obstruction is affected by the duration, the degree, the patient's age, baseline renal function, collecting system compliance, and infection.

16. Chronic ureteral obstruction leads to renal inflammation, increased extracellular matrix formation, tubulointerstitial fibrosis, and apoptosis of renal tubules, thus limiting the potential for return of renal function.

17. Ureteral obstruction may result in prolonged decreases in concentrating ability, urinary acidification, and electrolyte transport long after the obstruction is released.

18. A Whitaker test requires a fixed rate of infusion of 10 mL/min into the renal pelvis. A catheter is placed in the bladder. After equilibration, a renal pelvic pressure less than 15 cm of water is considered normal. A pressure greater than 22 cm of water is considered obstructed, and a pressure of 15 to 22 cm of water is equivocal.

19. For diuretic renograms a half-time of less than 10 min is normal; a half-time greater than 20 min is obstructed, and between 10 and 20 min is equivocal.

20. Postobstructive diuresis is a result of (1) a physiologic diuresis that involves volume expansion and solute accumulation and (2) a pathologic diuresis that involves derangements of the medullary gradient and transport processes for solutes in the renal tubule.

21. Distended bladders should be expeditiously decompressed. There is no role for gradual decompression, because this does not limit hematuria or postobstructive diuresis.

22. Retroperitoneal fibrosis usually extends from the renal hilum to the pelvic brim. It is composed of a fibrous component and a cellular component with lymphocytes, macrophages, plasma cells, and eosinophils in varying degrees of abundance. It is more common in males than females, with a 3:1 ratio, and an underlying malignancy must always be ruled out. Ureters are deviated medially.

23. An F-18 FDG-PET scan may be helpful in indicating the degree of inflammation in the retroperitoneal process, which would then predict a better response to therapy.

24. Medications that have been used for treatment of retroperitoneal fibrosis include tamoxifen, azathioprine, and cyclophosphamide along with steroids.

25. Pelvic lipomatosis occurs predominantly in blacks, with a strong male predisposition.

26. Proliferative cystitis and cystitis glandularis are frequently found in patients with pelvic lipomatosis.

27. Obstruction in pregnancy is more common on the right and is due to mechanical compression, as well as the hormonal influence of progesterone.

28. Aneurysms may cause obstruction of the ureter due to perianeurysmal fibrosis and inflammation. When the aneurysm is repaired, the inflammatory process may resolve spontaneously, thus relieving the obstruction.

Management of Upper Urinary Tract Obstruction

Stephen Y. Nakada, MD ● Thomas H.S. Hsu, MD

QUESTIONS

1. Ureteropelvic junction (UPJ) obstruction in the neonate is most frequently found as a result of:
   a. maternal-fetal ultrasonography.
   b. voiding cystourethrography.
   c. diuretic renography.
   d. abdominal radiography.
   e. physical examination.

2. Which study is diagnostic for functional obstruction at the UPJ?
   a. Retrograde pyelography
   b. Three-dimensional helical CT
   c. Diuretic renography
   d. Renal ultrasound
   e. Renal angiography

3. A 62-year-old man presents with left flank pain. Intravenous pyelography reveals delayed excretion and hydronephrosis to the level of a 2.5-cm calculus at the UPJ. Percutaneous stone extraction is accomplished without difficulty, but a postextraction nephrostogram reveals hydronephrosis to the level of the UPJ without residual stone. A follow-up nephrostogram 1 week later is unchanged. The best next step is:
   a. removal of the nephrostomy tube.
   b. diuretic renography.
   c. CT angiography.
   d. antegrade endopyelotomy.
   e. Whitaker pressure-perfusion test.

4. The condition most predictive of failure after percutaneous endopyelotomy is:
   a. renal ptosis.
   b. ipsilateral stones.
   c. ipsilateral renal function.
   d. moderate to severe hydronephrosis.
   e. chronic flank pain.

5. A 27-year-old woman has right flank pain, and her diuretic renography reveals UPJ obstruction and a differential renal function of 75:25 (L:R). The next best step is:
   a. CT angiography.
   b. stent placement.

   c. endopyelotomy.
   d. laparoscopic pyeloplasty.
   e. laparoscopic nephrectomy.

6. The highest failure rate in treating UPJ obstruction is associated with:
   a. antegrade endopyelotomy.
   b. retrograde ureteroscopic endopyelotomy.
   c. balloon dilation.
   d. pyeloplasty.
   e. cautery balloon incision.

7. The most appropriate location for endoscopic incision of a proximal ureteral stricture is:
   a. lateral.
   b. anterior.
   c. medial.
   d. posterior.
   e. anterolateral.

8. The best treatment option for a patient with a functional left ureteroenteric anastomotic stricture is:
   a. metallic stent.
   b. balloon dilation.
   c. laser endoureterotomy.
   d. cautery wire balloon incision.
   e. open repair.

9. The most common cause of retroperitoneal fibrosis is:
   a. methysergide.
   b. infection.
   c. lymphoma.
   d. breast cancer.
   e. immune-mediated aortitis.

10. Retrocaval ureter results from:
    a. persistence of posterior cardinal veins.
    b. persistence of anterior cardinal veins.
    c. duplication of inferior vena cava.
    d. aberrance of lumbar veins.
    e. retroaortic renal veins.

11. Transperitoneal laparoscopic pyeloplasty:
    a. is used rarely compared with retroperitoneal approach.
    b. does not require water-tight, tension-free anastomosis.

c. provides more working space than that in the retroperitoneal approach.

d. provides unfamiliar anatomy.

e. does not require an external surgical drain.

12. Surgical repair of ureteropelvic junction obstruction requires:

a. a funnel-shaped transition between the renal pelvis and ureter.

b. dependent drainage.

c. water-tight anastomosis.

d. tension-free anastomosis.

e. all of the above.

13. Contraindications for transureteroureterostomy include a history of:

a. retroperitoneal fibrosis.

b. urothelial malignancy.

c. nephrolithiasis.

d. a, b, and c.

e. b and c.

14. A 25-year-old man presents with right flank pain. He underwent a laparoscopic pyeloplasty, which failed within 1 year. Consequently, he underwent failed endopyelotomy. A CT scan shows moderate cortical loss in the right kidney with a normal-appearing left kidney. A renogram reveals 35% differential function on the affected side, and a diuretic study demonstrates functional obstruction ($T_{1/2}$ > 30 min). The next step is:

a. chronic internal ureteral stent.

b. ileal ureter.

c. Davis intubated ureterotomy.

d. ureterocalicostomy.

e. renal autotransplantation.

15. Spiral flap procedures for UPJ obstruction are used:

a. to bridge a shorter length stenosis.

b. to treat crossing vessels.

c. to bridge a longer length stenosis.

d. for a small, intrarenal pelvis.

e. only in the presence of greater than 30% ipsilateral renal function.

16. Foley Y-V plasty is a suitable approach when encountering:

a. high ureteral insertion.

b. small intrarenal pelvis.

c. anterior crossing vessel.

d. duplication of collecting system.

e. redundant renal pelvis.

17. Which type of pyeloplasty is suitable when there is an aberrant crossing vessel?

a. Foley Y-V plasty

b. Culp-DeWeerd spiral flap

c. Dismembered pyeloplasty

d. Scardino-Prince vertical flap

e. Ligation and transection of the crossing vessel

18. Ileal ureter can be performed in the face of:

a. renal insufficiency (serum creatinine >2 mg/dL).

b. inflammatory bowel disease.

c. bladder dysfunction.

d. radiation enteritis.

e. small intrarenal pelvis.

19. A 55-year-old woman underwent left transperitoneal laparoscopic dismembered pyeloplasty over an internal ureteral stent. An abdominal drain was placed at surgery, and there was minimal drain output during the first 24 hours after surgery. Within 3 hours after Foley catheter removal, the patient's nurse noted a significant amount of fluid coming out of the drain site. The next step is to:

a. change dressings frequently and continue observation.

b. replace the urethral catheter.

c. restrict fluid intake.

d. remove the surgical drain.

e. change the ureteral stent.

20. In performing a psoas hitch, additional bladder mobility can be achieved by transection of the:

a. contralateral superior vesical artery.

b. ipsilateral inferior vesical artery.

c. contralateral inferior vesical artery.

d. ipsilateral superior vesical artery.

e. ipsilateral gonadal artery.

21. A 40-year-old woman with a history of hypertension and recurrent nephrolithiasis presents with a 5-cm proximal right ureteral stricture following an iatrogenic injury in a recent abdominal surgery. She has had an indwelling right nephrostomy tube for more than 6 months. Her baseline serum creatinine is 2.5 mg/dL. Renal scan shows split function of 65% in the right kidney. Her bladder capacity is found to be less than 300 mL. The next step is:

a. ureteroureterostomy.

b. Boari flap.

c. transureteroureterostomy.

d. ileal ureteral substitution.

e. autotransplantion.

22. During a psoas hitch, the structure particularly susceptible to injury is the:

a. obturator nerve.

b. iliohypogastric nerve.

c. ilioinguinal nerve.

d. sacral nerve.

e. genitofemoral nerve.

23. The technique that does not require normal bladder capacity, drainage, and function is the:

a. ileal ureteral substitution.

b. psoas hitch.

c. ureteroneocystostomy.

d. endoscopic incision of transmural ureter.

e. Boari flap.

Imaging

1. See Figure 41–1.

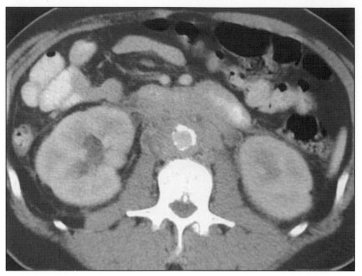

Figure 41–1.

A 72-year-old man with malaise has this CT scan. The serum creatinine is mildly elevated. What is the best diagnosis?

a. Retroperitoneal fibrosis
b. Retroperitoneal hematoma
c. Tuberculosis
d. Retroperitoneal sarcoma
e. Perianeurysmal fibrosis

ANSWERS

1. **a. maternal-fetal ultrasonography.** The current widespread use of maternal ultrasonography has led to a dramatic increase in the number of asymptomatic newborns being diagnosed with hydronephrosis, many of whom are subsequently found to have ureteropelvic junction obstruction.

2. **c. Diuretic renography.** Provocative testing with a diuretic urogram may allow accurate diagnosis of UPJ obstruction. Renal ultrasound, CT scan, and retrograde pyelogram give anatomic assessments of the UPJ without quantitatively assessing urinary drainage and function.

3. **e. Whitaker pressure-perfusion test.** When there remains doubt as to the clinical significance of a dilated collecting system, placement of percutaneous nephrostomy allows access for pressure perfusion studies. In the pressure perfusion test, as first described by Whitaker in 1973 and then modified in 1978, the renal pelvis is perfused with normal saline or dilute radiographic contrast solution and the pressure gradient across the presumed area of obstruction is determined. Renal pelvic pressures in excess of 15 to 22 cm are highly suggestive of a functional obstruction. Although diuretic renography is useful for diagnosis as well, the Whitaker test is ideal for this situation because a nephrostomy tube is already in situ.

4. **d. moderate to severe hydronephrosis.** Consideration of any of the less invasive alternatives to open operative intervention must take into account individual anatomy including, but not limited to, the degree of hydronephrosis, overall and ipsilateral renal function, and, in some cases, the presence of crossing vessels or concomitant calculi. One

study found that endopyelotomy success rates were less than 50% when significant hydronephrosis and crossing vessels were identified preoperatively.

5. **b. laparoscopic pyeloplasty.** Evidence indicates that crossing vessels lower the success rate of endopyelotomy from several investigators. When such patients were culled from the pool of candidates available for treatment of UPJ obstruction, endopyelotomy success rates improved in most studies. A CT angiography would be necessary to assess this. However, laparoscopic pyeloplasty would be a straightforward minimally invasive option for this young patient. The kidney has too much function to remove at this stage.

6. **c. balloon dilation.** McClinton reported long-term follow-up data on balloon dilation of the UPJ, finding a success rate of only 42%, which was significantly lower than the initial publications would indicate.

7. **c. lateral.** Proximal ureteral strictures are incised laterally, similar to UPJ strictures. Posterior incision is offered to UPJ obstruction patients who have failed open pyeloplasty. Distal strictures are incised anteriorly, as are strictures of the middle ureter.

8. **e. open repair.** Several studies have linked poor outcomes with endoscopic management of left ureteroenteric strictures. This may be a result of diminished blood flow to the ureter because the left ureter requires more mobilization than the right side at the time of diversion. Although metallic stents show promise in limited studies, using open repair, reports demonstrate an 80% success.

9. **e. immune-mediated aortitis.** Growing evidence indicates that the majority of cases of retroperitoneal fibrosis are, in fact, immune-mediated aortitis. Regardless, the other conditions are relatively rare causes of retroperitoneal fibrosis.

10. **a. persistence of posterior cardinal veins.** Retrocaval ureter results from the persistence of the posterior cardinal veins.

11. **c. it provides more working space than that in the retroperitoneal approach.** Transperitoneal laparoscopic pyeloplasty provides a larger working space relative to a retroperitoneoscopic approach. Together with more familiar anatomy, the transperitoneal approach is used most commonly in the laparoscopic urologic community to date.

12. **e. all of the above.** For any surgical repair of UPJ obstruction, the resultant anastomosis should be widely patent and completed in a watertight fashion without tension. In addition, the reconstructed UPJ should allow a funnel-shaped transition between the pelvis and the ureter that is in a position of dependent drainage.

13. **d. a, b and c.** Relative contraindications include history of nephrolithiasis, retroperitoneal fibrosis, urothelial malignancy, chronic pyelonephritis, and abdominopelvic radiation.

14. **d. ureterocalicostomy.** Direct anastomosis of the proximal ureter to the lower calyceal system is a well-accepted salvage technique for the failed pyeloplasty and small renal pelvis.

15. **c. to bridge a longer length stenosis.** Flap procedures can be useful in situations involving a relatively long segment of ureteral narrowing or stricture. Of the various flap procedures, a spiral flap can bridge a strictured or narrow area of longer length. The flap procedures are not appropriate in the setting of crossing vessels.

16. **a. high ureteral insertion.** The Foley Y-V-plasty is designed for repair of a UPJ obstruction secondary to a high ureteral insertion. It is specifically contraindicated when transposition of lower pole vessels is necessary. In situations requiring concomitant reduction of redundant renal pelvis, this technique is also of little value.

17. **c. Dismembered pyeloplasty.** In the presence of crossing aberrant or accessory lower pole renal vessels associated with UPJ obstruction, a dismembered pyeloplasty is the only method to allow transposition of the UPJ in relation to these vessels.

18. **e. small intrarenal pelvis.** In ileal segment usage, a small intrarenal pelvis is not contraindicated and an ileocalycostomy can be performed successfully.

19. **b. replace the urethral catheter.** If the drain output increases following the removal of the Foley catheter, the catheter should be replaced for several days to avoid vesicoureteral reflux up the stent in the operated ureter and decrease urinary extravasation.

20. **a. contralateral superior vesical artery.** In psoas hitch, transection of the contralateral superior vesical artery can be helpful to bridge the gap to the ipsilateral ureteral end, thereby achieving tension-free anastomosis.

21. **e. autotransplant.** Ureteroureterostomy is inappropriate for a 5-cm upper ureteral defect. Boari flap is inappropriate for a small bladder capacity. Transureteroureterostomy is contraindicated in the patient with a history of recurrent nephrolithiasis. Ileal ureter is contraindicated in the presence of elevated serum creatinine above 2 mg/dL. Autotransplant is appropriate for this particular patient.

22. **e. genitofemoral nerve.** The genitofemoral nerve courses over the psoas muscle.

23. **d. endoscopic incision of transmural ureter.** Normal bladder function without significant outlet obstruction is crucial to the success of ileal ureteral substitution, psoas hitch, Boari flap, and ureteroneocystostomy.

Imaging

1. **a. Retroperitoneal fibrosis.** There is increased soft tissue in the retroperitoneum, which obscures and effaces the planes between the inferior vena cava and the aorta. Tuberculosis causes calcification and stricturing in the kidneys and collecting systems, and tuberculous iliopsoas abscess extends along the iliopsoas muscles. Retroperitoneal hematoma and sarcoma are not centered solely around the aorta and the IVC. In perianeurysmal fibrosis, a retroperitoneal fibrosis-like picture occurs in association with an abdominal aortic aneurysm; the aorta is of normal caliber in this case.

Additional Study Points

1. Intrinsic UPJ obstruction is a result of an aperistaltic segment in which the normal spiral arrangement of the muscle bundles is replaced by longitudinal muscle bundles and fibrous tissue.

2. A crossing vessel has the most detrimental effect on the success of an endopyelotomy.

3. UPJ obstruction may coexist with vesicoureteral reflux.

4. A multicystic kidney is distinguished from a UPJ obstruction on ultrasound by the "cyst" being connected in hydronephrosis as opposed to being distinct in a multicystic dysplastic kidney.

5. A Whittaker test is performed by perfusing the renal pelvis at 10 mL/minute. Pressures less than 15 cm of water suggest a nonobstructed system. Pressures greater than 22 cm of water suggest an obstructed system, and pressures between the two are indeterminate.

6. The indications for repair of a UPJ include symptoms, impairment of renal function, stones, infection, and hypertension.

7. In neonates, unilateral hydronephrosis when carefully followed results in 7% of patients requiring a pyeloplasty.

8. Generally, kidneys with less than 15% function are not salvageable in adult patients.

9. A long segment stricture (>2 cm) is generally not successfully managed by the endopyelotomy method. An endopyelotomy cannot be performed safely by any route until access across the UPJ is established.

10. The majority of endopyelotomy failures occur within the first year. Success rates for endopyelotomy range between 60% and 80%.

11. High-grade hydroureteronephrosis and crossing vessels have a detrimental effect on the success rate of endopyelotomy.

12. When bleeding occurs following an endopyelotomy, one should have a low threshold to precede to angiography to thrombose the severed vessel.

13. Seventy percent of failures following laparoscopic pyeloplasty occur in the first 2 years.

14. When repairing a retrocaval ureter, the ureter is transected and relocated ventral to the vena cava.

15. Lower ureteral strictures are incised in an anterior medial direction; upper ureteral strictures are incised in a lateral or posterior lateral direction.

16. With ureteral strictures, one must always rule out malignancy.

17. There is no significant difference in preserving renal function in the adult when reimplanting the ureter into the bladder by either a refluxing or antirefluxing method.

18. Most patients with long-term urinary conduits will have an element of hydronephrosis that is not secondary to obstruction.

19. Retroperitoneal fibrosis secondary to malignancy is often indistinguishable from idiopathic retroperitoneal fibrosis and can be identified only with appropriate biopsy that identifies islands of tumor cells.

20. The initial management of retroperitoneal fibrosis is generally with steroids. Steroids are more likely to be beneficial if there is evidence of active inflammation as indicated by an elevated erythrocyte sedimentation rate, leukocytosis, and infiltration of lymphocytes on biopsy.

21. In addition to steroids, azathioprine, cyclophosphamide, cyclosporine, colchicine, and tamoxifen have been used with some success.

Upper Urinary Tract Trauma

Richard A. Santucci, MD • Leo R. Doumanian, MD

QUESTIONS

1. What method is used to perform "one-shot" intraoperative intravenous pyelography (IVP) in a 50-kg woman?
   a. Inject a 50-mL bolus of intravenous contrast agent followed by a full IVP series including abdominal compression to evaluate the ureters.
   b. Inject a 100-mL bolus of intravenous contrast agent followed in exactly 10 minutes by a flat plate of the abdomen on the operating room table.
   c. Inject a 50-mL bolus of intravenous contrast agent followed in exactly 10 minutes by a flat plate of the abdomen on the operating room table.
   d. Determine the patient's serum creatinine level before administration of intravenous contrast agent to make sure that he or she will not experience renal failure as a result of reaction to the contrast agent.
   e. Inject 100 mL of intravenous contrast and obtain a kidney, ureter, bladder (KUB) film 20 minutes following injection.

2. What is the best option for repair of midureteral transection after a stab wound?
   a. Ureteroureterostomy
   b. Transureteroureterostomy
   c. Boari flap
   d. Nephrectomy
   e. Cutaneous ureterostomy

3. When ureteroureterostomy is performed, which of the following is required?
   a. Postoperative retroperitoneal penrose drain
   b. Postoperative nephrostomy drain
   c. Spatulated, watertight repair
   d. Nonabsorbable sutures
   e. Intraperitonealization of the ureteral anastomosis

4. Which maneuver is cited as a cause of ureteral injury during stone basketing?
   a. Ureteroscopy without dilating the ureteral orifice first
   b. Ureteroscopy in nondilated systems

   c. Use of the holmium laser
   d. Pulsatile saline irrigation to assist visualization
   e. Persistence in stone basketing attempts in the face of a ureteral tear

5. Which of the following is a contraindication to transureteroureterostomy for repair of significant lower ureter injury?
   a. History of urolithiasis
   b. History of ureteral trauma
   c. Obesity
   d. Neurogenic bladder
   e. Spinal fracture

6. What is the treatment of choice for a ureteral contusion by a high-velocity bullet?
   a. Observation
   b. Ureteral stent placement
   c. Transureteroureterostomy
   d. Ureteroureterostomy
   e. Oversewing the contusion with healthy ureteral tissue

7. Which imaging technique is most useful for detecting ureteral injuries after trauma?
   a. CT without use of contrast material
   b. CT with use of contrast agent, obtained immediately after injection of the contrast agent
   c. CT with the use of contrast material, obtained 20 minutes after injection of the contrast agent
   d. Intravenous pyelography
   e. Furosemide (Lasix) renography

8. Which of the following statements is TRUE about ureteral injuries during laparoscopy?
   a. The total number of injuries has stayed steady over the years.
   b. Surgery for endometriosis greatly increases the risk.
   c. Bipolar cautery use during tubal ligation eliminates risk.
   d. Most ureteral injuries are recognized immediately.
   e. Indigo carmine dye eliminates the risk of injury.

Imaging

1. See Figure 42–1.

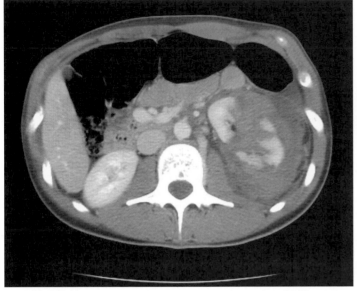

Figure 42–1.

A 22-year-old woman has this CT scan after a motor vehicle accident. Her vital signs are stable, and there are no other significant injuries.

The next step is:

a. open surgical repair of the kidney.

b. delayed imaging to evaluate the collecting system.

c. left nephrectomy to avoid future complications.

d. renal artery embolization.

e. intravenous urogram.

2. See Figure 42–2.

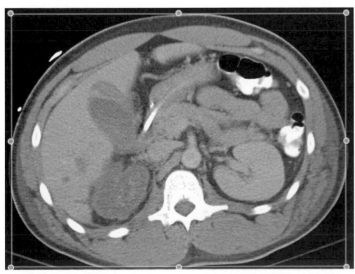

Figure 42–2.

A 24-year-old man undergoes this CT scan 36 hours after a motor vehicle accident. The most likely diagnosis is:

a. ureteral injury.

b. segmental renal artery transection.

c. main renal artery occlusion.

d. ureteropelvic junction disruption.

e. traumatic renal vein occlusion.

3. See Figure 42–3.

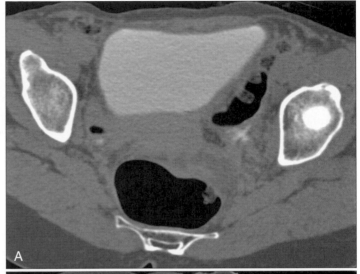

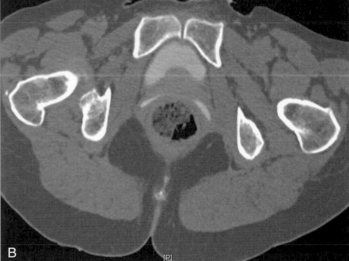

Figure 42–3.

A 36-year-old woman presents with increased vaginal discharge 3 weeks after an abdominal hysterectomy. On the axial CT images in the delayed excretory phase, the most likely diagnosis is:

a. vesico vaginal fistula.

b. ureterovaginal fistula.

c. colovesical fistula.

d. ureteral duplication.

e. vesicocutaneous fistula.

ANSWERS

1. **b. Inject a 100-mL bolus of intravenous contrast agent followed in exactly 10 minutes by a flat plate of the abdomen on the operating room table.** Only a single film is taken 10 minutes after intravenous injection (IV push) of 2 mL/kg of contrast material.

2. **a. Ureteroureterostomy.** Ureteroureterostomy, so-called end-to-end repair in injuries to the upper two thirds of the

ureter, is common (up to 32% of one large series) and has a reported success rate as high as 90%.

3. **c. Spatulated, watertight repair.** Repair ureters under magnification with spatulated, tension-free, stented, watertight anastomosis and place a retroperitoneal closed suction drain.

4. **e. Persistence in stone basketing attempts in the face of a ureteral tear.** One factor cited as a cause of injury was the persistence in stone basket attempts after recognition of a ureteral tear. Current recommendations are to stop and place a ureteral stent.

5. **a. History of urolithiasis.** This operation is contraindicated in patients with a history of urothelial calculi.

6. **d. Ureteroureterostomy.** Ureteral contusions, although the most "minor" of ureteral injuries, often heal with stricture or break down later if microvascular injury results in ureteral necrosis. Severe or large areas of contusion should be treated with excision and ureteroureterostomy.

7. **c. CT with the use of contrast material, obtained 20 minutes after injection of the contrast agent.** Because modern helical CT scanners can obtain images before intravenous contrast dye is excreted in the urine, delayed images must be obtained (5 to 20 minutes after contrast material injection) to allow contrast material to extravasate from the injured collecting system, renal pelvis, or ureter.

8. **b. Surgery for endometriosis greatly increases the risk.** A large percentage of ureteral injuries after gynecologic

laparoscopy occur during electrosurgical or laser-assisted lysis of endometriosis.

Imaging

1. **b. delayed imaging to evaluate the collecting system.** When blunt renal trauma results in deep parenchymal lacerations, delayed imaging at the time of the CT is essential to evaluate the collecting system for injury. In a stable patient with this type of injury, neither surgical repair nor angiographic embolization is indicated. Most renal injuries heal well with conservative and expectant management, making options a and c incorrect. Intravenous urography no longer plays a role in the acute evaluation of blunt renal trauma.

2. **c. main renal artery occlusion.** There is complete absence of enhancement of the entire right kidney, which is caused only by main renal artery occlusion. Segmental occlusion would cause abnormality only in a portion of the right renal nephrogram. Ureteral injury and UPJ disruption may cause delay in the nephrogram but not complete absence of enhancement.

3. **b. ureterovaginal fistula.** There is extraluminal contrast around the left distal pelvic ureter with contrast opacification of the vagina on the lower image. The bladder is normal in appearance with no contrast extravasation, making options a, c, and e incorrect. Ureteral duplication does not have this appearance.

Additional Study Points

1. See Table 42–1 in *Campbell-Walsh Urology, 10th edition* for the classification of renal injuries by grade.
2. The initial evaluation and treatment of a trauma patient involves the following priorities of care and may be remembered as "abcde": (a) airway with cervical spin protection, (b) breathing, (c) circulation, (d) disability (neurologic status), and (e) exposure and environment.
3. Rapid deceleration involving high-velocity impact may result in injuries at points of fixation such as the ureteral pelvic junction and the renal hilum (renal artery intimal disruption).
4. The degree of hematuria and the severity of renal injury are not consistently correlated.
5. Criteria for radiologic imaging include (a) all penetrating trauma, (b) high-impact rapid deceleration trauma, (c) all blunt trauma with gross hematuria, (d) all blunt trauma with hypotension, and (e) all pediatric patients with microscopic hematuria.
6. Adult patients with microscopic hematuria without shock may be observed without imaging studies.
7. Findings suggestive of a major renal injury on CT include medial hematoma, medial urinary extravasation, and lack of contrast enhancement of the entire kidney.
8. Nonoperative management for renal injuries is preferred in the hemodynamically stable patient, particularly with grades I to III renal injuries.
9. Obligatory exploration of renal gunshot wounds is no longer mandatory. Those patients with grade IV parenchymal lacerations with well-contained hematomas who are hemodynamically stable may be observed expectantly.
10. Absolute indications for renal exploration are (a) hemodynamic instability with shock, (b) expanding pulsatile hematoma, (3) suspected renal pedicle avulsion, and (4) ureteral pelvic junction disruption.
11. Surgical exploration of the acutely injured kidney is best performed through a transabdominal incision with early isolation of the renal artery to the affected kidney.
12. "Damage control" involves packing the wound around the injured kidney with laparotomy pads to control bleeding and a planned return to the operating room in 24 hours. This is rarely indicated but is a management strategy in the multiply injured patient in whom an attempt to salvage the kidney is necessary when the additional time required to do this is inadvisable during initial post-trauma exploration.
13. Hypertension as a result of renal trauma is due to renal vascular injury or compression of the renal parenchyma by a circumferential hematoma (Page kidney).
14. When repairing ureteral injuries, the ureteral tissue should be debrided back to bleeding tissue to remove all traumatized microvascular damaged tissue.
15. Placement of a vascular graft anterior to the ureter and aneurysms may cause a periureteral inflammatory reaction and ureteral injury/stenosis.
16. In emergent situations where a ureteral repair in the multiply traumatized patient cannot be adequately performed, the ureter may be tied off and postoperatively the kidney drained through a percutaneous nephrostomy with planned reconstruction at a later date.

Renal Failure and Transplantation

43

Etiology, Pathogenesis, and Management of Renal Failure

David A. Goldfarb, MD ● Emilio D. Poggio, MD

QUESTIONS

1. Creatinine clearance overestimates glomerular filtration rate (GFR) in renal insufficiency because:
   a. tubular creatinine reabsorption is increased.
   b. creatinine production is decreased.
   c. the proportion of tubular creatinine secretion is increased.
   d. total body creatinine is increased.
   e. Glomerular creatinine selectivity is increased.

2. In patients with occult renal artery stenosis, angiotensin-converting enzyme (ACE) inhibitors cause acute renal failure (ARF) due to:
   a. sodium retention.
   b. increased antidiuretic hormone.
   c. afferent arteriolar vasoconstriction.
   d. efferent arteriolar vasodilation.
   e. decreased sympathetic nervous system activity.

3. Six days after partial nephrectomy in a solitary kidney the patient is oliguric. Large amounts of fluid are coming from the flank drain. The serum creatinine increases from 1.7 to 3.2 mg/dL. The next step in management is:
   a. renal angiography.
   b. CT scan with intravenous contrast.
   c. renal scan.
   d. immediate surgical exploration.
   e. MRI.

4. After a 7-hour, complex urethral reconstruction performed in the extended lithotomy position, a patient has severe thigh and buttock pain. The creatine phosphokinase (CPK) is dramatically elevated. The next step is:
   a. dopamine infusion.
   b. plasmapheresis.
   c. dobutamine infusion.
   d. forced alkaline diuresis.
   e. dialysis.

5. The sentinel cellular change in renal ischemic injury is:
   a. loss of cell polarity.
   b. depletion of ATP.
   c. alteration of Na^+ metabolism.
   d. increased intracellular Ca^{2+}.
   e. increased oxidant stress.

6. The renal structure at greatest risk for ischemic injury is the:
   a. afferent arteriole.
   b. cortical collecting duct.
   c. juxtaglomerular apparatus.
   d. straight segment (S3) proximal tubule.
   e. distal convoluted tubule.

7. A patient with acute kidney injury has a urinary sodium of 10 mEq/L, urinary osmolality of 650, and renal failure index of less than 1. Urinalysis shows 10 to 20 red blood cell (RBC)/high-power field (HPF), 3 to 5 WBC/HPF, 2+ proteinuria, and RBC casts. The most likely diagnosis is:
   a. acute tubular necrosis.
   b. prerenal azotemia.
   c. acute glomerulonephritis.
   d. acute interstitial nephritis.
   e. obstruction.

8. When acute kidney injury is first recognized in a patient, the initial therapeutic intervention should be to:
   a. begin low-dose dopamine.
   b. administer a cardiac inotropic agent.
   c. restore adequate circulating blood volume.
   d. administer a loop diuretic.
   e. begin a mannitol infusion.

9. Loop diuretics are of benefit in the management of acute kidney injury (AKI) due to:
   a. improved patient survival.
   b. decreasing metabolic demand.
   c. decreasing hypoxic cell swelling.
   d. free radical scavenging.
   e. increased renal vascular resistance.

10. The major risk of MRI with gadolinium in patients with advanced chronic kidney disease (CKD) is:
    a. nephrotoxicity.
    b. anaphylaxis.
    c. nephrogenic systemic fibrosis.
    d. seizures.
    e. hepatotoxicity.

11. Dopamine therapy in acute kidney injury:
    a. causes efferent arteriolar vasodilation.
    b. is recommended for routine use after renal transplantation.
    c. is effective due to improved cardiac function.
    d. is an unproven treatment.
    e. improves patient survival.

12. A patient with AKI after partial nephrectomy has a serum potassium of 6.9 mEq/L and widening of the QRS complex on electrocardiogram. The initial step in management should be:
    a. intravenous calcium.
    b. intravenous insulin and glucose.
    c. sodium polystyrene sulfonate resin (Kayexalate).
    d. intravenous furosemide.
    e. dialysis.

13. A patient with a serum creatinine of 2.7 mg/dL requires renal angiography. The best way to protect renal function is:
    a. saline diuresis.
    b. prestudy mannitol.
    c. furosemide before study.
    d. dopamine throughout the study.
    e. atrial natriuretic factor before study.

14. In response to a reduction in renal mass, a number of events occur within the kidney. These include all of the following EXCEPT:
    a. activation of the sympathetic nervous system.
    b. hyperfiltration.
    c. glomerular hypertrophy.
    d. intrarenal vascular occlusion.
    e. interstitial fibrosis.

15. A 65-year-old man has a radical nephrectomy. The estimated GFR by the Modification of Diet in Renal Disease equation is 52 mL/min. Follow-up should include:
    a. low-protein diet.
    b. renal transplant evaluation.
    c. nephrology consult for stage 3 CKD.
    d. reassessment of kidney function every few months.
    e. loop diuretics.

16. A hypertensive patient with CKD should take an ACE inhibitor drug to:
    a. improve renal function.
    b. prevent progressive kidney disease.
    c. improve cardiac ejection fraction.
    d. enhance glycemic control.
    e. control blood lipids.

17. The most common cause for ESRD in the United States is:
    a. focal segmental glomerulosclerosis.
    b. membranoproliferative glomerulonephritis (type 2).
    c. membranous glomerulonephritis.
    d. autosomal dominant polycystic kidney disease.
    e. diabetes mellitus.

18. The most accurate monitoring tool for assessment of progression of renal failure is:
    a. urinary creatinine clearance.
    b. the Cockcroft-Gault formula.
    c. serum creatinine.
    d. the MDRD study equation.
    e. iothalamate GFR measurement.

19. A hypertensive 38-year-old man has a serum creatinine of 2.4 mg/dL. The urinalysis has 10 to 20 RBC/HPF, 3+ protein, and RBC casts. Ultrasound shows echogenic kidneys without hydronephrosis. The best way to achieve a diagnosis is:
    a. renal angiography.
    b. renal biopsy.
    c. retrograde pyelography.
    d. magnetic resonance imaging.
    e. spiral CT scan.

20. In addition to an ACE inhibitor, patients with CKD would benefit from which drug to help slow the progression of renal disease?
    a. α blockers
    b. Thiazide diuretics
    c. HMG-CoA reductase inhibitors (statins)
    d. β blockers
    e. Nitrates

21. CKD patients treated with an ACE inhibitor may experience a decrease in residual renal function in the setting of:
    a. partial nephrectomy for renal cell carcinoma.
    b. concomitant treatment with an α blocker.
    c. aquired renal cystic disease.
    d. left ventricular hypertrophy.
    e. autosomal dominant polycystic kidney disease with cysts larger than 10 cm.

22. The best renal replacement therapy for an otherwise healthy 37-year-old woman with chronic interstitial nephritis is:
    a. pre-emptive transplantation.
    b. stabilize with hemodialysis 1 year, then transplant.
    c. stabilize with peritoneal dialysis 1 year, then transplant.
    d. home hemodialysis.
    e. peritoneal dialysis with an automated cycler.

23. On the basis of the National Kidney Foundation K/DOQI Clinical Guidelines, dialysis should be initiated in CKD patients EXCEPT when:
    a. the weekly KrT/V urea is less than 2.
    b. the patient has greater than 6% involuntary reduction of edema free water.
    c. body weight less than 90% of standardized body weight for NHANES II.
    d. reduction of albumin by greater than 0.3 g/dL.
    e. hematocrit is greater than 25%.

24. Late referral for dialysis is associated with:
    a. hematocrit less than 20%.
    b. Kt/V greater than 2.
    c. increased mortality.

d. vascular access problems.

e. increased edema-free body weight.

25. The strongest predictor of hospitalization in chronic dialysis patients is:

a. African-American race.

b. hematocrit less than 30%.

c. glomerulonephritis.

d. poor nutritional status.

e. age younger than 30 years.

Imaging

1. See Figure 43–1.

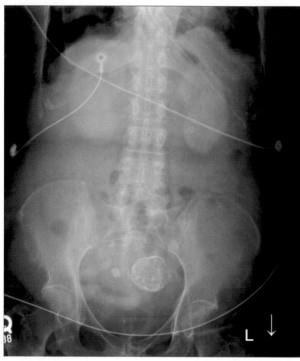

Figure 43–1.

A 55-year-old woman has this abdominal radiograph 1 day after a contrast-enhanced CT scan done for abdominal pain. Her creatinine before the CT scan was 1.9 mg/dL. The most likely diagnosis is:

a. normal film.

b. acute tubular necrosis.

c. renal artery occlusion.

d. hypertensive kidneys.

e. nephrocalcinosis.

ANSWERS

1. **c. the proportion of tubular creatinine secretion is increased.** Serum creatinine is produced at a constant rate by muscle and reflects the GFR. When renal function deteriorates, tubular secretion represents an increasing proportion of creatinine excretion. Therefore creatinine clearance may overestimate the GFR as renal function slowly declines when measured in the steady state.

2. **d. efferent arteriolar vasodilatation.** Angiotensin II has selectively greater vasoconstrictor effects on the efferent than on the afferent arteriole, whereas vasodilatory prostaglandins cause afferent arteriolar vasodilatation. Drugs that block angiotensin II synthesis (ACE inhibitors), block angiotensin II receptor binding (angiotensin II receptor antagonists), or inhibit vasodilatory prostaglandin synthesis (nonsteroidal anti-inflammatory drugs) may cause ARF in selected clinical settings.

3. **c. renal scan.** There are several ways to confirm urinary extravasation. These include assessment of drain fluid for creatinine, intravenous administration of a vital dye excreted by the kidneys (such as indigo carmine or methylene blue), and radiographic demonstration of a fistula (isotope renography, retrograde pyelography, cystography, computed tomography). Renal scan can assess perfusion and also demonstrate extravasation.

4. **d. forced alkaline diuresis.** The combination of renal hypoperfusion and the nephrotoxic insult of myoglobin within the proximal tubule may result in acute tubular necrosis (ATN). Early recognition of this disorder is crucial, because a forced alkaline diuresis is indicated to minimize nephrotoxicity.

5. **b. depletion of ATP.** The sentinel biochemical event in renal ischemia is the depletion of ATP, which is the major energy currency for cellular work.

6. **d. straight segment (S3) proximal tubule.** The S3 segment of the proximal tubule is associated with the greatest ischemic damage. Other structures that sustain injury in this region include the medullary thick ascending limb, which is metabolically active and rich in the energy-requiring Na^+,K^+-ATPase.

7. **c. acute glomerulonephritis.** A low fractional excretion of sodium (or renal failure index) may be associated with either prerenal azotemia or acute glomerulonephritis. These entities could be separated clinically by examination of the urine. Conditions associated with prerenal azotemia would have a bland urinalysis, whereas proteinuria, RBCs, and RBC casts would be seen with acute glomerulonephritis.

8. **c. restore adequate circulating blood volume.** During the initial stages, a trial of parenteral hydration with isotonic fluids may correct ARF secondary to prerenal causes.

9. **b. decreasing metabolic demand.** They decrease active NaCl transport in the thick ascending limb of Henle and thereby limit energy requirements in the metabolically active segment, which often bears the greatest ischemic insult.

10. **c. nephrogenic systemic fibrosis.** Recently, gadolinium-based contrast agents have been associated with the development of nephrogenic systemic fibrosis. At-risk patients include those with advanced CKD. It is important that these compounds only be given to these patients after careful consideration of the indication for the study.

11. **d. is an unproven treatment.** Results of clinical studies have not conclusively proved that dopamine infusion improves ARF.

12. **a. intravenous calcium.** Priorities for treatment of acute hyperkalemia with electrocardiographic changes include stabilizing the electrical membrane of the cardiac conduction system, which may be accomplished with the use of intravenous calcium salts. These have an immediate effect and a rather short duration of action.

13. **a. saline diuresis.** A study by Solomon and colleagues confirmed that prestudy intravenous hydration with saline was crucial in limiting the nephrotoxic effect of

radiocontrast agents in patients with preexisting azotemia. The addition of either a loop diuretic or mannitol did not improve outcome.

14. **d. intrarenal vascular occlusion.** In response to reduced nephron mass, a mosaic of events occurs linking sympathetic nervous system activation, renal structural remodeling, altered gene expression and regulation, and several regulatory mechanisms for progression.

15. **c. nephrology consult for stage 3 CKD.** According to the National Kidney Foundation (K/DOQI) guidelines, this patient indeed has stage 3 CKD. A nephrologist should follow this patient and institute appropriate preventive strategies for preservation of kidney function and to minimize the impact of comorbidities.

16. **b. prevent progressive kidney disease.** ACE inhibitors work by hemodynamic and nonhemodynamic mechanisms to slow the progression of renal disease.

17. **e. diabetes mellitus.** Diabetes mellitus and hypertension account for the greatest percentage of cases, followed by glomerular diseases (e.g., FSGS, membranous glomerulonephritis) and then secondary glomerulonephritis associated with systemic diseases (e.g., systemic lupus erythematosus, Wegener granulomatosis).

18. **e. iothalamate GFR measurement.** The iothalamate GFR assay is the "gold standard" for measuring renal function, but it requires a dedicated staff and laboratory to carry out the tests.

19. **b. renal biopsy.** For definitive diagnosis, a renal biopsy is required to aid prognosis and therapy decisions, especially in the setting of abnormal renal function.

20. **c. HMG Co-A reductase inhibitors (statins).** Evidence now supports the role of statin drugs in reducing fibrosis and mesangial proliferation. They should be incorporated into renal protective strategies.

21. **e. autosomal dominant PKD with cysts larger than 10 cm.** Individuals with bilateral renal artery stenosis and autosomal dominant PKD patients with cyst size greater than 10 cm may also experience a decrease in residual renal function while being given ACE inhibitor therapy.

22. **a. performing pre-emptive transplantation.** A comparison of outcomes suggests that renal transplantation is the best overall treatment for ESRD patients.

23. **e. the hematocrit is higher than 25%.** The K/DOQI guidelines recommend that dialysis be initiated when the weekly renal Krt/Vurea decreases to less than 2, unless all three of the following criteria are met: (1) stable or increased edema-free body weight, (2) randomized protein equivalent of total nitrogen appearance greater than 0.8, and (3) absence of clinical symptoms and signs attributable to uremia. The patient should begin renal replacement therapy if Krt/Vurea is less than 2 and more than 6% involuntary reduction of edema-free weight exists or the patient weighs less than 90% of standard body weight from the National Health and Nutrition Examination Survey III standard, or there is a reduction in albumin by greater than or equal to 0.3 g/dL.

24. **c. increased mortality.** Historically, mortality among late referrals for dialysis is consistently higher than among those with more timely initiated renal replacement therapy patterns.

25. **d. poor nutritional status.** The strongest predictors of the number of hospitalizations per year of patients at risk include low serum albumin, decreased activity level, diabetes mellitus as a primary cause of ESRD, peripheral vascular disease, white race, increasing age, and congestive heart failure. Both nutritional status (levels of serum albumin, creatinine, transferrin, prealbumin, and lean body mass) and inflammatory response (e.g., C-reactive protein) are independent predictors of hospitalization in chronic hemodialysis patients.

Imaging

1. **b. acute tubular necrosis.** Both kidneys are diffusely dense 24 hours after contrast administration (persistent nephrogram), with no excretion into the collecting system, making option b the best diagnosis. The process is likely related to contrast-induced nephropathy. Renal artery occlusion is usually a unilateral process, and the nephrogram is absent in the affected kidney due to the lack of perfusion. The kidneys are small in patients with severe hypertension, and the nephrogram would have washed out at 24 hours rather than be persistent. No calcifications are seen in the kidneys, making nephrocalcinosis an unlikely diagnosis.

Additional Study Points

1. ARF is divided into prerenal, intrarenal, and postrenal.
2. Prerenal failure is the result of decreased renal blood flow or increased nitrogen load. The serum blood urea nitrogen–to-creatinine ratio is greater than 10:1. Urine volume is generally low, osmolality high, and sodium content very low.
3. Intrarenal failure is due to parenchymal disease. It may involve the glomerulus as in acute glomerulonephritis, the tubule as in ATN, or the interstitium as in acute interstitial nephritis. The serum blood urea nitrogen–to-creatinine ratio is 10:1. Urine output is variable, and urinary sodium is generally above 20 mEq/L. If the cause is ATN, urinary sodium is generally greater than 40 mEq/L.
4. Postrenal failure is due to obstruction of the entire nephron mass. Patients who are anuric should be suspected of having complete urinary tract obstruction, acute cortical necrosis, or bilateral vascular occlusion. The serum blood urea nitrogen–to-creatinine ratio is 10:1.
5. In acute tubular necrosis, renal blood flow is reduced by 50% or more with the perfusion defect most marked in the outer medulla. Tubule permeability is also increased.
6. The use of mannitol before an ischemic insult has been shown to be of benefit.
7. Hyperkalemia as evidenced on the electrocardiogram by peaked T-waves, a prolonged PR interval, and widening of the QRS complex is initially treated with IV calcium salts to stabilize the myocardium and then transiently lower serum potassium with IV glucose and insulin or IV sodium bicarbonate, as well as to permanently lower the potassium with either Kayexalate or dialysis.
8. The indications for initiation of dialysis include volume overload, severe hyperkalemia, severe metabolic acidosis, pericarditis, selected poisonings, and uremic symptomatology.
9. Peritoneal dialysis is less stressful hemodynamically.

10. The mortality rate for patients with acute tubular necrosis approximates 50%. Of those who survive ATN, 5% will require chronic dialysis.

11. Patients who are to receive IV contrast and are at risk for renal failure should be given IV hydration with saline and acetyl cysteine before the use of nonionic IV contrast.

12. CKD is defined as a GFR less than 60 mL/min.

13. Hyperfiltration results when a decreased number of nephrons are called on to perform the entire workload. This results in elevated glomerular hydrostatic pressure, which is a major contributor to decreased renal function.

14. A family history of ESRD is a strong predictor of future risk for renal failure.

15. The Cockcroft Gault formula, MDRD equation, and the CKD-EPI equation are all used to estimate GFR from serum creatinine. These equations are inaccurate for patients who have changing renal function, are at the extremes of age or body size, are obese, have decreased muscle mass, or are sick with moderately advanced renal failure.

16. Cystatin-C, a serum protein, may be more predictive of renal function than creatinine.

17. Mortality rates secondary to sepsis are one to several hundred times higher in dialysis patients.

Renal Transplantation

John Maynard Barry, MD ● Michael Joseph Conlin, MD, FACS

QUESTIONS

1. The incidence of patients starting renal replacement therapy for end-stage renal disease (ESRD) in the United States is between that of which two cancers?
   a. Breast and prostate
   b. Prostate and bladder
   c. Bladder and kidney
   d. Kidney and testis
   e. Bladder and testis

2. ESRD in adults is usually defined as an irreversible glomerular filtration rate (GFR) of less than how many milliliters per minute or a serum creatinine level of greater than how many milligrams per deciliter?
   a. 5 mL/min, 10 mg/dL
   b. 10 mL/min, 8 mg/dL
   c. 15 mL/min, 6 mg/dL
   d. 20 mL/min, 5 mg/dL
   e. 20 mL/min, 4 mg/dL

3. The most common form of treatment for adults with ESRD is:
   a. kidney transplantation.
   b. chronic ambulatory peritoneal dialysis.
   c. hemodialysis.
   d. medical management.
   e. in-center peritoneal dialysis.

4. When was the first human-to-human kidney transplantation performed?
   a. 1908
   b. 1926
   c. 1933
   d. 1951
   e. 1954

5. Which of the following renal diseases has a high probability of recurrence in patients with a kidney transplant, resulting in failure of the kidney graft?
   a. Chronic glomerulonephritis
   b. Focal segmental glomerulosclerosis
   c. IgA nephropathy
   d. Alport syndrome
   e. Autosomal dominant polycystic kidney disease

6. Lymphoproliferative disorders are most commonly associated with which of the following viruses?
   a. Herpes simplex virus type 1
   b. Varicella-zoster virus
   c. Epstein-Barr virus (EBV)
   d. Cytomegalovirus virus (CMV)
   e. Cocksackie virus

7. To reduce the risk of cancer recurrence, a minimum waiting time of how many cancer-free years from the time of last cancer treatment is recommended for patients who have had invasive malignancies?
   a. 1
   b. 2
   c. 3
   d. 4
   e. 5

8. A disadvantage of gastric augmentation cystoplasty in an anephric hemodialysis patient is:
   a. hyperkalemia.
   b. hypernatremia.
   c. metabolic acidosis.
   d. bladder ulceration.
   e. mucus.

9. Pretransplant nephrectomy is indicated for:
   a. hypertension controlled with medication.
   b. prior renal infection.
   c. renal stones unsuitable for minimally invasive procedures.
   d. 200 mg/dL proteinuria.
   e. most polycystic kidneys.

10. The best renal imaging protocol for a living renal donor to define renal anatomy and renal vasculature and to rule out renal stones is:
    a. kidney, ureter, bladder (KUB) radiography and selective renal arteriography.
    b. magnetic resonance nephrotomography and angiography.

c. helical CT without and with intravenous contrast.

d. helical CT without and with intravenous contrast and KUB radiograph.

e. renal ultrasonography and selective renal arteriography.

11. After living donor nephrectomy, the renal donor is expected to have what level of total renal function?

a. 50%

b. 60%

c. 75%

d. 90%

e. 95%

12. A 25-year-old woman has recovered uneventfully after donating a kidney to her sister. How long should she delay pregnancy?

a. not at all

b. 3 months

c. 6 months

d. 12 months

e. 24 months

13. Kidney transplant survival rates are poorest for which of the following donor categories?

a. Sibling

b. Parent

c. Spouse

d. Standard criteria deceased

e. Expanded criteria deceased

14. The initial goals of resuscitation of the brain-dead cadaver donor are systolic blood pressure of what level and urinary output exceeding how many milliliters per kilogram per hour?

a. 100 mm Hg, 0.25 mL/kg/hr

b. 60 mm Hg, 0.5 mL/kg/hr

c. 90 mm Hg, 0.5 mL/kg/hr

d. 90 mm Hg, 0.3 mL/kg/hr

e. 80 mm Hg, 0.4 mL/kg/hr

15. Which of the following is required for the cellular sodium-potassium pump to maintain a high intracellular concentration of potassium and a low intracellular concentration of sodium?

a. ADP

b. ATP

c. CMP

d. CTP

e. Nitric oxide

16. The best solution for preservation of all abdominal organs is:

a. EuroCollins.

b. Collins 2.

c. Sach solution.

d. University of Wisconsin (UW) solution.

e. Histidine-tryptophan-ketogluterate (HTK).

17. A cadaver kidney transplant recipient receives points on the national waiting list for all of the following EXCEPT:

a. time on the waiting list.

b. age younger than 18 years.

c. panel reactive antibody (PRA) level greater than 80%.

d. histocompatibility.

e. full-time employment.

18. In the absence of significant recipient arteriosclerosis, the renal artery is usually anastomosed to the:

a. aorta.

b. inferior mesenteric artery.

c. common iliac artery.

d. internal iliac artery.

e. internal pudendal artery.

19. The renal vein is usually anastomosed to the recipient's:

a. inferior vena cava.

b. common iliac vein.

c. external iliac vein.

d. posterior gluteal vein.

e. internal iliac vein.

20. The standard method of urinary tract reconstruction during renal transplantation is:

a. ureteropyelostomy.

b. ureteroureterostomy.

c. ureteroneocystostomy.

d. vesicopyelostomy.

e. cutaneous ureterostomy.

21. The usual intravenous solution for urine volume replacement after renal transplantation is:

a. 0.25% saline.

b. 0.45% saline.

c. 0.45% saline in D5W.

d. 0.90% saline.

e. D5W.

22. A woman wishes to donate a kidney to her husband who has ESRD. She is ABO blood type A, and he is ABO blood type O. Each of the following is a possible solution to this problem EXCEPT:

a. plasmapheresis.

b. immunoadsorption.

c. immunoglobulin administration.

d. anti-CD 37 antibody administration.

e. a paired kidney exchange.

23. The risk of a hyperacute rejection after kidney transplantation is high when which of the following is positive?

a. B-cell flow cross match

b. T-cell flow cross match

c. B-cell microlymphocytotoxicity cross match

d. T-cell microlymphocytotoxicity cross match

e. DR-cell cross match

24. Which of the following immunosuppressants inhibits cell cycle progression?
    a. Azathioprine
    b. Mycophenolate mofetil
    c. Cyclosporine
    d. Tacrolimus
    e. Sirolimus

25. Which of the following paired immunosuppressants have similar mechanisms of action and toxicity?
    a. Azathioprine and cyclosporine
    b. Azathioprine and tacrolimus
    c. Basiliximab and mycophenolate mofetil
    d. Tacrolimus and cyclosporine
    e. Muromonab CD3 and mycophenolate mofetil

26. Which of the following two drugs have been used to reduce calcineurin inhibitor dosing and cost while maintaining blood levels and immunosuppressive effect?
    a. Diltiazem and ketoconazole
    b. Prednisone and azathioprine
    c. Basiliximab and daclizumab
    d. Equine antilymphocyte globulin and azathioprine
    e. Mycophenolate mofetil and azathioprine

27. Steroid-resistant rejection is often treated with:
    a. rabbit antithymocyte globulin.
    b. higher doses of glucocorticoids.
    c. sirolimus.
    d. daclizumab.
    e. mycophenolate mofetil.

28. Prophylaxis against *Pneumocystis* infection is best achieved with:
    a. trimethoprim-sulfamethoxazole.
    b. erythromycin.
    c. ciprofloxacin.
    d. cephalexin.
    e. minocycline.

29. Prophylaxis against cytomegalovirus infection is best done with:
    a. trimethoprim-sulfamethoxazole.
    b. erythromycin.
    c. ganciclovir.
    d. basiliximab.
    e. minocycline.

30. Five years after successful renal transplantation, a 55-year-old man is referred to you because of total gross hematuria. Each of the following is an important part of the workup EXCEPT:
    a. urine cytology.
    b. urine PCA3 determination.
    c. images of the native kidneys.
    d. images of the kidney transplant.
    e. cystourethroscopy.

31. A deceased donor kidney transplant recipient has a plasma creatinine level of 1.9 mg/dL. A large, asymptomatic perigraft fluid collection is aspirated, and the creatinine level is 2.0 mg/dL. What is the most likely diagnosis?
    a. Hydrocele
    b. Lymphocele
    c. Perinephric abscess
    d. Hematoma
    e. Urinoma

32. Which of the following interferes with the tubular secretion of creatinine and can cause an increase in serum creatinine levels?
    a. Azathioprine
    b. Trimethoprim
    c. Mycophenolate mofetil
    d. Tacrolimus
    e. Basiliximab

33. Oral fluconazole is prescribed to treat cystitis caused by yeast. Which of the following medications will need to have the dose reduced?
    a. Muromonab CD3
    b. Prednisone
    c. Tacrolimus
    d. Azathioprine
    e. Mycophenolate mofetil

34. Hemorrhagic cystitis in an immunosuppressed patient has been most commonly associated with which of the following viruses?
    a. Cytomegalovirus
    b. Adenovirus
    c. Herpes simplex virus type 1
    d. Herpes simplex virus type 2
    e. Polyoma virus

35. Which of the following antihypertensive agents is least likely to cause erectile dysfunction?
    a. Propranolol
    b. Clonidine
    c. Methyldopa
    d. Labetalol
    e. Lisinopril

36. A successful kidney transplant recipient and his wife desire to have a child. What is the recommended length of time between transplantation and impregnation?
    a. 3 months
    b. 6 months
    c. 9 months
    d. 12 months
    e. 24 months

37. At what frequency would preterm delivery be expected in a pregnant kidney transplant recipient?
    a. 10%
    b. 20%

c. 30%

d. 40%

e. 50%

38. The most common cancer after kidney transplantation is:

a. skin.

b. cervix.

c. Kaposi sarcoma.

d. thyroid.

e. breast.

39. A kidney transplant recipient has recurrent superficial transitional cell carcinoma of the urinary bladder. Each of the following treatments is acceptable EXCEPT:

a. fulguration.

b. thiotepa instillation

c. mitomycin instillation.

d. BCG instillation.

e. doxorubicin hydrochloride (Adriamycin) instillation.

40. Hyperlipidemia is most often associated with which of the following three-drug combinations?

a. Prednisone, cyclosporine, sirolimus

b. Equine antithymocyte globulin, tacrolimus, mycophenolate mofetil

c. Mycophenolate mofetil, tacrolimus, basiliximab

d. Cyclosporine, tacrolimus, mycophenolate mofetil

e. Caclizumab, mycophenolate mofetil, azathioprine

ANSWERS

1. **b. Prostate and bladder.** The estimated number of patients starting renal replacement therapy each year for ESRD in the United States is about 360 per million population. The two most common urologic cancers, in order, are prostate and bladder, and the incidence of ESRD is between them.

2. **b. 10 mL/min, 8 mg/dL.** Permanent renal failure in adults is commonly defined as an irreversible GFR of less than 10 mL/min or a serum creatinine level of greater than 8.0 mg/dL. Patients with symptomatic uremia are considered on an individual basis.

3. **c. hemodialysis.** Hemodialysis is the predominant form of therapy for adults with ESRD. In the United States, it accounts for about 65% of all treated ESRD patients.

4. **c. 1933.** The first human renal allograft was performed by Voronoy in the Ukraine. The recipient was a 26-year-old woman who had attempted suicide by ingesting mercuric chloride. The donor was a 66-year-old man whose kidney had been removed 6 hours after death.

5. **b. Focal segmental glomerulosclerosis.** Patients with focal segmental glomerulosclerosis, hemolytic-uremic syndrome, or primary oxalosis should be counseled about the significant probability of disease recurrence and the risk of secondary graft failure.

6. **c. Epstein-Barr virus (EBV).** EBV titers are determined in children, and, for the EBV-seronegative child, a kidney from an EBV-seronegative donor is preferred to reduce the risk of a post-transplant lymphoproliferative disorder, the most common de novo malignancy in pediatric organ transplant recipients.

7. **b. 2.** To reduce the risk of cancer recurrence, a waiting time of 2 to 5 cancer-free years from the time of last cancer treatment is recommended for patients who have had invasive malignancies. Individual cases may be managed with the application of nomograms and calculations of expected remaining lifetime after transplantation.

8. **d. bladder ulceration.** The gastric flap continues to secrete acid, and this can be especially problematic in the anuric patient.

9. **c. renal calculi unsuitable for minimally invasive procedures.** The generally accepted recommendations for pretransplant nephrectomy, as outlined in the table, include the following: renal stones not cleared by minimally invasive techniques or lithotripsy; solid renal tumors with or without acquired renal cystic disease; polycystic kidneys that are symptomatic, extend below the iliac crest, have been infected, or have solid tumors; persistent antiglomerular basement membrane antibody levels; significant proteinuria not controlled with medical nephrectomy or angio-ablation; recurrent pyelonephritis; and grade 4 or 5 hydronephrosis.

10. **d. helical CT with and without intravenous contrast and a KUB radiograph.** Three-dimensional CT angiography with and without intravenous contrast followed by a radiograph of the abdomen has been widely accepted for use with living renal donors because it satisfactorily excludes stone disease, demonstrates renal and vascular anatomy, and defines the urinary collecting system, all with minimal donor morbidity and at reasonable expense.

11. **c. 75%.** Hyperfiltration injury has not been a problem for living renal donors. Endogenous creatinine clearance rapidly approaches 70% to 80% of the preoperative level, and this has been shown to be sustained for more than 10 years. The development of late hypertension is nearly the same as that for the general population, and the development of proteinuria is negligible.

12. **d. 12 months.** It is recommended that women wait at least a year after kidney donation before becoming pregnant.

13. **e. Expanded criteria deceased.** Kidney transplant survival rates are poorest when the quality of the kidney is the worst. Expended criteria deceased kidney donors are older than the age of 60 years or are older than the age of 50 years and have two of the following: death from cerebrovascular accident, hypertension, or serum creatinine greater than 1.5 mg/dL.

14. **c. 90 mm Hg, 0.5 mL/kg/hr.** The initial goals of resuscitation of the brain-dead cadaver donor are a systolic blood pressure of 90 mm Hg and a urinary output exceeding 0.5 mL/kg/hr.

15. **b. ATP.** ATP is required for the cellular sodium-potassium pump to maintain a high intracellular concentration of potassium and a low intracellular concentration of sodium.

16. **d. University of Wisconsin (UW) solution.** The UW solution minimizes cellular swelling with the impermeable solutes lactobionate, raffinose, and hydroxyethyl starch. Phosphate is used for its hydrogen ion buffering qualities, adenosine is for ATP synthesis during reperfusion, glutathione is a free radical scavenger, allopurinol inhibits xanthine oxidase and the generation of free radicals, and magnesium and dexamethasone are membrane-stabilizing

agents. A major advantage of this preservation solution has been its utility as a universal preservation solution for all intra-abdominal organs.

17. **e. full-time employment.** A point system that has evolved in the United States for the selection of cadaver kidney transplant recipients includes the following variables: waiting time; human leukocyte antigen panel reactive antibody greater than 80%; age younger than 18 years; donor of kidney, liver segment, lung segment, partial pancreas, or small bowel segment; and histocompatibility.

18. **d. internal iliac artery.** The renal artery is usually anastomosed to the end of the internal iliac artery or to the side of the external iliac artery.

19. **c. external iliac vein.** The renal vein, with or without an extension, is usually anastomosed end-to-side to the external iliac vein.

20. **c. ureteroneocystostomy.** Urinary tract reconstruction is usually by antireflux ureteroneocystostomy, of which there are several techniques.

21. **b. 0.45% saline.** Intravenous fluid that contains 5% dextrose is given to replace estimated insensible losses, and 0.45% saline without dextrose is given at a rate equal to the previous hour's urinary output. This is to prevent hyperglycemia and an osmotic diuresis when the urinary output is high.

22. **d. anti-CD 37 antibody administration.** Plasmapheresis and immunoadsorption are used to remove antibodies. Immunoglobulin administration and anti CD-20 antibody (not anti CD-37 antibody) are used to prevent antibody reformation. Paired kidney exchange is an inexpensive way to deal with the problem.

23. **d. T-cell microlymphocytotoxicity cross match.** Hyperacute rejection is rare when the T-cell microlymphocytotoxicity cross match between recipient serum and donor lymphocytes is negative.

24. **e. Sirolimus.** Sirolimus (formerly called *rapamycin*) inhibits cell cycle progression. Azathioprine and mycophenolate mofetil are purine antagonists, and they prevent lymphocyte proliferation. Tacrolimus and cyclosporine are calcineurin inhibitors. They inhibit the production of calcineurin and interleukin-2.

25. **d. Cyclosporine and tacrolimus.** Cyclosporine and tacrolimus have similar mechanisms of action, effectiveness, and cost but slightly different side effect profiles, and they are not used together.

26. **a. Diltiazem and ketoconazole.** Diltiazem and ketoconazole have been used to reduce calcineurin inhibitor dosing and cost while maintaining blood levels and immunosuppressive effect.

27. **a. rabbit antithymocyte globulin.** Conventional treatment for acute renal allograft rejection is high-dose pulses of glucocorticoids. Treatment of steroid-resistant rejection is with lymphocyte-depleting antibody preparations such as muromonab CD3, rabbit antithymocyte globulin, and alemtuzumab.

28. **a. trimethoprim-sulfamethoxazole.** Commonly used regimens to prevent infections and peptic ulcer disease include trimethoprim-sulfamethoxazole for 3 months for prophylaxis against *Pneumocystis* pneumonia.

29. **c. gancyclovir.** Prophylaxis against cytomegalovirus disease is possible with ganciclovir, acyclovir, valacyclovir, or cytomegalovirus immune globulin.

30. **urine PCA3 determination.** Urine PCA3 determinations have been used to screen for prostate cancer, not renal cell carcinoma or urothelial carcinomas.

31. **b. Lymphocele.** Lymph, urine, and blood can be differentiated from each other by creatinine and hematocrit determinations. Lymph has a creatinine concentration that is the same as plasma, urine has a creatinine concentration higher than that of plasma and approaching that of bladder urine, and blood has a high hematocrit level when compared with the other two fluids.

32. **b. Trimethoprim.** Trimethoprim interferes with the tubular secretion of creatinine, and this can cause an increase in serum creatinine levels.

33. **c. Tacrolimus.** Cyclosporine and tacrolimus doses usually have to be reduced when fluconazole or ketoconazole is given because these drugs interfere with the metabolism of both of those immunosuppressants via the cytochrome P-450 system.

34. **b. Adenovirus.** Hemorrhagic cystitis can be caused by adenovirus. The disease is usually self-limited and resolves within a few weeks.

35. **e. Lisinopril.** Erectile dysfunction can be due to any one or a combination of factors. Included are the antihypertensives clonidine, methyldopa, propranolol, and labetalol. Angiotensin-converting enzyme (ACE) inhibitors, calcium channel blockers, and α blockers are relatively less likely to cause erectile dysfunction than are the other antihypertensive medications. Lisinopril is an ACE inhibitor.

36. **d. 12 months.** Among male recipients who have fathered children, there has been no increase in congenital abnormalities in the offspring. However, it is recommended that impregnation be delayed for at least 1 year after transplantation.

37. **e. 50%.** Successful renal transplantation usually restores female fertility. In a report based on thousands of pregnancies in renal transplant recipients, Davison and Milne noted, among other findings, that 50% of the deliveries were preterm.

38. **a. skin.** Immunosuppressed patients are more likely to develop cancer than age-matched control subjects in the general population. Among several thousand tumors that occurred in renal transplant recipients, the common cancers, in order, were skin, lymphoma, Kaposi sarcoma, carcinomas of the cervix, renal tumors, and carcinomas of the vulva and perineum.

39. **d. BCG instillation.** BCG should be avoided for the treatment of superficial transitional cell carcinoma of the bladder in immunosuppressed kidney transplant recipients because of the risk of systemic infection and the likelihood of diminished therapeutic response.

40. **a. Prednisone, cyclosporine, sirolimus.** Prednisone, cyclosporine, and sirolimus all result in hyperlipidemia.

Additional Study Points

1. The most common causes of ESRD in order are diabetes, hypertension, glomerulonephritis, and renal cystic disease.
2. ESRD in children may result in growth failure, poor nutrition, and psychiatric problems.
3. The major causes of death for patients with ESRD who are on dialysis or who have received a transplant are heart disease, sepsis, and stroke.
4. A defunctionalized bladder usually regains normal volume within weeks of transplantation.
5. Clean intermittent catheterization when necessary has been successfully used in transplant recipients.
6. Surgical treatment of the bladder outlet should not be performed in the anuric patient. If the native kidneys are producing no urine and a procedure on the bladder outlet is deemed necessary, bladder cycling should be instituted.
7. The quality of early graft function is directly correlated with cold ischemia time.
8. The routine use of a ureteral stent for all cases of renal transplantation has been shown to reduce the incidence of ureteral complications.
9. The histo compatibility antigens of greatest importance are ABO blood group and the major histo compatibility complex (MHC).
10. Class-1 antigens are HLA-A, HLA-B, and HLA-C.
11. Class-2 antigens are HLA-DR, HLA-DQ, and HLA-DP.
12. The MHC antigens generally tested for are the HLA-A, B, C, and DR.

Urinary Lithiasis and Endourology

Urinary Lithiasis: Etiology, Epidemiology, and Pathogenesis

Margaret S. Pearle, MD, PhD ● Yair Lotan, MD

QUESTIONS

1. The ethnic/racial group with the highest prevalence of stone disease is:
   a. African-Americans.
   b. Hispanics.
   c. Caucasians.
   d. Asians.
   e. American Indians.

2. The geographic area in the United States associated with the highest incidence of calcium oxalate stone disease is the:
   a. Northeast.
   b. Southeast.
   c. Southwest.
   d. West.
   e. Northwest.

3. Which of the following occurs when the concentration product of urine falls in the metastable range?
   a. Urine is supersaturated.
   b. Homogeneous nucleation occurs.
   c. Solubility product is reduced.
   d. Urinary inhibitors decrease the formation product.
   e. Nucleation never occurs.

4. The process by which nucleation occurs in pure solutions is:
   a. homogeneous nucleation.
   b. heterogeneous nucleation.
   c. epitaxy.
   d. aggregation.
   e. agglomeration.

5. The proteinaceous component of stones is composed of:
   a. concentric lamination.
   b. protein-crystal complex.
   c. matrix.
   d. nephrocalcin.
   e. osteocalcin.

6. Citrate inhibits calcium oxalate stone formation by:
   a. binding urinary inhibitors.
   b. lowering urine magnesium levels.
   c. increasing urinary saturation of sodium urate.

d. complexing calcium.
   e. lowering urine pH.

7. Stone-forming propensity is best described by:
   a. formation product.
   b. ionic activity.
   c. saturation index.
   d. solubility product.
   e. relative saturation ratio.

8. The most common abnormal urinary finding in patients undergoing Roux-en-Y gastric bypass surgery is:
   a. hypercalciuria.
   b. low urine pH.
   c. low urine volume.
   d. hypocitraturia.
   e. hyperoxaluria.

9. The vitamin D metabolite that stimulates intestinal calcium absorption is:
   a. 7-dehydrocholesterol.
   b. cholecalciferol.
   c. 25-dihydroxyvitamin D_3.
   d. 1,25-dihydroxyvitamin D_3.
   e. calcitonin.

10. Which of the following factors increases intestinal oxalate absorption?
    a. High dietary calcium intake
    b. Low dietary calcium intake
    c. *Oxalobacter formigenes* colonization in the colon
    d. *Helicobacter pylori* colonization in the stomach
    e. Irritable bowel syndrome

11. The primary determinant of urinary citrate excretion is:
    a. acid-base status.
    b. urinary sodium excretion.
    c. citric acid intake.
    d. insulin sensitivity.
    e. urinary calcium excretion.

12. Absorptive hypercalciuria is associated with:
    a. hypercalcemia.
    b. low to normal PTH levels.

c. elevated PTH levels.

d. fasting hypercalciuria.

e. suppressed 1,25-dihyroxyvitamin D_3.

13. The underlying abnormality of renal hypercalciuria is:

a. enhanced calcium filtration.

b. enhanced calcium secretion.

c. enhanced calcium reabsorption.

d. primary renal wasting of calcium.

e. primary renal storage of calcium.

14. Accumulation of which metabolite is expected in patients with primary hyperoxaluria type 1?

a. Glyoxylate

b. Hydroxypyruvate

c. L-glycerate

d. Glycolate

e. Pyruvate

15. Hypercalciuria associated with sarcoidosis is a result of:

a. absorptive hypercalciuria.

b. renal hypercalciuria.

c. resorptive hypercalciuria.

d. acidosis.

e. medical induction.

16. Enteric hyperoxaluria occurs as a result of:

a. excessive intake of oxalate.

b. reduced excretion of oxalate.

c. increased dietary fat.

d. low calcium intake.

e. fat malabsorption.

17. The most likely mechanism accounting for low urinary pH in uric acid stone formers with type 2 diabetes mellitus is:

a. defective ammoniagenesis.

b. impaired urinary bicarbonate excretion.

c. lactic acidosis.

d. glucosuria.

e. ketoacidosis.

18. In idiopathic calcium oxalate stone formers, Randall plaques originate in the:

a. basement membrane of the thin loops of Henle.

b. terminal collecting ducts.

c. medullary interstitium.

d. vasa recta.

e. papillary tip.

19. In calcium oxalate stone formers, Randall plaques are composed of:

a. calcium oxalate.

b. brushite.

c. calcium carbonate.

d. calcium apatite.

e. uric acid.

20. How is urinary saturation of calcium oxalate determined?

a. Primarily by urinary calcium concentration

b. Primarily by urinary oxalate concentration

c. Equally by urinary calcium and oxalate concentrations

d. Primarily by urinary pH

e. Primarily by urinary volume

21. O. formigenes reduces urinary oxalate by:

a. reducing intestinal calcium absorption, leading to decreased luminal free oxalate and reduced oxalate absorption.

b. degrading urinary oxalate in infected urine.

c. increasing urinary oxalate reabsorption.

d. inhibiting the intestinal oxalate transporter.

e. using oxalate as a substrate in the intestine, thereby reducing intestinal oxalate absorption.

22. Which of the following organisms is most likely to produce urease?

a. Staphylococcus aureus

b. Escherichia coli

c. Streptococcus pneumoniae

d. Serratia marcescens

e. Chlamydia

23. The mechanism responsible for type 1 (distal) renal tubular acidosis (RTA) is:

a. impaired bicarbonate reabsorption in the proximal tubule.

b. defective H+-ATPase in the distal tubule that is unable to excrete excess acid.

c. defective ammoniagenesis.

d. impaired excretion of nontitratable acids.

e. hypoaldosteronism.

24. Patients with Lesch-Nyhan syndrome treated with high doses of allopurinol are at risk for formation of stones of which of the following compositions?

a. Hypoxanthine

b. Uric acid

c. Xanthine

d. 2,8-Dihydroxyadenine

e. Calcium apatite

25. The etiology of ammonium acid urate stone formation in patients abusing laxatives is:

a. recurrent infections with urease-producing bacteria.

b. chronic dehydration and excessive uric acid excretion.

c. increased ammoniagenesis.

d. urinary phosphate deficiency and intracellular acidosis.

e. chronic dehydration, intracellular acidosis, and low urinary sodium.

26. The primary mechanism of action of citrate in preventing stone formation is:

a. reducing urinary calcium excretion.

b. reducing urinary oxalate excretion.

c. complexing calcium in urine.

d. complexing oxalate in urine.

e. complexing phosphate in urine.

27. Type 1 (distal) RTA is characterized by which abnormality?
    a. Hyperkalemia
    b. Hypochloremia
    c. Alkalosis
    d. Hypercitraturia
    e. Hypokalemia

28. The primary defect in type 2 (proximal) RTA is failure of bicarbonate reabsorption in the:
    a. glomerulus.
    b. proximal tubule.
    c. loop of Henle.
    d. distal tubule.
    e. collecting duct.

29. The most common abnormality identified in patients with uric acid stones is:
    a. acidic urine.
    b. alkaline urine.
    c. low uric acid concentration.
    d. high uric acid concentration.
    e. distal renal tubular acidosis.

30. The etiology of stone formation in patients with cystic fibrosis is:
    a. absorptive hypercalciuria.
    b. renal leak hypercalciuria.
    c. renal tubular acidosis.
    d. reduced or absent *O. formigenes*.
    e. chronic diarrheal syndrome.

31. Carbonic anhydrase inhibitors are associated with formation of stones composed of:
    a. calcium oxalate.
    b. calcium phosphate.
    c. struvite.
    d. cystine.
    e. uric acid.

32. Which of the following physiologic changes occurs in the kidney during pregnancy?
    a. Decreased uric acid excretion
    b. Decreased citrate excretion
    c. Increased calcium excretion
    d. Decreased glomerular filtration rate (GFR)
    e. Increased magnesium excretion

ANSWERS

1. **c. Caucasians.** The highest prevalence of stone disease in both men and women occurs in Caucasians. In men the lowest prevalence occurs in African-Americans, whereas Asian women have been found to have the lowest prevalence in one series.

2. **b. Southeast.** According to hospital discharge rates among U.S. veterans, calcium oxalate stone disease is most prevalent in the Southeast.

3. **a. Urine is supersaturated.** The solubility product refers to the point of saturation where dissolved and crystalline components in solution are in equilibrium. Addition of any more crystals to the solution will result in precipitation of crystals. In this supersaturated urine (metastable state), crystallization can occur on preexisting crystals but spontaneous crystallization occurs only when the concentration product exceeds the formation product. In the metastable state, the presence of inhibitors prevents or delays crystallization.

4. **a. homogeneous nucleation.** The process by which nuclei form in pure solutions is called *homogeneous nucleation*. Heterogeneous nucleation occurs when microscopic impurities or other constituents in the urine promote nucleation by providing a surface on which the crystal components can grow.

5. **c. matrix.** Depending on their type, kidney stones contain between 2.5% and 65% of noncrystalline material or matrix. Extensive investigations have characterized matrix as a derivative of several of the mucoproteins of urine and serum.

6. **d. complexing calcium.** Citrate inhibits stone formation by complexing calcium, thereby lowering urinary saturation of calcium oxalate. In addition it inhibits spontaneous precipitation of calcium oxalate and agglomeration of calcium oxalate crystals. It also inhibits calcium oxalate and calcium phosphate crystal growth, with its effect on calcium phosphate crystal growth more pronounced than on calcium oxalate crystal growth. Lastly, it prevents heterogeneous nucleation of calcium oxalate by monosodium urate.

7. **c. saturation index.** The state of saturation of the urine with respect to particular stone-forming salts indicates the stone-forming propensity of the urine. The state of saturation is determined by pH and the ionic strength of the major ions in solution. Relative saturation ratio, determined by the EQUIL 2 computer program, has been the standard for determining stone-forming propensity. However, the newer, *JESS* computer program takes into account several soluble complexes not recognized by the EQUIL 2 program and is likely a more accurate measure of stone-forming propensity, although it has not yet gained widespread use.

8. **e. hyperoxaluria.** Hyperoxaluria has been described in both stone-forming and non–stone-forming patients who have undergone Roux-en-Y gastric bypass surgery, with urinary oxalate levels in some patients exceeding 100 mg/day. Although a mild decrease in urinary calcium compared with stone-forming control subjects has been described by some investigators, no difference compared with normal individuals was found.

9. **d. 1,25-dihydroxyvitamin D_3.** It is generally accepted that 1,25-dihydroxyvitamin D_3 is the vitamin D metabolite that is the most potent stimulator of intestinal calcium absorption. The other metabolites, except for calcitonin, are precursors of 1,25-dihydroxyvitamin D_3.

10. **b. Low dietary calcium intake.** Intestinal oxalate absorption is modulated by dietary oxalate and calcium intake and by the presence or absence of *O. formigenes*. In the setting of a high calcium intake, oxalate absorption decreases, and during calcium restriction, oxalate absorption increases due to reduced formation of a soluble calcium oxalate complex and increased availability of oxalate for absorption. *H. pylori*, which can colonize the stomach, has no effect on intestinal oxalate absorption. *O. formigenes*, an oxalate-degrading bacterium, uses oxalate as a substrate in the intestinal lumen, thereby reducing oxalate absorption.

Irritable bowel syndrome, unless it is associated with chronic diarrhea, does not affect intestinal oxalate absorption.

11. **a. acid-base status.** Acid-base status determines urinary citrate excretion. Metabolic acidosis reduces citrate excretion by augmenting citrate reabsorption and mitochondrial oxidation, whereas alkalosis enhances citrate excretion. Citric acid intake has a limited effect on urinary citrate excretion because only a small portion of dietary citrate is excreted into the urine unmetabolized. The majority of absorbed citrate is metabolized to bicarbonate, which is neutralized by the free proton from citric acid, thereby providing no net alkali load that would increase urinary citrate excretion.

12. **b. low to normal PTH levels.** The underlying pathophysiologic abnormality in absorptive hypercalciuria is overabsorption of calcium from the intestine, resulting in a transient increase in serum calcium, which suppresses PTH secretion. The increased filtered load of calcium and the suppressed PTH lead to increased urinary excretion of calcium. Serum calcium concentration remains normal because the increased intestinal absorption of calcium is matched by increased renal excretion. Fasting hypercalciuria may occur in severe cases of absorptive hypercalciuria type 1 but is more typical of renal calcium leak or resorptive hypercalciuria.

13. **d. primary renal wasting of calcium.** In this condition, the underlying abnormality is a primary renal leak of calcium due to impaired renal tubular calcium reabsorption.

14. **d. Glycolate.** Primary hyperoxaluria type 1 is due to a defect in the enzyme alanine glyoxylate aminotransferase (AGT), which converts glyoxylate, a direct precursor of oxalate, to glycine. With a defect in AGT, the metabolic pathway favors formation of oxalate and glycolate, which is formed from glyoxylate through the GRHPR enzyme.

15. **a. absorptive hypercalciuria.** The sarcoid granuloma produces 1,25-dihydroxyvitamin D_3, causing increased intestinal calcium absorption, hypercalcemia, and hypercalciuria.

16. **e. fat malabsorption.** Malabsorption from any cause including small bowel resection, intrinsic disease, or jejunoileal bypass increases luminal fatty acids and bile salts. Calcium, which normally complexes with oxalate forming a soluble complex that is lost in the stool, instead binds to fatty acids, thereby increasing luminal oxalate available for absorption. In addition, poorly absorbed bile salts increase colonic permeability to oxalate, further increasing oxalate absorption.

17. **a. defective ammoniagenesis.** Patients with type 2 diabetes mellitus typically exhibit characteristics of the metabolic syndrome including insulin resistance. Although peripherally, insulin resistance leads to typical symptoms of diabetes, insulin resistance at the level of the kidney leads to impaired ammoniagenesis, by way of reduced production of ammonia from glutamine and reduced activity of the Na^+/H^+ exchanger in the proximal tubule that is responsible for either the direct transport or trapping of ammonium in the urine. The result is reduced urinary ammonium and low urine pH.

18. **a. basement membrane of the thin loops of Henle.** In idiopathic calcium oxalate stone formers, Randall plaques have been found to originate in the basement membrane of the thin loops of Henle. From there, they extend through the medullary interstitium to a subepithelial location, where they serve as an anchoring site for calcium oxalate stone formation.

19. **d. calcium apatite.** Randall plaques are invariably composed of calcium apatite, which serve as an anchoring site onto which calcium oxalate crystals can adhere and grow.

20. **c. Equally by urinary calcium and oxalate concentrations.** Urinary saturation of calcium oxalate is strongly, positively correlated with urinary calcium and oxalate concentrations. Both contribute equally to urinary saturation of calcium oxalate. Urinary volume and pH are inversely correlated with urinary saturation of calcium oxalate.

21. **e. using oxalate as a substrate in the intestine, thereby reducing intestinal oxalate absorption.** *O. formigenes* is an oxalate-degrading bacterium found in the intestinal lumen that uses oxalate as an energy source, thereby reducing luminal oxalate and intestinal oxalate absorption. *Oxalobacter* is not found in urine.

22. **a. *Staphylococcus aureus.*** Although *Proteus* species are most commonly associated with struvite stones, more than 90% of *S. aureus* organisms produce urease and are therefore associated with struvite stone formation.

23. **b. defective H^+-ATPase in the distal tubule that is unable to excrete excess acid.** A defective H^+-ATPase in the distal tubule has been implicated in the inability to excrete excess acid in the presence of an oral acid load among patients with distal RTA. Type 2, or proximal RTA, is characterized by impaired bicarbonate reabsorption in the proximal tubule, and type 4 RTA is common in diabetics with chronic renal damage who demonstrate aldosterone resistance.

24. **c. Xanthine.** Patients with Lesch-Nyhan syndrome suffer from an inherited deficiency of the purine salvage enzyme hypoxanthine-guanine phosphoribosyltransferase, which leads to the accumulation of hypoxanthine, which is ultimately converted to uric acid. Allopurinol inhibits xanthine oxidase, which is responsible for converting hypoxanthine to xanthine and xanthine to uric acid. High doses of allopurinol in these patients lead to the accumulation of hypoxanthine and xanthine, but because xanthine is less soluble in urine than hypoxanthine, xanthine stones form.

25. **e. chronic dehydration, intracellular acidosis, and low urinary sodium.** Subjects who abuse laxatives are chronically dehydrated, resulting in intracellular acidosis. In addition, urinary sodium is low from sodium loss as a result of the laxatives. In this environment, urate preferentially complexes with the abundant ammonium rather than sodium and produces ammonium acid urate stones.

26. **c. complexing calcium in urine.** The primary mechanism of action of citrate is as a complexing agent for calcium, thereby reducing ionic calcium and urinary saturation of calcium oxalate.

27. **e. Hypokalemia.** Distal RTA is characterized by hypokalemic, hyperchloremic, non–anion gap metabolic acidosis and a urinary pH consistently above 6.0.

28. **b. proximal tubule.** The primary defect in type 2 or proximal RTA is a failure of bicarbonate reabsorption in the

proximal tubule, leading to excessive urinary bicarbonate excretion and metabolic acidosis.

29. **a. acidic urine.** Patients with uric acid stones often have prolonged periods of acidity in the urine.

30. **d. reduced or absent *O. formigenes*.** Cystic fibrosis patients on chronic antibiotic therapy have been shown to have reduced or absent *O. formigenes* colonization, which potentially leads to increased intestinal oxalate absorption and reduced secretion.

31. **b. calcium phosphate.** Carbonic anhydrase inhibitors such as acetazolamide and topiramate block reabsorption of bicarbonate in the renal proximal and distal tubules,

thereby preventing urinary acidification and inducing a metabolic acidosis. Similar to RTA, carbonic anhydrase inhibition results in the formation of calcium phosphate stones due to the high urine pH, hypercalciuria, and hypocitraturia.

32. **c. Increased calcium excretion.** During pregnancy, increased renal blood flow increases GFR, thereby increasing the filtered load of calcium, sodium, and uric acid. Placental production of 1,25 dihydroxyvitamin D_3 increases intestinal calcium absorption, further increasing urinary calcium.

Additional Study Points

1. Renal calculi are two to three times more common in men than women and in this country whites have the highest prevalence. They are uncommon before the age of 20, and the peak incidence occurs in the fourth to sixth decades of life.

2. The prevalence and incidence of stone disease is directly correlated with body mass index; patients with high body mass index excrete increased levels of oxalate, uric acid, sodium, and phosphorus and are more likely to have urinary supersaturation for uric acid.

3. Concentration product is the product of the concentrations of the chemical components.

4. Solubility product is the concentration at which precipitation of the components occurs.

5. A solution is saturated when the solubility product is exceeded.

6. When the solubility product is exceeded and precipitation does not occur, the solution is said to be metastable. When precipitation occurs, the concentration at that point is called *formation product*.

7. Magnesium and citrate inhibit crystal aggregation; nephrocalcin inhibits nucleation, growth, and aggregation; Tamm-Horsfall glycoprotein inhibits aggregation; and uropontin inhibits crystal growth.

8. Nanobacteria have been implicated in calcifying nanoparticles and serving as a nidus for stone formation.

9. Most stone-forming salts are found in the urine in a supersaturated state. Inhibitors keep them in solution.

10. The noncrystalline component of stones is called *matrix* and generally accounts for about 2.5% of the weight of the stone. It is composed of muco proteins, carbohydrates, and urinary inhibitors.

11. Parathormone increases renal calcium reabsorption and enhances phosphate excretion.

12. Patients with small bowel disease or a history of intestinal resection and an intact colon have an increased oxalate absorption.

13. Calcium absorption occurs primarily in the small intestine at a rate that is dependent on calcium intake.

14. Calcium oxalate accounts for 60% of stones; mixed calcium oxalate and hydroxyapatite, 20%; brushite, 2%; uric acid, 10%; struvite, 10%; and cystine, 1%.

15. Hypercalciuria is the most common abnormality identified in calcium stone formation. Hypercalciuria is defined as a urinary excretion greater than 4 mg/kg/day.

16. Absorptive hypercalciuria is defined as an increased urinary calcium excretion after an oral calcium load and is due to increased intestinal absorption of calcium. It is divided into type 1 in which urinary calcium remains high despite a low calcium diet and type 2 in which urinary calcium normalizes with a restricted calcium intake.

17. Renal hypercalciuria is due to impaired renal tubular reabsorption of calcium and leads to secondary hyperparathyroidism.

18. Reabsorptive hypercalciuria is due to hyperparathyroidism. The administration of thiazides to patients with primary hyperparathyroidism exacerbates hypercalcemia. Parathormone-like hormone resulting in hypercalcemia is produced by lung, breast, renal, penile, and head and neck tumors; lymphoma; and myeloma.

19. Hyperoxaluria is defined as greater than 40 mg/day excreted in the urine. Foods that are oxalate rich include nuts, chocolate, brewed tea, spinach, broccoli, strawberries, and rhubarb.

20. Hyperuricosuria is defined as urinary uric acid excretion exceeding 600 mg/day.

21. Urate formation promotes calcium oxalate stone formation through heterologous nucleation.

22. Citrate inhibits stone formation by complexing with calcium and thereby preventing spontaneous nucleation of calcium oxalate; it inhibits agglomeration and growth of the crystal, and it enhances the inhibitory effect of Tamm-Horsfall glycoprotein.

23. Hypocitraturia is defined as urinary citrate excretion less than 320 mg/day.

24. Renal tubular acidosis, type 1 (distal tubular RTA) is characterized by calcium phosphate stone formation, hypercalciuria, hypocitraturia, and an increased urinary pH.

25. Low magnesium levels result in reduced inhibitory activity and are often associated with decreased urinary citrate levels.

26. Cystine stones form due to a defect in the transport of four amino acids: cystine, lysine, ornithine, and arginine. It is inherited as an autosomal recessive and accounts for up to 10% of stones in children. There are two genes involved in the inheritance of the disease.

27. Stones of infection (struvite stones) are composed of magnesium ammonium phosphate and may contain carbonate apatite; they occur in association with urea-splitting

bacteria. Urease-producing pathogens include *Proteus, Klebsiella, Pseudomonas,* and *Staphylococcus.*

28. The cause of stones associated with horseshoe kidneys and ureteropelvic junction obstructions is due to the anatomic abnormality resulting in stasis and an underlying metabolic abnormality.

29. Medullary sponge kidney is characterized by ectasia of the renal collecting ducts and leads to stones through renal acidifying defects, hypercalciuria, and hypocitraturia.

30. Most stones in pregnancy pass spontaneously.

31. The most important determinate of uric acid stone formation is low urinary pH. Low urinary pH in uric acid stone formers is likely due to impaired ammoniagenesis associated with insulin resistance.

Evaluation and Medical Management of Urinary Lithiasis

Michael N. Ferrandino, MD ● Paul K. Pietrow, MD ● Glenn M. Preminger, MD

QUESTIONS

1. Patients with enteric hyperoxaluria are most likely to form stones composed of:
   a. calcium phosphate.
   b. calcium oxalate.
   c. magnesium ammonium phosphate.
   d. uric acid.
   e. cystine.

2. The risk factor most associated with recurrent stone formation in patients with inflammatory bowel disease is:
   a. hyperabsorption of oxalate in the jejunum.
   b. hyperexcretion of calcium from the distal tubule.
   c. diminished citrate absorption in the terminal ileum.
   d. hyperabsorption of calcium in the small bowel.
   e. increased colonic absorption of free oxalate.

3. Hypocitraturia in patients with inflammatory bowel disease or chronic diarrhea syndrome is due to:
   a. persistent bicarbonate losses.
   b. hypokalemia.
   c. metabolic acidosis.
   d. intracellular acidosis.
   e. all of the above.

4. The optimum treatment for patients with enteric hyperoxaluria includes:
   a. calcium supplements, potassium citrate, and increased oral fluid intake.
   b. dietary restriction of oxalate.
   c. thiazides and potassium citrate.
   d. allopurinol.
   e. pyridoxine.

5. The most important factor predisposing patients to gouty diathesis is:
   a. hypercalciuria.
   b. low urinary pH.
   c. hypocitraturia.
   d. low urine volumes.
   e. hyperuricosuria.

6. The initial laboratory test that provides the most important diagnostic clue in patients with uric acid calculi is:
   a. urine pH.
   b. serum uric acid levels.
   c. urine sodium.
   d. urine calcium.
   e. urine uric acid levels.

7. The most appropriate medical treatment of a patient with gouty diathesis is:
   a. allopurinol.
   b. thiazides.
   c. increased fluids.
   d. dietary calcium restriction.
   e. potassium citrate.

8. A patient with recurrent uric acid calculi is placed on oral medical treatment and returns for follow-up 3 months later. He is noted to have significantly elevated urinary uric acid levels as compared with his first 24-hour urine collection. This finding is due to:
   a. increased production of endogenous uric acid.
   b. failure to avoid high-sodium foods.
   c. increased solubility of uric acid.
   d. increased consumption of red meat.
   e. inhibition of xanthine oxidase.

9. A patient with uric acid calculi is placed on alkali therapy but returns 1 year later having passed two calcium phosphate stones. A repeat 24-hour urine demonstrates a urine pH of 7.4, a urinary citrate of 450 mg/day, and a urinary uric acid of 875 mg/day. The most likely cause for recurrent stone formation is:
   a. cessation of potassium citrate.
   b. increase in oral purine intake.
   c. decrease in solubility of uric acid.
   d. excess alkalization.
   e. increase in saturation of oxalate.

10. A patient with gouty diathesis is started on sodium bicarbonate therapy, and urinary pH is maintained between 6.3 and 6.7. Calcium oxalate stones may form due to:
    a. sodium inhibiting calcium reabsorption in the proximal tubule.
    b. homogeneous nucleation of calcium oxalate.
    c. undiagnosed hypercalciuria.
    d. lack of allopurinol in medical management regimen.
    e. reduction in monosodium urate.

11. A 58-year-old Hispanic female with a history of recurrent urinary tract infections treated three to four times in the past 18 months is seen by her family physician. At present she is asymptomatic. She has no history of nephrolithiasis. Renal ultrasound demonstrates moderate left hydronephrosis and a large density within the renal pelvis with posterior shadowing. A kidney-ureter-bladder (KUB) view with tomography reveals a poorly opacified dendritic stone in the renal pelvis and lower pole calyces. Prior urine cultures have *Proteus* and *Klebsiella* species. The stone composition of this patient is most likely:
    a. calcium oxalate.
    b. uric acid.
    c. magnesium ammonium phosphate.
    d. cystine.
    e. hydroxyapatite.

12. The most significant factor contributing to stone formation in patients with struvite calculi is:
    a. gouty diathesis.
    b. recurrent urinary tract infections.
    c. family history.
    d. hyperoxaluria.
    e. hypercalciuria.

13. The most common cause of recurrent stone disease in a patient having undergone "sandwich" therapy for a staghorn calculus is:
    a. hypomagnesuria.
    b. hyperoxaluria.
    c. retained stone fragments.
    d. renal tubular acidosis.
    e. hypercalciuria.

14. Which of the following treatments is contraindicated for patients with recurrent struvite calculi?
    a. Orthophosphate
    b. Fluoroquinolones
    c. Thiazide diuretics
    d. Acetohydroxamic acid
    e. Calcium channel blockers

15. Acetohydroxamic acid contributes to reducing infection stone formation by:
    a. reversing associated metabolic defects.
    b. preventing recurrent urinary tract infections.
    c. alkalization of the urine.

    d. irreversibly inhibiting urease.
    e. all of the above.

16. A 12-year-old boy is seen for evaluation of recurrent nephrolithiasis. He has spontaneously passed three stones over the previous 4 years and has recently undergone shock wave lithotripsy twice without success. He has been treated in the past with an unknown medication, but this was discontinued because the parents believed it was of no benefit. Urinalysis demonstrates hexagonal crystals. The likely metabolic diagnosis contributing to this patient's recurrent stone formation is:
    a. hypocitraturia.
    b. hyperoxaluria.
    c. low urine volumes.
    d. gouty diathesis.
    e. cystinuria.

17. First-line medical treatment for the prevention of recurrent cystine stones would be aimed at:
    a. urinary acidification.
    b. increasing the solubility of cystine.
    c. decreasing urinary sodium.
    d. decreasing the solubility of cystine.
    e. binding of cystine within the intestines.

18. α-Mercaptopropionylglycine (α-MPG, Thiola) may be helpful in the management of cystinuria because it:
    a. acts as a diuretic, further decreasing urinary cystine concentration.
    b. is significantly more effective than D-penicillamine.
    c. can be used as both an oral and intrarenal chemolytic agent.
    d. has equivalent efficacy at increasing solubility with reduced toxicity as compared with D-penicillamine.
    e. adequately alkalizes the urine, obviating the need for potassium citrate.

19. Three years after initiating treatment for cystine stones with α-MPG, 800 mg/day, a patient returns with a follow-up, 24-hour urine collection demonstrating a significant reduction in cystine excretion from 740 to 250 mg/day. Urine volume is 775 mL/day. He has two additional stones. The reason for recurrent stone formation is:
    a. increased age, thereby exacerbating the disorder.
    b. decreased efficacy of α-MPG.
    c. continued supersaturation of urinary cystine.
    d. continued hypocitraturia.
    e. increased urine acidity.

20. A 19-year-old white woman with a 6-year history of recurrent stone disease is found to have multiple bilateral renal calculi by renal ultrasound during an evaluation for recurrent flank pain. She reports having passed more than 10 stones in the previous 2 years. Review of the renal ultrasound indicates no evidence of hydronephrosis. KUB film and tomograms demonstrate five stones on the left and eight stones on the right, all less than 4 mm. She has a strong family history of stones with three first-degree relatives and two cousins with nephrolithiasis. Urine pH is consistently above 6.8. Stone compositions have been mixed

calcium phosphate and calcium oxalate. The most definitive test to identify this disorder would demonstrate:

a. decreased serum parathyroid hormone (PTH) levels.
b. persistently elevated urine calcium.
c. inability to reduce the urine pH below 5.3.
d. normalization of hypercalciuria.
e. marked increase in urinary uric acid levels with initiation of treatment.

21. Which of the following is NOT a cause of hypocitraturic calcium nephrolithiasis?
a. Thiazide-induced hypocitraturia
b. Absorptive hypercalciuria type I
c. Distal renal tubular acidosis
d. Metabolic acidosis
e. Chronic diarrheal syndrome

22. The most appropriate treatment for patients with renal tubular acidosis is:
a. thiazides.
b. allopurinol.
c. sodium alkali.
d. acetohydroxamic acid.
e. potassium alkali.

23. Renal tubular acidosis may be associated with nephrolithiasis due to:
a. hypercalciuria and hypocitraturia.
b. hyperoxaluria and hypercalcemia.
c. hyperuricosuria.
d. hypocitraturia with normal urine magnesium.
e. hypercitraturia and hypercalciuria.

24. Chronic metabolic acidosis may cause:
a. increased PTH levels.
b. significantly reduced bone density.
c. hypercalcemia.
d. increased intestinal calcium absorption.
e. all of the above.

25. To accurately diagnose a patient with renal leak hypercalciuria, one must identify both:
a. increased intestinal calcium absorption and hyperthyroidism.
b. renal leak of calcium and normal intestinal calcium absorption.
c. hypoparathyroidism and increased intestinal calcium absorption.
d. secondary hyperparathyroidism and renal calcium leak.
e. primary hyperparathyroidism and increased intestinal calcium absorption.

26. Which of the following findings would support the diagnosis of renal leak hypercalciuria?
a. Hypocitraturia
b. Diminished urinary cyclic AMP excretion
c. Normocalciuria on a calcium-restricted diet
d. Decreased urinary sodium with thiazide challenge
e. Low or low/normal radial bone density

27. The primary abnormality in patients with renal leak hypercalciuria is considered to be:
a. impairment of renal tubular reabsorption of calcium.
b. excessive mobilization of calcium from bone.
c. increased 1,25-$(OH)_2$ vitamin D levels.
d. elevation of serum PTH levels.
e. hyperabsorption of intestinal calcium.

28. Which of the following mechanisms explains the effectiveness of thiazides in treating patients with renal leak hypercalciuria? Thiazides:
a. bind calcium in the intestinal tract.
b. cause intracellular volume depletion.
c. correct the renal leak of calcium by augmenting calcium reabsorption in the proximal tubule.
d. directly inhibit calcium absorption.
e. restore normal serum 1,25-$(OH)_2$ vitamin D levels.

29. Which of the following medications is contraindicated in this renal leak hypercalciuria disorder because it will cause a negative calcium balance?
a. Trichlormethiazide
b. Sodium cellulose phosphate
c. Orthophosphate
d. Acetohydroxamic acid
e. Allopurinol

30. The primary defect in patients with absorptive hypercalciuria is considered to be:
a. primary hyperabsorption of intestinal calcium.
b. hypersecretion of PTH.
c. renal leak of calcium.
d. bone disease.
e. excessive dietary intake of calcium-containing foods.

31. The most appropriate initial treatment for patients with absorptive hypercalciuria is:
a. sodium cellulose phosphate.
b. allopurinol.
c. potassium citrate.
d. limited dietary calcium.
e. phosphate binders.

32. Which of the following is NOT a potential complication of sodium cellulose phosphate?
a. Hyperoxaluria
b. Hyperuricosuria
c. Hypomagnesuria
d. Negative calcium balance with secondary hyperparathyroidism
e. Gastrointestinal upset

33. After 18 months of chlorthalidone treatment, a patient with hypercalciuria is doing well with no further stone formation. However, 8 months later, while still on thiazides, she passed a small stone. The most likely cause of her recurrent stone formation is:
a. excessive intake of dietary calcium.
b. inappropriate fluid management.

c. excessive sodium intake.

d. thiazide-induced hypocitraturia.

e. cessation of medications.

34. A patient with absorptive hypercalciuria is continued on chlorthalidone and potassium citrate without problems for 18 months and then passes two stones spontaneously. She claimed that she was still on her medications. The most likely cause of her continued stone formation is:

a. excessive calcium intake.

b. heterogeneous nucleation of calcium oxalate.

c. high dietary sodium intake.

d. bone mobilization of calcium.

e. exacerbation of intestinal calcium absorption.

35. The metabolic condition in a patient with absorptive hypercalciuria type II is:

a. a less severe form of absorptive hypercalciuria type I.

b. controlled by a calcium-restricted diet.

c. not characterized by a renal leak of calcium.

d. characterized by an increased intestinal absorption of calcium.

e. all of the above.

36. The most appropriate treatment in a patient with absorptive hypercalciuria type II may include all of the following EXCEPT:

a. moderate intake of high calcium-containing foods.

b. limit sodium intake.

c. increase fluids to maintain urine volumes greater than 2 L/day.

d. restrict dietary oxalate.

e. intake of potassium citrate.

Imaging

1. A 50-year-old woman with chronic left back pain undergoes an intravenous urogram (IVU) depicted in Figure 46–1.

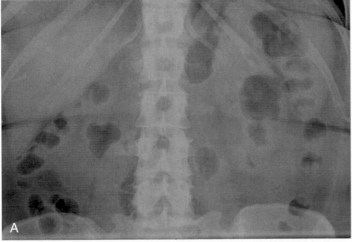

Scout

Figure 46–1.

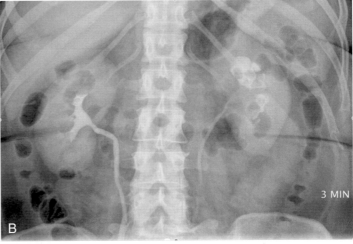

Excretory phase

Figure 46–1, cont'd.

A spiral CT scan (not shown) shows the filling defects depicted to measure 400 Hounsfield units. These findings are most suggestive of:

a. urothelial carcinoma.

b. uric acid calculi.

c. calcium oxalate calculi.

d. blood clots.

e. drug calculi.

ANSWERS

1. **b. calcium oxalate.** Patients with enteric hyperoxaluria are more likely to form calcium oxalate stones, owing to increased urinary excretion of oxalate and decreased inhibitory activity from hypocitraturia, secondary to chronic metabolic acidosis and hypomagnesuria. In addition, fluid losses from persistent diarrhea from inflammatory bowel disease may cause an extremely concentrated environment suitable for stone formation.

2. **e. increased colonic absorption of free oxalate.** Intestinal hyperabsorption of oxalate in patients with enteric hyperoxaluria is the most significant risk factor leading to recurrent calculus formation. Intestinal transport of oxalate is primarily increased because of the effects of bile salts and fatty acids on the permeability of colonic intestinal mucosa to oxalate. The total amount of oxalate absorbed may also be increased because of an enlarged intraluminal pool of oxalate available for absorption. Intestinal fat malabsorption characteristic of ileal disease will exaggerate calcium soap formation, limit the amount of "free" calcium to complex to oxalate, and thereby raise the oxalate pool available for absorption.

3. **e. all of the above.** Acid-base status is probably the most important factor in the renal handling of citrate. Hypokalemia with its induced intracellular acidosis (caused by bicarbonate loss from chronic diarrhea) will reduce urinary citrate both by enhancing renal tubular resorption and reducing the synthesis of citrate. Therefore in patients with enteric hyperoxaluria in whom bicarbonate loss and hypokalemia both contribute to metabolic acidosis, the hypocitraturia is often profound.

4. **a. calcium supplements, potassium citrate, and increased oral fluid intake.** The initial goals of medical

management are to rehydrate and reverse metabolic acidosis. Hydration is at times difficult in some patients because an increase in oral fluids may exacerbate diarrhea. Hydration and potassium citrate will contribute to the reversal of the metabolic acidosis, as well as enhance the excretion of citrate to increase its inhibitory effects on stone formation. Calcium supplements will bind excess oxalate within the intestine, thereby reducing intestinal oxalate absorption. Calcium citrate may offer an ideal calcium supplement in this condition because it should reduce urinary oxalate and increase urinary citrate. Thiazides may worsen metabolic acidosis and hypokalemia through their diuretic effects and renal potassium losses. Colon resection may be of benefit in those patients refractory to medical management because the primary site of intestinal absorption of oxalate is the large bowel.

5. **b. low urinary pH.** Although low urine volumes and hyperuricosuria contribute to the possibility of uric acid stone formation, the most critical determinant of the crystallization of uric acid remains urinary pH. In addition, uric acid stones may be formed in patients with primary gout with associated severe hyperuricosuria and other secondary causes of purine overproduction such as myeloproliferative states, glycogen storage disease, and malignancy.

6. **a. urine pH.** Patients with gouty diathesis and uric acid stones will characteristically have urinary pH lower than the dissociation constant for uric acid (5.5). In fact, many will have a urine pH consistently close to 5. Whereas serum and urine uric acid levels may be elevated in patients with uric acid calculi, the urine pH remains the most cost-effective means of screening for this condition and monitoring therapy.

7. **e. potassium citrate.** Allopurinol will decrease the production of uric acid by inhibiting xanthine oxidase in the purine metabolic pathway but is most effective in patients with extremely elevated levels of uric acid (urinary uric acid >1500 mg/day). In addition, increasing total urine volume will decrease the concentration of uric acid to assist in preventing stone formation. However, raising the urinary pH above the dissociation constant of uric acid is the key to preventing recurrent uric acid stone formation and correcting gouty diathesis. The urine pH should be maintained between 6.0 and 6.5. Thiazides and calcium restriction have limited roles in the medical treatment of uric acid stone patients.

8. **c. increased solubility of uric acid.** With adequate alkali therapy, this patient has been able to raise the urine pH above the dissociation constant of uric acid. The solubility of uric acid is more than 10 times greater at a pH of 7 than at a pH of 5. Therefore patients may initially present with low/normal 24-hour urinary uric acid levels because the uric acid will precipitate out of solution in the acid urinary environment. Once the urine has been alkalized, all of the uric acid will come back into solution, causing a significant increase in the urinary uric acid.

9. **d. excess alkalization.** Excessive alkalization with urinary pH values above 7.0 may result in calcium phosphate stone formation. Alkali therapy with potassium citrate should aim to keep the urinary pH between 6.5 and 7.0 when treating patients with gouty diathesis.

10. **a. sodium inhibiting calcium reabsorption in the proximal tubule.** Patients treated with sodium alkali will occasionally begin forming calcium oxalate stones due to an excess sodium load that will inhibit reabsorption of calcium in the proximal tubule, thereby causing hypercalciuria. In addition, heterogeneous nucleation of calcium oxalate induced by monosodium urate may occur in those individuals with hyperuricosuria. Thus potassium-based alkali, usually in the form of potassium citrate, is the treatment of choice for patients with gouty diathesis.

11. **c. magnesium ammonium phosphate.** Ascending urinary tract infections with urea-splitting organisms such as *Proteus* species will metabolize urea to ammonia. Ammoniuria, in conjunction with a matrix composed of organic compounds, carbonate apatite, inflammatory cells, and bacteria, results in the rapid formation of an "infection" calculus, eventually progressing into a mineralized, dense stone. Bacteria trapped within the stone perpetuate the recurrent urinary tract infections, and further stone formation eventually develops into the classic staghorn calculus.

12. **b. recurrent urinary tract infections.** Etiologic factors involved with infection calculi include a history of recurrent urinary tract infections and potential anatomic or physiologic abnormalities. It is important to remember that these patients may also have underlying metabolic disorders such as hypercalciuria, which could contribute to the stone formation. These disorders are most commonly found in patients with mixed stone composition (i.e., struvite and calcium calculi). A comprehensive metabolic evaluation is warranted in these patients.

13. **c. retained stone fragments.** After removal of an infected struvite calculus, the most common cause of recurrent stone formation is failure to completely eradicate the calculus. Surgical therapy may leave retained fragments of infected stone within calyces, thus allowing infection to persist. Underlying metabolic disorders may also contribute to recurrent stone formation, but persistent calculus remains the most important risk factor.

14. **a. Orthophosphate.** "Struvite stones," "infection stones," or "triple-phosphate stones" all refer to calculi composed of magnesium ammonium phosphate or carbonate apatite. Because phosphate is a major component of these two salts, phosphate therapy would be contraindicated in cases of infection calculi because this medication may promote further stone formation.

15. **d. irreversibly inhibiting urease.** Acetohydroxamic acid (AHA), a competitive inhibitor of the bacterial enzyme urease, will reduce the urinary saturation of struvite and retard stone formation. When given at a dose of 250 mg orally three times a day, this medication can prevent the recurrence of new stones and inhibit the growth of existing stones in patients with chronic urea-splitting infections. AHA can also cause dissolution of small stones. However, up to 30% of patients will experience minor side effects including headache, nausea, vomiting, anemia, rash, or alopecia. In addition, 15% of patients have developed deep venous thrombosis while on long-term treatment. Therefore careful monitoring is required when using this medication.

16. **e. cystinuria.** Cystinuria is a complex autosomal recessive disorder of amino acid transport involving cystine, ornithine, lysine, and arginine (COLA). Supersaturation of the urine will occur in patients with the homozygous state. Therefore it is unusual to see a family history with cystine

stones, and the age at onset is often in the first or second decade.

17. **b. increasing the solubility of cystine.** Increasing the solubility of cystine is the mainstay of treating this disorder. Therefore medical therapy is aimed at dissociating cystine into cysteine, which is 200 times more soluble than cystine. Solubility increases dramatically when this disulfide exchange occurs, effectively preventing further stone formation.

18. **d. has equivalent efficacy at increasing solubility with reduced toxicity as compared with D-penicillamine.** D-Penicillamine and α-MPG are equally effective in their ability to decrease urinary cystine levels. However, studies have demonstrated that α-MPG is significantly less toxic than D-penicillamine. Moreover, the side effects that may occur with α-MPG are also less severe. However, if a patient has been doing well on D-penicillamine with no significant complications, there is no need to switch medications.

19. **c. continued supersaturation of urinary cystine.** The primary goal of medical therapy is to reduce the urinary cystine concentration below the solubility limit of 200 to 250 mg/L of urine. Because many of these patients present at a young age, compliance may be difficult. Even though this patient's cystine excretion has been reduced to 250 mg/day by the α-MPG therapy, his cystine concentration remains greater than 300 mg/L. Therefore a combination of medication along with an increased urine output is essential to reduce the urinary cystine concentration. Long-term follow-up is necessary to ensure urinary cystine beneath the saturation concentration.

20. **c. inability to reduce the urine pH below 5.3.** Renal tubular acidosis is a clinical syndrome of chronic metabolic acidosis resulting from renal tubular abnormalities while glomerular filtration is relatively well preserved. Although patients may present with many different symptoms and physical findings, renal stone formation is a well-recognized manifestation of distal renal tubular acidosis (dRTA). Patients with the incomplete form of dRTA are not persistently acidemic despite their inability to lower urinary pH with an acid load. These patients are able to compensate for their acidification defect and remain in acid-base balance by increasing ammonia synthesis and ammonium excretion as a buffering mechanism. The initial identification of incomplete dRTA is often a chance finding. Many of these patients will present with recurrent nephrolithiasis or may be referred for evaluation after the discovery of nephrocalcinosis after routine abdominal radiographs. Most patients will have normal serum electrolytes, yet they will have a high-normal urine pH along with significant hypocitraturia. The diagnosis of incomplete dRTA can be confirmed by inadequate urinary acidification after an ammonium chloride loading test.

21. **b. Absorptive hypercalciuria type I.** Urinary citrate is a potent inhibitor of stone formation, particularly in excess of 600 mg/day on a 24-hour urine collection. Hypocitraturia can be a result of any acidotic state because acidosis will cause both decreased endogenous renal citrate production and increased renal tubular absorption of citrate. Hypokalemia induced by thiazide wasting of potassium will cause intracellular metabolic acidosis, thus using citrate and reducing excretion in a manner similar to metabolic acidosis. Chronic diarrheal syndromes promote intestinal loss of alkali and dehydration, resulting in metabolic acidosis and reduced urinary citrate levels.

22. **e. potassium alkali.** In the past, sodium alkali has been the treatment of choice for chronic therapy in patients with distal renal tubular acidosis. It was given either in the form of sodium bicarbonate or Shohl solution (a combination of sodium citrate and citric acid). Although sodium alkali is beneficial in correcting the acidosis, excess sodium may be detrimental to calcium metabolism, especially with respect to nephrolithiasis. Sodium alkali therapy has been complicated by the development of calcium stones (calcium phosphate or calcium oxalate), especially when the urinary pH is above 7. Potassium citrate has been shown to reduce the excretion of urinary calcium, whereas sodium alkali has no effect on urinary calcium. Therefore potassium alkali, usually in the form of potassium citrate (Poly Citra K or Urocit-K), is the recommended first-line therapy.

23. **a. hypercalciuria and hypocitraturia.** Hypocitraturia, commonly seen in patients with distal renal tubular acidosis, promotes the formation of nephrolithiasis due to reduced inhibitory action of urinary citrate. In addition, hypercalciuria will occur due to mobilization of calcium from bone and impaired renal tubular absorption of calcium, both as a result of chronic acidosis.

24. **b. significantly reduced bone density.** It is well established that metabolic acidosis may cause a negative calcium balance as a result of impaired renal tubular reabsorption of calcium in the proximal tubule, leading to excessive renal loss of calcium. In addition, intestinal calcium absorption is diminished in patients with persistent acidosis. Slow dissolution of bone mineral can also be identified as calcium and phosphate act as buffering mechanisms to correct the acidosis. Chronic acidosis has been cited as a major factor in the genesis of bone disease.

25. **d. secondary hyperparathyroidism and renal calcium leak.** To confirm the diagnosis of renal hypercalciuria, evidence for secondary hyperparathyroidism and renal leak of calcium must be present. Both of these values can be obtained during the fasting urinary calcium test. Before arrival at the physician's office, it is essential that patients have adhered to a calcium- and sodium-restricted diet for at least 12 hours before testing to eliminate the effects of absorbed calcium on fasting calcium excretion. Three hundred milliliters of distilled water is consumed 12 and 9 hours before the fasting urine collection to ensure adequate hydration. At 7 AM, patients empty their bladder completely, discard the urine, and drink another 600 mL of distilled water. Urine is then collected as a pooled sample for a 2-hour period (7 AM to 9 AM). A fasting serum blood is obtained at the end of the 2-hour period. The serum sample is analyzed for PTH levels. The fasting urine sample is assayed for calcium and creatinine. Fasting urinary calcium is expressed as milligrams per deciliter of glomerular filtrate because it is reflective of renal function. To obtain this value, urinary calcium in milligrams per milligram of creatinine is multiplied by serum creatinine in milligrams per deciliter. Normal fasting urinary calcium is less than 0.11 mg/dL glomerular filtrate.

26. **e. Low or low/normal radial bone density.** Patients with renal hypercalciuria may display a low or low/normal radial bone density. The diminished bone density is a result of the secondary hyperparathyroidism, which causes

stimulation of parathormone (PTH) and subsequent production of 1,25-$(OH)_2$ vitamin D. Both PTH and vitamin D will act on bone to mobilize calcium and cause a loss in bone density. Calcium restriction has no effect in managing renal hypercalciuria.

27. **a. impairment of renal tubular reabsorption of calcium.** The primary abnormality in renal hypercalciuria is an impairment in proximal renal tubular calcium reabsorption. This urinary calcium wasting and subsequent reduction in serum calcium concentration stimulates the production of PTH. As a result, vitamin D synthesis in the kidney is stimulated. Both PTH and vitamin D will increase bone resorption and absorption of intestinal calcium, increasing the circulating concentration and filtered load of calcium. This often causes significant hypercalciuria. Unlike primary hyperparathyroidism, serum calcium is normal and the state of hyperparathyroidism is secondary.

28. **c. correct the renal leak of calcium by augmenting calcium reabsorption in the proximal tubule.** Thiazide is the primary medical treatment of renal hypercalciuria and has been shown to correct the renal leak of calcium by augmenting the calcium reabsorption in the distal tubule. In addition, thiazides cause extracellular volume depletion, thereby stimulating proximal tubular reabsorption of calcium. A positive calcium balance ensues, with correction of the secondary hyperparathyroidism.

29. **b. Sodium cellulose phosphate.** Sodium cellulose phosphate is a calcium-binding resin that inhibits the absorption of calcium in the intestine. This medication will further exaggerate secondary hyperparathyroidism in patients with renal hypercalciuria by binding the intestinal calcium being absorbed to compensate for the renal calcium loss. Therefore sodium cellulose phosphate should only be used in cases of absorptive hypercalciuria, in which the object of treatment is to reduce the primary defect of intestinal calcium hyperabsorption.

30. **a. primary hyperabsorption of intestinal calcium.** The basic abnormality in absorptive hypercalciuria type I is the intestinal hyperabsorption of calcium. The consequent increase in the circulating concentration of calcium enhances the renal filtered load and suppresses parathyroid function. Hypercalciuria results from the combination of increased filtered load and reduced renal tubular reabsorption of calcium, a function of parathyroid suppression. The excessive renal loss of calcium compensates for the high calcium absorption from the intestinal tract and helps to maintain serum calcium in the normal range.

31. **e. phosphate binders.** Sodium cellulose phosphate (SCP) does not correct the primary intestinal defect in this condition. However, SCP will bind calcium within the gut, making it less available for absorption. Complications of SCP treatment may include induction of hyperoxaluria and hypomagnesemia because sodium cellulose phosphate will bind cations other than calcium. In addition, sodium cellulose phosphate, if used in patients with other types of hypercalciuria, can perpetuate a negative calcium balance by parathyroid stimulation. SCP should be used only in patients with severe type I absorptive hypercalciuria. Although widely used to treat this condition, thiazides are not considered selective medical therapy for type I absorptive hypercalciuria. Thiazides do not correct the basic abnormality of increased calcium intestinal absorption but will augment calcium reabsorption in the distal tubule. In addition, extracellular volume depletion indirectly stimulates proximal tubular reabsorption of calcium.

32. **b. Hyperuricosuria.** Sodium cellulose phosphate will bind calcium in the intestinal tract to aid in correcting hypercalciuria of type I absorptive hypercalciuria. This may result in excess filtered load of oxalate because calcium is no longer available to bind oxalate in the gut for excretion. Sodium cellulose phosphate will bind other cations, causing hypomagnesemia due to intestinal losses. In addition, sodium cellulose phosphate, if used in patients with other types of hypercalciuria, can perpetuate a negative calcium balance by parathyroid stimulation and further calcium wasting. A common adverse effect of sodium cellulose phosphate is gastrointestinal upset, occasionally causing cessation of therapy.

33. **d. thiazide-induced hypocitraturia.** Intracellular acidosis resulting from thiazide-induced hypokalemia will augment renal tubular reabsorption of citrate with resultant hypocitraturia. The reduction in the inhibitory effects of hypocitraturia may promote further stone formation. Therefore potassium repletion is necessary if long-term thiazide treatment is anticipated. Our potassium supplement of choice is potassium citrate, either in pill or liquid preparations.

34. **c. high dietary sodium intake.** A high dietary sodium intake has two deleterious effects in this case. An excess sodium load will inhibit reabsorption of calcium in the proximal tubule, thereby causing hypercalciuria. Moreover, sodium will block the hypocalciuric action of thiazides. Therefore patients placed on thiazide diuretics for management of hypercalciuria should also be placed on a dietary sodium restriction.

35. **e. all of the above.** Absorptive hypercalciuria type II is believed to be a less severe form of absorptive hypercalciuria type I. Placing a patient on a calcium-restricted diet will normalize his or her urinary calcium excretion. However, patients with hypercalciuria type I have a high urinary calcium excretion despite dietary modifications. Appropriate therapy for absorptive hypercalciuria type II would be to moderate calcium intake and maintain a high fluid intake to maintain urine output greater than 2 L/day. A severe dietary calcium restriction is not indicated because significant dietary modifications may exacerbate stone disease.

36. **d. restrict dietary oxalate.** Initial treatment of patients diagnosed with absorptive hypercalciuria type II includes moderating dietary calcium intake to reduce the filtered calcium load, increasing fluid intake to maintain urine output greater than 2 L/day, limiting sodium intake to reduce the calciuric effects of sodium on proximal tubular reabsorption of calcium, and initiating potassium citrate to alkalize the urine and reduce calcium stone formation.

Imaging

1. **b. uric acid calculi.** The scout radiograph from the IVU (X1-1) shows no densely radiopaque calculi. On the excretory images (X1-2), there are well-demarcated filling defects with a staghorn configuration in the left renal pelvis and detached round calculi in the mildly hydronephrotic upper pole calyces. Calcium oxalate or cystine calculi should be much

more radiopaque on the scout radiograph and would have Hounsfield units above 600. Uric acid calculi are often not seen on a KUB and have densities in the 400 to 600 Hounsfield range, thus making b the most likely possibility. Urothelial carcinoma will not have a smooth and rounded

configuration to the filling defects in the collecting system, and their density will be similar to tissue. Drug calculi occur in patients on protease inhibitor therapy for HIV infections. They tend to be tiny in size, cause ureteral obstruction, and are unlikely to be visible on an IVU.

Additional Study Points

1. First-time stone formers are at a 50% risk for recurrence. Males have both a higher instance of calculi and a higher recurrence rate.

2. Infection calculi may contain large quantities of endotoxin.

3. A complete urine collection is confirmed by the 24-hour excretion of creatinine. On average 1 mg/kg/hour is excreted.

4. As the phosphate content of the stone increases from calcium oxalate to calcium oxalate/calcium apatite to calcium apatite, the incidence of renal tubular acidosis increases from 5% to 39% and the incidence of primary hyperthyroidism from 2% to 10%. Thus higher phosphate content in stones correlates with an increased incidence of renal tubular acidosis and primary hyperparathyroidism.

5. Obesity increases the risk of nephrolithiasis.

6. Hypercalciuria not associated with hypercalcemia may be subdivided into (1) excess gastrointestinal absorption, (2) renal tubular leak, or (3) normocalcemic hyperparathyroidism.

7. Patients with hyperuricosuria have increased calcium oxalate urolithiasis due to heterogeneous nucleation.

8. Increased protein intake increases the likelihood of renal stones due to increased urinary calcium, oxalate, and uric acid excretion. Moderate calcium ingestion and a reduced sodium diet when combined with animal protein restriction reduce calcium stone episodes by approximately 50%.

9. Thiazides may unmask primary hyperparathyroidism by causing a marked rise in serum calcium.

10. Indinavir stones may not be visible on CT.

11. Furosemide-induced nephrolithiasis should always be considered in neonates who develop nephrolithiasis.

12. Children with stones should always be worked up because inborn errors of metabolism may be responsible for the stones in a significant number of patients. The inborn errors of metabolism most commonly found in this circumstance include cystinuria, renal tubular acidosis, and primary hyperoxaluria.

Percutaneous Approaches to the Upper Urinary Tract Collecting System

J. Stuart Wolf, Jr., MD, FACS

QUESTIONS

1. Percutaneous nephrostomy is not indicated for:
   a. instillation of bacillus Calmette-Guérin.
   b. a Whitaker test.
   c. urinary retention.
   d. ureteral obstruction.
   e. calyceal obstruction.

2. Relative to retrograde ureteral stent placement, percutaneous nephrostomy:
   a. requires less anesthesia.
   b. has a lower success rate.
   c. is less commonly complicated by bacteriuria.
   d. is associated with better health-related quality-of-life scores.
   e. is preferred in most cases of ureteral obstruction owing to malignancy.

3. Which of the following is correct regarding the orientation of the kidney?
   a. The left kidney is slightly inferior to the right kidney.
   b. The longitudinal axis is 45 degrees from vertical, with the lower pole lateral to the upper pole.
   c. The longitudinal axis is 45 degrees from vertical, with the lower pole anterior to the upper pole.
   d. The apposition of the colon to the kidney is greatest on the right side and at the lower pole.
   e. Immediately posterior to the kidneys are the quadratus lumborum muscle, the psoas muscle, and the diaphragm.

4. Which of the following is correct regarding the intrarenal collecting system?
   a. There are 8 to 16 minor calyces.
   b. Compound calyces are most common in the lower pole.
   c. Most kidneys have three distinct infundibula: the upper, middle, and lower.
   d. Paired anterior and posterior calyces enter about 90 degrees from each other.
   e. There is a consistent relationship between anterior and posterior calyces and their medial-lateral position on anterior-posterior radiography.

5. The correct order of the division of the intrarenal branches of the renal artery is:
   a. segmental, interlobar (infundibular), arcuate, interlobular.
   b. segmental, arcuate, interlobar (infundibular), interlobular.
   c. segmental, arcuate, interlobular, interlobar (infundibular).
   d. interlobular, segmental, interlobar (infundibular), arcuate.
   e. segmental, interlobular, interlobar (infundibular), arcuate.

6. To reduce the risk of infectious complications from percutaneous renal surgery:
   a. urine cultures should be obtained on all patients.
   b. urine must be sterile before the procedure.
   c. all patients should receive prophylactic antimicrobials.
   d. gentamicin is an acceptable single agent for antimicrobial prophylaxis.
   e. ampicillin/sulbactam is not an acceptable single agent for antimicrobial prophylaxis.

7. An advantage of the supine over the prone position for percutaneous renal surgery is:
   a. improved pulmonary mechanics.
   b. a large horizontal working surface.
   c. easier entry into posterior calyces.
   d. reduced pressure in the collecting system.
   e. easier entry into upper pole calyces.

8. Access into which site provides the best balance of versatility and safety for percutaneous renal surgery in the prone position?
   a. Upper pole posterior calyx
   b. Lower pole anterior calyx
   c. Renal pelvis
   d. Upper pole infundibulum
   e. Middle calyceal compound calyx

9. Techniques for retrograde assistance for percutaneous renal access include all of the following EXCEPT:
   a. straight ureteral catheter to inject air.
   b. ureteral access sheath to facilitate drainage.
   c. ureteroscopy to retrieve guidewire.

d. retrograde approach to percutaneous access.

e. retrograde placement of externalized (single pigtail) ureteral stent for drainage.

10. Compared with an 18-gauge needle, the 21-gauge needle for percutaneous renal access:

a. requires a 0.025-inch guidewire.

b. cannot be directed as easily.

c. is more traumatic.

d. should not be used by inexperienced operators.

e. entails less risk of loss of access.

11. Compared with ultrasonography, fluoroscopy for percutaneous renal access:

a. is more portable.

b. provides more rapid evaluation of the entire kidney.

c. visualizes the access needle better.

d. cannot be used to monitor tract dilation.

e. is preferred in transplant kidneys.

12. The "eye-of-the-needle" technique for fluoroscopic percutaneous renal access:

a. cannot be performed in morbidly obese patients.

b. increases radiation exposure to the operator's hands compared with the "triangulation" technique.

c. is not as dependent on retrograde assistance as the "triangulation" technique

d. can be used to place a needle at any useful location and angle.

e. continuously monitors the depth of needle penetration.

13. Dilation of the tract for percutaneous renal surgery is:

a. most effective with a balloon dilator.

b. least expensive with metal dilators.

c. safest with semirigid dilators.

d. most rapid with metal dilators.

e. easiest with a one-shot semirigid dilator.

14. When considering percutaneous renal surgery in horseshoe kidneys:

a. lower hemorrhage rates than in normal kidneys can be expected.

b. upper pole access is dangerous.

c. CT can be misleading.

d. lower pole access is preferred in most cases.

e. the puncture site is more lateral than in normal kidneys.

15. When considering percutaneous renal surgery in transplant kidneys:

a. fluoroscopy is more useful than ultrasonography for initial access.

b. semirigid plastic dilators should not be used.

c. retrograde assistance is difficult.

d. the typical hypermobility renders tract dilation difficult.

e. secondary procedures are usually required.

16. Foley catheters for postprocedure nephrostomy drainage:

a. do not need to be secured at the skin.

b. can have a ureteral catheter passed through the end.

c. should have the balloon filled with dilute contrast material.

d. stay more securely in the kidney than Malecot catheters.

e. are less likely to become infected than Malecot catheters.

17. The Cope retention mechanism:

a. is used in internal ureteral stents.

b. is more secure than a balloon catheter.

c. is functionally equivalent to a pigtail retention mechanism.

d. requires cutting the tube to disengage.

e. is used in nephro-ureteral stents.

18. A postoperative nephrostomy tube:

a. reduces postoperative bleeding.

b. offers greater assurance of upper urinary tract drainage than an internal ureteral stent.

c. does not maintain the percutaneous access tract unless it is greater than 18 French.

d. should be placed in the dilated access site.

e. is associated with pain unrelated to tube diameter.

19. Alternatives to a nephrostomy tube after percutaneous renal surgery include all of the following EXCEPT:

a. maintenance of the working sheath.

b. an internal ureteral stent that is removed cystoscopically.

c. an internal ureteral stent with an attached string that exits out the flank.

d. a ureteral stent externalized out the urethra.

e. no drainage tube at all.

20. Adjuncts intended to enhance hemostasis of the percutaneous tract include all EXCEPT:

a. direct cauterization of the tract.

b. cryotreatment of the tract.

c. radiofrequency ablation of the tract.

d. insertion of oxidized cellulose.

e. instillation of fibrin glue.

21. Compared with internal ureteral stents after percutaneous renal surgery, nephrostomy tubes are associated with:

a. the need for a second procedure for removal.

b. greater technical success rates.

c. fewer complications.

d. greater narcotic use, more so if the nephrostomy tube is of large caliber.

e. less urinary leakage from skin entry site.

22. Following an unremarkable percutaneous nephrolithotomy, there is nonpulsatile bleeding from the tract when the sheath is removed around an 8.5-Fr Cope nephrostomy tube. The next step is to:

a. irrigate the nephrostomy tube.

b. occlude the nephrostomy tube and apply pressure to the incision.

c. replace the nephrostomy tube with a ureteral stent and suture the skin.

d. replace the nephrostomy tube with an 18-Fr Malecot catheter.

e. replace the nephrostomy tube with a Kaye nephrostomy tamponade balloon.

23. During a percutaneous resection of a 2-cm upper pole urothelial neoplasm, there is sudden hemorrhage from the resection site. The next step is to:
a. continue if vision is adequate.
b. instill gelatin granules plus thrombin into the collecting system.
c. insert a percutaneous nephro-ureteral stent.
d. place an 18-Fr Councill catheter with the balloon inflated at the injury site.
e. prepare the patient for selective angio-embolization.

24. A 52-year-old woman calls the office 1 week after percutaneous nephrolithotomy complaining of bright red blood in the urine on her past two urinations. She denies light-headedness. The next step in management should be to:
a. force fluids and call back if bleeding persists.
b. check the percutaneous access site and come to the hospital if there is external bleeding.
c. apply pressure to the percutaneous access site.
d. take amino-caproic acid (Amicar).
e. admit to the hospital.

25. Which of the following has *not* been reported to cause renal pelvic perforation in association with percutaneous renal surgery?
a. Wire passage
b. Tract dilation
c. Use of resectoscope
d. Ultrasonic lithotripsy
e. Massive hemorrhage

26. Two days after percutaneous endopyelotomy in a 45-year-old man, a nephrostogram reveals contrast entering the colon. The next step is to:
a. maintain a nephrostomy tube in place and insert a ureteral stent.
b. maintain a nephrostomy tube in place and insert a colostomy tube.
c. back out the nephrostomy tube into the colon and insert a new nephrostomy tube.
d. start parenteral feeding after appropriate tube insertions.
e. do exploratory laparotomy.

27. Which of the following is TRUE regarding pleural injuries in association with percutaneous renal surgery?
a. Access below the 12th rib results in hydrothorax/pneumothorax in 1% to 2% of cases.
b. Supra-12th rib punctures (the 11th intercostal space) result in hydrothorax/pneumothorax in 20% to 40% of cases.
c. Supra-11th rib punctures (the 10th intercostal space) result in hydrothorax/pneumothorax in 50% to 75% of cases.
d. Combined with distal ureteral obstruction, a nephropleural fistula can occur.
e. Thoracostomy to water seal drainage and suction is recommended.

28. Irrigation fluid during percutaneous renal surgery:
a. should be normal saline except during percutaneous nephrolithotomy.
b. is not absorbed systemically unless there is significant venous injury.
c. should not be glycine.
d. will not create a defined extrarenal collection.
e. can have fatal consequences.

29. A 75-year-old woman has an oral temperature of 38.9° C on the first night after an uncomplicated percutaneous nephrolithotomy for a partial staghorn renal calculus. A nephrostomy tube is in place. She is hemodynamically stable. The preoperative urine culture had grown *Proteus* sp. sensitive to oral trimethoprim sulfamethoxazole, which she received for 2 weeks preoperatively. One gram of cefazolin had been administered on call to the operating room. The next step is to:
a. observe the patient.
b. administer broad-spectrum antibiotics.
c. culture urine and blood, obtain a chest radiograph, and administer broad-spectrum antibiotics.
d. culture aspirate from the nephrostomy tube and irrigate the tube.
e. conduct Doppler ultrasonography of the lower extremities and/or pulmonary embolus–protocol CT scan.

30. Following percutaneous renal surgery, loss of renal function is:
a. approximately 5% of the ipsilateral function per access site.
b. minimal in the absence of vascular injury.
c. greater than after shock wave lithotripsy.
d. less in the ectopic compared with orthotopic kidneys.
e. greater in solitary compared with nonsolitary kidneys.

ANSWERS

1. **c. urinary retention.** Obstruction of the lower urinary tract is best treated by drainage of the bladder rather than the kidney, unless secondary obstruction of the upper tract has developed that is refractory to vesical drainage. The other indications are appropriate ones for percutaneous nephrostomy.

2. **a. requires less anesthesia.** Percutaneous nephrostomy can be done under local anesthesia, as opposed to retrograde ureteral stent placement, which usually requires general or regional anesthesia. Percutaneous nephrostomy has a greater initial success rate than retrograde ureteral stent placement, at least when the collecting system is dilated. Percutaneous nephrostomy is commonly associated with bacteriuria and has health-related quality-of-life scores that are equivalent to those associated with retrograde ureteral stent placement. Ureteral stents provide satisfactory drainage in most cases of ureteral obstruction owing to malignancy.

3. **e. Immediately posterior to the kidneys are the quadratus lumborum muscle, the psoas muscle, and the diaphragm.** The upper poles are anterior to attachments of the diaphragm. It is the right kidney that is slightly inferior to the left one. The second two statements are correct except that the angulation is 30 degrees rather than 45 degrees. The apposition of the colon to the kidney

varies with location; it is greatest on the left side and at the lower pole.

4. **d. Paired anterior and posterior calyces enter about 90 degrees from each other.** There are 5 to 14 minor calyces in each kidney. Compound calyces are common in the lower pole but are almost always present in the upper pole. In about two thirds of kidneys, there are only two major calyceal systems (upper and lower). Because variation is considerable, the lateral-medial orientation of the calyces on anteroposterior radiography cannot be used to reliably determine which calyces are posterior.

5. **a. segmental, interlobar (infundibular), arcuate, interlobular.**

6. **c. all patients should receive prophylactic antimicrobials.** The American Urological Association recommends periprocedural antimicrobial prophylaxis for all cases of percutaneous renal surgery. Urine cultures are considered standard only in patients where bacteriuria is likely; in other cases a screening urinalysis might be adequate, with urine culture when the urinalysis is suspicious. The urine cannot be sterilized in some patients, especially in the presence of an externalized urinary catheter or an infected calculus, and the goal in these situations is only to suppress the bacterial count before to intervention. Aminoglycosides (e.g., gentamicin) are acceptable for antimicrobial prophylaxis when combined with another agent. Ampicillin/sulbactam, first- and second-generation cephalosporins, and fluoroquinolones are acceptable single agents for antimicrobial prophylaxis.

7. **d. reduced pressure in the collecting system.** The angle of the sheath is more horizontal in the supine compared with the prone position for percutaneous renal surgery, which reduces pressure in the collecting system (the volume also is reduced, which is a disadvantage). When padding is appropriate, pulmonary mechanics are better in the prone position. The prone position also provides a large horizontal working surface and easier entry into posterior and upper pole calyces compared with the supine position.

8. **a. Upper pole posterior calyx.** This offers the most versatile access to the intrarenal collecting system, and as long as the entry is below the 11th rib the advantages generally outweigh the risks. In the prone position an anterior calyx offers little access to the rest of the kidney. Percutaneous access into an infundibulum or the renal pelvis poses a greater risk of vascular injury than calyceal entry. Middle calyces are rarely compound, and middle calyceal access usually does not provide good access to the upper and lower calyces.

9. **e. retrograde placement of externalized (single pigtail) ureteral stent for drainage.** This can be performed at the conclusion of the procedure for drainage as an alternative to a nephrostomy tube, but it is not useful before access because the pigtail might interfere with the procedure and it would not have any advantage over a straight ureteral catheter or an occlusion balloon catheter. The other choices are all well-described techniques of retrograde assistance for percutaneous renal access.

10. **b. cannot be directed as easily.** A 21-gauge needle requires a 0.018-inch guidewire, and because of this extra step (exchanging the 0.018-inch guidewire for a 0.035-inch guidewire) there is a greater risk of loss of access. Compared with an 18-gauge needle, the 21-gauge needle is less

traumatic; this is its primary advantage, and it is for this reason that the 21-gauge needle should be used when the operator is less experienced or if minimizing trauma is paramount.

11. **c. visualizes the access needle better.** It is easier to see a needle and monitor tract dilation with fluoroscopy than with ultrasonography. Ultrasonography is more portable, can more rapidly evaluate different views of the kidney, and is preferred in settings in which retrograde access cannot be attained or is difficult to attain (kidneys above urinary diversions, transplanted kidneys, kidneys above a completely obstructed ureter, etc.)

12. **d. can be used to place a needle at any useful location and angle.** The "eye-of-the-needle" technique can be used to place the access needle at any useful location and angle. If the fluoroscopy field is collimated down and the needle is held with a hemostat, sponge forceps, or purpose-built needle holder, then radiation exposure to the operator's hands can be avoided. Retrograde assistance is useful with any fluoroscopic percutaneous renal access. The "triangulation" technique monitors depth of needle placement in all fluoroscopic views, whereas the "eye-of-the-needle" technique assesses depth only at the final step.

13. **b. least expensive with metal dilators.** Metal dilators are least expensive on a per-case basis because they are reusable. The metal dilators are also the most effective dilators. The safest dilators, at least in terms of association with less hemorrhage in most comparative series, are the balloon dilators. The balloon dilators are also more rapid than sequential passage of metal or semirigid dilators. The one-shot semirigid dilator technique requires considerable manual force to create the tract.

14. **a. lower hemorrhage rates than in normal kidneys can be expected.** The rate of major hemorrhagic complications during percutaneous renal surgery in horseshoe kidneys (4.3%) is less than in normal kidneys (6% to 20%). Upper pole access is useful, and direct lower pole access is usually not possible. Cross-sectional imaging is useful in assessing the anatomy of horseshoe kidneys. The initial entry into a horseshoe kidney is usually more medial than in normal kidneys.

15. **c. retrograde assistance is difficult.** Owing to the site of ureteral implantation in the bladder, retrograde assistance for percutaneous renal surgery in transplant kidneys is difficult. Given this, ultrasonography is more useful than fluoroscopy for guiding initial access. Semirigid plastic and metal dilators are often more useful than balloon dilators owing to the perinephric scarring, which makes the transplant kidney quite fixed in place rather than hypermobile. Despite the challenges, percutaneous renal surgery in transplant kidneys has a high success rate and secondary procedures are usually not required.

16. **d. stay more securely in the kidney than Malecot catheters.** Malecot tubes are the easiest to pull out, and circle nephrostomy tubes are the hardest. All tubes should be secured at the skin to reduce the risk of at least one mechanism of tube removal. A ureteral catheter can be passed through the end hole of a Councill catheter; a Foley catheter does not have this end hole. Water should be used to inflate the balloon because the more viscous contrast material might hinder emptying of the balloon when removal is attempted. All nephrostomy tubes, even ones with robust internal retention devices, should be fixed to

the skin externally with a suture or other mechanism. There is no evidence that Foley and Malecot catheters differ in propensity for infection.

17. **e. is used in nephro-ureteral stents.** The Cope retention mechanism is used in the renal pelvic portion of nephro-ureteral stents. According to one study, the Cope retention mechanism is more secure than Malecot wings but does not retain as well as a balloon. It is more secure than a passive pigtail retention mechanism owing to the string that holds the coil in place. Although cutting the tube is one way of releasing the string, this can also be achieved by loosening the locking mechanism.

18. **b. offers greater assurance of upper urinary tract drainage than an internal ureteral stent.** Drainage of the upper urinary tract after percutaneous renal surgery is adequate with an internal ureteral stent in most cases (or with no tube at all in selected cases), but when hemorrhage occurs the larger caliber of a nephrostomy tube provides better drainage of the upper urinary tract collecting system than an internal ureteral stent. Although redilation may be required, any external nephrostomy tube maintains the percutaneous access tract. The nephrostomy tube does not have to be placed in the dilated access site (i.e., it can be placed at a new site), although that is common practice. Most studies suggest that the pain associated with nephrostomy tubes is related to tube diameter, with smaller-caliber tubes causing less pain.

19. **a. maintenance of the working sheath.** The stiff working access sheath would be a poor choice for postprocedure collecting system drainage. The other options have all been described.

20. **c. radiofrequency ablation of the tract.** Radiofrequency ablation of the tract would be difficult with current instruments. The other options have all been described. Other hemostatic agents that have been inserted/instilled into the tract include gelatin sponge and gelatin granules plus thrombin.

21. **d. greater narcotic use, more so if the nephrostomy tube is of large caliber.** Most randomized controlled trials comparing internal ureteral stents to large-caliber nephrostomy tubes after percutaneous renal surgery have shown reduced narcotic use in the stented patients. The difference is less significant when a small-caliber nephrostomy tube is used. A small caliber nephrostomy tube can be removed at the bedside after a period of clamping to assess clinically for distal ureteral obstruction, without a need for nephrostography. Randomized controlled trials comparing internal ureteral stents to nephrostomy tubes have not revealed any difference in technical success rates, complication rates, or incidence of urinary leakage from the skin entry site.

22. **b. occlude the nephrostomy tube and apply pressure to the incision.** The first step in this situation is to occlude the nephrostomy tube and apply pressure to the incision. Let the collecting system clot off, and do not irrigate until the following morning. This management is successful in the majority of cases. If bleeding persists, then insert a Kaye nephrostomy tamponade balloon. An 18-Fr Malecot catheter will be no more effective than the 8.5-Fr Cope nephrostomy tube, and removing the nephrostomy tube altogether is ill-advised.

23. **a. continue if vision is adequate.** If the procedure can be safely continued, then the blood loss cannot be great. If vision is lost, however, then the procedure must be aborted. If so, then inserting and occluding a nephrostomy tube, as well as applying pressure to the incision such that the collecting system clots off, will suffice in most cases. If this is not successful, then place a Councill catheter and attempt to inflate the balloon at the injury site. Instillation of gelatin granules plus thrombin into the collecting system can create a clot that is difficult to manage. Selective angio-embolization is required only when an arterial injury does not respond to less intensive management or if the injury is obviously a significant one that will not respond to these maneuvers.

24. **e. admit to the hospital.** Any report of bright red blood in the urine after percutaneous renal surgery should prompt hospital admission. This woman likely has an arteriovenous fistula or arterial pseudoaneurysm. The conservative measures are not likely to be helpful, and amino-caproic acid (Amicar) is contraindicated in the setting of upper tract hemorrhage.

25. **e. Massive hemorrhage.** The renal pelvis would clot off before the pressure from hemorrhage could rupture it. Any manipulation during percutaneous renal surgery can cause renal pelvic perforation.

26. **c. back out the nephrostomy tube into the colon and insert a new nephrostomy tube.** The main principle of care of a colon injury associated with percutaneous renal surgery is prompt and separate drainage of the colon and urinary collecting system. If detected post-operatively, the simplest management is to back the nephrostomy tube out of the kidney and into colon to serve as a colostomy, and then obtain separate access to the upper urinary tract, either with a new percutaneous access that does not traverse the colon or a retrograde-placed ureteral stent. Parenteral feeding is usually not required, and for the typical extraperitoneal injury open surgical repair usually is needed only if the patient develops peritonitis or sepsis.

27. **d. Combined with distal ureteral obstruction, a nephropleural fistula can occur.** Nephropleural fistula (urinothorax) is a direct and persistent communication between the intrarenal collecting system and the intrathoracic cavity, which can follow percutaneous renal access of the upper urinary tract in the setting of pleural transgression. Some degree of distal ureteral obstruction usually contributes to the problem. The rates of pleural injuries for infra-12th rib, supra-12th rib, and supra-11th rib punctures are approximately less than 0.5%, 5%, and 25%, respectively. Thoracostomy is not necessary for all patients with hydrothorax. If one is necessary, then a small-caliber tube with a Heimlich valve is all that is required in the absence of lung injury.

28. **e. can have fatal consequences.** Intravascular hemolysis from the extravasated water irrigant can be fatal. The irrigant for percutaneous renal surgery should be saline, with the exception of glycine or similar nonelectrolytic isotonic fluids when monopolar electrocautery is used. Intravascular or extravascular extravasation of fluid from continued irrigation in the setting of a large venous injury or collecting system perforation can lead to clinically significant sequelae including volume overload and extrarenal fluid collections that require drainage.

29. **a. observe the patient.** Preoperative and perioperative management of this patient has been appropriate. In this setting, most patients with fever after percutaneous

nephrolithotomy do not have infection. If the fever is an isolated postoperative one, then standard postoperative care (e.g., early ambulation, use of incentive spirometry) is all that is necessary. If the fever does not resolve promptly, then appropriate diagnostic evaluation and initiation of antimicrobial therapy and other supportive care are indicated.

30. **b. minimal in the absence of vascular injury.** The kidney suffers little permanent damage after uncomplicated percutaneous renal surgery. If there is significant loss of function, it is usually owing to disastrous vascular injury or the angio-embolization used to treat hemorrhage. Loss of renal function associated with percutaneous renal surgery is less than or equal to the loss associated with shock wave lithotripsy. There is no evidence that damage to the kidney is any more or less in ectopic, orthotopic, solitary, or nonsolitary kidneys.

Additional Study Points

1. Percutaneous nephrostomy and retrograde ureteral stents are generally equivalent in their capacity to resolve fever in patients with upper urinary tract obstruction.
2. The colon can be lateral or posterior to the right and left kidney.
3. A guidewire that enters the kidney percutaneously and exits the urethra via the meatus (through and through access) may be the only guidewire used when operating on the upper urinary tract. However, in all other situations, two guidewires—a safety and working guidewire—are required. No matter what the access, it is always prudent to have a safety guidewire in addition to the working guidewire.
4. It is imperative that the dilators do not pass too far into the collecting system because this results in renal pelvic injury.
5. Percutaneous nephrostomy is generally the preferred approach for endoscopy of the obstructed collecting system in the transplanted kidney.
6. Approximately 1% of percutaneous procedures are complicated by delayed hemorrhage. Delayed hemorrhage is usually due to arteriovenous fistulas or arterial pseudo-aneurysms. The preferred management is selective angio-embolization.

48

Surgical Management of Upper Urinary Tract Calculi

Brian R. Matlaga, MD, MPH ● James E. Lingeman, MD

QUESTIONS

1. The best predictor of post–percutaneous nephrolithotomy (PNL) urosepsis is:
   a. preoperative bladder urine culture.
   b. intraoperative bladder urine culture.
   c. stone culture.
   d. preoperative blood culture.
   e. intraoperative blood culture.

2. What is the risk of mortality from an untreated struvite staghorn stone?
   a. Less than 10%
   b. 10% to 30%
   c. 30% to 50%
   d. 50% to 70%
   e. Greater than 70%

3. The increased risk of residual fragments after extracorporeal shockwave lithotripsy (SWL) of large-volume calculi is of particular importance for patients with stones composed of:
   a. brushite.
   b. uric acid.
   c. struvite.
   d. calcium oxalate monohydrate.
   e. calcium oxalate dihydrate.

4. What is the single most important factor when choosing among SWL, ureteroscopic stone removal, and PNL for renal calculi?
   a. Stone composition
   b. Stone location
   c. Anatomic abnormalities
   d. Stone burden
   e. Body habitus

5. What is the preferred treatment for a known brushite stone former harboring a lower pole renal calculus 25 mm in diameter?
   a. SWL
   b. SWL with ureteral stenting

   c. Flexible ureteroscopy with holmium laser lithotripsy
   d. PNL
   e. Laparoscopic pyelolithotomy

6. What is the preferred initial treatment for staghorn calculi?
   a. SWL with ureteral stenting
   b. Flexible ureteroscopy with holmium laser lithotripsy
   c. PNL
   d. Extended pyelolithotomy
   e. Anatrophic nephrolithotomy

7. Which of these is the most difficult stone composition to fragment with SWL?
   a. Calcium oxalate dihydrate
   b. Calcium oxalate monohydrate
   c. Struvite
   d. Hydroxyapatite
   e. Uric acid

8. What is the preferred treatment approach for a symptomatic 1.5-cm stone in a lower pole calyceal diverticulum?
   a. SWL
   b. Flexible ureteroscopy
   c. PNL
   d. PNL with fulguration of the diverticulum
   e. Laparoscopic diverticulectomy

9. What is the preferred initial treatment for a 10-mm stone in the renal pelvis of a horseshoe kidney with minimal hydronephrosis?
   a. SWL
   b. Flexible ureteroscopy
   c. PNL
   d. Laparoscopic pyelolithotomy
   e. Symphysiotomy with pyelolithotomy

10. What is the preferred treatment approach for a 10-mm renal calculus in a patient who weighs 375 lb?
    a. SWL
    b. Flexible ureteroscopy
    c. PNL

d. SWL using the "blast path" technique

e. Open surgery

11. What is the preferred treatment option for a patient with a symptomatic 1.5-cm renal calculus and a coagulopathy?

a. SWL

b. SWL after administration of fresh-frozen plasma

c. Indwelling ureteral stent

d. Flexible ureteroscopy

e. PNL

12. Residual fragments after SWL have been associated with which of the following?

a. Hypertension

b. An increased rate of recurrent stones

c. A decreased rate of recurrent stones

d. Perinephric hematomas

e. Hematuria

13. What is the most sensitive test for identifying residual fragments after PNL?

a. Nephrotomography

b. MRI

c. Ultrasonography

d. Noncontrast CT

e. Contrast-enhanced CT

14. Factors affecting the probability of spontaneous passage of ureteral calculi include all of the following EXCEPT:

a. stone size.

b. stone location at presentation.

c. stone composition.

d. degree of hydronephrosis.

e. duration of symptoms.

15. Irreversible loss of renal function can occur within what time period when a completely obstructing ureteral stone is present?

a. 1 week

b. 2 to 4 weeks

c. 4 to 6 weeks

d. More than 6 weeks

e. 3 months

16. A first-time stone former is diagnosed with a 4-mm proximal ureteral calculus. The best initial management is:

a. ureteroscopic laser lithotripsy.

b. ureteral stent placement.

c. SWL.

d. expectant management.

e. SWL with ureteral stent placement.

17. Large-volume matrix calculi, which form as a consequence of urinary tract infection, are:

a. effectively fragmented with SWL.

b. best approached in a ureteroscopic fashion.

c. generally sterile.

d. radiopaque and well visualized on plain radiographic studies.

e. most efficiently treated with PNL.

18. Ureteral stent placement when SWL is performed for ureteral stones is appropriate for all of the following reasons EXCEPT:

a. solitary kidney.

b. relief of severe symptoms.

c. enhancement of stone fragmentation.

d. relief of obstruction.

e. aid in localization of difficult-to-visualize stones.

19. The preferred single agent for medical expulsive therapy for distal ureteral calculi is:

a. nifedipine.

b. tamsulosin.

c. Solu-Medrol.

d. ibuprofen.

e. terazosin.

20. The treatment modality associated with the greatest stone-free rates and the least morbidity for patients with distal ureteral stones of any size is:

a. PNL.

b. SWL.

c. ureteroscopy.

d. open ureterolithotomy.

e. laparoscopic ureterolithotomy.

21. Renal colic during pregnancy is associated with which of the following?

a. Increased risk of pre-term delivery

b. Urinary tract infection

c. Renal dysfunction

d. Increased rate of spontaneous stone passage

e. A lack of clinical symptoms

22. Metabolic changes associated with pregnancy that are relevant to urolithiasis include all of the following EXCEPT:

a. absorptive hypercalciuria.

b. hypercalcemia.

c. hyperuricosuria.

d. increased citrate excretion.

e. increased magnesium excretion.

23. What is the preferred initial diagnostic study for suspected urolithiasis in pregnant patients?

a. Kidney, ureter, and bladder radiograph (KUB)

b. Tailored intravenous pyelography (i.e., two or three films)

c. Renal ultrasonography

d. Spiral CT

e. MRI

24. All of the following treatments of an obstructing ureteral calculus in a pregnant woman are acceptable EXCEPT:

a. ureteroscopy.

b. placement of a double-J ureteral stent.

c. placement of a nephrostomy drain.

d. SWL.

e. All of the above are acceptable interventions.

25. The risk of ureteral perforation is greatest with which of the following intracorporeal lithotripsy technologies?

a. Electrohydraulic lithotripsy (EHL)

b. Holmium laser

c. Pulsed-dye laser

d. Ultrasonic lithotripsy

e. Ballistic lithotripsy

26. The risk of retrograde stone propulsion is greatest with which of the following intracorporeal lithotripsy technologies?

a. EHL

b. Holmium laser

c. Pulsed dye laser

d. Ultrasonic lithotripsy

e. Ballistic lithotripsy

27. What are the preferred initial power settings for holmium laser lithotripsy of ureteral stones?

a. 0.6 J, 6 Hz

b. 0.6 J, 10 Hz

c. 1.0 J, 10 Hz

d. 1.2 J, 10 Hz

e. 1.0 J, 15 Hz

28. Which intracorporeal lithotripsy technology will most efficiently fragment and evacuate renal calculi?

a. Ultrasonic lithotripsy

b. Ballistic lithotripsy

c. Combination ultrasonic/ballistic lithotripsy

d. Holmium laser

e. EHL

29. Which intracorporeal lithotripsy technology has the least risk of ureteral perforation?

a. Ultrasound

b. Ballistic

c. Holmium laser

d. EHL

e. Erbium laser

30. Energy sources for SWL include all of the following EXCEPT:

a. electrohydraulic.

b. holmium laser.

c. piezoelectric.

d. electromagnetic.

e. microexplosive.

31. What is a major disadvantage of ultrasound imaging for SWL?

a. Inability to visualize ureteropelvic junction (UPJ) stones

b. Exposure to ionizing radiation

c. Inability to visualize radiolucent stones

d. Expense of ultrasonography systems

e. Inability to visualize ureteral stones

32. Factors influencing the amount of pain during SWL include all but which of the following?

a. Power level applied

b. Stone composition

c. Type of shockwave generator

d. Shockwave energy density at the point of skin penetration

e. Stone location

33. Which lithotripter produces the highest stone-free rates?

a. Wolf Piezolith 2300

b. Siemens Lithostar

c. Modified Dornier HM3

d. Unmodified Dornier HM3

e. HealthTronics LithoTron

34. Possible mechanisms producing stone fragmentation during SWL include all of the following EXCEPT:

a. compression fracture.

b. spallation.

c. acoustic cavitation.

d. dynamic fatigue.

e. vaporization.

35. What percentage of kidneys experience trauma during SWL?

a. 0% to 20%

b. 20% to 40%

c. 40% to 60%

d. 60% to 80%

e. 80% to 100%

36. Risk factors that will enhance the bioeffects of shockwaves include all of the following EXCEPT:

a. patient's age older than 60 years.

b. pediatric age.

c. stone burden.

d. preexisting hypertension.

e. reduced renal mass.

37. The primary insult to the kidney exposed to shockwaves occurs in which of the following tissues?

a. Blood vessels

b. Proximal tubule

c. Renal papillae

d. Glomerulus

e. Renal capsule

38. Which anesthetic technique is associated with the greatest likelihood of a successful SWL treatment outcome?

a. General endotracheal

b. Intravenous sedation

c. Epidural

d. Sedation

e. Topical anesthetic

39. Which of the following is an absolute contraindication to PNL?
    a. Morbid obesity
    b. Uncorrected coagulopathy
    c. Neurogenic bladder
    d. Pelvic kidney
    e. Horseshoe kidney

40. Which treatment maneuver will reduce the likelihood of SWL-induced renal injury?
    a. Begin treatment at a high energy level
    b. Treat at a rate of 120 shocks per minute
    c. Treat with a topical local anesthetic
    d. Pretreat the targeted kidney at a low-energy level and then ramp up treatment to a high-energy level
    e. Pretreat the contralateral kidney at a high-energy level and then ramp up treatment of the target kidney to a high-energy level

41. What is the most common secondarily infecting organism after percutaneous stone removal?
    a. *Proteus mirabilis*
    b. *Klebsiella oxytoca*
    c. *Pseudomonas aeruginosa*
    d. *Staphylococcus epidermidis*
    e. *Enterococcus (Streptococcus) faecalis*

42. Which of the following is the antimicrobial of choice for ureteroscopy?
    a. First-generation cephalosporin
    b. Second-generation cephalosporin
    c. Aminoglycoside
    d. Fluoroquinolone
    e. Nitrofurantoin

43. What is the preferred site of puncture into the renal collecting system during access for PNL?
    a. Upper pole infundibulum
    b. Anterior lower pole calyx
    c. Posterior lower pole calyx
    d. Upper pole calyx
    e. Renal pelvis

44. Risk factors for colon injury during PNL include all of the following EXCEPT:
    a. horseshoe kidney.
    b. kyphoscoliosis.
    c. access lateral to the posterior axillary line.
    d. previous jejunoileal bypass for obesity.
    e. upper pole puncture.

45. To minimize the risk of lung and pleura injury during supracostal upper pole access for PNL:
    a. the puncture should be performed during full expiration.
    b. the puncture should be performed during full inspiration.
    c. CO_2 should be injected through the ureteral catheter to identify the upper pole calyx.
    d. the puncture should be done with local anesthesia.
    e. the puncture should be performed by a radiologist.

46. Indications for supracostal access during PNL include all of the following EXCEPT:
    a. predominant stone distribution in the upper pole.
    b. access to the UPJ or proximal ureter required.
    c. cystine stones.
    d. multiple lower pole infundibula and calyces containing stone material.
    e. horseshoe kidneys.

47. When performing PNL and endopyelotomy in the same setting, the optimal point of entry is:
    a. posterior upper pole calyx.
    b. posterior lower pole calyx.
    c. anterior upper pole calyx.
    d. anterior lower pole calyx.
    e. renal pelvis.

48. During access for PNL, what is the preferred initial wire?
    a. Amplatz Super-stiff
    b. Benson
    c. Hydrophilic glide
    d. Lunderquist
    e. J-tipped movable core

49. What is the most common serious error in PNL access?
    a. Not using an Amplatz sheath
    b. Overadvancement of the dilator/sheath
    c. Anterior calyceal puncture
    d. Ultrasonographically guided puncture
    e. The use of telescoping metal dilators

50. What is the appropriate irrigating solution for PNL?
    a. 3% sorbitol
    b. Sterile water
    c. Glycine
    d. Dilute contrast material
    e. 0.9% saline

51. Middle or upper pole access for PNL in horseshoe kidneys is preferred for all of the following reasons EXCEPT:
    a. a higher incidence of retrorenal colon.
    b. malrotation of the renal collecting system.
    c. incomplete ascent of horseshoe kidneys.
    d. anterior medial location of lower pole calyces.
    e. facilitated access to the UPJ or upper ureter.

52. What is the most significant complication of PNL?
    a. Hemorrhage
    b. Extravasation of irrigation fluid
    c. Incomplete stone removal
    d. Urinary tract infection
    e. Pleural effusion

53. What is the risk of arteriovenous fistula formation after PNL?
    a. 1 in 10
    b. 1 in 100
    c. 1 in 200
    d. 1 in 500
    e. 1 in 1000

54. If uncontrolled bleeding persists after nephrostomy tube placement after PNL, what would the preferred approach be?
    a. Insertion of a double-J stent
    b. Administration of furosemide (Lasix) to promote diuresis
    c. Surgical exploration
    d. Immediate angiography
    e. Insertion of a Kaye tamponade balloon

55. If a retroperitoneal injury to the colon is diagnosed after PNL, what is the preferred management?
    a. Surgical exploration and repair
    b. Diverting colostomy with later definitive repair
    c. Leaving the nephrostomy tube in for 2 weeks to allow the tract to mature
    d. Insertion of a double-J stent and withdrawal of the nephrostomy tube into the colon
    e. Immediate removal of the nephrostomy tube

56. The use of double-J stents to reduce the risk of steinstrasse after SWL has been demonstrated to be beneficial for what size of stones?
    a. Greater than 5 mm
    b. Greater than 10 mm
    c. Greater than 15 mm
    d. Greater than 20 mm
    e. Greater than 25 mm

57. Proper management of a stone trapped in a basket, with an avulsed ureter all in continuity and no safety guidewire in place, is:
    a. immediate surgical exploration and primary repair.
    b. cystoscopy to place a guidewire and ureteral stent.
    c. placement of a percutaneous nephrostomy drain.
    d. immediate ureteral reimplantation.
    e. immediate ileal ureter.

58. During the course of a ureteroscopic laser lithotripsy procedure for a 1-cm proximal ureteral stone, a ureteral perforation is noted after fragmentation and removal of the calculus. On inspection of the perforation, a stone fragment is noted outside the ureter in the retroperitoneum. The most appropriate management is to:
    a. terminate the procedure and place a ureteral stent.
    b. advance the ureteroscope into the retroperitoneum and remove the stone fragment with a basket device.
    c. place a nephrostomy tube.
    d. perform laparoscopic exploration and removal of the residual fragment.

e. advance the ureteroscope into the retroperitoneum and fragment the stone with the holmium:YAG laser.

ANSWERS

1. **c. stone culture.** The best predictor of post-PNL urosepsis is stone culture or renal pelvic urine culture results.
2. **b. 10% to 30%.** The 10-year mortality rate of untreated staghorn stones was 28%, versus 7.2% in patients treated with surgery.
3. **c. struvite.** Struvite stones must be removed completely to minimize the risk of continued urea-splitting bacteriuria.
4. **d. Stone burden.** Stone burden (size and number) is perhaps the single most important factor in deciding the appropriate treatment modality for a patient with kidney calculi.
5. **d. PNL.** The Lower Pole Stone Study Group compared ureteroscopy and PNL for patients with 10- to 25-mm lower pole stones and found a significant difference in stone clearance, with only 40% of the ureteroscopic cohort stone free at 3 months versus 76% of the PNL cohort.
6. **c. PNL.** The management of staghorn stones with a combined approach must be viewed as primarily percutaneous, with SWL being used only as adjunct to minimize the number of accesses required.
7. **b. Calcium oxalate monohydrate.** Cystine and brushite are the stones most resistant to SWL, followed by calcium oxalate monohydrate. Next, in descending order, are hydroxyapatite, struvite, calcium oxalate dihydrate, and uric acid stones.
8. **d. PNL with fulguration of the diverticulum.** The percutaneous approach for the management of patients with calyceal diverticular stones provides the patient with the best chance of becoming stone and symptom free. Fulguration of the diverticulum will reduce the risk of recurrence of the diverticulum.
9. **a. SWL.** SWL can achieve satisfactory results in properly selected patients, such as those with small stones (<1.5 cm) in the presence of normal urinary drainage. For larger stones or when there is evidence of poor urinary drainage, PNL should be used as the primary approach.
10. **b. Flexible ureteroscopy.** Retrograde ureteroscopic intrarenal surgery may be the preferred modality of treatment for morbidly obese patients when the stone burden is not excessively large.
11. **d. Flexible ureteroscopy.** When anticoagulation cannot be temporarily discontinued, the use of ureteroscopy in combination with holmium laser lithotripsy is preferred. One study reported that even when patients' coagulopathies were not fully corrected the stones could be successfully treated with no increase in hemorrhagic complications.
12. **b. An increased rate of recurrent stones.** At follow-up (1.6 to 85.4 months), 43% of the patients with residual fragments had a significant symptomatic episode or required intervention.
13. **d. Noncontrast CT.** Although flexible nephroscopy is often considered the "gold standard" for assessing residual stones after PNL, the routine use of flexible nephroscopy has been challenged by studies showing the high sensitivity of noncontrast CT in detecting residual stones. Noncontrast CT had 100% sensitivity for detecting residual stones after PNL

in 36 patients evaluated by both CT and flexible nephroscopy.

14. **c. stone composition.** One study analyzed 75 patients with ureteral calculi and found that the interval to stone passage was highly variable and dependent on stone size, location, and side. Stones that were smaller, more distal, and on the right side were more likely to pass spontaneously. In another study, duration of symptoms before presentation was the most influential factor, followed by the degree of hydronephrosis.

15. **b. 2 to 4 weeks.** Even with complete ureteral obstruction, irreversible loss of renal function does not occur for more than 2 weeks but can progress to total renal unit loss at up to 6 weeks.

16. **d. expectant management.** The majority of ureteral stones less than 5 mm will pass spontaneously and therefore can be treated with expectant management.

17. **e. most efficiently treated with PNL.** Matrix stones are most effectively treated with PNL. SWL is usually ineffective because of the stone's gelatinous nature, and ureteroscopy may be compromised by the large volume of stone material present.

18. **c. enhancement of stone fragmentation.** Although early reports supported the routine use of a ureteral stent to bypass ureteral stones before SWL, data analyzed by the American Urological Association Ureteral Calculi Guidelines Panel showed no improvement in fragmentation with stenting, and therefore routine stent placement before SWL was discouraged. However, ureteral stent placement is appropriate for other indications, such as management of pain, relief of obstruction, and stones that are difficult to visualize, and is mandatory in a patient who has a solitary obstructed kidney.

19. **b. tamsulosin.** Tamsulosin, a selective α-adrenergic blocker, is the preferred agent for medical expulsive therapy, owing to its reported efficacy and superior side effect profile.

20. **c. ureteroscopy.** The stone-free rate for distal ureteral stones approached with ureteroscopy was 91% in the American Urological Association/European Association of Urology Ureteral Stones Guidelines document, an outcome superior to SWL.

21. **a. Increased risk of pre-term delivery.** Pregnant women who require admission and require treatment for renal colic have a greater risk of preterm delivery compared with pregnant women who do not suffer from renal calculi.

22. **b. hypercalcemia.** Pregnancy induces a state of absorptive hypercalciuria and mild hyperuricosuria that is offset by increased excretion of urinary inhibitors such as citrate and magnesium, as well as increased urinary output. The metabolic changes in pregnancy do not influence the rate of new stone occurrence. However, paradoxically, it has been suggested that metabolic alterations in urine may contribute to accelerated encrustation of stents during pregnancy.

23. **c. Renal ultrasonography.** To avoid the small risk of radiation, ultrasonography has become the first-line diagnostic study for urolithiasis in pregnancy.

24. **d. SWL.** Shockwave lithotripsy is not an appropriate treatment for a pregnant woman and should not be performed.

25. **a. EHL.** The major disadvantage of EHL is its propensity to damage the ureteral mucosa and its association with ureteral perforation.

26. **e. Ballistic lithotripsy.** Ballistic lithotripsy is accompanied by a relatively high rate of stone propulsion of between 2% and 17% when ureteral stones are treated. The holmium laser has been associated with a reduced potential for causing retropulsion owing to the weak shockwave that is typically induced during holmium laser lithotripsy.

27. **a. 0.6 J, 6 Hz.** It is recommended to begin treatment using low-pulse energy (i.e., 0.6 J) with a pulse rate of 6 Hz and increase the pulse frequency (in preference to increasing the pulse energy) as needed to speed fragmentation.

28. **c. Combination ultrasonic/ballistic lithotripsy.** Combination ultrasonic and ballistic lithotrites have been reported to provide greater stone clearance rates than do conventional ultrasonic or ballistic lithotrites.

29. **b. Ballistic.** When compared with EHL or ultrasonic or laser lithotripsy, ballistic devices have a significantly lower risk of ureteral perforation.

30. **b. holmium laser.** There are three primary types of shockwave generators: electrohydraulic (Spark Gap), electromagnetic, and piezoelectric. Microexplosive generators have also been produced but have not gained mainstream acceptance.

31. **e. Inability to visualize ureteral stones.** Sonographic localization of a kidney stone requires a highly trained operator. Furthermore, localization of stones in the ureter is difficult or impossible.

32. **b. Stone composition.** The discomfort experienced during SWL is related directly to the energy density of the shockwave as it passes through the skin as well as the size of the focal point, parameters that are affected by all of the choices listed except for stone composition.

33. **d. Unmodified Dornier HM3.** To date, despite the proliferation of lithotripters and the variety of solutions devised for stone targeting and shockwave delivery, no other lithotripter system has convincingly equaled or surpassed the results produced by the unmodified Dornier HM3 device.

34. **e. vaporization.** Several potential mechanisms for SWL stone breakage have been described: (1) spall fracture, (2) squeezing, (3) shear stress, (4) superfocusing, (5) acoustic cavitation, and (6) dynamic fatigue.

35. **e. 80% to 100%.** SWL is now known to induce acute structural changes in the treated kidney in a majority, if not all, patients. Morphologic studies using both MRI and quantitative radionuclide renography have suggested that 63% to 85% of all SWL patients treated with an unmodified Dornier HM3 lithotripter exhibit one or more forms of renal injury within 24 hours of treatment.

36. **c. stone burden.** Patients with existing hypertension are at increased risk for the development of perinephric hematomas as a consequence of SWL. Age is a factor on both ends of the scale in that children and the elderly both appear to be at a greater risk for structural and functional changes after exposure to shockwaves. These responses are probably related to a reduction in the large renal reserve present in most healthy adult patients.

37. **a. Blood vessels.** Macroscopically, the acute changes noted in dog and pig kidneys treated with a clinical dose of shockwaves are strikingly similar to those described for

patients. This lesion is predictable in size, is focal in location, and is unique in the types of injuries (primarily vascular insult) induced. Regions of damage reveal rupture of nearby thin-walled veins, walls of small arteries, and glomerular and peritubular capillaries, which correlates with the vasoconstriction measured in both treated and untreated kidneys. These observations show that both the microvasculature and the nephron are susceptible to shockwave damage; however, the primary injury appears to be a vascular insult.

38. **a. General endotracheal.** Patients undergoing SWL with general endotracheal anesthesia experience a significantly greater stone-free outcome than do patients undergoing SWL with alternative anesthetics.

39. **b. Uncorrected coagulopathy.** Uncorrected coagulopathy and an active, untreated urinary tract infection are two absolute contraindications to PNL.

40. **d. Pretreat the targeted kidney at a low-energy level and then ramp up treatment to a high-energy level.** A number of studies have demonstrated that pretreating the target kidney with low-energy shockwaves, followed by a full clinical treatment dose, will attenuate the renal injury associated with SWL.

41. **d. *Staphylococcus epidermidis*.** Cephalosporins are the most appropriately used antibiotics for prophylaxis of surgical procedures in noninfected stone cases, because the most common secondarily infecting organism is *S. epidermidis*.

42. **d. Fluoroquinolone.** The prophylactic antimicrobial agent of choice for ureteroscopy is a fluoroquinolone.

43. **c. Posterior lower pole calyx.** Because the posterior calyces are generally oriented so that the long axis points to the avascular area of the renal cortex, a posterolateral puncture directed at a posterior calyx would be expected to traverse through the avascular zone.

44. **e. upper pole puncture.** A puncture placed too laterally may injure the colon. The position of the retroperitoneal colon is usually anterior or anterolateral to the lateral renal border. Therefore, risk of colon injury is usually only with a very lateral (lateral to the posterior axillary line) puncture. Posterior colonic displacement is more likely in thin female patients with very little retroperitoneal fat and/or elderly patients, as well as in patients with jejunoileal bypass resulting in an enlarged colon. Other factors increasing the risk of colon injury include anterior calyceal puncture, previous extensive renal operation, horseshoe kidney, and kyphoscoliosis. A retrorenal colon is more frequently noted on the left side.

45. **a. the puncture should be performed during full expiration.** A supracostal puncture should be performed only during full expiration.

46. **c. cystine stones.** A supracostal puncture is indicated when the predominant distribution of stone material is in the upper calyces, when there is an associated UPJ stricture requiring endopyelotomy, in cases of multiple lower pole infundibula and calyces containing stone material or an associated ureteral stone, in staghorn calculi with substantial upper pole stone burden, and in horseshoe kidneys.

47. **a. posterior upper pole calyx.** A posterior upper pole calyx puncture, typically through a supracostal approach, aligns the axis of puncture with the UPJ. This allows the

treating urologist to perform endopyelotomy with a rigid nephroscope, while exerting minimal torque on the instrument.

48. **c. Hydrophilic glide.** The hydrophilic glide wire is preferred for entering the collecting system, because it is the most flexible and maneuverable wire available.

49. **b. Overadvancement of the dilator/sheath.** Overadvancement of the dilator/sheath is the most common serious error in access for PNL and may result in significant trauma to the renal collecting system and/or excessive hemorrhage.

50. **e. 0.9% saline.** Physiologic solutions should be used for irrigation during PNL to minimize the risk of dilutional hyponatremia in the event of large-volume extravasation.

51. **a. a higher incidence of retrorenal colon.** The optimal point of entry for a horseshoe kidney is through a posterior calyx, which is typically more medial than in the normal kidney because of the altered renal axis and rotation associated with the midline fusion. An upper pole collecting system puncture is often appealing, because the entire kidney is usually subcostal. In most cases the lower pole calyces are anterior and inaccessible percutaneously.

52. **a. Hemorrhage.** Bleeding is the most significant complication of PNL, with transfusion rates varying from less than 1% to 10%.

53. **c. 1 in 200.** Bleeding from an arteriovenous fistula or pseudoaneurysm requiring emergency embolization is seen in less than 0.5% of patients.

54. **e. Insertion of a Kaye tamponade balloon.** If bleeding is not controlled by nephrostomy tube placement and clamping, a Kaye nephrostomy tamponade balloon catheter should be placed (Cook Urological, Spencer, IN). The Kaye nephrostomy tube incorporates a low-pressure 12-mm balloon that may be left inflated for prolonged periods to tamponade bleeding from the nephrostomy tract.

55. **d. Insertion of a double-J stent and withdrawal of the nephrostomy tube into the colon.** Colonic injury is an unusual complication often diagnosed on a postoperative nephrostogram. Typically, the injury is retroperitoneal; thus signs and symptoms of peritonitis are infrequent. If the perforation is extraperitoneal, management may be expectant with placement of a ureteral catheter or double-J stent to decompress the collecting system and by withdrawing the nephrostomy tube from an intrarenal position to an intracolonic position, thus serving as a colostomy tube. The colostomy tube is left in place for a minimum of 7 days and is removed after a nephrostogram or a retrograde pyelogram showing no communication between the colon and the kidney.

56. **d. Greater than 20 mm.** Stents may be particularly advantageous with stones larger than 20 mm.

57. **c. placement of a percutaneous nephrostomy drain.** Should a ureteral avulsion occur, the patient should undergo immediate diversion of the renal unit with the placement of a percutaneous nephrostomy drain.

58. **a. terminate the procedure and place a stent.** When an extruded stone is noted outside the ureter, the procedure should be terminated and a ureteral stent placed.

Additional Study Points

1. Determinants of poor stone clearance rates after SWL include large renal calculi, dependent or obstructed portions of the collecting system, very hard stones, and obesity.

2. Most calyceal stones in the absence of intervention are likely to increase in size and cause pain or infection.

3. If left untreated, staghorn calculi are likely to be associated with a progressive decrease in renal function.

4. Patients with cystinuria are more likely to have decreased renal function than other stone formers.

5. There is a linear correlation between Hounsfield units (density) and success of SWL.

6. Complete stone clearance from lower pole calyces is less likely than from other calyces for reasons that are not totally clear.

7. Spontaneous passage of a distal ureteral stone is more likely than that of a proximal ureteral stone.

8. For patients with proximal ureteral stones there is no difference between treating the stone in situ or pushing it back into the renal pelvis when utilizing SWL.

9. In the human there is no clear time threshold for irreversible damage in complete ureteral obstruction. It is clear, however, that patients with compromised vasculature, decreased renal reserve, poor nutrition, and other comorbid diseases such as diabetes tolerate obstruction less well than do patients with normal kidneys.

10. Transvaginal ultrasonography may be used in the pregnant female to observe the lower ureters.

11. Fifty to 80 percent of pregnant patients will spontaneously pass the calculus.

12. EHL produces a hydraulic shockwave and cavitation bubble. It may be used in normal saline solutions.

13. Holmium laser lithotripsy causes stone vaporization by a photothermal mechanism, and when it is used the stone should be painted.

14. Cyanide may be produced when the holmium laser is used to fragment uric acid calculi. To date no untoward effects due to this have been reported.

15. Ultrasound breaks the stone by causing the stone to resonate at a high frequency. Considerable heat may develop at the interface.

16. Stone comminution occurs by two basic mechanisms: mechanical stresses produced by the incident shockwave and collapse of cavitation bubbles adjacent to the surface of the stone.

17. The entire ureter can be more easily accessed in the female with a rigid ureteroscope.

18. For uncomplicated ureteroscopies, a ureteral stent may be safely omitted.

Neoplasms of the Upper Urinary Tract

chapter 49

Malignant Renal Tumors

Steven C. Campbell, MD, PhD ● Brian R. Lane, MD, PhD

QUESTIONS

1. Postoperative radiographic surveillance after radical nephrectomy for T1N0M0 RCC should comprise which studies?

    a. No imaging studies

    b. Chest radiograph yearly

    c. Chest radiograph and abdominal CT scan yearly

    d. Chest radiograph yearly and abdominal CT scan every 2 years

    e. Chest radiograph and abdominal CT scan every 2 years

2. All of the following are advantages of partial nephrectomy compared with radical nephrectomy for localized stage 1 RCC in the setting of a normal contralateral kidney EXCEPT:

    a. lower likelihood of perioperative renal failure.

    b. improved long-term renal function.

    c. reduced risk of cardiovascular events on a longitudinal basis.

    d. lower incidence of local tumor recurrence.

    e. similar cancer-specific survival.

3. After partial nephrectomy for T2N0M0 RCC, it is necessary to perform surveillance abdominal CT with what frequency?

    a. Never

    b. Every 6 months

    c. Every year

    d. Every 2 years

    e. Every 4 years

4. After partial nephrectomy of a solitary kidney, what is the most effective method of screening for hyperfiltration nephropathy?

    a. Urinary dipstick test for protein

    b. 24-Hour urinary protein measurement

    c. Iothalamate glomerular filtration rate (GFR) measurement

    d. Serum creatinine measurement

    e. Renal biopsy

5. The most accurate practical assessment of renal function for routine use after nephrectomy is:

    a. serum creatinine measurement.

    b. urinary dipstick test for protein.

    c. 24-hour urinary protein measurement.

    d. iothalamate GFR measurement.

    e. serum creatinine-based estimation of GFR, such as MDRD equation.

6. What is an important prerequisite for successful laparoscopic cryoablation of a renal tumor?

    a. Slow freezing

    b. Rapid thawing

    c. A single freeze-thaw cycle

    d. A double freeze-thaw cycle

    e. Freezing of tumor to a temperature of –10° C

7. Which two imaging modalities are preferred for demonstrating the presence and extent of an inferior vena caval tumor thrombus?

    a. Abdominal ultrasonography and CT

    b. MRI and renal artery angiography

    c. CT and MRI

    d. MRI and contrast venacavography

    e. Contrast venacavography and transesophageal ultrasonography

8. In patients undergoing complete surgical excision of an RCC, the lowest 5-year survival rate is associated with:

    a. perinephric fat involvement.

    b. microvascular renal invasion.

    c. subdiaphragmatic inferior vena caval involvement.

    d. intra-atrial tumor thrombus.

    e. lymph node involvement.

9. A 45-year-old man has a 5-cm RCC in the upper pole of a solitary left kidney and a single 2-cm left lower lung metastasis. What is the best treatment?

    a. Initial immunotherapy, then partial nephrectomy

    b. Partial nephrectomy, then immunotherapy

    c. Staged partial nephrectomy and pulmonary lobectomy

    d. Simultaneous partial nephrectomy and pulmonary lobectomy

    e. Simultaneous radical nephrectomy and pulmonary lobectomy

10. A healthy 79-year-old man is referred after renal biopsy of a 3.0-cm centrally located renal mass. The biopsy is definitive for renal oncocytoma. The other kidney is normal, the serum creatinine level is 1.0 mg/dL, and there is no evidence of metastatic disease. What is the best next step?
    a. Open radical nephrectomy
    b. Laparoscopic nephroureterectomy
    c. Percutaneous thermal ablation
    d. Partial nephrectomy
    e. Observation with follow-up renal imaging in 6 to 12 months

11. Tuberous sclerosis is similar to von Hippel-Lindau disease in which of the following respects?
    a. Propensity toward development of seizure disorders
    b. Similarity of cutaneous lesions
    c. Common development of adrenal tumors
    d. Frequent involvement of cerebral cortex with vascular lesions
    e. Mode of genetic transmission

12. A 48-year-old woman with a history of seizure disorder presents with recurrent gross hematuria and left flank pain. Abdominal CT shows a large left perinephric hematoma associated with a 3.0-cm left renal angiomyolipoma. There are also multiple right renal angiomyolipomas ranging from 1.5 to 6.5 cm. What is the best management of the left renal lesion?
    a. Selective embolization
    b. Radical nephrectomy
    c. Observation
    d. Partial nephrectomy
    e. Laparoscopic exposure and renal cryoablative therapy

13. Which of the following statements is TRUE regarding cystic nephromas occurring in adults?
    a. They are complex cystic lesions that are typically classified as Bosniak II to III.
    b. They are malignant 2% to 5% of the time.
    c. They are more common in men than in women.
    d. When suspected, they should be treated by radical nephrectomy.
    e. They are readily differentiated from cystic RCC on the basis of appropriate imaging studies.

14. Which environmental factor is most generally accepted as a risk factor for RCC?
    a. Radiation therapy
    b. Antihypertensive medications
    c. Tobacco use
    d. Diuretics
    e. High-fat diet

15. Which of the following manifestations is restricted to certain families with von Hippel-Lindau disease?
    a. RCC
    b. Pancreatic cysts or tumors

    c. Epididymal tumors
    d. Pheochromocytoma
    e. Inner ear tumors

16. RCC develops in what percentage of patients with von Hippel-Lindau disease?
    a. 0% to 20%
    b. 21% to 40%
    c. 41% to 60%
    d. 61% to 80%
    e. 81% to 100%

17. What is the most common cause of death in patients with von Hippel-Lindau disease?
    a. Renal failure
    b. Cerebellar hemangioblastoma
    c. Unrelated medical disease
    d. Pheochromocytoma
    e. RCC

18. The von Hippel-Lindau disease tumor suppressor protein regulates the expression of which of the following mediators of biologic aggressiveness for RCC?
    a. Basic fibroblast growth factor
    b. Vascular endothelial growth factor (VEGF)
    c. Epidermal growth factor receptor (EGFR)
    d. Hepatocyte growth factor (scatter factor)
    e. P-glycoprotein (multiple drug resistance efflux protein)

19. What do hereditary papillary RCC syndrome and von Hippel-Lindau disease have in common?
    a. The mode of genetic transmission
    b. Chromosome 3 abnormalities
    c. A propensity toward tumor formation in multiple organ systems
    d. Inactivation of a tumor suppressor gene
    e. Nearly complete penetrance

20. Mutation of the c-MET proto-oncogene in hereditary papillary RCC leads to:
    a. increased expression of hepatocyte growth factor.
    b. increased sensitivity to VEGF.
    c. inactivation of a tumor suppressor gene that regulates cellular proliferation.
    d. constitutive activation of the receptor for hepatocyte growth factor.
    e. increased expression of VEGF.

21. P-glycoprotein is a transmembrane protein that is involved in:
    a. immunotolerance.
    b. resistance to high-dose interleukin-2 therapy.
    c. resistance to cisplatin therapy.
    d. resistance to radiation therapy.
    e. efflux of large hydrophobic compounds, including many cytotoxic drugs.

22. What is the primary proangiogenic molecule in clear cell RCC?
    a. Basic fibroblast growth factor
    b. Hepatocyte growth factor
    c. VEGF
    d. Epidermal growth factor
    e. Transforming growth factor-β

23. Which of the following is most likely to demonstrate an infiltrative growth pattern?
    a. Clear cell RCC
    b. Sarcomatoid variants of RCC
    c. Papillary RCC
    d. Chromophobe RCC
    e. Oncocytoma

24. What is the most common mutation identified in sporadic clear cell RCC?
    a. Activation of the c-*MET* proto-oncogene
    b. Activation of the von Hippel-Lindau tumor suppressor gene
    c. Inactivation of the von Hippel-Lindau tumor suppressor gene
    d. Inactivation of *TP53*
    e. Inactivation of genes on chromosome 9

25. Which of the following cytogenetic abnormalities is among those commonly associated with papillary RCC?
    a. Trisomy of chromosome 7
    b. Trisomy of the Y chromosome
    c. Loss of chromosome 17
    d. Loss of all or parts of chromosome 3
    e. Loss of chromosome 7

26. What percentage of RCCs are chromophobe cell carcinomas?
    a. 0% to 2%
    b. 4% to 5%
    c. 8% to 10%
    d. 12% to 15%
    e. 18% to 25%

27. Most renal medullary carcinomas are:
    a. found in patients with sickle cell disease.
    b. diagnosed in the fifth decade of life.
    c. responsive to high-dose chemotherapy.
    d. genetically and histologically similar to papillary RCC.
    e. metastatic at the time of diagnosis.

28. Which paraneoplastic syndrome associated with RCC can often be managed or palliated medically?
    a. Polycythemia
    b. Stauffer syndrome
    c. Neuropathy
    d. Hypercalcemia
    e. Cachexia

29. A healthy 64-year-old man is found to have a 6.0-cm solid, heterogeneous mass in the hilum of the right kidney. CT of the abdomen and pelvis shows interaortocaval lymph nodes enlarged to 2.5 cm. A chest radiograph and a bone scintiscan are negative, and the contralateral kidney is normal. The serum creatinine level is 1.0 mg/dL. What is the next best step?
    a. Right radical nephrectomy and regional or extended lymph node dissection
    b. Abdominal exploration, sampling of the enlarged lymph nodes, and possible radical nephrectomy pending frozen section analysis
    c. CT-guided percutaneous biopsy of the lymph nodes
    d. CT-guided percutaneous biopsy of the tumor mass
    e. Systemic therapy followed by radical nephrectomy

30. Which of the following patients would be the best candidate for percutaneous biopsy of a renal mass?
    a. A 42-year-old man with a 2.5-cm Bosniak III complex renal cyst
    b. An 88-year-old man with angina and a 1.7-cm solid, enhancing renal mass
    c. A 32-year-old woman with bilateral solid, enhancing renal masses ranging from 1.5 to 4.0 cm
    d. A 48-year-old woman with a 3.5-cm solid, enhancing renal mass with fat density present
    e. A 38-year-old woman with a fever, a urinary tract infection, and a 3.5-cm solid, enhancing renal mass

31. A 67-year-old man undergoes radical nephrectomy and inferior vena caval thrombectomy (level 2 tumor thrombus). The primary tumor is otherwise confined to the kidney, and the lymph nodes are not involved. What is the approximate 5-year cancer-free survival rate?
    a. 15% to 25%
    b. 26% to 35%
    c. 36% to 45%
    d. 46% to 60%
    e. 61% to 75%

32. Which of the following is NOT a predictor of cancer-specific survival after nephrectomy for RCC?
    a. Pathologic stage
    b. Tumor size
    c. Fuhrman nuclear grade
    d. Patient age
    e. Histologic necrosis

33. Which of the following statements about renal lymphoma is TRUE?
    a. Five to 10 percent of all lymphomas involving the kidney are primary tumors.
    b. The radiographic patterns manifested by renal lymphoma are diverse and can be difficult to differentiate from RCC.
    c. Percutaneous biopsy is rarely indicated if renal lymphoma is suspected.
    d. Renal failure associated with renal lymphoma is most often due to extensive parenchymal replacement by the malignancy.
    e. The most common pattern of renal involvement is from direct extension from adjacent retroperitoneal lymph nodes.

34. The main limitation of renal mass biopsy is:
    a. Risk of needle tract seeding
    b. Difficulty differentiating the eosinophilic variants of RCC from renal oncocytoma
    c. Risk of pneumothorax
    d. Risk of hemorrhage
    e. High incidence of inadequate tissue sampling

35. A common and pathogenic cytogenetic finding in children with RCC is:
    a. *VHL* mutation.
    b. c-*MET* oncogene mutation.
    c. *TP53* mutation.
    d. *TFE3* gene fusions.
    e. *PTEN* mutations.

36. The central mediator for loss of VHL protein function is:
    a. HIF-α.
    b. PEGF.
    c. erythropoietin.
    d. VEGF.
    e. TP53.

37. Most tumors at various sites in patients with von Hippel Lindau disease share what following characteristic?
    a. Malignant behavior
    b. Hypervascularity
    c. Rapid growth rate
    d. High nuclear grade
    e. Symptomatic presentation

38. One major difference between hereditary papillary RCC syndrome and von Hippel-Lindau disease is:
    a. pattern of genetic inheritance.
    b. age at onset.
    c. gender distribution.
    d. incidence of metastasis.
    e. incidence of associated tumors in nonrenal organ systems.

39. Which disease/syndrome is most likely to exhibit aggressive behavior of RCC?
    a. von Hippel-Lindau disease
    b. Hereditary papillary RCC syndrome
    c. Hereditary leiomyomatosis and RCC syndrome
    d. Birt-Hogg-Dubé syndrome
    e. Familial oncocytosis

40. Spontaneous pneumothorax is occasionally observed in which of the following?
    a. von Hippel-Lindau disease
    b. Hereditary papillary RCC syndrome
    c. Hereditary leiomyomatosis and RCC syndrome
    d. Birt-Hogg-Dubé syndrome
    e. Familial oncocytosis

41. Chromophobe RCC shares many characteristics with:
    a. oncocytoma.
    b. type 2 papillary RCC.
    c. clear cell RCC.
    d. mesoblastic nephroma.
    e. mixed epithelial and stromal tumor of the kidney.

42. A finding that is diagnostic for collecting duct carcinoma is:
    a. central location and infiltrative growth pattern.
    b. aggressive clinical course.
    c. *TP53* mutation.
    d. positive staining for *Ulex europaeus* lectin.
    e. sensitivity to chemotherapy.

43. Sarcomatoid differentiation is most commonly observed with which histologic subtypes of RCC?
    a. Clear cell and papillary
    b. Papillary and chromophobe
    c. Clear cell and collecting duct
    d. Clear cell and chromophobe
    e. Chromophobe and collecting duct

44. Which of the following factors has greatest utility for predicting bone metastasis from RCC?
    a. Tumor size
    b. Tumor grade
    c. Performance status
    d. Elevated alkaline phosphatase concentration
    e. Invasion of the perinephric fat

45. The prognosis for a 3-cm tumor infiltrating the renal sinus fat is:
    a. similar to that of a pT1bN0 tumor.
    b. similar to a that of a pT2N0 tumor.
    c. similar to that of a pT3a tumor with invasion of the perinephric fat laterally.
    d. worse than that of a pT3a tumor with invasion of the perinephric fat laterally.
    e. similar to that of a tumor with ipsilateral adrenal involvement.

46. The single most important prognostic factor for RCC is:
    a. tumor size.
    b. tumor grade.
    c. tumor stage.
    d. histologic subtype.
    e. performance status.

47. The most accurate assessment of prognosis for patients with RCC is usually provided by:
    a. tumor size.
    b. clinician judgment.
    c. tumor stage.
    d. integrated analysis of prognostic factors.
    e. performance status.

48. Which choice indicates a tumor that is NOT correctly staged according to the 2010 TNM staging system for RCC?
    a. Localized RCC, 8.5 cm: pT2a
    b. RCC with direct ipsilateral adrenal involvement: pT3a
    c. RCC with metastatic involvement of the adrenal gland: pM1
    d. RCC with tumor thrombus within a segmental branch of the renal vein: pT3a
    e. RCC with three lymph node metastases: pN1

49. Risk of local recurrence is highest in which of the following situations?
    a. A pT3b tumor after radical nephrectomy and IVC thrombectomy
    b. Patient with von Hippel-Lindau disease after partial nephrectomy with wedge resection of a single tumor
    c. A 4.5-cm tumor after partial nephrectomy with focal positive parenchymal margin
    d. A 3.5-cm tumor after cryoablation
    e. A 2.5 cm centrally located tumor after radiofrequency ablation

50. What is the most common form of renal sarcoma?
    a. Liposarcoma
    b. Rhabdosarcoma
    c. Fibrosarcoma
    d. Leiomyosarcoma
    e. Angiosarcoma

51. The most useful prognostic factors for renal sarcoma are:
    a. tumor size and grade.
    b. tumor stage and grade.
    c. histologic subtype and stage.
    d. tumor stage and ploidy status.
    e. margin status and grade.

52. Which of the following renal tumors has the best prognosis?
    a. Sarcoma
    b. Carcinoid
    c. Adult Wilms tumor
    d. Primitive neuroectodermal tumor
    e. Small cell carcinoma

53. Patients with which RCC subtype are most likely to benefit from immunotherapy?
    a. Papillary RCC
    b. Clear cell RCC
    c. Renal medullary carcinoma
    d. Collecting duct carcinoma
    e. Chromophobe RCC

54. Standard postoperative management for patients at high risk of recurrence after nephrectomy includes which of the following?
    a. High-dose interleukin-2
    b. Targeted molecular therapy
    c. Autologous tumor vaccine
    d. Observation
    e. Interferon-α

55. Agents targeting which of the following signaling pathways in clear cell RCC have significant antitumor effects in patients with metastatic disease?
    a. VEGF and EGFR
    b. TP53 and EGFR
    c. VEGF and mTOR
    d. mTOR and TGF-β
    e. All of the above

56. The greatest determinant of renal function after partial nephrectomy is:
    a. surgical approach.
    b. tumor size.
    c. absence of a functioning contralateral kidney.
    d. renal function before partial nephrectomy.
    e. gender.

57. Which of the following statements is TRUE regarding chronic kidney disease (CKD)?
    a. The increasing prevalence of CKD in the elderly indicates that CKD is a part of the natural aging process.
    b. A serum creatinine concentration below 1.4 mg/dL excludes the possibility of CKD.
    c. CKD can be diagnosed based on a single estimated GFR value less than 60 mL/min/1.73 m^2.
    d. Increasing CKD stage has been associated with an increase in morbid cardiovascular events.
    e. Choice of intervention for localized renal malignancy has little impact on development or progression of CKD.

58. Which of the following is an indication for adrenalectomy at the time of partial nephrectomy?
    a. A 6-cm upper pole renal tumor
    b. A 4-cm adrenal lesion measuring −20 Hounsfield units on noncontrast CT scan
    c. Bilateral adrenal hyperplasia
    d. A 3-cm renal tumor adjacent to the adrenal gland on CT scan but readily separable from the adrenal gland at surgery
    e. A 1-cm adrenal lesion that is bright on T2-weighted MRI

Pathology

1. A 48-year-old man undergoes a right radical nephrectomy and adrenalectomy for a 6-cm upper pole mass. The pathology is depicted in Figure 49–1.

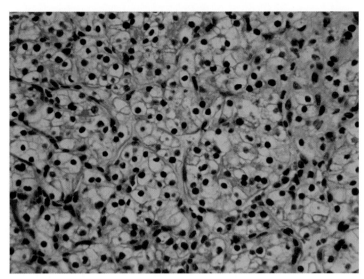

Figure 49–1.   (From Bostwick DG, Cheng L. Urologic surgical pathology. 2nd ed. Edinburgh: Mosby; 2008.)

The diagnosis is:

a. normal adrenal.

b. clear cell carcinoma.

c. metastatic carcinoma to the kidney.

d. papillary carcinoma.

e. adrenocortical carcinoma.

2. A 48-year-old woman has gross hematuria. CT reveals a 4-cm midcentral lesion. A radical nephrectomy is performed and the pathology is depicted in Figure 49–2.

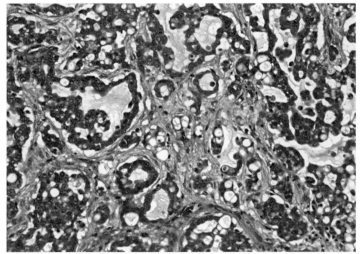

Figure 49–2.   (From Bostwick DG, Cheng L. Urologic surgical pathology. 2nd ed. Edinburgh: Mosby; 2008.)

Based on the histology this patient likely has:

a. metastases.

b. a hematologic malignancy.

c. a perineoplastic syndrome.

d. sickle cell disease.

e. a gastrointestinal malignancy.

Imaging

1. See Figure 49–3.

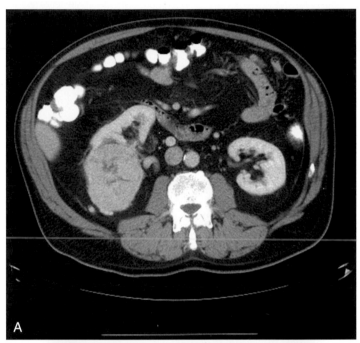

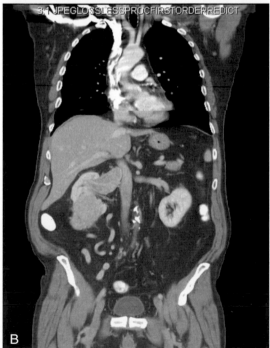

Figure 49–3.

A 55-year-old man with hematuria has this contrast-enhanced CT scan for evaluation. The most appropriate therapy is:

a. laparoscopic nephron-sparing surgery.

b. radical nephrectomy.

c. open nephron-sparing surgery.

d. radiofrequency ablation.

e. cryoablation.

2. See Figure 49–4.

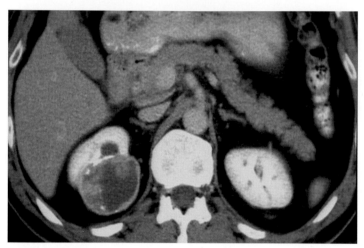

Figure 49–4.

A 45-year-old man with no urinary symptoms has this axial contrast-enhanced CT scan. What is the most likely diagnosis?

a. Bosniak IIF lesion—short interval imaging follow up

b. Bosniak IV—cystic RCC

c. Bosniak II cyst

d. Bosniak III cyst

e. Bosniak I cyst

ANSWERS

1. **a. No imaging studies.** Surveillance for recurrent malignancy after radical nephrectomy for RCC can be tailored according to the initial pathologic tumor stage. All patients should be evaluated with a medical history, physical examination, and selected blood studies on a yearly or twice-yearly basis. For patients with T1N0M0 tumors, routine postoperative radiographic imaging is not necessary because of the low risk of recurrent malignancy.

2. **d. lower incidence of local tumor recurrence.** The major disadvantage of nephron-sparing surgery is the risk of postoperative local tumor recurrence in the operated kidney, which has occurred in up to 5% to 10% of patients. On the other hand there is also a 2% to 3% risk of tumor recurrence in the contralateral kidney, at which point the patient would have tumor in a solitary kidney if a radical nephrectomy was performed for the first tumor. The current American Urological Association guidelines stress the importance of using a nephron-sparing approach whenever possible based on the improved renal function and comparable oncologic outcomes with these approaches when applied to small renal masses.

3. **d. Every 2 years.** Surveillance for recurrent malignancy after nephron-sparing surgery for RCC can be tailored according to the initial pathologic tumor stage. A yearly chest radiograph is recommended after nephron-sparing surgery for T2N0M0 tumors because the lung is the most common site of postoperative metastasis. Abdominal or retroperitoneal tumor recurrence is uncommon in the latter group, particularly early after nephron-sparing surgery, and these patients require only occasional follow-up abdominal CT; the authors recommend that this be done every 2 years.

4. **b. 24-Hour urinary protein measurement.** Patients who undergo nephron-sparing surgery for RCC may be left with a relatively small amount of renal tissue. These patients are at risk for developing long-term renal functional impairment from hyperfiltration renal injury. Because proteinuria is the initial manifestation of the phenomenon, a 24-hour urinary protein measurement should be obtained yearly in patients with a solitary remnant kidney to screen for hyperfiltration nephropathy.

5. **e. Serum-creatinine based estimation of GFR, such as MDRD formula.** At the present time there are several formulas in clinical use, including the MDRD, Cockcroft-Gault, and CKD-EPI formulas, each of which is an improvement over using the serum creatinine concentration alone for identification of patients with or at risk for chronic kidney disease. Serum levels of creatinine are dependent on gender, muscle mass, and other factors and can therefore lead to an underappreciation of kidney disease in certain populations, such as thin, elderly women. Urinary creatinine concentration measurement is impractical and provides only marginally more valuable information than serum creatinine concentration measurement. Urinary protein measurement can identify patients with early signs of kidney disease (proteinuria) but is not the best screening test. Direct measurement of GFR using iothalamate (or other agents) is costly and not routinely available; it is therefore impractical in most settings.

6. **d. A double freeze-thaw cycle.** Renal cryosurgery is an ablative nephron-sparing treatment option for RCC that can be performed percutaneously under radiographic guidance or laparoscopically under direct vision and ultrasound guidance. The aim of cryosurgery is to ablate the same predetermined volume of tissue that would have been removed had a conventional surgical excision been performed. Established critical prerequisites for successful cryosurgery include rapid freezing, gradual thawing, and a repetition of the freeze-thaw cycle.

7. **c. CT and MRI.** Both CT and MRI are noninvasive and accurate modalities for demonstrating both the presence and the distal extent of vena caval involvement. Although MRI had been recommended as the test of choice at most centers, several recent studies have demonstrated that multiphase CT also provides sufficient information necessary for surgical planning and has become the preferred diagnostic study at many centers.

8. **e. lymph node involvement.** In most studies the presence of lymph node or distant metastases has carried a dismal prognosis that is much more profound than the other distractors.

9. **d. Simultaneous partial nephrectomy and pulmonary lobectomy.** The subset of patients with metastatic RCC and a solitary metastasis, estimated at

between 1.6% and 3.2% of patients, may derive benefit from nephrectomy with resection of the metastatic lesion. This patient also needs partial nephrectomy to preclude the need for dialysis.

10. **e. Observation with follow-up renal imaging in 6 to 12 months.** Renal mass biopsy is only occasionally performed for those with a small renal mass, in part based on the difficulty in differentiating oncocytoma from eosinophilic variants of RCC. For those in whom nonextirpative options are being considered, biopsy can provide important information such as a definitive nonmalignant diagnosis (as in this example). Given the benign nature of renal oncocytomas, the best answer is observation with follow-up imaging in 6 to 12 months.

11. **e. Mode of genetic transmission.** Approximately 20% of angiomyolipomas are found in patients with the tuberous sclerosis syndrome, an autosomal dominant disorder characterized by mental retardation, epilepsy, and adenoma sebaceum, a distinctive skin lesion. Tuberous sclerosis, similar to von Hippel-Lindau disease, is transmitted in an autosomal dominant manner.

12. **a. Selective embolization.** Most patients with acute or potentially life-threatening hemorrhage will require total nephrectomy if exploration is performed; if the patient has tuberous sclerosis, bilateral disease, preexisting renal insufficiency, or other medical or urologic disease that could affect renal function in the future, selective embolization should be considered. In such circumstances selective embolization can temporize hemorrhage and in many cases will prove to be definitive treatment.

13. **a. They are complex cystic lesions that are typically classified as Bosniak II to III.** Cystic nephromas are benign renal neoplasms that occur most commonly in middle-aged women. They appear to be genetically related to mixed epithelial/stromal tumors but generally have a somewhat different radiographic appearance. Unlike mixed epithelial/stromal tumors, which contain a solid stromal component and often appear as solid or Bosniak IV lesions on cross-sectional imaging, cystic nephromas are typically characterized as complex cystic lesions without a solid component. Multiloculated cystic nephromas occurring in children are now considered a distinct pathologic entity.

14. **c. Tobacco use.** The most generally accepted environmental risk factor for RCC is tobacco use, although the relative associated risks have been modest, ranging from 1.4 to 2.3 when compared with controls. All forms of tobacco use have been implicated, with risk increasing with cumulative dose or pack-years. Other well-established risk factors include obesity and hypertension.

15. **d. Pheochromocytoma.** The familial form of the common clear cell variant of RCC is von Hippel-Lindau disease. Major manifestations include the development of RCC, pheochromocytoma, retinal angiomas, and hemangioblastomas of the brain stem, cerebellum, or spinal cord. Penetrance for all of these traits is far from complete, and some, such as pheochromocytomas, tend to be clustered in certain families but not in others.

16. **c. 41% to 60%.** RCC develops in about 50% of patients with von Hippel-Lindau disease and is distinctive for early age at onset, often developing in the third, fourth, or fifth decades of life, and for bilateral and multifocal involvement.

17. **e. RCC.** With improved management of the central nervous system manifestations of the disease, RCC has now become the most common cause of mortality in patients with von Hippel-Lindau disease.

18. **b. Vascular endothelial growth factor (VEGF).** Inactivation or mutation of the von Hippel-Lindau gene leads to dysregulated expression of hypoxia-inducible factor-1, an intracellular protein that plays an important role in regulating cellular responses to hypoxia, starvation, and other stresses. This in turn leads to a severalfold upregulation of the expression of VEGF, the primary proangiogenic growth factor in RCC, contributing to the pronounced neovascularity associated with this carcinoma.

19. **a. The mode of genetic transmission.** Studies of families with hereditary papillary RCC have demonstrated an autosomal dominant mode of transmission, similar to those with von Hippel-Lindau disease, which is caused by inactivation or mutation of a tumor suppressor gene, whereas hereditary papillary RCC is caused by activation of an oncogene.

20. **d. constitutive activation of the receptor for hepatocyte growth factor.** Missense mutations of the c-*MET* proto-oncogene at 7q31 were found to segregate with the disease, implicating it as the relevant genetic locus. The protein product of this gene is the receptor tyrosine kinase for the hepatocyte growth factor (also known as scatter factor), which plays an important role in regulating the proliferation and differentiation of epithelial and endothelial cells in a wide variety of organs, including the kidney. Most of the mutations in hereditary papillary RCC have been found in the tyrosine kinase domain of *MET* and apparently lead to constitutive activation.

21. **e. efflux of large hydrophobic compounds, including many cytotoxic drugs.** P-glycoprotein is a 170-kD transmembrane protein expressed by 80% to 90% of RCCs that acts as an energy-dependent efflux pump for a wide variety of large hydrophobic compounds, including several cytotoxic drugs.

22. **c. VEGF.** The primary angiogenesis inducer in clear cell RCC appears to be VEGF, which is suppressed by the wild-type von Hippel-Lindau protein under normal conditions and is dramatically upregulated during tumor development.

23. **b. Sarcomatoid variants of RCC.** Most RCCs are round to ovoid and circumscribed by a pseudocapsule of compressed parenchyma and fibrous tissue rather than a true histologic capsule. Unlike upper tract transitional cell carcinomas, most RCCs are not grossly infiltrative, with the notable exception of some sarcomatoid variants.

24. **c. Inactivation of the von Hippel-Lindau tumor suppressor gene.** Chromosome 3 alterations and von Hippel-Lindau mutations are common in conventional RCC, and mutation or inactivation of this gene has been found in over 75% of sporadic cases.

25. **a. Trisomy of chromosome 7.** The cytogenetic abnormalities associated with papillary RCC are characteristic and include trisomy of chromosomes 7 and 17 and loss of the Y chromosome.

26. **b. 4% to 5%.** Chromophobe cell carcinoma is a distinctive histologic subtype of RCC that appears to be derived from the cortical portion of the collecting duct. It represents 4% to 5% of all RCCs.

27. **e. metastatic at the time of diagnosis.** Renal medullary carcinoma is a rare histologic subtype of RCC

that occurs almost exclusively in association with sickle cell trait. It is typically diagnosed in young African-Americans, often in the third decade of life. Many cases are both locally advanced and metastatic at the time of diagnosis. Most patients do not respond to therapy and succumb to their disease in a few to several months.

28. **d. Hypercalcemia.** Hypercalcemia has been reported in up to 13% of patients with RCC and can be due to either paraneoplastic phenomena or osteolytic metastatic involvement of the bone. The production of parathyroid hormone–like peptides is the most common paraneoplastic etiology, although tumor-derived 1,25-dihydroxyvitamin D_3 and prostaglandins may contribute in a minority of cases. Medical management includes vigorous hydration followed by diuresis with furosemide and the selective use of bisphosphonates, corticosteroids, and/or calcitonin.

29. **a. Right radical nephrectomy and regional or extended lymph node dissection.** An aggressive surgical approach is still preferred because it will prolong survival and represents the only realistic chance for a cure. Lymph nodes in this size range are most likely malignant, and this patient will likely need to consider adjuvant clinical trials.

30. **e. A 38-year-old woman with a fever, urinary tract infection, and a 3.5-cm solid, enhancing renal mass.** Patients with flank pain, a febrile urinary tract infection, and a renal mass may be considered for percutaneous biopsy or aspiration to establish a diagnosis of renal abscess rather than malignancy.

31. **d. 46% to 60%.** Venous involvement was once thought to be a poor prognostic finding for RCC, but more recent studies suggest that most patients with tumor thrombi can be salvaged with an aggressive surgical approach. These studies document 45% to 69% 5-year survival rates for patients with venous tumor thrombi as long as the tumor is otherwise confined to the kidney.

32. **d. Patient age.** Although patient age and comorbidity are important predictors of overall survival in patients with RCC and greatly impact the choice of treatment in these patients, they do not impact the likelihood of dying of cancer-specific causes. Each of the other factors has been incorporated into one or more RCC prognostic algorithms for cancer-specific outcomes.

33. **b. The radiographic patterns manifested by renal lymphoma are diverse and can be difficult to differentiate from RCC.** Five different radiographic patterns have been described for lymphoma involving the kidney, including a solitary mass that can be difficult to differentiate from RCC.

34. **b. Difficulty differentiating the eosinophilic variants of RCC from renal oncocytoma.** The main limitation of renal mass biopsy is difficulty differentiating renal oncocytoma, the most common benign renal mass, from eosinophilic variants of conventional, papillary, and chromophobe RCC on biopsy material. The risk of complications is low in the modern era with the use of smaller-gauge needles, and needle tract seeding with RCC appears to be a rare event.

35. **d. *TFE3* gene fusions.** Mutations or translocations resulting in *TFE3* gene fusions are common in RCC, occurring in the pediatric population. Although these cancers often present with advanced stage, the t(X;17) variant frequently follows an indolent course whereas t(X;1) cancers can recur with late lymph node metastases.

36. **a. HIF-α.** Inactivation of the VHL protein or loss of its function allows HIF-1α to accumulate, leading to a variety of downstream events, including upregulation of VEGF, erythropoietin, and PEGF. HIF-α is the primary mediator of these events.

37. **b. Hypervascularity.** Tumors in patients with von Hippel-Lindau disease include adrenal pheochromocytoma, retinal angiomas, cerebellar and brain stem hemangioblastoma, RCC, and others. Most are relatively slow growing and asymptomatic if patients are evaluated and screened in a proactive manner. The common feature is that almost all are hypervascular.

38. **e. incidence of associated tumors in nonrenal organ systems.** The incidence of nonrenal tumors is low in the familial papillary RCC syndrome in contrast to patients with von Hippel-Lindau disease, who commonly develop tumors in the eyes, spinal cord, cerebellum, adrenals, inner ear, epididymis, and pancreas.

39. **c. Hereditary leiomyomatosis and RCC syndrome.** Malignant behavior is particularly common in the hereditary leiomyomatosis and RCC syndrome, and proactive and aggressive management is recommended.

40. **d. Birt-Hogg-Dubé syndrome.** Lung cysts and spontaneous pneumothoraces are well described and relatively common findings in the Birt-Hogg-Dubé syndrome.

41. **a. oncocytoma.** Both chromophobe RCC and renal oncocytoma are derived from the distal tubules and both are commonly observed in the Birt-Hogg-Dubé syndrome. There are also some overlapping cytogenetic changes, all suggesting a potential relationship between these renal tumors.

42. **d. positive staining for *Ulex europaeus* lectin.** *Ulex europaeus* lectin is expressed by the normal collecting duct, and tumor staining suggests origin from this structure. Most collecting ducts are centrally located and exhibit an infiltrative growth pattern and aggressive clinical course, but this is also true for poorly differentiated transitional cell carcinomas of the renal pelvis or centrally located sarcomatoid RCC.

43. **d. Clear cell and chromophobe.** Sarcomatoid differentiation is most commonly found in association with clear cell and chromophobe RCC.

44. **c. Performance status.** Poor performance status (PS) can be used to segregate patients when deciding whether to obtain a bone scintiscan for metastatic RCC. Shvarts and colleagues (2004) have shown that patients with good performance status (ECOG performance status = 0), no evidence of extraosseous metastases, and no bone pain had extremely low risk for bone metastasis and did not benefit from bone scintigraphy. They recommended a bone scintiscan for all other patients, and the incidence of bone metastasis in this group was more than 15% (Shvarts et al, 2004).*

45. **d. worse than that of a pT3a tumor with invasion of the perinephric fat laterally.** Invasion of the perinephric fat medially has been shown to be a poor prognostic sign. Medial invasion places the tumor in proximity to the venous system and likely increases the risk

---

*Sources referenced can be found in *Campbell-Walsh Urology*, 10th *Edition*, on the Expert Consult website.

of metastatic dissemination. Ipsilateral adrenal involvement is even worse.

46. **c. Tumor stage.** Although not truly a single factor, because it combines tumor size with several other pieces of information obtained from final pathologic analysis, tumor stage is the most powerful individual predictor of oncologic outcomes. When incorporated into a multiple-predictor analysis such as a nomogram or other multivariable analysis, its predictive ability increases further.

47. **d. integrated analysis of prognostic factors.** Integrated analysis of a variety of factors such as tumor stage and grade, performance status, tumor necrosis, and histologic subtype has yielded the most accurate prognostication for RCC. Several studies have documented that nomograms and other algorithms outperform traditional staging systems, clinical opinion, individual risk factors, and chance.

48. **b. RCC with direct ipsilateral adrenal involvement: pT3a.** Several studies have demonstrated that RCC directly invading the adrenal gland is associated with poorer prognosis than RCC with perinephric or renal sinus fat invasion. Direct ipsilateral adrenal involvement is now grouped with other RCCs that extend beyond the Gerota fascia as pathologic stage T4 (pT4). These patients have a high risk for disease recurrence or progression.

49. **b. Patient with von Hippel-Lindau disease after partial nephrectomy with wedge resection of a single tumor.** Local recurrence after partial nephrectomy for VHL disease is common if patients are followed long-term owing to multifocal tumor diathesis. These kidneys have been shown to harbor several hundred incipient tumors, and the risk of local recurrence is thus high during longitudinal follow-up.

50. **d. Leiomyosarcoma.** Leiomyosarcoma is the most common histologic subtype of renal sarcoma, accounting for 50% to 60% of such tumors. The most common type of sarcoma in the retroperitoneum is liposarcoma.

51. **e. margin status and grade.** Margin status and tumor grade are the primary prognostic factors for sarcoma. Patients with high-grade disease are at risk for systemic metastasis and those with low-grade disease are at risk for local recurrence. Wide local excision with negative margins is essential for minimizing the risk of recurrence for sarcomas because these tumors are derived from the mesenchymal tissues and are typically infiltrative and thus do not respect natural barriers.

52. **b. Carcinoid.** All of these tumor types have a relatively poor prognosis except for renal carcinoid, which tends to be associated with good outcomes in most patients.

53. **b. Clear cell RCC.** Immunotherapy, and high-dose interleukin-2 in particular, can provide a durable and complete cure in about 5% of patients with metastatic RCC. Almost all objective responses have been observed in individuals with clear cell RCC. Very few patients with non–clear cell histology derive any benefit from this highly toxic treatment.

54. **d. Observation.** All randomized postoperative adjuvant trials in patients with resected RCC have failed to demonstrate an improvement in survival or time to progression. Several ongoing clinical trials are evaluating whether targeted molecular therapy will show a benefit, but the results are not available at the present time. The standard of care continues to be surveillance with periodic radiographic and clinical observations, although enrollment in a clinical trial is highly preferred.

55. **c. VEGF and mTOR.** Several recent clinical trials indicate that agents targeting VEGF signaling, including sunitinib and sorafenib, and mTOR pathway signaling, including temsirolimus and everolimus, demonstrate substantial tumor responses or significant improvement in progression-free survival.

56. **d. renal function before partial nephrectomy.** When compared with radical nephrectomy, partial nephrectomy has been associated with better renal functional outcomes. Duration of regional ischemia appears to be the greatest modifiable risk factor for loss of function; however, initial renal function is the main determinant of postoperative renal function.

57. **d. Increasing CKD stage has been associated with an increase in morbid cardiovascular events.** Increasing CKD stage has been associated with an increase in morbid cardiovascular events, hospitalization, and death on a longitudinal basis.

58. **e. A 1-cm adrenal lesion that is bright on T2-weighted MRI.** Several pathologic adrenal lesions can be diagnosed based on their radiographic characteristics without histologic confirmation. Lesions that are bright on T2-weighted MRI are suggestive of pheochromocytomas and should be surgically removed. Careful preoperative and intraoperative management are essential for safe management in this circumstance.

Pathology

1. **b. clear cell carcinoma.** Notice the clear cytoplasm due to the glycogen content.
2. **a. metastases.** This is a collecting duct carcinoma that is often metastatic at the time of diagnosis.

Imaging

1. **b. radical nephrectomy.** The images demonstrate a large mass in the lower pole of the right kidney, with tumor extension into the right renal vein, extending to the junction of the right renal vein with the inferior vena cava. The renal vein is enlarged, and tumor vessels are seen within the thrombus in the renal vein. These findings make radical nephrectomy the best option.
2. **b. Bosniak IV—cystic RCC.** There are enhancing nodules in the cystic lesion, with foci of dystrophic calcification. These findings indicate a malignant cystic RCC. Bosniak I cyst is a simple renal cyst. Bosniak II and IIF cysts are minimally complicated whereas Bosniak III lesions are more complicated in their appearance. However, the presence of enhancing nodules makes cystic RCC the most likely diagnosis.

Additional Study Points

1. A solid mass on CT scan that enhances more than 15 Hounsfield units is suggestive of RCC.
2. Twenty percent of small solid enhancing masses on CT are benign.
3. Clear cell RCCs originate from the proximal tubule; oncocytomas and chromophobe RCCs originate from the distal tubule.
4. There is ample evidence for impaired immune surveillance in RCC.
5. Bilateral involvement in RCC either synchronously or metachronously occurs in 2% to 4% of patients.
6. RCC pathologically is classified as clear cell: 70% to 80%; papillary: 10% to 15%; chromophobe: 3% to 5%; collecting duct: less than 1%; and medullary: rare.
7. Stauffer syndrome is a perineoplastic syndrome associated with RCC that results in elevated liver function tests. If hepatic function does not normalize after nephrectomy, persistent hepatic dysfunction is indicative of persistent disease.
8. Enlarged perirenal lymph nodes noted on CT may be inflammatory, particularly if they are less than 2 cm in diameter. Lymph nodes larger than 2 cm generally contain metastases.
9. RCC involving the vena cava that infiltrates the wall of the vena caval has an extremely poor prognosis.
10. A patient with a tumor thrombus involving the vena cava associated with metastatic regional nodal disease has a very poor prognosis.
11. A patient with a tumor thrombus involving the vena cava in which the nodes are negative and there is no invasion of the vein wall (except the ostia) has a good prognosis.
12. Ipsilateral adrenalectomy as part of a radical nephrectomy is not necessary unless there is CT evidence of adrenal involvement, contiguous spread of the tumor to the adrenal, or large upper pole renal masses that are adjacent to the adrenal gland.
13. The risk for developing recurrent malignant disease is greatest in the first 3 years after surgery.
14. In a partial nephrectomy the amount of renal parenchyma taken with the tumor appears to be immaterial provided the margin itself is negative.
15. RCCs less than 3.5 cm in general grow less than a 0.5 cm per year; some may grow up to a 1 cm a year.
16. Incomplete excision of a large primary tumor or debulking is rarely indicated.
17. Sarcomas typically have a pseudocapsule that cannot be relied on for a plane of dissection because tumor will be left behind.
18. Metastatic tumors to the kidney are common, appearing in 12% of patients who die of other cancers; the most common primary lesions are those of the lung, breast, or gastrointestinal tract, melanoma, or hematologic.

chapter 50

Treatment of Advanced Renal Cell Carcinoma

Ramaprasad Srinivasan, MD, PhD ● W. Marston Linehan, MD

QUESTIONS

1. What is the approximate overall objective response rate to interleukin-2 (IL-2) monotherapy in patients with metastatic renal cell carcinoma (RCC)?
   a. 5%
   b. 10%
   c. 15%
   d. 25%
   e. 35%

2. Which of the following regarding IL-2 therapy for metastatic RCC is TRUE?
   a. IL-2 has demonstrable efficacy in clear cell as well as papillary RCC.
   b. Randomized studies have demonstrated a survival benefit associated with high-dose IL-2.
   c. Low-dose subcutaneous and high-dose intravenous IL-2 have comparable efficacy.
   d. Durable complete responses are seen in a small proportion of patients receiving high-dose IL-2.
   e. Newer formulations have led to better tolerability of high-dose IL-2.

3. In the Memorial Sloan-Kettering Cancer Center prognostic scheme for patients with metastatic RCC undergoing therapy with cytokine or chemotherapy, which of the following is not a predictor of poor outcome?
   a. Karnofsky performance score greater than 80%
   b. Elevated lactate dehydrogenase
   c. Elevated calcium
   d. Decreased hemoglobin
   e. Absence of prior nephrectomy

4. In which of the following patients with metastatic RCC is cytoreductive nephrectomy most appropriate?
   a. A 50-year-old man with an Eastern Cooperative Oncology Group (ECOG) performance status of 0, a large 12-cm right renal mass, and four small pulmonary metastases
   b. A 67-year-old woman with an ECOG performance status of 0, a 7-cm left renal mass, retroperitoneal adenopathy, and hepatic metastases that have doubled in size over 4 weeks
   c. An 81-year-old man with an asymptomatic 6 cm right renal mass and multiple hepatic metastases who has declined systemic therapy
   d. A 72-year-old man with an ECOG performance status of 2, a 5-cm right renal mass, and mild dyspnea associated with numerous pulmonary metastases
   e. None of the above

5. The rationale for cytoreductive nephrectomy followed by immunotherapy with cytokines in patients with synchronous metastatic RCC includes all of the following EXCEPT:
   a. removal of tumor burden.
   b. removal of source of tumor-associated immunosuppressive factors.
   c. reversal of acquired immune dysfunction.
   d. improved tolerance to cytokine therapy.
   e. improved T-lymphocyte function.

6. Which of the following statements about cytokine therapy for metastatic RCC is TRUE?
   a. Lymphokine activated killer (LAK) cells augment the efficacy of both interferon-α and IL-2.
   b. Randomized trials have demonstrated a significant survival advantage for combined IL-2 and interferon over either agent given as monotherapy.
   c. The combination of IL-2 and interferon leads to higher overall response rates than either agent alone.
   d. The complete response rate with interferon-α monotherapy is 10%.
   e. All of the above

7. Which of the following metastatic RCC tumors is most likely to benefit from cytokine therapy?
   a. Papillary carcinoma
   b. Clear cell carcinoma
   c. Medullary carcinoma
   d. Collecting duct carcinoma
   e. Chromophobe carcinoma

8. A 58-year-old woman had a nephrectomy 6 years previously for a grade 2 clear cell carcinoma. She was incidentally found to have three left-sided pulmonary nodules (two <1.0 cm, another of 2.5 cm). A physical examination is normal, as are results of all blood chemistries. CT of the brain, lungs, abdomen, and pelvis show three pulmonary nodules with no associated hilar or mediastinal adenopathy, and a bone scintiscan is normal. Which of the following is the most appropriate next step in her management?

a. Therapy with high dose IL-2

b. Biopsy of a pulmonary nodule

c. Mediastinoscopy followed by resection of the pulmonary nodules

d. Observation

e. IFN-α therapy

9. The sirolimus analogues temsirolimus and everolimus act primarily on which of the following pathways?

a. VEGF

b. PDGF

c. Raf-1

d. mTOR

e. c-*MET*

10. The overall Response Evaluation Criteria in Solid Tumors (RECIST) response rate in metastatic clear cell RCC patients receiving front-line therapy with sunitinib is:

a. 15% to 20%.

b. 30% to 40%.

c. 60% to 70%.

d. less than 10%.

e. more than 70%.

11. In patients with previously untreated metastatic clear cell RCC, sunitinib is

a. associated with a higher response rate compared with interferon-α.

b. associated with a longer progression-free survival compared with interferon-α.

c. associated with a better quality of life compared with interferon-α.

d. All of the above

e. None of the above

12. Which of the following agents has been shown to prolong progression-free survival in patients with metastatic clear cell RCC who have progressed on first-line therapy with VEGFR antagonists?

a. Axitinib

b. Bevacizumab + interferon-α

c. High-dose IL-2

d. Everolimus

e. Low-dose subcutaneous IL-2

13. Randomized trials in patients with previously untreated metastatic clear cell RCC have demonstrated that sorafenib is:

a. associated with better overall survival compared with interferon-α.

b. associated with a longer progression-free survival compared with interferon-α.

c. associated with a better quality of life compared with interferon-α.

d. All of the above

e. None of the above

14. Which of the following agents has been shown in randomized phase 3 trial to prolong survival in "poor risk" metastatic RCC patients?

a. IL-2

b. Sunitinib

c. Sorafenib

d. Temsirolimus

e. Interferon-α

15. Which of the following molecules is not known to be upregulated as a consequence of VHL dysfunction?

a. VEGF

b. PDGF

c. TGF-α

d. Glut-1

e. raf-1

16. In what proportion of sporadic clear cell tumors are mutations or promoter hypermethylation of the *VHL* gene seen?

a. 70% to 90%

b. 10% to 20%

c. 100%

d. Less than 10%

17. A 47-year-old man presents with multiple metastatic lesions to the lungs and liver 8 months after a radical nephrectomy for a 9-cm papillary type I renal tumor. Which of the following statements about his systemic treatment options is TRUE?

a. Sunitinib is associated with a 30% to 40% overall RECIST response rate in this subtype of RCC.

b. Sorafenib is associated with better long-term outcomes than sunitinib in papillary type I RCC.

c. mTOR inhibitors improve survival in patients with metastatic papillary RCC.

d. Enrollment on a phase 2 trial evaluating a novel inhibitor of c-*MET* activity is a reasonable consideration in this patient.

e. None of the above

18. Which of the following statements about agents targeting components of the VHL pathway is TRUE in patients with metastatic clear cell RCC?

a. The combination of sunitinib and temsirolimus is associated with higher progression-free and overall survival than use of sunitinib alone.

b. The addition of interferon-α to bevacizumab has been shown in randomized trials to improve progression-free survival compared with bevacizumab alone.

c. Overlapping toxicity may limit maximal tolerated doses when two agents targeting this pathway are combined.

d. c-*MET* is an important target in clear cell RCC due to the presence of c-*MET* mutations in approximately 90% of clear cell renal tumors.

e. None of the above

ANSWERS

1. **c. 15%.** Although response rates of 30% or more were reported in early phase 2 studies with IL-2, the overall response rate with this agent was determined to be approximately 15% in larger studies and meta-analysis.

2. **d. Durable complete responses are seen in a small proportion of patients receiving high-dose IL-2.** Complete responses are seen in 7% to 9% of metastatic clear cell RCC patients receiving high-dose IL-2, with the majority of these remaining free of disease for long periods. The efficacy of IL-2 has not been adequately evaluated in patients with non–clear cell histologies, and the use of this agent is largely restricted to patients with clear cell RCC. There are no randomized phase 3 studies demonstrating survival benefit with IL-2.

3. **a. Karnofsky performance score greater than 80%.** A Karnofsky performance score of less than 80% was determined to be an adverse prognostic feature and is one of the factors used to predict outcome in the Memorial Sloan-Kettering Cancer Center prognostic system for patients with metastatic RCC. All other factors listed have been associated with poor outcome.

4. **a. A 50-year-old man with an Eastern Cooperative Oncology Group (ECOG) performance status of 0, a large 12-cm right renal mass, and four small pulmonary metastases.** Cytoreductive nephrectomy is most likely to benefit patients who are good surgical candidates as well as candidates for postnephrectomy systemic therapy, such as those with a good performance status, relatively slow rate of disease progression, and those with relatively low metastatic burden (as demonstrated in a randomized phase 3 study in which interferon was offered post nephrectomy). Patients described in b to d are less likely to benefit from this approach because they do not satisfy one or more of the above criteria.

5. **d. improved tolerance to cytokine therapy.** Studies suggest patients with synchronous metastatic RCC have a high frequency of acquired immune dysfunction involving T lymphocytes. The abnormalities described include increased T-cell apoptosis, impaired proliferative responses, and tumor-associated immunosuppressive factors. Cytoreductive nephrectomy may improve these abnormalities. No data demonstrate better patient tolerance to cytokine therapy.

6. **c. The combination of IL-2 and interferon leads to higher overall response rates than either agent alone.** In a randomized phase III study, the combination of IL-2 and interferon was associated with a higher response rate than either agent given alone, although this did not translate to an improved long-term outcome (overall survival) in the combination arm. The addition of LAK cells to cytokine therapy does not appear to improve outcome.

7. **b. Clear cell carcinoma.** Clear cell RCC is the histology most likely to respond to cytokine therapy. Although there are inadequate data to make definitive determinations about the activity of cytokines such as IL-2 or interferons in other histologic subtypes, these agents do not appear particularly effective in non–clear cell RCC variants.

8. **c. Mediastinoscopy followed by resection of the pulmonary nodules.** Patients with metachronous pulmonary nodules related to remote renal tumors may have prolonged survival after resection of the nodule(s), as demonstrated by several retrospective studies.

9. **d. mTOR.** mTOR (mammalian target of rapamycin) is the primary target of sirolimus (rapamycin) and its analogues.

10. **b. 30% to 40%.** Objective overall RECIST response rates in metastatic clear cell RCC patients undergoing sunitinib therapy is 30% to 40%, as demonstrated in a randomized phase 3 study comparing sunitinib to interferon.

11. **d. All of the above.** A randomized phase 3 study demonstrated that sunitinib was associated with a higher response rate, longer progression-free survival, and better quality of life compared with interferon-α in the front-line treatment of patients with metastatic clear cell RCC.

12. **d. Everolimus.** In a randomized phase 3 trial, everolimus has been shown to prolong progression-free survival compared with placebo (median 4.0 vs. 1.9 months) in patients with metastatic clear cell RCC who have progressed on sunitinib and/or sorafenib.

13. **e. None of the above.** In a randomized phase 2 study, sorafenib was not superior to interferon-α in previously untreated patients with metastatic clear cell RCC.

14. **d. Temsirolimus.** In a randomized phase 3 study, temsirolimus was associated with better overall survival than interferon-α (median 10.9 vs. 7.3 months) in metastatic RCC patients presenting with three or more predefined factors predictive of poor prognosis.

15. **e. raf-1.** raf-1 is a mediator of growth factor signaling pathways but has not been shown to be upregulated in RCC as a consequence of VHL inactivation/HIF upregulation.

16. **a. 70% to 90%.** Based on numerous recent studies, it is estimated that VHL inactivation by mutation or promoter hypermethylation occurs in 70% to 90% of clear cell renal tumors.

17. **d. Enrollment on a phase 2 trial evaluating a novel inhibitor of c-*MET* activity is a reasonable consideration in this patient.** There is no conclusive evidence suggesting that standard agents with activity in clear cell RCC (including VEGF pathway inhibitors and mTOR inhibitors) have a favorable impact on outcome in patients with metastatic papillary RCC, and patients with these tumors are appropriate candidates for rational targeted therapy approaches. The presence of activating c-*MET* mutations in some papillary tumors has kindled interest in the evaluation of c-*MET* pathway antagonists in this patient population.

18. **c. Overlapping toxicity may limit maximal tolerated doses when two agents targeting this pathway are combined.** Agents targeting different components of the VHL/HIF pathway often share an overlapping adverse event profile and dictate the need for dose reduction of individual agents when used in combination. Although this is an area under active investigation there is currently no evidence to suggest that combined therapy with VEGF pathway and mTOR antagonists is superior to either class of agents administered alone. c-*MET* mutations have been identified in some papillary tumors but not in clear cell RCC.

Additional Study Points

1. Metastatic RCC is almost always fatal with a 10-year survival of less than 5%.

2. In patients with metastatic RCC, long-term survival is generally associated with a long time interval between the initial diagnosis and the appearance of metastatic disease and the development of limited sites of metastatic disease.

3. Nephrectomy as the sole treatment for metastatic RCC is unlikely to affect survival.

4. Isolated pulmonary nodules are the most common metastatic site amenable to resection with curative intent.

5. After nephrectomy, the incidence of spontaneous regression of metastases is less than 1%.

6. High dose IL-2 causes the vascular leak syndrome.

7. Patients who overexpress carbonic anhydrase IX are most likely to benefit from IL-2 therapy.

8. The *VHL* gene is a tumor suppressor gene. Mutations of it promote accumulation of hypoxia-inducible factor, which upregulates a variety of growth factors.

9. Conventional cytotoxic chemotherapy is generally ineffective for metastatic RCC.

10. Hormonal therapy for metastatic RCC has no role.

11. Targeted chemotherapy in clear cell RCC is directed at vascular endothelial growth factor.

chapter 51

Benign Renal Tumors

Vitaly Margulis, MD ● Surena F. Matin, MD ● Christopher G. Wood, MD

QUESTIONS

1. The most accurate imaging study for characterizing a renal mass is:
   a. intravenous pyelography.
   b. ultrasonography.
   c. CT with and without contrast enhancement.
   d. MRI.
   e. renal arteriography.

2. A hyperdense renal cyst may also be termed a:
   a. probable malignancy.
   b. Bosniak II cyst.
   c. Bosniak III cyst.
   d. Bosniak IV cyst.
   e. probable angiomyolipoma.

3. The primary indication for fine-needle aspiration of a renal mass is which suspected clinical diagnosis?
   a. Renal cell carcinoma
   b. Renal oncocytoma
   c. Renal adenoma
   d. Renal metastasis
   e. Renal angiomyolipoma

4. All of the following statements are TRUE about renal cysts EXCEPT:
   a. They are the most common benign renal lesions found in the kidney.
   b. They are best characterized using the Bosniak criteria to assess risk of harboring a malignancy.
   c. They are best imaged using ultrasound to allow classification using the Bosniak criteria.
   d. They can harbor internal septa, calcifications, and internal debris and still be considered benign according to the Bosniak classification.
   e. They rarely require treatment.

5. Which of the following is TRUE about renal adenoma?
   a. There is uniform agreement regarding the clinical and pathologic classification of renal adenoma.
   b. Recent studies suggest that renal adenoma may be a premalignant precursor of papillary renal cell carcinoma (RCC).

   c. They are most common in young females.
   d. They can be high grade or low grade, as long as they are less than 3 cm.
   e. They are usually of clear cell histology but can also be found with chromophobe and papillary cells as well.

6. A diagnosis of renal adenoma:
   a. can be made primarily on the basis of histologic criteria.
   b. can be rendered only if tumor size is less than 1.0 cm.
   c. is commonly made at autopsy.
   d. requires specific immunohistochemical staining.
   e. can be confirmed by electron microscopy.

7. A healthy 62-year-old man is scheduled to undergo surgery for a 3.0-cm enhancing renal mass; CT shows it to be interpolar, exophytic, and with a central stellate scar. Which of the following best describes the most appropriate surgical strategy?
   a. A radical nephrectomy with adrenalectomy
   b. A radical nephrectomy without adrenalectomy
   c. Renal exploration with biopsy and intraoperative frozen section analysis determining radical versus partial nephrectomy
   d. Renal exploration, partial nephrectomy with intraoperative frozen section analysis of histology (if malignant, a radical nephrectomy)
   e. Partial nephrectomy

8. A 48-year-old woman with a history of seizure disorder presents with recurrent gross hematuria and left flank pain. Abdominal CT shows a large left perinephric hematoma associated with a 3.0-cm left renal angiomyolipoma. There are also multiple right renal angiomyolipomas ranging from 1.5 to 6.5 cm. The next best step in management of the left renal lesion is:
   a. selective embolization.
   b. radical nephrectomy.
   c. observation.
   d. partial nephrectomy.
   e. laparoscopic exposure and renal cryoablation.

9. Which of the following statements is TRUE regarding multiloculated cystic nephromas?
   a. They are complex cystic lesions that are typically classified as Bosniak II.

b. They are malignant 2% to 5% of the time.

c. They are more common in men than in women.

d. They are characterized by bimodal age distribution.

e. They are readily differentiated from RCC on the basis of appropriate imaging studies.

10. Metanephric adenoma is differentiated from RCC based on all the following features EXCEPT:

a. female predominance.

b. benign clinical course.

c. specific pattern on immunostain marker panel.

d. characteristic appearance on MRI.

e. peak incidence in the fifth decade of life.

11. Which of the following would be considered diagnostic for renal angiomyolipoma?

a. Hyperechoic pattern on ultrasonography

b. Enhancement of more than 30 Hounsfield units (HU) on CT

c. Small area of less than –20 HU on nonenhanced CT

d. Aneurysmal changes on renal arteriogram

e. Positive signal on T2-weighted images of MRI

12. Which of the following features is typically required for the diagnosis of renal adenoma in a clinical setting?

a. Tumor size less than 3 cm

b. Low to moderate grade

c. Papillary architecture

d. Nonconventional histology

e. Noncentral location

13. Which of the following tumors is most likely to be a malignant RCC?

a. A 2.5-cm hyperechoic complex cyst, with no enhancement after intravenous administration of a contrast agent

b. A 6.0-cm complex cyst with four thin septa

c. A 5.0-cm cyst with thin, curvilinear calcification

d. An 11-cm cyst with water density and a homogeneous nature

e. A 3.0-cm tumor with fat associated with calcification

14. A reliable finding for the diagnosis of renal oncocytoma is:

a. trisomy of chromosomes 7 and 17.

b. central, stellate scar on CT.

c. a spoke-wheel pattern on renal angiography.

d. multiple mitochondria on electron microscopy.

e. hypervascular pattern.

15. A distinctive finding for renal angiomyolipoma is:

a. positive staining for vimentin.

b. a unique cytokeratin expression pattern.

c. positive staining for HMB-45.

d. multiple microsomes on electron microscopy.

e. occasional aneuploidy.

16. All of the following statements accurately describe mixed epithelial and stromal tumors of the kidney EXCEPT:

a. There is a female predilection.

b. They are associated with estrogen replacement therapy in women or with androgen ablation therapy in men.

c. Radiologic diagnostic criteria exist for reliable differentiation from RCC.

d. Nephron sparing with partial nephrectomy when technically feasible is appropriate.

e. A benign clinical course is expected.

17. A 44-year-old man undergoes left laparoscopic partial nephrectomy for a 2-cm exophytic renal mass. Final pathologic review reveals intersecting fascicles of smooth muscle with no evidence of hypercellularity, pleomorphism, or mitotic activity. Surgical margins are negative. The next step in management is:

a. completion radical nephrectomy.

b. adjuvant chemotherapy.

c. adjuvant targeted therapy.

d. observation.

e. retroperitoneal external-beam radiation therapy.

Pathology

1. A nephrectomy is performed in a 67-year-old man for a solid renal mass; the gross specimen is depicted in Figure 51–1A and the microscopic findings are shown in Figure 51–1B.

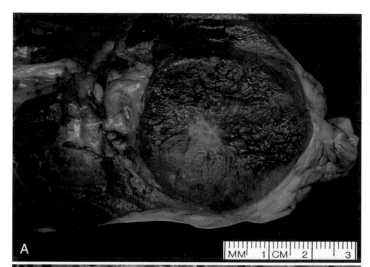

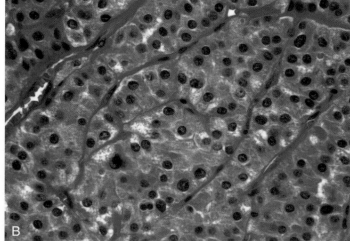

Figure 51–1. (From Bostwick DG, Cheng L. Urologic surgical pathology. 2nd ed. Edinburgh: Mosby; 2008. **A,** Courtesy of Philip Bomeisl, MD.)

The most likely diagnosis is:

a. metastatic lymphoma.

b. oncocytoma.

c. RCC, chromophobe type.

d. angiomyolipoma.

e. pheochromocytoma.

2. A 15-year-old boy has a renal mass incidentally discovered. He is asymptomatic and he has a left nephrectomy. Pathologic findings are depicted in Figure 51–2.

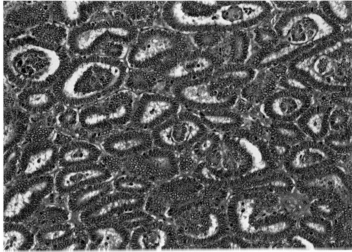

Figure 51–2. (From Bostwick DG, Cheng L. Urologic surgical pathology. 2nd ed. Edinburgh: Mosby; 2008.)

The diagnosis is:

a. neuroblastoma.

b. Wilms tumor.

c. metanephric adenoma.

d. lymphoma.

e. papillary RCC.

Imaging

1. See Figure 51–3.

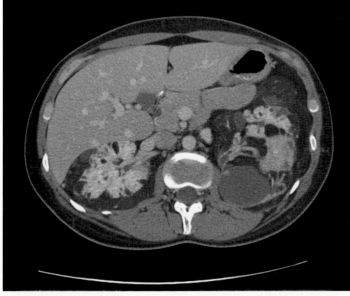

Figure 51–3.

CT is obtained in a 23-year-old woman with hematuria. In this patient:

a. selective renal embolization may be indicated in symptomatic lesions.

b. there is an associated high risk for urothelial neoplasms.

c. the renal lesions contain microscopic fat.

d. the renal lesions commonly calcify.

e. the renal lesions are premalignant.

ANSWERS

1. **c. CT with and without contrast enhancement.** A dedicated (thin-slice) renal CT scan remains the single most important radiographic image for delineating the nature of a renal mass. In general, any renal mass that enhances with administration of intravenous contrast material on CT should be considered an RCC until proved otherwise.

2. **b. Bosniak II cyst.** Category II lesions are minimally complicated cysts that are benign but have some radiologic findings that cause concern. Classic hyperdense renal cysts are small (<3 cm), round, and sharply marginated and do not enhance after administration of contrast material.

3. **d. Renal metastasis.** Fine-needle aspiration or biopsy is of limited value in the evaluation of renal masses. The major problem with this technique is the high incidence of false-negative findings in patients with renal malignancy. The primary indication for needle aspiration or biopsy of a renal mass occurs when a renal abscess or infected cyst is suspected or when differentiating RCC from metastatic malignancy or renal lymphoma.

4. **c. They are best imaged using ultrasound to allow classification using the Bosniak criteria.** Contrast enhancement using imaging that utilizes contrast (CT, MRI) is critical to the Bosniak classification criteria.

5. **b. Recent studies suggest that renal adenoma may be a premalignant precursor of papillary renal cell carcinoma.** Recent immunohistochemical studies suggest that renal adenomas are commonly associated with papillary RCC and may represent a premalignant precursor along a biologic continuum.

6. **c. is commonly made at autopsy.** Small, evidently benign, solid renal cortical lesions have been found at autopsy with an incidence of 7% to 23% and have been designated renal adenomas.

7. **e. Partial nephrectomy.** Most renal oncocytomas cannot be differentiated from malignant RCCs on the basis of clinical or radiographic means, nor can they be reliably differentiated on frozen section at the time of surgery. Given these uncertainties about a diagnosis, and the excellent outcomes obtained with partial nephrectomy of either benign or malignant tumors, most authors have emphasized the need to treat these tumors with nephron-sparing surgery depending on the clinical circumstances.

8. **a. selective embolization.** Most patients with acute or potentially life-threatening hemorrhage will require total nephrectomy if exploration is done. If the patient has tuberous sclerosis, bilateral disease, preexisting renal insufficiency, or other medical or urologic disease that could affect renal function in the future, selective embolization should be considered. In such circumstances, selective embolization can temporize and in many cases will prove to be definitive treatment.

9. **d. They are characterized by bimodal age distribution.** Multiloculated cystic nephroma is a characteristic renal lesion with a bimodal age distribution and a benign clinical course.

10. **d. characteristic appearance on MRI.** Metanephric adenoma is radiographically indistinguishable from RCC and is typically a diagnosis made postoperatively. All other answers are distinguishing features of metanephric adenoma.

11. **c. Small area of less than −20 HU on nonenhanced CT.** The presence of even a small focus of fat, as evidenced by less than −20 HU on a nonenhanced CT scan, is diagnostic for angiomyolipoma. The findings described in a, b, and d are all suggestive but not diagnostic for renal angiomyolipoma.

12. **c. Papillary architecture.** Most pathologists will not make the diagnosis of renal adenoma in a nonautopsy setting unless the lesion is low grade, small (<1.0 cm), and of papillary architecture.

13. **e. A 3.0-cm tumor with fat associated with calcification.** Tumors with calcification associated with fat are uncommon but are almost always malignant RCC. In this setting the fat is thought to be a reactive process related to tumor necrosis. Calcification is virtually never seen in association with angiomyolipoma. The lesions described in a to c are Bosniak II renal cysts, with risk of malignancy of less than 10%. The lesion described in d is a simple cyst and highly likely to be benign despite its large size.

14. **d. multiple mitochondria on electron microscopy.** A distinctive and diagnostic feature of renal oncocytoma is the presence of multiple mitochondria on electron microscopy. Suggestive radiographic findings including a central stellate scar on CT or spoke-wheel pattern on renal angiography have been described but can be seen with RCC and are absent in many oncocytomas. Trisomy of chromosomes 7 and 17 is found in papillary RCC, not renal oncocytoma.

15. **c. positive staining for HMB-45.** Angiomyolipoma will stain positive for HMB-45 in most cases, and this can be used to confirm the diagnosis in challenging cases. This antigen, which was originally found in association with melanoma, is expressed by most angiomyolipomas.

16. **c. Radiologic diagnostic criteria exist for reliable differentiation from RCC.** Conclusive differentiation of mixed epithelial/stromal tumor from RCC or cystic Wilms tumor is not possible based on current imaging modalities. The other answers are characteristic for mixed epithelial/stromal tumors.

17. **d. observation.** Pathologic diagnosis is of renal leiomyoma with a benign clinical course. Observation is appropriate.

Pathology

1. **b. oncocytoma.** Notice the central scar on the gross specimen and the eosinophilic cytoplasm and also the low mitotic activity on the photomicrograph. These are the hallmarks of oncocytoma.

2. **c. metanephric adenoma.** Notice the uniformity of the cells, scant cytoplasm, and no nuclear mitotic activity. The three elements of a Wilms tumor are not present. Sheets of small cells that are seen in a neuroblastoma also are not present.

Imaging

1. **a. selective renal embolization may be indicated in symptomatic lesions.** The CT scan demonstrates multiple bilateral low-attenuation lesions. The attenuation of the majority of the lesions is similar to the low density of retroperitoneal fat and lower than the fluid in the gallbladder. This indicates that the lesions are composed of macroscopic fat and represent angiomyolipomas. There are also large cysts in the left kidney. Calcification in angiomyolipomas is unusual, and bilateral angiomyolipomas are often seen in patients with tuberous sclerosis. There is no association with urothelial neoplasms. Angiomyolipomas that are larger than 4 cm have a propensity to bleed spontaneously, and angiographically directed selective embolization of such lesions is indicated when such lesions are symptomatic. Microscopic fat is not visible on CT.

Additional Study Points

1. See Table 51–1 in *Campbell-Walsh Urology, 10th Edition* for the Bosniak classification.
2. Simple renal cysts increase in both size and number over time. The risk factors for development of cysts include age, male gender, hypertension, and renal insufficiency.
3. There is a higher incidence of RCC in acquired renal cystic disease.
4. The diagnosis of oncocytoma may be made on biopsy with reasonable assurance if the features are classic; however, on occasion it may be difficult to differentiate an RCC with oncocytic features from an oncocytoma. Under these circumstances, the lesion should be treated as though it were an RCC.
5. Oncocytomas are derived from distal renal tubule cells. Chromophobe RCCs also originate from distal renal tubule cells.
6. Angiomyolipomas may be difficult to differentiate from RCCs when they are fat poor and appear more solid on CT.

chapter 52

Retroperitoneal Tumors

Thomas J. Guzzo, MD, MPH ● Stanley Bruce Malkowicz, MD

QUESTIONS

1. The most common histologic subtype of retroperitoneal sarcoma is:
   a. fibrosarcoma.
   b. liposarcoma.
   c. rhabdomyosarcoma.
   d. leiomyosarcoma.
   e. gastrointestinal stromal tumor.

2. In what group is pelvic lipomatosis most commonly found?
   a. African-American women
   b. White women
   c. White men
   d. African-American men
   e. Asian women

3. What is the most common clinical presentation in patients with retroperitoneal sarcoma?
   a. Lower extremity edema
   b. Hematuria
   c. Neurologic symptoms
   d. Uncontrolled hypertension
   e. Abdominal pain and palpable mass

4. What is the most important predictor of prognosis for patients with retroperitoneal sarcomas?
   a. Complete surgical resection with negative margins
   b. Histologic subtype and tumor grade
   c. Patient age
   d. Tumor size
   e. Administration of neoadjuvant chemotherapy

5. What is the most common organ that requires resection at the time of surgery for retroperitoneal sarcomas?
   a. Distal pancreas
   b. Colon
   c. Kidney
   d. Spleen
   e. Adrenal gland

6. What percentage of patients with retroperitoneal sarcomas present with metastatic disease?
   a. 5%
   b. 10%
   c. 20%
   d. 40%
   e. More than 50%

7. Which chemotherapeutic agent or regimen is most commonly used for patients with advanced retroperitoneal sarcoma?
   a. Cisplatin
   b. Methotrexate/vinblastine/doxorubicin/cisplatin
   c. Bleomycin/etoposide/platinum
   d. Doxorubicin
   e. Imatinib

8. Which of the following statements is FALSE?
   a. The incidence of retroperitoneal sarcoma has been rising steadily over the past 30 years.
   b. Retroperitoneal sarcomas account for 15% of all soft tissue sarcomas.
   c. The most common age at presentation for a retroperitoneal sarcoma is in the sixth decade.
   d. Retroperitoneal sarcomas are slightly more common in men.
   e. Retroperitoneal sarcomas comprise less than half of all tumors presenting in the retroperitoneum.

9. What is the most common sarcoma associated with prior radiation treatment?
   a. Fibrosarcoma
   b. Liposarcoma
   c. Rhabdomyosarcoma
   d. Leiomyosarcoma
   e. Malignant fibrous histiocytoma

10. Which of the following statements is TRUE?
    a. The risk of local recurrence after resection of a retroperitoneal sarcoma is very low.

b. All patients require computed tomographic–guided biopsy before surgical resection.

c. The average 5-year survival for completely resected retroperitoneal sarcoma is approximately 50%.

d. Neoadjuvant chemotherapy is the standard of care for retroperitoneal sarcoma.

e. The peak incidence of retroperitoneal sarcoma is in the third decade.

ANSWERS

1. **b. liposarcoma.** Classically, liposarcoma is the most common histologic variant of retroperitoneal sarcoma, followed by leiomyosarcoma and fibrosarcoma, followed by other histologies. Many tumors previously described as variants of fibrosarcoma or liposarcoma have been reclassified as malignant fibrous histiocytoma. Therefore, fibrosarcoma has been replaced in order of frequency by this condition.

2. **d. African-American men.** Approximately two thirds of cases of pelvic lipomatosis occur in African-Americans. Pelvic lipomatosis is more common in men than women.

3. **e. Abdominal pain and palpable mass.** A palpable abdominal mass and abdominal pain are present in 60% to 80% of patients presenting with retroperitoneal sarcomas. Because of their anatomic location within the retroperitoneum, these tumors can grow quite large before a patient experiences symptoms.

4. **a. Complete surgical resection with negative margins.** Complete resection of the tumor with negative soft tissue margins is the most important predictor of prognosis and recurrence for retroperitoneal sarcomas.

5. **c. Kidney.** To achieve a negative margin, other organs adjacent to a retroperitoneal sarcoma often require resection. In order of decreasing frequency the most common resected organs are kidney (32% to 46%), colon (25%), adrenal gland (18%), pancreas (15%), and spleen (10%).

6. **c. 20%.**

7. **d. Doxorubicin.** Doxorubicin is the foundation for chemotherapy in advanced sarcoma. The general response rate is 20% to 25%, but sustained complete responses are uncommon. Median survival is 7.7 to 12 months.

8. **a. The incidence of retroperitoneal sarcoma has been rising steadily over the past 30 years.** The incidence of retroperitoneal sarcoma is 2.7 cases per 100,000 individuals and has been stable over the past 3 decades.

9. **e. Malignant fibrous histiocytoma.** Approximately one tenth of a percent of patients who receive radiation therapy may develop a sarcoma at the treatment site.

10. **c. The average 5-year survival for completely resected retroperitoneal sarcoma is approximately 50%.** On the average the 5-year survival for patients with completely resected retroperitoneal sarcoma is 54% compared with 17% for incomplete resections; at 10 years this difference is 45% to 17%. Thus a nearly 40% survival advantage is seen at 5 to 10 years in those patients with complete surgical resection of their lesion.

Additional Study Points

1. Gastrointestinal stromal tumors demonstrate c-*KIT* mutations, suggesting a role for targeted therapy using tyrosine kinase inhibitors.
2. Pelvic lipomatosis is a hyperplastic rather than a neoplastic process.
3. Myelolipoma usually occurs in the adrenal gland but may be found in the retroperitoneum.
4. Sarcomas have a tendency to recur in part owing to pseudoencapsulation and the false gross appearance of complete surgical resection.
5. Rhabdomyosarcomas are classified as embryonal, alveolar, and pleomorphic.
6. Tumor involvement of neural foramina suggests unresectability.

Urothelial Tumors of the Upper Urinary Tract and Ureter

Arthur I. Sagalowsky, MD • Thomas W. Jarrett, MD • Robert C. Flanigan, MD

QUESTIONS

1. Which factor is the major determinant of the type of treatment for upper tract urothelial tumors?
   a. Size
   b. Number
   c. Stage and grade
   d. Contralateral renal function
   e. Level of lesion

2. What is (are) the most common symptom(s) of localized upper tract tumors?
   a. None, inasmuch as such tumors are incidental findings
   b. Flank pain
   c. Frequency
   d. Dysuria and hematuria
   e. Weight loss and fatigue

3. Which of the following statements is TRUE regarding flank pain in patients with upper tract tumors?
   a. It is rare.
   b. It signifies invasive disease.
   c. It indicates invasion into adjacent structures.
   d. It correlates with stage.
   e. None of the above

4. In patients with upper tract tumors, what is the most common finding on imaging studies of the urinary tract?
   a. A mass
   b. A filling defect
   c. Hydronephrosis
   d. Nonfunction
   e. Delayed function

5. The majority of renal pelvis tumors are:
   a. papillary and invasive.
   b. papillary and noninvasive.
   c. sessile and invasive.
   d. sessile and noninvasive.
   e. mixed papillary and sessile.

6. Most ureteral tumors are:
   a. sessile.
   b. high grade and noninvasive.
   c. low grade and noninvasive.
   d. medium grade and low stage.
   e. low grade and invasive.

7. What is the most common location of ureteral tumors?
   a. Ureteropelvic junction
   b. Proximal
   c. Middle
   d. Distal
   e. Intramural

8. After complete conservative treatment of a ureteral tumor (i.e., segmental excision or endoscopic ablation), which of the following is TRUE?
   a. Ipsilateral recurrence is common.
   b. Recurrence is rare.
   c. Recurrence most likely is contralateral.
   d. Recurrence signifies incomplete initial therapy.
   e. Recurrence in the renal pelvis is common.

9. What is the major factor predisposing to recurrence of upper tract tumors?
   a. Incomplete therapy
   b. Multifocal field change
   c. Implantation during instrumentation
   d. Normal ureteral peristalsis
   e. Periureteral spread

10. What is the best predictor of outcome in patients with multifocal upper tract tumors?
    a. Stage
    b. Early radical surgery
    c. Grade
    d. Rate of recurrence
    e. Extent of surgery

11. What is the single most important determinant of outcome in the treatment of upper tract tumors?
    a. Grade
    b. Stage
    c. Early diagnosis
    d. Extent of surgery
    e. Size and focality of lesion

12. What is the earliest site of spread of proximal ureteral tumors?
    a. Lung and bone
    b. Liver and bone
    c. Lung and liver
    d. Pelvic nodes
    e. Para-aortic nodes

13. Reasons to consider nephron-sparing surgery for patients with upper tract tumors include all of the following EXCEPT:
    a. bilateral tumors.
    b. unreliable follow-up.
    c. Balkan nephropathy.
    d. diabetic nephropathy.
    e. solitary kidney.

14. A 60-year-old diabetic man is diagnosed with a 4-cm, grade 2 to 3/3 transitional cell carcinoma (TCC) of the renal pelvis. Serum creatinine concentration is 2.2 mg/dL. The best treatment is:
    a. ureteroscopic ablation.
    b. antegrade percutaneous resection.
    c. pyelotomy and tumor excision,
    d. radical nephroureterectomy.
    e. ileal ureteral substitution.

15. A 57-year-old man with a grade 3, stage T2 tumor of the proximal ureter is undergoing radical nephroureterectomy. Correct management of the ureter requires which of the following?
    a. Ligation and division as far as exposure allows
    b. Ureterectomy in continuity with the kidney
    c. Ligation and division at the juxtavesical portion
    d. Complete distal ureterectomy with a bladder cuff
    e. Ligation and division 4 cm distal to the tumor and a negative margin on frozen section

16. Lymphadenectomy in conjunction with radical nephroureterectomy:
    a. should not be performed.
    b. is helpful for determining prognosis.
    c. is associated with a high morbidity rate.
    d. decreases the occurrence of distant relapse.
    e. is therapeutic.

17. A 46-year-old woman has a 2.5-cm stage Ta, grade 2 TCC of the midureter. Initial treatment consists of "complete" ureteroscopic laser ablation of the tumor. Six months later there is a recurrent 2-cm tumor of the same stage and grade at the same location in the ureter. The next best step in management is:

    a. segmental ureterectomy.
    b. nephroureterectomy.
    c. ureteroscopic ablation.
    d. antegrade resection.
    e. antegrade resection followed by instillation of mitomycin.

18. A 38-year-old man has a brief episode of gross hematuria. His initial evaluation included bladder wash cytology, intravenous urography, cystoscopy, bladder biopsy, urethral biopsy, and bilateral retrograde pyelography, all of which were normal. The upper tract cytologic findings are positive for the right and negative for the left. The next step in management is:
    a. repeat upper tract cytology in 6 months.
    b. ureteropyeloscopy.
    c. right nephroureterectomy.
    d. intravesical bacille Calmette-Guérin (BCG).
    e. right nephrostomy and infusion of BCG.

19. After radical nephroureterectomy for a stage T3 TCC of the renal pelvis:
    a. local relapse is the main limitation to survival.
    b. adjuvant radiation decreases local relapse.
    c. adjuvant chemotherapy increases survival.
    d. adjuvant radiation does not improve survival.
    e. adjuvant radiation plus chemotherapy increases survival.

20. Which of the following statements is TRUE regarding metastatic TCC of the upper urinary tract?
    a. It is not chemosensitive.
    b. It responds to the same chemotherapy as that used for bladder cancer.
    c. It is uniquely sensitive to taxanes.
    d. It is uniquely sensitive to interleukin-2.
    e. It responds best to debulking surgery plus chemotherapy.

21. A 46-year-old man is diagnosed with a 2-cm grade 3 tumor of the left renal pelvis. He is otherwise healthy. Acceptable treatment options include which of the following?
    a. Ureteroscopic ablation of the tumor
    b. Percutaneous resection of the tumor followed by BCG therapy
    c. Laparoscopic nephroureterectomy
    d. Open nephroureterectomy
    e. Both c and d

22. After a proper laparoscopic nephroureterectomy, surveillance is best accomplished by:
    a. interval cystoscopy and ureteroscopy of the stump.
    b. cystoscopy with retrograde pyelography of the stump.
    c. cystoscopy and ureteral stump cytology.
    d. radiographic imaging with CT.
    e. cystoscopy and voided urine cytology.

23. When endoscopic treatment of TCC of the upper urinary tract is used, ureteroscopy is best employed for:
    a. small papillary tumors of the renal pelvis or ureter.
    b. large-volume tumors of the renal pelvis.
    c. small papillary tumors in the upper tracts of patients with previous urinary diversion.

d. large bulky tumors of the lower pole of the kidney.

e. large parenchymal invasive tumors of the renal pelvis.

24. Which of the following is NOT a distinct advantage of the ureteroscopic approach?

a. Decreased morbidity when compared with percutaneous renal surgery

b. Maintenance of a closed system without exposure of nonurothelial surfaces to tumor cells

c. Higher risk of tumor implantation outside the urinary tract

d. Ease of access to the entire urinary tract without extensive dilatation of the ureteral orifice

e. Usually can be done on an outpatient basis

25. A 60-year-old man who had undergone prior urinary diversion and a right nephroureterectomy is diagnosed with a grade 1 tumor of the lower pole collecting system of his solitary kidney. What is the optimal approach for this patient?

a. Ureteroscopy with laser therapy of the lower pole tumor

b. Nephroureterectomy

c. Open lower pole partial nephrectomy

d. Placement of a nephrostomy tube and BCG therapy

e. Percutaneous access and resection of the lower pole tumor

26. Which of the following statements regarding adjuvant therapy for upper tract TCC is the most accurate?

a. Adjuvant therapy with BCG has shown a definite advantage with regard to survival and tumor recurrence rates.

b. Adjuvant therapy with mitomycin has shown a definite improvement with regard to survival and tumor recurrence rates.

c. Although many studies have shown responses to instillation therapy, no significant improvement in survival or recurrence rate has been demonstrated.

d. The most common complication of instillation therapy is systemic absorption of the agent.

e. Granulomatous disease of the kidney is rare after upper tract BCG therapy.

27. An otherwise healthy 50-year-old man has a grade 1 tumor of the intramural ureter. The endoscopic approach or approaches that are acceptable options are:

a. ureteroscopic treatment.

b. transurethral resection of the ureteral orifice and distal ureter.

c. percutaneous antegrade ureteroscopy.

d. placement of a ureteral stent and BCG therapy.

e. both a and b.

28. Which of the following statements is NOT true regarding follow-up after treatment of upper urinary tract TCC?

a. Patients undergoing conservative (organ-sparing) therapy need interval endoscopy of the ipsilateral urinary tract for tumor recurrence.

b. Follow-up should be identical for all patients regardless of tumor stage or grade.

c. Efficient and cost-effective follow-up should be based on tumor grade and stage.

d. Cross-sectional imaging with CT or MRI is necessary with high-grade and high-stage tumors to assess for local recurrence and metastatic spread.

e. All patients need interval evaluation of the contralateral urinary tract to assess for bilateral disease.

29. A 67-year-old patient with a solitary kidney has a large tumor of the renal pelvis. His urinary cytology is negative, and CT shows no evidence of invasive disease. What is the best course of action?

a. Radical nephroureterectomy and hemodialysis

b. Single-stage percutaneous access and resection of the entire tumor

c. Single-stage ureteroscopic treatment of the entire tumor

d. Endoscopic evaluation and biopsy with continued endoscopic therapy only if the pathologic evaluation shows a low potential for tumor progression

e. Laparoscopic nephroureterectomy and hemodialysis

30. All of the following statements regarding the percutaneous approach to upper tract TCCs are true EXCEPT:

a. The nephrostomy should be maintained for postoperative surveillance nephroscopy of the tract for tumor implantation.

b. Tumor seeding of the nephrostomy tract is a common complication.

c. Adjuvant therapy with BCG can be given through the established nephrostomy.

d. The larger endoscopes used for percutaneous removal of TCC allow for tumor staging as well as grading.

e. Percutaneous tumor resection has a higher morbidity rate when compared with a ureteroscopic approach.

Pathology

1. A 38-year-old woman has right flank pain and microscopic hematuria. Her cytology is atypical. Cystoscopy is negative. Her past medical history is significant in that she has had intermittent chronic pelvic pain and has been unable to achieve a pregnancy. A CT scan shows a mass in the distal ureter with significant hydronephrosis. Ureteroscopy is unsuccessful. The distal ureter is excised and the pathology is depicted in Figure 53–1.

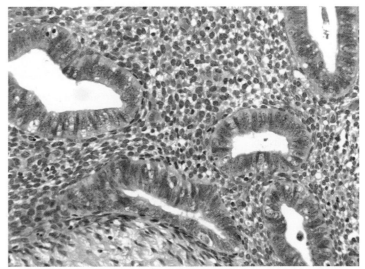

Figure 53–1. (From Bostwick DG, Cheng L. Urologic surgical pathology. 2nd ed. Edinburgh: Mosby; 2008.)

The diagnosis is:

a. adenocarcinoma of the ureter.

b. inverted papilloma.

c. endometriosis.

d. von Brunn nest.

e. cystitis glandularis.

2. A 60-year-old man has microscopic hematuria. Cytology is atypical. CT scan is negative. Cystoscopy and retrograde pyelography show a distal 2-cm filling defect in the left ureter. The lesion is excised and shown in Figure 53–2.

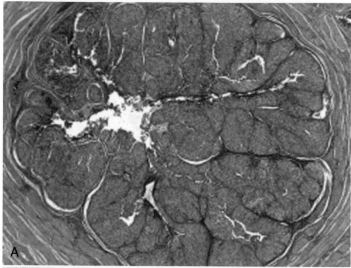

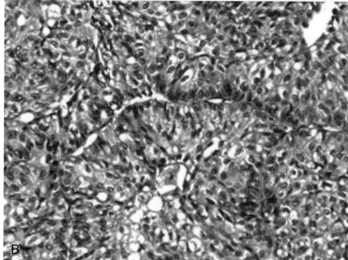

Figure 53–2.   (From Bostwick DG, Cheng L. Urologic surgical pathology. 2nd ed. Edinburgh: Mosby; 2008.)

The diagnosis is:

a. endometriosis of the ureter.

b. high-grade invasive TCC.

c. low-grade noninvasive TCC.

d. inverted papilloma.

e. nephrogenic adenoma.

Imaging

1. See Figure 53–3.

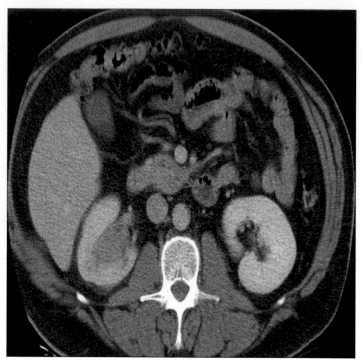

Figure 53–3.

A CT scan of a 62-year-old man with hematuria is shown. The most likely diagnosis is:

a. renal cell carcinoma.

b. urinary obstruction.

c. urothelial carcinoma.

d. lymphoma.

e. metastatic disease.

ANSWERS

1. **c. Stage and grade.** Treatment may be based primarily on the risk the tumor poses and the efficacy of specific treatment rather than on other considerations.

2. **d. Dysuria and hematuria.** The common symptoms of localized disease (hematuria and dysuria) and advanced upper tract tumors (weight loss, fatigue, anemia, and bone pain) are similar in type and frequency to those of bladder cancer.

3. **e. None of the above.** Flank pain caused by obstruction by tumor or clot is more prevalent in upper tract tumors, being reported in 10% to 40% of cases. Flank pain in patients with upper tract tumors does not correlate with either locally advanced tumor stage or worse prognosis, as is the case with bladder cancer.

4. **b. A filling defect.** A filling defect is the most common finding on imaging studies.

5. **a. papillary and invasive.** Approximately 85% of renal pelvis tumors are papillary; the remainder are sessile. In contrast to the majority of bladder tumors being noninvasive, 50% to 60% of renal pelvis tumors are invasive.

6. **c. low grade and noninvasive.** Although invasion is still more common among ureteral tumors than among bladder tumors, 55% to 75% of ureteral tumors are low grade and low stage.

7. **d. Distal.** Ureteral tumors occur in the distal, middle, or proximal segment in 70%, 25%, and 5% of cases, respectively.

8. **a. Ipsilateral recurrence is common.** After conservative treatment, ipsilateral upper tract tumor recurrence is common in a proximal to distal direction and is seen in 33% to 55% of cases.

9. **b. Multifocal field change.** The high rate of ipsilateral recurrence is due in part to a multifocal field change.

10. **a. Determined mainly by stage.** Tumor multifocality per se does not lessen patient survival independent of stage.

11. **b. Stage.** The single most important determinant of outcome is tumor stage.

12. **e. Para-aortic nodes.** Renal pelvis and upper ureteral tumors spread initially to para-aortic and paracaval nodes, whereas distal ureteral tumors spread to pelvic nodes.

13. **b. unreliable follow-up.** Reasons to consider nephron sparing include the presence of a tumor in a solitary kidney, synchronous bilateral tumors, or a predisposition to form multiple recurrences, as in endemic Balkan nephropathy.

14. **d. radical nephroureterectomy.** Radical nephroureterectomy with excision of a bladder cuff is recommended for large, high-grade, invasive tumors of the renal pelvis and proximal ureter.

15. **d. Complete distal ureterectomy with a bladder cuff.** The role of complete distal ureterectomy with excision of a bladder cuff in radical nephroureterectomy for upper tract tumors is well established. The risk of tumor recurrence in a retained ureteral stump is 30% to 75%.

16. **b. it is helpful for determining prognosis.** The rationale for continuing regional lymphadenectomy is that it adds little time or morbidity to the surgery, is important for prognosis, and may occasionally have therapeutic value.

17. **a. segmental ureterectomy.** Segmental ureterectomy and ureteroureterostomy are indicated for noninvasive grade 1 and 2 tumors of the proximal ureter or midureter that are too large for complete endoscopic ablation and for grade 3 or invasive tumors when nephron sparing for preservation of renal function is a factor. Repeated endoscopic ablation of the tumor is not categorically incorrect. However, the rapid and large tumor recurrence is a matter of concern and favors segmental ureterectomy.

18. **b. ureteropyeloscopy.** Occasionally, one is faced with a patient who has an isolated positive cytologic result from the upper urinary tract. By definition, the patient should have negative results from intravenous urography and retrograde pyelography, cystoscopy, and biopsy from the bladder and urethra. Ureteropyeloscopy is indicated in such cases, because the yield for direct visualization of small lesions is superior to that of retrograde pyelography.

19. **d. adjuvant radiation does not improve survival.** In one series of patients with tumor stages of T2, T3, or N+, all patients with local relapse also had distant relapse, leading the authors of the report to conclude that adjuvant radiation is not beneficial. Another retrospective review of patients with stage T3 disease with or without adjuvant radiation found that radical nephroureterectomy alone provides a high rate of local control. Adjuvant radiation for high-stage disease does not decrease local relapse or protect against a high rate of distant failure.

20. **b. It responds to the same chemotherapy as that used for bladder cancer.** The systemic chemotherapy regimens offered for treatment of patients with metastatic urothelial tumors of the upper urinary tract are the same as those used for TCC of the bladder.

21. **e. Both c and d.** Percutaneous management is acceptable in patients with low-grade (grade 1) disease regardless of the status of the contralateral kidney. Patients with grade 3 disease do poorly regardless of the modality chosen but should probably undergo nephroureterectomy to maximize cancer therapy (provided that they are medically fit). Radical nephroureterectomy with excision of a bladder cuff is recommended for large, high-grade invasive tumors of the renal pelvis and proximal ureter. Nephroureterectomy can be performed either completely laparoscopically or assisted with an open incision in the lower abdomen. The indications for laparoscopic nephroureterectomy are the same as those for open nephroureterectomy.

22. **e. cystoscopy and voided urine cytology.** No surveillance of the ureter stump is needed because it has been removed in identical manner to the open surgical counterpart. Cystoscopy is indicated in follow-up to exclude new bladder tumor.

23. **a. small papillary tumors of the renal pelvis or ureter.** The ureteroscopic approach to tumors is generally favored for ureteral and smaller renal tumors. Tumors of the upper urinary tract can be approached in a retrograde or antegrade manner. The approach chosen depends largely on the tumor location and size. In general, a retrograde ureteroscopic approach is used for low-volume ureteral and renal tumors. An antegrade percutaneous approach is preferred for larger tumors of the upper ureter or kidney or those that cannot be adequately manipulated in a retrograde approach because of location (i.e., lower pole calyx) or previous urinary diversion.

24. **c. Higher risk of tumor implantation outside the urinary tract.** The advantages of a ureteroscopic approach are lower morbidity than the percutaneous and open surgical counterparts and the maintenance of a closed system. With a closed system, nonurothelial surfaces are not exposed to the possibility of tumor seeding.

25. **e. Percutaneous access and resection of the lower pole tumor.** A percutaneous approach may avoid the limitations of flexible ureteroscopy, especially when working in complicated calyceal systems or areas that are difficult to access such as the lower pole calyx or the upper urinary tract of patients with urinary diversion.

26. **c. Although many studies have shown responses to instillation therapy, no significant improvement in survival or recurrence rate has been demonstrated.** Many studies have described small retrospective uncontrolled series of patients undergoing therapy with thiotepa, mitomycin, and BCG. Although the cumulative experience appears encouraging, no individual study has shown statistical improvement with relation to survival and recurrence rates.

27. **e. Both a and b.** When a tumor protrudes from the ureteral orifice, complete ureteroscopic ablation of the tumor or aggressive transurethral resection of the entire most distal ureter can be performed with acceptable results.

28. **b. Follow-up should be identical for all patients regardless of tumor stage or grade.** All patients should be assessed at 3-month intervals the first year after they are rendered free of tumor by endoscopic or open surgical approaches. If an organ-sparing approach is chosen, the

ipsilateral urinary tract must be assessed as well as the remainder of the urinary tract. The frequency and duration of the follow-up depend largely on the grade and stage of the lesion but are usually every 6 months for several years and then annually. Metastatic restaging is required in all patients at significant risk for disease progression to local or distant sites. This group includes those with high-grade and/or high-stage disease, who should be assessed by use of cross-sectional imaging, chest radiography, liver function tests, and selective use of bone scintigraphy.

29. **d. Endoscopic evaluation and biopsy with continued endoscopic therapy only if the pathologic evaluation shows a low potential for tumor progression.** Endoscopic management is completed only after the pathologic evaluation shows that the patient is an acceptable candidate for continued minimally invasive endoscopic management. If the tumor is high grade or invasive, the patient should proceed to nephroureterectomy and dialysis, provided that he or she is medically fit.

30. **b. Tumor seeding of the nephrostomy tract is a common complication.** A major concern of the percutaneous approach is potential seeding of nonurothelial

surfaces with tumor cells. Although there have been several reported cases of nephrostomy tract infiltration with high-grade tumors, there were no reported occurrences in the three largest series. Tract seeding is a possibility but appears to be an uncommon event.

Pathology

1. **c. endometriosis.** Notice the endometrial tissue that is in the ureteral wall.
2. **c. low-grade noninvasive TCC.** Notice the papillary architecture, orderly nature of the cells with low mitotic numbers, and lack of ureteral wall invasion.

Imaging

1. **c. urothelial carcinoma.** There is an enhancing mass centered in the renal sinus. The appearance is typical for a urothelial neoplasm of the renal pelvis. Parenchymal tumors such as renal cell carcinoma are rounder in configuration and distort the renal contour. Urinary obstruction would cause hydronephrosis, which is of low attenuation on a CT scan. Lymphoma and metastatic disease cause renal parenchymal masses and are not confined to the renal sinus.

Additional Study Points

1. Upper tract urothelial tumors are rarely diagnosed at autopsy; they present clinically during the patient's lifetime much as bladder tumors do.
2. Upper tract recurrence is more likely with high-grade tumors and those associated with carcinoma in situ.
3. Upper tract tumors develop in 2% to 4% of patients with bladder cancer. Patients with upper tract tumors develop bladder cancer 30% of the time.
4. Bilateral upper tract tumors occur either synchronously or meticulously in 2% to 6% of patients.
5. In renal pelvic tumors, parenchyma invasion is the most significant predictor of metastases.
6. Inverted papillomas may be associated with upper tract tumors; it is not likely that cancers arise from them.
7. Squamous cell carcinoma and adenocarcinoma, although rare in the upper tract, are usually associated with long-term obstruction, inflammation, and occasionally calculi.
8. Lymphovascular invasion is a predictor of poor prognosis.

9. A significant problem with ureteroscopic biopsy is that grade may be accurate but accurate staging can be extremely difficult.
10. There is a 30% to 50% recurrence rate in ureteral tissue left distal to an invasive ureteral cancer.
11. Upper tract ureteral tumors after radial cystectomy for bladder cancer occur in 4% to 7% of patients.
12. Patients with Balkan nephropathy, those with analgesic abuse, and those who have ingested arsenic in endemic regions of Taiwan have a higher tendency for multiple and bilateral recurrences than do those with sporadic tumors.
13. Patients with T3 tumors located in the renal pelvis have a better survival than those with T3 tumors located in the ureter.
14. An adrenalectomy is not indicated for patients undergoing a nephroureterectomy for upper tract tumors.
15. After percutaneous resection of a tumor of the renal pelvis the nephrostomy is left indwelling to allow for revisualization several weeks later to be certain that all tumors have been removed.

Contemporary Open Surgery of the Kidney

Patrick A. Kenney, MD ● Chad Wotkowicz, MD ● John A. Libertino, MD

QUESTIONS

1. Please match the following innovations in open renal surgery to the year and author:
   1. Earliest case series of radical nephrectomy patients
   2. First planned partial nephrectomy for hydronephrosis
   3. First cavotomy to extirpate caval thrombus
   4. Caval resection/reimplant opposite renal vein
   5. Renal hypothermia surgery
   a. 1870 (Gustav Simon)
   b. 1913 (Berg)
   c. 1960 (Klotz and Kerr)
   d. 1969 (Robson)
   e. 1922 (Rehn)

2. A 45-year-old healthy man with no family history of cancer is found to have a 6-cm enhancing mass in the upper pole of his right kidney. A 2-cm solitary nodule is noted on preoperative chest radiography. CT confirms a solitary nodule in the lower lobe of the right lung. What is the most appropriate treatment course?
   a. Systemic chemotherapy alone
   b. Radical right nephrectomy and postoperative chemotherapy
   c. Biopsy of pulmonary nodule
   d. Radical nephrectomy and simultaneous pulmonary metastectomy
   e. Radical nephrectomy with staged resection of pulmonary nodule 6 weeks postoperatively.

3. What is the preferred technique for radical nephrectomy and removal of tumor thrombus above the level of the diaphragm in the absence of significant metastatic disease?
   a. Flank incision with extensive liver mobilization and removal of tumor through an incision in the diaphragm
   b. Flank incision with cardiopulmonary bypass and deep hypothermic circulatory arrest (CPB-DHCA)
   c. Chevron incision with CPB-DHCA
   d. Chevron incision with Pringle maneuver
   e. Midline incision with CPB-DHCA

4. Deep hypothermic circulatory arrest (DHCA) can have irreversible neurologic effects after what period of time?
   a. 10 minutes
   b. 20 minutes
   c. 40 minutes
   d. 60 minutes
   e. 90 minutes

5. In a 45-year-old man with a normal contralateral kidney and no family history of kidney cancer, in which of the following clinical scenarios would partial nephrectomy be indicated?
   a. Two tumors less than 3 cm each in the upper and lower pole
   b. Single 8-cm tumor in the upper pole
   c. Single 2-cm tumor in a hilar location with small renal vein tumor thrombus
   d. Single 4-cm tumor in any location
   e. All of the above

6. What is the ideal surgical approach to repair a 2-cm renal artery aneurysm occurring at the anterior and posterior segmental arteries just beyond their branch points from the main renal artery in a 30-year-old hypertensive woman with normal contralateral renal function?
   a. Hepatorenal bypass with autogenous saphenous vein interposition
   b. In-vivo primary resection and autogenous vein patch angioplasty
   c. Ex-vivo repair with autogenous vein patch angioplasty times two and autotransplant
   d. Ex-vivo repair with autogenous internal iliac artery and autotransplant
   e. Ex-vivo repair with autogenous internal iliac artery and reanastomoses to native aorta and inferior vena cava

7. What is the strongest modifiable risk factor for renal insufficiency after partial nephrectomy?
   a. Duration of renal ischemia
   b. Surgical approach

c. Administration of nephrotoxins

d. Resection margin

e. Administration of heparin

8. During a posterior right lumbotomy approach what is the order of appearance of the renal artery, renal vein, and renal pelvis?

a. Artery, renal pelvis, vein

b. Artery, vein, renal pelvis

c. Renal pelvis, artery, vein

d. Vein, renal pelvis, artery

e. Renal pelvis, vein, artery

9. What is the optimal surgical approach for removal of a 12-cm right renal mass with tumor thrombus at the confluence of the right renal vein and inferior vena cava?

a. Right supra-11th flank incision without CPB-DHCA

b. Right subcostal incision without CPB-DHCA

c. Anterior midline incision with CPB-DHCA

d. Chevron incision with CPB-DHCA

e. Right thoracoabdominal incision without CPB-DHCA

10. Match the following T stage with the tumor characteristics:
    1. T3b
    2. T1a
    3. T3a
    4. T4
    5. T2

a. Greater than 7.0 cm confined to capsule

b. Less than 4 cm confined to capsule

c. 6 cm invading adrenal gland

d. 5 cm with renal vein thrombus

e. 13 cm invading the liver

11. Five days after left partial nephrectomy for a hilar tumor there is persistent drainage from the Penrose drain site. Laboratory analysis of the drain fluid demonstrates elevated amylase levels. Imaging studies demonstrate small bowel dilation consistent with ileus and fluid around the tail of pancreas. What is the ideal management?

a. Antibiotics

b. Immediate surgical exploration

c. Percutaneous drain placement

d. Nasogastric tube placement, parenteral nutrition, and conservative management

e. Nasogastric tube placement, low fat diet, and conservative management

12. Which segmental branch of the renal artery is most consistent and supplies 25% of the arterial supply to the renal unit?

a. Apical (superior) segmental artery

b. Anterior superior segmental artery

c. Posterior segmental artery

d. Anterior inferior segmental artery

e. The basilar (inferior) segmental artery

13. In which scenario is partial nephrectomy contraindicated?

a. 8-cm hilar tumor in a solitary kidney

b. Two 3-cm tumors (upper and lower pole) in a solitary kidney

c. 10-cm lower pole tumor in a patient with prior contralateral heminephrectomy

d. 7-cm tumor in solitary kidney with single pulmonary metastatic deposit

e. 6-cm hilar tumor in solitary kidney with multiple biopsy-proven metastatic deposits

14. What maneuver refers to the reflection of the second and third portions of the duodenum in a medial direction to expose the right renal vessels and ventral inferior vena cava?

a. Cattell maneuver

b. Langenbeck maneuver

c. Sorcini maneuver

d. Kocher maneuver

e. Pringle maneuver

15. Which form of renovascular disease is most amenable to endovascular treatment?

a. 3-cm renal artery aneurysm

b. Intimal fibrous dysplasia

c. Medial fibrous dysplasia

d. Nonostial atherosclerosis

e. Ostial atherosclerosis

16. What partial nephrectomy technique should be used as a last resort in a solitary kidney?

a. Enucleation

b. Wedge resection

c. Cryotherapy

d. Polar resection

e. Extracorporeal repair and autotransplantation

17. The subcostal nerve may be inadvertently transected during an anterior subcostal incision for a radical nephrectomy. Between what two layers does this nerve run?

a. Posterior peritoneum and transversalis fascia

b. Scarpa fascia and external oblique muscle

c. External oblique and internal oblique

d. Internal oblique and transversalis

e. Gould and Wszolek fascia

18. What is the motor deficit resulting from transaction of the subcostal nerve?

a. Winged scapula

b. Hemidiaphragmatic paralysis

c. Paresis of the flank musculature and flank bulge

d. Inability to flex ipsilateral adductor muscle

e. Weakness of contralateral rectus abdominis muscle

19. What percentage of patients have multiple renal arteries?

a. 0% to 2%

b. 2% to 10%

c. 10% to 20%

d. 20% to 30%

e. More than 30%

20. Which of the following is not an indication for simple nephrectomy?

a. Nonfunctional chronically infected kidney

b. Nonfunctional persistently hydronephrotic kidney causing pain

c. Renovascular hypertension refractory to medical and nephron-sparing surgical intervention

d. Polycystic kidney with minimal function and recurrent infections

e. Kidney with 8-cm enhancing upper pole hilar mass

21. Two days after cardiopulmonary bypass and circulatory arrest (20 minutes) for an extensive right-sided renal mass with thrombus extending into the atrium, using traditional median sternotomy, a relatively healthy 36-year-old patient is unable to be extubated and has no purposeful right-sided movement. Imaging reveals a large left-sided cerebrovascular infarct. What clinical scenario can explain this event?

a. Pulmonary air embolism

b. Cerebral ischemia from bypass and circulatory arrest

c. Tension pneumothorax

d. Right main stem bronchial intubation

e. Unrecognized paradoxical embolism

22. Which of the following is *not* a benefit of using hypothermic perfusate, heparin and mannitol during renal autotransplantation?

a. Prevents graft thrombosis

b. Limits free radical accumulation from ischemia

c. Shrinks renal parenchyma to better expose intrarenal vasculature

d. Limits membrane transport metabolism

e. Allows operative times to exceed 10 hours of cold ischemia

23. Which form of therapy has been considered the "gold standard" for localized renal cell carcinoma?

a. Chemotherapy

b. Immunotherapy

c. Radiation

d. Hormonal therapy

e. Surgical resection

24. On postoperative day 2 after radical nephrectomy for a 14-cm complex left renal tumor using an anterior midline incision there are overt signs of peritonitis. The patient is 72 years old with significant atherosclerotic disease. At exploration the entire small bowel is necrotic and nonviable. What artery was inadvertently ligated?

a. Celiac

b. Left gastric

c. Inferior mesenteric

d. Superior mesenteric

e. Right gastroepiploic

25. During resection of a large right renal mass the main renal artery is identified, ligated, and divided but the renal vein fails to decompress. What is the most likely explanation for this?

a. Renal vein tumor thrombus

b. Subclinical renal arteriovenous malformation

c. Bleeding disorder

d. Arterial collateral branch vessels

e. Extensive venous collateral obstruction

26. What is the preferred interposition graft during a splenorenal bypass in a 60-year-old man with significant atherosclerosis?

a. Cephalic vein

b. Saphenous vein

c. Hypogastric artery

d. Gore-Tex

e. Brachial artery

27. What is most appropriate setting for a thoracoabdominal incision?

a. Large right upper pole renal mass with tumor thrombus in the renal vein

b. 5-cm right renal tumor in a hilar location

c. Large left lower pole tumor with extensive lymphadenopathy

d. Large right renal mass with tumor thrombus to the retrohepatic level

e. A 10-cm right lower pole tumor with arteriovenous malformation

28. Which renovascular disease is best managed medically due to the low rates of complete renal artery occlusion and ischemic nephropathy?

a. Perimedial fibroplasia

b. Segmental pseudoaneurysms

c. Atherosclerosis

d. Intimal fibroplasia

e. Medial fibroplasia

29. What is the most common complication associated with performing CPB-DHCA for the removal of large renal cell tumor thrombus?

a. Pulmonary air emboli

b. Intestinal ischemia

c. Bleeding and coagulopathy

d. Lower extremity tumor emboli

e. Tumor emboli

30. Which of the following is NOT a positive predictor of renal function return after revascularization of a totally occluded renal artery?

a. Angiographic demonstration of a nephrogram

b. Proximal occlusion and retrograde filling of distal circulation by perihilar collateral vessels

c. Intraoperative back-bleeding from a renal arteriotomy distal to the occlusion

d. Demonstration on intraoperative frozen section or preoperative biopsy of an intact glomerular architecture

e. A 5-cm kidney

31. Which of the following is NOT a proposed benefit of renal artery embolization (RAE)?

a. Shrinkage of an arterialized tumor thrombus to ease surgical removal

b. Reduced blood loss

c. Facilitation of dissection due to tissue plane edema

d. Ability to ligate the renal vein before the renal artery at time of nephrectomy

e. Modulation of the immune response

f. None of the above

32. What is the most common complication after RAE?

a. Groin hematoma from puncture site

b. Paraplegia from spinal artery occlusion

c. Coil migration

d. Postinfarction syndrome (pain, nausea, and fever)

e. Adrenal insufficiency

33. A 65-year-old man with left renal artery stenosis and significant atheromatous disease of the abdominal aorta undergoes splenorenal arterial bypass. Which of the following is NOT a component of the procedure?

a. Splenectomy

b. Division of the splenic artery distally

c. End-to-end splenorenal anastomosis

d. Use of reverse saphenous vein interposition graft

e. Preoperative aortography to assess the celiac axis

34. What is the most common complication after partial nephrectomy for nonexophytic renal masses?

a. Hemorrhage

b. Renal failure

c. Rhabdomyolysis

d. Hydronephrosis

e. Urinary leak

35. Ten days after a left partial nephrectomy for a 4.5-cm hilar tumor there is persistent fluid output from the surgical drain. No ureteral stent was placed at the time of surgery, and a small opening in the collecting system was oversewn. The creatinine concentration of the drain fluid is 34.5 mg/dL, consistent with urine. Despite conservative management the volume fails to decline. A retrograde pyelogram demonstrates a moderate amount of contrast extravasation confirming the urinary fistula. What is the most appropriate management at this time?

a. Immediate reexploration and repair

b. Percutaneous nephrostomy tube placement

c. Removal of surgical drain

d. Internalized ureteral stent placement

e. Internalized ureteral stent placement, continued surgical drain monitoring, and placement of Foley catheter.

ANSWERS

1. **a: 2; b: 3; c: 5; d: 1; e: 4.**

2. **d. Radical nephrectomy and simultaneous pulmonary metastectomy.** This patient would be best managed with a radical nephrectomy and removal of the pulmonary nodule using a thoracoabdominal incision. Systemic therapy is not a primary treatment unless there is extensive metastatic disease at presentation. Given his age and lack of medical problems there is no reason to delay the removal of his kidney and the pulmonary nodule. The tumor location and pulmonary nodule both can be accessed through one incision.

3. **c. Chevron incision with CPB-DHCA.** CPB-DHCA has been established as the most prudent course for the removal of these tumor thrombi. The chevron incision provides the

best exposure. Alternatives to CPB, including extensive liver mobilization and intrapericardial resection, carry an increased risk of bleeding.

4. **c. 40 minutes.** The duration of DHCA can vary depending on the degree of tumor thrombus. Vena cava resection and substitution can add additional time if there is significant tumor invasion into the wall of the vena cava. Studies have suggested that irreversible neurologic effects may be observed after 40 minutes of DHCA.

5. **d. Single 4-cm tumor in any location.** In patients with a normal contralateral kidney the current literature supports elective partial nephrectomy for single T1 tumors.

6. **d. Ex-vivo repair with autogenous internal iliac artery and autotransplant.** An ex-vivo approach will offer the best exposure to repair these aneurysms. Using an arterial patch will provide a more durable outcome and minimize the risk of recurrent aneurysm formation associated with venous patch systems.

7. **a. Duration of renal ischemia.** Duration of renal ischemia is the strongest modifiable risk factor for renal insufficiency after partial nephrectomy.

8. **c. Renal pelvis, artery, vein.** The renal pelvis is the first structure one encounters with the posterior right lumbotomy incision, followed by the artery and vein. This approach can be used to repair ureteropelvic junction obstruction, especially in children or patients with multiple prior abdominal and/or flank surgeries.

9. **e. Right thoracoabdominal incision without CPB-DHCA.** The right thoracoabdominal incision provides exposure of the anterior vena caval wall after mobilization of the ascending colon and a Kocher maneuver. There should be enough room to isolate the right and left renal veins. The vena cava also needs to be partially mobilized above and below the renal vein confluence in case the thrombus cannot be milked back into the renal vein.

10. **a: T2; b: T1a; c: T3a; d: T3b; e: T4.**

11. **d. Nasogastric tube placement, parenteral nutrition, and conservative management.** Conservative management of a pancreatic fistula should be the first approach in this patient. Initial nasogastric tube placement can help resolve the ileus. Parenteral nutrition will limit any pancreatic secretions from oral intake.

12. **c. Posterior segmental artery.** The posterior division is the first and most consistent branch point of the renal artery and supplies roughly one fourth of the blood supply.

13. **e. 6-cm hilar tumor in solitary kidney with multiple biopsy-proven metastatic deposits.** Multiple distant metastases are a contraindication to partial nephrectomy. There are ongoing clinical trials studying debulking nephrectomy with immunotherapy. Patient performance status must be reasonable prior to enrollment in most of these studies.

14. **d. Kocher maneuver.** Mobilization of the second and third portions of the duodenum is referred to as a Kocher maneuver. The Pringle maneuver is the temporary occlusion of the porta hepatis. The Langenbeck maneuver is the division of the coronary and right triangular ligaments providing medial rotation of the right lobe of the liver and exposure of the suprarenal inferior vena cava.

15. **d. Nonostial atherosclerosis.** Success rates for nonostial lesions are up to 90% using endovascular intervention.

16. **e. Extracorporeal repair and autotransplantation.** All patients with solitary kidneys are high-risk candidates

for partial nephrectomy and may have transient renal impairment postoperatively. The degree and duration of renal impairment may be increased owing to risks associated with renal autotransplantation (hemorrhage, thrombosis, lymphocele, stenosis).

17. **d. Internal oblique and transversalis.** The subcostal nerve runs between these two layers. Caution must be taken not to severe this nerve during flank incisions.

18. **c. Paresis of the flank musculature and flank bulge.** Damage to the subcostal nerve results in denervation and paresis of the flank musculature, leading to chronic postoperative pain or flank bulge.

19. **d. 20% to 30%.** Multiple postmortem and radiographic studies estimate that 25% of the general population have supernumerary renal arteries.

20. **e. Kidney with 8-cm enhancing upper pole hilar mass.** There should be little reservation about performing a radical nephrectomy for an enhancing mass especially in the upper pole. Almost all nonmalignant disease affecting the kidney can be treated via a simple approach.

21. **e. Unrecognized paradoxical embolism.** This rare but devastating clinical situation occurs in patients with a patent foramen ovale. An embolism may originate from tumor thrombus manipulation or from deep venous thromboembolism.

22. **e. Allows operative times to exceed 10 hours of cold ischemia.** Operative times should be limited to 4 hours maximum.

23. **e. Surgical resection.** There have been numerous studies to suggest that surgical resection is the mainstay of therapy for kidney cancer.

24. **d. Superior mesenteric.** Ligation of the superior mesenteric artery produces ischemia in the bowel distribution above. The superior mesenteric artery can be mistaken for the left renal artery from the anterior approach. Visualizing the artery from a posterior position as it enters the hilum will help to minimize this complication.

25. **d. Arterial collateral branch vessels.** Failure of the renal vein to decompress after ligation of the main renal artery indicates additional arterial inflow, which may be secondary to a missed lower or upper pole artery or extensive collateral arteries.

26. **b. Saphenous vein.** Patients with significant atherosclerotic disease often will have disease in the iliac system, precluding a hypogastric graft. A reversed saphenous vein graft is a durable option in this instance.

27. **a. Large right upper pole renal mass with tumor thrombus in the renal vein.** The thoracoabdominal incision is ideal for larger tumors involving the upper pole.

The incision is also ideal for managing tumor thrombus extending into the renal vein. The inferior vena cava can be nicely exposed via this approach.

28. **e. Medial fibroplasia.** Medial fibroplasias can often be managed without surgical intervention due to low progression rates.

29. **c. Bleeding and coagulopathy.** Intraoperatively the administration of heparin in addition to hypothermia leads to significant coagulopathy. The bleeding from heparin is typically limited to an "ooze" intraoperatively and should not consume time and energy during the operation. After tumor removal the rewarming process helps to promote coagulation.

30. **e. A 5-cm kidney.** The lower limit of acceptable size is 7 to 9 cm for revascularization of a totally occluded renal artery.

31. **f. None of the above.** Proposed benefits of preoperative RAE include shrinkage of an arterialized tumor thrombus to ease surgical removal, reduced blood loss, facilitation of dissection due to tissue plane edema, ability to ligate the renal vein before the renal artery at time of nephrectomy, and modulation of the immune response.

32. **d. Postinfarction syndrome (pain, nausea, and fever).** The triad of fever, flank pain, and nausea occurs in up to 75% of patients after angioembolization. Fevers can often exceed 39.4° C (103° F) and are best managed with antipyretics.

33. **a. Splenectomy.** Removal of the spleen is usually not necessary because it receives adequate blood flow from the short gastric arteries.

34. **e. Urinary leak.** Partial nephrectomy for nonexophytic masses has an increased risk of entering the collecting system. Even when the collecting system is closed under direct vision there may still be extravasation of urine that collects in the perirenal space. The use of postoperative surgical drains is imperative in the management of these collections to reduce the risk of infections. In addition, the drain output volume can be observed to determine if collections are resolving. Renal failure is rare unless operating on a solitary kidney or on a patient with marginal renal function. Rhabdomyolysis can be encountered secondary to patient positioning and increased body mass index.

35. **e. Internalized ureteral stent placement, continued surgical drain monitoring, and placement of Foley catheter.** Placement of a ureteral stent can promote urine drainage into the bladder. Keeping a Foley catheter in place reduces urine reflux.

Additional Study Points

1. The right renal artery is posterior to the inferior vena cava.
2. Renal arteries are end arteries; ligation results in infarction of the segment that they supply.
3. The renal venous network intercommunicates.
4. Lumbar veins often enter the left renal vein and not infrequently the right renal vein. They enter posteriorly. Care must be taken when encircling the renal vein not to tear one of these lumbar veins.
5. There is no conclusive evidence that renal artery embolization has any immunologic therapeutic benefit.
6. The renal artery is always ligated before the renal vein when performing a nephrectomy; each vessel is ligated individually.
7. Intimal fibroplasia is generally a disease of children and young adults. Medial fibroplasia usually occurs in females

between 25 and 50 years of age, and perimedial fibroplasia is a rare disease.

8. Percutaneous transluminal angioplasty for the treatment of fibromuscular dysplasia is the treatment of choice because the results are excellent.

9. Transesophageal echocardiography is an excellent modality to determine the level of the vena cava tumor thrombus immediately before the surgical event.

10. In patients with vena cava tumor thrombi cephalad to the hepatic venous outflow who require CPB either mild hypothermia and no circulatory arrest or significant hypothermia with circulatory arrest may be done. Each technique has its advantages and disadvantages. The method used is at the discretion of the surgeon.

11. The addition of a lymphadenectomy to a radical nephrectomy for renal cell carcinoma has a questionable impact on progression-free and overall survival.

12. Ligation of the right renal vein will result in failure of the right renal unit due to lack of venous collateral vessels.

13. Ligation of the left renal vein is possible because collateral venous drainage may occur through lumbar and gonadal vessels.

Laparoscopic Surgery of the Kidney

Louis R. Kavoussi, MD, MBA ● Michael J. Schwartz, MD ● Inderbir S. Gill, MD, MCh

QUESTIONS

1. All of the following statements are true regarding renal laparoscopy in obese patients EXCEPT:
   a. Location of trocar sites may require lateral shift.
   b. Longer instrumentation may be needed.
   c. Higher intra-abdominal pressure should be used to counter the weight of the pannus.
   d. Laparoscopy carries a higher risk of open conversion compared with nonobese patients.
   e. Rhabdomyolysis may occur in prolonged cases or with insufficient patient padding.

2. Hand assistance for renal laparoscopy may be valuable for which of the following scenarios?
   a. Encountering dense perinephric adhesions
   b. Bilateral nephrectomy for autosomal-dominant polycystic kidney disease (ADPKD)
   c. Vascular injury
   d. A novice laparoscopic surgeon
   e. All of the above

3. Which of the following would not be recommended in the treatment of cystic renal disease?
   a. Retrograde instillation of methylene blue to ensure collecting system integrity after cyst decortication in a 65-year-old woman
   b. Aspiration of simple peripelvic cysts and instillation of sclerosing agent in a 47-year-old man with intermittent flank pain
   c. Laparoscopic cyst unroofing for a 62-year-old woman with a large symptomatic renal cortical cyst, one prior failed aspiration, and sclerosing agent instillation
   d. Laparoscopic partial nephrectomy for a 51-year-old man with a Bosniak III cyst
   e. Laparoscopic bilateral radical nephrectomy for a 49-year-old female transplant recipient with recurrent urinary tract infections, ADPKD, and positive cultures from the right native ureter

4. The most common complication secondary to laparoscopic renal biopsy is:
   a. hemorrhage.
   b. inadequate tissue sampling.
   c. intraoperative bowel injury.
   d. arteriovenous fistula.
   e. urine leak.

5. When compared with open radical nephrectomy, laparoscopic radical nephrectomy results in:
   a. superior cosmesis.
   b. equivalent long-term oncologic outcomes.
   c. less pain medication requirement.
   d. shorter convalescence.
   e. all of the above.

6. Risk factors for port-site recurrence include all of the following EXCEPT:
   a. high-grade tumor.
   b. direct contact between incision and tumor.
   c. wound closure technique.
   d. immunosuppression.
   e. tumor spillage.

7. After failed ablative therapy for a 3-cm exophytic renal mass, a laparoscopic partial nephrectomy is planned. The patient should be counseled:
   a. no differently from a patient undergoing primary surgery.
   b. that a biopsy of the cryolesion is necessary prior to proceeding.
   c. that selective renal embolization would be recommended prior to surgery.
   d. that there is an increased risk of radical nephrectomy or open conversion.
   e. about all of the above.

8. All of the following measures should be taken to minimize the impact of laparoscopy on long-term renal function EXCEPT:
   a. pneumoperitoneum should not be maintained at pressures above 20 mm Hg.
   b. use of helium gas insufflation when anticipating a long procedure time.
   c. duration of insufflation should not exceed 6 hours.
   d. clamp time during laparoscopic partial nephrectomy should be minimized.
   e. all of the above.

9. A 76-year-old man has a 3-cm exophytic renal mass. His past medical history is significant for severe chronic obstructive pulmonary disease (COPD). After obtaining medical clearance for surgery, a laparoscopic partial nephrectomy is planned. During the procedure, significant hypercarbia is noted by the anesthesiologist. The first step is:

   a. reduce the intra-abdominal pressure.
   b. switch to helium insufflation.
   c. convert to radical nephrectomy.
   d. place a chest tube to evacuate the pneumothorax.
   e. all of the above.

10. A 24-year-old female patient presents with intermittent renal colic (worse after drinking alcohol), which is relieved after lying down. Nuclear renal scan shows no obstruction. The next step is:

    a. renal sonography.
    b. laparoscopic pyeloplasty.
    c. supine and erect intravenous pyelography.
    d. observation.
    e. laparoscopic nephropexy.

11. Compared with laparoscopic partial nephrectomy, laparoscopic renal ablative therapies are:

    a. associated with a higher risk of progression to metastatic disease.
    b. associated with a higher risk of recurrence.
    c. associated with an equivalent risk of treatment failure.
    d. contraindicated for endophytic lesions.
    e. associated with all of the above.

12. Absolute contraindications to laparoscopic renal surgery include:

    a. dilated loops of bowel.
    b. multiple prior abdominal surgeries.
    c. prior ipsilateral renal surgery.
    d. uncorrected coagulopathy.
    e. body mass index greater than 50.

13. A 47-year-old man presents to the emergency room on postoperative day 4 after laparoscopic right radical nephrectomy with nausea, low-grade fever, and localized abdominal pain. A CT scan with oral contrast demonstrates extravasation of contrast from the ascending colon. The most likely etiology of the injury is:

    a. trocar placement.
    b. blunt dissection.
    c. sharp dissection.
    d. bowel ischemia.
    e. electrocautery.

14. A 61-year-old woman presents to the emergency room with gross hematuria, tachycardia, and mild hypotension 7 days after left laparoscopic partial nephrectomy. Her hematocrit is 22%. The next step after initial fluid resuscitation is:

    a. a CT scan with contrast.
    b. broad-spectrum antibiotics.
    c. an echocardiogram.

d. renal angiography with embolization.
e. ICU admission and blood transfusion.

15. On postoperative day 2 after laparoscopic cyst ablation, drain output is noted to be 150 cc/day, and drain creatinine concentration is 15 mg/dL (serum: 1.3 mg/dL). The patient is afebrile, and his blood pressure and heart rate are normal. The next step is:

    a. ureteral stent placement.
    b. ureteral stent placement and Foley catheter placement.
    c. percutaneous nephrostomy tube.
    d. a CT scan of the abdomen and pelvis.
    e. observation.

16. A 55-year-old man presents with 4+ proteinuria and intermittent milky-white urine. Retrograde pyelogram demonstrates a lymphorenal fistula. Further history is mostly likely to reveal:

    a. prior renal surgery.
    b. foreign travel.
    c. positive purified protein derivative (PPD).
    d. vasculitis.
    e. polycystic kidney disease.

17. Compared with a traditional laparoscopic approach, hand-assisted laparoscopy is associated with increased risk of:

    a. bowel injury.
    b. vascular injury.
    c. wound infection.
    d. port-site metastasis.
    e. none of the above.

18. Laparoendoscopic single site surgery (LESS) of the kidney has been shown to have which of the following benefits when compared with conventional laparoscopy?

    a. Less analgesic requirement
    b. Shorter length of stay
    c. Shorter operative time
    d. Shorter return to convalescence
    e. None of the above

19. Intraoperatively identified deep injuries to the pancreas during left-sided renal surgery are best managed by:

    a. drain placement and observation.
    b. use of biologic glue or sealant.
    c. isolation of the injured segment with the gastrointestinal anastomosis (GIA) stapler.
    d. observation and somatostatin.
    e. observation and postoperative parenteral nutrition.

20. During a laparoscopic radical nephrectomy, urine output is noted to be 30 cc after 2 hours of surgery. Blood pressure and heart rate are normal. The patient has been given 1200 cc of lactated Ringer solution over the course of the procedure, and estimated blood loss is 175 cc. The next step is:

    a. continue the surgery.
    b. administer a bolus of intravenous fluids.
    c. check the Foley catheter placement.

d. administer blood transfusion.

e. administer 12.5 g of mannitol.

ANSWERS

1. **c. higher intra-abdominal pressure should be used to counter the weight of the pannus.** Although it may be true that the weight of the pannus may decrease intra-abdominal working space, higher intra-abdominal pressures should not be used to counter this effect. Intra-abdominal pressures above 20 mm Hg have been shown to cause renal cortical hypoperfusion, increased venous outflow resistance, and put the patient at risk for temporary renal insufficiency. In addition, obesity combined with pneumoperitoneum may cause significant elevation of airway pressures, making it difficult to ventilate the patient. All of the other answers are true of the obese patient population.

2. **e. All of the above.** Hand assistance may be of use for the novice laparoscopic surgeon making a transition from open surgery. The hand provides tactile feedback, is helpful for retraction, and may be particularly valuable in cases with dense adhesions or scar tissue around the kidney, such as ADPKD or xanthogranulomatous pyelonephritis. In cases of laparoscopic vascular injury, a hand port may also be useful to help control bleeding and avoid open conversion.

3. **b. Aspiration of simple peripelvic cysts and instillation of sclerosing agent in a 47-year-old man with intermittent flank pain.** Instillation of a sclerosing agent into peripelvic cysts is not recommended, because fibrosis has been reported to occur by several authors. Retrograde instillation of methylene blue may be used to assess the integrity of the collecting system at surgery. The other options are all indicated surgical options based on the individual clinical scenarios.

4. **a. hemorrhage.** Published series of laparoscopic renal biopsy show hemorrhage to be the most common complication of the surgery. Careful hemostasis using the argon beam coagulator or other adjuvant hemostatic agents should be obtained in every case and caution used with anticoagulation postoperatively. Adequate tissue is obtained in 96% of patients. Bowel injury, arteriovenous fistula, and urine leakage are all rare complications of laparoscopic renal biopsy.

5. **e. all of the above.** All of the above are now well-established benefits of laparoscopy compared with open surgery for radical nephrectomy.

6. **c. wound closure technique.** Numerous factors have been studied for their relationship to port-site recurrence. Modifiable risk factors include tumor spillage and direct contact between incision and tumor, both of which have been shown to correlate with port-site recurrence. Routine vigilance in specimen handling, especially with cystic masses will minimize likelihood of spillage. Use of an entrapment sac eliminates potential contact been tumor and incision. Immunosuppression and high-grade tumor are nonmodifiable risk factors that have also been shown to be risk factors for port-site recurrence. Wound closure technique is irrelevant and has been specifically shown to not be associated with risk of recurrence.

7. **d. that there is an increased risk of radical nephrectomy or open conversion.** Salvage laparoscopic partial nephrectomy after failure of primary cryoablation is difficult to complete successfully due to the extensive adhesions and scar tissue that form around the kidney. The patient should be thoroughly counseled that either open conversion or radical nephrectomy are necessary in approximately 40% of patients. There is no need of biopsy prior to surgery if follow-up imaging demonstrates persistent enhancement or an enlarging lesion. There is no indication for selective angioembolization in this setting.

8. **b. use of helium gas insufflation when anticipating a long procedure time.** All of the above factors, with the exception of helium insufflation, have been shown to help minimize the effect of laparoscopy on long-term renal function. Choice of helium or carbon dioxide does not impact this outcome. However, patients with significant COPD may benefit from the use of helium because it will minimize the potential for hypercarbia.

9. **a. reduce the intra-abdominal pressure.** The first step for any patient with significant hypercarbia undergoing laparoscopic surgery is to decrease the intra-abdominal pressure. This will lessen carbon dioxide absorption and improve ventilation. Helium insufflation may help decrease the hypercarbia but is not the first step. Converting to a radical nephrectomy may speed the procedure, but will not provide the patient with any immediate benefit. There is no evidence of pneumothorax in this patient, such as a billowing diaphragm or sudden change in the ability to ventilate the patient.

10. **c. supine and erect intravenous pyelography.** Ptotic kidneys often present with a history similar to that of a ureteropelvic junction obstruction. The exception may be that the pain is relieved after a period of lying down such that the renal descent no longer causes either transient renal ischemia or obstruction. Obtaining supine and erect intravenous pyelograms will help rule out a ptotic kidney. Erect renal scan or power Doppler sonography performed in both the supine and erect positions may also help in this case. Nephropexy should not proceed before definitively establishing the diagnosis of ptotic kidney.

11. **b. associated with a higher risk of recurrence.** A multi-institutional evaluation of ablative therapy outcomes has found recurrence rates of 13.4% and 3.9% for radiofrequency ablation and cryotherapy, respectively. Meta-analysis of patients undergoing partial nephrectomy versus ablative therapies found the relative risk of recurrence to be 7.45 and 18.23, respectively, for cryotherapy and radiofrequency ablation when compared with partial nephrectomy. However, there was no increased association between treatment modality and progression to metastatic disease.

12. **d. uncorrected coagulopathy.** Uncorrected coagulopathy is the only true contraindication to laparoscopic renal surgery of the listed choices. Multiple prior abdominal surgeries may influence approach (retroperitoneal vs. transperitoneal), but is not a contraindication. Similarly, prior ipsilateral renal surgery may make dissection and identification of landmarks more challenging but is not a contraindication. Dilated loops of bowel and morbidly obese patients should both be approached with caution but are not a contraindication to surgery.

13. **e. electrocautery.** Although blunt dissection, sharp dissection, and electrocautery are each responsible for approximately equal proportions of bowel injuries, electrocautery is the most frequent cause of unrecognized

bowel injury. Electrocautery may lead to delayed necrosis and perforation of the bowel wall, leading to atypical or delayed presentation. Trocar placement and bowel ischemia are both infrequent causes of bowel injury.

14. **d. renal angiography with embolization.** A patient who has recently undergone laparoscopic partial nephrectomy presenting with gross hematuria and hemodynamic changes will most likely have a postoperative bleed. Although a CT scan with contrast will help diagnose and localize a postoperative bleed, this will ultimately delay treatment in this case. Immediate renal angiogram with embolization to diagnose, localize, and treat a postoperative bleed is indicated.

15. **e. observation.** Urinary extravasation after laparoscopic cyst ablation or partial nephrectomy will almost always resolve with observation. If the drain output does not decrease, then ureteral obstruction is likely to be present, and placement of a ureteral stent is indicated with or without a Foley catheter. There is no indication at this point for either a CT scan or nephrostomy tube.

16. **b. foreign travel.** The most common cause of chyluria is filariasis caused by *Wuchereria bancrofti* or *Brugia malayi*. Nonparasitic causes are rare, although prior renal surgery, tuberculosis, and vasculitis are all reported causes of chyluria. There is no known association between polycystic kidney disease and chyluria.

17. **c. wound infection.** There is no difference in oncologic outcome or incidence of port-site metastasis between standard laparoscopy and a hand-assisted approach for the treatment of renal malignancy. However, it has been shown that patients undergoing hand-assisted laparoscopy had more postoperative pain and a higher wound complication rate (hernia and wound infection). There is no difference in the incidence of bowel or vascular injury.

18. **e. None of the above.** Few comparative studies have been performed to date between laparoendoscopic single site surgery and standard laparoscopy, but those studies, to date, have shown no advantage in any of the listed outcomes.

19. **c. isolation of the injured segment with the gastrointestinal anastomosis (GIA) stapler.** Deep injuries to the pancreas should be intraoperatively addressed as pancreatic leak may lead to significant postoperative morbidity. The distal pancreas is most often manipulated during the medial mobilization of the spleen, pancreas, and descending colon during transperitoneal left-sided kidney or adrenal surgery. The best approach is typically to isolate the injury and seal it using an endovascular GIA stapling device. This is the same approach used with much success during intentional distal pancreatectomy and closes both the pancreatic stump and duct, if injured. Use of a biologic glue or sealant may be used as an adjuvant, but should not be the primary means of addressing the injury. Drain placement and observation may be used for superficial but not deep pancreatic injuries.

20. **a. continue the surgery.** Oliguria is extremely common during laparoscopic surgery, even in cases with fairly aggressive IV fluid administration such as donor nephrectomy. In the setting of minimal blood loss and hemodynamic stability, the surgery should be continued. Excessive intravenous fluids may lead to volume overload, prolonging postoperative recovery. Patients with diminished cardiac reserve may also develop congestive heart failure with excessive IV fluids.

Additional Study Points

1. Obesity is associated with an increased risk of open conversion.
2. Transperitoneal laparoscopy provides the largest working space with greater versatility of angles.
3. When performing a laparoscopic nephrectomy, the renal artery should be divided first then followed by division of the renal vein. The vascular stapler will provide three rows of staples left on the stump.
4. In obese patients, intraoperative ultrasonography may be helpful in localizing the kidney.
5. One must be careful not to mistake the inferior vena cava for the renal vein.
6. En bloc hilar stapling (artery and vein together) over the short term does not result in arterial venous fistula formation.
7. In patients undergoing partial nephrectomy, both open and laparoscopic, there is no significant difference in long-term outcome for those who have positive surgical margins and those who do not.
8. Patients with unrecognized bowel injury following laparoscopy typically present with persistent and increased trocar-site pain at the site closest to the bowel injury.

Ablative Therapy for Renal Tumors

Wesley M. White, MD ● Jihad H. Kaouk, MD

QUESTIONS

1. Nephron-sparing surgery (partial nephrectomy):
   a. is the predominant treatment modality employed in the United States for the management of small renal masses.
   b. offers equivalent cancer-specific and overall survival when compared with radical nephrectomy.
   c. when performed laparoscopically is associated with fewer complications than radiofrequency ablation (RFA) or cryoablation.
   d. offers metastatic recurrence-free survival and cancer-specific survival similar to that of radiofrequency ablation and cryoablation.
   e. was not impacted by the advent of hand-assisted laparoscopic radical nephrectomy.

2. The critical treatment temperature threshold during cryoablation at which irreparable cell damage is achieved is:
   a. 0° C
   b. −60° C
   c. −20° C
   d. −40° C
   e. −19.4° C

3. Critical parameters for successful renal cryosurgery include:
   a. a double freeze-thaw cycle.
   b. achieving a critical target temperature.
   c. treatment under real-time image guidance.
   d. treatment to beyond 1 cm of the targeted lesion.
   e. all of the above.

4. Compared with renal cryoablation, the primary disadvantage of RFA is:
   a. higher risk of hemorrhage following RFA.
   b. inability to use RFA laparoscopically.
   c. inability to monitor treatment under image guidance.
   d. inferior cancer-specific survival.
   e. none of the above.

5. Recent meta-analyses have demonstrated:
   a. higher local recurrence rates with ablative technologies when compared with partial or radical nephrectomy.
   b. conflicting results regarding the superiority of cryoablation versus RFA.
   c. a lack of uniformity regarding evaluation, patient selection, treatment, and follow-up of patients undergoing renal tumor ablation.
   d. comparable or fewer complications with renal tumor ablation compared with extirpative treatments.
   e. all of the above.

6. The most important technique to increase the size of RF lesions is:
   a. using higher RF currents.
   b. applying RF currents faster to achieve better heating.
   c. clamping hilar vessels.
   d. reducing impedance by improving current conductivity.
   e. using bipolar electrodes.

7. Regarding high-intensity focused ultrasonography (HIFU), which of the following is TRUE?
   a. Preliminary data suggests equivalent oncologic outcomes with HIFU when compared with alternative ablative technologies or extirpative options.
   b. HIFU acts through local thermal and cavitary processes to generate tissue temperatures in excess of 65° C.
   c. Animal and human studies have demonstrated consistent tissue necrosis following treatment.
   d. The most commonly cited complication following HIFU for the treatment of renal lesions is post-treatment hemorrhage.
   e. Because renal HIFU is performed under real-time image guidance, targeting is not significantly impacted by respiratory movement.

8. Following tumor ablation, the most reliable method of documenting treatment success is:
   a. biopsy of the treatment area with hematoxylin and eosin (H&E) staining.
   b. biopsy of the treatment area with reduced nicotinamide adenine dinucleotide (NADH) diaphorase staining.
   c. follow-up CT or MRI with contrast that demonstrates complete loss of contrast enhancement and stable or decreased size of the treated area.

d. follow-up CT or MRI without contrast that demonstrates a decrease in size of the treated area.

e. all of the above.

9. Regarding stereotactic radiosurgery, which of the following is FALSE?

a. Renal cell carcinoma (RCC) is radioresistant, and stereotactic radiosurgery has consistently demonstrated poor outcomes with treatment of RCC.

b. Stereotactic radiosurgery employs 3-dimensional coordinates to target and focally ablate tissue using high-dose external beam radiation.

c. Stereotactic treatment systems compensate for respiratory movement and radiation scatter by automatically tracking, detecting, and correcting for tumor and/or organ movement without interrupting the treatment or repositioning the patient.

d. Radiation scatter is minimized, and higher doses may therefore be applied in a focal manner that effectively ablates masses in the kidney without compromising overall renal function.

e. Its use in the management of renal cell carcinoma remains investigational and should be performed under protocol.

10. In-situ renal tumor ablation is appropriate for all of the following patients except:

a. a 74-year-old man with a 2.5-cm enhancing renal mass oriented posterior to the axis of the kidney. The patient has multiple comorbidities and desires a minimally invasive treatment approach.

b. an otherwise healthy 81-year-old woman with a 3.2-cm lower pole enhancing renal mass that is anterior to the axis of the kidney. The patient desires treatment.

c. a 47-year-old man who is otherwise healthy and demonstrates a 3.1-cm mesophytic enhancing lesion of the right kidney.

d. a 54-year-old man who has undergone prior left nephrectomy, right partial nephrectomy, and prior right tumor ablation for pathologically proven RCC. He now presents with an independent 2-cm enhancing renal lesion abutting the psoas muscle.

e. a 64-year-old woman with a 1.7-cm enhancing mass concerning for RCC in her transplant allograft. She has previously undergone bilateral native nephrectomy.

ANSWERS

1. **d. offers metastatic recurrence-free survival and cancer-specific survival similar to that of radiofrequency ablation and cryoablation.** Nephron-sparing surgery is considered the gold standard treatment for small renal masses but is underused in the United States. Partial nephrectomy offers equivalent oncologic outcomes when compared with radical nephrectomy and demonstrates superior renal functional preservation. Laparoscopic partial nephrectomy offers excellent cancer-specific end points but is technically challenging and is associated with significant complications. Cryoablation and radiofrequency ablation are associated with significantly fewer complications than laparoscopic partial nephrectomy. There is no significant difference in metastatic recurrence-free survival between

extirpative and ablative treatments. Cancer-specific survival (CSS) following RFA is comparable to laparoscopic partial nephrectomy. CSS is comparable between open partial nephrectomy and both RFA and cryoablation. Preliminary studies suggest that the technical ease and minimal morbidity of hand-assisted laparoscopic nephrectomy may ultimately lead to fewer nephron-sparing procedures.

2. **d. −40° C.** Experimental evidence suggests that irreversible cellular damage is achieved in normal renal parenchyma at −19.4° C. However, tumor cells require lower treatment temperatures to achieve uniform cellular necrosis. The recommended treatment temperature during renal cryosurgery is −40° C.

3. **e. all of the above.** Animal studies have demonstrated that a single freeze-thaw cycle is inferior to a double freeze-thaw cycle with respect to adequacy of tissue ablation and local tumor control. As mentioned, complete cellular necrosis is consistently achieved at a targeted temperature of −40° C. Campbell and colleagues (1998)* demonstrated that the aforementioned threshold temperature of −40° C was achieved 3.1 mm inside the edge of the evolving ice ball. To guarantee that the tumor is completely ablated with a margin of normal tissue, the ice ball is generally carried 5 to 10 mm beyond the edge of the tumor when viewed under real-time imaging.

4. **c. inability to monitor treatment under image guidance.** The primary disadvantage when employing RFA for the treatment of renal lesions is difficulty in monitoring treatment under real-time image guidance. The risk of hemorrhage is higher with cryoablation. RFA may be employed laparoscopically, percutaneously, or openly. Cancer-specific survival is equivalent between RFA and cryoablation.

5. **e. all of the above.** Three recent meta-analyses evaluated outcomes following partial nephrectomy, radical nephrectomy, cryoablation, and RFA for the treatment of small renal masses. Both RFA and cryoablation demonstrated higher local recurrence rates when compared with partial or radical nephrectomy. However, the majority of published studies on cryoablation and RFA have enrolled small numbers of patients and employed disparate operative and follow-up protocols, pathology is either not obtained or is difficult to interpret, and the reliability of radiographic imaging remains unknown. Although the aggregate duration of follow-up is too short to derive irrefutable conclusions, treatment outcomes with cryoablation and RFA appear comparable. In general, complications occur with equal or less frequency with tumor ablation when compared with partial or radical nephrectomy.

6. **d. reducing impedance by improving current conductivity.** The electrically conductive agent facilitates the delivery of energy from the electrode to surrounding tissue, rendering it a much larger, "virtual" electrode. Impedance remains lower, and larger volumes are ablated.

7. **b. HIFU acts through local thermal and cavitary processes to generate tissue temperatures in excess of 65° C.** The use of HIFU in the treatment of small renal masses remains investigational. Experimental data has demonstrated "skip" lesions following treatment, which have been attributed to targeting obstacles, including

---

*Sources referenced can be found in *Campbell-Walsh Urology*, 10th Edition, on the Expert Consult website.

acoustic interference and respiratory movement. Skin burns have been reported in as many as 10% of patients.

8. **c. follow-up CT or MRI with contrast that demonstrates complete loss of contrast enhancement and stable or decreased size of the treated area.** Complete loss of contrast enhancement on follow-up CT or MRI has been considered a sign of complete tissue destruction. Following cryoablation, the treated area demonstrates a decrease in size of approximately 50% in the year following treatment. Following RFA, the treated area may not demonstrate a decrease in size. Any increase in size following treatment should be viewed as an ominous sign, and intervention should be directed accordingly. Postablative biopsy, although helpful, yields ambiguous results following RFA. Its use and interpretation remain controversial.

9. **a. Renal cell carcinoma (RCC) is radioresistant, and stereotactic radiosurgery has consistently demonstrated poor outcomes with treatment of RCC.** Although RCC is widely considered "radioresistant," it is unclear if this assertion is justifiable. It remains unclear if poor outcomes with radiation therapy for RCC are due to an inherent resistance to radiation or due to limitations with radiation delivery. Conventional external beam radiation systems are inadequately designed to deliver high doses in a focal manner without significant radiation scatter and attendant damage to adjacent tissues. Stereotactic radiosurgery allows focal delivery of high-dose radiation without attendant scatter. Experimental studies have demonstrated favorable results. Use of sterotactic radiosurgery for the treatment of small renal masses remains investigational but promising.

10. **c. a 47-year-old man who is otherwise healthy and demonstrates a 3.1-cm mesophytic enhancing lesion of the right kidney.** Although the indications for in-situ tumor ablation are expanding, young patients who are otherwise healthy are better served with the gold standard, a partial nephrectomy. Patients with multiple comorbidities, or those of advanced age who desire treatment, may be appropriate candidates for tumor ablation percutaneously or laparoscopically. In patients with a solitary kidney and recurrent RCC, in-situ ablation often affords favorable cancer-specific outcomes while sparing the kidney. The use of RFA and cryoablation has been previously reported in transplant patients that demonstrate lesions concerning for RCC. Outcomes have been favorable.

Additional Study Points

1. Currently, a double freeze-thaw cycle is suggested for cryotherapy with a period of time during each cycle in which the temperature is maintained at a −40° C.
2. Radiofrequency waves generate heat by causing ionic agitation in the tissue through which they pass; charring at the probe tip prevents adequate conduction of the wave from the probe into tissue; and to prevent heat at the probe becoming excessive with resultant charring, the probes are cooled.
3. Successful cryoablation on follow-up imaging often reveals a reduction in size of the lesion. Similarly, RF ablation followed over the long term often shows both a reduction in size and cavitation.
4. A major difficulty in comparing reports of ablative therapy is that the pathologic diagnosis of the lesion being treated is either benign or unknown in up to 40% of the patients studied making an assessment of cancer control difficult.
5. The most common complication following cryoablation is hemorrhage; a serious complication following radiofrequency ablation is ureteral/collecting system injury.
6. High-intensity focused ultrasonography generates heat by focusing the ultrasound waves at a point; unfortunately skin burns are a common complication of this technology.

The Adrenals

Pathophysiology, Evaluation, and Medical Management of Adrenal Disorders

Alexander Kutikov, MD • Paul L. Crispen, MD • Robert G. Uzzo, MD

QUESTIONS

1. At birth the adrenal cortex:
   a. is completely developed.
   b. weighs half as much as the adrenal cortex in adults.
   c. is composed of fetal and adult components.
   d. will continue to enlarge until 12 months of age.
   e. is composed of a single histologic zone.

2. Adrenal rest tissue within the testis can mimic testicular cancer in patients with:
   a. neuroblastoma.
   b. pheochromocytoma.
   c. primary aldosteronism.
   d. congenital adrenal hyperplasia.
   e. cryptorchidism.

3. In cases of renal agenesis, the ipsilateral adrenal gland is typically:
   a. absent.
   b. in the normal location.
   c. located at the level of the 8th thoracic vertebral body.
   d. located at the level of the 1st lumbar vertebral body.
   e. at a location dependent on the cause of renal agenesis.

4. The most abundant product of the adrenal cortex is:
   a. mineralocorticoids.
   b. glucocorticoids.
   c. adrenal androgens.
   d. catecholamines.
   e. adrenocorticotropic hormone (ACTH).

5. Aldosterone synthase (CYP11B2) is unique to:
   a. the zona glomerulosa.
   b. the zona fasciculata.
   c. the zona reticularis.
   d. the adrenal medulla.
   e. the distal renal tubule.

6. The only zone of the adrenal cortex that does not atrophy upon pituitary failure is:
   a. the zona glomerulosa.
   b. the zona fasciculata.
   c. the zona reticularis.
   d. the adrenal medulla.
   e. none of the above.

7. Presence of the phenylethanolamine-N-methyl transferase (PNMT) enzyme in the adrenal medulla is significant because:
   a. the enzyme catalyzes degradation of catecholamines to metanephrines.
   b. the enzyme catalyzes conversion of catecholamines to vanillylmandelic acid (VMA).
   c. the enzyme converts tyrosine to dopamine.
   d. the enzyme catalyzes the conversion of norepinephrine to epinephrine.
   e. of all of the above.

8. Metanephrines:
   a. refers to the term used for catecholamines and their byproducts.
   b. refers to the combined term for methylated metabolites of norepinephrine (normetanephrine) and epinephrine (metanephrine).
   c. refers to precursors to normetanephrines.
   d. are rarely helpful in establishing a diagnosis of pheochromocytoma.
   e. refers to the term used to describe epinephrine and norepinephrine in the context of pheochromocytoma symptomatology.

9. The term free metanephrines:
   a. is interchangeable with the term total metanephrines.
   b. is interchangeable with the term fractionated metanephrines.
   c. refers to normetanephrine and metanephrine that are not conjugated by a sulfate moiety.

d. refers to normetanephrine and metanephrine that are not bound to albumin.

e. refers to all of the above.

10. The most common cause of Cushing syndrome (exclusive of exogenous steroid intake) is:

a. Cushing disease.

b. a cortisol-producing adrenal adenoma.

c. ectopic ACTH production by a lung malignancy.

d. an adrenal carcinoma.

e. a pheochromocytoma.

11. What common urologic ailment can be found in up to 50% of patients with Cushing syndrome?

a. Testicular cancer

b. Torsion of the appendix testis

c. Urolithiasis

d. Fournier gangrene

e. Stress urinary incontinence

12. How does one perform a low-dose dexamethasone (LDDST) suppression test?

a. Admit the patient and measure q6hr serum cortisol levels while the patient is on a dexamethasone drip.

b. Measure the patient's saliva cortisol level at midnight.

c. Obtain a 24-hour urine cortisol measurement after the patient receives 1 mg of dexamethasone with the first void.

d. Have the patient take 10 mg of dexamethasone at 11 PM and measure urinary cortisol the next morning.

e. Have the patient take 1 mg of dexamethasone at 11 PM and measure serum cortisol the next morning.

13. TRUE or FALSE: The adrenal surgeon plays no role in the management of Cushing disease.

a. True

b. False

14. What percentage of patients presenting with primary aldosteronism are hypokalemic?

a. 5% to 12%

b. 9% to 37%

c. 33% to 50%

d. 55% to 75%

e. 63% to 91%

15. Elevated aldosterone in patients with familial hyperaldosteronism type I is mediated by:

a. renin.

b. sodium.

c. angiotensin II.

d. cortisol.

e. ACTH.

16. What percentage of patients with a positive screening test will be diagnosed with primary aldosteronism after confirmatory testing?

a. 2% to 10%

b. 20% to 40%

c. 30% to 50%

d. 50% to 70%

e. 75% to 90%

17. What is the most common subtype of primary aldosteronism?

a. Idiopathic hyperplasia

b. Aldosterone-producing adenoma

c. Unilateral adrenal hyperplasia

d. Familial hyperaldosteronism type I

e. Adrenocortical carcinoma

18. The primary determinant of potentially surgically correctable primary aldosteronism is:

a. blood pressure.

b. patient age.

c. demonstration of lateralized aldosterone secretion.

d. response to medical therapy.

e. plasma aldosterone levels.

19. Which class of antihypertensives is contraindicated during the evaluation of primary aldosteronism?

a. Calcium channel blockers

b. Alpha blockers

c. Beta blockers

d. Aldosterone-receptor blockers

e. Angiotensin-converting enzyme inhibitors

20. What percentage of patients with incidental adrenal masses prove to have pheochromocytoma?

a. 1%

b. 5%

c. 10%

d. 25%

e. 35%

21. What subtype is assigned to patients with a von Hippel-Lindau (VHL) mutation and a history of pheochromocytoma but no other stigmata of the VHL syndrome?

a. Type 1

b. Type 2A

c. Type 2B

d. Type 2C

e. None of the above

22. What genetic abnormality is strongly linked with malignant pheochromocytoma?

a. *RET* mutation

b. *VHL* mutation

c. *SDHB* mutation

d. *SDHD* mutation

e. All of the above

23. What test is considered the cornerstone for modern pheochromocytoma biochemical testing?

a. Plasma catecholamines

b. Plasma–free metanephrines or fractionated urinary metanephrines

c. Vanillylmandelic acid testing

d. Fasting morning urinary norepinephrine

e. Adrenal vein sampling for catecholamines

24. With regard to preoperative pheochromocytoma blockade, β-blockers should be started:

    a. 2 weeks prior to adrenalectomy.

    b. at least several days prior to α blockers.

    c. to control tachycardia and arrhythmias that can result upon initiation of α blockade.

    d. in conjunction with metyrosine.

    e. never, because β blockers can be lethal in patients with pheochromocytomas.

25. Patients with adrenal crisis can exhibit all of the following symptoms EXCEPT:

    a. hypotension unresponsive to fluid resuscitation.

    b. abdominal pain.

    c. nausea.

    d. fever.

    e. priapism.

26. All of the following lesions can be extra-adrenal EXCEPT:

    a. myelolipoma.

    b. ganglioneuroma.

    c. aldosteronoma.

    d. pheochromocytoma.

    e. oncocytoma.

27. A 25-year-old woman is diagnosed with a left adrenal mass, with abundant stippled calcifications, that exhibits imaging features inconsistent with adrenal adenoma. The patient complains of a severe bout of diarrhea that started approximately 8 months ago. Adrenalectomy reveals a ganglioneuroma. At her postoperative visit she is grateful, because her gastrointestinal (GI) complaints vanished following surgery. The substance responsible for diarrhea in this patient is most likely:

    a. metanephrine.

    b. epinephrine.

    c. norepinephrine.

    d. vanillylmandelic acid (VMA).

    e. vasoactive intestinal polypeptide (VIP).

28. What percentage of adrenal cysts is associated with malignancy in surgical series?

    a. 1%

    b. 3%

    c. 7%

    d. 12%

    e. 15%

29. Adrenocortical carcinoma in children:

    a. has a more favorable 5-year survival rate compared with adults.

    b. uses the same pathologic staging system as adults.

    c. is rarely associated with virilization.

    d. has an equal female to male incidence in children greater than 10 years of age.

    e. is frequently metastatic to the central nervous system.

30. The most common hormone secreted by adrenocortical carcinoma is:

    a. aldosterone.

    b. testosterone.

    c. dehydroepiandrosterone (DHEA).

    d. cortisol.

    e. androstenedione.

31. The Weiss criteria for identifying malignant adrenal tumors should be applied with caution in tumors with:

    a. necrosis.

    b. high mitotic index.

    c. inferior vena cava (IVC) invasion.

    d. liver metastasis.

    e. oncocytic features.

32. In patients presenting with metastatic adrenocortical carcinoma, the systemic agent of choice is:

    a. valrubicin.

    b. mitotane alone or in combination with additional cytotoxic agents.

    c. gemcitabine and cisplatin.

    d. Taxotere.

    e. bleomycin, etoposide, and cisplatin.

33. In the treatment of pathologically localized adrenocortical carcinoma:

    a. adjuvant radiation therapy decreases systemic progression.

    b. complete surgical excision offers the best chance of cure.

    c. increased Ki-67 expression has been associated with improved survival.

    d. the tumor's functional status is an independent predictor of survival.

    e. adjuvant therapy with mitotane has no proven benefit.

34. A 50% false-positive rate can be seen during low-dose dexamethasone suppression testing in:

    a. men with testicular cancer.

    b. women taking oral contraceptives.

    c. men with history of orchiopexy.

    d. patients with brain malignancy.

    e. patients with pheochromocytoma.

35. TRUE or FALSE: The adrenal gland should be resected whenever one performs a radical nephrectomy.

    a. True

    b. False

36. What common over-the-counter medication can produce a false-positive result during plasma–free metanephrine testing?

    a. Ibuprofen

    b. Aspirin

    c. Omeprazole

    d. Diphenhydramine

    e. Acetaminophen

37. A 55-year-old woman presents for the evaluation of an adrenal mass. Past medical history is significant for severe hypertension requiring four oral medications for adequate blood pressure control. A noncontrast CT scan of the abdomen reveals a 3-cm left adrenal mass, with an average attenuation of 7 Hounsfield units (HU). Appropriate initial screening should include:

a. free–fractionated plasma metanephrines, plasma aldosterone concentration, and plasma renin activity.

b. low-dose dexamethasone suppression test and serum catecholamines.

c. late-night salivary cortisol test, plasma aldosterone concentration, plasma renin activity, and plasma–free metanephrines.

d. plasma aldosterone concentration and plasma renin activity.

e. 24-hour urinary–fractionated metanephrines and serum cortisol concentration.

38. A 62-year-old man presents for postoperative surveillance of renal cell carcinoma. Three years prior, a right nephrectomy was performed for T2N0M0 grade III clear cell renal cell carcinoma. A current abdominal CT scan reveals a 3.5-cm right adrenal mass with an average attenuation of 32 HU prior to contrast administration. A CT washout study is performed, and absolute percent washout is calculated to be 52%. No other suspicious lesions are noted within the chest, abdomen, or pelvis. The next step in management should be:

a. observation.

b. adrenalectomy.

c. percutaneous biopsy.

d. initiation of an oral tyrosine kinase inhibitor.

e. assessment of the adrenal tumor's functional status

39. A 58-year-old woman has been diagnosed with primary aldosteronism based upon appropriate screening and confirmatory testing. A CT scan of the abdomen reveals a 1.0-cm left adrenal mass. Adrenal vein sampling is performed with the results outlined below. Results of adrenal vein sampling:

   Right cortisol gradient   2.7 : 1

   Left cortisol gradient   3.4 : 1

   Aldosterone ratio (left : right)   2.5 : 1

The next step in management would be:

a. repeat adrenal vein sampling with ACTH stimulation.

b. counseling for left adrenalectomy.

c. counseling for right adrenalectomy.

d. initiation of medical management based on diagnosis of bilateral adrenal hyperplasia.

e. ^{131}I-iodomethyl-norcholesterol (NP-59) scintigraphy to confirm lateralization.

40. A 43-year-old woman undergoes an uneventful right laparoscopic adrenalectomy for a 4.5-cm pheochromocytoma. The pathology report states that the lesion is benign and that the margins are negative. On postoperative day 1, she is ready for discharge and wants to

know if any additional follow-up is necessary. You inform her that the following is required.

a. Consideration of genetic screening

b. Repeat metabolic testing in 2 weeks

c. Cross-sectional imaging in 6 months

d. Biochemical testing in 6 months and then lifelong biochemical testing

e. All of the above

Pathology

1. A 60-year-old woman is noted to have a 4-cm left adrenal mass on an abdominal CT scan. The endocrine workup is negative, and the mass is excised laparoscopically. The pathology is depicted in Figure 57–1.

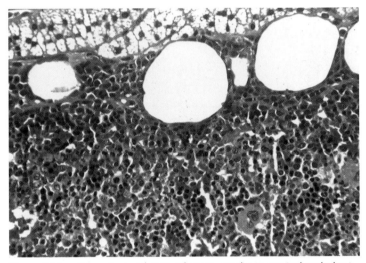

Figure 57–1. (From Bostwick DG, Cheng L. Urologic surgical pathology. 2nd ed. Edinburgh: Mosby; 2008.)

The next step in management is:

a. no additional therapy is indicated because this is a benign tumor.

b. a full metastatic workup should ensue with bone marrow aspiration to rule out neuroblastoma.

c. the patient should receive mitotane.

d. the patient should be followed carefully for development of hypertension.

e. a metaiodobenzylguanidine (MIBG) scan should be obtained.

2. A 45-year-old man has an incidentally discovered 6-cm adrenal mass. Hormonal workup is negative. The mass is laparoscopically removed. The pathology is depicted in Figure 57–2.

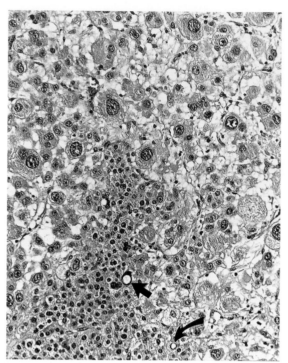

Figure 57–2.   (From Bostwick DG, Cheng L. Urologic surgical pathology. 2nd ed. Edinburgh: Mosby; 2008.)

On separate stains the lesion stains positive for Ki-67. The diagnosis is:

a. adrenal adenoma.

b. pheochromocytoma.

c. myolipoma.

d. adrenal corticocarcinoma.

e. neuroblastoma.

Imaging

1. See Figure 57–3.

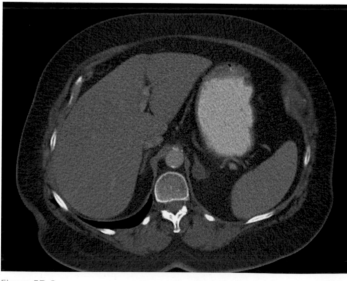

Figure 57–3.

A 42-year-old man with lung cancer has this CT scan. The right adrenal nodule has attenuation measurements of 7 HU. The most likely diagnosis is:

a. adrenal adenoma.

b. adrenal metastasis.

c. indeterminate adrenal nodule.

d. pheochromocytoma.

e. adrenal myelolipoma.

ANSWERS

1. **c. is composed of fetal and adult components.** The adrenal gland weighs twice as much as the adult gland and begins to atrophy at birth. Development of the gland continues during the first 3 years of life, with the zona reticularis developing last.

2. **d. congenital adrenal hyperplasia.** Testicular adrenal rests must be remembered when evaluating patients with congenital adrenal hyperplasia and testicular masses to avoid an unnecessary orchiectomy.

3. **b. in the normal location.** Reports of adrenal agenesis are extremely rare.

4. **c. adrenal androgens.** Although adrenal androgens are arguably the least physiologically significant compounds produced by the adrenals, the glands produce greater than 20 mg of these compounds per day. Meanwhile, only 100 to 150 mcg/day of aldosterone and approximately 10 to 20 mg/day of cortisol are produced by the glands.

5. **a. zona glomerulosa.** The zona glomerulosa cells are the sole source of aldosterone in humans.

6. **a. the zona glomerulosa.** Production of aldosterone in the zona glomerulosa is primarily regulated by angiotensin II through the renin-angiotensin-aldosterone system and potassium levels. Elevation of ACTH can also increase aldosterone secretion, but this is a much less potent stimulus. Therefore in pituitary failure, when ACTH levels fall, the zona glomerulosa fails to atrophy.

7. **d. the enzyme catalyzes the conversion of norepinephrine to epinephrine.** PNMT is virtually unique to the adrenal medulla (the brain and organ of Zuckerkandl also express the protein). Therefore the presence of PNMT results in epinephrine being virtually a unique product of the adrenal gland.

8. **b. refers to the combined term for methylated metabolites of norepinephrine (normetanephrine) and epinephrine (metanephrine).** The enzyme catechol-*O*-methyltransferase catalyzes the methylation of norepinephrine to normetanephrine and epinephrine to metanephrine. The term normetanephrines is not used.

9. **c. refers to normetanephrine and metanephrine that are not conjugated by a sulfate moiety.** See Figure 57–4 in *Campbell-Walsh Urology, 10th Edition* for a summary of appropriate terminology. Free metanephrines are unsulfonated normetanephrine and metanephrine, while total metanephrines refers to both conjugated and free compounds. The term fractionated metanephrines refers to laboratory reports that differentiate between metanephrine and normetanephrine concentrations (i.e., instead of only reporting metanephrine concentration, state the concentration of metanephrine and normetanephrine separately).

10. **a. Cushing disease.** See Figure 57–6 in *Campbell-Walsh Urology, 10th Edition.* Cushing disease, which describes

overproduction of ACTH by the pituitary, accounts for some 70% of endogenous Cushing syndrome.

11. **c. Urolithiasis.** Urolithiasis is seen in up to 50% of patients with Cushing syndrome; therefore stone formers with cushinoid features deserve a hypercortisolemia workup. The astute urologist should also remember that Cushing patients can also exhibit hypogonadal hypogonadism and should have a low threshold for a hypercortisolism workup in men with low testosterone and low gonadotropin levels.

12. **e. Have the patient take 1 mg of dexamethasone at 11 PM and measure serum cortisol the next morning.** Despite its intimidating name and rather complex physiologic underpinnings, the test is remarkably simple to administer. Write the patient a prescription for 1 mg of dexamethasone and ask that it be taken by mouth at 11 PM. The next morning determine the patient's serum cortisol level. If the cortisol level is 5 mcg/dL or higher (i.e., not suppressed), then the patient likely has hypercortisolemia. Beware that women on birth control will have false-positive results.

13. **b. False.** ACTH-secreting pituitary adenomas are treated with transsphenoidal surgical resection. However, a cure is seen in only 60% to 80% of patients. Among those who are cured, there is approximately 25% relapse. One option for patients who are refractory to neurosurgical treatment is a bilateral adrenalectomy. However, this treatment should not be performed hastily. It is crucial that a thoughtful multidisciplinary decision is made. Up to 30% of patients with Cushing disease who undergo bilateral adrenalectomy may develop Nelson syndrome—progressive growth of the pituitary adenoma causing increased intracranial pressure and compression of the ocular chiasm.

14. **b. 9% to 37%.** Although hypokalemia has been classically described as a common finding in primary aldosteronism, only 9% to 37% of newly diagnosed patients are hypokalemic.

15. **e. ACTH.** Due to the chimeric fusion of the promoter region of 11β-hydroxylase and the coding region of aldosterone synthase, aldosterone production is mediated by ACTH in familial hyperaldosteronism type I.

16. **d. 50% to 70%.** Fifty to 70 percent of patients with a positive screening test will be diagnosed with primary aldosteronism following confirmatory testing.

17. **a. idiopathic hyperplasia.** This subtype of primary aldosteronism accounts for ≈60% of cases.

18. **c. demonstration of lateralized aldosterone secretion.** Lateralization of aldosterone secretion is the primary determinant of successful surgical treatment of primary aldosteronism.

19. **d. Aldosterone-receptor blockers.** Aldosterone-receptor blockers (spironolactone and eplerenone) are contraindicated during the evaluation of primary aldosteronism. Patients requiring these agents for blood pressure control should be transitioned to other medications during testing for at least 6 weeks.

20. **b. 5% (approximately).** Incidentally discovered lesions account for 10% to 25% of all pheochromocytomas.

21. **d. Type 2C.** Type 1 = VHL patient with no evidence or family history of pheochromocytoma. Type 2 patients are those with evidence or family history of pheochromocytoma. Type 2 is further subdivided. Type 2A = patients with concomitant RCC; type 2B = no evidence of renal malignancy; type 2C = patients with

pheochromoctyoma and evidence of a *VHL* gene mutation but no other stigmata of VHL.

22. **c. SDHB mutation.** Patients with multiple endocrine neoplasia (type 2A and 2B) possess a mutation in the *RET* proto-oncogene. Approximately half of these patients develop pheochromocytoma, but only about 3% of those with pheochromocytoma exhibit malignant potential. Ten to 20 percent of patients with VHL develop pheochromocytomas, but only 5% of those with pheochromocytoma have malignant disease. Pheochromocytoma among patients with neurofibromatosis type 1 is rare (1%), but malignant disease can be seen in greater than 10%. Familial paraganglioma syndrome type 4 (*SDHB* mutation) carries the highest risk of malignancy (30% to 50%) among patients with the condition who develop pheochromocytoma (≈20%). Its pathologic cousin, familial paraganglioma syndrome type 1 (*SDHD* mutation) carries a negligible risk (<3%) of malignancy among patients who develop pheochromocytomas (≈20%).

23. **b. Plasma–free metanephrines or fractionated urinary metanephrines.** Methylated metabolites of catecholamines are known as metanephrines. Therefore normetanephrine (from norepinephrine) and metanephrine (from epinephrine) are collectively known as metanephrines. The vast majority of the methylation occurs within the adrenal medulla or pheochromocytoma, when present. Because this conversion of catecholamines to metanephrines is an uninterrupted process within pheochromocytomas, testing for these compounds is a much more sensitive means for tumor detection than the measurement of catecholamine levels, which may be paroxysmal. Furthermore, measurement of levels of metanephrines is rather specific (see *Campbell-Walsh Urology, 10th Edition*). Controversy exists regarding whether measurement of plasma–free metanephrines versus fractionated urinary metanephrine should be used as the initial test (see *Campbell-Walsh Urology, 10th Edition*). The term "free" indicates that the metanephrines being measured are not conjugated by a sulfate moiety, while the term "fractionated" simply indicates that normetanephrine and metanephrine levels are reported as separate values.

24. **c. to control tachycardia and arrhythmias that can result upon initiation of α blockade.** Beta-blockade should never be started prior to appropriate α blockade. In the absence of α blockade, β antagonists cause a potentiation of the action of epinephrine on the α_1 receptor, due to blockade of the arteriolar dilation at the β_2 receptor. Nevertheless, β blockade is at times necessary to control reflex tachycardia and arrhythmias that can result from α blockade.

25. **e. priapism.** Patients with adrenal crisis are easily misdiagnosed with an acute abdomen. Children can exhibit hypoglycemic seizures. Persistent painful erections are generally not associated with adrenal insufficiency.

26. **c. aldosteronoma.** All listed lesions, other than an aldosterone-producing adenoma, can develop outside of the adrenal gland.

27. **e. vasoactive intestinal polypeptide (VIP).** Ganglioneuromas are rare lesions that can arise in the adrenal glands and can secrete the vasoactive intestinal polypeptide (VIP), causing profound diarrhea in some patients. Nevertheless, most ganglioneuromas are asymptomatic.

28. **c. 7%.** In a meta-analysis accounting for 515 adrenal cysts, the incidence of associated adrenal malignancy was 7%.

29. **a. has a more favorable 5-year survival rate compared with adults.** The 5-year survival rate in children with adrenal cortical carcinoma is 54% compared with only 20% to 47% in adults.

30. **d. cortisol.** Up to 74% of functional adrenocortical tumors produce excess cortisol.

31. **e. oncocytic features.** The Weiss criteria should be applied with caution in pediatric cases and in those with oncocytic features.

32. **b. mitotane alone or in combination with additional cytotoxic agents.** Mitotane has adrenolytic activity and is the first-line agent of choice in patients with metastatic adrenocortical carcinoma. The addition of streptozotocin or etoposide, doxorubicin, and cisplatin to mitotane is potentially beneficial and is currently being investigated in a randomized trial.

33. **b. complete surgical resection** (including en bloc resection of locally advanced disease) **offers the best chance of cure.** Adjuvant radiation therapy has demonstrated a decreased rate of local recurrence but has not been shown to improve overall survival. Adjuvant mitotane therapy has been shown to significantly improve recurrence-free and overall survival. The impact of a tumor's functional status has not been consistently demonstrated to impact survival.

34. **b. women taking oral contraceptives.** The urologist must be aware that the low-dose dexamethasone suppression test can yield as high as a 50% false-positive rate in women using oral contraceptives, because the contraceptives increase total (but not bioavailable) cortisol levels by raising the patient's cortisol-binding globulin concentrations.

35. **b. False.** The classical description by Robson in the 1950s suggested that radical nephrectomy should include adrenalectomy. Today, however, adrenalectomy is believed to be necessary only for large (T2) upper pole tumors, in cases where an abnormality in the gland can be seen on preoperative imaging and in cases where a vein thrombus is present to the level of the adrenal gland.

36. **d. Diphenhydramine.** Prior to plasma–free metanephrine testing, ideally patients should not consume food or liquids after midnight. Caffeinated beverages, especially, must be avoided. Acetaminophen can produce a false-positive result due to cross reactivity in the assay and should be stopped for at least 5 days prior to testing. Tricyclic antidepressants and phenoxybenzamine should also be stopped, because these have been shown to be responsible for false-positive results (Eisenhofer et al, 2003).* Usual antihypertensive therapy can be continued. Although β blockade can potentially result in a false-positive test result, the current

---

*Sources referenced can be found in *Campbell-Walsh Urology, 10th Edition,* on the Expert Consult website.

recommendation is to stop the medication only on repeat testing (Eisenhofer et al, 2003). Ideally, the serum sample should be drawn in the supine position following at least 20 minutes of supine rest. Position is especially important if a positive result has been obtained and confirmatory testing is being performed.

37. **c. late-night salivary cortisol test, plasma aldosterone concentration, plasma renin activity, and plasma-free metanephrines.** All patients presenting with an adrenal mass should be evaluated for cortisol and catecholamine hypersecretion. Given the patient's history of hypertension, evaluation of primary aldosteronism should also be undertaken. Choice c is the best answer.

38. **e. assessment of the adrenal tumor's functional status.** Although there is a high probability that the adrenal lesion, in this case, represents a recurrence of the patient's renal cell carcinoma, the functional status of the adrenal mass should be assessed. A pheochromocytoma may always be lurking.

39. **b. counseling for left adrenalectomy.** Both the right and left cortisol gradients suggest proper catheter placement for adrenal vein sampling. The aldosterone ratio of 2.5 : 1 demonstrates left lateralization of autonomous aldosterone secretion, and counseling for left adrenalectomy is appropriate.

40. **e. All of the above.** The patient is less than 50 years old; therefore genetic screening is recommended. Up to 25% of patients who appear to have sporadic pheochromocytoma on presentation turn out to have germline mutations upon genetic testing (see Fig. 57–19 in *Campbell-Walsh Urology, 10th Edition*). Repeat metabolic testing at 2 weeks after resection is prudent. Most experts recommend additional biochemical testing at 6 months, followed by annual lifelong screening. More than 15% of patients will demonstrate recurrence of pheochromocytoma in the first 10 years after a successful resection. Recurrent disease has been reported more than 15 years following adrenalectomy; therefore lifelong annual biochemical screening is advised. Although cross-sectional imaging is not absolutely required in the face of a negative biochemical workup, most surgeons obtain at least one study at some point during the postoperative follow-up.

Pathology

1. **a. no additional therapy is indicated because this is a benign tumor.** This is a benign myolipoma. Notice that it consists of fat mixed with hematopoietic elements.

2. **d. adrenal corticocarcinoma.** The marked nuclear variability, increased mitotic figures, and positive staining for Ki-67 all strongly suggest adrenal corticocarcinoma.

Imaging

1. **a. adrenal adenoma.** Adrenal nodules that are less than 10 HU in density are almost always benign nodules, most often adrenal adenomas.

Additional Study Points

1. The right adrenal gland is triangular in shape; the left is crescent shaped.

2. The zona glomerulosa secrets mineralocorticoids; the zona fasciculata secretes glucocorticoids; and the zona reticularis secretes sex steroids.

3. The production of cortisol is circadian, with the majority being produced in the early morning.

4. Adrenal androgens are under the control of ACTH.

5. Ectopic ACTH production almost always originates from malignant tissue.

6. Renin release is stimulated by low renal perfusion pressure, increased renal sympathetic nervous activity, and low sodium.

7. Mineralocorticoid production results in sodium retention and volume expansion initially; however, with continued production the kidney escapes from the sodium retentive action of the hormone.

8. Sodium loading reduces endogenous aldosterone and renin production in those patients who do not have autonomous aldosterone secretion, i.e., from tumors.

9. The predictors of persistent hypertension following adrenalectomy for primary aldosteronism include (1) age greater than 50 years, (2) the requirement for more than two antihypertensive agents preoperatively, (3) a first-degree relative with hypertension, (4) prolonged duration of hypertension prior to adrenalectomy, and (5) renal insufficiency.

10. Ki-67 staining of adrenal tissue is perhaps the best indicator of malignancy.

11. Chromogranin A elevation in the serum has been used as a confirmatory test in patients with pheochromocytoma.

12. Restoration of intravascular volume is the most important component of preoperative preparation in patients with pheochromocytoma.

13. The most frequent cause of adrenal insufficiency in the United States is autoimmune adrenalitis; in the third world, it is tuberculosis.

14. Patients with congenital adrenal hyperplasia have a high risk for developing benign adrenal corticoadenomas.

15. The Weiss criteria distinguish benign from malignant adrenal tumors. The presence of three or more of the Weiss criteria is associated with malignancy.

16. An attenuation of less than 10 Hounsfield units on unenhanced CT scan is strongly suggestive of an adrenal adenoma.

17. There are four histologic types of adrenal cysts: (1) pseudocyst, (2) endothelial, (3) epithelial, and (4) parasitic.

Surgery of the Adrenal Glands

George K. Chow, MD ● Michael L. Blute, Sr., MD

QUESTIONS

1. Which statement is FALSE?
   a. The right adrenal gland rests higher than the left adrenal gland.
   b. The right adrenal gland tends to lie in a retrocaval position.
   c. The right adrenal vein usually drains into the vena cava directly.
   d. The left adrenal gland receives arterial branches from the left inferior phrenic artery, aorta, and left renal artery.
   e. None of the above

2. Absolute contraindications for laparoscopic adrenalectomy include:
   a. bleeding diathesis.
   b. adrenal mass size greater than 12 cm.
   c. adrenocortical carcinoma with adrenal vein thrombus.
   d. a and c.
   e. a, b, and c.

3. All of the following statements are true regarding adrenal cortical carcinoma EXCEPT:
   a. Adrenal masses larger than 6 cm are always a carcinoma.
   b. CT may distinguish infiltrative from well-encapsulated tumors.
   c. Adrenal cortical carcinoma is a relative contraindication for laparoscopic surgery.
   d. Removal should not be attempted through the posterior lumbodorsal open approach.
   e. All of the above are true.

4. Intraoperative ultrasonography helps laparoscopic adrenalectomy by:
   a. locating the adrenal gland.
   b. identifying the adrenal vein.
   c. locating an adrenal mass.
   d. a and c.
   e. a, b, and c.

5. During a right adrenalectomy, severe bleeding occurs. The most likely causes include all the following EXCEPT:
   a. right adrenal vein avulsion at origin on vena cava.
   b. avulsion of the right hepatic vein branch.
   c. disruption of the adrenal capsule.
   d. inadvertent ligation of upper pole renal artery.
   e. all of the above.

6. Which of the following statements is TRUE regarding laparoscopic partial adrenalectomy?
   a. The adrenal vein can be taken without compromising the adrenal glands venous drainage.
   b. Enucleation of a mass can be performed with an ultrasonic scalpel.
   c. Laparoscopic partial adrenalectomy is facilitated by intraoperative ultrasonography.
   d. a and c are true.
   e. a, b, and c are true.

7. Which of the following statements about postoperative addisonian crisis is TRUE?
   a. It is the result of contralateral adrenal activation.
   b. It can occur with fever and hypotension.
   c. It is managed by administration of spironolactone.
   d. It occurs only after laparoscopic adrenalectomy.
   e. All of the statements are true.

8. A pregnant woman has the acute onset of hypertension. Pheochromocytoma may be distinguished from PIH (pregnancy-induced hypertension, or "pre-eclampsia") by the observation that:
   a. PIH is never paroxysmal, whereas pheochromocytoma-related hypertension can be.
   b. proteinuria occurs with PIH not pheochromocytoma.
   c. the hypertension of PIH typically occurs in the first trimester, whereas pheochromocytoma hypertension can occur at any stage of pregnancy.
   d. a and b are true.
   e. a, b, and c are true.

9. Clinical indications for partial adrenalectomy include all of the following EXCEPT:
   a. a solitary adrenal gland.
   b. bilateral adrenal tumors.
   c. von Hippel-Lindau disease.
   d. multiple endocrine neoplasia type I.
   e. multiple endocrine neoplasia type IIA.

ANSWERS

1. **e. None of the above.** The right adrenal gland sits in a retrocaval position and lies in a more cephalad position than its left confrere. The venous drainage of the right adrenal gland can be variable but typically drains directly into the vena cava. In contrast, the left renal vein receives tributaries from the left adrenal vein and left gonadal vein. In some instances, a lumbar vein can drain directly into the left renal vein. Arterial supply is often more numerous and variable than the venous drainage. The adrenal glands receive arterial branches from the aorta, renal artery, and phrenic arteries.

2. **d. a *and* c.** With improvements in technical skill and equipment, larger adrenal masses are being approached laparoscopically. There is no clear limit to the size of an adrenal that can be removed laparoscopically. Various size limits have been suggested in the past. However, case reports continue to be published describing ever larger masses that have been removed laparoscopically. Therefore size should be a relative contraindication for laparoscopic surgery, and a surgeon's experience and skill must be factored into the decision-making process. Larger masses are more likely to be adrenocortical carcinoma that can directly invade surrounding organs, rendering them very difficult to resect laparoscopically. However, adrenocortical carcinomas can be resected laparoscopically as long as there is no suspicion of tumor extension into surrounding structures. The presence of an adrenal vein tumor thrombus should be considered an absolute contraindication to the laparoscopic approach. Finally, severe coagulopathy should be considered an absolute contraindication for laparoscopic surgery.

3. **a. adrenal masses larger than 6 cm are always a carcinoma.** As was noted in the answer to question 3, there is no definite size that correlates absolutely with an adrenocortical carcinoma. Many forms of adrenal pathology can exceed 6 cm, including adrenal cysts, pheochromocytomas, adrenal hemorrhage, and so on. An adrenocortical carcinoma is not a contraindication for laparoscopic surgery. However, certain conditions that can exist with an adrenocortical carcinoma (organ invasion, tumor thrombus) are. Cross-sectional imaging (CT and MRI) are critical for making such distinctions.

4. **e. a, b, *and* c.** Intraoperative ultrasonography can assist with the identification of important structures during laparoscopy. This is especially true when operating on morbidly obese patients with lots of retroperitoneal fat. The direct localization of an adrenal mass can assist with ablative therapy or partial adrenalectomy.

5. **d. inadvertent ligation of upper pole renal artery.** All of the noted vascular injuries cause bleeding, except ligation of an upper pole renal artery. Ligation of this artery would result in upper pole devascularization, not hemorrhage.

6. **e. a, b, *and* c are true.** Although the adrenal vein is the principal route of venous drainage, in most instances there are smaller vessels that can be relied on to drain the adrenal should the adrenal vein be ligated. Laparoscopic partial adrenalectomy has been described using a laparoscopic stapler and enucleation with an ultrasonic scalpel. Intraoperative ultrasonography is an invaluable tool for localizing the tumor during partial adrenalectomy.

7. **b. It can occur with fever and hypotension.** Addisonian crisis, or acute adrenal insufficiency, can occur after adrenalectomy or be due to other nonsurgical causes (e.g., adrenal hemorrhage and tuberculosis). Patients can present with back/abdominal pain, nausea, vomiting, diarrhea, hypotension, fever, hypoglycemia, and hyperkalemia. Removal of an adrenal gland can trigger addisonian crisis if there has been endocrine suppression (not activation) of the contralateral adrenal gland. Addisonian crisis is usually managed by steroid replacement, both glucocorticoid and mineralocorticoid (fludrocortisone).

8. **d. a *and* b are true.** PIH typically occurs in the third trimester and is distinguished from pheochromocytoma by the presence of proteinuria and the absence of paroxysmal symptoms.

9. **d. multiple endocrine neoplasia type I.** All of the answers correspond to strong clinical reasons to consider partial adrenalectomy, namely, conditions that result in solitary adrenal gland or multifocal/bilateral adrenal disease. Multiple endocrine neoplasia type I is not associated with adrenal tumors and therefore is not a reason for considering partial adrenalectomy.

Additional Study Points

1. The right adrenal vein enters the inferior vena cava in a posterior lateral position. When torn, the cava must be rotated to gain access to suture the defect.
2. Local regional recurrence in the adrenal cortical carcinoma occurs in 60% of cases.
3. It is important to note that the tail of the pancreas can lie adjacent to the upper pole of the kidney and adrenal. Care must be taken not to injure this organ.
4. In a thoracoabdominal incision, the diaphragm should not be incised radially but, rather, circumferentially because the former results in a phrenic nerve injury with an atonic diaphragm lateral to the incision.
5. An addisonian crisis is most commonly seen after excision of an adrenal tumor that secretes cortisol as the contralateral adrenal is suppressed.
6. In removing large adrenal masses, it is important to be careful not to ligate an upper pole renal artery branch because this will result in an infarction of the renal segment that is served by this artery.

Urine Transport, Storage, and Emptying

chapter
59

Physiology and Pharmacology of the Renal Pelvis and Ureter

Robert M. Weiss, MD

QUESTIONS

1. During development, the ureteral lumen is obliterated and then recanalizes. Which of the following substances appears to be involved in this recanalization process?
   a. Prostaglandin E_2
   b. c-KIT
   c. Angiotensin
   d. Calcitonin gene–related peptide (CGRP)
   e. Acetylcholine

2. Caspases are involved in:
   a. smooth muscle relaxation.
   b. smooth muscle contraction.
   c. hysteresis.
   d. apoptosis.
   e. calcium sequestration.

3. The resting membrane potential is primarily determined by the distribution of which of the following ions across the cell membrane and the preferential permeability of the cell membrane to that ion?
   a. Potassium
   b. Sodium
   c. Calcium
   d. Chloride
   e. Barium

4. With excitation of the ureteral muscle cell, an action potential is formed. Which of the following pairs of ions are primarily responsible for the upstroke of the action potential?
   a. Potassium and calcium
   b. Sodium and chloride
   c. Calcium and sodium
   d. Potassium and sodium
   e. Calcium and chloride

5. Which of the following must be phosphorylated for smooth muscle contraction to occur?
   a. Actin
   b. Myosin

   c. Calmodulin
   d. Calcium
   e. Troponin

6. The primary site for intracellular storage of calcium is:
   a. mitochondria.
   b. caveolae.
   c. the nucleolus.
   d. actin.
   e. the endoplasmic reticulum.

7. The second messenger involved in β-adrenergic agonist–induced ureteral relaxation is:
   a. cyclic AMP.
   b. cyclic GMP.
   c. nitric oxide.
   d. inositol 1,4,5-triphosphate (IP_3).
   e. diacylglycerol (DG).

8. The enzyme that degrades cyclic GMP is:
   a. guanylyl cyclase.
   b. myosin light-chain kinase.
   c. phosphodiesterase.
   d. phospholipase C.
   e. nitric oxide synthase (NOS).

9. The enzyme that degrades cyclic AMP is:
   a. adenylyl cyclase.
   b. myosin light-chain kinase.
   c. phosphodiesterase.
   d. phospholipase C.
   e. NOS.

10. Nitric oxide causes smooth muscle relaxation. In doing so, it activates which of the following enzymes?
    a. Guanylyl cyclase
    b. Myosin light-chain kinase
    c. Phosphodiesterase
    d. Phospholipase C
    e. NOS

11. The substrate for NOS is:
    a. cyclic AMP.
    b. cyclic GMP.
    c. GTP.
    d. L-arginine.
    e. L-citrulline.

12. Inducible NOS (iNOS) is:
    a. nicotinamide adenine dinucleotide phosphate (NADPH) independent and calcium independent.
    b. NADPH independent and calcium dependent.
    c. NADPH dependent and calcium independent.
    d. NADPH dependent and calcium dependent.
    e. nitric oxide dependent and calcium dependent.

13. The enzyme involved in the formation of DG is:
    a. adenylyl cyclase.
    b. guanylyl cyclase.
    c. phosphodiesterase.
    d. protein kinase C.
    e. phospholipase C.

14. DG increases the activity of which enzyme?
    a. Adenylyl cyclase
    b. Guanylyl cyclase
    c. Phosphodiesterase
    d. Protein kinase C
    e. Phospholipase C

15. An agent that prevents reuptake of norepinephrine in nerve terminals and thus potentiates and prolongs the activity of norepinephrine is:
    a. tyrosine.
    b. monoamine oxidase.
    c. imipramine.
    d. tetramethylammonium.
    e. tetraethylammonium.

16. Norepinephrine is synthesized from:
    a. tyrosine.
    b. arginine.
    c. choline.
    d. cocaine.
    e. imipramine.

17. Which of the following inhibits ureteral and renal pelvic contractile activity?
    a. Substance P
    b. Neurokinin A
    c. Neuropeptide K
    d. Neuropeptide Y
    e. CGRP

18. Which of the following collagen types is associated with ureteral obstruction?
    a. Type I collagen
    b. Type II collagen
    c. Type III collagen

    d. Type IV collagen
    e. Type V collagen

19. The enzyme involved in prostaglandin synthesis is:
    a. phospholipase C.
    b. cyclooxygenase.
    c. protein kinase C.
    d. phosphodiesterase.
    e. ATPase.

20. With ureteral obstruction, prostaglandins are involved in a process that aids in the preservation of renal function. What is this process?
    a. Afferent arteriole vasoconstriction
    b. Afferent arteriole vasodilatation
    c. Efferent arteriole vasoconstriction
    d. Efferent arteriole vasodilatation
    e. Glomerular vasoconstriction

21. Which of the following agents could theoretically cause urinary retention?
    a. Bethanechol
    b. BAY K 8644
    c. Prostaglandin $F_{2\alpha}$
    d. Verapamil
    e. Substance P

22. Which of the following is a β-adrenergic agonist?
    a. Cromakalim
    b. Physostigmine
    c. Propranolol
    d. Phenoxybenzamine
    e. Isoproterenol

23. Which of the following conditions must be present for urine to pass efficiently from the ureter into the bladder?
    a. Intraluminal ureteral contractile pressure must be above 40 cm H_2O.
    b. The ureterovesical junction must relax.
    c. Intraluminal ureteral contractile pressures must be greater than intravesical baseline pressures.
    d. Intravesical contractile pressures must be less than 40 cm H_2O.
    e. The bladder must relax just before contraction of the ureter.

24. What is normal baseline or resting ureteral pressure?
    a. 0 to 5 cm H_2O
    b. 5 to 10 cm H_2O
    c. 10 to 15 cm H_2O
    d. 15 to 20 cm H_2O
    e. 20 to 25 cm H_2O

25. The Laplace equation expresses the relationship between the variables that affect intraluminal pressure. Which of the following conforms to the Laplace relationship?
    a. Tension = (radius × wall thickness)/pressure
    b. Tension = (radius × pressure)/wall thickness
    c. Tension = (wall thickness × pressure)/radius

d. Pressure = (radius × wall thickness)/tension

e. Pressure = (radius × tension)/wall thickness

26. Factors that facilitate ureteral stone passage include:

a. increased hydrostatic pressures proximal to the calculus and relaxation of the ureter in the region of the stone.

b. increased hydrostatic pressures proximal to the calculus and contraction of the ureter in the region of the stone.

c. decreased hydrostatic pressures proximal to the calculus and relaxation of the ureter in the region of the stone.

d. decreased hydrostatic pressures proximal to the calculus and contraction of the ureter in the region of the stone.

e. decreased contractile pressures proximal to the calculus and contraction of the ureter in the region of the stone.

27. Which of the following hormones inhibits ureteral contractility?

a. Bombesin

b. Thyroxine

c. Estrogen

d. Aldosterone

e. Progesterone

28. A drug that has efficacy in managing ureteral colic is:

a. bethanechol.

b. prostaglandin $F_{2\alpha}$.

c. physostigmine.

d. indomethacin.

e. ephedrine.

29. Which of the following is a calcium-binding protein that plays a role in smooth muscle contraction?

a. Connexin43

b. Calmodulin

c. Cromakalim

d. Survivin

e. Myosin

30. In the ureter, the resting or the contractile force developed at any given length depends on the direction in which the change in length is occurring. This is referred to as:

a. viscoelasticity.

b. creep.

c. hysteresis.

d. stress relaxation.

e. compensatory relaxation.

31. Which of the following is noted to be expressed before initiation of ureteral peristaltic activity?

a. Prostanoids

b. Nitric oxide

c. c-KIT

d. Myosin light chain

e. Phosphodiesterase

32. Ureteral pacemaker activity is amplified by:

a. prostanoids.

b. norepinephrine.

c. CGRP.

d. cyclic GMP.

e. potassium channel openers.

33. Which cells are the primary pacemaker cells for ureteral peristalsis?

a. Interstitial cells of Cajal-like cells (ICC-like cells)

b. c-KIT–positive mast cells

c. c-KIT–negative typical smooth muscle cells

d. Atypical smooth muscle cells

e. Caveolae-containing smooth muscle cells

ANSWERS

1. **c. Angiotensin.** At a point during development, the ureteral lumen is obliterated and then recanalizes. It appears that angiotensin, acting through the AT2 receptor, is involved in the recanalization process. Knockout mice for the ATR2 gene have congenital anomalies of the kidney and urinary tract, which include multicystic dysplastic kidneys, megaureters, and ureteropelvic junction obstructions.

2. **d. apoptosis.** Programmed cell death, or apoptosis, is involved in branching of the ureteric bud and subsequent nephrogenesis, and inhibitors of caspases, which are factors in the signaling pathway of apoptosis, inhibit ureteral bud branching.

3. **a. Potassium.** When a ureteral muscle cell is in a nonexcited or resting state, the electrical potential difference across the cell membrane, the transmembrane potential, is referred to as the resting membrane potential (RMP). The RMP is determined primarily by the distribution of potassium ions (K^+) across the cell membrane and by the permeability of the membrane to potassium ions.

4. **c. Calcium and sodium.** When the ureteral cell is excited, its membrane loses its preferential permeability to K^+ and becomes more permeable to calcium ions (Ca^{2+}) that move inward across the cell membrane, primarily through L-type Ca^{2+} channels, and give rise to the upstroke of the action potential.

5. **b. Myosin.** The most widely accepted theory suggests that phosphorylation of myosin is involved in the contractile process.

6. **e. the endoplasmic reticulum.** Calcium release from tightly bound storage sites (i.e., the endoplasmic or sarcoplasmic reticulum) increases the Ca^{2+} concentration in the sarcoplasm.

7. **a. cyclic AMP.** Cyclic AMP is believed to mediate the relaxing effects of β-adrenergic agonists in a variety of smooth muscles.

8. **c. phosphodiesterase.** Another cyclic nucleotide, cyclic GMP, also can cause smooth muscle relaxation. Cyclic GMP is synthesized from GTP by the enzyme guanylyl cyclase and is degraded to 5′-GMP by a phosphodiesterase.

9. **c. phosphodiesterase.** Phosphodiesterase activity that can degrade both cyclic AMP and cyclic GMP has been demonstrated in the canine ureter, and various inhibitors can preferentially inhibit the breakdown of one or the other cyclic nucleotide.

10. **a. Guanylyl cyclase.** Nitric oxide released from the nerve activates the enzyme guanylyl cyclase in the smooth muscle cell, with the resultant conversion of guanosine triphosphate to cyclic GMP, thus with the resultant smooth muscle relaxation (see Fig. 59–11 in *Campbell-Walsh Urology*, 10th Edition).

11. **d. L-arginine.** NOS converts L-arginine to nitric oxide and L-citrulline in a reaction that requires nicotinamide adenine dinucleotide phosphate (NADPH).

12. **c. NADPH dependent and calcium independent.** An inducible NOS isoform, iNOS, is NADPH dependent but Ca^{2+} independent and has been identified in ureteral smooth muscle.

13. **e. phospholipase C.** Some actions of α_1-adrenergic and muscarinic cholinergic agonists and a number of other hormones, neurotransmitters, and biologic substances are associated with an increase in intracellular Ca^{2+} and are related to changes in inositol lipid metabolism. These agonists combine with a receptor on the cell membrane, and the agonist-receptor complex, in turn, activates an enzyme, phospholipase C, that leads to the hydrolysis of polyphosphatidylinositol 4,5-bisphosphate, with the formation of two second messengers: IP_3 and DG (see Fig. 59–12 in *Campbell-Walsh Urology, 10th Edition*).

14. **d. Protein kinase C.** DG binds to an enzyme, protein kinase C, causes its translocation to the cell membrane, and, by reducing the concentration of Ca^{2+} required for protein kinase C activation, results in an increase in this enzyme's activity.

15. **c. imipramine.** The greatest percentage of the norepinephrine is actively taken up (reuptake or neuronal uptake) into the neuron. Neuronal reuptake regulates the duration that norepinephrine is in contact with the innervated tissue and thus regulates the magnitude and duration of the catecholamine-induced response. Agents such as cocaine and imipramine (Tofranil), which inhibit neuronal uptake, potentiate the physiologic response to norepinephrine.

16. **a. tyrosine.** Norepinephrine, the chemical mediator responsible for adrenergic transmission, is synthesized in the neuron from tyrosine.

17. **e. CGRP.** Tachykinins and CGRP are neurotransmitters released from peripheral endings of sensory nerves. Tachykinins stimulate contractile activity and CGRP inhibits contractile activity.

18. **c. Type III collagen.** Increased amounts of type III collagen are seen in a variety of obstructed ureteral states.

19. **b. cyclooxygenase.** The "primary" prostaglandins, PGE_1, PGE_2, and $PGF_{2\alpha}$, are synthesized from the fatty acid arachidonic acid by enzymatic reactions involving two cyclooxygenase (COX) isoforms, COX-1 and COX-2.

20. **b. Afferent arteriole vasodilatation.** Indomethacin has been employed in the management of ureteral colic. The beneficial effects are probably due to indomethacin's inhibition of the prostaglandin-mediated vasodilatation that occurs subsequent to obstruction. The vasodilatation theoretically would result in an increase in glomerular capillary pressure and subsequent increase in pelviureteral pressure.

21. **d. Verapamil.** The calcium channel blockers verapamil, D-600 (a methoxy derivative of verapamil), diltiazem, and nifedipine have been shown to inhibit ureteral activity. These inhibitory effects are accompanied by decreases in action potential duration, number of oscillations on the plateau of the guinea pig action potential, excitability, and rate of rise and amplitude of the action potential. High concentrations of verapamil and D-600 cause a complete cessation of electrical and mechanical activity. Similar inhibition of bladder activity can occur.

22. **e. Isoproterenol.** Isoproterenol, a β-adrenergic agonist, depresses contractility.

23. **c. Intraluminal ureteral contractile pressures must be greater than intravesical baseline pressures.** The theoretical aspects of the mechanics of urine transport within the ureter were described in detail by Griffiths and Notschaele in 1983*; these are depicted in Figure 59–18 in *Campbell-Walsh Urology, 10th Edition*. At normal flow rates, as the renal pelvis fills, a rise in renal pelvic pressure occurs, and urine is extruded into the upper ureter, which is initially in a collapsed state. The contraction wave originates in the most proximal portion of the ureter and moves the urine in front of it in a distal direction. The urine that had previously entered the ureter is formed into a bolus. To propel the bolus of urine efficiently, the contraction wave must completely coapt the ureteral walls, and the pressure generated by this contraction wave provides the primary component of what is recorded by intraluminal pressure measurements. The bolus that is pushed in front of the contraction wave lies almost entirely in a passive, noncontracting part of the ureter.

24. **a. 0 to 5 cm H_2O.** Baseline or resting ureteral pressure is approximately 0 to 5 cm H_2O.

25. **b. Tension = (radius × pressure)/wall thickness.** The Laplace equation expresses the relationship between the variables that affect intraluminal pressure: pressure = (tension × wall thickness)/radius. The Laplace law: T = PR , where T is tension, P is pressure and R is radius.

26. **a. increased hydrostatic pressures proximal to the calculus and relaxation of the ureter in the region of the stone.** Two factors that appear to be most useful in facilitating stone passage are an increase in hydrostatic pressure proximal to a calculus and relaxation of the ureter in the region of the stone.

27. **e. Progesterone.** Several studies have shown an inhibitory effect of progesterone on ureteral function. Progesterone has been noted to increase the degree of ureteral dilatation during pregnancy and to retard the rate of disappearance of hydroureter in postpartum women.

28. **d. indomethacin.** Indomethacin, by reducing pelviureteral pressure and thus pelviureteral wall tension, might eliminate some of the pain of renal colic that is dependent on distention of the upper urinary tract.

29. **b. Calmodulin.** With excitation, there is a transient increase in the sarcoplasmic Ca^{2+} concentration from its steady-state concentration of 10^{-8} to 10^{-7} M to a concentration of 10^{-6} M or higher. At this higher concentration, Ca^{2+} forms an active complex with the calcium-binding protein calmodulin. Calmodulin without Ca^{2+} is inactive (see Fig. 59–7 in *Campbell-Walsh Urology, 10th Edition*). The calcium-calmodulin complex activates a calmodulin-dependent enzyme, myosin light-chain kinase (see Fig. 59–7 in *Campbell-Walsh Urology, 10th Edition*). The activated myosin light-chain kinase, in turn, catalyzes the phosphorylation of the 20,000-dalton light chain of myosin (see Fig. 59–8 in *Campbell-Walsh Urology, 10th Edition*). Phosphorylation of the myosin light chain allows activation by actin of myosin Mg^{2+}-ATPase activity, leading to hydrolysis of ATP and the development of smooth muscle

---

*Sources referenced can be found in *Campbell-Walsh Urology, 10th Edition*, on the Expert Consult website.

tension or shortening (see Fig. 59–9 in *Campbell-Walsh Urology, 10th Edition*).

30. **c. hysteresis.** Because the ureter is a viscoelastic structure, the resting or contractile force developed at any given length depends on the direction in which change in length is occurring and on the rate of length change. This is referred to as hysteresis; for the ureter, at any given length, the resting force is less and contractile force is greater when the ureter is allowed to shorten than when the ureter is being stretched (see Fig. 59–13 in *Campbell-Walsh Urology, 10th Edition*).

31. **c. c-KIT.** This tyrosine kinase receptor is important in the development of pacemaker activity and peristalsis of the gut (Der-Silaphet et al, 1998). Pezzone and colleagues (2003) identified c-KIT–positive cells in the mouse ureter. The expression of c-KIT was noted to be upregulated in the embryonic murine ureter before its development of unidirectional peristaltic contractions (David et al, 2005). Incubation of isolated cultured embryonic murine ureters with antibodies that neutralize c-KIT activity alters ureteral morphology and inhibits unidirectional peristalsis. c-KIT–positive cells have been identified in the human ureter (Metzger et al, 2004).

32. **a. prostanoids.** The ionic conduction underlying pacemaker activity in the upper urinary tract is due to the opening and slow closure of voltage-activated L-type Ca^{2+} channels, which are amplified by prostanoids (Santicioli et al, 1995a). This is opposed by the opening and closure of voltage and Ca^{2+}-dependent K^+ channels.

It has been suggested that prostaglandins and excitatory tachykinins, released from sensory nerves, help maintain autorhythmicity in the upper urinary tract through maintenance of Ca^{2+} mobilization. Tetrodotoxin and blockers of the autonomic nervous system, both parasympathetic and sympathetic, have little effect on peristalsis, suggesting that autonomic neurotransmitters play little role in maintaining pyeloureteral motility.

33. **d. Atypical smooth muscle cells.** Atypical smooth muscle cells give rise to pacemaker activity in the rat and guinea pig ureter. In contrast to typical smooth muscle cells, they have less than 40% of their cellular area occupied by contractile elements and demonstrate sparse immunoreactivity for smooth muscle and actin (Klemm et al, 1999; Lang et al, 2001). ICC-like cells in the upper urinary tract do not appear to be primary pacemaker cells but rather may provide for preferential conduction of electrical signals from pacemaker cells to typical smooth muscle cells of the renal pelvis and ureter (Klemm et al, 1999). In the mouse ureteropelvic junction c-KIT–positive ICC-like cells have been identified that showed high frequency spontaneous transient inward currents that often occurred in bursts to sum and produce long-lasting large inward currents (Lang et al, 2007b). It is postulated that in the absence of a proximal pacemaker drive that these ICC-like cells could act as pacemaker cells and trigger contractions in adjacent smooth muscle cells in the ureteropelvic junction. Thus both atypical smooth muscle cells and ICC-like cells both may play a pacemaker role in the initiation and propagation of pyeloureteric peristalsis (Lang et al, 2006, 2007a).

Additional Study Points

1. Efficient propulsion of the urinary bolus depends on the ability of the walls of the ureter to co-apt.
2. Autonomic neurotransmitters play little role in maintaining pyeloureteral motility.
3. Ureteral muscle fibers are arranged in a longitudinal, circumferential, and spiral configuration.
4. The ureter is a syncytial type of smooth muscle without discrete neuromuscular junctions.
5. Ureteral peristalsis can occur without innervation; however the nervous system does play at least a modulating role in ureteral peristalsis, particularly the sympathetic nervous system.
6. Alpha-adrenergic stimulation increases ureteral activity. Beta-adrenergic stimulation inhibits ureteral and renal pelvic activity.
7. Ureteral pressures can be as high as 20 to 80 cm of water during a contraction.
8. Pressure within the bladder during the storage phase is of paramount importance in determining the efficiency of urine transport across the ureterovesical junction (UVJ).
9. Ureteral obstruction causes a gradual increase in ureteral length and diameter.
10. Infection impairs urine transport and reduces compliance at the UVJ, which may permit reflux.
11. The obstruction of pregnancy is primarily due to mechanical factors and secondarily due to the hormonal effects of progesterone.

chapter 60

Physiology and Pharmacology of the Bladder and Urethra

Naoki Yoshimura, MD, PhD ● Michael B. Chancellor, MD

QUESTIONS

1. Sacral-evoked response testing measures nerve conduction time by which pathways?

AFFERENT	EFFERENT
a. Somatic	Sympathetic
b. Somatic	Somatic
c. Sympathetic	Somatic
d. Sympathetic	Parasympathetic
e. Parasympathetic	Sympathetic

2. During the resting state, bladder smooth muscle electrical activity is characterized by:

   a. a concentration of K^+ ions that is higher on the outside of the cell membrane.

   b. a concentration of Na^+ ions that is higher on the inside of the cell membrane.

   c. a cell membrane that is preferentially permeable to K^+.

   d. a cell membrane that is preferentially permeable to Na^+.

   e. the inside of the cell membrane being positive with respect to the outside.

3. Two weeks following complete C6 spinal cord injury a 31-year-old woman has a urodynamic study that demonstrates detrusor areflexia. The most likely urodynamic finding two years later is:

   a. detrusor overactivity.

   b. detrusor areflexia.

   c. detrusor overactivity with detrusor-sphincter dyssynergia.

   d. detrusor areflexia with decreased bladder compliance.

   e. detrusor areflexia with detrusor-sphincter dyssynergia.

4. Urinary tract smooth muscle contractility is inhibited by:

   a. propranolol.

   b. nifedipine.

   c. phenylephrine.

   d. acetylcholine.

   e. substance P.

5. Phosphodiesterase inhibitors cause smooth muscle relaxation by inhibiting:

   a. calmodulin binding.

   b. production of cGMP.

   c. production of cAMP.

   d. degradation of phospholipase C.

   e. degradation of cGMP.

6. The most common urodynamic finding in sacral level spinal cord injury is:

   a. detrusor overactivity.

   b. detrusor overactivity with detrusor-external sphincter dyssynergia.

   c. detrusor areflexia.

   d. decreased detrusor compliance.

   e. normal urodynamic study.

7. During physiologic filling bladder compliance is most affected by:

   a. perivesical ganglia activity.

   b. peripheral nerve activity.

   c. sacral spinal cord activity.

   d. suprasacral spinal cord activity.

   e. bladder wall viscoelasticity.

8. Increased bladder wall tension is directly related to:

   a. decreased bladder size.

   b. increased bladder size.

   c. decreased intravesical pressure.

   d. increased intravesical pressure.

   e. thin bladder wall.

9. When the hypogastric nerve is stimulated, what is the primary neurotransmitter released at the ganglionic level?

   a. Acetylcholine

   b. Adenosine triphosphate

   c. Dopamine

   d. Norepinephrine

   e. Prostaglandin $F_{2\alpha}$

10. Pudendal nerve block may be useful in the treatment of neuropathic bladder dysfunction in patients with:

    a. lower motor lesions with spastic bladder.

    b. lower motor lesions with spastic sphincter.

    c. upper motor lesions with atonic bladder.

    d. upper motor lesions with spastic sphincter.

    e. upper motor lesions with vesicoureteral reflux.

11. Postganglionic sympathetic nerve fibers to the bladder release:
    a. acetylcholine.
    b. epinephrine.
    c. nitric oxide.
    d. norepinephrine.
    e. vasoactive intestinal polypeptide (VIP).

12. The bladder contraction and simultaneous urethral relaxation during voiding are coordinated by a reflex center located in:
    a. the hypothalamus.
    b. the basal ganglia.
    c. the medulla.
    d. the pons.
    e. the thoracic cord.

13. The sudden rise in detrusor pressure seen at the onset of carbon dioxide cystometry is due to:
    a. tonic contraction of the bladder.
    b. phasic contraction of the bladder.
    c. viscoelastic properties of the bladder.
    d. sacral reflex arc.
    e. bladder-urethral reflex arc.

14. The first event to occur with normal micturition is:
    a. relaxation of the bladder neck.
    b. relaxation of the prostate and prostatic capsule.
    c. relaxation of the external striated sphincter.
    d. contraction of the bladder body.
    e. contraction of the bladder trigone.

15. In patients with hypersensitive bladder dysfunction, intravesical capsaicin instillation may potentially benefit the patient by blockade of:
    a. glycosaminoglycan receptor.
    b. serotonin reuptake.
    c. Aδ fiber afferents.
    d. C-fiber afferents.
    e. tachykinin receptor.

16. Bladder painful sensations are conveyed by which nerve(s)?
    a. Hypogastric
    b. Pelvic
    c. Pudendal
    d. Pelvic and hypogastric
    e. Pelvic and pudendal

17. Smooth muscle contraction results from phosphorylation of which protein?
    a. Actin
    b. Caldesmon
    c. Desmin
    d. G protein
    e. Myosin

18. Which of the following is NOT a characteristic of detrusor interstitial cells?
    a. Participates in spontaneous activity of the bladder
    b. Linked by gap junctions

    c. Located in the suburothelial space between urothelium and nerve endings
    d. Similar to myofibroblasts (urothelial interstitial cells)
    e. Triggers bladder pain

19. Neurally mediated relaxation of the urethra during voiding occurs by release of:
    a. nitric oxide from sympathetics.
    b. nitric oxide from parasympathetics.
    c. VIP from sympathetics.
    d. VIP from parasympathetics.
    e. neuropeptide Y from sympathetics.

20. Influx of which ion/chemical is responsible for generation of action potential by bladder smooth muscle cells?
    a. Calcium
    b. Potassium
    c. Sodium
    d. Chloride
    e. Nitric oxide

21. The decrease in bladder compliance is due to what change in a connective tissue component?
    a. Decreased elastin
    b. Decreased type I collagen
    c. Decreased type II collagen
    d. Increased type III collagen
    e. Increased type V collagen

22. Acetylcholine binds predominately to which of the five muscarinic receptor(s) to induce bladder contraction?
    a. M_1
    b. M_2
    c. M_1 and M_2
    d. M_2 and M_3
    e. M_2 and M_4

23. Which adrenergic receptor participates in human detrusor muscle relaxation during the storage phase?
    a. β_1
    b. β_2
    c. β_3
    d. α_1
    e. α_2

24. Substance P is located in which types of nerves?
    a. Afferent
    b. Efferent
    c. Afferent and efferent
    d. Aδ fibers
    e. Spinal cord interneurons

25. Which hormone increases α-adrenergic receptors' density in the urethra?
    a. Luteinizing hormone–releasing hormone (LHRH)
    b. Dihydrotestosterone
    c. Testosterone
    d. Estrogen
    e. Testosterone and estrogen

26. Which is the most important excitatory neurotransmitter in the central nervous system to facilitate micturition?
    a. Acetylcholine
    b. γ-Aminobutyric acid (GABA)
    c. Norepinephrine
    d. Glutamate
    e. Serotonin

27. Which central nervous system neurotransmitter inhibits micturition?
    a. Acetylcholine
    b. Substance P
    c. Norepinephrine
    d. Glutamate
    e. Serotonin

28. What is the function of delta and mu opioid receptors in the spinal cord?
    a. Opioid receptors do not participate in the micturition reflex
    b. Enhance bladder sensation
    c. Inhibit descending potine spinal signaling
    d. Stimulate bladder contraction
    e. Inhibit bladder contraction

29. Which nerve or nerves initiate normal micturition reflex?
    a. Sympathetic nerves
    b. Myelinated Aδ afferent nerves
    c. Unmyelinated C afferent nerves
    d. Both Aδ- and C-fiber afferent nerves
    e. None of the above

30. Which nerve triggers uninhibited bladder contractions induced by a spinal micturition reflex in the cat model of chronic spinal cord transection?
    a. Sympathetic
    b. Aδ
    c. C fiber
    d. Both Aδ and C fibers

31. Botulinum toxin relaxes detrusor muscle tone by:
    a. antagonizing vanilloid receptors.
    b. blocking synaptosome-associated membrane receptor (SNARE) proteins.
    c. enhancing nitric oxide release.
    d. presynaptic neurovesical reuptake inhibition.
    e. postsynaptic neurovesical antagonist.

32. Resiniferatoxin and capsaicin act on a C-fiber sensory nerve as:
    a. TRPM8 receptor agonists.
    b. TRPM8 receptor antagonists.
    c. TRPV1 receptor agonists.
    d. TRPV1 receptor antagonists.
    e. TRPM1 receptor antagonists.

33. Experimental models of chronic partial obstruction of the urethra commonly induce:
    a. increased muscle hypertrophy.
    b. decreased denervation supersensitivity.

c. decreased nerve growth factors.
d. increased myofilaments.
e. decreased detrusor overactivity.

34. Experimental models of chronic bladder inflammation induce:
    a. increased threshold for bladder afferent nerve.
    b. decreased neurotrophic factors.
    c. increased myofilaments.
    d. decreased expression of the early-immediate gene c-FOS in the lumbosacral spinal cord.
    e. decreased prostaglandins in urine and the bladder wall.

ANSWERS

1. **b. Somatic/Somatic.** Sacral-evoked response testing or measurement of sacral latency is accomplished by electrical stimulation of the skin of the penis while recording activity of the bulbocavernosus muscle. Both the afferent and efferent limbs of this reflex arc are somatic nerves. At present, no clinically validated neurophysiologic study exists that directly measures nerve conduction over autonomic nerves which supply the lower urinary tract or penis but research is underway using electrodes mounted on catheters using low- and high-frequency stimulation to assess conduction in myelinated and unmyelinated afferent nerve fibers.

2. **c. a cell membrane is preferentially permeable to K^+.** The tendency of K^+ is to move from the inside of the cell where it is more concentrated to the outside of the cell membrane. This outward migration of potassium creates an electrical gradient across the cell membrane with the inside of the cell membrane being negative with respect to the outside.

3. **c. detrusor overactivity with detrusor-sphincter dyssynergia.** After spinal cord injury (SCI), patients generally develop a spinal shock phase that lasts approximately 4 weeks. During spinal shock, the detrusor is areflexic. In patients with complete high SCI, the long-term urodynamic manifestation is most commonly neurogenic detrusor overactivity with detrusor-sphincter dyssynergia. Incomplete SCI generally demonstrates neurogenic detrusor overactivity with or without detrusor-sphincter dyssynergia. In up to 10% to 15% of cervical SCI, acontractile detrusor may be a permanent finding. The variability of urodynamic findings in SCI emphasizes the need for careful urodynamic evaluation and follow-up in all SCI patients.

4. **b. nifedipine.** Phenylephrine is an α-adrenergic agonist; acetylcholine is a muscarinic cholinergic agonist; and substance P is a tachykinin. All three agents stimulate smooth muscle contractility. Propranolol is a β-adrenergic antagonist and blocks the inhibitory effects of β-adrenergic agonists such as isoproterenol. Nifedipine is a calcium channel blocker and inhibits the inward movement of calcium across the cell membrane that is needed for the upstroke of the smooth muscle action potential and for supplying the calcium that is required for contractility.

5. **e. degradation of cGMP.** cGMP is a second messenger for nitric oxide that activates protein kinases promoting smooth muscle relaxation. cGMP is degraded to GMP by phosphodiesterase. A phosphodiesterase inhibitor potentiates the effect of cGMP. Ca^{2+} binding to calmodulin

is the first step in the initiation of smooth muscle contraction that activates myosin light-chain kinase.

6. **c. detrusor areflexia.** Sacral level spinal injury most commonly results in cauda equina injury. This lower motor neuron injury presents as paralysis of bladder. Only a minority of patients with detrusor areflexia have decreased detrusor compliance.

7. **e. bladder wall viscoelasticity.** The elastic and viscoelastic properties of the bladder are the main determinate of compliance during filling. Although neurogenic influences may be operative in late stages of filling, it is clear these passive properties are the main determinate of the pressure/volume curve. When these properties are destroyed, as in fibrosis of the bladder wall, markedly decreased compliance occurs.

8. **d. increased intravesical pressure.** The Laplace law states that there is a direct relationship between wall tension (T) and intravesical pressure (P) and bladder size (R = radius). $T = P \times R/2$. Large increases in intravesical pressure, especially a hypertrophic, small-capacity bladder, can dramatically elevate bladder wall tension.

9. **a. Acetylcholine.** All preganglionic efferent autonomic fibers release acetylcholine, whether or not they are anatomically parasympathetic or sympathetic. The term cholinergic refers to all those receptor sites where acetylcholine is a primary neurotransmitter, including the autonomic ganglion cells, neuromuscular junctions of somatic nerve fibers, and the junction of all postganglionic parasympathetic fibers. Cholinergic receptor sites are divided into two major classes: muscarinic and nicotinic. Muscarinic sites include all autonomic effector cells. The term nicotinic is applied to the receptor sites on autonomic ganglia, such as those referred to in this question and the motor end plates of skeletal muscle.

10. **d. upper motor lesions with spastic sphincter.** The pudendal nerve innervates the striated muscle sphincter. Temporary [lidocaine] or permanent block [alcohol] of the pudendal nerve may inhibit detrusor-sphincter dyssynergia. This form of treatment has not been popular, however, because complete bilateral blockade of the pudendal nerves is not easy and has the side effect of impotence.

11. **d. norepinephrine.** Postganglionic sympathetic nerves are traditionally noradrenergic and release norepinephrine. Other substances released include neuropeptide Y (NPY) and adenosine triphosphate (ATP). Vasoactive intestinal polypeptide (VIP) often coexists with acetylcholine in parasympathetic postganglionics. However, "sympathetic" does not ALWAYS mean "noradrenergic" because in some tissues (e.g., sweat glands) sympathetics release acetylcholine.

12. **d. pons.** The center for integration and coordination of bladder and urethral activity during voiding is located in the pons (the pontine micturition center), based on animal electrophysiology studies and studying lesion locations or PET scans in humans. The basal ganglia and medulla seem to be involved in modulation of detrusor activity and perhaps in facilitation of detrusor contractility but not integration of bladder and urethral response.

13. **c. viscoelastic properties of the bladder.** Sudden stretch of detrusor muscle strips (in-vivo preparations or human bladder) during cystometry causes a sudden rise in pressure that is entirely due to passive viscoelastic properties of the bladder. Clinically, this rise in pressure may stimulate a detrusor contraction. Because the phenomenon is a passive one, it does not require intact innervation.

14. **c. relaxation of the external striated sphincter.** Synchronous pressure/flow/EMG studies have demonstrated that the initiation of micturition reflex is characterized by a sudden and complete relaxation of the striated external sphincter followed by detrusor contraction, opening of the bladder neck, and uroflow.

15. **d. C-fiber afferents.** Capsaicin inhibits C-fiber afferent activity, because vanilloid receptors that bind to capsaicin are predominantly located in C fibers. Although there are animal studies of capsaicin blockade of bladder inflammation, clinical data are scant. Only uncontrolled trials suggest that bladder hypersensitivity and pain are mediated by C-fiber afferents and that the symptoms are improved with intravesical capsaicin therapy.

16. **d. Pelvic and hypogastric.** Bladder pain due to overdistention is mediated by the hypogastric nerve. Bladder pain from inflammatory stimuli is mediated by pelvic nerves.

17. **e. Myosin.** Phosphorylation of myosin by myosin light-chain kinase results in smooth muscle contraction. This process is critical for contraction of the ureter, vas deferens, bladder, and corporeal smooth muscle.

18. **e. Triggers bladder pain.** Interstitial cells or myofibroblasts have been identified in the suburethral space and are unique cells linked by gap junctions. Interstitial cells may play a pacemaker role in initiating or participating in the generation or propagation of spontaneous bladder activity. Interstitial cells have not been linked with triggering bladder pain.

19. **b. nitric oxide from parasympathetics.** During voiding, active contraction of the bladder occurs through parasympathetically mediated cholinergic contraction. In addition, parasympathetically mediated urethral smooth and striated muscle relaxation occurs. An abundance of experimental data indicates that nitric oxide is responsible for this relaxation.

20. **a. Calcium.** Influx of calcium results in action potential generation in smooth muscle cells.

21. **d. Increased type III collagen.** An increase in type III collagen results in decreased bladder compliance.

22. **d. M_2 and M_3.** Binding of acetylcholine to predominately M_2 and M_3 muscarinic receptors results in bladder contraction.

23. **c. $β_3$.** Stimulation of $β_3$-adrenergic receptors in the human detrusor results in the direct relaxation of the detrusor smooth muscle. β-Adrenoceptor–mediated relaxation of the human detrusor was not blocked by selective $β_1$ and/or $β_2$-adrenoceptor antagonists but is blocked by selective $β_3$-adrenoceptor antagonists. $β_3$ agonists are under evaluation for treatment of the overactive bladder.

24. **a. Afferent.** Substance P is located exclusively in afferent nerves.

25. **d. Estrogen.** Only estrogen has been shown to increase the number of α-adrenergic receptors. However, there is no convincing clinical evidence that estrogen supplementation benefits stress or urgency urinary incontinence.

26. **d. Glutamate.** Glutamate plays an essential role as an excitatory neurotransmitter in the central nervous system to facilitate voiding. Glutamate is facilitatory at the levels of bladder afferents, spinal neurons, descending projection from the pons, within the pons, and in the brain.

27. **e. Serotonin.** Serotonin acts as a neurotransmitter in the spinal cord to inhibit micturition.
28. **e. Inhibit bladder contraction.** Delta and mu opioid receptors in the spinal cord and the brain regulate micturition threshold volume and inhibit bladder contraction.
29. **b. Myelinated Aδ afferent nerves.** Aδ myelinated pelvic nerve afferents are responsible for triggering normal micturition. C fibers are unmyelinated afferent nerves.
30. **c. C fiber.** After spinal cord transection, unmyelinated C-fiber afferents in the pelvic nerve trigger a spinal micturition reflex in the cat. In the rat, C-fiber afferents are responsible for nonvoiding uninhibited bladder contractions, although voiding bladder contractions are still dependent on Aδ-fiber afferent nerves.
31. **b. blocking synaptosome-associated membrane receptor SNARE proteins.** Botulinum toxin inhibits neurotransmitter release at the neuromuscular junction by cleaving the neuron-terminal cytosolic translocation SNARE proteins, thus preventing neurovesical fusion with the plasma membrane.
32. **c. TRPV1 receptor agonists.** Capsaicin and its ultrapotent analog resiniferatoxin (RTX) are vanilloids that stimulate and desensitize a specific population of sensory nerves (unmyelinated C fibers) to produce pain and release neuropeptides. Capsaicin and RTX activate nociceptive sensory nerve fibers through an ion channel known as TRPV1. The TRPV1 receptor is a nonselective cation channel with a limited selectivity for calcium. Capsaicin and RTX are TRPV1 receptor agonists that induce slowly activating but persistent currents in dorsal root ganglia (DRG) neurons. This induces a prolonged desensitization of the C fiber.
33. **a. increased muscle hypertrophy.** After chronic partial obstruction of the urethra, the bladder enlarges and the growth is mainly accounted for by muscle hypertrophy. Gap junctions between hypertrophic muscle cells are virtually absent. Bladder outlet obstruction often produces detrusor overactivity. Obstruction-induced detrusor overactivity with irritative voiding symptoms has been attributed to denervation supersensitivity, because increased contractile responses of the bladder smooth muscle to cholinergic agonists and electrical stimulation have been observed. Nerve growth factor (NGF) content is increased in obstructed bladders in animals and in humans.
34. **a. increased threshold for bladder afferent nerve.** Inflammation of the urinary bladder is accompanied by a reduction in the threshold for bladder afferents. After chemical or mechanical inflammation of the rat urinary bladder, increased expression of the early-immediate gene c-FOS has been detected within the lumbosacral spinal cord. Cyclooxygenase 2 and prostaglandins are increased in the bladder and afferent neurons in lumbosacral DRG, innervating the bladder with bladder inflammation. With use of a rat model of chronic cystitis, increased expression of neurotrophic growth factors such as NGF occurs. Studies also demonstrated that exogenous NGF can induce bladder nociceptive responses and bladder overactivity in rats when it is applied acutely into the bladder lumen or chronically to the bladder wall or intrathecal space.

Additional Study Points

1. The bladder has two parts: the body, which lies above the ureteral orifices, and the base, consisting of a trigone and bladder neck.
2. In men, the bladder neck is rich in adrenergic innervation. In women, there is little adrenergic innervation at the bladder neck.
3. A very low outflow resistance at the bladder neck can result in high flow rates with low detrusor pressures. This is seen in women.
4. Smooth muscle is able to adjust its length over a much wider range than can skeletal muscle. Thus an empty bladder has a small intravesical space despite the amount of smooth muscle it contains.
5. Bladder mucosal blood flow is reduced by distention.
6. In noncompliant bladders, there is a greater-than-normal decrease in blood flow with distention.
7. The GAG layer may have importance in bacterial anti-adherence and prevention of urothelial damage by large macromolecules, but there is no evidence that the glycosaminoglycan (GAG) layer acts as a primary epithelial barrier.
8. The umbrella cells are the primary barrier between lumen and bladder submucosa.
9. The striated urethral sphincter is horseshoe shaped, with the opening facing dorsal.
10. The vascular filling of the urethra lamina propria is an important mechanism of urethra coaptation, which contributes to urinary continence.
11. The hammock hypothesis of urinary continence suggests that the urethra has a fixed dorsal surface due to its attachments to the pubis, pelvic muscles, and fascia, which allows ventral wall compression of the urethra against the fixed dorsal wall.
12. The external urethral sphincter has two parts: the periurethral striated muscle of the pelvic floor musculature and the striated muscle of the sphincter itself.
13. Pelvic parasympathetic nerves excite the bladder and relax the urethra.
14. Sympathetic nerves inhibit the bladder body and excite the bladder base and urethra.
15. The pudendal nerve excites the external urethral sphincter.
16. Irritation of one organ can affect another; colonic irritation can sensitize the bladder.
17. During chronic inflammation of the bladder, there is recruitment of C fibers, and a new functional pathway develops.
18. In women with mixed incontinence, leakage of urine into the urethra can stimulate afferents and induce detrusor overactivity. Thus when the incontinence is repaired and leakage of urine into the urethra is prevented during filling, overactivity of the detrusor in some patients disappears.
19. Neonatal pathways responsible for bladder overactivity do not disappear with growth and development, but rather there is increasing cerebral maturation that actively inhibits them.

20. The ice-water test has been used as a diagnostic tool to detect hyperexcitability of C-fiber bladder afferent pathways.

21. Botulinum neurotoxin inhibits the release of acetylcholine from efferent nerve terminals, suppresses afferent activity, and inhibits the release of neurotransmitters, such as substance P and CGRP from afferent nerves.

22. Cystitis may induce chemical changes in the spinal cord.

23. Aging appears to induce hypofunction of the bladder and urethra due, in part, to reduced activity of efferent and afferent nerves innervating the bladder.

Pathophysiology and Classification of Lower Urinary Tract Dysfunction: Overview

Alan J. Wein, MD, PhD (Hon)

QUESTIONS

1. Which of the following best describes normal bladder behavior during the filling-storage phase of the micturition cycle?
   a. Low compliance due to elastic properties
   b. High compliance due to elastic properties
   c. Low compliance due to elastic and viscoelastic properties
   d. High compliance due to elastic and viscoelastic properties
   e. High compliance due to a low relaxation coefficient of the lamina propria

2. A patient who has significantly and urodynamically dangerous decreased compliance because of a replacement by collagen of other components of the stroma is generally best managed by:
   a. pharmacologic regimen.
   b. hydraulic distention.
   c. nerve section.
   d. augmentation cystoplasty.
   e. neuromodulation.

3. The "guarding reflex" refers to the:
   a. abrupt increase in striated sphincter activity seen with a cough during normal bladder filling/storage.
   b. spinal sympathetic inhibition of parasympathetic ganglion activity.
   c. gradual increase in striated sphincter activity seen during normal bladder filling/storage.
   d. gradual inhibition of the pontine-mesencephalic micturition center by the cerebral cortex during normal bladder filling/storage.
   e. gradual inhibition of the sacral spinal cord ventral nuclei by the pontine-mesencephalic brainstem during normal bladder filling/storage.

4. The primary effect of the spinal sympathetic reflexes that are evoked in animals during bladder filling and that facilitate bladder filling/storage is:
   a. neurally mediated stimulation of the α-adrenergic receptors in the area of the smooth sphincter.
   b. neurally mediated stimulation of the β-adrenergic receptors in the bladder body smooth musculature.
   c. direct inhibition of detrusor motor neurons in the sacral spinal cord.
   d. neurally mediated inhibition of cholinergic receptors in the area of the bladder body.
   e. neurally mediated sympathetic modulation of cholinergic ganglionic transmission.

5. The organizational center for the micturition reflex in an intact neural axis is the:
   a. pontine mesencephalic formation in the brainstem.
   b. frontal area of the cerebral cortex.
   c. parietal area of the cerebral cortex.
   d. cerebellum.
   e. sacral spinal cord.

6. Involuntary bladder contractions are most commonly seen in association with:
   a. sacral spinal cord neurologic disease or injury.
   b. infrasacral neurologic disease or injury.
   c. suprasacral neurologic disease or injury.
   d. peripheral nerve neurologic disease or injury.
   e. interstitial cystitis.

7. Using the functional classification system, the usual lower urinary tract dysfunction seen after a stroke would be categorized as:
   a. failure to store because of the bladder (overactivity).
   b. combined deficit (failure to store because of the bladder, failure to empty because of striated sphincter dyssynergy).
   c. combined deficit (failure to store because of the bladder, failure to empty because of a nonrelaxing outlet).
   d. failure to store because of the bladder (hypersensitivity).
   e. failure to store because of the outlet.

8. In the International Continence Society (ICS) classification system, the disorder described in question 7 would be characterized as:

a. during storage, overactive neurogenic detrusor activity increased sensation, low bladder capacity, and incompetent urethral closure mechanism and during voiding, normal detrusor activity and abnormal urethral function (dysfunctional voiding).

b. during storage, normal detrusor function, increased sensation, low bladder capacity, and normal urethral closure mechanism and during voiding, normal detrusor activity and abnormal urethral function (dysfunctional voiding).

c. during storage, overactive neurogenic detrusor activity, normal sensation, normal bladder capacity, and incompetent urethral closure mechanism and during voiding, normal detrusor activity and normal urethral function.

d. during storage, stable detrusor activity, reduced sensation, low bladder capacity, and normal urethral closure mechanism and during emptying, normal detrusor activity and abnormal urethral function (dysfunctional voiding).

e. during storage, overactive neurogenic detrusor activity, normal sensation, low capacity, normal compliance, and normal urethral closure function and during emptying, normal detrusor activity and normal urethral function.

9. In the ICS current terminology, "detrusor hyperreflexia" has been replaced by:

a. detrusor instability.

b. idiopathic detrusor overactivity.

c. hyperactive bladder.

d. neurogenic detrusor overactivity.

e. neurogenic detrusor instability.

10. In the Krane-Siroky urodynamic classification system, a patient with postcerebrovascular accident voiding dysfunction characterized by urgency, frequency, and urge incontinence would most commonly be characterized as having:

a. detrusor areflexia, striated sphincter dyssynergia, and smooth sphincter dyssynergia.

b. detrusor hyperreflexia, striated sphincter synergia, and smooth sphincter dyssynergia.

c. detrusor hyperreflexia, striated sphincter dyssynergia, and smooth sphincter synergia.

d. detrusor areflexia, striated sphincter synergia, and smooth sphincter dyssynergia.

e. detrusor hyperreflexia, striated sphincter synergia, and smooth sphincter dyssynergia.

11. In the Lapides classification system, a patient with postcerebrovascular accident voiding dysfunction characterized by urgency, frequency, and urge incontinence would most commonly be characterized as having:

a. sensory neurogenic bladder.

b. motor paralytic bladder.

c. uninhibited neurogenic bladder.

d. reflex neurogenic bladder.

e. autonomous neurogenic bladder.

12. A reflex neurogenic bladder, as described in the Lapides system classification, is characteristically seen in which of the following?

a. Traumatic spinal cord injury between the sacral spinal cord and the brainstem

b. Traumatic spinal cord injury between the sacral spinal cord and conus medullaris

c. Cerebrovascular accident and insulin-dependent diabetes mellitus

d. Non-insulin-dependent diabetes mellitus

e. Multiple sclerosis

13. In the Bors-Comarr system of classification, the term unbalanced, when applied to a patient with an upper motor neuron (UMN) lesion, implies:

a. cerebellar lesion.

b. involuntary bladder contractions during filling.

c. areflexic bladder.

d. decreased bladder compliance during filling.

e. sphincter dyssynergia.

14. In the Bors-Comarr system, a patient with postcerebrovascular accident voiding dysfunction characterized by urgency, frequency, and urge incontinence would most commonly be characterized as having:

a. a UMN lesion, complete, and balanced.

b. a UMN lesion, complete, and imbalanced.

c. a lower motor neuron (LMN) lesion, complete, and imbalanced.

d. an LMN lesion, incomplete, and balanced.

e. a UMN lesion/LMN lesion, complete, and balanced.

15. Which of the following is an absolute requirement for a patient to be included in the symptom syndrome of overactive bladder (multiple answers possible)?

a. Nocturia

b. Urinary frequency

c. Urgency

d. Urgency incontinence

e. Detrusor overactivity

16. Which of the following pathophysiologic factors is (are) shared by men and women with urinary incontinence (failure to store) due to outlet underactivity (multiple answers possible):

a. Bladder neck hypermobility

b. Intrinsic sphincter dysfunction

c. Proximal urethral hypermobility

d. Nonrelaxing striated sphincter

e. Bladder neck dysfunction

ANSWERS

1. **d. High compliance due to elastic and viscoelastic properties.** The normal adult bladder response to filling at a physiologic rate is an almost imperceptible change in intravesical pressure. During at least the initial stages of bladder filling, after unfolding of the bladder wall from its collapsed state, this high compliance ($\Delta V/\Delta P$) of the bladder is due primarily to its elastic and viscoelastic properties. Elasticity allows the constituents of the bladder wall to

stretch to a certain degree without any increase in tension. Viscoelasticity allows stretch to induce a rise in tension followed by a decay (stress relaxation) when the filling (stretch stimulus) slows or stops.

2. **d. augmentation cystoplasty.** The viscoelastic properties of the stroma (bladder wall less smooth muscle and epithelium) and the urodynamically relaxed detrusor muscle account for the passive mechanical properties and normal bladder compliance seen during filling. The main components of stroma are collagen and elastin. When the collagen component increases, compliance decreases. This can occur with various types of injury, chronic inflammation, bladder outlet obstruction, and neurologic decentralization. Once decreased compliance occurs because of a replacement by collagen of other components of the stroma, it is generally unresponsive to pharmacologic manipulation, hydraulic distention, or nerve section. Most often, under those circumstances, augmentation cystoplasty is required to achieve satisfactory reservoir function.

3. **c. gradual increase in striated sphincter activity seen during normal bladder filling/storage.** There is a gradual increase in urethral pressure during bladder filling, contributed to by at least the striated sphincter element and perhaps by the smooth sphincteric element as well. The rise in urethral pressure seen during the filling/storage phase of micturition can be correlated with an increase in efferent pudendal nerve impulse frequency and in electromyographic activity of the periurethral striated musculature. This constitutes the efferent limb of a spinal somatic reflex, the so-called guarding reflex, which results in a gradual increase in striated sphincter activity during normal bladder filling and storage.

4. **e. neurally mediated sympathetic modulation of cholinergic ganglionic transmission.** Does the nervous system affect the normal bladder response to filling? At a certain level of bladder filling, spinal sympathetic reflexes facilitatory to bladder filling/storage are clearly evoked in animals, a concept developed over the years by deGroat and colleagues, who have also cited indirect evidence to support such a role in humans. This inhibitory effect is thought to be mediated primarily by sympathetic modulation of cholinergic ganglionic transmission. Through this reflex mechanism, two other possibilities exist for promoting filling/storage. One is neurally mediated stimulation of the predominantly α-adrenergic receptors in the area of the smooth sphincter, the net result of which would be to cause an increase in resistance in that area. The second is neurally mediated stimulation of the predominantly β-adrenergic receptors (inhibitory) in the bladder body smooth musculature, which would cause a decrease in bladder wall tension. McGuire has also cited evidence for direct inhibition of detrusor motor neurons in the sacral spinal cord during bladder filling that is due to increased afferent pudendal nerve activity generated by receptors in the striated sphincter. Good evidence also seems to exist to support a tonic inhibitory effect of other neurotransmitters on the micturition reflex at various levels of the neural axis. Bladder filling and consequent wall distention may also release autocrine-like factors that influence contractility (e.g., nitric oxide, prostaglandins, peptides).

5. **a. pontine mesencephalic formation in the brainstem.** Although the origin of the parasympathetic neural outflow to the bladder, the pelvic nerve, is in the sacral spinal cord, the actual organizational center for the micturition reflex in an intact neural axis is in the brainstem, and the complete neural circuit for normal micturition includes the ascending and descending spinal cord pathways to and from this area and the facilitatory and inhibitory influences from other parts of the brain.

6. **c. suprasacral neurologic disease or injury.** Involuntary contractions (IVCs) are most commonly seen associated with suprasacral neurologic disease or after suprasacral neurologic injury; however, they may also be associated with aging, inflammation, or irritation of the bladder wall, bladder outlet obstruction, or stress urinary incontinence, or they may be idiopathic.

7. **a. failure to store because of the bladder (overactivity).** The classic symptoms of poststroke lower urinary tract dysfunction are urgency, frequency, and possible urgency incontinence. The urodynamic findings are generally detrusor overactivity during filling/storage with normal sensation and synergic sphincter activity during voluntary or involuntary emptying, unless the patient attempts to inhibit the involuntary contractions with striated sphincter contraction. This translates simply in the functional system to a failure to store because of the bladder. See Tables 61–1 and 61–5 in *Campbell-Walsh Urology, 10th Edition.*

8. **e. during storage, overactive neurogenic detrusor activity, normal sensation, low capacity, normal compliance, and normal urethral closure function and during emptying, normal detrusor activity and normal urethral function.** The micturition dysfunction of a stroke patient with urgency incontinence would most likely be classified during storage as overactive neurogenic detrusor function, normal sensation, low capacity, normal compliance, and normal urethral closure function. During voiding, the dysfunction would be classified as normal detrusor activity and normal urethral function, assuming that no anatomic obstruction existed. See Table 61–6 in *Campbell-Walsh Urology, 10th Edition.*

9. **d. neurogenic detrusor overactivity.** The Standardization Subcommittee of the ICS made some changes in definitions of terms (published as a committee report in 2002). One change was to eliminate the terms *detrusor hyperreflexia* and *instability* and replace them with *neurogenic detrusor overactivity* and *idiopathic detrusor over-activity* (Abrams P et al, 2003).*

10. **b. detrusor hyperreflexia, striated sphincter synergia, and smooth sphincter dyssynergia.** When exact urodynamic classification is possible, this system provides a truly precise description of the voiding dysfunction that occurs. If a normal or hyperreflexic detrusor exists with coordinated smooth and striated sphincter function and without anatomic obstruction, normal bladder emptying should occur.

    Detrusor hyperreflexia is most commonly associated with neurologic lesions above the sacral spinal cord. Striated sphincter dyssynergia is most common after complete suprasacral spinal cord injury, following the period of spinal shock. Smooth sphincter dyssynergia is seen most classically in autonomic hyperreflexia, when it is characteristically

---

*Sources referenced can be found in *Campbell-Walsh Urology, 10th Edition,* on the Expert Consult website.

associated with detrusor hyperreflexia and striated sphincter dyssynergia.

Detrusor areflexia may be secondary to bladder muscle decompensation or to various other conditions that produce inhibition at the level of the brainstem micturition center, sacral spinal cord, bladder ganglia, or bladder smooth muscle. Patients with a voiding dysfunction secondary to detrusor areflexia generally attempt bladder emptying by abdominal straining, and their continence status and the efficiency of their emptying efforts are determined by the status of their smooth and striated sphincter mechanisms.

11. **c. uninhibited neurogenic bladder.** Lapides contributed significantly to the classification and care of the patient with neuropathic voiding dysfunction by slightly modifying and popularizing a system originally proposed by McLellan in 1939. Lapides' classification differs from that of McLellan's in only one respect, and that is the division of the group "atonic neurogenic bladder" into sensory neurogenic bladder and motor neurogenic bladder. This remains one of the most familiar systems to urologists and nonurologists because it describes in recognizable shorthand the clinical and cystometric conditions of many types of neurogenic voiding dysfunction. An uninhibited neurogenic bladder was described originally as resulting from injury or disease to the "corticoregulatory tract." The sacral spinal cord was presumed to be the micturition reflex center, and this corticoregulatory tract was believed to normally exert an inhibitory influence on the sacral micturition reflex center. A destructive lesion in this tract would then result in overfacilitation of the micturition reflex. Cerebrovascular accident, brain or spinal cord tumor, Parkinson disease, and demyelinating disease were listed as the most common causes in this category. The voiding dysfunction is most often characterized symptomatically by frequency, urgency, and urge incontinence, as well as urodynamically by normal sensation with IVC at low filling volumes. Residual urine is characteristically low unless anatomic outlet obstruction or true smooth or striated sphincter dyssynergia occurs. The patient can generally initiate a bladder contraction voluntarily but is often unable to do so during cystometry because sufficient urine storage cannot occur before the IVC is stimulated.

12. **a. Traumatic spinal cord injury between the sacral spinal cord and the brainstem.** Reflex neurogenic bladder describes the post–spinal shock condition that exists after complete interruption of the sensory and motor pathways between the sacral spinal cord and the brainstem. Most commonly, this occurs in traumatic spinal cord injury and transverse myelitis, but it may occur with extensive demyelinating disease or any process that produces significant spinal cord destruction as well. Typically, there is no bladder sensation and there is inability to initiate voluntary micturition. Incontinence without sensation generally results because of low-volume IVC. Striated sphincter dyssynergia is the rule. This type of lesion is essentially equivalent to a complete UMN lesion in the Bors-Comarr system.

13. **e. sphincter dyssynergia.** This system applies only to patients with neurologic dysfunction and considers three factors: (1) the anatomic localization of the lesion; (2) the neurologic completeness or incompleteness of the lesion; and (3) a designation as to whether lower urinary tract

function is balanced or unbalanced. The latter terms are based solely on the percentage of residual urine relative to bladder capacity. Unbalanced signifies the presence of greater than 20% residual urine in a patient with a UMN lesion or 10% in a patient with an LMN lesion. This relative residual urine volume was ideally meant to imply coordination (synergy) or dyssynergia between the smooth and striated sphincters of the outlet and the bladder, during bladder contraction or during attempted micturition by abdominal straining or the Credé method.

14. **a. a UMN lesion, complete, and balanced.** In this system, UMN bladder refers to the pattern of micturition that results from an injury to the suprasacral spinal cord after the period of spinal shock has passed, assuming that the sacral spinal cord and the sacral nerve roots are intact and that the pelvic and pudendal nerve reflexes are intact. LMN bladder refers to the pattern resulting if the sacral spinal cord or sacral roots are damaged and the reflex pattern through the autonomic and somatic nerves that emanate from these segments is absent. This system implies that if skeletal muscle spasticity exists below the level of the lesion, the lesion is above the sacral spinal cord and is by definition a UMN lesion. This type of lesion is characterized by IVCs during filling. If flaccidity of the skeletal musculature below the level of a lesion exists, an LMN lesion is assumed to exist, implying detrusor areflexia. Exceptions occur and are classified in a mixed lesion group characterized either by IVCs with a flaccid paralysis below the level of the lesion or by detrusor areflexia with spasticity or normal skeletal muscle tone neurologically below the lesion level. UMN lesion, complete, and imbalanced implies a neurologically complete lesion above the level of the sacral spinal cord that results in skeletal muscle spasticity below the level of the injury. IVC occurs during filling, but a residual urine volume of greater than 20% of the bladder capacity is left after bladder contraction, implying obstruction in the area of the bladder outlet during the involuntary detrusor contraction. This obstruction is generally due to striated sphincter dyssynergia, typically occurring in patients who are paraplegic and quadriplegic with lesions between the cervical and the sacral spinal cord. Smooth sphincter dyssynergia may be seen as well in patients with lesions above the level of T6, usually in association with autonomic hyperreflexia. LMN lesion, complete, and imbalanced implies a neurologically complete lesion at the level of the sacral spinal cord or of the sacral roots, resulting in skeletal muscle flaccidity below that level. Detrusor areflexia results, and whatever measures the patient may use to increase intravesical pressure during attempted voiding are not sufficient to decrease residual urine to less than 10% of bladder capacity.

15. **c. Urgency.** Overactive bladder is defined (ICS) as urgency, with or without urinary urgency incontinence, usually with frequency and nocturia. One third of the patients have incontinence, but two thirds do not. Frequency and nocturia are usually but not always present. Detrusor overactivity is a urodynamic term indicating an involuntary bladder contraction. Urgency may or may not be associated with DO on a urodynamic study.

16. **b. Intrinsic sphincter dysfunction.** Failure to store because of outlet underactivity in the female is due to a combination of a failure of support, generally accompanied by hypermobility of the bladder outlet and intrinsic

sphincter dysfunction. It is impossible to have effort-related incontinence in the woman without some element of ISD. Outlet-related incontinence in the male is most commonly seen after prostatectomy, and there is no pathophysiologic factor of hypermobility involved. The condition is essentially intrinsic sphincter dysfunction. A nonrelaxing striated sphincter would not produce urinary incontinence, nor would bladder neck dysfunction.

Additional Study Points

1. Please see Table 61–2 in *Campbell-Walsh Urology, 10th Edition*.
2. The micturition cycle is divided into two phases: (1) bladder filling/urine storage and (2) bladder empting/voiding.
3. There are two urethral sphincters: (1) the smooth urethral sphincter is the smooth musculature of the bladder neck and proximal urethra; the smooth sphincter is not under voluntary control and (2) the striated sphincter, which has two parts—the striated intramural sphincter called the rhabdosphincter and the external striated sphincter, which is part of the levator musculature; this sphincter is under voluntary control.
4. As collagen content of the bladder wall increases, compliance decreases.
5. There is increased afferent input when inflammation or irritation occurs, causing hypersensitivity to pain.
6. The hammock hypothesis of continence proposes that there is a fixed dorsal portion of the urethra due to fascial attachments against which the ventral aspect of the urethra is compressed.

Urodynamic and Video-Urodynamic Evaluation of the Lower Urinary Tract

Victor W. Nitti, MD

QUESTIONS

1. Indications for urodynamics (UDS) are:
   a. supported by high-quality, level 1 evidence for most conditions.
   b. better defined for men versus women.
   c. best defined by the clinician who has clear-cut reasons for performing the study and who will use the information obtained to guide treatment.
   d. of little value in assessing a patient with neuropathic voiding dysfunction.
   e. a and b.

2. Before performing a UDS study the clinician should:
   a. decide on questions to be answered for a particular patient.
   b. for consistency, be prepared to perform the study the same way, no matter what the circumstances.
   c. prepare patients telling them why the test is being done, how the results may affect treatment, and what to expect during the actual UDS test.
   d. a and c
   e. a, b, and c

3. Which of the following tests do not assess the emptying phase of micturition?
   a. Uroflowmetry
   b. Cystometrogram
   c. Micturitional urethral pressure profile
   d. Postvoid residual volume
   e. Voiding pressure flow study

4. Detrusor pressure:
   a. can be measured directly via a transurethral catheter.
   b. should remain low (near zero) during bladder filling.
   c. rises abruptly and does not return to baseline with detrusor overactivity.
   d. rises before the external sphincter relaxes in normal voluntary micturition.
   e. is characterized by a and b.

5. Detrusor overactivity can be seen in all of the following conditions EXCEPT:
   a. an acontractile bladder.
   b. bladder outlet obstruction.
   c. normal asymptomatic men and women.
   d. spinal cord injury.
   e. overactive bladder.

6. Which of the following is not a UDS risk factor for upper tract damage?
   a. Impaired compliance
   b. Detrusor-external sphincter dyssynergia
   c. Poor emptying with high storage pressures
   d. A high detrusor leak point pressure (>40 cm H_2O)
   e. A high abdominal leak point pressure (>100 cm H_2O)

7. The hallmark of bladder outlet obstruction is:
   a. incomplete bladder emptying.
   b. low pressure, low-flow voiding dynamics.
   c. high pressure, low-flow voiding dynamics.
   d. impaired detrusor contractility.
   e. a and b.

8. The external urethral sphincter should normally:
   a. relax with an involuntary bladder contraction in a neurologically normal person.
   b. relax before a voluntary detrusor contraction in a neurologically normal person.
   c. progressively relax as the bladder fills.
   d. contract when the detrusor contracts in cases of detrusor-external sphincter dyssynergia.
   e. b and d.

9. Video-urodynamics (VUDS) is:
   a. the most precise measure of lower urinary tract function and should be used in all cases where UDS is to be performed.
   b. the only way to assess obstruction in a man.
   c. the procedure of choice for documenting bladder neck dysfunction in men and women.

d. too difficult to perform in spinal cord–injured patients.

e. of no value in the pediatric population.

10. Urethral function tests like abdominal leak point pressure (ALPP) and maximum urethral closure pressure (MUCP):

    a. can precisely define intrinsic sphincter deficiency.

    b. must be done routinely before all surgery for stress incontinence, as supported by the literature.

    c. are the most important part of the UDS assessment of women with stress urinary incontinence.

    d. should not be used as a single factor to grade the severity of incontinence.

    e. are characterized by a and b.

11. The accurate measurement of compliance may be affected by all of the following EXCEPT:

    a. filling rate.

    b. involuntary detrusor contractions.

    c. presence of vesicoureteral reflux.

    d. bladder outlet obstruction.

    e. none of the above.

12. According to the Fourth International Consultation on Incontinence, which of the following is not a recommended role for UDS in clinical practice?

    a. To identify or rule out factors contributing to lower urinary tract dysfunction

    b. To predict consequences of lower urinary tract dysfunction on the upper tract

    c. To distinguish between neuropathic and non-neuropathic voiding dysfunction

    d. To predict the outcome of specific treatments

    e. To confirm the effects of intervention

13. According to the Functional Classification System, the symptom of incontinence may be classified as:

    a. failure to store secondary to an overactive bladder outlet.

    b. failure to empty secondary to an overactive bladder.

    c. failure to store secondary to an underactive bladder outlet.

    d. failure to empty secondary to an underactive bladder outlet.

    e. all of the above.

14. Intra-abdominal pressure can be measured by:

    a. a rectal catheter.

    b. a vaginal catheter.

    c. a bladder catheter.

    d. a and c.

    e. all of the above.

15. For women with stress incontinence, UDS has its most useful role:

    a. in women who are considering surgical correction and have mixed incontinence symptoms or emptying difficulty.

    b. in predicting outcomes of surgery for women with pure stress incontinence.

    c. in predicting the likelihood of voiding dysfunction in women with pure stress incontinence

    d. in predicting outcomes of conservative, nonsurgical treatments for women with mixed incontinence.

    e. in any women considering surgical treatment.

16. The role of UDS in men with lower urinary tract symptoms who are considering surgery for bladder outlet obstruction can best be stated as:

    a. All men who are considering invasive therapy for BOO should have UDS to rule out detrusor overactivity.

    b. There is little role for UDS in predicting outcomes of invasive therapy for BOO.

    c. Almost all evidence for the advantages of UDS before invasive therapy for BOO is level 1 and allows a grade A recommendation in support of its use.

    d. Almost all evidence for the advantages of UDS before invasive therapy for BOO is level 3 and allows a grade B recommendation in support of its use.

    e. Almost all evidence for the advantages of UDS before invasive therapy for BOO is level 3 and allows a grade B recommendation against its use.

ANSWERS

1. **c. best defined by the clinician who has clear-cut reasons for performing the study and who will use the information obtained to guide treatment.** UDS has been used for decades, yet clear-cut, level 1, evidence-based "indications" for its use are surprisingly lacking. There are a number of reasons for this. It is difficult to conduct proper randomized controlled trials on UDS for conditions where lesser levels of evidence and expert opinion strongly suggest clinical utility and where "empiric treatment" is potentially harmful or even life threatening (e.g., neurogenic voiding dysfunction). Additionally, symptoms can be caused by a number of different conditions and it is difficult to study pure or homogeneous patient populations. Given the current state of evidence for UDS studies, what is most important is that the clinician has clear-cut reasons for performing the study and that the information obtained will be used to guide treatment of the patient. Despite having established nomograms for BOO in men, the indications for UDS in men are no more clear-cut than they are in women. UDS probably has its most important role in the diagnosis and management of patients with neuropathic voiding dysfunction.

2. **d. a and c.** All patients are not alike and therefore each urodynamic evaluation may be different depending on the information needed to answer the questions relevant to a particular patient. Therefore in many cases the study must be customized to answer specific questions for a given patient.

3. **b. Cystometrogram.** All of the tests assess some aspect of bladder emptying except the cystometrogram, which assesses the bladder's response to filling only.

4. **b. should remain low (near zero) during bladder filling.** Detrusor pressure normally remains low during filling as the bladder is highly compliant. It cannot be measured directly with a transurethral catheter but must be obtained via subtraction of abdominal pressure from vesical pressure. With detrusor overactivity, pressure usually returns to baseline after the involuntary contraction abates.

5. **a. an acontractile bladder.** Detrusor overactivity has been reported in all conditions mentioned, even in

asymptomatic men and women. An acontractile detrusor, by definition, should not display any contractility.

6. **e. A high abdominal leak point pressure (>100 cm H$_2$O).** Upper tract damage occurs as a result of high intravesical pressures during storage. Abdominal leak point pressure measures outlet resistance and in continent patients cannot be demonstrated (i.e., it is well over 100 cm H$_2$O).

7. **c. high pressure, low-flow voiding dynamics.** Obstruction is defined by high-pressure, low-flow voiding. It may or may not be accompanied by incomplete bladder emptying. Impaired detrusor contractility may sometimes, but not always, be a long-term consequence of obstruction.

8. **e. b and d.** In a neurologically normal person the external sphincter progressively contracts with bladder filling and will also contract during an involuntary bladder contraction (guarding reflex). External sphincter relaxation is the first step in the micturition cycle and precedes the detrusor contraction. In DESD the external sphincter contracts when the detrusor contracts.

9. **c. the procedure of choice for documenting bladder neck dysfunction in men and women.** Although VUDS provides the most precise evaluation of voiding function and dysfunction and is particularly useful when anatomic structure and function are important, it is neither practical nor necessary for all centers to have VUDS capabilities. VUDS is useful for a number of conditions when an accurate diagnosis cannot otherwise be obtained (e.g., by conventional UDS) including complicated voiding dysfunction or known or suspected neuropathic voiding dysfunction (adults and children), unexplained urinary retention in women, prior radical pelvic surgery, urinary diversion, prerenal or postrenal transplant, or prior pelvic radiation. VUDS is the procedure of choice for documenting bladder neck dysfunction in men and women.

10. **d. should not be used as a single factor to grade the severity of incontinence.** Urethral function tests like ALPP and MUCP have not been shown to be consistently useful in defining "ISD" or outcomes of treatments for SUI.

They may be useful for some clinicians but are by no means mandatory. According to the International Continence Society, "Urethral function measurements of leak point pressures and urethral closure pressures are not used as a single factor to grade the severity of incontinence."

11. **d. bladder outlet obstruction.** Bladder outlet obstruction can cause a decrease in compliance but should not affect its accurate measurement. Filling rate and IDCs can make compliance look worse than it actually is, and pop-off mechanisms like vesicoureteral reflux can make compliance look better than it actually is.

12. **c. To distinguish between neuropathic and non-neuropathic voiding dysfunction.** Although UDS can certainly help to determine the effects of neurologic and non-neurologic conditions on the lower urinary tract, it is not meant to specifically diagnose neurologic diseases.

13. **c. failure to store secondary to an underactive bladder outlet.** Incontinence is a symptom caused by failure to store urine. It can be caused by an overactive bladder and/or an underactive bladder outlet.

14. **e. all of the above.** Rectal, vaginal, and total vesical pressure are all ways of measuring abdominal pressure. Total vesical pressure equals intra-abdominal pressure in the absence of a detrusor contraction.

15. **a. in women who are considering surgical correction and have mixed incontinence symptoms or emptying difficulty.** The value of UDS in stress incontinence has not been clearly established on the basis of level 1 evidence, although there is increasing evidence that it is less useful in predicting any outcomes for women with pure SUI and no voiding difficulties.

16. **d. Almost all evidence for the advantages of UDS before invasive therapy for BOO is level 3 and allows a grade B recommendation in support of its use.** Although there is not a large body of level 1 evidence for the use of UDS before invasive treatment for BOO, almost all studies provide good-quality, retrospective "case-control studies" or "case series" that allow a grade B recommendation in support of its use.

Additional Study Points

1. UDS is performed in an unnatural setting and therefore does not always predict the findings with normal activity.
2. Normal uroflow is a bell-shaped curve.
3. EMG patch electrodes measure perineal muscle function with the assumption that it is reflective of urethral external sphincter function.
4. To specifically measure external sphincter function, needle electrodes must be used.
5. Mean values for compliance are 40 to 120 mL/cm of water.
6. Measurement of compliance is difficult to interpret; therefore pressures during filling are more often used to predict outcome.
7. There are two types of leak point pressures: (a) abdominal leak point pressure, which is defined as the intravesical pressure at which urine leakage occurs due to increased abdominal pressure; and (b) detrusor leak point pressure, which is a measure of detrusor pressure at which urine leakage occurs in the absence of a detrusor contraction or increased abdominal pressure. This measure is generally used in patients with decreased compliance or lower motor neuron disease.
8. Detrusor leak point pressures that are sustained above 40 cm of water lead to deterioration of the upper tracts.
9. Maximum urethra closure pressure is defined as the difference between peak urethral pressure and intravesical pressure.
10. Bladder outlet obstruction index is defined by the equation: BOOI = Pdet Qmax − 2(Qmax). A value greater than 40 is considered obstructed; a value less than 20 is considered unobstructed.
11. A uroflow less than 12 mL/sec and Pdet greater than 25 cm of water predicts outlet obstruction in women.
12. Detrusor external sphincter dyssynergia can be due to a neurologic lesion or a learned disorder. The latter is considered dysfunctional voiding.
13. Internal sphincter dyssynergia must be diagnosed by VUDS.

chapter 63

Urinary Incontinence and Pelvic Prolapse: Epidemiology and Pathophysiology

Christopher R. Chapple, MD, FRCS (Urol), FEBU ● Ian Milsom, MD, PhD

QUESTIONS

1. The function of the lower urinary tract is best considered as:
   a. predominantly dependent on the bladder.
   b. predominantly dependent on the sphincter mechanisms.
   c. a single functional unit.
   d. related to effective voiding of urine.
   e. directly reflected by associated lower urinary tract symptoms (LUTS).

2. LUTS are:
   a. useful in making a specific diagnosis of lower urinary tract dysfunction.
   b. more useful than signs.
   c. a quantitative indicator of lower urinary tract dysfunction.
   d. purely subjective in nature.
   e. most troublesome when they affect voiding.

3. Overactive bladder is:
   a. an accurate clinical diagnosis.
   b. a collection of storage symptoms characterized by frequency.
   c. a urodynamic diagnosis.
   d. a nonspecific symptomatic diagnosis.
   e. part of the diagnosis of "mixed symptoms" when associated with urgency incontinence.

4. In women with a sphincteric weakness:
   a. 40% will have a significant cystocele.
   b. a history of leakage associated with raised intra-abdominal pressure is diagnostic.
   c. incontinence is not affected by associated prolapse.
   d. bladder overactivity occurs in less than 15%.
   e. urinary leakage is a symptom and a sign but not a diagnosis.

5. Bladder compliance:
   a. describes the relationship between change in bladder volume and change in detrusor pressure.
   b. is often low during slow bladder filling.
   c. is associated with little or no pressure change as the bladder fills.
   d. of high value denotes an abnormal volume-pressure relationship.
   e. is rarely seen in neurologic patients.

6. Urethral sphincter dysfunction is accurately assessed by:
   a. urethral pressure profilometry.
   b. abdominal leak point pressures.
   c. detrusor leak point pressures.
   d. surface electromyographic (EMG) studies.
   e. concentric needle EMG studies.

7. It is uncommon for patients with severe pelvic floor prolapse to:
   a. develop voiding dysfunction.
   b. experience fecal soiling.
   c. have occult incontinence.
   d. have stable detrusor function.
   e. experience sexual dysfunction.

8. Urinary continence relies on the following:
   a. Storing a continuously increasing amount of urine at gradually increasing pressure
   b. A low degree of "tonus" within the bladder
   c. Positive influences of the higher centers acting on the pontine micturition center
   d. Gradually increasing afferent traffic back to the brain
   e. Voluntary control of micturition

9. The following factor is often not important in maintaining continence in women:
   a. Watertight apposition of the urethral lumen
   b. Compression of the wall around the lumen
   c. Structural support to keep the proximal urethra from moving during increases in pressure
   d. A strong bladder neck mechanism
   e. A means of compensating for abdominal pressure changes (pressure transmission)

10. Intrinsic sphincter deficiency can be most reliably assessed by:
    a. Q tip test
    b. cystoscopy.
    c. detrusor leak point pressure.
    d. cystography.
    e. clinical examination.

11. Important connective tissue support mechanisms to the bladder base and urethra do not include the:
    a. pubo-urethral ligament.
    b. urethro-pelvic ligament.
    c. ileo-pectineal ligament.
    d. pubo-cervical fascia.
    e. arcus tendineus.

12. Muscular pelvic floor support is not dependent on:
    a. puborectalis muscle.
    b. pubococcygeus muscle.
    c. the intact pudendal nerve.
    d. iliococcygeus muscle.
    e. type I muscle fibers alone.

13. The maintenance of continence has clearly been established to be due to:
    a. equal transmission of increased intra-abdominal pressure to both bladder and urethra.
    b. the hammock theory.
    c. the "integral" hypothesis.
    d. the provision of a "backplate."
    e. a combination of all of the above.

14. Risk factors for the development of urinary incontinence do not include:
    a. pregnancy.
    b. body mass.
    c. menopause.
    d. diabetes.
    e. genetics.

15. Urinary incontinence in men:
    a. has been as well characterized as for women.
    b. is predominantly stress in type.
    c. occurs in up to 57% of men after radical prostatectomy.
    d. does not increase if there are preexisting symptoms.
    e. is not related to age at the time of radical prostatectomy.

16. An increased prevalence of pelvic organ prolapse (POP) is associated with:
    a. prior hysterectomy.
    b. an increased prevalence in African-American women.
    c. caesarean section.
    d. urgency incontinence.
    e. a lower incidence in a twin when the other twin has POP.

ANSWERS

1. **c. a single functional unit.** The lower urinary tract comprises the bladder and urethra and should be considered as a single functioning vesicourethral unit required to store urine and empty efficiently. Most of the bladder's functional time is spent in storing urine.

2. **d. purely subjective in nature.** *Symptoms* are the subjective indicator of a disease or change in condition as perceived by the patient, caregiver, or partner and may lead him or her to seek help from health care professionals. They may be volunteered or described during the patient interview. They are usually qualitative. In general, LUTS cannot be used to make a definitive diagnosis. LUTS can also indicate pathologies other than lower urinary tract dysfunction such as urinary infection.

    Signs are observed by the physician including simple means to verify symptoms and quantify them. For example, a classical sign is the observation of leakage on coughing. Observations from frequency volume charts, pad tests, and validated symptom and quality of life questionnaires are examples of other instruments that can be used to verify and quantify symptoms.

3. **d. a nonspecific symptomatic diagnosis.** Overactive bladder (OAB), or the urgency-frequency symptom syndrome, comprises urgency, with or without urgency incontinence, usually with frequency and nocturia. Urgency is widely held to be a key symptom driving the clinical sequence as demonstrated in Figure 63–1 in *Campbell-Walsh Urology, 10th Edition.*

    Mixed urinary symptoms refers to the presentation of a patient with a combination of OAB dry (without urgency incontinence) and stress incontinence (see Fig. 63–2 in *Campbell-Walsh Urology, 10th* Edition).

4. **a. 40% will have a significant cystocele.** More than 40% of women with urethral sphincter incompetence will have a significant cystocele (Cardozo, 1980).* Conversely, a history of stress incontinence associated with a mild or moderate cystocele is not specific for diagnosing genuine stress incontinence (Summitt, 1992). "Occult," or "latent," incontinence is urethral sphincteric incompetence masked by the presence of pelvic prolapse (Rosenzweig, 1992a, 1992b). Not infrequently, incontinent women may note the decrease or disappearance of stress incontinence episodes as the degree of prolapse worsens. The sign of occult stress incontinence is facilitated by the use of a speculum or pessary to reduce the prolapse while a stress maneuver is performed. The method to reduce vaginal prolapse to evaluate latent incontinence is not universally agreed upon or standardized at this time.

5. **a. describes the relationship between change in bladder volume and change in detrusor pressure.** Bladder compliance describes the relationship between change in bladder volume and change in detrusor pressure. The observation of reduced bladder compliance during conventional filling cystometry is often related to relatively fast bladder filling: The incidence of reduced compliance is markedly lower if the bladder is filled at physiologic rates, as in ambulatory urodynamics.
    - Compliance is calculated by dividing the volume change (ΔV) by the change in detrusor pressure ($\Delta Pdet$) during that change in bladder volume ($C = \Delta V. \Delta Pdet$). It is expressed in mL/cm H_2O.

---

*Sources referenced can be found in *Campbell-Walsh Urology, 10th Edition,* on the Expert Consult website.

- A variety of means of calculating bladder compliance have been described. The ICS recommends that two standard points should be used for compliance calculations. The investigator may wish to define additional points. The standards points are:
  1. the detrusor pressure at the start of bladder filling and the corresponding bladder volume (usually zero).
  2. the detrusor pressure (and corresponding bladder volume) at cystometric capacity or immediately before the start of any detrusor contraction that causes significant leakage (and therefore causes the bladder volume to decrease, affecting compliance calculation). Both points are measured excluding any detrusor contraction.

6. **e. concentric needle EMG studies.** Accurate electromyographic evaluation of the urethral sphincter is only possible with a concentric needle electrode, but it is a painful investigation and cannot be carried out during voiding.

7. **d. have stable detrusor function.** Patients with severe prolapse may develop voiding symptoms as a result of urethral kinking, leading to obstruction that is worsened during straining effort (Richardson, 1983). For instance, a moderate or severe cystocele may promote urethral compression and kinking, pressure dissipation, and an increase in maximum urethral closure pressures (Bergman, 1998; Versi, 1998). Clearly a number of storage urinary symptoms may occur in combination with prolapse. Risk factors contributing to the symptoms of urgency and frequency include age and urogenital atrophy. One study found that women with mild cystoceles had a 20% incidence of detrusor overactivity, and the incidence increased to 52% in those with moderate to severe cystoceles (Enhorning, 1961).

8. **a. Storing a continuously increasing amount of urine at gradually increasing pressure.** The function of the lower urinary tract is to temporarily store a continuously increasing amount of urine at low pressure and expel it under appropriate circumstances. This is dependent on the coordinated activity of smooth and striated muscles in the bladder, urethra, and pelvic floor. The bladder and the urethra constitute a functional unit, which is controlled by a complex interplay between the central and peripheral nervous systems and local regulatory factors (Andersson and Wein, 2004).

9. **d. A strong bladder neck mechanism.** Females are much more likely to suffer from urinary incontinence due to sphincteric deficiency than males, due to the much less powerful sphincteric mechanisms. The bladder neck is a far weaker structure than the male bladder neck and is often incompetent, even in nulliparous young women (Chapple, 1989) The bladder neck is poorly defined with the muscle fibers having a mainly longitudinal orientation.

Urinary continence is usually reliant on the integrity of the distal urethral sphincteric mechanism in females, which, like the male distal mechanism, is composed of a longitudinal intrinsic urethral smooth muscle and a larger extrinsic striated muscle component. This sphincter extends throughout the proximal two thirds of the urethra, being most developed in the middle one third of the urethra. Damage to the innervation of the urethral sphincter (in particular the pudendal nerve) by obstetric trauma reduces the effectiveness of this mechanism and predisposes to stress urinary incontinence.

10. **d. cystography.** An integrated approach involving anatomy and physiology is essential to an improved understanding of pathophysiology. Clearly a continent bladder outlet in the females depends on multiple factors (resting tone, active contraction, external compression, pressure transmission, integrity of configuration), and the focal point appears to be the midpoint of the urethra. In patients with stress incontinence there is clearly a spectrum between the two components of intrinsic sphincter deficiency and urethral hypermobility. Clearly, some patients have primary sphincteric problems, whereas others have an adequately functioning sphincter but significant hypermobility, and the majority lie somewhere between these two extremes.

In recent years there has been a gradual change from this dichotomic classification of stress incontinence: hypermobility or ISD. ISD alone is rare, and urethral hypermobility may occur commonly without significant ISD, but usually there is a combination of both of them in individual patients.

This evolution in our understanding in part followed the development of the concept of Valsalva leak point pressure (VLPP) introduced by McGuire in 1995 and also from analysis of long-term results of incontinence surgery. Despite lacking standardization of recording methods, as well as lacking consensus on how to deal with any associated prolapse, low VLPP (less than 60 cm H_2O has been suggested) has been widely considered as an indicator of ISD. There is considerable variability in the reports in the literature to the extent of correlation between VLPP and outcome. Similarly, urethral pressure profilometry has been extensively studied in this context, but there is a similar lack of correlation both in terms of predictive value and outcome. For instance, a low-pressure urethra may not leak, whereas the high-pressure urethra may. Also, a number of studies have failed to show any correlation between postoperative UPP and outcome. Cystography, although an invasive technique requiring radiologic input, provides a reproducible and easily interpreted technique that allows the relative contribution of both sphincteric weakness and hypermobility to be assessed (Blaivas and Olsson, 1988).

11. **c. ileo-pectineal ligament.** The pubo-urethral ligament attaches the midurethra to the inferior side of the pubic symphysis and prevents downward its rotational descent (Zacharin, 1963). It works in conjunction with the pubo-urethralis muscle, a subdivision of the levator ani muscle that forms a sling around the proximal urethra. Together they form the midurethral complex. In particular it has been postulated that an elongation of the posterior pubo-urethral ligaments may be a significant contributory factor to the loss of urethral support seen in stress incontinence. A major fascial support for the urethra is provided by the urethro-pelvic ligament, which attaches the urethra to the tendinous arc (Rovner et al, 1997).

In addition, the vesico-pelvic fascia or pubo-cervical fascia, extending between the bladder and the vagina, suspends and attaches the vagina and cervix to the pelvic sidewall, to each arcus tendineus fascia pelvis, thereby offering posterior support to the bladder and bladder neck. It has two surfaces, the perivesical fascia on the vaginal side and the endopelvic fascia on the abdominal side. Its upper zone supports the bladder above the cervix, the middle zone supports the trigone, and the lower zone supports the bladder neck. Laxity of the fascia in each of the zones will result in uterine prolapse, cystocele and urethrocele, respectively (DeLancey, 2001).

The arcus tendineus fasciae pelvis are tensile structures located bilaterally on either side of the urethra and vagina that act like the ropes of a suspension bridge and provide the necessary support needed to hang the urethra on the anterior vaginal wall. They originate as fibrous bands from the pubic bone and broaden out as aponeurotic structures moving dorsally to insert into the ischial spine.

The cardinal ligaments and the more medially placed utero-sacral ligaments support the uterus and cervix; their relaxation results in uterine prolapse.

12. **e. type I muscle fibers alone.** The pelvic floor musculature, represented by the levator ani muscles, carries the weight of the pelvic contents and prevents the abdominal pressure from stretching the ligamentous support structures. The levator ani includes the puborectalis muscle, which surrounds the rectum connecting the pubic bones anteriorly in a U-shaped configuration; the pubococcygeus muscle, which crosses from the pubis to the coccyx; and iliococcygeus muscle. The last one arises laterally from the arcus tendineus levator ani and forms a horizontal sheet that spans the posterior opening of the pelvis, providing a shelf on which the pelvic organs lie. The urethra and vagina pass through an aperture in the levator musculature, the urogenital hiatus. The levator ani contains not only type I fibers providing resting tone but also type II (fast-twitch) fibers that, under stress, maintain the urethral closure and prevent stretching of the pelvic ligaments.

The constant muscle tone (Critchley et al, 1980) maintained by predominantly type I (slow-twitch) striated muscle fibers compresses the vagina and urethra anteriorly toward the pubic bone and keeps the hiatus closed (DeLancey and Hurd, 1998).

The pudendal nerve provides somatic innervation to the striated muscle of levator ani, as well as to the striated muscle within the external anal and urethral sphincters. The intrapelvic somatic fibers travel along the anterior vaginal wall from the sacral segments S2-S4 to provide a somatic nerve supply to the pelvic floor (Borirakchanyavat et al, 1997). Neuromuscular injuries have been proposed as an important factor in predisposing to pelvic floor dysfunction. Childbirth and age are often considered as the two major factors predisposing to pelvic floor denervation (Smith et al, 1989). Other factors include pelvic surgery (rectal and vaginal surgery with extensive pelvic dissection), radiotherapy, and congenital neurologic conditions such as spina bifida and muscular dystrophy.

13. **e. a combination of all of the above.** The most commonly held view of the pathophysiology of stress incontinence secondary to urethral hypermobility is based on DeLancey's theory of urethral support, the so-called hammock theory (DeLancey, 1994). In anatomic specimens in which increases in abdominal pressure were simulated, he found that the urethra lies in a position where it can be compressed against a hammock-like musculofascial layer on which the bladder and urethra rest (DeLancey, 1994). In this model, it is the stability of this supporting layer rather than the position of the urethra that determines stress continence.

14. **c. menopause.** Urinary incontinence (UI) is a common symptom that may affect women at all ages, and there is a wide range of severity and nature of symptoms. UI is not a life-threatening disease, but the symptoms may seriously influence the physical, psychologic, and social well-being of the affected individuals.

Pregnancy, labor, and vaginal delivery (vs. caesarean section) are significant risk factors for later UI, but the strength of this association diminishes substantially with age (level 1 evidence).

Although several specific parturition factors such as instrumental delivery and birth weight are risk factors for UI in the postpartum period, their association with UI in later life is weak or nonexistent, suggesting that changes in birthing practices in developed countries are unlikely to affect UI in older age (level 2 evidence).

Additional evidence has now established body mass as an important, modifiable risk factor for UI (level 1 evidence).

Physical function also appears to be an independent risk factor for UI in older women. Whether improvement in physical function leads to a reduction in UI remains to be established (level 2 evidence).

Evidence from two blinded, randomized, controlled trials indicate that oral estrogen, with or without progestogen, is a significant risk factor for UI in women age 55 and older (level 1 evidence).

Diabetes is a risk factor for UI in most studies. Although diabetic neuropathy and/or vasculopathy are possible mechanisms by which diabetes could lead to UI, no mechanism has been established, nor is it clear whether prevention or treatment of diabetes, separate from weight reduction, will reduce the risk of UI (level 2 evidence).

Menopause, as generally defined, does not appear to be an independent risk factor for stress UI (level 2 evidence).

Hysterectomy remains a possible risk factor for later UI, but the evidence is inconsistent (level 2 evidence).

Moderate to severe dementia in older women is a moderate to strong independent risk factor for UI (level 2 evidence). Whether interventions to maintain or improve cognitive functioning also reduce UI has not been evaluated.

Mild loss of cognitive function in community-dwelling women, separated from physical function and other factors, increases the risk of UI slightly if at all, but may increase the impact of UI (level 2 evidence).

Data from twin studies suggest that there is a substantial genetic component to UI (level 1 evidence).

Other potential risk factors including smoking, diet, depression, constipation, UTIs, and exercise, although associated with UI, have not been established as etiologic risk factors and are in fact difficult to study with observational data because of the potential for unmeasured confounding and questions of direction of the association (level 3 evidence).

15. **c. occurs in up to 57% of men after radical prostatectomy.** The epidemiology of UI in men has not been investigated to the same extent as for females. But it appears that UI is at least twice as prevalent in women as compared with men. There seems to be a more steady increase in prevalence with increasing age than for women.

16. **a. prior hysterectomy.** A number of studies suggest that hysterectomy and other pelvic surgery may increase the risk for pelvic organ prolapse (level 2 evidence).

Additional Study Points

1. Pelvic organ prolapse may mask incontinence.
2. Fecal incontinence occurs in 17% of women with pelvic organ prolapse.
3. The female bladder neck is weaker than the male bladder neck and is often incompetent.
4. In women the majority of the urethra should be considered an active area of sphincter control; however, in the female the most important portion of continence is the midurethra.
5. A Valsalva leak point pressure of less than 60 cm of water indicates but does not confirm intrinsic sphincter dysfunction (ISD).
6. Twelve percent of men report terminal dribbling.
7. Rates of overactive bladder increase with age.

64

Evaluation of Patients with Urinary Incontinence and Pelvic Prolapse

Kathleen C. Kobashi, MD

QUESTIONS

1. Pelvic floor disorders include:
   a. stress urinary incontinence.
   b. urinary urgency.
   c. fecal incontinence.
   d. pelvic organ prolapse.
   e. all of the above.

2. Risk factors for the development of pelvic floor disorders include all of the following EXCEPT:
   a. advanced age.
   b. parity.
   c. low body mass index.
   d. genetic predisposition.
   e. smoking.

3. All of the following statements are true regarding local hormone replacement therapy EXCEPT:
   a. It can be helpful in the treatment of urgency incontinence.
   b. It can make stress urinary incontinence worse.
   c. It has the same effect on stress urinary incontinence as systemic hormone replacement therapy.
   d. It is more effective in treating urgency urinary incontinence than systemic replacement therapy.
   e. It should be used routinely in the treatment of all types of urinary incontinence.

4. Diuretics:
   a. have direct effects on the bladder.
   b. do not increase urine production.
   c. can aggravate urinary incontinence problems.
   d. do not have any effect on the lower urinary tract.
   e. can be used to treat urinary incontinence.

5. Which of the following is NOT a true statement?
   a. Sympathomimetics can decrease detrusor contractility and precipitate urinary retention.

   b. Sympathomimetics can increase outlet resistance and exacerbate obstructive symptoms.
   c. Sympathomimetics can exacerbate overactive bladder symptoms.
   d. Sympatholytics can decrease outlet resistance and exacerbate stress urinary incontinence.
   e. Anticholinergics can contribute to retention by paradoxically increasing outlet resistance.

6. Which of the following statements is INCORRECT regarding the assessment of a patient with pelvic floor disorders?
   a. Medicare specifies precise requirements to fulfill various levels of a physical examination.
   b. Family history is not a pertinent part of the assessment of patients with pelvic floor disorders.
   c. Past surgical history, with particular attention to previous pelvic floor reconstruction or anti-incontinence procedures, is important in patients with pelvic floor disorders.
   d. It is important to review hormone replacement history because both systemic and local exogenous hormone replacement therapy, either past or current, can increase the risk of stress incontinence.
   e. Numerous medical conditions can affect continence.

7. The POP-Q (Pelvic Organ Prolapse Quantification) system:
   a. is a simple six-point quantification system for pelvic prolapse.
   b. was created in an effort to quantify pelvic organ prolapse and urinary incontinence.
   c. includes six specific points of position measurement in relation to the introitus.
   d. includes a simplified five-level staging system that does not require listing each of the points specifically.
   e. includes measurement of the total vaginal length performed without reduction of the prolapse.

8. The bulbocavernosus reflex (BCR):
   a. represents sacral nerve roots 2 to 4.
   b. is negative in 30% of normal females.

c. should be positive in all normal males.

d. is a and c.

e. is all of the above.

9. Which of the following statements is TRUE regarding voiding diaries?

a. They do not provide accurate information regarding voiding symptoms.

b. They have both diagnostic and therapeutic advantages.

c. They are no more accurate than patient recall.

d. A minimum of a 3-day diary should be used to gather accurate information.

e. They are a good substitute for more invasive studies.

10. Regarding pad tests:

a. The International Consultation on Incontinence (ICI) considers up to 1.3 g/24 hours to be normal.

b. Pad tests are simple to perform and should be a routine part of the evaluation of patients with pelvic floor disorders.

c. Up to 8 g/24 hours may be considered normal.

d. The International Continence Society (ICS) method requires patients to perform exercise following instillation of 500 mL of Na-free fluid into the bladder.

e. a and c apply.

11. Multichannel urodynamics:

a. is the most accurate diagnostic tool available for the evaluation of incontinence.

b. should be used in all patients with incontinence.

c. includes three directly measured values: detrusor pressure (Pdet), vesical pressure (Pves), and abdominal pressure (Pabd).

d. is not helpful in determining if a patient is at risk of developing upper tract deterioration.

e. is all of the above.

12. Urodynamics should be considered in which of the following circumstances?

a. In patients in whom conservative measures have failed

b. In patients in whom the clinical picture is unclear

c. In patients in whom the symptoms cannot be confirmed by the clinician

d. In patients who have undergone previous pelvic floor reconstruction

e. All of the above

13. Electromyelogram:

a. should be performed in all patients undergoing urodynamics.

b. should be silenced during the voiding phase.

c. should not show recruitment during coughing.

d. should be silent with BCR.

e. is b and d.

14. Factors that indicate increased risk for development of upper tract deterioration include all of the following EXCEPT:

a. young age at development of urinary incontinence.

b. elevated storage pressures, particularly greater than 40 cm H_2O.

c. vesicoureteral reflux.

d. active EMG during voiding.

e. compromised compliance.

15. All of the following statements regarding overactive bladder treatment are true EXCEPT:

a. Antimuscarinic agents function via competitive inhibition of the cholinergic receptors of the detrusor.

b. The pudendal afferents to the spinal cord inhibit the overactive supraspinal voiding stimulus, and sacroneuromodulation is thought to function by inhibition of afferent processing of sensory stimulation in the spinal cord.

c. Available studies have only supported the use of botulinum toxin A injection of the bladder for neurogenic detrusor overactivity and not idiopathic detrusor overactivity.

d. Botulinum toxin A appears to function on a variety of pathways in addition to the cholinergic pathway.

e. The urothelial and interstitial cells may play a key role in bladder sensation.

ANSWERS

1. **e. all of the above.**

2. **c. low body mass index.** High body mass index (BMI) is a risk factor for development of pelvic floor disorders.

3. **e. It should be used routinely in the treatment of all types of urinary incontinence.** Recent evidence shows that exogenous hormones, both systemic and local, can exacerbate stress incontinence such that local hormone replacement therapy should no longer be considered as part of the routine treatment for stress incontinence. However, local hormone replacement therapy can be helpful in the treatment of urgency incontinence.

4. **c. can aggravate urinary incontinence problems.** Diuretics increase urine production and can therefore aggravate incontinence symptoms. They do not have a direct effect on the bladder or lower urinary tract function.

5. **e. Anticholinergics can contribute to retention by paradoxically increasing outlet resistance.** Sympathomimetics can cause urinary retention by decreasing detrusor contractility and/or increasing bladder outlet resistance. Sympatholytics can contribute to stress incontinence by decreasing outlet resistance. The mechanism by which anticholinergics contribute to retention is by decreasing detrusor contractility.

6. **b. Family history is not a pertinent part of the assessment of patients with pelvic floor disorders.** Because genetic predisposition has been shown to be a risk factor for pelvic floor disorders, family history is an important part of the evaluation of patients with incontinence and pelvic organ prolapse.

7. **d. includes a simplified five-level staging system that does not require listing each of the points specifically.** POP-Q is a nine-point system that was created for the assessment of pelvic organ prolapse. It measures six specific points in relation to the hymen. The remaining three points include the total vaginal length, measured with the vagina completely reduced, the perineal body, and the genital hiatus. It has been simplified into a five-stage system that does not require listing of each of the nine points.

8. **e. is all of the above.** BCR represents S2-4 and is present in all normal males and 70% of normal females.

9. **b. They have both diagnostic and therapeutic advantages.** Voiding diaries have been shown to be more accurate than patient recall and provide accurate information regarding voiding pattern and symptoms. Twenty-four-hour diaries provide useful information and can be helpful both diagnostically and therapeutically because they often make patients aware of simple behavioral issues that may affect their symptomatology. Voiding diaries, however, are not a substitute for a more thorough examination when indicated.

10. **e. a and c apply.** Although the ICI considers up to 1.3 g/24 hours to be normal, other groups have allowed up to 8 g/24 hours. Pad tests are tedious and difficult to perform and reproduce. The ICS method requires patients to drink 500 mL of Na-free liquid followed by a 30-minute resting period before the recommended activity. This method does not result in a standardized bladder volume.

11. **a. is the most accurate diagnostic tool available for the evaluation of incontinence.** Multichannel urodynamics is currently the most accurate diagnostic tool available for the evaluation of urinary incontinence. Whether it is necessary in the assessment of all patients with urinary incontinence remains controversial. Findings on urodynamics, which include direct measurements of vesical and abdominal pressures (Pves and Pabd, respectively) and a calculated measure of detrusor pressure (Pdet), can provide helpful information including findings such as elevated Pdet, which may suggest a patient is at increased risk of developing upper tract deterioration.

12. **e. All of the above.** Any patient with a picture complicated by issues such as previous pelvic or anti-incontinence surgery, radiation therapy, neurologic disease, or difficult or unclear diagnosis should be considered for urodynamics.

13. **b. should be silenced during the voiding phase.** EMG should be used in selected patients. Recruitment should occur with increased intra-abdominal pressure such as with coughing and with BCR. It should be silent during voiding.

14. **a. young age at development of urinary incontinence.** Any situation in which the detrusor pressures are elevated such as vesicoureteral reflux, elevated storage pressures (particularly sustained pressures >40 cm H_2O), poor compliance, detrusor overactivity, and detrusor-sphincter dyssynergia, may put an individual at increased risk for developing upper tract deterioration. Although children with incontinence may potentially have any of a number of risk factors for upper tract deterioration, young age at onset of incontinence alone has not been determined to be a risk factor.

15. **c. Available studies have only supported the use of botulinum toxin A injection of the bladder for neurogenic detrusor overactivity and not idiopathic detrusor overactivity.** Botulinum toxin A has been shown to be successful in the treatment of refractory urgency incontinence and overactive bladder symptoms in both neurologic and idiopathic detrusor overactivity.

Additional Study Points

1. Pelvic organ prolapse is categorized according to affected compartment: anterior (cystocele), posterior (rectocele), apical (descent of the uterus or bowel—enterocele).
2. Hypermobility is defined as a Q tip angle of greater than 30 degrees from horizontal on abdominal straining.
3. In the pelvic organ prolapse quantification system, positions cephalad to the hymen are considered negative. Positions caudad to the hymen are considered positive.
4. Pad use per day is an unreliable indicator of the quantity of incontinence.
5. A postvoid residual of less than 50 mL represents adequate emptying. Ninety percent of normal individuals will have a PVR less than 100. A PVR greater than 200 represents inadequate emptying.
6. Stress urinary incontinence may be unmasked by the reduction of prolapse.
7. Apical prolapse is treated with uterosacral ligament suspension or a sacrospinous ligament fixation.

Neuromuscular Dysfunction of the Lower Urinary Tract

Alan J. Wein, MD, PhD (Hon) ● Roger R. Dmochowski, MD, FACS

QUESTIONS

1. What is the general pattern of voiding dysfunction secondary to neurologic lesions above the level of the brainstem?
   a. Involuntary bladder contractions, smooth sphincter dyssynergia, striated sphincter synergy
   b. Involuntary bladder contractions, smooth sphincter synergy, striated sphincter synergy
   c. Involuntary bladder contractions, smooth sphincter synergy, striated sphincter dyssynergia
   d. Detrusor hypocontractility, smooth sphincter synergy, striated sphincter synergy
   e. Detrusor areflexia, smooth sphincter synergy, striated sphincter synergy

2. What is the general pattern of voiding dysfunction that results from complete lesions of the spinal cord above the level of S2 after recovery from spinal shock?
   a. Involuntary bladder contractions, smooth sphincter dyssynergia, striated sphincter synergy
   b. Involuntary bladder contractions, smooth sphincter synergy, striated sphincter synergy
   c. Involuntary bladder contractions, smooth sphincter synergy, striated sphincter dyssynergia
   d. Detrusor hypocontractility, smooth sphincter synergy, striated sphincter synergy
   e. Detrusor areflexia, smooth sphincter synergy, striated sphincter synergy

3. Which of the following is the most common long-term expression of lower urinary tract dysfunction after a cerebrovascular accident (CVA)?
   a. Detrusor areflexia
   b. Lack of sensation of filling
   c. Impaired bladder contractility
   d. Striated sphincter dyssynergia
   e. Detrusor overactivity

4. Urinary incontinence is most likely to occur in a patient after a CVA if which of the following areas is affected?
   a. Internal capsule
   b. Basal ganglia
   c. Thalamus
   d. Cerebellum
   e. Hypothalamus

5. In a post-CVA patient who exhibits urgency and frequency but no incontinence, the state of striated sphincter activity can most commonly be best described as:
   a. uninhibited relaxation.
   b. dyssynergia.
   c. fixed voluntary tone.
   d. pseudodyssynergia.
   e. myotonus.

6. A 65-year-old man who has sustained a stroke but is otherwise in good health has symptoms of hesitancy, straining to void, urgency, and frequency. The optimal next step in management is:
   a. anticholinergic therapy.
   b. transurethral resection of the prostate (TURP).
   c. transurethral incision of the bladder neck and prostate.
   d. clean intermittent catheterization.
   e. full urodynamic evaluation.

7. When considering the subject of voiding dysfunction associated with brain tumors, which of the following areas is more likely to be associated with urinary retention than with urinary incontinence?
   a. Pituitary gland
   b. Cerebellum
   c. Posterior fossa
   d. Hypothalamus
   e. Frontal cortex

8. The most common pattern of micturition in children and adults who have cerebral palsy (CP) and no other complicating neurologic condition is:
   a. abnormal filling/storage because of detrusor overactivity; normal emptying.
   b. normal filling/storage; normal emptying.
   c. normal filling/storage; abnormal emptying because of smooth sphincter dyssynergia.
   d. normal filling/storage; abnormal emptying because of striated sphincter dyssynergia.
   e. abnormal filling/storage because of detrusor overactivity; abnormal emptying because of striated sphincter dyssynergia.

9. The most common urodynamic findings in those individuals with cerebral palsy who do exhibit lower urinary tract dysfunction are:
   a. detrusor areflexia, coordinated sphincters.
   b. detrusor overactivity, smooth sphincter dyssynergia, striated sphincter dyssynergia.
   c. detrusor overactivity, smooth sphincter synergy, striated sphincter dyssynergia.
   d. decreased detrusor compliance, coordinated sphincters.
   e. detrusor overactivity, coordinated sphincters.

10. Deficiency of which of the following compounds in the nigrostriatal pathway accounts for most of the classic clinical motor features of Parkinson disease (PD)?
    a. Dopamine
    b. Norepinephrine
    c. Acetylcholine
    d. Serotonin
    e. L-Dopa

11. The most common urodynamic abnormality found in patients with voiding dysfunction secondary to PD is:
    a. impaired sensation during filling.
    b. striated sphincter dyssynergia.
    c. striated sphincter bradykinesia.
    d. detrusor overactivity.
    e. impaired detrusor contractility.

12. Which of the following is more common in patients with PD than in patients with multiple system atrophy (MSA)?
    a. Intrinsic sphincter deficiency
    b. Evidence of striated sphincter denervation on an electromyogram
    c. Decreased compliance
    d. Incontinence after TURP
    e. Disease diagnosis preceding voiding and erectile symptoms

13. The lesions seen in multiple sclerosis most commonly affect which of the following locations in the nervous system?
    a. Thoracic spinal cord
    b. Sacral spinal cord
    c. Cervical spinal cord
    d. Lumbar spinal cord
    e. Midbrain

14. Which of the following urodynamic findings is least common in patients with multiple sclerosis and voiding dysfunction?
    a. Detrusor overactivity
    b. Detrusor areflexia
    c. Impaired detrusor contractility
    d. Striated sphincter dyssynergia
    e. Smooth sphincter dyssynergia

15. The incidence of upper urinary tract deterioration is greatest in which of the following?
    a. Multiple sclerosis
    b. Multiple system atrophy
    c. PD
    d. Spinal cord injury (SCI)
    e. Diabetes

16. Which of the following most accurately reflects the number of patients with HIV/AIDS, overall, with moderate or severe voiding problems?
    a. 15% or less
    b. 15% to 25%
    c. 25% to 40%
    d. 40% to 60%
    e. 60% to 80%

17. The sacral spinal cord terminates in the cauda equina at approximately the spinal column level of:
    a. T10.
    b. L1.
    c. L2.
    d. L3.
    e. S1.

18. In spinal shock, findings generally include all of the following EXCEPT:
    a. acontractile bladder.
    b. areflexic bladder.
    c. open bladder neck.
    d. absent guarding reflex.
    e. maximal urethral closure pressure above normal.

19. All of the following are risk factors for upper urinary tract deterioration in a patient with a suprasacral SCI EXCEPT:
    a. high-pressure storage.
    b. high detrusor leak-point pressure.
    c. chronic bladder overdistention.
    d. high abdominal leak-point pressure.
    e. vesicourethral reflux with infection.

20. The presence of true detrusor–striated sphincter dyssynergia implies a neurologic lesion between the:
    a. pons and the sacral spinal cord.
    b. cerebral cortex and the pons.
    c. cervical and the sacral spinal cord.
    d. sacral spinal cord and the striated sphincter.
    e. cauda equina and the striated sphincter.

affect micturition generally result in involuntary bladder contractions with smooth and striated sphincter synergy. Sensation and voluntary striated sphincter function are generally preserved. Areflexia may occur either initially or as a permanent dysfunction.

2. **c. Involuntary bladder contractions, smooth sphincter synergy, striated sphincter dyssynergia.** Patients with complete lesions of the spinal cord between spinal cord levels T6 and S2, after they recover from spinal shock, generally exhibit involuntary bladder contractions without sensation of the contraction, smooth sphincter synergy, but striated sphincter dyssynergia. Those with lesions above T6 may experience, in addition, smooth sphincter dyssynergia and autonomic hyperreflexia.

3. **e. Detrusor overactivity.** The most common long-term expression of lower urinary tract dysfunction after a CVA is detrusor hyperreflexia. Sensation is variable but is classically described as generally intact, and thus the patient has urgency and frequency with hyperreflexia.

4. **a. Internal capsule.** Previous descriptions of the voiding dysfunction after a CVA have all cited the preponderance of detrusor hyperreflexia with coordinated sphincter activity. It is difficult to reconcile this with the relatively high incontinence rate that occurs, even considering the probability that a percentage of these patients had an incontinence problem before the CVA. Tsuchida and colleagues (1983)* and Khan and colleagues (1990) made early significant contributions in this area by correlating the urodynamic and CT pictures after CVA. They reported that patients with lesions in only the basal ganglia or thalamus have normal sphincter function. This means that when an impending involuntary contraction or its onset was sensed, these patients could voluntarily contract the striated sphincter and abort or considerably lessen the effect of an abnormal micturition reflex. The majority of patients with involvement of the cerebral cortex and/or internal capsule were unable to forcefully contract the striated sphincter under these circumstances.

5. **d. pseudodyssynergia.** Some authors have described striated sphincter dyssynergia in 5% to 21% of patients with brain disease and voiding dysfunction. This is incompatible with accepted neural circuitry. The authors agree with those who believe that true detrusor-striated sphincter dyssynergia does not occur in this situation. Pseudodyssynergia may indeed occur during urodynamic testing of these patients. This refers to an EMG sphincter "flare" during filling cystometry, which is secondary to attempted inhibition of an involuntary bladder contraction by voluntary contraction of the striated sphincter.

6. **e. full urodynamic evaluation.** Poor flow rates and high residual urine volumes in a male with pre-CVA symptoms of prostatism generally indicate prostatic obstruction, but a full urodynamic evaluation is advisable before committing a patient to mechanical outlet reduction primarily to exclude detrusor hyperactivity with impaired contractility as a cause of symptoms.

7. **c. Posterior fossa.** The areas that are most frequently involved with associated micturition dysfunction are the superior aspects of the frontal lobe. When voiding dysfunction occurs, it generally consists of detrusor

*Sources referenced can be found in *Campbell-Walsh Urology*, *10th Edition*, on the Expert Consult website.

hyperreflexia and urinary incontinence. These individuals may have a markedly diminished awareness of all lower urinary tract events and, if so, are totally unable to even attempt suppression of the micturition reflex. Smooth and striated sphincter activity is generally synergic. Pseudodyssynergia may occur during urodynamic testing. Fowler (1999) reviewed the literature on frontal lobe lesions and bladder control. She cited instances of resection of a tumor relieving the micturition symptoms for a period of time, raising the question of whether the phenomenon of tumor-associated bladder hyperreflexia was a positive one (activating some system) rather than a negative one (releasing a system from control). Urinary retention has also been described in patients with space-occupying lesions of the frontal cortex, in the absence of other associated remarkable neurologic deficits. Posterior fossa tumors may be associated with voiding dysfunction (32% to 70%, based on references cited by Fowler). Retention or difficulty voiding is the rule, with incontinence being rarely reported.

8. **b. normal filling/storage; normal emptying.** Most children and adults with only CP have urinary control and what seems to be normal filling/storage and normal emptying. The actual incidence of voiding dysfunction is somewhat vague because the few available series report findings predominantly in those who present with voiding symptoms. One study estimated that a third or more of children with CP are so affected. When an adult with CP presents with an acute or subacute change in voiding status, however, it is most likely unrelated to CP.

9. **e. detrusor overactivity, coordinated sphincters.** In those individuals with CP who exhibit significant dysfunction, the type of damage that one would suspect from the most common urodynamic abnormalities seems to be localized above the brainstem. This is commonly reflected by detrusor overactivity and coordinated sphincters. Spinal cord damage can occur, however, and probably accounts for those individuals with CP who seem to have evidence of striated sphincter dyssynergia.

10. **a. Dopamine.** PD is a neurodegenerative disorder of unknown cause that affects primarily the dopaminergic neurons of the substantia nigra but also heterogeneous populations of neurons elsewhere. The most important site of pathology is the substantia nigra pars compacta, the origin of the dopaminergic nigrostriatal tract to the caudate nucleus and putamen. Dopamine deficiency in the nigrostriatal pathway accounts for most of the classic clinical motor features of PD.

11. **d. detrusor overactivity.** The most common urodynamic finding is detrusor overactivity. The pathophysiology of detrusor overactivity most widely proposed is that the basal ganglia normally have an inhibitory effect on the micturition reflex, which is abolished by the cell loss in the substantia nigra.

12. **e. Disease diagnosis preceding voiding and erectile symptoms.** One study compared the clinical features of 52 patients with probable MSA and 41 patients with PD. Of patients with MSA, 60% had their urinary symptoms precede or present with their symptoms of parkinsonism. Of patients with PD, 94% had been diagnosed for several years before the onset of urinary symptoms. In patients with MSA, urinary incontinence was a significant complaint in 73%, whereas 19% had only frequency and urgency without incontinence. Sixty-six percent of the patients with MSA

had a significant postvoid residual volume (100 to 450 mL). In patients with PD, frequency and urgency were the predominant symptoms in 85% and incontinence was the primary complaint in 15%. In only 5 of 32 patients with PD in whom residual urine volume was measured was it significant. Ninety-three percent of the men with MSA questioned about erectile function reported erectile failure, and in 13 of 27 of these the erectile dysfunction preceded the diagnosis of MSA. Seven of the 21 men with PD had erectile failure, but in all these men the diagnosis of erectile dysfunction followed the diagnosis of PD by 1 to 4 years. The initial urinary symptoms of MSA are urgency, frequency, and urge incontinence, occurring up to 4 years before the diagnosis is made, as does erectile failure. Cystourethrography or video-urodynamic studies generally reveal an open bladder neck (intrinsic sphincter deficiency), and many patients exhibit evidence of striated sphincter denervation on motor unit electromyography. The smooth and striated sphincter abnormalities predispose women to sphincteric incontinence and make prostatectomy hazardous in men.

13. **c. Cervical spinal cord.** The demyelinating process most commonly involves the lateral corticospinal (pyramidal) and reticulospinal columns of the cervical spinal cord.

14. **e. Smooth sphincter dyssynergia.** Detrusor overactivity is the most common urodynamic abnormality detected, occurring in 34% to 99% of cases in reported series. Of the patients with overactivity, 30% to 65% have coexistent striated sphincter dyssynergia. Up to 60% of those with overactivity may have impaired detrusor contractility, a phenomenon that can considerably complicate treatment efforts. Bladder areflexia may also occur; reports of its frequency vary but generally average from 5% to 20%. Generally, the smooth sphincter is synergic.

15. **d. Spinal cord injury (SCI).** Progressive neurologic diseases cause upper tract damage much less commonly than SCI, even when associated with severe disability and spasticity (Wyndaele et al, 2005).

16. **a. 15% or less.** How common are voiding problems overall in patients with HIV infection and AIDS? One study prospectively investigated voiding function in 77 men and 4 women with HIV infection or AIDS consecutively attending an outpatient clinic. Eight of these (10%) had moderate subjective voiding problems, whereas two (2%) had severe problems. The authors thought that in only 4% of patients did the nature of the disturbance warrant urodynamic examination and concluded that urinary voiding symptoms are only a modest problem; overall in an HIV/AIDS population, neuropathic bladder dysfunction is rare and mostly occurs in the late stages of the disease (Gyrtrup et al, 1995).

17. **c. L2.** Spinal column (bone) segments are numbered by the vertebral level, and these have a different relationship to the spinal cord segmental level at different locations. The sacral spinal cord begins at about spinal column level T12-L1. The spinal cord terminates in the cauda equina at approximately the spinal column level of L2.

18. **c. open bladder neck.** Spinal shock includes a suppression of autonomic activity and somatic activity, and the bladder is acontractile and areflexic. Radiologically, the bladder has a smooth contour with no evidence of trabeculation. The bladder neck is generally closed and competent unless there has been prior surgery or, in some cases, thoracolumbar and presumably sympathetic injury. The smooth sphincter mechanism seems to be functional. Some EMG activity may be recorded from the striated sphincter, and the maximum urethral closure pressure is lower than normal but still maintained at the level of the external sphincter zone; however, the normal guarding reflex is absent and there is no voluntary control.

19. **d. high abdominal leak-point pressure.** As with all patients with neurologic impairment, a careful initial evaluation and periodic follow-up evaluation must be performed to identify and correct the following risk factors and potential complications: bladder overdistention, high pressure storage, high detrusor leak-point pressure, vesicoureteral reflux, stone formation (lower and upper tracts), and complicating infection, especially in association with reflux.

20. **a. pons and the sacral spinal cord.** A diagnosis of striated sphincter dyssynergia implies a neurologic lesion that interrupts the neural axis between the pontine-mesencephalic reticular formation and the sacral spinal cord.

21. **a. Cervical.** Autonomic hyperreflexia represents an acute massive disordered autonomic (primarily sympathetic) response to specific stimuli in patients with SCI above the level of T6 to T8 (the upper level of the sympathetic outflow). It is more common with cervical (60%) than thoracic (20%) injuries.

22. **d. Tachycardia.** Symptomatically, autonomic hyperreflexia is a syndrome of exaggerated sympathetic activity in response to stimuli below the level of the lesion. The symptoms are pounding headache, hypertension, and flushing of the face and body above the level of the lesion with sweating. Bradycardia is a usual accompaniment, and an arrhythmia may be present.

23. **b. decreased compliance.** In autonomic hyperreflexia, the urodynamic picture is that of a suprasacral SCI. Smooth sphincter dyssynergia is generally found as well, at least in men.

24. **b. β-Adrenergic blockade.** Acutely the hemodynamic effects may be managed with parenteral ganglionic or α-adrenergic blockade. Any endoscopic procedure in susceptible patients ideally should be done with the patient under spinal or carefully monitored general anesthesia.

25. **a. Ureteral reimplantation.** The best initial treatment for reflux in a patient with voiding dysfunction secondary to neurologic disease or injury is to normalize lower urinary tract urodynamics as much as possible. Depending on the clinical circumstances, this may be by pharmacotherapy, urethral dilatation (in the myelomeningocele patient), neuromodulation, deafferentation, augmentation cystoplasty, or sphincterotomy. If this fails, the question of whether to operate on such patients for correction of the reflux or to correct the reflux while performing another procedure (e.g., augmentation cystoplasty) is not an easy one because correction of reflux in an often thickened bladder may not be an easy task.

26. **e. neurologic evaluation initially and yearly for an indefinite period.** All but e were specific recommendations (Linsenmeyer and Culkin, 1999).

27. **e. Maximum bladder capacity decreased.** One must remember the potential artifact that significant reflux can introduce into urodynamic studies. Measured bladder capacity may be more, and measured pressures at given

chapter
68

Pharmacologic Management of Lower Urinary Tract Storage and Emptying Failure

Karl-Erik Andersson, MD, PhD ● Alan J. Wein, MD, PhD (Hon)

QUESTIONS

1. The effects of administration of antimuscarinic agent to an individual with an overactive bladder (OAB) include all EXCEPT:
   a. increased total bladder capacity.
   b. depressed amplitude of involuntary bladder contractions.
   c. increased outlet resistance.
   d. increased volume to the first involuntary bladder contraction.
   e. increased mean volume voided.

2. Which of the following muscarinic receptor subtypes is the most common in human detrusor smooth muscle?
   a. M_1
   b. M_2
   c. M_3
   d. M_4
   e. M_5

3. Which of the following muscarinic receptor subtypes is predominantly responsible for the mediation of bladder contraction in human detrusor smooth muscle?
   a. M_1
   b. M_2
   c. M_3
   d. M_4
   e. M_5

4. The use of antimuscarinic agents to treat OAB is limited by their lack of uroselectivity. Which of the following is not a recognized side effect of antimuscarinic agents?
   a. Dry mouth
   b. Constipation
   c. Cognitive dysfunction
   d. Bradycardia
   e. Blurred vision

5. Which of the following characteristics increases the possibility for an antimuscarinic agent to pass the blood-brain barrier? (Multiple answers are possible.)
   a. High lipophilicity
   b. Large molecular size
   c. Low electrical charge
   d. Quaternary ammonium structure
   e. Small molecular size

6. As a therapeutic antimuscarinic agent, propantheline bromide is:
   a. receptor specific.
   b. tissue specific.
   c. poorly absorbed from the gastrointestinal tract.
   d. a tertiary ammonium compound.
   e. more effective than oxybutynin.

7. Oxybutynin exerts its clinical effects on the urinary bladder primarily by:
   a. calcium channel blockade.
   b. local anesthetic activity.
   c. inhibition of norepinephrine uptake.
   d. M_3 receptor blockade.
   e. M_1 receptor blockade.

8. The Committee on Pharmacologic Treatment of the Fourth (2008) International Consultation on Incontinence assessed agents according to the Oxford Guidelines, according to level of evidence and grade of recommendation with respect to treatment of detrusor overactivity (DO). Which of the following (multiple answers are possible) did not receive a level of evidence rating of 1 and a grade of recommendation of A?
   a. Dicyclomine
   b. Flavoxate
   c. Trospium
   d. Tolterodine
   e. Oxybutynin

9. The pharmacologic characteristics of which class of drugs would suggest that they may be active during the filling/storage phase of micturition and effective in abolishing DO, yet with no effect on normal bladder contraction?
   a. Calcium antagonists
   b. Antimuscarinics
   c. Cyclooxygenase inhibitors
   d. Potassium channel openers
   e. β-Adrenoreceptor antagonists

10. Which of the following pharmacologic actions is most probably responsible for the effects of oxybutynin when given systemically?
    a. Antimuscarinic, direct muscle relaxant, and local anesthetic actions
    b. Direct muscle relaxant effect alone
    c. Direct muscle relaxant effect and local anesthetic action
    d. Antimuscarinic and direct muscle relaxant effects
    e. Antimuscarinic effect

11. Which two of the following muscarinic receptor subtypes are not known to be involved in the potential antimuscarinic side effects of dry mouth, constipation, tachycardia, drowsiness, and blurred vision?
    a. M_1
    b. M_2
    c. M_3
    d. M_4
    e. M_5

12. The primary adverse event reported with the usage of oxybutynin-transdermal has been:
    a. tachycardia.
    b. dry mouth.
    c. constipation.
    d. application site reactions.
    e. blurred vision.

13. Which of the following agents is relatively selective for M_3 receptor blockade?
    a. Darifenacin
    b. Oxybutynin
    c. Solifenacin
    d. Tolterodine
    e. Trospium

14. Which of the following drugs have a theoretical advantage for causing less cognitive dysfunction and why? (Multiple answers are possible.)
    a. Darifenacin
    b. Oxybutynin
    c. Solifenacin
    d. Tolterodine
    e. Trospium

15. Of the following agents, which is actively excreted by the kidney in the proximal convoluted tubules?
    a. Darifenacin
    b. Oxybutynin

c. Solifenacin
d. Tolterodine
e. Trospium

16. Which of the following pharmacologic actions of imipramine is least prominent?
    a. Sedative, on a central basis
    b. Block reuptake of norepinephrine in presynaptic nerve endings
    c. Block reuptake of serotonin in presynaptic nerve endings
    d. Antihistaminic, by blocking H_1 receptors
    e. Direct antimuscarinic effects on bladder smooth muscle

17. Which of the following is NOT listed as a common side effect of imipramine?
    a. Peripheral antimuscarinic effects
    b. Weakness, fatigue
    c. Priapism
    d. Cardiac arrhythmia
    e. Hepatic dysfunction

18. Resiniferatoxin, as compared with capsaicin, exhibits which of the following properties?
    a. Has greater desensitization at lower concentrations
    b. Has more early noxious side effects when administered intravesically
    c. Has more late side effects when administered intravesically
    d. Blocks only Aδ fiber–mediated contraction
    e. Acts on nonvanilloid receptors

19. When used as an intradetrusor injection for DO, botulinum toxin A (Botox) appears to exert its effects within what time frame and last for what time frame before reinjection is necessary?
    a. 3 weeks and 4 to 6 months
    b. 3 days and 6 to 9 months
    c. 2 hours and 6 to 9 months
    d. 1 week and 6 to 9 months
    e. 2 weeks and 4 to 6 months

20. α-Adrenergic agonists, in general, produce all but which of the following?
    a. An increase in maximum urethral pressure
    b. An increase in maximum urethral closure pressure
    c. A contraction of urethral smooth muscle
    d. A decrease in maximum bladder capacity
    e. An increase in bladder outlet resistance

21. The side effects of the α-adrenergic agonists include all of the following EXCEPT:
    a. tremor.
    b. palpitations.
    c. hypertension.
    d. somnolence.
    e. respiratory difficulties.

22. Which of the following agents has been reported to increase stroke risk in young women within 3 days of taking their first dose?

a. Phenylpropanolamine

b. Ephedrine

c. Pseudoephedrine

d. Midodrine

e. Clenbuterol

23. In theory, which of the following agents, from the standpoint of potential efficacy and safety, would be preferred for the treatment of stress urinary incontinence (SUI) in a hypertensive individual?

a. Ephedrine

b. Propranolol

c. Phenylpropanolamine

d. Pseudoephedrine

e. Clenbuterol

24. Which of the following statements is NOT true with respect to duloxetine hydrochloride?

a. It significantly increases sphincteric muscle activity during filling/storage in an animal model.

b. It is a serotonin-norepinephrine reuptake inhibitor.

c. It is lipophilic and well absorbed.

d. It is effective in decreasing SUI episodes in women.

e. It is not metabolized by the liver.

25. Which of the following statements is FALSE with respect to desmopressin?

a. It is classically used to treat nocturnal enuresis.

b. It is classically used to treat diabetes insipidus.

c. It can be given orally or intranasally at the same doses.

d. It suppresses urine production for 7 to 12 hours.

e. It can be used in both children and adults.

26. A 75-year-old man placed on intranasal desmopressin therapy 3 days previously presents with a change of mental status and mental confusion. The most likely cause is:

a. cognitive dysfunction due to antimuscarinic effect.

b. hyponatremia.

c. hypernatremia.

d. hypokalemia.

e. hyperkalemia.

27. With regard to bethanechol chloride, the least objective evidence exists to support which of the following statements?

a. It has relatively selective in-vitro action on urinary bladder and bowel.

b. It has little or no nicotinic action.

c. It is cholinesterase resistant.

d. It causes in-vitro contraction of bladder smooth muscle.

e. It facilitates bladder emptying.

28. What oral dose of bethanechol chloride is required to produce the same urodynamic effects, at least in a denervated bladder, at the subcutaneous dose of 5 mg?

a. 200 mg

b. 100 mg

c. 50 mg

d. 25 mg

e. 10 mg

29. Prostaglandins have been hypothesized to affect bladder activity through all of the following actions EXCEPT:

a. neuromodulation of efferent and afferent neurotransmission.

b. sensitization to sensory stimuli (activation occurs with a lower degree of filling).

c. activation of certain sensory nerves.

d. potentiation of acetylcholine release from cholinergic nerve terminals.

e. potentiation of adenosine triphosphate release from urothelial mucosa.

30. With respect to α-adrenergic receptors versus β-adrenergic receptors in the lower urinary tract, all of the following statements are true EXCEPT:

a. The α-adrenergic receptors are more prominent in the bladder base than are β-adrenergic receptors.

b. The α_1-adrenergic receptors are more common than α_2-adrenergic receptors.

c. The α-adrenergic receptors are less prominent in the bladder body than are β-adrenergic receptors.

d. Bladder smooth muscle contraction is mediated predominantly by α_1-adrenergic receptors.

e. Urethral smooth muscle contraction is mediated predominantly by α_1-adrenergic receptors.

31. Which of the following α-adrenergic blocking agents has significant antagonistic properties at both α_1 and α_2 receptor sites?

a. Prazosin

b. Terazosin

c. Phenoxybenzamine

d. Doxazosin

e. Tamsulosin

32. Available data suggest that which of the following side effects is more common with tamsulosin than with either terazosin or doxazosin?

a. Dizziness

b. Asthenia

c. Postural hypotension

d. Palpitations

e. Retrograde ejaculation

33. Which of the following agents or classes of agents, when administered systemically, will selectively relax the striated musculature of the pelvic floor?

a. Benzodiazepines

b. Dantrolene

c. Baclofen

d. Botulinum toxin

e. None of the above

34. Which of the following is the most widely distributed inhibitory neurotransmitter in the mammalian central nervous system?

a. γ-Aminobutyric acid (GABA)

b. Glycine

c. Glutamate

d. Dopamine

e. Norepinephrine

35. Baclofen (Lioresal) acts to decrease striated sphincter activity by which of the following mechanisms?

a. Facilitating neuronal hyperpolarization through the $GABA_A$ receptor.

b. Activating the $GABA_B$ receptor and depressing monosynaptic and polysynaptic excitation of motor neurons and interneurons in the spinal cord.

c. Inhibiting excitation-contraction coupling in skeletal muscle by decreasing calcium release from the sarcoplasmic reticulum.

d. Inhibiting excitation-contraction coupling by preventing calcium entry into the cell.

e. Inhibiting acetylcholine release at the neuromuscular junction.

36. All of the following statements are true with regard to botulinum toxin EXCEPT:

a. It has been reported to be useful in the treatment of striated sphincter dyssynergia via direct sphincteric injection.

b. It has been reported to be useful in the treatment of DO by direct intradetrusor injection.

c. It inhibits the release of acetylcholine and other transmitters at the neuromuscular junction of somatic nerve and striated muscle and the autonomic nerves in smooth muscle.

d. It has been reported to be of use, via periurethral striated muscle injections, in the treatment of SUI.

e. The immunologic subtype utilized for urologic use has primarily been type A.

37. All of the following statements are true regarding the action of atropine and atropine-like agents (antimuscarinic agents) in patients with OAB and DO EXCEPT:

a. Volume to first involuntary contraction increases.

b. Total bladder capacity increases.

c. Heart rate decreases.

d. Urgency episodes decrease.

e. Amplitude of the DO contractions decreases.

38. Which of the following statements is FALSE with respect to atropine resistance?

a. It is secondary to release of norepinephrine from pelvic nerve in addition to acetylcholine.

b. It is of little importance in normal human detrusor function.

c. Its importance in treatment of DO in humans remains to be established.

d. It applies to the response of the whole bladder to pelvic nerve stimulation but not to the response of the detrusor to exogenous cholinergic stimulation.

e. It is commonly invoked as a cause for only partial clinical improvement in the treatment of OAB with antimuscarinic agents.

39. Which statement is FALSE regarding M_3 receptors?

a. They are less common than M_2 receptors in detrusor smooth muscle.

b. They are more common than M_2 receptors in urothelium.

c. They are the most important muscarinic receptor for detrusor contraction.

d. They are blocked by atropine.

e. When activated they lead to an increase in intracellular calcium in detrusor smooth muscle cells.

40. All of the following are well-known potential adverse events of antimuscarinic therapy EXCEPT:

a. constipation.

b. cognitive dysfunction.

c. increased heart rate.

d. blurred vision.

e. hyperhidrosis.

41. Match the side effects with the predominant muscarinic receptor subtype:

    1. M_1
    2. M_2
    3. M_3
    4. M_4
    5. M_5
    6. None

a. Constipation

b. Dry mouth

c. Cognitive dysfunction

d. Increased heart rate

e. Increased QT interval

42. When used for the treatment of OAB in a patient who is not on clean intermittent catheterization, antimuscarinic agents act primarily by (more than one response may be correct):

a. reducing detrusor voiding contraction.

b. decreasing activity in C fibers.

c. decreasing activity in Aδ fibers.

d. reducing the micromotions caused by release of small packets of acetylcholine.

e. reducing excitation of afferent nerves from the urothelium and detrusor.

43. An 80-year-old man has OAB-wet and cognitive dysfunction. The drug that has the least blood-brain barrier penetration is:

a. solifenacin.

b. oxybutynin ER.

c. fesoterodine.

d. trospium.

e. tolterodine.

44. Activation of detrusor smooth muscle by both acetylcholine and adenosine triphosphate requires:

a. increase in intracellular potassium concentration.

b. decrease in intracellular potassium concentration.

c. increase in intracellular calcium concentration.

d. increase in intracellular cyclic guanosine monophosphate.

e. increase in intracellular cyclic adenosine monophosphate.

45. Which of the following have 1A or 1B ratings (modified Oxford System) for treatment of DO? (Multiple answers are possible.)
    a. Flavoxate
    b. Dicyclomine
    c. Estrogen
    d. Tamsulosin
    e. Tolterodine
    f. Fesoterodine
    g. Darifenacin
    h. Solifenacin
    i. Propiverine
    j. Oxybutynin
    k. Trospium

46. Which of the following drugs can produce or aggravate SUI in a woman (multiple answers are possible)?
    a. Alfuzosin
    b. Nifedipine
    c. Tamsulosin
    d. Oxybutynin
    e. Propantheline
    f. Flavoxate
    g. Fesoterodine
    h. Duloxetine

47. Intravesical DMSO is (multiple answers are possible):
    a. generally used in a 70% solution.
    b. generally used in a 50% solution.
    c. useful for the treatment of neurogenic DO.
    d. useful for the treatment of bladder pain syndrome (interstitial cystitis).
    e. useful for the treatment of idiopathic DO.

48. Regarding the vanilloids, which of the following is/are TRUE? (Multiple answers are possible.)
    a. They act primarily to render C fibers insensitive.
    b. They act primarily to render Aδ fibers insensitive.
    c. When delivered intravesically they cause a biphasic (excitation then blockade) effect.
    d. Resiniferatoxin is much more potent than capsaicin for desensitization but proportionately less so for excitation.
    e. Capsaicin is more potent than resiniferatoxin desensitization.

49. A 30-year-old paraplegic man is wet between intermittent catheterizations (catheterizes five times per day). He is on solifenacin 10 mg daily and reports moderate dry mouth and increased difficulty in his bowel regimen. A reasonable next step in treatment is:
    a. to increase dose of solifenacin.
    b. to add oxybutynin ER 10 mg daily.
    c. to add darifenacin 7.5 mg daily.
    d. to add darifenacin 15 mg daily.
    e. to use intradetrusor botulinum toxin.

50. Generally, treatment with intradetrusor botulinum toxin (multiple answers are possible):
    a. must be repeated every 3 to 12 months.
    b. improves quality of life in patients incontinent due to neurogenic DO.
    c. loses efficacy with repeat treatments.
    d. can cause urinary retention.
    e. requires general anesthesia.

51. The HERS, Womens Health Initiative, and Nurses Health Study compositely showed (multiple answers are possible):
    a. oral estrogen + progesterone worsened urinary incontinence in older postmenopausal women with incontinence.
    b. oral estrogen + progesterone increased the incidence of SUI and urgency urinary incontinence in those continent at baseline.
    c. oral estrogen and progesterone worsened the frequency of incontinence in those incontinent at baseline.
    d. transvaginal estrogen improves SUI in postmenopausal women.
    e. the risk of developing incontinence was increased in postmenopausal women taking estrogen alone or estrogen with progestin.

52. Estrogen treatment in postmenopausal women (multiple answers are possible):
    a. if unopposed increases the risk of endometrial cancer.
    b. causes a twofold to threefold increase in gallbladder disease.
    c. with progesterone causes no increase in the risk of endometrial cancer.
    d. if unopposed causes an increased risk of breast cancer.
    e. causes an increased risk of thromboembolic disease.

53. Adrenergically induced smooth muscle contraction in the human lower urinary tract is mediated primarily by which receptor?
    a. α_{1D}
    b. β_3
    c. β_2
    d. α_{1A}
    e. α_2

ANSWERS

1. **c. increased outlet resistance.** Atropine and atropine-like agents will depress normal bladder contractions and involuntary bladder contractions of any cause. In such patients the volume to the first involuntary bladder contraction will generally be increased, the amplitude of the involuntary bladder contraction decreased, and the total bladder capacity increased. Outlet resistance, at least as reflected by urethral pressure measurements, does not seem to be clinically affected.

2. **b. M_2.** On the basis of existing knowledge it is now recommended that the designations M_1 to M_5 be used to describe both the pharmacologic subtypes and the molecular subtypes of muscarinic acetylcholine receptors. The human urinary bladder smooth muscle contains a mixed population of M_2 and M_3 subtypes, with M_2 receptors being

predominant (M_2 receptors predominate at least $3:1$ over M_3 receptors not only on detrusor cells but also on other bladder structures, which may be of importance for detrusor activation).

3. **c. M_3.** The minor population of M_3 receptors is generally accepted at this time as being primarily responsible for the mediation of bladder contraction.

4. **d. Bradycardia.** In general, drug therapy for lower urinary tract dysfunction is hindered by a concept that can be expressed in one word: uroselectivity. The clinical utility of available antimuscarinic agents is limited by their lack of selectivity, responsible for the classic peripheral antimuscarinic side effects of dry mouth, constipation, blurred vision, tachycardia, and effects on cognitive function.

5. **a, c, *and* e.** High lipophilicity, small molecular size, and low electrical charge increase the possibilities for an antimuscarinic agent to pass the blood-brain barrier. Quaternary ammonium compounds pass into the central nervous system to a limited extent.

6. **c. poorly absorbed from the gastrointestinal tract.** Propantheline bromide (Pro-Banthine, others) was the classically described oral agent for producing an antimuscarinic effect in the lower urinary tract. It is a nonselective muscarinic antagonist. Propantheline is a quaternary ammonium compound and is poorly absorbed after oral administration. There seems to be little difference between the antimuscarinic effects of propantheline on bladder smooth muscle and the effects of other classic antimuscarinic agents.

7. **d. M_3 receptor blockade.** Although the agents with mixed actions do relax smooth muscle in vitro by musculotropic activity and do have some local anesthetic properties, it is generally accepted that the clinical effects, at least of oxybutynin, occur solely through muscarinic blockade, because the other effects occur at much higher concentrations than its antimuscarinic actions. Oxybutynin chloride (Ditropan) is a potent muscarinic receptor antagonist with some degree of selectivity for M_3 and M_1 receptors.

8. **a *and* b.** A level of evidence of 1 implies the presence of systematic reviews, meta-analyses, and good quality randomized controlled clinical trials. A grade of recommendation of A means that the agent is highly recommended, based on level 1 evidence. Dicyclomine received a level of evidence of 3, meaning that only case-controlled studies and case series existed as evidence for efficacy, and a grade of recommendation of C, meaning that only level 4 studies (based on only expert opinion) or majority evidence existed. Flavoxate received a level of evidence of 2, meaning that either randomized control trials and/or good quality prospective cohort studies existed regarding its usage, but a grade of recommendation of D, meaning that no recommendation for usage is possible because of inconsistent/inconclusive evidence. The complete listing of the Oxford Guidelines and the committee recommendations can be found in Tables 68–1 and 68–2 in *Campbell-Walsh Urology, 10th Edition.*

9. **d. Potassium channel openers.** Opening of potassium channels and subsequent efflux of potassium will produce hyperpolarization of various smooth muscles, including the detrusor. This leads to a decrease in calcium influx with subsequent relaxation or inhibition of contraction.

Theoretically, such drugs may be active during the filling/storage phase of micturition, abolishing DO with no effect on normal bladder contraction. Unfortunately, the first generation of potassium channel openers were found to be more potent as inhibitors of vascular than of detrusor muscle; and in clinical trials performed with these drugs, no bladder effects were found at doses that lowered blood pressure. However, new drugs with potassium/adenosine triphosphate channel opening properties have been described that may prove to be useful for the treatment of DO.

10. **e. Antimuscarinic effect.** Oxybutynin has several pharmacologic effects, some of which seem difficult to relate to its effectiveness in the treatment of DO. It has antimuscarinic, direct muscle relaxant, and local anesthetic actions. The local anesthetic action and direct muscle relaxant effect may be of importance when the drug is administered intravesically but probably play no role when it is given orally. In vitro, oxybutynin was shown to be 500 times weaker as a smooth muscle relaxant than as an antimuscarinic agent. Most probably, when given systemically, oxybutynin acts mainly as an antimuscarinic drug.

11. **d *and* e.** The M_3 receptor has a primary role in salivation, bowel motility, and visual accommodation. The M_1 receptor is thought to be involved in cognition. The M_2 receptor is the primary cholinergic receptor in the heart, causing bradycardia when activated and, potentially, tachycardia, when blocked. The M_4 and M_5 receptors do not at this time seem to have a primary role in any of these organ systems.

12. **d. application site reactions.** The transdermal delivery of oxybutynin alters oxybutynin metabolism, reducing production of the primary metabolite, responsible for most of the side effects, to an even greater extent than extended-release oxybutynin. The primary adverse event for this preparation has been application site reaction: pruritus in 14% and erythema in 8.3%.

13. **a. Darifenacin.** Darifenacin is relatively selective for M_3 receptor blockade, meaning that, in vitro, the affinity for M_3 receptors is greater than for the other muscarinic receptors. This is only a relative selectivity, however, and whether this translates into either greater efficacy or greater tolerability has yet to be established.

14. **a, d, *and* e.** The currently accepted theory as to why some antimuscarinic agents may cause cognitive dysfunction is antagonism of M_1 receptor activity in the brain. Theoretically, to have this side effect, an agent must be able to cross rather freely the blood-brain barrier and affect M_1 receptors to a significant extent. Darifenacin is relatively selective for M_3 receptor blockade, although it does cross the blood-brain barrier freely. Tolterodine, because of its low lipophilicity, relatively large molecular size, and charge status, is thought to have limited passage across the blood-brain barrier in a normal individual. Trospium, by virtue of its quaternary amine status, has limited passage across the blood-brain barrier in a normal individual.

15. **e. Trospium.** Darifenacin, oxybutynin, solifenacin, and tolterodine are all actively metabolized in the liver by the cytochrome P450 enzyme system. Trospium chloride is not metabolized to any significant degree in the liver. It is actively excreted by the proximal convoluted tubules in the kidney.

16. **e. Direct antimuscarinic effects on bladder smooth muscle.** All of these agents possess various degrees of at

least three major pharmacologic actions: (1) they have central and peripheral antimuscarinic effects at some, but not all, sites; (2) they block the active transport system in the presynaptic nerve ending, which is responsible for the reuptake of the released amine neurotransmitters norepinephrine and serotonin; and (3) they are sedatives, an action that occurs presumably on a central basis but is perhaps related to antihistaminic properties. Imipramine has prominent systemic antimuscarinic effects but has only a weak antimuscarinic effect on bladder smooth muscle. A strong direct inhibitory effect on bladder smooth muscle does exist, however, that is neither antimuscarinic nor adrenergic.

17. **c. Priapism.** The most frequent side effects of the tricyclic antidepressants are those attributable to their systemic antimuscarinic activity. Allergic phenomena (including rash), hepatic dysfunction, obstructive jaundice, and agranulocytosis may also occur, but rarely. Central nervous system side effects may include weakness, fatigue, parkinsonian effect, fine tremor noted most in the upper extremities, manic or schizophrenic picture, and sedation, probably from an antihistaminic effect. Postural hypotension may also be seen, presumably on the basis of selective blockade (a paradoxical effect) of α_1-adrenergic receptors in some vascular smooth muscle. Tricyclic antidepressants can also cause excess sweating of obscure cause and a delay of orgasm or orgasmic impotence, whose cause is likewise unclear. They can also produce arrhythmias and interact in deleterious ways with other drugs, and so caution must be observed in their use in patients with cardiac disease.

18. **a. Has greater desensitization at lower concentrations.** Resiniferatoxin is an analogue of capsaicin that is approximately 1000 times more potent for desensitization but only a few hundred times more potent for excitation. Although both may have effects on Aδ fibers, this is speculative, and their primary action is to render sensitive primary afferents (C fibers) resistant to activation by natural stimuli.

19. **e. 2 weeks and 4 to 6 months.**

20. **d. A decrease in maximum bladder capacity.** The bladder neck and proximal urethra contain a preponderance of α_1-receptor sites, which, when stimulated, produce smooth muscle contraction. The static infusion urethral pressure profile is altered by such stimulation, which produces an increase in maximum urethral pressure and maximum urethral closure pressure. Various orally administered pharmacologic agents are available that produce α-adrenergic stimulation. Generally, outlet resistance is increased to a variable degree by such an action.

21. **d. somnolence.** Potential side effects of all of these agents include blood pressure elevation, anxiety, and insomnia due to stimulation of the central nervous system; headache; tremor; weakness; palpations; cardiac arrhythmias; and respiratory difficulties. They should be used with caution in patients with hypertension, cardiovascular disease, or hyperthyroidism.

22. **a. Phenylpropanolamine.** The U.S. Food and Drug Administration (FDA) originally asked manufacturers to stop selling phenylpropanolamine-containing drugs and to replace the ingredient with a safe alternative. Subsequently, it was taken off the market in the United States. The

original request was based on a study reported by Kernan and colleagues (2000).* In commenting on this article, the *Medical Letter* (Abramowicz and Zuccotti, 2000) noted that no case-control studies were available on the safety of phenylephrine, ephedrine, or pseudoephedrine but did note that case reports have associated ephedra alkaloids with hypertension, stroke, seizures, and death. The *Medical Letter* concluded: "Phenylpropanolamine may not be the only alpha-adrenergic agonist that can cause serious adverse effects when taken systemically in over-the-counter products marketed for nasal congestion or weight loss."

23. **b. Propranolol.** Theoretically, β-adrenergic blocking agents might be expected to "unmask" or potentiate an α-adrenergic effect, thereby increasing urethral resistance. Such treatment has been suggested as an alternative treatment to α-adrenergic agonists in patients with sphincteric incontinence and hypertension.

24. **e. It is not metabolized by the liver.** Duloxetine hydrochloride is a serotonin-norepinephrine reuptake inhibitor that has been shown, in an animal model, to significantly increase urethral sphincteric muscle activity during the filling/storage phase of micturition. It is lipophilic, well absorbed, and extensively metabolized by the liver. Its effectiveness in the treatment of SUI in the female has been documented. At the time of this writing it was withdrawn from the FDA approval process and has not been resubmitted, but it has been approved for use in Europe.

25. **c. It can be given orally or intranasally at the same doses.** The synthetic antidiuretic hormone peptide analog DDAVP (1-deamino-8-d-arginine vasopressin), now more commonly known as desmopressin, has been utilized for the symptomatic relief of refractory nocturnal enuresis in both children and adults. The drug can conveniently be administered by intranasal spray at bedtime (10 to 40 μg) or as an oral preparation (100 to 400 μg) and effectively suppresses urine production for 7 to 12 hours.

26. **b. hyponatremia.** Side effects are relatively uncommon during desmopressin treatment, but there is a risk of water retention and hyponatremia, such that it is recommended that serum sodium concentration should be measured in elderly patients before and after a few days of treatment.

27. **e. It facilitates bladder emptying.** Many acetylcholine-like drugs exist, but only bethanechol chloride (Urecholine, Duvoid, others) exhibits a relatively selective in-vitro action on the urinary bladder and gut with little or no nicotinic action. Bethanechol chloride is cholinesterase resistant and causes an in-vitro contraction of smooth muscle from all areas of the bladder. Although it has been reported to increase gastrointestinal motility and has been used in the treatment of gastroesophageal reflux, and although anecdotal success in specific patients with voiding dysfunction seems to occur, there is no evidence to support its success in facilitating bladder emptying in a series of patients when the drug was the only variable.

28. **a. 200 mg.** It is generally agreed that, at least in a "denervated" bladder, an oral dose of 200 mg is required to produce the same urodynamic effects as a subcutaneous dose of 5 mg.

---

*Sources referenced can be found in *Campbell-Walsh Urology, 10th Edition,* on the Expert Consult website.

29. **e. Potentiation of adenosine triphosphate release from urothelial mucosa.** Prostanoids are synthesized both locally in bladder muscle and mucosa, with synthesis being initiated by various physiologic stimuli such as detrusor muscle stretch, mucosal injury, neural stimulation, directly by adenosine triphosphate, and by mediators of inflammation. Prostanoids have been reported to be useful in facilitating bladder emptying, with intravesical administration. Possible roles include (1) neuromodulators of efferent and afferent transmission; (2) sensitization; (3) activation of certain sensory nerves; and (4) potentiation of acetylcholine release from cholinergic nerve terminals through prejunctional prostanoid receptors.

30. **b. The α_1-adrenergic receptors are more common than α_2-adrenergic receptors.** The smooth muscle of the bladder base and proximal urethra contains predominantly α-adrenergic receptors, although β-adrenergic receptors are present. The bladder body contains both varieties of adrenergic receptors, with the β-adrenergic variety being more common. The human lower urinary tract contains more α_2- than α_1-adrenergic receptors, but prostatic smooth muscle contraction and human lower urinary tract smooth muscle contraction are mediated largely, if not exclusively, by α_1-adrenergic receptors.

31. **c. Phenoxybenzamine.** Phenoxybenzamine (Dibenzyline) was the α-adrenolytic agent originally used for the treatment of voiding dysfunction. It and phentolamine have blocking properties at both α_1-adrenergic and α_2-adrenergic receptor sites. Prazosin hydrochloride (Minipress) was the first potent selective α_1-adrenergic antagonist used to lower outlet resistance. Terazosin (Hytrin) and doxazosin (Cardura) are two highly selective postsynaptic α_1-adrenergic blockers. Most recently, alfuzosin and tamsulosin (Flomax), both highly selective α_1-adrenergic blockers, have appeared and are marketed solely for the treatment of benign prostatic hyperplasia because of some reports suggesting preferential action on prostatic rather than vascular smooth muscle.

32. **e. Retrograde ejaculation.** Available data suggest that retrograde ejaculation and rhinitis are more common with tamsulosin, whereas dizziness and asthenia are more common with terazosin and doxazosin.

33. **e. None of the above.** There is no class of pharmacologic agents that will selectively relax the striated musculature of the pelvic floor.

34. **a. γ-Aminobutyric acid (GABA).** GABA and glycine have been identified as major inhibitory transmitters in the central nervous system. GABA is the most widely distributed inhibitory neurotransmitter in the mammalian central nervous system. It appears to mediate the inhibitory actions of local interneurons in the brain and presynaptic inhibition within the spinal cord.

35. **b. Activating the GABA$_B$ receptor and depressing monosynaptic and polysynaptic excitation of motor neurons and interneurons in the spinal cord.** Benzodiazepines potentiate the action of GABA by facilitating neuronal hyperpolarization through the GABA$_A$ receptor. Baclofen (Lioresal) depresses monosynaptic and polysynaptic excitation of motor neurons and interneurons in the spinal cord by activating GABA$_B$ receptors. Dantrolene (Dantrium) exerts its effects by a direct peripheral action on skeletal muscle. It is thought to inhibit the excitation-induced release of calcium ions from the sarcoplasmic reticulum of striated muscle fibers, thereby inhibiting excitation-contraction coupling and diminishing the mechanical force of contraction. Botulinum A toxin (Botox) is an inhibitor of acetylcholine release at the neuromuscular junction of somatic nerves on striated muscle.

36. **d. It has been reported to be of use, via periurethral striated muscle injections, in the treatment of SUI.** Intersphincteric injections of botulinum toxin A were first reported useful in the treatment of striated sphincter dyssynergia in 1990. The toxin blocks the release of acetylcholine and other transmitters from presynaptic nerve endings by interacting with the protein complex necessary for docking vesicles. This results in decreased muscle contractility and muscle atrophy at the injection site. The drug has been reported to be of use as well in the treatment of neurogenic DO and cases of non-neurogenic DO. There are seven immunologically distinct antigenic subtypes. Types A and B are in clinical use in urology, but most studies and treatments have been carried out with botulinum toxin type A (Botox). Intrasphincteric injections of botulinum toxin are not useful for SUI. In fact, they can cause SUI in females.

37. **c. Heart rate decreases.** Those with an M$_2$ receptor blockade profile can increase heart rate, but the clinical significance of this is unknown.

38. **a. It is secondary to release of norepinephrine from pelvic nerve in addition to acetylcholine.** The most common neurotransmitter mentioned as the prime alternate in atropine resistance is adenosine triphosphate. Norepinephrine is released by postganglionic sympathetic nerves (e.g., hypogastric) not by parasympathetic ones (e.g., pelvic).

39. **b. They are more common than M$_2$ receptors in urothelium.** M$_2$ receptors outnumber M$_3$ in urothelium.

40. **e. hyperhidrosis.** If anything, antimuscarinic agents can cause decreased sweating. All the others are antimuscarinic side effects.

41. **a: 3; b: 3; c: 1; d: 2; e: 6.** Increased QT interval, caused by some antimuscarinic compounds, is not an antimuscarinic property. All the others are and are caused primarily by blockade of the indicated receptor subtype.

42. **b, c, d, and e.** At the doses employed for OAB treatment antimuscarinic agents do not cause significant reduction in the voiding contraction of voluntary micturition. They have been implicated in all the others. C and Aδ fibers refer to afferent nerves carrying noxious and "normal" stimuli, respectively.

43. **d. trospium.** Trospium, as a quaternary amine, is lipophobic and does not penetrate well through the blood-brain barrier. The others, all tertiary amines, and do pass the blood-brain barrier to a greater extent.

44. **c. increase in intracellular calcium concentration.** This occurs through extracellular influx and mobilization of intracellular calcium.

45. **e, f, g, h, i, j, and k.** See Table 68–2 in *Campbell-Walsh Urology*, 10th *Edition*.

46. **a and c.** The α-adrenergic antagonists can decrease outlet resistance and thereby irritate or worsen SUI. Nifedipine is a calcium antagonist; fesoterodine and propantheline are anticholinergic agents; duloxetine is a serotonin-norepinephrine reuptake inhibitor; oxybutynin is primarily an antimuscarinic agent with some direct smooth muscle relaxant effects on the bladder; and flavoxate has mixed actions and questionable effects.

47. **b *and* d.** DMSO is a naturally occurring compound with multiple pharmacologic actions used in a 50% solution for the treatment of bladder pain syndrome (including interstitial cystitis). It is not useful for the treatment of DO.

48. **a, c, *and* d.** It is possible that they have some effects on Aδ fibers as well. They cause an initial excitation followed by a long-lasting blockade. Resiniferatoxin is 1000 times more potent than capsaicin for desensitization and a few hundred times more potent for excitation.

49. **e. to use intradetrusor botulinum toxin.** Adding or increasing antimuscarinic medication will simply increase the severity of the adverse events already experienced. Intradetrusor botulinum toxin, although not approved in the United States, has been shown to be very effective in neurogenic DO and should be considered if allowing failure of, or intolerance to, antimuscarinic therapy.

50. **a, b, *and* d.** Repeat injections (2 to 9) have not lost efficacy over time. The injections can be done without general anesthesia (local). Intravesical BONTA is effective in reducing neurogenic DO and does improve quality of life in such patients. It is not approved for use in the United States.

51. **a, b, c, *and* e.** a is from the HERS Study, b and c from the WHI, and e from the Nurses Health Study. Although many clinicians prescribe transvaginal estrogen or estrogen + progestin cream for symptoms of OAB or/and SUI, there is no real evidence that estrogen, with or without progesterone, is useful in the treatment of urinary incontinence.

52. **a, b, c, *and* e.** Unopposed use in women without a uterus may actually decrease the relative risk of breast cancer. For

a, the increased risk is 5 to 15 times (prevented if progestin is added); for e, the increase in stroke and pulmonary embolism has been cited as an increase of 8/10,000 for each.

53. **d.** α_{1A}. More α_2 than α_1 receptors are present, but adrenergically induced contraction is mediated largely by the α_{1A} (and in the detrusor, α_{1D}). β receptors cause smooth muscle relaxation. The β_3 variety is predominant in the human detrusor.

Additional Study Points

1. The major neurohumoral stimulus for physiologic bladder contraction is acetylcholine-induced stimulation of postganglionic parasympathetic muscarinic cholinergic receptor sites in the bladder.
2. The muscarinic receptor functions may be changed in different urologic disorders without an overt neurogenic cause.
3. Behavioral therapy should always be used in conjunction with drug therapy for OAB.
4. Calcium channel antagonists are not effective in treating OAB.
5. Potassium channel openers available today do not work.
6. The use of estrogens to treat SUI has resulted in worsening of preexisting urinary incontinence in those with SUI and urgency urinary incontinence and new-onset incontinence in those who have not had it.
7. Intravesical oxybutynin has shown some efficacy in treating OAB as well as treating intestinal augmented OABs.

Conservative Management of Urinary Incontinence: Behavioral and Pelvic Floor Therapy, Urethral and Pelvic Devices

Christopher K. Payne, MD

QUESTIONS

1. The consequences of urinary incontinence (UI) include an increased risk of all of the following EXCEPT:

   a. pressure ulcers.

   b. renal failure.

   c. urinary tract infections.

   d. admission to nursing homes.

   e. falls and fractures.

2. According to the National Institutes of Health (NIH) report to the U.S. Congress, which of the following statements is TRUE?

   a. NIH research spending on UI as a percentage of direct costs of disease is less than one tenth that of most other common diseases.

   b. NIH research spending for a percentage of direct costs of disease is approximately equal for most common diseases.

   c. The cost of HIV/AIDS is 10 times that of UI.

   d. The cost of UI is about 10 times that of cerebrovascular disease/stroke.

   e. The total NIH research funding for UI was almost 10 times that for Alzheimer disease or asthma.

3. Which of the following is NOT an example of behavioral therapy?

   a. Use of an incontinence dish to treat stress urinary incontinence (SUI)

   b. Using a group session to teach patients about lower urinary tract anatomy and function

   c. Using "quick flicks" to inhibit urinary urgency

   d. Keeping a frequency-volume chart or bladder diary

   e. Discontinuing caffeinated beverages

4. Which of the following is the most appropriate therapy for a cognitively impaired, institutionalized patient with UI?

   a. Prompted voiding

   b. Timed voiding

   c. Pelvic floor biofeedback

   d. Anticholinergic agents given on an "as needed" basis

   e. Extracorporeal magnetic stimulation

5. Which of the following statements is TRUE?

   a. Epidemiologic studies show increased risk of SUI and urgency urinary incontinence (UUI) for all smokers.

   b. A dose-response relationship has been established for UI and smoking in men and women.

   c. It is not known whether smoking cessation reduces UI.

   d. The risk of smoking for UI is limited to those with exposure greater than two packs per day.

   e. The risk of smoking for UI is limited to SUI in patients who have chronic cough.

6. Which of the following statements about UI and beverage consumption is TRUE?

   a. Instructing patients to decrease fluid intake by 25% to 50% from baseline resulted in statistically significant improvements in UI.

   b. Cross-sectional population studies show a dose-response relationship between caffeine consumption and UI.

   c. Coffee consumption is strongly correlated with UI but tea intake shows an inverse association.

   d. Increasing free water intake to 6 to 8 glasses per day has been shown to improve UI.

   e. There is strong statistical relationship between alcohol intake and UI.

7. Which of the following statements about obesity and UI is TRUE?

   a. Moderate weight loss in obese patients (body mass index >25) produced statistically significantly improvement in overall UI and SUI.

   b. The threshold for improving SUI with weight loss begins around two thirds of excess body weight.

   c. Although obesity has been shown to correlate with UI, the only prospective data showing that weight loss improves UI come from extreme cases with bariatric surgery.

    d. Although obesity is strongly correlated with incident UI there is as yet no evidence that weight loss can reverse the condition.

    e. The primary mechanism by which weight loss improves continence is by improving diabetes and reversing prediabetes.

8. Which of the following statements accurately assesses risk factors for developing UI?

    a. Increasing levels of physical activity are correlated with lower risk of developing UI.

    b. After adjustment for other comorbidities there is a stepwise increase in all forms of UI with age.

    c. Depression is the primary cause of UI in the elderly.

    d. Diabetes increases the risk (odds ratio) of UI threefold.

    e. Type 2 diabetes is primarily associated with increased SUI.

9. The prevalence of UI increases with age because:

    a. of the increasing comorbidities associated with aging.

    b. loss of urethral neuronal function increases SUI.

    c. diminished tight junctions in the aging bladder increase overactive bladder/UUI.

    d. Women do not continue to practice pelvic floor muscle training (PFMT).

    e. Surgical therapy has only a short-term positive effect.

10. Which of the following does NOT accurately describe PFMT?

    a. Daily exercise is essential to a positive outcome.

    b. The effect is not directly related to increase in muscle bulk.

    c. Biofeedback was an essential part of the exercise program as originally described by Kegel.

    d. "Training" was added to emphasize the need for a commitment to exercising over time.

    e. Programs taught by health care professionals show superior outcomes to self-directed exercise.

11. In preventing UI, the evidence supports routine use of PFMT in which of the following groups?

    a. All primiparous women, before delivery

    b. Primiparous women, after instrumented delivery

    c. All pregnant women, before delivery

    d. a and b

    e. All of the above

12. In long-term follow-up studies of PFMT:

    a. 50% of women who complete 12 weeks of PFMT will still be exercising at least weekly after 15 years.

    b. results at 10 years are equivalent to surgical therapy for women with SUI.

    c. biofeedback training is essential to long-term success of PFMT.

    d. more than two thirds of women with SUI who initially respond to PFMT eventually go on to surgical therapy.

    e. the majority of women remain satisfied with their level of improvement from PFMT.

13. Which of the following is NOT a form of biofeedback for UI?

    a. The NeoControl device

    b. Digital palpation

    c. Vaginal cones

    d. Pressure perineometry

    e. Perineal patch electrodes

14. Which of the following statements is NOT true regarding electrical stimulation in the treatment of UI?

    a. Bulk in the pelvic floor muscles begins to increase within 2 weeks and clinical benefit begins within 8 weeks.

    b. High-frequency stimulation (50 to 200 Hz) is used for SUI.

    c. Low frequency stimulation (5 to 20 Hz) is used for OAB.

    d. Published reports comprise a selected patient population because many patients will not accept this treatment modality.

    e. Every-other-day therapy is as effective as daily therapy.

15. Prospective trials of posterior tibial nerve stimulation (PTNS) show:

    a. over half of patients treated for UUI continued to respond to therapy over 1 year.

    b. superior outcomes to the use of tolterodine in treatment of UUI.

    c. equal outcomes to the use of surgery for SUI.

    d. 50% response rate in treatment of urinary retention.

    e. three times a week appears to be the optimal frequency for treatment.

16. In comparing magnetic stimulation to electrical stimulation, which of the following is FALSE?

    a. Superior results in the treatment of SUI

    b. No internal probe: increased patient acceptance

    c. Patient can wear street clothes: convenience

    d. Operated by a technician with minimal training

    e. No supervision required

17. Which of the following statements about the use of vaginal support devices for patients with SUI is FALSE?

    a. Over 90% of patients do not leak with a device in place.

    b. They can be used in patients with mixed UI to estimate the response to surgery.

    c. They can cause vaginitis and vaginal bleeding in one fourth of patients.

    d. They can be used on an "as needed" basis.

    e. They should not affect voiding efficiency.

18. Vaginal support devices (pessaries):

    a. may unmask occult SUI in 50% of patients with a cystocele.

    b. can be used to determine if lower-grade prolapse is symptomatic.

    c. can be used to identify reversible urinary retention related to prolapse.

    d. All of the above

    e. None of the above

19. Which of the statements about urethral inserts is FALSE?
    a. The most common adverse event is gross hematuria.
    b. A new device is inserted after each void.
    c. More than half of women surveyed do not feel comfortable using such devices.
    d. The devices are not intended to treat UUI.
    e. An uncommon but serious adverse event is migration of the device into the bladder.

20. Patient satisfaction has been shown to be correlated to:
    a. expectations.
    b. setting goals.
    c. goal achievement.
    d. surgical cure of SUI.
    e. anatomic cure of pelvic organ prolapse.

21. The key information for planning use of conservative therapies comes from:
    a. incontinence type, bladder diary, pelvic examination/muscle assessment.
    b. bladder diary, urodynamics, cystoscopy.
    c. incontinence type, bladder diary, cystoscopy.
    d. bladder diary, urodynamics, pelvic examination/muscle assessment.
    e. incontinence type, pelvic examination/muscle assessment, cystoscopy.

22. The bladder diary is valuable for all of the following EXCEPT:
    a. it correlates with urodynamic bladder capacity.
    b. it predicts successful interval for bladder training program.
    c. it involves the patient in behavioral therapy.
    d. it provides a means of assessing response to therapy.
    e. it predicts the likelihood of response to PFMT.

23. Considering pelvic floor muscle strength/control:
    a. patients with absent/poor muscles and SUI should always initiate therapy with PFMT.
    b. patients with absent/poor muscles and UUI respond better to electrical stimulation than to biofeedback/PFMT.
    c. patients with SUI who have decreased strength who can isolate muscle function should be treated with biofeedback.
    d. patients with strong pelvic floor muscles and UUI should be treated with anticholinergic medications.
    e. patients with strong pelvic floor muscles and SUI should not undergo surgery until all alternatives have been exhausted.

24. In prospective trials of PFMT for patients considering surgical therapy for SUI:
    a. 40% to 50% of those undergoing PFMT ultimately choose not to undergo surgery.
    b. 40% to 50% of those undergoing PFMT have a complete response and are dry to stress.
    c. 90% of those initially satisfied with PFMT cross over to surgery within 1 year.
    d. in randomized trials the 1-year cure/improve rate is identical between PFMT and surgery.

    e. only patients with weak/absent pelvic muscle contractions should undergo PFMT.

25. In considering treatment of OAB/UUI, which of the following statements is TRUE?
    a. PFMT, bladder training, and anticholinergic medications are all equally effective.
    b. Bladder training should always be used when anticholinergic medications are prescribed.
    c. Anticholinergic medications should always be used when PFMT is prescribed.
    d. PFMT is the most effective therapy for the majority of patients.
    e. Anticholinergic medications should be considered to be a lifelong therapy.

26. Which statement is FALSE in describing the treatment of patients with refractory OAB?
    a. The patient should be reevaluated for correctable causes of UI.
    b. Botulinum toxin (Botox) bladder injections provide permanent relief of UI for approximately a third of patients.
    c. Neuromodulation is approved by the U.S. Food and Drug Administration for treatment for such patients.
    d. Botox injections cost less than neuromodulation and may be effective when neuromodulation fails.
    e. The main drawback of Botox therapy is the risk of urinary retention requiring catheterization.

27. In considering patients with mixed urinary incontinence:
    a. surgical therapy may be more effective when the bladder diary demonstrates the patient has a good functional capacity.
    b. urodynamic studies are critical for treatment planning.
    c. electrical stimulation is ineffective.
    d. support of the bladder neck with a pessary will exacerbate the SUI component.
    e. SUI surgery is indicated when medical therapy is ineffective.

ANSWERS

1. **b. renal failure.** In contrast to the other responses, UI does not commonly affect the upper urinary tracts. Lower urinary tract dysfunction can lead to renal failure when there are high storage pressures in the bladder. Incontinence can rarely coexist with high storage pressures in certain disorders such as neurogenic bladder with external sphincter dyssynergia and retention due to bladder outlet obstruction, but these cases represent a small fraction of the incontinent population.

2. **a. NIH research spending on UI as a percentage of direct costs of disease is less than one tenth that of most other common diseases.** Despite the high prevalence and significant costs associated with incontinence there has been inadequate funding of research into the condition.

3. **a. Use of an incontinence dish to treat SUI.** An incontinence dish provides mechanical support to the bladder neck. All the other options use education about bodily function or habits to decrease leakage.

4. **a. Prompted voiding.** Cognitively impaired individuals need assistance and/or a reminder to void before incontinence occurs; this is referred to as "prompted voiding." Timed voiding is used in the cognitively intact population. Biofeedback cannot be used in the cognitively impaired. Anticholinergic agents have increased side effects in this population and are only potentially indicated for the subset with OAB/UUI. There is no evidence supporting the use of magnetic stimulation in this population.

5. **c. It is not known whether smoking cessation reduces UI.** Although smoking has many negative effects on health, including an increased risk for bladder cancer, the epidemiology of smoking and UI is not consistent. There are no trials showing that smoking cessation improves continence.

6. **a. Instructing patients to decrease fluid intake by 25% to 50% from baseline resulted in statistically significant improvements in UI.** A randomized crossover trial demonstrated reduced UI with fluid restriction and worsening with increased fluids. However, the epidemiology of various types of fluids has not shown consistent findings.

7. **a. Moderate weight loss in obese patients (body mass index >25) produced statistically significantly improvement in overall UI and SUI.** A randomized controlled trial showed significant improvement in incontinence with average weight loss of less than 20 pounds. Weight loss improves health in a variety of manners, but it is not clear what are the most important factors in the change.

8. **a. Increasing levels of physical activity are correlated with lower risk of developing UI.** Although it has been postulated that vigorous exercise and straining may produce UI the epidemiologic data show decreased UI with increasing levels of activity. Diabetes is weakly associated with UI, mainly by increased UUI. Depression and UI are associated, but it is not the main cause of UI in the elderly. Although the prevalence of UI increases steadily with age it is primarily due to the presence of other disorders.

9. **a. of the increasing comorbidities associated with aging.** Although the prevalence of UI increases steadily with age it is primarily due to the presence of many other disorders that increase with age. When these disorders are accounted for, the prevalence of UI is not increased in the elderly.

10. **a. Daily exercise is essential to a positive outcome.** The current teaching from exercise physiology is that every-other-day exercise of specific muscle groups is most effective and that training the muscles by long-term exercise is essential. Kegel originally described teaching exercises with a pressure perineometer that could also be used to measure improvement. Whereas written instructions for bladder training and exercise are an inexpensive way to improve continence, superior results are achieved with professional instruction. Improvement in continence clearly occurs before, and is not dependent on, measurable increase in muscle bulk.

11. **d. a and b.** PFMT are recommended as first-line therapy for established incontinence and for prevention of incontinence in selected cases. PFMT have proven efficacy for prevention in primiparous women and women after high-risk deliveries such as instrumental delivery or delivery of a large neonate. There are no data yet to prove effectiveness in preventing incontinence for all pregnant women.

12. **e. the majority of women remain satisfied with their level of improvement from PFMT.** We have inadequate long-term data about most forms of treatment for UI, including PFMT. Three published studies suggest that most women who initially respond to PFMT remain satisfied at 10 to 15 years, although few continued to exercise regularly and the level of improvement deteriorated with time. In one study, half of women with SUI went on to surgical therapy but in another less than 10% did so.

13. **a. The NeoControl device.** Biofeedback can be used in many different forms including digital palpation with verbal instructions, vaginal cones, auditory, visual, and so on. The NeoControl device (Neotonus Corporation, Marietta, GA) delivers passive magnetic stimulation and is not a form of biofeedback.

14. **a. Bulk in the pelvic floor muscles begins to increase within 2 weeks and clinical benefit begins within 8 weeks.** The mechanism of response to electrical stimulation is not completely clear but definitely does not depend on increased muscle bulk. The frequency ranges listed are the most commonly used, and many clinicians use combination therapy for mixed UI. There are many patients with UI who will not accept a vaginal or anal probe. A randomized trial showed that equivalent results were achieved with every-other-day therapy compared with daily treatment.

15. **a. Over half of patients treated for UUI continued to respond to therapy over 1 year.** Two multicenter trials and another report of 1-year follow-up of patients from one of the trials show that PTNS is clearly superior to sham therapy and is competitive with anticholinergic medical therapy. The response was approximately the same as with tolterodine 4 mg daily but without the typical side effects. It has not been shown to be effective for SUI or urinary retention. An earlier trial showed approximately equal results with weekly versus thrice weekly therapy.

16. **a. Superior results in the treatment of SUI.** Randomized trials have not shown efficacy for women with SUI; the other statements are all potential advantages of magnetic stimulation.

17. **a. Over 90% of patients do not leak with a device in place.** A variety of bladder neck support devices have been developed to treat women with SUI. Approximately 60% of patients are dry with the device in place. The devices can be used for the short term as a test to estimate response to surgical therapy, on an "as needed" basis for infrequent leakage, in the intermediate term for women who have chosen surgery but need to delay treatment, or for the long term for those patients who are satisfied. The devices specifically developed for SUI usually do not affect voiding, but it is appropriate to fit patients with a half-full bladder and then test them for effectiveness against cough and make sure they can then urinate well.

18. **d. All of the above.** Pelvic relaxation can cause local discomfort, voiding dysfunction/urinary retention, and SUI. Use of a pessary to restore normal anatomy can help predict when surgical correction will successfully relieve symptoms and identify cases in which prolapse actually hides SUI.

19. **a. The most common adverse event is gross hematuria.** Urethral inserts are intended for the treatment

of SUI and in some series have exacerbated urgency. They are intended for single use, and women must be willing to learn to insert the device in the urethra; many will not consider such therapy. However, they are very effective for properly selected patients. Approximately one third of women using the devices will have a urinary tract infection within 1 year of follow-up. Gross hematuria and device migration into the bladder are much less common side effects.

20. **c. goal achievement.** In prospective studies, patient satisfaction is not correlated with objective cure of SUI or pelvic prolapse but is related to achieving specific goals.

21. **a. incontinence type, bladder diary, pelvic examination/muscle assessment.** Treatment planning for women with UI can usually be done after classifying the type of UI, performing a pelvic examination and assessing muscle function, and reviewing a bladder diary. Urodynamics are reserved for complicated cases and treatment failures. Cystoscopy is not part of the routine evaluation of UI but may be necessary to evaluate other problems such as hematuria.

22. **e. predicts likelihood of response to PFMT.** The bladder diary is an extremely useful tool, but it has not been shown to predict response to PFMT; in fact, little is known about which patients will respond best to PFMT.

23. **d. patients with strong pelvic floor muscles and UUI should be treated with anticholinergic medications.** Unless PFMT can be delivered by a skilled therapist with face-to-face instruction and the opportunity to evaluate response as in clinical trials there is little reason to assume that patients who cannot identify and contract the muscles on an initial examination will respond. They should have biofeedback or passive stimulation. At this time the optimal treatment for patients who can isolate the muscles but who have a weak contraction is unknown. Nothing has been shown to be superior to PFMT. Patients with strong pelvic muscles are good candidates for medical therapy for UUI and surgical treatment for SUI.

24. **a. 40% to 50% of those undergoing PFMT ultimately choose not to undergo surgery.** Approximately 70% of women with SUI improve with PFMT, 40% to 50% improve enough to decide against surgical therapy, and perhaps 20% become totally dry. Surgical therapy is still superior, but women who are willing should be encouraged to try PFMT because the results are reasonable and most women who initially respond will remain satisfied over time.

25. **b. Bladder training should always be used when anticholinergic medications are prescribed.** Bladder training, PFMT, and anticholinergic medications are all complementary treatments for the patient with OAB/UUI. PFMT and anticholinergic medications are approximately equally effective. Bladder training should always be prescribed when medications are used because the medications do not eliminate unstable contractions; they only delay and diminish them. When patients have a complete response to therapy it is reasonable to try titrating off the medications.

26. **b. Botulinum toxin bladder injections provide permanent relief of UI for approximately a third of patients.** When patients do not respond to standard therapy for OAB/UUI it is important to reassess them with attention to other correctable causes such as SUI, prolapse, voiding dysfunction, or specific bladder lesions. If no cause is found, sacral neuromodulation has been FDA approved since 1997. Botox injections are not yet FDA approved but are clearly effective for some patients, even some who fail neuromodulation, but can cause prolonged urinary retention in 5% to 10% of cases.

27. **a. surgical therapy may be more effective when the bladder diary demonstrates a good functional capacity.** Patients with mixed incontinence require a thoughtful approach. Surgical therapy is appropriate whenever the SUI component is clearly the most bothersome part and has been objectively demonstrated. Urodynamics may be useful but are not mandatory; a bladder diary showing a large capacity at rest (overnight) is a clue to good bladder storage function, and the patient is a good candidate for surgery. Electrical stimulation can theoretically improve both types of UI and is reasonable for motivated patients. A bladder neck support device may relieve the SUI component and give an approximation of the result of surgical treatment.

Additional Study Points

1. UUI affects quality of life more than SUI because of its unpredictable nature.
2. When taking a conservative approach to UI, invasive testing is rarely required before initiating treatment.
3. Caffeine promotes detrusor overactivity.
4. Abdominal leak point pressures appear to be volume dependent.
5. Weight loss is an effective treatment for UI in the obese patient.
6. Epidemiologic data support a link between consumption of carbonated beverages and UI.
7. In PFMT, half of the patients are unable to perform a proper contraction with simple instruction.
8. Pessaries used only to treat prolapse should be fitted with an empty bladder.
9. Pessaries used to treat SUI should be fitted with the bladder at a comfortable volume.
10. The use of devices for SUI is most successful in patients with very predictable episodic SUI; for example, when it occurs only during sporting activities.
11. To plan treatment for conservative management of SUI it is imperative to know three things: (a) the type of incontinence, (b) a baseline voiding diary, and (c) an assessment of the anatomy with particular emphasis on pelvic floor muscle strength and function.
12. Voided volume on a diary has been shown to correlate with cystometric capacity.
13. There is no accepted objective method for evaluating pelvic floor strength.
14. Patients who have no voluntary pelvic muscle contractions should be offered biofeedback training or passive stimulation.

Electrical Stimulation and Neuromodulation in Storage and Emptying Failure

Sandip P. Vasavada, MD ● Raymond Robert Rackley, MD

QUESTIONS

1. The current approved indications for sacral neuromodulation include all of the following EXCEPT:
   a. urinary urgency.
   b. urinary frequency.
   c. urgency urinary incontinence.
   d. interstitial cystitis.
   e. idiopathic nonobstructive urinary retention.

2. Which patient is not well suited for current neuromodulation therapies?
   a. A 65-year-old insulin-dependent diabetic man with bladder areflexia and nonobstructive urinary retention
   b. A 67-year-old woman status post cerebrovascular accident and now with urinary urgency and frequency
   c. A 41-year-old woman with urgency urinary incontinence
   d. A 55-year-old woman status post vaginal sling surgery and urgency urinary incontinence
   e. A 36-year-old woman with a history of interstitial cystitis with minimal pain who voids between 20 and 25 times per day

3. What reflex or reflexes are responsible for modulation of bladder function?
   a. Guarding
   b. Bladder afferent loop
   c. Bladder bladder
   d. Bladder urethral
   e. a and b

4. Which of the following is(are) considered the major clinical concern(s) associated with performing a sacral rhizotomy?
   a. Pelvic pain
   b. Creation of bladder areflexia
   c. Abnormal sexual function
   d. Pelvic and lower extremity sensory or motor abnormalities
   e. c and d

5. The S3 sensory and motor response pattern to electrical stimulation is best described as having which one of the following?
   a. Plantarflexion of the entire foot with sensation in the leg and buttock
   b. Levator reflex (bellows reflex) and sensations in the leg and buttock
   c. Dorsiflexion of the great toe and bellows reflex and pulling sensation in the rectum, scrotum, or vagina
   d. Plantarflexion of the first three toes of the foot and sensation of pulling in the rectum or vagina
   e. Bellows reflex (levator contraction) and sensation of pulling of the rectum

6. What is the main concern of performing magnetic resonance imaging (MRI) in the setting of neuromodulation and pacemaker type devices?
   a. Potential of dislodgement of the pacemaker
   b. Heating of the electrical leads
   c. Heating of the pacemaker itself
   d. Potentially fatal arrhythmias
   e. Significant neuromuscular injury risk

7. Which of the following represents the best clinical scenario in using neuromodulation therapy in a patient with multiple sclerosis (MS)?
   a. Detrusor sphincter dyssynergy
   b. Bedridden with significant functional incontinence
   c. Mild symptoms with no potential need for future MRI
   d. A poorly compliant bladder
   e. Areflexic bladder

8. What skeletal landmarks are associated with the S3 nerve foramen?
   a. 9 cm from the tip of the coccyx
   b. 11 cm from the tip of the coccyx
   c. 13 cm from the tip of the coccyx
   d. The inferior aspect of the sacral iliac joints
   e. a and d

9. Perhaps the main reason why neuromodulation devices are not currently approved for use in the United States by the Food and Drug Administration in pediatric patients is due to:
   a. lack of efficacy.
   b. potential worsening of neuromuscular function due to bony abnormalities (spina bifida and myelomeningocele).
   c. lack of data on growth of the spinal cord and nerve roots in the setting of neuromodulation devices.
   d. worsening of bowel function (Hinman bladder syndrome).
   e. excellent results with noninvasive therapies (transcutaneous electrical nerve stimulation) and therefore no reason to perform more invasive sacral neuromodulation in the long term.

10. The best option for a patient who has undergone a failed stage I sacral neuromodulation for severe refractory urgency urinary incontinence (Medtronic InterStim stage I) is:
    a. anticholinergic therapy.
    b. bilateral stimulation.
    c. radical cystectomy and ileal conduit.
    d. vaginal sling procedure.
    e. bladder augmentation.

11. Which of the following statements is FALSE about the dorsal genital nerve?
    a. Specific branches include the dorsal nerve of the penis in males and clitoral nerve in females.
    b. It is an afferent nerve that carries sensory information.
    c. Proximally, it carries sensory information from the hypogastric nerve.
    d. It is a pure sensory afferent nerve branch of the pudendal nerve.
    e. It has been proposed as a contributor to the pudendal pelvic nerve reflex.

12. An implantable pulse generator (IPG) infection would be best treated by:
    a. intravenous antibiotics.
    b. oral antibiotics.
    c. irrigation of the pocket.
    d. removal of the entire device.
    e. a and b.

13. Which of the following statements about impedances is FALSE?
    a. Impedance is best described as the resistance of flow of electrons through a circuit.
    b. If there is too much resistance, no current will flow (open).
    c. If there is too little resistance, excessive current will flow.
    d. If there is a broken circuit, electrons cannot flow and this will result in low impedance measurements.
    e. Unipolar measurements are most useful for identifying open circuits during impedance testing.

14. Which of the following statements is False about the Brindley device?
    a. It requires intact neuron pathways between the sacral cord and nuclei, pelvic nerve, and bladder to function.

b. It works best in a state of long-term areflexic bladder function.
c. It is used most often in patients with insufficient or nonreflex micturition after spinal cord injury.
d. It is usually coupled with sacral posterior rhizotomy.
e. Electrodes are applied extradurally to S2, S3, and S4 nerve roots.

15. Direct electrical stimulation of the bladder often results in all of the following EXCEPT:
    a. pelvic musculature contraction.
    b. erection.
    c. defecation.
    d. bladder neck opening.
    e. ejaculation.

16. Which one the following statements regarding the use of the Brindley device is FALSE?
    a. It requires intact neural pathways between the sacral cord and the bladder.
    b. Sacral posterior rhizotomy is generally performed.
    c. Myogenic decompensation is a contraindication.
    d. Electrodes are applied extradurally to sacral roots S2 to S4.
    e. It utilizes the principle of post-stimulation voiding.

17. Which of the following statements regarding neurostimulation or neuromodulation is FALSE?
    a. The desired effect of neurostimulation is through direct stimulation of nerves and muscles.
    b. Neurostimulation is mainly reserved for neurogenic conditions.
    c. Neurostimulation produces a delayed clinical response.
    d. The effect of neuromodulation is achieved through alteration of neurotransmission processes.
    e. Neuromodulation may be useful for neurogenic as well as non-neurogenic conditions.

18. Which of the following studies is(are) the most useful in predicting which patients will or will not respond to sacral neuromodulation?
    a. Uroflow/postvoid residual monitoring
    b. Voiding diary
    c. Urodynamics/electromyography
    d. Percutaneous lead placement and trial stimulation
    e. c and d

19. Which of the following is(are) relative clinical contraindications for excluding potential candidates for neuromodulation and neurostimulation therapies?
    a. Patients with significant anatomic abnormalities in the spine or sacrum may present challenges to gaining access
    b. Patients who cannot manage their device or judge the clinical outcome due to mental incapacitation
    c. Patients with physical limitations that prevent them from achieving normal pelvic organ function such as functional urinary incontinence
    d. Patients who are noncompliant
    e. All of the above

20. Which of the following statements best characterizes bilateral S3 nerve root stimulation for sacral neuromodulation therapy?

    a. It is a rational consideration for salvage therapy or added benefit as the bladder receives bilateral innervation.

    b. It is an approach alternative to failed unilateral stimulation in patients with urinary retention.

    c. Initial basis for this approach produced in spinal cord–injured animal models suggests this may be a potential approach in humans.

    d. All of the above

    e. a and c only

21. Potential sites of selective nerve stimulation other than the S3 sacral root for neuromodulation therapies for pelvic health conditions include which of the following?

    a. S4 sacral root

    b. Pudendal nerve

    c. Dorsal genital nerve

    d. Posterior tibial nerve

    e. All of the above

22. When troubleshooting the complication of IPG site discomfort or pain, which of the following statements best describes the necessary action(s) needed?

    a. Rule out IPG site infection by physical examination.

    b. Turn off the device and ask the patient if the discomfort is still present to differentiate IPG pocket site issues from IPG electrical output-related causes.

    c. If the IPG discomfort is output related, check whether bipolar stimulation is better than unipolar stimulation.

    d. If IPG site discomfort is output related, check impedances because a current leak may be present from the neuroelectrode to extension lead connection.

    e. All of the above

23. When patients report recurrent symptoms after having achieved reduction or improvement of symptoms with sacral neuromodulation therapy, which of the following should be undertaken to evaluate the reason for the loss of clinical efficacy?

    a. Check the device settings for inadvertent on/off changes and battery performance.

    b. Evaluate the stimulation perception and anatomic localization for changes.

    c. Check for intermittent stimulation perception via positional changes of the patient because this may suggest lead migration or a loose lead connection.

    d. Obtain a radiograph to detect macro changes in the neuroelectrode position if findings in b and c are evident.

    e. All of the above

ANSWERS

1. **d. interstitial cystitis.** Although used commonly for interstitial cystitis (IC) symptoms, urgency/frequency IC is not truly an indication for the sacral neuromodulation devices. Several groups have seen benefits of sacral neuromodulation in IC patients and there may be an expanding indication for this in the future.

2. **a. A 65-year-old insulin-dependent diabetic man with bladder areflexia and nonobstructive urinary retention.** It is implied that the end organ response (bladder in this case) should have good function for sacral neuromodulation and, for that matter, any form of neuromodulation to work. Neurostimulation may be different, but even if neurostimulation were used then simultaneous relaxation of the outlet would be required for a coordinated contraction and emptying phase to ensue.

3. **e. a and b.** Two important reflexes may play an important role in modulation of bladder function: the guarding reflex and the bladder afferent loop reflex. Both reflexes promote urine storage under sympathetic tone. The guarding reflex guards or prevents urine loss from times of cough or other physical stress that would normally trigger a micturition episode. Suprapontine input from the brain turns off the guarding reflex during micturition to allow efficient and complete emptying. The bladder afferent reflex works through sacral interneurons that then activate storage through pudendal nerve efferent pathways directed toward the urethral sphincter. Similar to the guarding reflex, the bladder afferent reflex promotes continence during periods of bladder filling and is quiet during micturition.

4. **e. c and d.** Bilateral anterior and posterior sacral rhizotomy or conusectomy converts a hyperreflexic bladder to an areflexic one. This alone may be inappropriate therapy because it also adversely affects the rectum, anal and urethral sphincters, sexual function, and the lower extremities. In an attempt to leave sphincter and sexual function intact, selective motor nerve section was originally introduced as a treatment to increase bladder capacity by abolishing only the motor supply responsible for involuntary contractions.

5. **c. Dorsiflexion of the great toe and bellows reflex and pulling sensation in the rectum, scrotum, or vagina.** The characteristic response of the S3 nerve distribution based on its lower innervation is to the levator musculature (bellows contraction) of the anus and ipsilateral great toe contraction. The other answers suggest either S2 stimulation (leg rotation) or S4 levator contraction.

6. **b. Heating of the electrical leads.** Although many concerns exist for MRI and pacemaker devices, it has been shown that the main concern is heating of the electrical leads. This may, in turn, traumatize blood vessels, nerve roots, or other structures that the leads, themselves, are next to. Currently, MRI is contraindicated in the presence of a pacemaker.

7. **c. Mild symptoms with no potential need for future MRI.** It is unknown whether subcategories of MS patients (delayed emptying/storage dysfunction, areflexia, poor compliance) would be very good candidates for sacral neuromodulation, although it is doubtful based on disease severity alone. A mildly symptomatic patient without functional issues (e.g., can get to the bathroom in time with no major mobility issues) probably makes sense as to the best patient.

8. **e. a and d.** The measurements for the rough vicinity of the S3 nerve foramen have been tested using the "cross hair" technique (Chai et al, 2000)* and simple measurements. The answers b and c are incorrect because they represent

---

*Sources referenced can be found in *Campbell-Walsh Urology, 10th Edition,* on the Expert Consult website.

measurements from the anal verge (11 cm), and 13 cm is too far in general from the coccyx and would likely place one near S2 or S1.

9. **c. lack of data on growth of the spinal cord and nerve roots in the setting of neuromodulation devices.** Pediatric patients have undergone sacral neuromodulation in off-label trials, but large-scale use has been limited by lack of data on the growth of the pediatric patient and the relation of the sacral lead with regard to the sacral nerve roots, and so on. Although noninvasive therapies have worked, they are limited by the need for continued repeat therapy to maintain durability of result.

10. **e. bladder augmentation.** The patient should have tried and failed anticholinergic therapy before having the sacral neuromodulation therapy. Scheepens and coworkers have shown that bilateral stimulation, although logical, has not shown in urgency incontinent patients to make much improvement (Scheepens et al, 2002). One could argue that contralateral lead placement should be attempted, but no prospective trials have shown that this makes a difference in outcomes. The vaginal sling procedure and radical cystectomy are not indicated per se in this condition (the vaginal sling is for stress urinary incontinence, and cystectomy is too radical).

11. **c. Proximally, it carries sensory information from the hypogastric nerve.** The dorsal genital nerve is a terminal branch of the pudendal nerve and is being investigated for functional neuromodulation outcomes via a percutaneous approach. It does not carry information directly from the hypogastric nerve.

12. **d. removal of the entire device.** Because an IPG is a foreign body it could harbor bacteria within a biofilm created by the infection. Accordingly, it is best to have it removed in its entirety. Antibiotics and irrigation for the most part are temporizing measures. Furthermore, there is a risk of an infection tracking along the sacral lead, which may create a sacral infection.

13. **d. If there is a broken circuit, electrons cannot flow and this will result in low impedance measurements.** Impedance describes the resistance to the flow of electrons through a circuit. Impedance or resistance is an integral part of any functioning circuit; however, if there is too much resistance, no current will flow (open). If there is too little resistance, excessive current flow resulting in diminished battery longevity occurs (short). If the circuit is broken somehow, electrons cannot flow. This is called an "open" circuit, and impedance measurements are high. Open circuits can be caused by a fractured lead or extension wires, loose connections, and so on.

14. **b. It works best in a state of long-term areflexic bladder function.** The chief applications of the Brindley device are in patients with inefficient or nonreflex micturition after spinal cord injury. Prerequisites for use are described by Fischer and associates (1993) as the following: (1) intact neural pathways between the sacral cord nuclei of the pelvic nerve and the bladder and (2) a bladder that is capable of contracting.

15. **d. bladder neck opening.** The spread of current to other pelvic structures whose stimulus thresholds are lower than that of the bladder has often resulted in (1) abdominal, pelvic, and perineal pain; (2) a desire to defecate or defecation; (3) contraction of the pelvic and leg muscles; and (4) erection and ejaculation in males. It has also been

noted that the increase in intravesical pressure was generally not coordinated with bladder neck opening or with pelvic floor relaxation and that other measures to accomplish voiding may be necessary.

16. **d. Electrodes are applied extradurally to sacral roots S2 to S4.** Prerequisites for such usage were described in one study as (1) intact neural pathways between the sacral cord nuclei of the pelvic nerve and the bladder and (2) a bladder that is capable of contracting. The chief application is in patients with inefficient or no reflex micturition after spinal cord injury. Simultaneous bladder and striated sphincter stimulation is obviated by sacral posterior rhizotomy, usually complete, which also (1) eliminates reflex incontinence and (2) improves low bladder compliance, if present. Electrodes are applied intradurally to the S2, S3, and S4 roots, but the pairs can be activated independently. The current Brindley stimulator utilizes the principle of *post-stimulus voiding,* a term first introduced by Jonas and Tanagho (1975). Relaxation time of the striated sphincter after a stimulus train is shorter than the relaxation time of the detrusor smooth muscle. Therefore, when interrupted pulse trains instead of continuous stimulus trains are used, post-stimulus voiding is achieved between the pulse trains due to the higher sustained intravesical pressure when compared with the striated sphincter.

17. **c. Neurostimulation produces a delayed clinical response.** In neurostimulation the use of electrical stimuli on nerves and muscles has mainly been developed for achieving immediate clinical responses in neurogenic conditions of pelvic organ dysfunction, whereas, in neuromodulation, the use of electrical stimuli to nerves has been developed for altering neurotransmission processes in cases of nonneurogenic as well as neurogenic conditions.

18. **d. Percutaneous lead placement and trial stimulation.** Despite all the studies done to date there are no defined preclinical factors such as urodynamic findings that can predict which patients will or will not have a response to sacral neuromodulation. Thus, a trial of stimulation via a temporary or percutaneous lead placement is the best predictor of long-term clinical responsiveness.

19. **e. All of the above.** Whereas most patients are considered candidates for neurostimulation and neuromodulation therapies who have failed more conservative therapies, all of the above clinical considerations for excluding patients from this therapy should be considered. Furthermore, relative contraindications for patients who may be considering or who have an implantable electrical stimulation device are the issues of MRI and pregnancy.

20. **d. All of the above.** Bilateral stimulation has been suggested as an alternative, particularly in failed unilateral lead placements, for potential salvage or added benefit as the bladder receives bilateral innervation. The initial basis to consider bilateral stimulation was based on animal studies that demonstrated bilateral stimulation yielded a more profound effect on bladder inhibition than did unilateral stimulation. Only one clinical study has been performed to demonstrate the potential differences in unilateral versus bilateral stimulation (Scheepens et al, 2002). This study showed no significant difference in outcomes for unilateral versus bilateral stimulation with regard to urgency urinary incontinence, frequency, or severity of leakage in the overactive bladder group, although, overall, results were impressive in both categories. The patients in the retention

group had better parameters of emptying (volume per void) in bilateral as compared with unilateral stimulation.

21. **e. All of the above.** The introduction of new stimulation methods as well as application of these methods to all the different nerve locations listed will continue to provide improved treatment alternatives, as shown in animal models and human applications. In addition, these innovations will provide the ability to further develop testable hypotheses of more basic questions on electrical neurostimulation, neuromodulation, and neurophysiology of the autonomic, somatic, and central pathways that regulate pelvic organ function.

22. **e. All of the above.** The probable causes of IPG site discomfort or pain are IPG pocket related or IPG output related. Pocket-related causes of discomfort include infection, pocket location (waistline), pocket dimension (too tight, too loose), seroma, and erosion. One should turn off the IPG and determine if the discomfort is still present to differentiate pocket-related from output-related cause. If the discomfort is persistent, the cause is not related to the IPG electrical output. In the absence of clinical signs of infection, IPG pocket-related causes such as pocket size, seroma, and erosion should be considered. If the discomfort disappears, the IPG electrical output is likely causing discomfort or pain. Output-related causes include sensitivity to unipolar stimulation if this mode is used or a current leak as demonstrated by abnormal impedances.

23. **e. All of the above.** When the patient presents with recurrent symptoms, one should evaluate the stimulation perception. The possibilities are that the patient perceives the stimulation in a wrong location as compared with baseline, has no stimulation, or has intermittent stimulation based on lead migration or mechanical issues related to a loose connection or elevated impedances.

Additional Study Points

1. The mechanism of neuromodulation may be activation of neurons that cause inhibition at spinal and supra-spinal levels.
2. For neuromodulation to work there must be at least some communication between sacral outflow and the pontine micturition center so as to allow for processing of reflexes that may be inhibited by the brain.
3. Neuromodulation has been used in fecal incontinence and constipation as well as bladder dysfunction.
4. The evidence suggests that neuromodulation works through supraspinal pathways.
5. The detrusor is usually innervated primarily by S3, rectal stimulation occurs in S2, S3, and S4, and erectile stimulation is mainly a function of S2.
6. Transcutaneous electrical stimulation demonstrates good efficacy but has a limited role because of the constant need to administer the therapy.

Retropubic Suspension Surgery for Incontinence in Women

Christopher R. Chapple, MD, FRCS (Urol), FEBU

QUESTIONS

1. Urodynamic stress urinary incontinence (SUI) refers to:
   a. incontinence that is demonstrated during a cough on clinical examination.
   b. incontinence occurring in the absence of urgency.
   c. incontinence occurring in combination with detrusor overactivity.
   d. incontinence associated on coughing in association with urgency and demonstrable detrusor overactivity.
   e. incontinence occurring on coughing in the absence of urgency and of urgency incontinence and with no demonstrable detrusor overactivity.

2. Anti-incontinence surgery via the retropubic route:
   a. is an effective approach for primary intrinsic sphincter deficiency.
   b. works by restoring the same mechanism of continence that was present before the onset of incontinence.
   c. aims to improve the support to the urethrovesical junction and correct deficient urethral closure.
   d. is the most effective form of anti-incontinence surgery.
   e. is carried out laparoscopically as effectively as via an open approach.

3. The most important determinant affecting the outcome of retropubic surgery is:
   a. increasing age.
   b. postoperative activity.
   c. coexisting medical morbidity.
   d. previous surgery.
   e. obesity.

4. Intrinsic sphincter deficiency is:
   a. present only in 30% of patients presenting with SUI.
   b. most likely present in the majority of women presenting with SUI.
   c. accurately identified on the basis of Valsalva leak point pressure.
   d. an absolute contraindication to a retropubic suspension procedure.
   e. clearly defined in the current literature.

5. Retropubic colposuspension procedures may act via which of the following mechanisms?
   a. Re-creating the normal continence mechanism.
   b. Elevating the anterior vaginal wall and paravesical tissues toward the iliopectineal line
   c. Anchoring the obturator internus fascia to the iliopectineal line
   d. Suspending the bladder onto the periosteum of the symphysis pubis
   e. Strengthening the pubourethral ligaments

6. In assessing the outcome of retropubic suspension surgery, which of the following is most important?
   a. Using objective urodynamic-based outcome criteria
   b. Improving symptoms from the patient's perspective
   c. Achieving complete continence
   d. Identifying the degree of improvement in the urethral closure pressure
   e. Having follow-up data of at least 6 months' duration

7. Which of the following is not an indication for retropubic repair of SUI?
   a. A patient who needs a concomitant hysterectomy that cannot be performed vaginally
   b. A patient with urethral descent with straining and SUI
   c. A patient with limited vaginal access
   d. A patient who frequently generates high intra-abdominal pressure due to a chronic cough
   e. A patient with inadequate vaginal length or mobility of the vaginal tissues

8. Which of the following statements is TRUE regarding retropubic procedures for incontinence?
   a. It is important to avoid dissecting the old retropubic adhesions from prior incontinence procedures because these may contribute to continence.
   b. Nonabsorbable sutures are better than absorbable sutures for retropubic suspension procedures.
   c. It may be necessary to open the bladder to facilitate identification of the bladder margins and bladder neck.
   d. A urethral Foley catheter is preferred for bladder drainage because it is more comfortable and associated with fewer

urinary tract infections and earlier resumption of voiding.

e. The retropubic space must be drained after the procedure to prevent bleeding.

9. Which of the following statements is TRUE regarding the Marshall-Marchetti-Krantz (MMK) procedure?

   a. It is important to elevate the midurethra and external sphincter in particular.

   b. It carries little risk of causing urethral obstruction.

   c. It is associated with osteitis pubis.

   d. A better than 90% cure rate can be expected in the long term.

   e. The sutures should incorporate a full thickness of the vaginal wall and lateral urethral wall.

10. Which of the following is TRUE of the Burch colposuspension?

    a. It is appropriate only for patients with adequate vaginal mobility and capacity.

    b. The repair is performed between the vagina and the arcus tendineus fasciae pelvis bilaterally.

    c. It is less effective than a tension-free vaginal tape procedure.

    d. It is less effective than a paravaginal repair.

    e. It is more effectively performed via a vaginal approach.

11. Laparoscopic retropubic colposuspension is advantageous over open colposuspension because:

    a. it is technically simple to perform.

    b. it provides access for repair of an associated central defect cystocele.

    c. it is more effective than an open colposuspension.

    d. it is associated with shorter hospitalization and recovery times.

    e. it is associated with shorter operating times.

12. Common complications specific to retropubic suspension procedures include:

    a. bladder denervation.

    b. detrusor sphincter dyssynergia.

    c. postoperative voiding difficulty.

    d. detrusor underactivity.

    e. genitourinary tract fistulae.

13. Postoperative voiding difficulty after a retropubic suspension procedure:

    a. is more likely if there is preexisting detrusor dysfunction.

    b. may be due to detrusor sphincter dyssynergia.

    c. is most likely to occur with undercorrection of the urethral axis.

    d. should be managed by urethrolysis within 1 month.

    e. occurs in less than 1% of patients.

14. Which of the following statements is TRUE regarding detrusor overactivity (DO) and retropubic suspension procedures?

    a. Preoperative DO is a contraindication to a retropubic suspension because it increases the risk of postoperative DO.

    b. New-onset DO after a suspension procedure performed for stress urinary incontinence invariably resolves within 3 months.

    c. DO occurs de novo, on average in less than 2% of the patients reported in the literature.

    d. A history of voiding symptoms and new-onset storage symptoms as well as a retropubically angulated urethra usually suggests obstruction.

    e. DO is not causally related.

15. Prolapse as a reported complication of retropubic repairs:

    a. is rarely associated with a central defect cystocele.

    b. results in genitourinary prolapse as a sequel to Burch colposuspension to occur in less than 10% of women.

    c. may aggravate posterior vaginal wall weakness, predisposing to enterocele.

    d. will be prevented by a synchronous hysterectomy.

    e. occurs only rarely after a paravaginal repair.

16. From comparative studies in the literature, which is correct about open retropubic colposuspension?

    a. It is not as effective as a pubovaginal sling.

    b. It is not effective in patients with a low leak point pressure.

    c. It is no more effective than an anterior colporrhaphy.

    d. It is less effective than a tension-free vaginal tape procedure.

    e. It is no more effective than a paravaginal repair.

ANSWERS

1. **e. incontinence occurring on coughing in the absence of urgency and of urgency incontinence and with no demonstrable detrusor overactivity.** Stress urinary incontinence (SUI) is the symptom of involuntary loss of urine during situations of increased intra-abdominal pressure such as coughing or sneezing. The International Continence Society defines *urodynamic stress incontinence* as the involuntary loss of urine during increased intra-abdominal pressure during filling cystometry, in the absence of detrusor (bladder wall muscle) contraction (Abrams et al, 2002).* Thus, urodynamic evaluation is a prerequisite for the diagnosis of urodynamic SUI. It is not clear, however, especially from the clinical management standpoint, whether a urodynamic diagnosis is imperative for successful treatment of SUI.

2. **c. aims to improve the support to the urethrovesical junction and correct deficient urethral closure.** Surgical procedures to treat SUI generally aim to improve the support to the urethrovesical junction and correct deficient urethral closure. There is disagreement, however, regarding the precise mechanism by which continence is achieved in the "normal asymptomatic female" and therefore not surprisingly how restoration of "normality" is reestablished via surgical manipulation. Anti-incontinence surgery is generally used to address the failure of normal anatomic support of the bladder neck and proximal urethra and intrinsic sphincter deficiency (ISD). Anti-incontinence surgery does not necessarily work by

---

*Sources referenced can be found in *Campbell-Walsh Urology,* 10th *Edition,* on the Expert Consult website.

restoring the same mechanism of continence that was present before the onset of incontinence. Rather, it works by a compensatory approach, creating a new mechanism of continence (Jarvis, 1994). The surgeon's preference, coexisting problems, and the anatomic features of the patient and her general health condition often influence the choice of procedure.

The current evidence would suggest that in adequately experienced hands there is no difference in overall safety and efficacy between laparoscopic and open colposuspension. Clearly, another concern is how generalizable the data are on laparoscopic colposuspension because the majority of reported studies are from expert laparoscopists or surgeons working in specialized units. The evidence base on both laparoscopic and open colposuspension is limited by relatively short-term follow-up (robust data are needed out to 5 years) and the tendency toward small numbers, and poor methodology limits the interpretation of most studies with the exception of those reported by Carey and coworkers (2006) and Kitchener and colleagues (2006).

3. **d. previous surgery.** Surgery for recurrent SUI has a lower success rate. One study has reported that Burch colposuspension has an 81% success rate after one previous surgical procedure has failed, but this drops to 25% after two previous repairs and 0% after three previous operations (Petrou and Frank, 2001). Other series report excellent results for colposuspension performed after prior failed surgery. Maher and associates (1999) and Cardozo and colleagues (1999) have both shown good objective (72% and 79%) and subjective (89% and 80%) success rates with repeat colposuspension at a mean follow-up of 9 months. Nitahara and coworkers (1999) reported a 69% subjective success at a mean follow-up of 6.9 years.

The evidence on the duration of symptoms as a predictor of outcome is conflicting. Age may not be a contraindication to colposuspension (with equivalent success rates in the elderly at long-term follow-up), although others reported less success with increasing age. Advice on the influence of levels of postoperative activity have been inadequately studied so that no recommendations can be made. There is limited evidence that medical comorbidity may impact on surgical outcomes depending on the outcomes selected. Obesity as a confounding variable is the subject of conflicting evidence in the literature and has not been studied in a prospective fashion. Approximately a fourth of women undergoing urodynamic study have mixed urodynamic SUI and detrusor overactivity. It is likely that the presence of concomitant detrusor overactivity lessens the success rate of surgery. There is no consensus in the literature as to whether the presence of intrinsic sphincter deficiency as assessed by urethral pressure profilometry has any influence in outcome of colposuspension.

4. **b. most likely present in the majority of women presenting with SUI.** Hypermobility of the bladder neck and proximal urethra results from a weakening or loss of the supporting elements (ligaments, fasciae, and muscles), which in turn may be consequent upon aging, hormonal changes, childbirth, and prior surgery. It seems likely that the majority of women with SUI will also have an element of intrinsic sphincteric weakness with a variable degree of loss of the normal anatomic support of the bladder neck and proximal urethra, resulting in hypermobility.

A standardized test is not however available to differentiate the relative contributions of intrinsic sphincter deficiency and hypermobility, and therefore few studies have been able to accurately differentiate their individual contributions to the incontinence. Retropubic procedures act to restore the bladder neck and proximal urethra to a fixed, retropubic position and are used when hypermobility is thought to be an important factor in the development of that woman's SUI. This may facilitate the function of a marginally compromised intrinsic urethral sphincter mechanism, but if significant intrinsic sphincter deficiency is present, SUI will persist despite efficient surgical repositioning of the bladder neck and proximal urethra.

5. **b. Elevating the anterior vaginal wall and paravesical tissues toward the iliopectineal line.** Retropubic colposuspension urethral repositioning can be achieved by three distinctly different procedure principles. These are all based on a similar underlying principle but in a spectrum in relation to the degree of the support/elevations they achieve, and their outcomes differ somewhat in the longer term.

The Burch colposuspension is the elevation of the anterior vaginal wall and paravesical tissues toward the iliopectineal line of the pelvic side wall using two to four sutures on either side (Burch, 1961). The vagino-obturator shelf repair aims to anchor the vagina to the obturator internus fascia and is a modification of a combination of the Burch colposuspension and paravaginal defect repair with placement of the sutures laterally anchored to the obturator internus fascia rather than hitching the vagina up to the iliopectineal line (Turner Warwick, 1986). The paravaginal defect repair aims to close a presumed fascial weakness laterally at the site of attachment of the pelvic fascia to obturator internus fascia (Richardson et al, 1976). The Marshall-Marchetti-Krantz procedure is the suspension of the vesicourethral junction (bladder neck) onto the periosteum of the symphysis pubis (Marshall et al, 1949). It aims to close the fascial defect rather than elevate the tissues in the paravesical area.

6. **b. Improving symptoms from the patient's perspective.** One or more high-quality validated symptom and quality of life instruments should be chosen at the outset of a clinical trial representing the patients viewpoint, accurately defining baseline symptoms as well as any other areas in which treatment may be beneficial and assessing the objective severity and subjective impact of bother. Although many, including the author, believe that urodynamic studies are helpful in helping define the underlying pathophysiology in cases with incontinence, these tests have not been proven to have adequate sensitivity, specificity, or predictive value (Chapple et al, 2005). The recent International Consensus Meeting on Incontinence concluded that although urodynamic studies such as frequency volume charts and pad tests were useful there was inadequate evidence to justify pressure-flow studies for routine testing as either entry criteria or outcome measures in clinical trials, and they recommended that most large-scale clinical trials should enroll subjects by carefully defined symptom-driven criteria when the treatment will be given on an empirical basis (Abrams et al, 2005).

7. **e. A patient with inadequate vaginal length or mobility of the vaginal tissues.** Although it has been suggested that a retropubic colposuspension should be

considered in patients who frequently generate high intra-abdominal pressure (e.g., those with chronic cough from obstructive pulmonary disease and women in strenuous occupations), it has also been argued that these patients may be better served by a pubovaginal sling as well. There may be specific indications for a retropubic approach for the correction of anatomic SUI, namely:

- A patient undergoing a laparotomy for concomitant abdominal surgery that cannot be performed vaginally.
- Where there is limited vaginal access.

Conversely, contraindications include:

- If there is a history of prior failed incontinence procedures the existence of significant sphincteric deficiency must be suspected, even if hypermobility exists, and consideration given to performing a pubovaginal sling.
- In cases with a pan–pelvic floor weakness a colposuspension should not be used in isolation but should be used as part of a comprehensive approach to the pelvic floor and be combined as appropriate with other alternative pelvic floor repair procedures. Although lateral defect cystocele and enterocele lend themselves to retropubic repair, central defect cystocele, rectocele, and introital deficiency do not.
- In cases in which there is an inadequate vaginal length or mobility of the vaginal tissues as for example after previous vaginal surgery or irradiation or after a previous vaginal incontinence procedure, a colposuspension should not be used.
- A retropubic colposuspension does not always adequately correct the associated vaginal prolapse that frequently coexists with bladder neck hypermobility.

8. **c. It may be necessary to open the bladder to facilitate identification of the bladder margins and bladder neck.** In open retropubic suspension procedures, good access to the retropubic space is crucial. This is best performed with the patient in the supine position with the legs abducted, in either a low or a modified dorsal lithotomy position using stirrups, allowing access to the vagina during the procedure and a perineoabdominal progression. A urethral Foley catheter is inserted; the catheter balloon is used for subsequent identification of the urethra and bladder neck and indeed is invaluable in allowing palpation of the edges of the bladder by appropriate manipulation. A Pfannenstiel or lower midline abdominal incision is made, separating the rectus muscles in the midline and sweeping the anterior peritoneal reflection off the bladder. It is essential to optimize the access to the retropubic space, and if a Pfannenstiel skin incision is made it is advisable to utilize the suprapubic V modification described by Turner-Warwick and colleagues (1974). Likewise, whatever incision is made, extra valuable access to the retropubic space is obtained by extending the division of the rectus muscles right down to the pubic bone and elevating the aponeurotic insertion of the rectus muscle right off the upper border of the pubic bone.

The retropubic space is then developed by teasing away the retropubic fat and underlying retropubic veins, from the back of the pubic bone. The bladder neck, anterior vaginal wall, and urethra are then easy to identify—often facilitated by the presence of the Foley catheter balloon. In patients who have had previous retropubic surgery, the dissection is performed sharply and it is important to take down all old retropubic adhesions, particularly in the presence of a prior failed repair. If difficulty is encountered in the identification of the bladder neck, the bladder may be partially filled or even opened to identify its limits; and an examining finger in the vagina is invaluable in aiding the dissection (Symmonds, 1972; Gleason et al, 1976).

It is important to identify the lateral limits of the bladder as it reflects off the vaginal wall, because only in this manner can one avoid inadvertent suturing of the bladder itself. Dissection over the bladder neck and urethra in the midline is to be avoided so as to not damage the intrinsic musculature. The lateral bladder wall may be "rolled off" medially and cephalad from the vaginal wall using a mounted swab and by using countertraction with a finger in the vagina. In the author's experience it is necessary to incise the endopelvic fascia. Occasional venous bleeding from the large vaginal veins is controlled by suture ligature, although it often resolves with tying of elevating sutures. To aid in the identification of the lateral margin of the bladder, it is helpful to displace the balloon of the Foley catheter into the lateral recess, where it can be easily palpated through the bladder wall.

Absorbable sutures were used in the original descriptions of the MMK procedure (chromic catgut), Burch colposuspension (chromic catgut), and vagino-obturator shelf procedure (polyglycolic acid or polydioxanone), whereas the original paravaginal repair used nonabsorbable sutures (silicon-coated Dacron). Fibrosis during subsequent healing is likely to be the most important factor in providing continued fixation of the perivaginal fascia to the suspension sites (Tanagho, 1996); nevertheless some surgeons believe that a nonabsorbable suture material is better because of the risk of suture dissolution before the development of adequate fibrosis (Penson and Raz, 1996). Clearly the choice of suspension suture material is a personal choice, but it must be remembered that nonabsorbent sutures eroding into the lumen of the bladder are a not uncommon complication and a not uncommon source of medical litigation (Woo et al, 1995).

Some degree of immediate postoperative voiding difficulty can be expected after retropubic suspensions (Lose et al, 1987; Colombo et al, 1996). Immediately postoperatively bladder drainage may take the form of a urethral or a suprapubic catheter, generally based on surgeon preference. A voiding trial is usually performed around the fifth day postoperatively. However, there is some evidence that a suprapubic catheter may be advantageous with respect to a lower incidence of asymptomatic and febrile urinary tract infection and earlier resumption of normal bladder function (Andersen et al, 1985; Bergman et al, 1987). In addition, the use of a suprapubic tube is generally more comfortable, allows the patient to participate in catheter management, and avoids the need for clean intermittent catheterization. Catheterization can be discontinued when efficient voiding has resumed, which is usually indicated by a postvoid residual volume either less than 100 mL or less than 30% of the functional bladder volume.

A tube drain may be placed in the retropubic space when there is concern about ongoing bleeding from perivaginal veins that may prove difficult to control with suture and electrocautery. Often, tying the suspension sutures is sufficient to stop this bleeding, but when it persists then drainage of the retropubic space is indicated. The drain is generally removed on the first to third day, when minimal output is noted.

9. **c. It is associated with osteitis pubis.** Complications occur in up to 21% of cases (Mainprize 1988), and the placement of sutures through the pubic symphysis incurs the risk of osteitis pubis, a potentially devastating complication of the MMK procedure that has been reported in 0.9% to 3.2% of patients (Lee et al, 1979; Mainprize 1988, Zorzos and Paterson, 1996). Patients usually present 1 to 8 weeks postoperatively with acute pubic pain radiating to the inner thighs and aggravated by moving. Physical examination reveals tenderness over the pubic symphysis, and radiography demonstrates haziness to the borders of the pubic symphysis and possibly lytic changes. Treatment is with bed rest, analgesics, and possibly corticosteroids (Lee et al, 1979).

10. **a. It is appropriate only for patients with adequate vaginal mobility and capacity.** The Burch retropubic colposuspension, which has undergone few modifications since its original description, is appropriate only if the patient has adequate vaginal mobility and capacity to allow the lateral vaginal fornices to be elevated toward and approximated to the Cooper ligament on either side.

11. **d. it is associated with shorter hospitalization and recovery times.** Proposed advantages to the laparoscopic approach include improved intraoperative visualization, less postoperative pain, shorter hospitalization, and quicker recovery times (Liu, 1993). Disadvantages include greater technical difficulty with resultant longer operating times and higher operating costs (Paraiso et al, 1999).

The last major publication in this field was a meta-analysis of all of the comparative studies published between 1995 and 2006 of laparoscopic versus open colposuspension (Tan et al, 2007). End points evaluated were operative outcomes and subjective/objective cure. A random-effect model was used and sensitivity analysis performed to account for bias in patient selection. Sixteen studies matched the selection criteria, reporting on 1807 patients, of whom 861 (47.6%) underwent laparoscopic and 946 (52.4%) underwent open colposuspension. Length of hospital stay and return to normal life were significantly reduced after laparoscopic surgery. These findings remained consistent on sensitivity analysis. Bladder injuries occurred more often in the laparoscopic group, but only with marginal statistical significance. Comparable bladder injury rates were found when studies were matched for quality, year, and randomized trials. Cure rates were similar between the two procedures at 2-year follow-up.

12. **c. postoperative voiding difficulty.** As with any major abdominal or pelvic surgical procedure, intraoperative and perioperative complications that may occur after a retropubic suspension include bleeding, injury to genitourinary organs (bladder, urethra, ureter), pulmonary atelectasis and infection, wound infection or dehiscence, abscess formation, and venous thrombosis/embolism. Other common complications more specific to retropubic suspension procedures include postoperative voiding difficulty, detrusor overactivity, and vaginal prolapse.

Nevertheless the reported incidence of these problems is relatively low. In their meta-analysis, Leach and associates (1997) noted a 3% to 8% transfusion rate for retropubic suspensions and no significant difference in the overall medical and surgical complication rates between retropubic suspensions, needle suspensions, anterior colporrhaphy, and pubovaginal slings.

Ureteral obstruction has been reported rarely after Burch colposuspension, and it usually results from ureteral kinking after elevation of the vagina and bladder base, although direct suture ligation of the ureter can occur (Applegate et al, 1987). If identified intraoperatively, it is best remedied by removal of the offending ligature and temporary placement of a ureteral stent. The so-called post-colposuspension syndrome, which has been described as pain in one or both groins at the site of suspension, has been noted in up to 12% of patients after a Burch colposuspension (Galloway et al, 1987). More recently Demirci and associates (2001) reported the occurrence of groin or suprapubic pain in 15 of 220 women (6.8%) after Burch colposuspension with a follow-up of 4.5 years.

13. **a. is more likely if there is preexisting detrusor dysfunction.** Postoperative voiding difficulty after any type of retropubic suspension is not uncommon, and undoubtedly its occurrence is more likely if there is preexisting detrusor dysfunction or denervation resulting from extensive perivesical dissection. In most cases, however, it is the result of overcorrection of the urethral axis, owing to sutures being inappropriately placed or excessively tightened. If they are placed too medially, sutures may also transfix the urethra or distort it.

Preoperatively, at-risk patients may be identified by their history of prior voiding dysfunction or episodes of urinary retention. Preoperatively these women should be counseled carefully about the potential for postoperative voiding difficulty and the possible need for self-catheterization. Their incontinence should be of sufficient magnitude that its correction offsets the risk of the need for self-catheterization.

Women with post-cystourethropexy voiding problems who have obstruction often do not exhibit the classic urodynamic features of obstruction. However, the history of postoperative voiding symptoms and associated new-onset bladder irritative symptoms and a finding of a retropubically angulated and fixed urethra generally indicate that obstruction does exist (Carr and Webster, 1997). In such cases, revision of the retropubic suspension by releasing the urethra into a more anatomic position resolves voiding symptoms in up to 90% of cases (Webster and Kreder, 1990; Nitti and Raz, 1994; Carr and Webster, 1997).

The meta-analysis by Leach and coworkers (1997) noted that the risk of temporary urinary retention lasting more than 4 weeks postoperatively was 5% for all retropubic suspensions, the risk for permanent retention was estimated to be less than 5%, and these risks were not significantly different from those for needle suspensions or pubovaginal slings.

14. **d. A history of voiding symptoms and new-onset irritative symptoms as well as a retropubically angulated urethra usually suggests obstruction.** Bladder hyperactivity commonly accompanies anatomic SUI, and its incidence preoperatively has been reported to be as high as 30% in patients undergoing either first correction or repeated operations (McGuire, 1981). Provided that it is considered as a diagnosis, urodynamic study is performed to show whether detrusor overactivity is present, an attempt at treatment of the related overactive bladder

symptoms has been made (with or without success), and the patient has been advised that the presence of detrusor overactivity will increase the risk of continuing storage symptoms postoperatively; then preoperative bladder overactivity does not contraindicate a retropubic suspension procedure, provided that anatomic SUI has also been demonstrated. In the majority of cases the bladder overactivity symptoms resolve after surgical repair (McGuire, 1988). Leach and coworkers' meta-analysis (1997) found the risk of urgency after a retropubic suspension was 66% if urgency and detrusor overactivity were present preoperatively, 36% if there was urgency but no documented overactivity preoperatively, and only 11% if there was neither urgency nor overactivity preoperatively. There was no significant difference in the incidence of postoperative urgency between retropubic suspensions, needle suspensions, and pubovaginal slings. Postoperative urgency was noted in only 0.9% of MMK procedures in Mainprize and Drutz's meta-analysis of 15 series (1988), although Parnell and associates (1982) reported that 28.5% of their patients developed postoperative storage symptoms. Jarvis' meta-analysis (1994) of Burch colposuspensions found the incidence of de novo bladder overactivity to be 3.4% to 18%. More recently Smith and associates quote a figure for postoperative detrusor overactivity of 6.6% for colposuspension (range 1.0% to 16.6%), whereas the incidence of postoperative urgency or urgency incontinence after the paravaginal/vagino-obturator shelf repair has been reported to be 0% to 6% (Shull and Baden, 1989; German et al, 1994; Colombo et al, 1996).

For those patients in whom postoperative storage symptoms persist, proven to be associated with detrusor overactivity and intractable to management with anticholinergic therapy and behavioral modification, surgical techniques including intravesical botulinum toxin therapy, neuromodulation, augmentation cystoplasty, or detrusor myectomy may be indicated.

Bladder storage symptoms arising de novo after retropubic suspension may be associated with bladder outlet obstruction. This premise is supported by the frequent coexistence of these symptoms with impaired voiding after suspension procedures and confirmed by the finding that urethrolysis, by freeing the urethra from an obstructed position, often resolves both storage and voiding symptoms (Raz, 1981; Webster and Kreder, 1990).

15. **c. May aggravate posterior vaginal wall weakness, predisposing to enterocele.** Retropubic suspensions alter vaginal and bladder base anatomy, and, thus, postoperative vaginal prolapse is a potential complication. Genitourinary prolapse has been reported as a sequel to Burch colposuspension in 22.1% of women (range 9.5% to 38.2%) by Smith and colleagues (2005) in their review of the literature. The Burch colposuspension, because of lateral vaginal elevation, may aggravate posterior vaginal wall weakness, predisposing to enterocele. The incidence varies between 3% and 17% (Burch, 1961, 1968; Galloway et al, 1987; Wiskind et al, 1992); and, because of this, prophylactic obliteration of the cul-de-sac of Douglas is sometimes considered when performing retropubic suspensions (Shull and Baden, 1989; Turner-Warwick and Kirby, 1993). However, simultaneous hysterectomy is not recommended prophylactically because it does not enhance the outcome of a retropubic suspension and should be

performed only if there is concomitant uterine pathology (Milani et al, 1985; Langer et al, 1988). Although the Burch colposuspension and paravaginal/vagino-obturator shelf repair both correct lateral defect cystourethroceles, recurrent cystourethroceles were noted in 11% and 39% of Burch colposuspensions and paravaginal repairs, respectively (Colombo et al, 1996). In Mainprize and Drutz's review (1988), postoperative cystocele was noted in only 0.4% of patients after an MMK procedure.

Wiskind and coworkers (1992) noted that 27% of patients who had undergone a Burch colposuspension developed prolapse requiring surgery: rectocele in 22%, enterocele in 11%, uterine prolapse in 13%, and cystocele in 2%. More recently it has been suggested that most women are asymptomatic and less than 5% have been reported to request further surgery (Smith et al, 2005). Ward and associates (2004) reported 4.8% of women needing a posterior repair whereas Kwon and coworkers (2003) reported 4.7% requiring subsequent pelvic reconstruction.

Because retropubic suspensions are unable to correct central defect cystoceles, patients must be carefully examined preoperatively to exclude their presence.

16. **a. It is not as effective as a pubovaginal sling procedure.** A total of 655 women were randomly assigned to study groups: 326 to undergo the sling procedure and 329 to undergo the Burch colposuspension; 520 women (79%) completed the outcome assessment (Aldo et al, 2007). At 24 months, success rates were higher for women who underwent the sling procedure than for those who underwent the Burch colposuspension for both the overall category of success (47% vs. 38%, $P = .01$) and the category specific to SUI (66% vs. 49%, $P < .001$). There was no significant difference between the sling and Burch colposuspension groups in the percentage of patients who had serious adverse events (13% and 10%, respectively; $P = .20$). However, more women who underwent the sling procedure had adverse events than in the Burch colposuspension group, with 415 events among 206 women in the sling group as compared with 305 events among 156 women in the Burch colposuspension group. This difference was due primarily to urinary tract infections: 157 women in the sling group (48%) had 305 events and 105 women in the Burch colposuspension group (32%) had 203 events. When urinary tract infections were excluded, although the rates of adverse events were similar in the two groups there was more difficulty voiding. The distribution of time to return to normal voiding differed significantly between the two groups: Voiding dysfunction was more common in the sling group than in the Burch colposuspension group (14% vs. 2%, $P < .001$). Consequently, surgical procedures to reduce voiding symptoms or improve urinary retention were performed exclusively in the sling group, in which 19 patients underwent 20 such procedures (63% vs. 47%, $P < .001$). Treatment satisfaction rates for the 480 subjects who answered the satisfaction question at 24 months were significantly higher in the sling group than in the Burch colposuspension group (86% vs. 78%, $P = .02$). A further analysis of this study focused on sexual activity as assessed by the Pelvic Organ Prolapse/Urinary Incontinence Sexual Questionnaire (PISQ-12) among those sexually active at baseline and 2 years after surgery (Brubaker et al, 2009). This report demonstrated that sexual function improves after

successful surgery and does not differ between Burch colposuspension and sling procedures.

It can therefore be reliably concluded that in specialist centers working in a standardized fashion, the autologous fascial sling results in a higher rate of successful treatment of SUI but also greater morbidity than the Burch colposuspension.

Comparisons between the MMK and the Burch colposuspension procedures have generally yielded similar results. Three articles that reviewed the literature on incontinence procedures all found retropubic suspensions to be more effective than either needle suspensions or anterior colporrhaphies (Jarvis, 1994; Black and Downs, 1996; Leach et al, 1997). Most studies in the literature have not demonstrated a significant difference in cure rates between retropubic suspensions (generally a Burch colposuspension) and pubovaginal slings (Jarvis, 1994; Black and Downs, 1996; Leach et al, 1997). The literature on the paravaginal repair is sparse. The only randomized study that compared the Burch colposuspension with a paravaginal repair found significantly greater subjective and objective cure with the Burch colposuspension (Colombo et al, 1996). At this point, the tension-free vaginal tape procedure appears to be at least equivalent to the Burch colposuspension.

Additional Study Points

1. Anti-incontinence surgery does not work by restoring the normal mechanism of continence but rather by a compensatory approach creating a new mechanism of continence.
2. Intrinsic sphincter deficiency is suggested by a leak point pressure less than 60 cm H_2O or a maximum urethral closure pressure of less than 20 cm H_2O.
3. Approximately 40% of nulliparous 30- to 49-year-old women experience some degree of incontinence with exercise.
4. The nonabsorbable sutures used in a retropubic suspension not uncommonly migrate into the bladder and serve as a foreign body nidus for stone formation and infection.
5. The postoperative risk of SUI in continent women undergoing an abdominal sacrocolpopexy is substantially reduced by the addition of a Burch colposuspension.
6. A maximum urethral closing pressure of less than 20 cm H_2O is a contraindication to the Burch colposuspension.
7. All patients prior to any colposuspension should be advised about the potential need for intermittent self-catheterization.
8. The Burch colposuspension is regarded as the standard open retropubic procedure for incontinence.

Vaginal and Abdominal Reconstructive Surgery for Pelvic Organ Prolapse

Jack Christian Winters, MD ● Joanna Maya Togami, MD ●
Christopher J. Chermansky, MD

QUESTIONS

1. Which of the following statements is FALSE?
   a. Pelvic organ prolapse occurs because of defects in the supporting tissues.
   b. Pelvic organ prolapse is a manifestation of discrete descent of the female pelvic viscera.
   c. Pelvic organ prolapse occurs as compartmental defects, and multiple compartments may be affected.
   d. The aim of surgical management is restoration of normal anatomy while maintaining visceral and sexual function.
   e. Pelvic organ prolapse essentially represents hernias within the pelvic floor.

2. Which structure does not insert onto the spinous process?
   a. Arcus tendineus fasciae pelvis
   b. Sacrospinous ligament
   c. Coccygeus muscle
   d. Arcus tendineus levator ani

3. With regard to three levels of vaginal support as described by DeLancey, which of the following is TRUE?
   a. Level I support provides a primarily vertical support of the upper vagina and cervix by the cardinal uterosacral ligament complex.
   b. Level II support includes the shortest fibers and anchors the midvagina.
   c. Level III support has intervening paracolpium and supports the most distal portion of the vagina.
   d. Level I support originates from the greater sciatic foramen, the medial sacrum, and the sacroiliac region.
   e. Level III support does not fuse the urethra anteriorly and the perineal body posteriorly.

4. Which statement about the endopelvic fascia is FALSE?
   a. The endopelvic fascia is a composite of fibrous tissues, embedded in a matrix.
   b. The tissues are supportive and contractile.
   c. The endopelvic fascia is easily divided into the various regions, which are readily identified at surgery.
   d. The endopelvic fascia lacks the organization of the fascial coverings of skeletal muscle.
   e. The endopelvic fascia has different regions that are specifically named.

5. Which structure does not attach to the perineal body?
   a. Rectovaginal fascia
   b. Levator ani muscles
   c. Transverse perinei muscles
   d. Pubocervical fascia
   e. External anal sphincter

6. Which of the following statements about apical compartment prolapse is FALSE?
   a. Vaginal vault prolapse can occur after hysterectomy if support is not reconstituted to the cardinal uterosacral ligament complex.
   b. An apical defect may result in uterine prolapse, vaginal vault prolapse, and prolapse of the peritoneum cul-de-sac.
   c. Failure to reconstitute the vaginal vault at the time of hysterectomy will lead to immediate vault prolapse.
   d. Total procidentia includes apical prolapse of the vagina in addition to multiple compartment defects.
   e. Enteroceles occur with or without vaginal vault prolapse.

7. Patient satisfaction is NOT highly correlated with which of the following?
   a. Patient readiness to undergo surgery
   b. Objective measures of surgical success
   c. Resolution of the symptoms of pelvic organ prolapse
   d. Lack of patient-perceived complications
   e. Achievement of patient-selected goals

8. Preoperative patient preparation does NOT include which of the following?
   a. Asking the patient to state what the planned procedure(s) is and its purpose

b. Administering preoperative antibiotics

c. Deep venous thrombosis prophylaxis

d. Local estrogen therapy

e. Routine use of vaginal douches

9. Which statement is FALSE regarding biologic and synthetic grafts?

a. Wound healing follows a stepwise cascade regardless of material type.

b. All synthetic grafts are biologically inert.

c. There is no ideal prosthetic implant.

d. Biologic grafts are classified as autologous, allografts, and xenografts.

e. Synthetic grafts may be absorbable.

10. Which statement is FALSE regarding wound healing and grafts/mesh?

a. The amount of foreign body reaction is proportional to the surface area of the material exposed to the host.

b. The degree of response and amount of tissue ingrowth is determined by the nature of the material.

c. The graft functions as a permanent mechanical support.

d. Host tissue integration leads to long-term graft function.

e. The graft/mesh acts as a scaffold to facilitate tissue ingrowth.

11. Which of the following processes must occur for long-term graft survival?

a. Rejection

b. Degeneration

c. Encapsulation

d. Absorption

e. Remodeling

12. Which tissue processing technique causes the least amount of variability in tissue quality of allografts and xenografts?

a. Tissue harvesting

b. Cross-linking

c. Freeze drying

d. Tissue fenestration

e. Solvent dehydration

13. The most important characteristic of a synthetic mesh is:

a. type of mesh (synthetic or absorbable).

b. pore size.

c. filament type (monofilament or multifilament).

d. mesh construct (woven or knitted).

e. flexibility.

14. Which of the following statements regarding anterior colporrhaphy is FALSE?

a. Anterior colporrhaphy is not used to treat stress incontinence.

b. Recent series report a 40% recurrence rate for standard anterior colporrhaphy.

c. The most likely contributing factor for failure of anterior compartment repairs is the concomitant presence of other compartmental defects.

d. Cystoscopy with indigo carmine is not routinely necessary.

e. Ensuring that the bladder is drained before perforating the endopelvic fascia may decrease bladder injuries.

15. Paravaginal repairs are used to repair which of the following anterior compartment defects?

a. Lateral

b. Central

c. Anterior

d. Posterior

e. Distal

16. Which of the following statements is FALSE regarding high-grade anterior compartment prolapse?

a. Urethral kinking or compression may occur.

b. Occult stress urinary incontinence may be unmasked by reducing the prolapse.

c. No method to reduce the prolapse is superior in evaluating occult stress urinary incontinence.

d. All women with high-grade anterior compartment prolapse should undergo a prophylactic anti-incontinence procedure.

e. Intervention for complications of midurethral slings equals the risk of having to perform a secondary sling.

17. A 50-year-old woman presents with symptoms of voiding difficulty and vaginal bulging. She has had no prior pelvic surgery. In the supine position she demonstrates anterior vaginal wall prolapse that extends 4 cm beyond the hymen. The cervix does not descend with straining during the supine examination. The least likely diagnosis is:

a. cystocele only.

b. uterine prolapse and cystocele.

c. uterine prolapse and enterocele.

d. uterine prolapse, enterocele, and cystocele.

e. uterine prolapse, widened genital hiatus, and enterocele.

18. Which statement is FALSE regarding apical defects?

a. Failure to recognize an apical defect at the time of prolapse repair will increase the risk of recurrence.

b. Apical defects may involve the bladder and rectum.

c. Hysterectomy with suspension of the vaginal apex to the cardinal uterosacral ligaments and attaching the pubocervical fascia to the rectovaginal fascia will ensure the apical support.

d. Enteroceles always contain small bowel.

e. Enteroceles are thought to occur by several mechanisms.

19. Which of the following statements is TRUE regarding uterosacral ligament suspensions?

a. The ureter courses closer to the uterosacral ligament proximally.

b. Suture placement in the most medial portion of the uterosacral ligament will avoid fibers of the sacral plexus.

c. The ureters are found consistently in the same location regardless of the degree of prolapse.

d. The sutures should be tied before performing a cystoscopy.

e. The suspensory sutures should be trimmed before the cystoscopy.

20. What method is NOT used to identify the cardinal uterosacral ligaments?

a. Traction of the dimples of the vaginal apex

b. Placing an Allis clamp at the 5-o'clock and 7-o'clock positions of the vaginal vault

c. Direct visualization

d. Tugging on the suture tied to the cardinal uterosacral ligaments at the time of hysterectomy

e. Randomly grasping a condensation of tissue along the pelvic side wall

21. Which of the following statements about apical repairs is TRUE?

a. Uterosacral suspension restores the vaginal apex.

b. With respect to durability, abdominal sacrocolpopexy has not been shown to be superior to sacrospinous ligament suspension.

c. Sacrospinous ligament suspension does not change the vaginal axis.

d. With abdominal uterosacral ligament suspension, one does not need to place as many sutures on the ligament.

e. Iliococcygeus repairs always foreshorten the vaginal length.

22. A disadvantage of sacrospinous ligament fixation is:

a. it requires a retroperitoneal approach.

b. the sacrospinous ligament is not a reliable structure on which to anchor the vaginal apex.

c. the procedure may only be approached anteriorly.

d. the hospital stay is equivalent compared with abdominal sacrocolpopexy.

e. there may be posterior or caudal displacement of the vagina.

23. Which structure is at risk of being injured with sacrospinous ligament suspensions?

a. Genitofemoral nerve

b. Pudendal nerve

c. Obturator vessels

d. Ilioinguinal nerve

e. Hypogastric vessels

24. Which statement is FALSE regarding the anatomy around the sacrospinous ligament?

a. The pudendal nerves and vessels are in close proximity as they course around the ischial spine.

b. The gluteal vessels course behind the sacrospinous ligament.

c. The highest concentration of sacral nerves is by the ischial spine.

d. The fibers of the sacrospinous ligament fan out closer to the sacrum.

e. The optimal position to place suture for fixation is 1.5 to 2 cm medial to the ischial spine.

25. Which of the following is FALSE regarding pain from the sacrospinous ligament suspension?

a. Gluteal pain generally resolves spontaneously in 2 to 3 months.

b. Injection of the nerve with local anesthetic can be done to relieve the pain.

c. Pudendal nerve entrapment causes gluteal pain.

d. Pain may occur in 15% of patients on the ipsilateral side.

e. Pain is musculoskeletal in origin.

26. All of the following statements regarding the iliococcygeus suspension are true EXCEPT:

a. The site of fixation may be approached either anteriorly or posteriorly.

b. Fixation is 1 cm distal to the ischial spine near the insertion of the arcus tendineus fasciae pelvis.

c. The dissection for the iliococcygeus suspension is as extensive as for the sacrospinous ligament fixation.

d. The iliococcygeus suspension maintains the vagina in the normal axis.

e. Neuropathy has been reported as a postoperative complication.

27. Key elements of the abdominal sacrocolpopexy do NOT include:

a. use of permanent monofilament mesh.

b. secure fixation to the sacral promontory.

c. secure fixation to the vaginal cuff.

d. use of a biologic graft.

e. complete enterocele reduction and culdoplasty.

28. Which structures are the sources of severe bleeding with the abdominal sacrocolpopexy?

a. Presacral veins

b. Internal iliac vein

c. Mesenteric veins

d. Middle sacral vein

e. a and d

29. Which statement is TRUE regarding culdoplasty?

a. Halban culdoplasty involves placing purse-string sutures.

b. Moschowitz culdoplasty involves placing longitudinal sutures.

c. The risk of the Moschowitz culdoplasty is ureteral obstruction due to angulation.

d. Culdoplasties prevent rectocele formation.

e. Downward retraction of the end-to end anastomosis sizer may help delineate the cul-de-sac.

30. Which of the following factors is FALSE regarding advantages of colpocleisis?

a. Shorter operative time

b. Ability to use either regional anesthesia or local anesthesia with sedation

c. Minimal complication rates

d. Appropriate choice for those wishing to maintain sexual activity

e. Decreased recuperative time

31. Which postoperative complication of both colpocleisis and partial colpocleisis, if identified preoperatively, may be reduced?

a. Stress urinary incontinence

b. Urinary retention

c. Regret over loss of sexual function

d. Recurrence

e. Infection

32. Uterine prolapse represents the loss of:
    a. apical support from the broad ligament.
    b. anterior support from the arcus tendineus fasciae pelvis.
    c. apical support from the cardinal uterosacral ligament.
    d. posterior support from the rectovaginal fascia.
    e. apical support from the round ligaments.

33. Contraindications to performing a vaginal hysterectomy do NOT include:
    a. endometriosis of unknown extent.
    b. obliteration of the cul-de-sac.
    c. size disproportion of the uterus to the introitus.
    d. grade II uterine prolapse or greater.
    e. malignancy of the uterus or ovaries.

34. Which maneuver performed during vaginal hysterectomy is essential to prevent recurrent prolapse?
    a. Leaving an adequate stump on the uterine artery
    b. Culdoplasty
    c. Leaving an adequate stump on the cardinal uterosacral ligament complex
    d. Closure of the cul-de-sac
    e. b and d

35. Which surgical technique of rectocele repair is most associated with postoperative dyspareunia?
    a. Levator plication
    b. Site-specific repair
    c. Site-specific repair with biologic interposition graft
    d. Transanal repair of rectocele
    e. Perineorrhaphy

36. Which symptom changes the least following site-specific posterior colporrhaphy?
    a. Dyspareunia
    b. Constipation
    c. Vaginal mass
    d. Splinting
    e. Vaginal pressure or pain

37. Which statement regarding vaginal kits is TRUE?
    a. There is ample evidence to support their use.
    b. The presence of mesh turns a single compartment repair into a multicompartmental repair.
    c. The volume of mesh used is less than that for traditional interposition repairs.
    d. The use of trocars reduces the complication rates.
    e. Complications associated with kit repairs are the same as those associated with traditional repairs.

38. Which structure is not used as a fixation point or point of reference for vaginal kits?
    a. Sacrospinous ligament
    b. Cardinal uterosacral ligament complex
    c. Ischial spine
    d. Obturator internus fascia
    e. Arcus tendineus fasciae pelvis

39. Complications that seem more likely when utilizing vaginal kits to repair pelvic organ prolapse include all of the following EXCEPT:
    a. pelvic hematoma.
    b. necrotizing fasciitis.
    c. vaginal extrusion of mesh.
    d. groin pain.
    e. visceral perforation.

40. Failure rate of standard anterior colporrhaphy approaches:
    a. 10%.
    b. 20%.
    c. 30%.
    d. 40%.
    e. 50%.

41. What Pelvic Organ Prolapse Quantification (POP-Q) stage is generally used to define anatomic failure in most modern series?
    a. Stage I or greater
    b. Stage II or greater
    c. Stage III or greater
    d. Stage IV
    e. Stage V

ANSWERS

1. **b. Pelvic organ prolapse is a manifestation of discrete descent of the female pelvic viscera.** Pelvic organ prolapse occurs because of defects within the support structures of the pelvic floor. Because the support is contiguous and boundaries are often difficult to delineate, conceptualizing the various regions of the vagina as compartments facilitates the current understanding of the pelvic floor. Multiple compartments are often involved in pelvic organ prolapse, and multiple defects can be seen in a single compartment.

2. **d. Arcus tendineus levator ani.** The spinous process serves as an anchoring point for the first three structures and is an important landmark for surgeons who operate on the pelvic floor.

3. **a. Level I support provides a primarily vertical support of the upper vagina and cervix by the cardinal uterosacral ligament complex.** Level I support originates from the greater sciatic foramen, the sacroiliac region, and the lateral sacrum. It has vertical support suspending the upper vagina and cardinal uterosacral ligament complex. Level II support has mid-length fibers and supports the mid vagina. Level III support has no intervening paracolpium, fuses the urethra anteriorly, and blends into the perineal body posteriorly.

4. **c. The endopelvic fascia is easily divided into the various regions, which are readily identified at surgery.** The endopelvic fascia is one contiguous unit, in which distinct areas are named. However, it is often difficult to identify where one region ends and the other begins. It should be considered as a unit. The challenge of the endopelvic fascia in its use as a supportive structure is that there is inherent weakness created by its structure of fibrous tissue embedded in a matrix in contrast to the fascial covering of skeletal muscle.

5. **d. Pubocervical fascia.** The perineal body is a condensation of fibromuscular tissue and collagen. It is located in the midline between the vagina and the anus. The pubocervical fascia is an anterior structure that does not insert into the perineal body.

6. **c. Failure to reconstitute the vaginal vault at the time of hysterectomy will lead to immediate vault prolapse.** The upper vagina is supported by two structures: the cardinal uterosacral ligament complex and the broad ligament. Therefore vaginal vault prolapse does not occur immediately after hysterectomy if the cardinal uterosacral ligaments are not reattached to the vaginal vault at the time of hysterectomy, owing to the support of the broad ligaments.

7. **b. Objective measures of surgical success.** In their study, Kenton and colleagues (2007)* found that patient perception of perioperative events and bother from recurrent symptoms resulted in dissatisfaction with prolapse surgery in the presence of high objective cure rates. Patient-perceived complications included postoperative pain, minor effects of anesthesia, hospital discharge with a catheter, constipation, and urgency incontinence. Preoperative counseling is a key time in which one may educate and affect postoperative patient satisfaction.

8. **e. Routine use of vaginal douches.** The Agency for Healthcare Research and Quality identified perioperative interventions to improve patient safety, which include asking the patient to recall and state what was discussed during informed consent, administering appropriate preoperative antibiotics, and deep venous thrombosis prophylaxis. Postmenopausal patients may be treated with local estrogen therapy, which may increase vascularity and promote wound healing. Most surgeons do not use vaginal douches preoperatively.

9. **b. All synthetic grafts are biologically inert.** Synthetic grafts are not biologically inert. All grafts will become involved in the wound healing process. Physical factors of each biologic graft or synthetic mesh will have different effects on the resultant scar tissue matrix.

10. **c. The graft functions as a permanent mechanical support.** Tissue incorporation must occur for long-term success of a biologic graft or synthetic mesh. The important concept is that the graft, synthetic or biologic, serves as a scaffold to facilitate tissue ingrowth, rather than functioning as permanent mechanical support.

11. **e. Remodeling.** Incorporation through a process called graft remodeling is needed for long-term graft survival.

12. **a. Tissue harvesting.** The other techniques can all induce variability in tissue strength and incorporation. Aldehyde cross-linking is cytotoxic in high concentrations, attracting gelatinases to the wound that may increase the rate of graft degradation. Fenestrations may decrease seroma formation and increase both angiogenesis and tissue ingrowth. Freeze drying demonstrated reduced maximum load to failure and stiffness of cadaveric fascia lata, in addition to variability of strength and stiffness throughout the graft.

13. **b. pore size.** Increased pore size results in greater flexibility. Pore size of 75 μm is the size that allows for the optimal tissue ingrowth with fibroblasts, blood vessels, and collagen fibrils. Monofilament knitted materials are able to assume a macroporous configuration.

14. **d. Cystoscopy with indigo carmine is not routinely necessary.** Cystoscopy after the administration of indigo carmine or methylene blue is recommended as a routine practice after anterior colporrhaphy. If blue-tinged urine is not seen effluxing from each ureteral orifice, catheterization may be considered before taking down the plication sutures. Appropriate steps must be performed to ensure ureteral patency, including takedown of the sutures.

15. **a. Lateral.** Lateral defects are repaired with paravaginal repairs. This defect may be approached transvaginally or transabdominally.

16. **d. All women with high-grade anterior compartment prolapse should undergo a prophylactic anti-incontinence procedure.** The risks and benefits of prophylactic anti-incontinence procedure on continent women should be reviewed with each patient. The literature supports selective use of an anti-incontinence procedure at the time of pelvic organ prolapse repair. All women with advanced-stage anterior compartment prolapse should be screened for occult stress urinary incontinence.

17. **a. cystocele only.** The patient has grade 4 anterior vaginal wall prolapse and the likelihood that the prolapse is bladder only is very low. She has a high likelihood of concomitant uterine prolapse.

18. **d. Enteroceles always contain small bowel.** Enteroceles may involve omentum and small bowel. Large vaginal vault prolapse may involve the bladder and rectum. Enteroceles can occur from causes that may be congenital, from pulsion, from traction, or iatrogenic.

19. **d. The sutures should be tied before performing a cystoscopy.** The sutures of the uterosacral ligament suspension should be tied before cystoscopy to evaluate the patency of the ureters. If cystoscopy is performed before tying the sutures, there may not be enough traction or compression from the sutures to appreciate ureteral obstruction. However, if the sutures need to be taken down, leaving them untrimmed until after the cystoscopy is practical because the tails will facilitate identification of the most lateral suture. They will need to be taken down one at a time until the offending suture is identified. As the ureter courses distally, it gets closer to the cardinal uterosacral ligament complex, becoming the closest at the level of the cervix. Location of the ureters may vary considerably depending on the degree of prolapse.

20. **e. Randomly grasping a condensation of tissue along the pelvic side wall.** The cardinal uterosacral ligament complex should be identified by tenting this structure either at the dimples of the vaginal apex or by placing Allis clamps at the vaginal vault or by tugging on the sutures. Alternatively, they can be directly visualized intra-abdominally. Random grasping of a condensation of tissue places the ureter at risk.

21. **a. Uterosacral suspension restores the vaginal apex.** The uterosacral suspension restores the normal anatomy of the vaginal apex. In contrast, right-sided unilateral sacrospinous ligament fixation often results in the vagina being displaced posteriorly and to the right. The abdominal sacrocolpopexy has been demonstrated to be superior to sacrospinous ligament suspension with respect to durability.

---

*Sources referenced can be found in *Campbell-Walsh Urology,* *10th Edition,* on the Expert Consult website.

Although the iliococcygeus repair may foreshorten the vagina, it does not always occur.

22. **e. there may be posterior or caudal displacement of the vagina.** The caudal displacement of the vagina is thought to potentially contribute to the rate of anterior prolapse recurrence. By displacing the vaginal apex posteriorly, the procedure places the anterior compartment at risk for recurrent prolapse.

23. **b. Pudendal nerve.** The pudendal nerve courses around the ischial spine. Medial placement of the sutures 1.5 cm away from the ischial spine will help to avoid entrapment of the pudendal nerve. The other structures are farther away from the sacrospinous ligament and are less likely to be injured.

24. **c. The highest concentration of sacral nerves is by the ischial spine.** The highest concentration of sacral nerves is closest to the sacrum.

25. **e. Pain is musculoskeletal in origin.** The pain from sacrospinous ligament suspension is either gluteal or radiates down the leg posteriorly. It is neuropathic, and it occurs in 15% of patients. The pain may last 2 to 3 months in patients who have delayed absorbable sutures. Injection of the nerve with local anesthetic has been described to alleviate the pain.

26. **c. The dissection for the iliococcygeus suspension is as extensive as for the sacrospinous ligament fixation.** The dissection for the iliococcygeus suspension is not as extensive as that used to access the sacrospinous ligament. Advantages include using either the anterior or posterior approach, maintaining the vagina in a near-normal axis.

27. **d. use of a biologic graft.** Permanent monofilament mesh has been shown to be superior to both cadaveric fascia lata graft (Culligan et al, 2005) and xenograft (Deprest et al, 2009). Secure fixation of the graft to both the sacral promontory and vaginal cuff, use of a monofilament mesh, and complete reduction of the enterocele with culdoplasty and tensioning so that the rectum is 2 fingerbreadths away from the mesh are key elements to the repair.

28. **e. a and d.** Severe bleeding can be encountered with shearing of the presacral and middle sacral veins. This may be avoided by placing sutures higher on the sacral promontory. Careful dissection is essential over the promontory. Sterile tacks may be used to stop the bleeding if encountered.

29. **c. The risk of the Moschowitz culdoplasty is ureteral obstruction due to angulation.** The Halban culdoplasty involves placing longitudinal sutures, and the Moschowitz culdoplasty involves placing purse-string sutures. The Moschowitz culdoplasty can result in ureteral angulation resulting in obstruction. A culdoplasty prevents enteroceles (not rectoceles) from forming. The end-to-end anastomosis sizer must be angled upward to see the cul-de-sac.

30. **d. Appropriate choice for those wishing to maintain sexual activity.** Both colpocleisis and partial colpocleisis are only considered for those patients who are not sexually active and do not wish to maintain the ability to be sexually active. Careful counseling is especially important with these procedures.

31. **a. Stress urinary incontinence.** Patients may give a history of stress urinary incontinence that improved over time as their pelvic organ prolapse worsened. Before undergoing colpocleisis, all women should be screened for occult stress urinary incontinence.

32. **c. apical support from the cardinal uterosacral ligament.** Loss of apical support from the cardinal uterosacral ligament complex leads to uterine prolapse. Because the broad ligament also provides a small amount of support, failure to reconstitute the support from the cardinal uterosacral ligament complex at the time of hysterectomy does not lead to immediate apical prolapse.

33. **d. grade II uterine prolapse or greater.** Endometriosis of unknown extent may make vaginal hysterectomy problematic. Obliteration of the cul-de-sac will preclude accessing the proper plane to identify the parametrium.

34. **e. b and d.** The key elements to prevent recurrent vaginal vault prolapse after vaginal hysterectomy is culdoplasty, which is a closure of the cul-de-sac. Attaching the pubocervical fascia to the rectovaginal fascia closes the cul-de-sac, thus preventing an enterocele. Attaching the vaginal apex to the cardinal uterosacral ligament complex reconstitutes the apical support.

35. **a. Levator plication.** Levator plication was associated with high rates of de novo postoperative dyspareunia. As such, it has largely been abandoned.

36. **b. Constipation.** Constipation may be associated with dysmotility disorders of the rectum that do not improve with an anatomic repair. The symptoms most likely to improve are dyspareunia, the need for vaginal splinting, vaginal mass, and pressure.

37. **b. The presence of mesh turns a single compartment repair into a multicompartmental repair.** The mesh placed with vaginal kits often supports both the vaginal apex and the anterior and posterior compartments, making direct comparisons between kits and traditional repairs challenging. The kits utilizing trocars have complications that are unique to those techniques. The volume of mesh used is more than the amounts used in traditional repairs.

38. **b. Cardinal uterosacral ligament complex.** The systems utilize the other structures as fixation points or references.

39. **c. vaginal extrusion of mesh.** Vaginal extrusion of mesh is not unique to the trocar kits. The other complications have been associated with kits involving trocars.

40. **d. 40%.** The current literature reports a 40% failure rate of standard anterior colporrhaphy (Sand et al, 2001; Weber et al, 2001).

41. **b. Stage II or greater.** Most modern series define anatomic failure as stage II or greater using the POP-Q. Some patients with recurrent stage II prolapse remain asymptomatic and do not require further surgical correction.

Additional Study Points

1. The iliococcygeus and the coccygeus muscles fuse in the midline and attach to the coccyx forming a complex called the levator plate that supports the upper vagina and cervix.

2. The urethra is fused to the anterior vaginal wall for much of its length.

3. Vaginal support is provided by the endopelvic connective tissues.

4. The cardinal and uterosacral ligaments provide level I support of the uterus and upper vagina; the endopelvic and pubocervical fascia provide level II support of the mid vagina as it attaches to the arcus tendineus fasciae pelvis; the distal vagina attaches to the levator ani muscles and perineal body to provide for level III support.

5. Pelvic organ prolapse is for the most part a quality of life issue.

6. Anterior compartment defects can be central, lateral, or both.

7. Anterior colporrhaphy and paravaginal repairs are both inefective alone in the treatment of stress urinary incontinence.

8. Sacrospinous ligament fixation may result in posterior displacement of the vaginal apex and increase the risk of anterior compartment prolapse.

9. If either the bladder or rectum is injured during pelvic organ prolapse repair, mesh should not be used.

Slings: Autologous, Biologic, Synthetic, and Midurethral

Roger R. Dmochowski, MD, FACS ● Priya Padmanabhan, MD, MPH ●
Harriette Miles Scarpero, MD

QUESTIONS

1. An autologous pubovaginal sling (PVS) is indicated in all of the following conditions EXCEPT:
   a. urethral incompetence in a T12 spinal cord injury.
   b. low urethral resistance with decreased bladder compliance.
   c. urethral incompetence and large urethral diverticulum.
   d. proximal urethral loss secondary to long-standing indwelling Foley catheter.
   e. refractory stress urinary incontinence (SUI) after failed midurethral sling and bulking agents.

2. Which of the statements about the normal female urethra and pelvic floor is TRUE?
   a. The female urethra is composed of four separate tissue layers, and the middle seromuscular layer is most important in enhancing the urethral sphincter mechanism during voiding.
   b. The Valsalva pressure of the bladder exceeds the resting closing pressure of the internal sphincter.
   c. The fast-twitch fibers of the external sphincter are responsible for sudden voluntary guarding reflex, and slow-twitch fibers provide passive control through the involuntary guarding reflex.
   d. The levator ani, urethropelvic ligament, and round ligament provide needed support to the bladder neck and undersurface of the bladder.
   e. The PVS is placed at the bladder neck to provide adequate urethral coaptation at rest and to decrease urethral responsiveness to abdominal pressure.

3. Which of the following statements regarding materials for bladder neck pubovaginal slings is FALSE?
   a. The ideal material has minimal tissue reaction and complete biocompatibility.
   b. Stiffness and maximal load failure are the same between freeze-dried fascia lata and solvent dehydrated and dermal grafts.
   c. The estimated risk of human immunodeficiency virus (HIV) transmission by an allograft sling is about 1 in 1,660,000.

   d. Porcine small intestinal submucosa has less tensile strength than cadaveric fascia lata.
   e. Synthetic materials are associated with high erosion rates during use for bladder neck PVS.

4. In outcomes associated with PVS procedures, which of the following is/are TRUE?
   a. Reported cure rates after an autologous PVS procedure are 50% to 97%.
   b. Preoperative Valsalva leak point pressure is a reliable predictor of outcomes after sling surgery.
   c. Bladder neck PVS slings should be utilized for refractory or recurrent SUI but are associated with worse outcomes.
   d. In the SiSTER trial, cure rates and voiding symptoms were greater for the pubovaginal sling than for the Burch colposuspension.
   e. a and d

5. Which of the following statements about erosion and PVS material is FALSE?
   a. Synthetic slings erode into the urethra 15 times more often than autologous, allograft, or xenograft slings.
   b. Urethral erosions are often associated with urinary retention and mixed urinary incontinence.
   c. There are only four cases of urethral erosion of an autologous PVS in the literature, and in most cases this may have been avoided by thorough cystoscopy.
   d. Erosion from synthetic slings requires removal of all visible and palpable sling material.
   e. The incidence of recurrent SUI in urethral erosions after use of a synthetic PVS is 74% to 100%.

6. Which one of the following statements is NOT associated with voiding dysfunction after a PVS procedure?
   a. Obstruction, detrusor overactivity, or impaired detrusor contractility are all manifestations of voiding dysfunction for iatrogenic PVS obstruction.
   b. Persistent urgency is more common than urinary retention in bladder outlet obstruction after a PVS procedure.

c. Fifty percent of affected patients have symptoms of overactive bladder, which can be avoided if sling lysis is performed within 2 weeks of PVS placement.

d. Urodynamic study is valuable in assessment and planning management.

e. There is up to a 20% recurrent SUI rate after urethrolysis.

7. Regarding the pathophysiology of incontinence:

a. hypermobility is the main underlying cause of SUI.

b. intrinsic sphincter deficiency (ISD) is rarely the primary cause of SUI.

c. ISD is the primary underlying cause of SUI for women, with hypermobility being a secondary finding.

d. the levator floor provides active compression to the proximal urethra.

e. the extrinsic urethral skeletal sphincter is the primary mechanism for urinary continence.

8. The integral theory regarding midurethral slings maintains that:

a. the midurethral continence mechanism is active both passively and during stress events.

b. the pubourethral ligaments are a secondary component of the complex.

c. the pubourethral ligaments and pubococcygeal muscles provide a central support point that, during stress events, function to kink or functionally hinge the urethra, rendering continence.

d. aging and childbirth have no effect on the midurethral support structures.

e. the midurethral mechanism is intrinsically involved with bladder neck support.

9. The tension-free vaginal tape (TVT or any midurethral sling) procedure incorporates all of the following EXCEPT:

a. insertion trocars are used to transpose the implanted material into position.

b. the synthetic material used is a wide porosity mesh.

c. loose tension is placed on the sling material.

d. the sling is sutured to the underlying tissues for fixation purposes.

e. cystoscopy is a crucial component of the procedure.

10. In review of the efficacy outcomes obtained with midurethral procedures, which of the following is TRUE?

a. Midurethral slings are less effective than open colposuspension procedures.

b. Midurethral slings produce inferior results compared with laparoscopic colposuspensions.

c. Postoperative voiding dysfunction is more common with midurethra procedures than with other types of suspension procedures.

d. Mixed incontinence results are superior to those of pure SUI.

e. Five-year results demonstrate durability similar to 1-year results.

11. In elderly patients, midurethral slings:

a. are less effective than in younger patients.

b. have rates of postoperative urgency higher than those in young patients.

c. have satisfaction rates lower than those in young patients.

d. have mixed incontinence resolution rates higher than those in young patients.

e. result in postoperative urinary retention occurring more frequently.

12. When midurethral slings are performed at the time of prolapse surgery:

a. risks of erosion and infection are higher than in cases in which only a sling is performed.

b. concomitant hysterectomy has an adverse effect on incontinence outcome.

c. rates of urethrolysis for postoperative retention are higher.

d. occult incontinence is not adequately addressed.

e. rates of retention are slightly higher than in those undergoing a sling procedure only.

13. When using midurethral slings as salvage procedures:

a. complication rates are higher than when midurethral slings are done primarily.

b. the technique needs to be altered when done as a primary procedure.

c. failure rates are unaffected by urethral hypermobility.

d. bladder perforation is less than in primary cases.

e. overall efficacy is similar to that of primary implantation.

14. Complications associated with midurethral slings include:

a. bladder perforation injury rates range up to 5%.

b. voiding dysfunction ranges from 4% to 20%.

c. de novo urgency occurs in up to 12% of patients.

d. wound healing is delayed in approximately 1%.

e. all of the above.

15. Material-related erosions associated with midurethral slings are:

a. decreased by the macroporous nature of the sling material.

b. unaffected by tension placed on the slings.

c. associated with vaginal erosions approximately 20% of the time.

d. associated with bladder erosion rates of 20%.

e. do not affect outcomes or satisfaction.

16. In regard to erosions associated with midurethral slings:

a. bladder erosions cannot be managed endoscopically in well-selected cases.

b. vaginal erosions cannot be managed conservatively.

c. erosions are not related to errant sling placement.

d. symptoms are not usually associated with erosion.

e. complete excision of exposed material should be performed.

17. Voiding dysfunction associated with midurethral slings is:

a. not associated with changes in urodynamic parameters.

b. predictable based on unique preoperative voiding parameters such as flow rate.

c. managed by immediate sling release.

d. managed initially conservatively, but sling release should be contemplated when persistent voiding trials are not successful.

e. resolved by complete excision of the sling.

18. Complications associated with midurethral slings include:

a. superficial vaginal material exposure.

b. vascular perforation.

c. intestinal perforation.

d. significant hemorrhage requiring transfusion.

e. all of the above.

19. Regarding the transobturator technique (TOT) the:

a. surgical placement of the tape requires insertion through the adductor longus tendon.

b. tape never traverses the gracilis or adductor magnus brevis muscles.

c. anterior branch of the obturator artery is located at the medial aspect of the obturator foramen.

d. the tape remains above the perineal membrane and outside the true pelvis and does not penetrate the levator ani group.

e. dorsal nerve of the clitoris is in close juxtaposition to the tape.

20. The TOT technique involves:

a. either outside-in or inside-out approaches.

b. no absolute requirement for cystoscopy.

c. no risk of lower urinary tract injury.

d. no risk of leg pain or dyspareunia.

e. similar meshes in all available kits.

21. Reported outcomes with the TOT:

a. appear to be relatively similar regardless of whether ISD is present preoperatively.

b. include bladder, but not urethral, injury being reported.

c. indicate that vaginal erosion is similar regardless of the type of tape used.

d. show that voiding dysfunction is significantly less with this technique as compared with the retropubic approach.

e. are not affected by the presence of urethral hypermobility.

22. Regarding the single incision midurethral slings:

a. tape is only appropriate in high-risk populations (e.g., prior urinary diversion, renal transplant).

b. the "hammock position" requires passage of trocars through the obturator externus muscle.

c. 1-year results demonstrate durability similar to the TVT and TOT approaches.

d. one benefit of this technique includes lack of need for cystoscopy after placement.

e. erosion and extrusion rates are higher.

ANSWERS

1. **b. low urethral resistance with decreased bladder compliance.** Decreased bladder compliance is of concern for upper tract deterioration. The addition of a PVS by increasing bladder outlet resistance would cause significant damage to the upper tracts. The compliance should be addressed before or concurrently to anti-incontinence measures. A PVS procedure is indicated for intrinsic sphincter deficiency (ISD) associated with urethral hypermobility, SUI presenting as concomitant cystoceles, SUI associated with urethral diverticulum, and SUI associated with urethral defects (e.g., urethrovaginal fistula) in which urethral reconstruction is required and in women with SUI and associated neurogenic conditions.

2. **c. The fast-twitch fibers of the external sphincter are responsible for sudden voluntary guarding reflex, and slow-twitch fibers provide passive control through the involuntary guarding reflex.** The female urethra is composed of four layers, with the middle muscular layer maintaining the resting urethral closure mechanism and the outer seromuscular layer augmenting this closing pressure. The levator ani, urethropelvic ligament, and pubocervical fascia provide support to the bladder neck and underside of the bladder. The round ligament provides support to the uterus. A PVS is placed at the bladder neck to provide adequate urethral coaptation for increasing urethral responsiveness to abdominal pressure.

3. **b. Stiffness and maximal load failure are the same between freeze-dried fascia lata and solvent dehydrated and dermal grafts.** Maximum load to failure, maximum load/graft width, and stiffness are significantly lower for the freeze-dried fascia lata group compared with the autologous, solvent-dehydrated, and dermal graft groups. The ideal graft material causes no tissue reaction, is completely biocompatible, leads to significant host fibroblast infiltration and neovascularization, and causes negligible erosion. The estimated risk of HIV transmission from an allograft is 1 in 1,667,600. The theoretical risk of developing Creutzfeldt-Jakob disease from a non-neural allograft is 1 in 3.5 million. Porcine small intestinal submucosa has less tensile strength than cadaveric fascia lata. Synthetic material is no longer used for bladder neck PVS owing to the exceedingly high erosion rates.

4. **e. a and d.** Cure rates reported in peer-reviewed literature for autologous PVS procedures are 46% to 97%. There are no risk factors that predict outcomes after PVS surgery for primary or recurrent SUI. The PVS is a valuable option for refractory and recurrent SUI and yields a cure rate of 86%. The SiSTER trial was a multicenter, randomized clinical trial (Albo et al, 2007)* that found higher cure rates for the PVS procedure than the Burch colposuspension, but also more associated voiding symptoms (urinary tract infection, difficulty voiding, and postoperative urge incontinence, $P < .001$).

5. **d. Erosion from synthetic slings requires removal of all visible and palpable sling material.** This includes sutures, bone anchors, and screws. Synthetic slings erode 15 times more often into the urethra and extrude 14 times more often into the vagina than autologous, allograft, and xenograft slings. Urethral erosion usually presents at a mean of 9 months as urinary retention, urgency, and mixed urinary incontinence. There are four cases of autologous PVS erosion in peer-reviewed literature caused by placement of

---

*Sources referenced can be found in *Campbell-Walsh Urology,* 10th Edition, on the Expert Consult website.

the PVS through the bladder, excessive tension, and traumatic urethral instrumentation after placement. The incidence of recurrent SUI after urethral erosions from a synthetic PVS is 74% to 100%, often necessitating placement of a secondary PVS.

6. **c. Fifty percent of affected patients have symptoms of overactive bladder, which can be avoided if sling lysis is performed within 2 weeks of PVS placement.** Transient urinary retention is common, and most patients return to spontaneous voiding within 10 days postoperatively. Obstructive symptoms may improve or resolve with time, which is the reason most physicians prefer waiting 3 months before considering surgical intervention. The incidence of voiding dysfunction after continence surgery varies from 2.5% to 35% and includes obstruction, detrusor overactivity, or impaired detrusor contractility. Persistent postoperative urgency incontinence and urgency present more commonly (8% to 25%) than frank retention. Although urodynamics do not preoperatively predict outcomes after anti-incontinence surgery or urethrolysis, it is useful in diagnosing and treating patients with obstruction after a PVS procedure. There is a 0% to 18% recurrent SUI rate after urethrolysis.

7. **c. ISD is the primary underlying cause of SUI for women, with hypermobility being a secondary finding.** Although urethral hypermobility is present in many women, most do not manifest incontinence and, therefore, ISD is considered to be the most important factor in women who experience urinary loss. The extrinsic urethral sphincter is not considered to be the primary mechanism for urinary continence in women. The ongoing debate regarding hypermobility and ISD is further compounded by the advent of midurethral slings, which clearly address hypermobility during stress events. Given the efficacy of midurethral slings, there has been some confusion regarding the role of hypermobility in promoting continence. However, most believe that the intrinsic urethral mechanism is of primary importance for urinary control.

8. **c. the pubourethral ligaments and pubococcygeal muscles provide a central support point that, during stress events, function to kink or functionally hinge the urethra, rendering continence.** The integral theory places significant emphasis on the role of the pubourethral ligaments and the pubococcygeal muscles as central to urethral support during stress events. These structures actively function to provide a fulcrum around which the urethra rotates and subsequently is compressed during the stress event. Aging and childbirth clearly have a detrimental effect on the midurethral support mechanism. The midurethral mechanism is believed to be separate from the proximal urethral and bladder neck component of continence, although the latter component is considered to still have some importance in the overall passive control of urine. The midurethral continence mechanism only functions during active events and not during passive events and therefore has no function at rest.

9. **d. the sling is sutured to the underlying tissues for fixation purposes.** The TVT procedure incorporates several specific technical components. Insertion trocars are used in either a suprapubic or a vaginal approach to assist in implantation of the material in the retropubic area. It is now well known that type 1 synthetic meshes are best

because of their wide porosity. In addition, this mesh should be monofilamentous. Most authorities recommend loose tension only being placed on the TVT, although some authorities now are placing greater tension on the TVT, with success being established in patients with lesser degrees of hypermobility. No suture fixation is necessary to the underlying periurethral fascia to anchor the sling. Cystoscopy is a vital component of this procedure to exclude urinary tract injury.

10. **e. Five-year results demonstrate durability similar to 1-year results.** Five-year (and now 7-year) longitudinal results have shown that midurethral slings have procedural durability in terms of efficacy. This efficacy is not substantially less than results obtained at 1 year. Randomized trials have demonstrated similar efficacy in patients undergoing either open colposuspensions or laparoscopic colposuspensions. Midurethral slings provide superior results compared with laparoscopic procedures. Although voiding dysfunction may be observed after any type of sling procedure, results suggest that midurethral slings are associated with less voiding dysfunction than either colposuspensions or bladder neck slings. Results with mixed incontinence are acceptable compared with other types of interventions for urinary incontinence but are less than those obtained in pure SUI.

11. **b. have rates of postoperative urgency that are higher than those in young patients.** Elderly patients experience higher rates of postoperative urgency associated with any sling material, and this is true for the midurethral sling as well. However, elderly patients have results similar to their younger peers, and therefore satisfaction rates are also similar to those of their younger peers. Mixed urinary incontinence resolution rates are similar to those of the younger population, and actual postoperative retention occurs to a similar degree as in younger patients, but postoperative voiding function may be slightly higher in the older population.

12. **d. occult incontinence is not adequately addressed.** Midurethral slings performed at the time of prolapse surgery have now been shown to be safe and efficacious. Risks of erosion and infection are no greater than when the midurethral sling is performed as a primary isolated procedure. Concomitant hysterectomy has been shown not to have an adverse effect on continence status associated with these procedures. Additionally, rates of postoperative urethrolysis are no greater when the midurethral sling technology is combined with a prolapse correction. Rates of retention are also not appreciably higher in this population as compared with those women undergoing isolated slings only.

13. **e. overall efficacy is similar to that of primary implantation.** As salvage procedures, midurethral slings have overall efficacy similar to their use in primary implantation procedures. Complications should be no higher than when done as primary procedures. The technique remains the same, and no alteration is required. Success does appear to be reliant on hypermobility, and patients with less hypermobility would appear to have less overall functional success than those patients with greater hypermobility. Rates of bladder perforation may be somewhat higher in this population than in primary cases.

14. **e. all of the above.** Complications with midurethral slings are an important part of informed consent. Bladder

perforation rates range up to 5% and in some studies are somewhat higher. Voiding function rates vary from 4% to 20%, and this variance is largely related to definitional reasons based on literature evidence. De novo urgency occurs with postoperative voiding dysfunction in up to 12% of patients, and wound healing can be affected in approximately 1% of patients; results represent dramatic improvement as compared with historic dense weave meshes.

15. **a. decreased by the macroporous nature of the sling material.** Erosion associated with midurethral slings is clearly decreased by the use of macroporous monofilament sling material (type 1). Tension may have a role in increasing erosion even in macroporous slings. Vaginal erosion rates and bladder erosion rates are very low and do not exceed 5% to 10% with newer sling materials. When material erosions do occur, however, they have an adverse impact on overall patient satisfaction.

16. **e. complete excision of exposed material should be performed.** Management of erosions is complex and must be individualized. Primarily, all exposed material, whether it be vaginal or within the urinary tract, must be removed or in some manner covered. There have been successful reports of bladder management endoscopically, although this is contingent on absolute excision of all exposed material. Some authors have reported successful management of vaginal erosions with conservative use of topical estrogens and delayed primary closure as well as simple secondary intention healing. Erosions are clearly linked to technique, and errant sling placement has a high significance in creating erosions. Symptoms are usually associated with erosions especially in the urinary tract, but even vaginal erosions are associated with voiding symptomatology as well as persistent vaginal discharge and dyspareunia.

17. **d. managed initially conservatively, but sling release should be contemplated when persistent voiding trials are not successful.** Voiding dysfunction associated with midurethral slings is substantially less than with bladder neck slings but still occurs. Timing of intervention is dependent on surgeon experience but is trending toward earlier intervention. Most experts recommend a period of conservative management of a few days to 1 month. Persistent obstruction will require intervention. Urodynamic parameters are often affected in cases of persistent obstruction. Unfortunately, no preoperative factors are predictive of postoperative voiding dysfunction. Immediate release is not recommended because a short period of observation usually results in resolution of the voiding dysfunction. When sling release occurs, midline incision of the sling is all that is required; the entire sling does not need to be excised.

18. **e. all of the above.** Complications of technique include injury to surrounding structures and significant hemorrhage due to laceration of perivesical vessels. Intestinal and vascular complications can cause substantial morbidity and mortality.

19. **d. the tape remains above the perineal membrane and outside the true pelvis and does not penetrate the levator ani group.** The TOT technique is unique because it avoids (when done correctly) entry into the true pelvis and the levator group. Errant sling placement through the adductor longus tendon can result in substantial pain. Smaller muscle groups such as the magnus brevis and gracilis are often traversed by this technique, without substantive complication. The obturator vessels are lateral and superior to the area of insertion of the device. The dorsal nerve of the clitoris is separated from the trajectory of the device by at least 1 to 2 cm.

20. **a. either outside-in or inside-out approaches.** The TOT technique can be performed by insertion of the passing needles from either vaginal or obturator approaches. Associated risks of device use include leg pain, dyspareunia, and injury to surrounding structures. Cystoscopy is a useful safety adjunct and should be performed as an integral and necessary part of the TOT. Different kits use different meshes, and not all meshes are similar. The kit to be used should be evaluated critically for this parameter.

21. **a. appear to be relatively similar regardless of whether ISD is present preoperatively.** TOT outcomes are relatively similar to those seen with the retropubic slings, regardless of urethral function. Any urinary tract structure can be injured by the TOT, including the urethra and bladder. Vaginal erosion is clearly related to mesh type. Voiding dysfunction is similar to retropubic techniques. Less urethral hypermobility probably militates against success rates with TOT, such as those reported in women with higher degrees of urethral hypermobility.

22. **c. 1-year results demonstrate durability similar to the TVT and TOT approaches.** This new technique has appeal in all types of patients, with avoidance of the retropubic space, decreased recovery time, and prevention of thigh pain. The "hammock position" fixes the implant into the obturator internus muscle. Cystoscopy should be performed after placement of all midurethral slings before removal of trocars. Erosion and extrusion rates have not been higher with this method.

Additional Study Points

1. Urethral slings are the procedure of choice for the surgical correction of female SUI.
2. Slings may be placed at either the bladder neck or midurethra.
3. Slings are particularly helpful in treating ISD.
4. The majority of patients who require clean intermittent catheterization after PVS placement had a neurogenic bladder preoperatively.
5. Persistent urgency incontinence or urgency are more common presenting symptoms for bladder outlet obstruction after a sling placement than is frank retention.
6. Maximum urethral closure pressure occurs at the level of the midurethra.
7. Success of midurethral slings is less in patients with a fixed urethra and/or a low leak point pressure.
8. Urethral mobility before midurethral sling procedures has been shown to be predictive of success; the more the proximal urethra moves during a Valsalva maneuver, the better the cure rate for incontinence.
9. For patients with persistently elevated residual urines and bothersome symptoms refractory to conservative management after a sling procedure, TVT release procedures consistently provide resolution of symptoms with maintenance of continence in the majority of patients.
10. Cystoscopy is an integral part of all urethral sling procedures to visualize any injury to the urethra or bladder.

Injection Therapy for Urinary Incontinence

Sender Herschorn, MDCM, FRCSC

QUESTIONS

1. Which of the following patient factors is a contraindication to the use of collagen as an injectable agent?
   a. Urethral hypermobility
   b. Detrusor overactivity
   c. Previous surgery
   d. Hypersensitivity
   e. Previous use of an injectable agent

2. The mechanism of action of injectable agents is:
   a. to augment urethral mucosa.
   b. not yet defined.
   c. to improve the hermetic seal.
   d. to create obstruction.
   e. to improve urethral coaptation.

3. Injectable agents are indicated for the treatment of stress urinary incontinence (SUI) due to intrinsic sphincter deficiency (ISD). Which of the following statements about urodynamics for ISD is TRUE?
   a. The diagnostic and predictive value of urethral pressure profilometry in characterizing ISD has been proved.
   b. The presence of hypermobility always raises the leak point pressure, thus excluding ISD.
   c. ISD is not present if the leak point pressure is greater than 90 cm H_2O.
   d. Many studies have not confirmed the value of leak point pressure measurement in quantifying ISD.
   e. A low urethral pressure point characteristically predicts the presence of ISD.

4. Which of the following statements about the usefulness of cystoscopy before injection is TRUE?
   a. The relative degree of ISD versus hypermobility can be ascertained.
   b. Adverse urethral factors such as scarring or diverticula can be assessed.
   c. The amount of SUI can be assessed.
   d. Bladder neck mobility, which contraindicates the use of injectable agents, can be measured.

   e. Cystoscopy should not be done before the use of injectable agents.

5. Which of the following statements about injection techniques is TRUE?
   a. Both the periurethral and transurethral techniques have shown similar results.
   b. The transurethral technique can be done only with cystoscopic monitoring.
   c. The periurethral technique always requires a general anesthetic.
   d. The transurethral technique is more painful for patients.
   e. The periurethral approach is more commonly done.

6. Which of the following injectable agents requires the use of a ratcheted injection gun?
   a. Silicone microimplants (Macroplastique)
   b. Carbon-coated zirconium beads (Durasphere)
   c. Bovine collagen
   d. Calcium hydroxylapatite (Coaptite)
   e. Hyaluronic acid detranomer (Deflux)

7. Which of the following statements regarding antibiotic prophylaxis for the use of injectable agents is TRUE?
   a. One week of a second-generation cephalosporin is required.
   b. An aminoglycoside should be given intravenously 1 hour before treatment.
   c. A fluoroquinolone or trimethoprim-sulfamethoxazole for 24 hours or less can be recommended.
   d. A 3-day course of a fluoroquinolone has been shown in randomized studies of injectable agents to be most effective.
   e. Prophylactic antibiotics are not effective for prevention of a urinary tract infection.

8. Which of the following statements about reinjections is TRUE?
   a. Reinjections rarely restore continence.
   b. Reinjections should always be done within 1 week.

c. The site of reinjection should always be away from the previous injection site.

d. Long-term reinjections are superior to short-term ones.

e. The minimum timing for reinjections is variable and depends on the agent.

9. Which of the following statements regarding long-term outcomes of injectable agents is TRUE?

a. Eliminating the failures from the denominator artificially raises the success rate.

b. The Stamey (0-3) Grading System has been subject to extensive epidemiologic testing.

c. Systematic reviews have confirmed efficacy versus pelvic floor muscle training.

d. Repeat injections usually fail to restore success.

e. Randomized trials with midurethral slings demonstrated superiority of injectable agents.

10. Which injectable agent requires skin testing before administration?

a. Porcine collagen

b. Silicone macroparticles

c. Carbon-coated zirconium beads

d. Bovine collagen

e. Autologous fat

11. Which of the following complications of collagen injections for SUI is least likely?

a. Urinary tract infection

b. Urethrovaginal fistula

c. Hematuria

d. Urgency incontinence

e. Retention

12. What is the minimum threshold for particle size that determines migration risk?

a. 20 μm

b. 40 μm

c. 60 μm

d. 80 μm

e. 100 μm

13. Which of the following complications were seen more frequently in the carbon-coated zirconium bead arm of collagen versus carbon-coated zirconium bead study?

a. Urgency and retention

b. Hematuria

c. Recurrent SUI

d. Mucosal prolapse

e. Particle migration

14. Which of the following agents showed a treatment benefit versus collagen in a randomized trial?

a. Zuidex (hyaluronic acid dextranomer)

b. Durasphere (carbon-coated zirconium bead)

c. Macroplastique (silicone microimplant)

d. Autologous fat

e. Coaptite (calcium hydroxyapatite)

15. Which of the following injectable agents are no longer used?

a. Teflon (polytetrafluoroethylene paste)

b. Zuidex (hyaluronic acid dextranomer with Implacer)

c. Autologous fat

d. Tegress (ethylene vinyl alcohol)

e. All of the above

16. Regarding the outcome of pelvic floor physiotherapy for post–radical prostatectomy incontinence, which statement is TRUE?

a. The treatment results are not seen until 18 months after surgery.

b. The outcome is independent of the postoperative starting time.

c. The results are equivalent to those of surgery.

d. At 12 months there is no difference compared with no treatment.

e. A combination of bulking agents and physiotherapy has been shown to be better than either alone.

17. Which statement about the outcome of injectable agents for post–radical prostatectomy incontinence is TRUE?

a. Multiple treatment sessions are usually required.

b. The results are similar to those of an artificial sphincter.

c. The combination of injectable agent and sling has been demonstrated to be superior to either modality alone.

d. Their noninvasive nature mandate their use in all patients.

e. Newer agents have been shown to be more effective than collagen.

18. Which of the following factors contribute to a poor response to injectable agents after prostatectomy?

a. Prior radiation

b. Stricture

c. High-grade SUI

d. Low abdominal leak point pressure

e. All of the above

19. Which of the following statements about results of the antegrade technique of collagen injection for postprostatectomy incontinence is TRUE?

a. The antegrade technique has extended the indications for the use of injectables.

b. The antegrade technique is best done under local anesthesia.

c. There is no advantage of the antegrade over the retrograde technique.

d. The antegrade technique results in less loss of injectable agent.

e. Patient satisfaction has been shown to be higher with the antegrade over the retrograde technique.

20. Which of the following is a recognized adverse factor for ProACT balloon success?

a. Slowly rising prostate-specific antigen level

b. Prior irradiation

c. Failed artificial sphincter

d. Detrusor overactivity

e. Urinary tract infection

ANSWERS

1. **d. Hypersensitivity.** Approximately 3% of patients will have a positive skin test reaction, with 70% showing the reaction within 3 days, indicating a preexisting sensitivity to bovine dermal collagen through dietary exposure. The remaining 30% do not respond until later so a 4-week period is required (Keefe et al, 1992).* A negative skin test does not preclude development of a hypersensitivity reaction to subsequent treatment and, although infrequently used, a second skin test has been recommended (Elson, 1989; Stothers and Goldenberg, 1998). Positive responders should be excluded.

2. **b. not yet defined.** It is generally thought that these agents improve intrinsic sphincter function, although the exact mechanism has not been defined (Smith et al, 2009). Bulking agents such as collagen have been reported (McGuire and Appell, 1994; Monga et al, 1995) to augment urethral mucosa and improve coaptation and intrinsic sphincter function, as evidenced by an increase in post-treatment abdominal leak pressure (Herschorn et al, 1992; Richardson et al, 1995; Winters and Appell, 1995). Bulking agents do not generally obstruct voiding after the initial post-treatment period.

3. **d. Many studies have not confirmed the value of leak point pressure measurement in quantifying ISD.** Because injectable agents are indicated for the ISD component of SUI, can urodynamic studies assess ISD? Two measures of urethral function have been used—maximum urethral closure pressure (MUCP) and abdominal leak point pressure (ALPP). An MUCP of 20 cm H_2O or less has been suggested as indicating clinically significant urethral weakness, but there is controversy regarding the diagnostic and predictive value of urethral pressure profilometry in characterizing ISD (Weber, 2001). Similarly, an ALPP of 60 cm H_2O or less was identified as an indicator of severe ISD (McGuire et al, 1993) but many studies have not confirmed the test's value in quantifying the degree of ISD (Koelbl et al, 2009). Previously, ALPP measurements of initially 65 cm H_2O or less and then 100 cm H_2O or less were used as indicators of ISD to justify the use of injectable agents (Appell and Winters, 2007). However, because ISD may be present in many patients with SUI with or without urethral hypermobility (Koelbl et al, 2009), the specific value of either the MUCP or ALPP may be of little importance in the clinical decision about the use of injectable agents. As with other patients with SUI who choose interventional therapy, urodynamic studies are helpful.

4. **b. Adverse urethral factors such as scarring or diverticula can be assessed.** Preinjection cystoscopy is helpful to make sure that there are no adverse factors or unexpected findings that may prevent or compromise the injection procedure such as extensive urethral scarring from previous surgery, irradiation, or trauma, foreign bodies, or urethral diverticula.

5. **a. Both the periurethral and transurethral techniques have shown similar results.** The periurethral and transurethral approaches for collagen were compared first by Faerber and colleagues (1998), who reported no significant difference in success rates and numbers of injections required in 24 patients with transurethral treatment versus 21 patients with a periurethral approach. However, significantly more collagen was required for the periurethral approach. Schulz and coworkers (2004) reported similar findings in 40 women randomly assigned to either technique. There was no difference in short-term success rate, but the 20 women assigned to the periurethral approach required more collagen than those assigned to the transurethral approach. The transurethral approach is now much more commonly reported than the periurethral approach.

6. **a. Silicone microimplants (Macroplastique).** Because of its high viscosity, Macroplastique injections require the use of a ratcheted injection gun. The injection needle is 7 Fr with a 10-mm 18-gauge needle tip.

7. **c. A fluoroquinolone or trimethoprim-sulfamethoxazole for 24 hours or less can be recommended.** Although randomized trials have not been done, prophylactic antibiotics with a fluoroquinolone or trimethoprim-sulfamethoxazole for 24 hours or less can be recommended (Wolf et al, 2008). An additional 2 to 3 days of therapy has also been suggested (Appell and Winters, 2007).

8. **e. The minimum timing for reinjections is variable and depends on the agent.** Although collagen can be reinjected within 7 days, most clinicians wait 4 weeks or longer to assess response of the urethra and the need for reinjection (Appell and Winters, 2007). Silicone microimplant (Macroplastique) injections can be repeated after 12 weeks. Carbon-coated zirconium beads (Durasphere) can be reinjected after a minimum of 7 days (Lightner et al, 2001), and calcium hydroxyapatite (Coaptite) can be reinjected after 1 month or less (Mayer et al, 2007).

9. **a. Eliminating the failures from the denominator artificially raises the success rate.** A number of pitfalls in reporting of injectable agent studies can lead to inflated success rates. Because use of injectable agents can be repeated if the first treatment is not a success, authors should specify whether that time point is after all treatments have been completed or whether it is from baseline. If durability is reported after all injections are administered, then an accurate picture of duration of efficacy can be conveyed. A Kaplan-Meier curve of efficacy has been useful in showing what happens to a patient's continence outcome over time (Herschorn and Radomski, 1997; Lightner et al, 2001). Nevertheless, some studies report duration of results from initial treatment ((Richardson et al, 1995) or do not specify it (Monga et al, 1995). This may overestimate success because patients who have treatment failure are re-treated and can be counted as successes within the follow-up period. Another pitfall is reporting success rates on cohorts of patients observed for the long term rather than on all patients treated from the start (Stenberg et al, 2003). If the patients in whom treatment failed or who were lost to follow-up are not included in the denominator, the success rate is higher.

10. **d. Bovine collagen.** All patients must undergo a skin test into the volar aspect of the forearm 30 days before

---

*Sources referenced can be found in *Campbell-Walsh Urology*, *10th Edition*, on the Expert Consult website.

treatment with bovine collagen. Approximately 3% of patients will have a positive skin test reaction, with 70% showing the reaction within 3 days, indicating a preexisting sensitivity to bovine dermal collagen through dietary exposure. The remaining 30% do not respond until later, so a 4-week period is required (Keefe et al, 1992). A negative skin test does not preclude development of a hypersensitivity reaction to subsequent treatment and, although infrequently used, a second skin test has been recommended (Elson, 1989; Stothers and Goldenberg, 1998). Positive responders should be excluded.

11. **b. Urethrovaginal fistula.** Vesicovaginal fistula occurring after collagen injections for SUI in two women after cystectomy and neobladder was described by Pruthi and colleagues (2000). Carlin and Klutke (2000) reported a urethrovaginal fistula in a woman who was on warfarin and its effects were not completely reversed. She had a postinjection hematoma that ultimately fistulized to the vagina.

12. **d. 80 μm.** The bead size of carbon-coated zirconium ranges from 212 to 500 μm, which is larger than the threshold for particle size migration of 80 μm (Malizia et al, 1984).

13. **a. Urgency and retention.** In the multicenter randomized trial of Durasphere versus collagen the adverse event profiles were similar (Lightner et al, 2001). However, more women had significantly more post-treatment urgency and acute retention with Durasphere versus collagen: 24.7% and 16.9% versus 11.9% and 3.4%, respectively.

14. **c. Macroplastique (silicone microimplant).** Ghoniem and colleagues (2009) reported results of North American multicenter randomized trial of Macroplastique versus collagen. After 1 year, 61.5% (75/122) with Macroplastique and 48% (60/125) with collagen had an improvement of at least one Stamey grade. This indicated that Macroplastique was noninferior to collagen ($P < .001$). The proportion of the patients who were dry was higher in the Macroplastique group at 36.9% versus 24.8% ($P < .05$). However, there were no significant differences in pad weight testing, quality of life scale, or adverse events.

15. **e. All of the above.** Despite the potential for complications with Teflon (polytetrafluoroethylene paste) the actual rate of reported problems is low. However, Teflon is not used as an injectable agent now. Lightner and colleagues (2009) reported 12-month outcomes of a North American prospective 2:1 randomized trial of Zuidex-Implacer versus collagen injected cystoscopically in 344 women. The study failed to demonstrate that Zuidex was equivalent to collagen. The proportion of women who achieved a 50% reduction in urinary leakage on provocation testing, the primary outcome, was achieved in 84% of collagen-treated women versus 65% of Zuidex-treated women. This negative trial prompted the company to withdraw the Zuidex product. Since the publication of the randomized trial of Lee and colleagues (2001) showing that fat was no more efficacious than saline, no further publications have appeared in the literature. Furthermore, the report of a death from fat embolism (Currie et al, 1997) most likely discouraged additional studies. Tegress (ethylene vinyl alcohol) is no longer available as an injectable and have been voluntarily withdrawn by C. R. Bard, Inc. (Hurtado et al, 2008).

16. **d. At 12 months there is no difference compared with no treatment.** Physiotherapy and pelvic floor rehabilitation have been shown to improve or enhance continence (decreased time to final continence level) in the postoperative period in two randomized studies, but only if such measures are instituted before or immediately after catheter removal (Van Kampen et al, 2000; Parekh et al, 2003). Maximum difference between physiotherapy and no treatment is achieved at 3 months, with almost no difference at 12 months. A randomized study in which randomization occurred 6 weeks after surgery showed no difference in continence at 6 months (Wille et al, 2003).

17. **a. Multiple treatment sessions are usually required.** All agents share the similar problems including the need for multiple injections and treatment sessions, deterioration of effect over time, and low cure rates. It remains to be seen if improvements in outcomes can be achieved with alternative agents or if the concept of urethral bulking has achieved its maximum benefit with currently available agents (Herschorn et al, 2010).

18. **e. All of the above.** Several authors have identified factors that negatively affect results including extensive scarring or stricture formation, previous irradiation, and high-grade stress incontinence and low abdominal leak point pressure (Aboseif et al, 1996; Sanchez-Ortiz et al, 1997; Smith et al, 1998; Cespedes et al, 1999).

19. **c. There is no advantage of the antegrade over the retrograde technique.** Unfortunately, the end points in most of these studies are subjectively based, making comparisons difficult; however, it is clear that cure rates (total dryness) are low, and multiple injections are required to achieve modest rates of subjective improvement. There is no advantage of delivery technique (retrograde vs. antegrade).

20. **b. Prior irradiation.** Reported risk factors for failure and complications were prior external beam irradiation (Lebret et al, 2008; Gregori et al, 2010) and severe preoperative incontinence (Gregori et al, 2010). Kocjanic and colleagues (2007) reported a continence rate of 67% in nonirradiated patients compared with 36% in irradiated patients.

Additional Study Points

1. Injection therapy has been shown to be effective in patients with intrinsic sphincter deficiency as well as hypermobility.
2. A maximum urethral closure pressure of less than or equal to 20 cm H_2O or an abdominal leak point pressure less than or equal to 60 cm H_2O have been used to diagnose intrinsic sphincter deficiency. However, when using these parameters the correlation with success after injectable therapy is not good.
3. The substance to be injected is injected at the bladder neck immediately beneath the mucosa at the 3- and 9-o'clock positions so as to coapt the mucosa.
4. A catheter is not routinely used after injection except in patients who have retention; if that is the case, then the catheter should be of a small caliber.
5. Sphincter and bladder dysfunction may coexist in a third of patients.
6. Injectable agents are not effective in a scarred membranous urethra.
7. Injections used for postprostatectomy incontinence have resulted in approximately 10% of patients being dry.

Other Therapies for Storage and Emptying Failure

R. Duane Cespedes, MD ● Jason L. Gerboc, DO

QUESTIONS

1. Acupuncture may exert its effects through all of the following EXCEPT:
   a. endorphinergic effects at the sacral spinal cord level.
   b. inhibitory somatovisceral reflexes.
   c. an increase in peripheral circulation.
   d. an increased level of parasympathetic stimulation.
   e. endorphinergic effects at the lumbar spinal cord level.

2. Which statement is TRUE regarding therapeutic overdistention of the bladder?
   a. It may be performed using local anesthesia.
   b. Significant improvement is often seen in neurogenic detrusor overactivity.
   c. The most consistent symptomatic improvement is seen in interstitial cystitis.
   d. Bladder rupture is seen in 10% to 15% of cases.
   e. Intravesical pressure during the procedure should be equal to diastolic pressure.

3. Reduction cystoplasty for high-capacity, myogenic decompensation may improve all the following parameters EXCEPT:
   a. capacity.
   b. postvoid residual.
   c. detrusor contractility.
   d. frequency of urinary tract infections (UTIs).
   e. the frequency of clean intermittent catheterization (CIC).

4. Which one of the following statements is FALSE regarding urethral compression devices in a male?
   a. Urethral pressure should be released at least twice per day.
   b. They should be removed while sleeping.
   c. Pressure-related injuries may occur in patients with altered cognition.
   d. The lowest pressure that relieves incontinence should be used.
   e. Patients with pure sphincteric incontinence will obtain the best results.

5. Condom catheters are preferred over long-term Foley drainage in neurologically impaired males because:
   a. they have a lower incidence of bacteriuria.
   b. fewer symptomatic urinary tract infections occur.
   c. they have a lower overall incidence of death.
   d. fewer infection stones develop.
   e. all of the above apply.

6. The Credé maneuver of emptying the bladder is relatively contraindicated in patients:
   a. with decreased outlet resistance.
   b. who are obese.
   c. with vesicoureteral reflux.
   d. with high-pressure detrusor overactivity.
   e. under the age of 2.

7. The advantages of an incontinent ileovesicostomy, or "bladder chimney," include all of the following EXCEPT:
   a. It avoids the complications of a long-term indwelling catheter.
   b. It maintains the ureteral antireflux mechanism.
   c. It maintains transurethral access to the upper tracts.
   d. It significantly decreases colonization of the lower urinary tract.
   e. It may be reversed or converted to an ileal conduit.

8. Incontinence-associated dermatitis (IAD) is associated with the following factors in the incontinent patient EXCEPT:
   a. It may be caused by infrequent pad changes.
   b. It is manifested by inflammation of the skin with redness and edema.
   c. It may lead to malignant lesions of the skin.
   d. It predominately occurs in skin folds.
   e. It promotes candidiasis and bacterial infections.

9. All of the following statements are TRUE regarding bladder outlet closure EXCEPT:
   a. Complete closure of the bladder neck is rarely necessary.
   b. The main indication is urethral destruction after prolonged catheter drainage.

c. An obstructing sling or artificial urinary sphincter (AUS) is rarely feasible, if less than 1 cm of urethra exists.

d. Reflex sphincteric activity may result in disruption of the bladder neck closure.

e. The transvaginal approach has decreased the postoperative fistula rate.

10. Which one of the following statements is FALSE regarding myoplasty for functional sphincteric replacement?

a. Unstimulated graciloplasty may require prolonged leg adduction.

b. A free, innervated flap of proximal gracilis muscle is more easily transposed around the urethra and has shown encouraging results in human studies.

c. Electrical stimulation can transform type 2 muscle fibers into type 1 fibers.

d. Unstimulated graciloplasty may cause significant passive obstruction.

e. Allogenic muscle-derived progenitor cells (MDPC) injected directly into the sphincter can improve the contraction amplitude.

11. A surgical sphincterotomy, when performed in patients with spinal cord injury, may have late failures due to all of the following EXCEPT:

a. fibrosis at the sphincterotomy site.

b. development of smooth sphincter dyssynergia.

c. changes in detrusor function.

d. an increase in outlet resistance due to prostatic obstruction.

e. segmental reinnervation and muscular regrowth of the sphincter.

12. Of the following statements, which one is FALSE regarding "trigger voiding" in spinal cord–injured patients?

a. Trigger voiding can be induced by digital rectal stimulation.

b. Reflex contractions can be generated by using somatic motor axons to innervate parasympathetic bladder ganglia cells.

c. Rhythmic suprapubic manual pressure is usually the most effective method for trigger voiding.

d. Trigger voiding induces a reflex decrease in outlet resistance in patients with detrusor-sphincter dyssynergia.

e. Trigger voiding can be induced by squeezing the clitoris.

ANSWERS

1. **d. an increased level of parasympathetic stimulation.** Bergstrom and associates (2000)* hypothesized that any one or a combination of (1) endorphinergic effects at the sacral spinal cord level or above, (2) inhibitory somatovisceral reflexes, and (3) increase in peripheral circulation as possible mechanisms of action for how acupuncture facilitates bladder storage and filling. The true nature of how acupuncture exerts its beneficial effects remains incompletely understood but appears to be a form of somatic sensory stimulation.

---

*Sources referenced can be found in *Campbell-Walsh Urology, 10th Edition,* on the Expert Consult website.

2. **c. The most consistent symptomatic improvement is seen in interstitial cystitis.** Therapeutic overdistention involves prolonged stretching of the bladder wall using hydrostatic pressure equal to systolic blood pressure. It is thought that improvement occurs due to ischemic changes in the nerve endings in the bladder wall. Potential complications include a 5% to 10% bladder rupture rate, hematuria, and urinary retention. Therapeutic overdistention is regarded as an ineffective procedure in patients with storage failure secondary to neurogenic detrusor overactivity but may provide substantial, but usually temporary, improvement to some patients with non-neurogenic storage symptoms who have failed medical therapy.

3. **c. detrusor contractility.** The simplicity of partial cystectomy to reduce bladder capacity and theoretically restore contractility is enticing; however, if urodynamic evaluation after prolonged Foley catheter drainage shows no spontaneous detrusor contractions, this procedure is unlikely to be successful. If contractility is proven, surgical reduction may be a useful option in the appropriate patient. A few studies have reported success in reducing the bladder capacity, reducing residual urine volume, and frequency of urinary infection without improving contractility in patients with preoperative areflexic bladders. When compared with properly performed CIC alone, reduction cystoplasty is unlikely to add to the patient's quality of life and should only be used in select patients with demonstrated detrusor contractility.

4. **a. Urethral pressure should be released at least twice per day.** These devices are primarily used to treat patients with pure sphincteric incontinence, most commonly postprostatectomy incontinence, because normal bladder capacity and storage pressures are a relative requirement. These devices should be unclamped regularly at 3- to 4-hour intervals, because prolonged or excessive compression can cause pressure-related injury to the penis. Additionally, these devices should not be worn during an erection or while sleeping. Pressure-related injuries may also be more prevalent in patients with impaired sensation or cognition; therefore, penile clamp usage in this population should be considered a relative contraindication. Although these devices manage sphincteric incontinence relatively well, they are rarely used today because they are inconvenient, and many minimally invasive options for male sphincteric incontinence now exist. These devices remain useful for patients who cannot undergo surgical therapy due to medical conditions and for patients who have severe leakage during the early postprostatectomy period while surgical treatment is contraindicated.

5. **e. all of the above apply.** Condom catheters are generally perceived as more comfortable, less painful, and less restrictive on daily activities than indwelling catheters. In a prospective, randomized, controlled trial of 75 hospitalized men requiring a urinary collection device, condom catheters were associated with a lower incidence of complications, including bacteriuria, symptomatic urinary tract infection, and death, than in patients with indwelling catheters. Condom catheters are unacceptable to some patients, because the device may be visible through their clothing and leakage of urine may cause odor issues. It is generally recommended that condom catheters be changed daily because the risk for UTI is increased when catheters

are changed less frequently. Other potential complications include allergic reactions, skin maceration, and/or penile edema.

6. **c. with vesicoureteral reflux.** The Credé maneuver (manual compression of the bladder) is most effective in patients with decreased bladder tone who can generate an intravesical pressure greater than 50 cm H_2O and have decreased bladder outlet resistance. The Credé maneuver requires good hand control, is easier in a thin individual than an obese one, and is more easily performed in a child than in an adult. Voiding by Credé is unphysiologic, because active opening of the bladder neck does not occur, and increases in outlet resistance by a reflex mechanism may actually occur. If complete emptying does not occur, treatment to decrease outlet resistance can be contemplated, or an alternative method to empty the bladder should be used. Vesicoureteral reflux is a relative contraindication to external compression and straining maneuvers, especially in patients capable of generating a high intravesical pressure.

7. **d. It significantly decreases colonization of the lower urinary tract.** The incontinent ileovesicostomy, or "bladder chimney," is an excellent method for managing patients with neurogenic bladder who are unable to perform CIC independently. This procedure avoids the complications of long-term indwelling catheters and maintains the native antireflux and urethral sphincteric mechanisms. In addition, this procedure may be reversed if necessary. The bladder is in indirect contact with the skin through the "chimney" and therefore is likely to be colonized; however, because this is a low-pressure system, significant infectious complications are unlikely to occur.

8. **c. It may lead to malignant lesions of the skin.** Prolonged exposure of the skin to a wet environment may lead to supersaturation and disruption of the skin's protective barriers, thus promoting skin maceration, dermatitis, and possibly infection. Incontinence-associated dermatitis (IAD) can be defined as inflammation of the surface of the skin with redness, edema, and, in some cases, bullae containing clear exudate. IAD predominately occurs in skin folds and may promote candidiasis or bacterial skin infections. IAD has not been associated with premalignant or malignant lesions of the skin.

9. **e. The transvaginal approach has decreased the postoperative fistula rate.** Complete closure of the bladder neck is rarely necessary, because a compressive bladder neck sling is more easily performed, is less morbid, and allows transurethral access if necessary. The main indication for bladder outlet closure is urethral destruction secondary to prolonged catheter drainage in neurogenic bladder patients. A case series using "tight" autologous pubovaginal sling and lower urinary tract reconstruction for urethras destroyed by long-term Foley use reported excellent results with minimal incontinence. The authors concluded that at least 1 cm of normal urethra was required for proper functioning of the sling. The risk of complications, specifically a vesicovaginal fistula, is relatively common and can be difficult to repair. It is important to remember that a bladder neck closure is much more difficult than a simple closure of the bladder wall. The bladder neck is usually hyperactive in patients with neurologic disease, and every voiding reflex includes active opening and closing of the bladder neck, which forcibly attempts to destroy the bladder

neck closure. To reduce this risk, postoperative suppression of the voiding reflex using prolonged continuous catheter drainage (three weeks) and liberal use of anticholinergics is imperative. In addition, to reduce the risk of fistula, the repair must be watertight from the beginning, and this requires a precise mucosal closure using a running suture and multiple additional layers of muscle to reinforce the strength of the repair.

10. **b. A free, innervated flap of proximal gracilis muscle is more easily transposed around the urethra and has shown encouraging results in human studies.** Unstimulated gracilis muscle wrapped around the urethra can be used to improve sphincteric continence but requires the patient to voluntarily contract (adduct) the leg for prolonged periods to provide outlet resistance. Problems with the unstimulated graciloplasty include (1) poor sustainability of the contraction due to the fast twitch, non–fatigue-resistant fibers of the gracilis; (2) high passive resistance resulting in urethral obstruction; (3) postsurgical changes resulting in the loss of resting tension and reduced contractility; and (4) the potential for fibrosis due to segmental vascularization. External stimulation of the gracilis using implanted electrodes in an electrical stimulation program can be used to transform fatigable type 2 skeletal muscle fibers to the slow type 1 fibers. Electrically stimulated gracilis muscle was an improvement over the unstimulated muscle; however, the bulky musculature and propensity for stricture formation caused an inherent passive obstruction. An animal model using a free but innervated flap of well-vascularized proximal gracilis muscle in dogs has been successful. The smaller size of the graft allowed it to be more easily transposed around the urethra while stimulation of the sphincter was carried out using the graft's own motor innervation; however, no human clinical study has been formed. A rat model in which the urethra was mechanically denervated and subsequently injected with allogenic muscle-derived progenitor cells (MDPC) dramatically improved fast-twitch muscle contraction amplitude from 8.8% to 87% compared with normal contraction.

11. **e. segmental reinnervation and muscular regrowth of the sphincter.** When early failure of a sphincterotomy occurs, it is generally attributable to an inadequate surgical procedure (either not deep enough or not extensive enough), inadequate detrusor function, and bladder neck or prostatic obstruction. Late failure may occur due to fibrosis within the length of the sphincterotomy, a change in bladder function, the development of prostatic obstruction, or a change in neurologic status such that smooth sphincter dyssynergia develops. Failure rates following sphincterotomy have been reported to be as high as 40% to 50% in some series. Failure has been defined as (1) the presence of large postvoid residual urine volumes associated with urinary tract infections, (2) autonomic hyperreflexia symptomatology associated with bladder overdistention or high voiding pressures, and/or (3) progressive upper tract deterioration from persistent reflux or poor bladder emptying.

12. **d. Trigger voiding induces a reflex decrease in outlet resistance in patients with sphincter dyssynergia.** In some types of spinal cord injury or bladder dysfunction characterized by detrusor hyperreflexia, manual pressure may sometimes be used to initiate a

reflexive bladder contraction—sometimes called "trigger voiding." The most effective method of initiating a reflex contraction is thought to be rhythmic suprapubic manual pressure, typically seven or eight compressions every 3 seconds. This rhythmic pressure is thought to produce a summation effect on the tension receptors in the bladder wall, resulting in an afferent neural discharge that activates the bladder reflex arc. Trigger voiding can also sometimes be induced by pulling the skin or hair of the pubis, scrotum, or thigh; squeezing the clitoris; or digital rectal stimulation. Surgical procedures to reduce outlet resistance should be considered, if significant obstruction or sphincter dyssynergia are present. In an animal model using neural rerouting, a detrusor contraction without striated sphincter dyssynergia could be initiated by scratching the skin or by percutaneous electrical stimulation in the L7 dermatome. The pathway was found to be mediated by cholinergic transmission at both ganglionic and peripheral levels. The importance of this experimental model is that somatic motor axons were able to innervate parasympathetic bladder ganglion cells and therefore transfer somatic reflex activity to the lower urinary tract.

Additional Study Points

1. Noncentral denervation proximal to the postganglionic neuron is properly termed decentralization.
2. In many cases, central denervation or decentralization often result in a variable restoration of neurologic function with an even less-desired result than was present originally.
3. Sacral rhizotomy may involve either sectioning the anterior (motor) or posterior (sensory) root.
4. Complete sacral rhizotomy often results in bladder areflexia that rarely persists and recurrent detrusor overactivity with adverse effects on the anal sphincter, urethral sphincter, and sexual function.
5. The anterior S3 nerve root is the dominant motor innervation of the bladder.
6. Dorsal rhizotomy of S2 through S5 nerve roots abolishes reflex erections, reflex ejaculation, sacral sensation, and can reduce reflex defecation.
7. Supratrigonal complete bladder transaction has not proven efficacious.
8. Patients with intrinsic sphincter deficiency are the best candidates for bulking agents (injectibles).
9. An artificial urinary sphincter should generally not be placed in patients with a neurogenic bladder, particularly in those with low-capacity or noncompliant bladders as the risk of renal deterioration is significant.
10. Bladder augmentation should only be considered in patients who have the capability for self intermittent catheterization.
11. In patients who employ intermittent catheterization or in those with chronic indwelling catheters, the presence of asymptomatic bacteriuria does not require treatment. Continued prophylactic antibiotics are rarely indicated in this group as well.
12. Lapedes proposed that high intravesical pressures with bladder overdistention reduces bladder blood flow and makes the bladder susceptible to bacterial invasion and significant UTIs.
13. CIC should be used cautiously in patients known to have autonomic dysreflexia.
14. The frequency of intermittent catheterization should be such that bladder volumes remain below 400 to 500 cc between catheterizations.
15. The advantage of a suprapubic cystostomy in males compared with continuous urethral catheterization is a lower incidence of epididymitis and urethral stricture disease, with preservation of sexual function.
16. When bladder neck incision is performed, it should occur at the 5- and 7-o'clock position and extend caudally just proximal to the verumontanum. This results in retrograde ejaculation about 30% to 50% of the time.
17. Sphincterotomy should be performed at the 12-o'clock position because that is least likely to cause significant hemorrhage.
18. Pudendal neurectomy results in an extremely high rate of impotence and may result in significant fecal and stress incontinence.
19. If improperly treated, complications from detrusor sphincter dyssynergia will occur in greater than 50% of men.

Geriatric Incontinence and Voiding Dysfunction

Neil M. Resnick, MD ● Stasa D. Tadic, MD, MS ● Subbarao V. Yalla, MD

QUESTIONS

1. In persons older than age 65, the prevalence of urinary incontinence (UI) is:
   a. 1% to 10%.
   b. 15% to 30%.
   c. 35% to 50%.
   d. 55% to 75%.
   e. 75% to 100%.

2. In demented elderly patients, incontinence:
   a. is inevitable.
   b. is virtually always due to detrusor hyperreflexia.
   c. is unlikely to respond to therapy.
   d. is multifactorial and often reversible.
   e. treatment should focus primarily on preventing skin breakdown.

3. Urinary incontinence in older people is usually:
   a. brought to a physician's attention by the patient.
   b. detected by the patient's primary physician.
   c. obvious to the urologist.
   d. detected by the physician but ignored.
   e. unknown to the patient's physician.

4. In older patients, involuntary bladder contractions:
   a. are rarely seen in asymptomatic patients.
   b. are primarily due to central nervous system (CNS) pathology.
   c. are almost always the cause of the patient's incontinence.
   d. are inevitable in demented patients.
   e. may not be the cause of the incontinence.

5. After the history and physical exam, evaluation of the incontinent older patient should include:
   a. cystoscopy.
   b. videourodynamics.
   c. postvoid residual assessment.
   d. urinary cytology.
   e. assessment of prostate size in a male.

6. Which one of the following occurs as part of *normal* aging?
   a. Urinary incontinence
   b. A small increase in serum creatinine concentration
   c. Uninhibited detrusor contractions
   d. Increase in bladder capacity
   e. Urinary flow rate is unchanged

7. The cornerstone of treatment for persistent urgency incontinence is:
   a. behavioral therapy.
   b. flavoxate.
   c. oxybutynin.
   d. tolterodine.
   e. solifenacin.

8. Acute urinary retention in an older man:
   a. indicates the need for surgical decompression.
   b. is treated effectively with α-adrenergic blockers.
   c. can be seen with detrusor hyperactivity with impaired contractility (DHIC).
   d. is treated effectively with bethanechol.
   e. requires treatment of the underlying urinary tract abnormality.

9. Incontinence management products (e.g., garments/pads):
   a. are reimbursed by insurance companies.
   b. should include menstrual pads.
   c. generally cost less than a dollar per day.
   d. should be chosen according to the type of incontinence rather than its severity.
   e. should be tailored to the individual.

10. The five-year probability of an untreated older man with prostatism developing acute urinary retention is:
    a. 5% to 10%.
    b. 15% to 25%.

c. 30% to 50%.

d. 55% to 75%.

e. 75% to 100%.

11. The voiding diary completed by an 83-year-old woman bothered by daytime incontinence discloses 800 mL output between 8:00 AM and 11:00 PM, and 1500 mL from 11:00 PM to 8:00 AM. The next step should be:

    a. to have her repeat it with a record of fluid intake.

    b. to take furosemide at 7:00 PM each evening to reduce nocturnal excretion.

    c. to use pressure-gradient stockings to minimize peripheral edema.

    d. to advise her to curtail fluid intake after dinner.

    e. none of the above.

12. TRUE or FALSE: Cystometry in a 78-year-old incontinent man reveals detrusor overactivity. If behavioral methods fail, the next step is to prescribe a bladder relaxant.

    a. True

    b. False

13. TRUE or FALSE: Anticholinergic agents (other than those prescribed for overactive detrusor) should always be discontinued or substituted in an older patient who presents with incontinence.

    a. True

    b. False

14. TRUE or FALSE: A bladder relaxant medication with anticholinergic properties is contraindicated in older patients with cognitive impairment.

    a. True

    b. False

15. TRUE or FALSE: A bladder relaxant medication with anticholinergic properties is contraindicated in an older person with cognitive impairment who is currently taking an acetylcholinesterase inhibitor (AChEI, e.g., donepezil [Aricept]).

    a. True

    b. False

16. Anticholinergic bladder relaxants may, ironically, actually exacerbate incontinence through all of the following mechanisms EXCEPT:

    a. causing/exacerbating confusion.

    b. causing/exacerbating impaired mobility.

    c. causing/exacerbating a dry mouth.

    d. causing/exacerbating subacute urinary retention.

    e. precipitating acute urinary retention.

17. TRUE or FALSE: Desamino-D-arginine vasopressin (DDAVP) is an excellent agent for an older person with nocturia, especially if it is associated with incontinence occurring predominantly at night.

    a. True

    b. False

18. Each of these agents has been proved effective for urinary urgency incontinence EXCEPT:

    a. oxybutyinin.

    b. hyoscyamine.

c. darifenacin.

d. fesoterodine.

e. trospium.

19. A 78-year-old woman with dementia has responded modestly to donepezil (Aricept, a cholinesterase inhibitor) for the past year. The recent onset of urgency incontinence led her primary physician to prescribe tolterodine last month while awaiting your assessment. Her incontinence has responded well. The next appropriate step is to:

    a. discontinue tolterodine due to its interaction with donepezil.

    b. discontinue donepezil because her cognitive function is stable.

    c. discontinue both drugs because she is stable and the urgency incontinence may reflect an adverse effect of the donepezil.

    d. continue both drugs and monitor her for deterioration in cognitive function.

    e. taper the tolterodine.

20. A 68-year-old obese woman with significant daily stress incontinence comes for a follow-up. Her bladder diary shows maximal voided volume of 125 mL during the daytime. Each of these measures is appropriate EXCEPT:

    a. adjustment of fluid excretion and voiding intervals.

    b. advise weight reduction.

    c. teach her postural maneuvers.

    d. consideration of surgical correction.

    e. pelvic floor muscle exercises.

21. A 72-year-old man has urinary urgency and postvoid residual (PVR) of 40 mL. He also has hypertension and aortic stenosis that has caused minimal symptoms. His friend suggested that he ask for terazosin because it helped him with similar symptoms. The most appropriate response is:

    a. to prescribe terazosin and see him again in 4 weeks.

    b. to prescribe alfuzosin instead, because it has a better side-effect profile.

    c. to obtain medical consultation before prescribing the drug.

    d. to perform urodynamic testing before deciding.

    e. to prescribe an anticholinergic agent.

ANSWERS

1. **b. 15% to 30%.** Although its prevalence increases with age, incontinence is abnormal at any age. Even in nursing home residents, where the average age is 85 and dementia and immobility affect more than half of residents, incontinence prevalence is 40% to 60%. More impressive is the fact that incontinence affects only slightly more than 50% of the most severely demented nursing home residents, provided they can transfer themselves from a bed to a chair and do not have other contributing factors; and even if they do, many of the factors fall into the category of transient incontinence and are reversible. Thus incontinence is never the norm, no matter how old or frail the individual.

2. **d. is multifactorial and often reversible.** As noted above, incontinence is never normal, even with dementia.

Detrusor overactivity (DO) is the most common type of lower urinary tract dysfunction among demented incontinent nursing home residents, but it is also the most common dysfunction among their dry peers. Moreover, incontinence in 40% of these individuals is not associated with DO but with obstruction (in men), stress incontinence (in women), or a combination of an outlet and a detrusor problem, and the cause does not correlate with either the presence or severity of dementia. Thus it is no longer tenable to attribute incontinence a priori to DO. Because incontinence in the elderly is usually multifactorial, involving urinary tract as well as non–urinary tract contributions, it is often treatable. Even among nursing home patients, studies have documented more than a 50% reduction in incontinent episodes overall and full daytime continence in nearly 40% of residents. Particularly among demented individuals, nonurinary factors are prevalent and commonly include medication use, depression, fecal impaction, UTI, atrophic vaginitis, and disorders of fluid excretion. It is important to prevent skin breakdown, but this should not be the primary approach to the incontinent nursing home resident.

3. **e. unknown to the patient's physician.** Despite the fact that incontinence is so common and amenable to therapy, most patients do not mention it to a physician. Reasons include embarrassment, misperception that it is a normal part of aging, belief that it is untreatable, fear of complications associated with its evaluation and treatment, or misconception that only major surgery can cure it. Moreover, when patients do mention it, most physicians either dismiss it as a normal part of aging or merely check a urinalysis. With newer undergarments and pads that better absorb and deodorize, the doctor may be unaware of the problem unless he/she asks about it.

4. **e. may not be the cause of the incontinence.** It is important to realize that involuntary bladder contractions are found commonly in even continent, neurologically-intact elderly; the prevalence ranges in various studies between 50% and 55%. This fact underscores the concept that such contractions are a risk factor for UI but not necessarily sufficient. Moreover, even when such contractions are the major contributor to UI, they may be due to a urethral abnormality. Over half of obstructed individuals and approximately 25% of those with stress incontinence have associated DO that usually remits with correction of the urethral abnormality alone. The proportion of elderly individuals in whom DO remits is likely lower, but clearly it is insufficient merely to identify involuntary contractions on cystometry and attribute the incontinence to them. To be considered the cause of the UI, such contractions must reproduce the patient's type of leakage, and urethral abnormalities must be excluded. This is particularly important because a bladder relaxant medication prescribed for DO that is actually due to obstruction may precipitate acute retention.

5. **c. postvoid residual assessment.** Determining the PVR is essential in all incontinent older individuals, not only because retention can mimic other causes of UI, but also because knowledge of the PVR will affect therapy. For instance, an older woman with DO and PVR of 250 mL would be approached differently from a woman with DO and PVR of 5 mL. The rest of the diagnostic evaluation depends on the need for diagnostic certainty. In many older adults, the empiric approach outlined in the chapter will be appropriate. However, if surgical correction is contemplated, or if the risk of empiric therapy exceeds the benefit, further testing is warranted. Cytology is indicated when bladder carcinoma is suspected and would be treated if found (i.e., not in a bedfast, demented patient). Cystoscopy has many indications, but it is not routinely required for evaluation of incontinence, nor is it alone sufficient to detect or exclude prostatic obstruction. Palpated prostate size correlates poorly with the presence of obstruction.

6. **c. Uninhibited detrusor contractions.** Incontinence is never part of normal aging; even at age 90, at least half of people are continent. Although renal function declines in most older adults, there is no change in serum creatinine owing to a concomitant and balanced decrease in muscle mass. Involuntary detrusor contractions are common in continent and even asymptomatic elderly, but are rarely seen during routine cystometry in younger people. Bladder capacity may decrease in the elderly, but there is no evidence for an increase. Flow rate declines, not only because obstruction becomes more likely in aging men, but also because detrusor contractility appears to decrease in both sexes.

7. **a. behavioral therapy.** Behavioral therapy is the cornerstone of treatment for detrusor overactivity, although the type of therapy must be tailored to the individual. Bladder retraining attempts to restore a normal voiding pattern by progressively lengthening the voiding interval. Scheduled toileting aims to reduce incontinence by frequent voiding, which reduces total bladder volume and the chance of triggering involuntary bladder contractions. Prompted voiding works by regularly and frequently reminding cognitively-impaired residents of the need to void. The role of medications is to supplement behavioral therapy, but only if needed. By reducing bladder irritability, such agents allow the bladder to hold more urine before the spasm occurs. However, even when continence is restored by these drugs, detrusor overactivity is still generally demonstrable. Furthermore, if the drug increases residual urine more than total bladder capacity, it may paradoxically decrease functional capacity, allowing the persistent involuntary contraction to occur at more frequent intervals. Thus before deciding that drug therapy has failed, PVR should be remeasured. Except for flavoxate, each of the agents listed has been proved effective in randomized controlled trials that included a substantial number of elderly patients.

8. **c. can be seen with detrusor hyperactivity with impaired contractility (DHIC).** The differential diagnosis for urinary retention extends beyond urethral obstruction, particularly in the elderly. Patients with underactive detrusor or detrusor hyperactivity with impaired contractility (DHIC) also may develop urinary retention. In addition, fecal impaction, pain (e.g., following hip replacement) and medications with urinary tract side effects (e.g., anticholinergics, sedating antihistamines, decongestants, and opiates) may induce acute urinary retention, particularly in patients with underlying bladder weakness or obstruction. Thus the bladder should be decompressed for at least a week while reversible causes are addressed; the larger the PVR, the longer should be the decompression. Decompression allows some restoration of detrusor strength, which also facilitates urodynamic testing

should it be necessary. Alpha-adrenergic blockers are effective for men with symptoms of prostatism, but clinical trials excluded patients with significant urinary retention. Bethanechol, although originally designed to improve bladder emptying in unobstructed patients, has not proved effective for this purpose (and likely not for nonobstructed patients either). Decompression in some elderly patients can reduce but not eliminate residual urine; provided it does not cause symptoms or renal compromise, subclinical retention need not necessarily be treated in all elderly patients, even if obstruction is present.

9. **e. should be tailored to the individual.** The cost of pads is rarely covered by insurance and can easily exceed $1/day. Menstrual pads, although often employed for incontinence, are usually inappropriate. They are designed to absorb small amounts of slowly leaking viscid fluid rather than rapid gushes of urine. From among the numerous types of pads and garments, selection should be tailored to the individual's needs and comorbidity; the type of incontinence matters less than severity.

10. **a. 5% to 10%.** Few studies have examined the issue, but the risk of developing acute urinary retention in men with prostatism appears to be quite low for at least 5 years. In the recent Medical Therapy of Prostatic Symptoms (MTOPS) trial, for instance (mean age = 63 years at baseline), the risk of acute retention was less than 5% over nearly 5 years. Predictors of retention included age greater than 62 years, PVR greater than 40 mL, PSA greater than 1.6 ng/mL, and total prostate volume greater than 31 mL, but these factors increased the risk only slightly (Crawford et al, 2006; Kaplan et al, 2008).*

11. **e. none of the above.** The patient's altered pattern of fluid excretion may occur for a variety of reasons. The most common one is accumulation of peripheral edema due to venous insufficiency, peripheral vascular disease, low albumin states (malnutrition, hepatic disease), congestive heart failure, or medications (e.g., nonsterioidal anti-inflammatory drugs [NSAIDs], dihydropyridine calcium channel blockers [e.g., nifedipine], or thiazolodinediones [e.g., rosiglitazone]). Each can be readily addressed. Before doing so, however, it is important to realize that the multiple pathologic conditions so often found in the elderly may be causal, contributory, a consequence, or unrelated to the condition for which the patient seeks help. In this individual, daytime leakage is the problem. Addressing the excess nocturnal excretion will not improve the daytime problem and, if it shifts the excess nocturnal excretion to the daytime (e.g., by use of pressure-gradient stockings), therapy may exacerbate the daytime leakage. If the nocturnal polyuria can be eliminated entirely (e.g., by substituting a drug that does not cause fluid retention), this should be done. If, however, therapy will only shift excretion to the daytime, one may elect not to treat if it is not dangerous (e.g., venous insufficiency). Evening furosemide risks inducing hypovolemia and increasing her risk of falls and fracture.

Daytime predominance of incontinence suggests that she has stress incontinence, or DO associated with bladder neck incompetence that is exacerbated when she is upright. Once the cause is sorted out, the appropriate intervention can be prescribed, but, in this individual, it should not include alteration of fluid intake: Her daytime output is too small to contribute to her daytime UI and, unless she is ingesting two liters after dinner, her intake is also likely unrelated to her nocturnal polyuria. Moreover, the older kidney generally takes twice as long to respond to fluid restriction as the younger one; so, restricting fluid after dinner is apt to do little. This case highlights the need to tailor the evaluation and treatment to the patient rather than to a given abnormality.

12. **b. False.** Cystometry provides information only on the bladder, not the outlet, and only during filling, not voiding. Thus it is insufficient to adequately characterize lower urinary tract dysfunction. Rather than being the primary cause of this patient's leakage, the detected DO may be incidental to aging and unrelated to his incontinence; in this instance, bladder relaxants may lead only to side effects. Alternatively, if DO is due to urethral obstruction or bladder neck incompetence following prostatic resection, a bladder relaxant will likely exacerbate both. Further historical information is necessary, as is characterization of urethral function. Often, simply addressing issues outside the urinary tract—such as cognition, mobility, depression, manual dexterity, or fluid excretion and toileting—is sufficient to restore continence in an older adult. Such an approach is beneficial for other reasons: It avoids medication side effects and cost, and it improves many of their other symptoms and quality of life.

13. **b. False.** Although anticholinergic agents can cause urinary incontinence, they do so by well-known mechanisms. In the absence of confusion, urinary retention, or excess fluid intake engendered by xerostomia, they should not be impugned as the etiology of the leakage, and the search for a cause should continue.

14. **b. False.** Incontinence is more common among patients with cognitive impairment than among their cognitively intact peers. The first approach should be to address all of the reversible causes, which are also more common in such patients, and to initiate a toileting regimen. If this fails, therapy with a bladder relaxant should be considered. All of the available bladder relaxants (oxybutynin, tolterodine, solifenacin, darifenacin, trospium, and fesoterodine) have anticholinergic properties, but concern that confusion will worsen with administration of a bladder relaxant has proved to be more theoretical than real, and even trials that have included cognitively impaired nursing home patients rarely report this as a problem. Nonetheless, mental status should be carefully monitored in such patients, and the drug should be stopped if mentation worsens without another identifiable cause.

15. **b. False.** Acetylcholine is an important neurotransmitter involved in memory. Because acetylcholinesterase inhibitors (AChEIs) are designed to increase the concentration of CNS acetylcholine, there is concern that an anticholinergic medication might attenuate or even reverse the benefit. However, AChEIs have proved to be of only modest efficacy and the improvement is experienced by only a minority of patients. So any attenuation of benefit may be minimal. In addition, there are only rare reports of deterioration when bladder relaxants are added to the regimen of these patients. Finally, given the impact of urgency incontinence, many patients and families are willing to take the small risk. Thus

*Sources referenced can be found in *Campbell-Walsh Urology, 10th Edition,* on the Expert Consult website.

it is best to inform the patient and/or caregiver about the possible risk and, if they consider the expected benefit on incontinence to be worth the risk, to prescribe the drug and monitor its effect on both continence and cognition. A simple test, such as the MiniMental State Exam, can be used for this purpose. It is best to involve the primary care physician as well.

16. **b. causing/exacerbating impaired mobility.** As noted above, all five of the currently available bladder relaxant medications have anticholinergic properties and thus can cause anticholinergic side effects. Confusion may result through the mechanism described in Answer No. 15. Dry mouth (xerostomia) results from the anticholinergic effect on the salivary and parotid glands. Even the M_3-specific agents have this effect, because M_3 receptors are the predominant receptor in these glands as well as in the bladder. Because bladder relaxants generally do not abolish the involuntary detrusor contractions, the xerostomia-mediated increased fluid intake results in the bladder filling more frequently to the volume at which detrusor contractions may be triggered. Bladder relaxants often impair detrusor contractility and can lead to subacute retention. If the increase in PVR is more than the increase in total bladder capacity, the effective bladder capacity will decrease. In turn, this could allow involuntary contractions to occur at a lower effective volume; an increase in incontinence frequency can ensue.

17. **b. False.** Nocturnal incontinence is common in the elderly and it has a broad differential diagnosis. As indicated in Table 76–5 in *Campbell-Walsh Urology, 10th Edition*, the causes of nocturia in older adults generally can be grouped into three categories: excess excretion (polyuria), conditions that disrupt sleep (including pain, anxiety, depression, congestive heart failure [CHF], and nocturnal bronchospasm), and conditions that result in impaired bladder storage. Similar to most geriatric symptoms, however, the causes may be multiple in a single person; so, evaluation and management must address each cause. Once this has been accomplished, the symptom may disappear or improve so substantially that the inconvenience, side effects, and cost of further therapy may not be desired. However, even if nocturia does not improve, treatment with DDAVP is generally not warranted for several reasons. In trials that included older adults, treatment with DDAVP was associated with a significant risk of hyponatremia, despite the restrictive enrollment criteria and meticulous evaluation and follow-up. The risk would likely be higher in clinical practice, where it is more difficult to identify contraindications and to monitor patients' renal, cardiac, and fluid status as closely. In addition, there is little evidence that DDAVP is actually effective for incontinence in older adults. Thus given the frequency and potential seriousness of DDAVP's adverse effects, the minimal evidence of its efficacy, and the considerable associated cost, use of DDAVP should be considered as a last option in an otherwise healthy patient who can be carefully assessed and followed with the help of a capable and willing internist.

18. **b. hyoscyamine.** All of these drugs except for hyoscyamine have been proved effective in randomized controlled clinical studies of urgency incontinence.

19. **d. continue both drugs and monitor her for deterioration in cognitive function.** Because cholinesterase inhibitors block the metabolism of acetylcholine, there is concern that they will provoke urgency incontinence, especially in older adults who already may have underlying age-related involuntary detrusor contractions that have not yet caused incontinence. However, despite prescription of these agents to millions of demented patients, there is little evidence that they cause incontinence. Moreover, because the benefits of these drugs for dementia are modest at best and not seen in the majority of patients who use them, patients and families may decide that the benefit of the bladder relaxant outweighs the risk. Particularly in this patient, who has already benefited from tolterodine without notable cognitive deterioration, it is worth continuing therapy and monitoring her cognitive status.

20. **a. adjustment of fluid excretion and voiding intervals.** Recent evidence suggests that weight loss will improve stress incontinence in obese women, and data support the use of postural maneuvers, pelvic floor muscle exercises, and surgical correction as well. Adjusting fluid excretion and voiding intervals can also be useful, especially for women with volume-dependent stress leakage. It can work particularly well for women with a threshold of at least 150 mL and best in those with a threshold greater than 250 mL. However, when the threshold is this low, the extent of fluid restriction required is usually not feasible and might even lead to dangerous dehydration.

21. **c. to obtain medical consultation before prescribing the drug.** Men with these lower urinary tract symptoms and a low PVR generally respond well to an α-adrenergic receptor blocker. However, many of these agents can reduce cardiac preload and thus impede adequate left ventricular filling and cardiac output, especially in individuals whose ventricular filling is already more difficult in the setting of LVH. The risk is exacerbated by the normal age-related decline that occurs in baroreflex sensitivity and further compounded in patients who take a β blocker and/or have aortic stenosis. Thus although the overall risks of orthostasis, falls, and fracture appear to be lower with the newer α-adrenergic agents, it would be prudent to obtain medical consultation before prescribing an α blocker in this clinical setting. Anticholinergic therapy can be used in men with urgency and a low PVR but, owing to the risk of inducing a tachycardia in a man with aortic stenosis and thereby also reducing left ventricular filling—combined with the potential risk of inducing urinary retention—prescription of an anticholinergic should not be the next step.

Additional Study Points

1. Bladder capacity does not change with age; however, bladder sensation, contractility, and ability to postpone voiding decline in both sexes with age.
2. Asymptomatic bacteriuria does not cause incontinence.
3. Detrusor overactivity is the most common type of lower urinary tract dysfunction in incontinent elderly of either sex.
4. Detrusor overactivity is divided into two subsets: (1) detrusor overactivity in which contractile function is preserved and (2) detrusor overactivity in which contractility is impaired.
5. Stress incontinence in women is usually associated with urethra hypermobility, but it may co-exist with impaired intrinsic sphincter function as well.
6. Normal creatinine levels in the elderly do not imply a normal glomerular flow rate (GFR).
7. Conservative measures used to treat excessive fluid output at night include compression stockings, alteration of the pattern of fluid intake, and administering a rapidly acting diuretic late in the afternoon or early evening.
8. Anticholinergic agents are one of the most common causes of delirium in the elderly, especially those with pre-existing cognitive, sensory, affective, or functional impairment.
9. Alpha 1a blockers, especially tamsulosin, increase the risk of serious ophthalmic events following iridectomy.

77

Urinary Tract Fistulae

Eric S. Rovner, MD

QUESTIONS

1. The most common cause of vesicovaginal fistula in the nonindustrialized, developing world is:
   a. cesarean section.
   b. surgical trauma during abdominal hysterectomy.
   c. surgical trauma during vaginal hysterectomy.
   d. obstructed labor.
   e. none of the above.

2. The most common type of acquired urinary fistula is:
   a. vesicovaginal fistula.
   b. ureterovaginal fistula.
   c. colovesical fistula.
   d. rectourethral fistula.
   e. vesicouterine fistula.

3. Vesicovaginal fistulae (VVF) may occur as a result of:
   a. locally advanced vaginal cancer.
   b. incidentally noted and repaired iatrogenic cystotomy during hysterectomy.
   c. radiotherapy for cervical cancer.
   d. cystocele repair with bladder neck suspension.
   e. all of the above.

4. Intraoperative consultation is requested by a gynecologist for a possible urinary tract injury during a difficult abdominal hysterectomy. There is clear fluid noted in the pelvis. The gynecologist is particularly worried about postoperative VVF formation. All of the following statements are correct regarding counseling this gynecologist EXCEPT:
   a. the incidence of iatrogenic bladder injury during hysterectomy is approximately 0.5% to 1.0%.
   b. approximately 0.1% to 0.2% of individuals undergoing hysterectomy develops a VVF.
   c. the risk of ureterovaginal fistula is greater than the risk of VVF in this setting.
   d. the absence of blue-stained fluid in the operative field following the administration of intravenous indigo carmine eliminates any possibility of a urinary tract injury.
   e. all of the above are true.

5. VVF due to obstructed labor are:
   a. the most common etiology of VVF in Nigeria.
   b. usually located at the vaginal apex.
   c. never associated with simultaneous rectovaginal fistula.
   d. typically found in multiparous women.
   e. usually smaller and simpler to repair than those associated with gynecologic surgery.

6. A 47-year-old woman presents with the new onset of constant urinary leakage 5 years after completing radiation therapy for locally advanced cervical carcinoma. All of the following may be considered part of the diagnostic evaluation EXCEPT:
   a. cystoscopy and possible biopsy.
   b. voiding cystourethrography (VCUG).
   c. CT scan of the abdomen and pelvis.
   d. urodynamics.
   e. ureteroscopy.

7. A 52-year-old woman with a history of an abdominal hysterectomy 2 months previously, presents for the evaluation of a constant clear vaginal discharge since the surgery. Following oral intake of pyridium, her pads continue to have a clear watery discharge. The most likely diagnosis is:
   a. vesicovaginal fistula.
   b. ureterovaginal fistula.
   c. peritoneovaginal fistula.
   d. vesicouterine fistula.
   e. urethrovaginal fistula.

8. In the industrialized world, postsurgical VVF are associated with ureteral injury in approximately:
   a. 0.01% of cases.
   b. 0.1% of cases.
   c. 10% of cases.
   d. 25% of cases.
   e. 50% of cases.

9. A 68-year-old woman presents with a 1-week history of vaginal leakage 6 months after completion of radiation therapy for locally advanced cervical cancer. VCUG reveals a VVF. On physical examination the fistula is irregular and

indurated, and approximately 3 mm in size. Cystoscopy reveals bullous edema surrounding the fistula, and biopsy of the fistula tract reveals only fibrosis without evidence of malignancy. There is no suggestion of recurrent malignancy on CT scan. She should be counseled that:

a. the optimal timing for repair of this fistula may be in 5 to 6 months.

b. the best chance to repair this fistula is with immediate surgical intervention.

c. a vaginal approach is not indicated.

d. the use of an adjuvant flap will not be necessary.

e. the success rate for the repair of this fistula is similar to that of a nonradiated VVF.

10. The abdominal approach to VVF repair:

a. is the preferred approach in all patients with VVF.

b. has a higher success rate than the vaginal approach.

c. is suitable for the use of an omental interpositional flap.

d. is associated with less morbidity and a shorter hospital stay than the vaginal approach.

e. is more often associated with postoperative vaginal shortening and dyspareunia than the vaginal approach.

11. The vaginal approach to an uncomplicated VVF repair:

a. is most often bolstered with use of a gracilis flap.

b. may be accomplished with a three- or four-layer closure.

c. requires the use of nonabsorbable suture.

d. is not indicated for obstetric-related fistula.

e. is contraindicated if the fistula tract is within 2 cm of the ureter.

12. Principles of urinary fistula repair include all of the following EXCEPT:

a. excision of the fistula tract.

b. tension-free closure.

c. use of well-vascularized tissue flaps.

d. watertight closure.

e. adequate postoperative urinary drainage.

13. Level I evidence (one or more randomized control trials) exists to support which of the following statements?

a. Preoperative administration of topical estrogens improves tissue quality prior to the repair of VVF.

b. Preoperative administration of topical estrogens improves the success rate of transvaginal VVF repair.

c. Preoperative administration of broad-spectrum intravenous antibiotics improves the success rate of all types of VVF repair.

d. Suprapubic bladder drainage is superior to urethral (Foley) catheter drainage in preventing surgical failure following VVF repair.

e. None of the above.

14. Vaginal repair of VVF is contraindicated in:

a. multiparous women.

b. large fistulae.

c. radiation-induced fistulae.

d. fistulae located at the vaginal cuff.

e. none of the above.

15. Potential complications of repair for a VVF following abdominal hysterectomy include all of the following EXCEPT:

a. stress urinary incontinence.

b. dyspareunia.

c. recurrence of the fistula.

d. urinary urgency and frequency.

e. ureteral injury.

16. Advantages of the transabdominal approach to VVF repair as compared with the transvaginal repair include all of the following EXCEPT:

a. ease of mobilization of the omentum as an interpositional flap.

b. decreased rate of intraoperative ureteral injury.

c. preservation of vaginal depth.

d. easier access to the apical VVF in individuals with high narrow vaginal canals.

e. ability to perform an augmentation cystoplasty through the same incision.

17. Seventeen days following a transvaginal VVF repair, a cystogram is performed. The bladder is filled to 100 cc with contrast medium and several images are taken. There is no evidence of a fistula on the filling images; however, the patient was unable to void during the study. A postvoid film was not obtained. This study:

a. demonstrates successful repair of the VVF, and the catheter should be removed.

b. is nondiagnostic, because it was done too soon following repair.

c. is nondiagnostic, because there are no voiding images or postvoid images.

d. is nondiagnostic, because the bladder was not filled to an adequate volume.

e. should be terminated and cystoscopy performed to examine for a persistent fistula.

18. Prior to surgical mobilization, the blood supply to a potential Martius flap (fibrofatty labial flap) is through the:

a. inferior hemorrhoidal artery.

b. external pudendal artery.

c. uterine artery.

d. inferior epigastric artery.

e. gonadal artery.

19. An interpositional flap of the greater omentum during VVF repair:

a. may be able to reach the deep pelvis without any mobilization in some patients.

b. is most commonly based on the superior mesenteric artery.

c. is contraindicated in the setting of inflammation or infection.

d. should not be divided or incised vertically in the midline because this may compromise the blood supply.

e. is most commonly used during a transvaginal approach.

20. A 39-year-old woman presents with constant vaginal leakage for 1 month following an abdominal hysterectomy. She describes symptoms of stress incontinence prior to the hysterectomy. She has no urgency and is voiding normally. Physical examination demonstrates no obvious fistula tract at the vaginal cuff. Oral phenazopyridine is given, and the bladder is filled with 100 cc of saline mixed with indigo carmine. A gauze pad is packed from the apex of the vagina proximally to the introitus distally, and the patient is told to ambulate for 90 minutes. Upon return, the pad is removed and examined. The most proximal portion of the pad is stained yellow-orange, and the most distal portion is blue. This is most consistent with:

   a. ureterovaginal fistula.
   b. vesicovaginal fistula.
   c. urethrovaginal fistula.
   d. a and b.
   e. a and c.

21. Ureterovaginal fistulae are:

   a. not associated with transvaginal hysterectomy.
   b. usually associated with normal voiding patterns.
   c. best diagnosed on VCUG.
   d. found more commonly following hysterectomy for malignancy than for benign indications.
   e. usually located in the middle one third of the ureter.

22. Two weeks following an emergent cesarean section for fetal distress during labor, a 28-year-old woman reports constant leakage per vagina. Analysis of the collected fluid reveals it to have a high creatinine level consistent with urine. Physical examination, including pelvic examination, reveals absolutely no abnormalities or surgical trauma to suggest a urinary fistula. There is no stress incontinence elicited on physical examination. Renal ultrasonography demonstrates no hydronephrosis, and the bladder is empty. The most likely diagnosis is:

   a. occult vesicovaginal fistula.
   b. occult ureterovaginal fistula.
   c. urethrovaginal fistula.
   d. vesicouterine fistula.
   e. peritoneovaginal fistula.

23. Vesicouterine fistulae occur most commonly due to:

   a. low-segment cesarean section.
   b. vaginal delivery.
   c. malignancy.
   d. conization of the cervix.
   e. myomectomy.

24. Potential options for therapy of vesicouterine fistula in a patient desiring long-term preservation of fertility include:

   a. observation.
   b. cystoscopy and fulguration of the fistula tract.
   c. hormonal therapy.
   d. surgical exploration and repair of the fistula with interpositional omental flap.
   e. all of the above.

25. Two months following resection of a large urethral diverticulum extending proximally beyond the bladder neck, a patient complains of urinary leakage. All of the following may be the source of this patient's symptoms EXCEPT:

   a. a urethrovaginal fistula.
   b. a vesicovaginal fistula.
   c. stress urinary incontinence.
   d. a recurrent urethral diverticulum.
   e. a vesicouterine fistula.

26. Urethrovaginal fistulae in the distal one third of the urethra:

   a. are often asymptomatic.
   b. are associated with significant bladder overactivity.
   c. cannot be repaired using a vaginal flap technique.
   d. can result in severe stress incontinence.
   e. are usually the result of malignant infiltration.

27. The most common cause of a colovesical fistula is:

   a. colon cancer.
   b. bladder cancer.
   c. prostate cancer.
   d. Crohn disease.
   e. diverticulitis.

28. CT scan findings suggestive of a colovesical fistula include:

   a. intravesical mass, air in the bladder, and bladder wall thickening.
   b. air in the bladder, bowel wall thickening adjacent to the bladder, and clear fluid in a bowel segment adjacent to the bladder.
   c. air in the bladder, bladder wall thickening adjacent to a loop of thickened bowel wall, and the presence of a colonic diverticula.
   d. air in the colon, colonic mass adjacent to the bladder, and debris within the bladder.
   e. air in the colon, bladder wall thickening, and an intravesical mass.

29. In the evaluation of a possible colovesical fistula, cystoscopy:

   a. has high diagnostic accuracy in revealing the cause of the fistula.
   b. has a high yield in identifying potential fistulae.
   c. should not be performed due to the risk of sepsis.
   d. is usually normal.
   e. most commonly reveals a large connection to the bowel.

30. A 62-year-old man presents with pneumaturia and recurrent urinary tract infections. A cystoscopy is performed revealing a bullous lesion on the posterior bladder wall. Two hours later, a CT scan is performed revealing air in the bladder. In this patient, air in the bladder:

   a. suggests colovesical fistula.
   b. may be due to a bacterial infection.
   c. may be due to instrumentation.
   d. is a nonspecific finding.
   e. all of the above.

31. The most common cause of a ureterocolic fistula is:
    a. locally extensive colon cancer.
    b. appendicitis with an associated abscess.
    c. diverticulitis.
    d. Crohn disease.
    e. tuberculosis.

32. The incidence of rectal injury during radical retropubic prostatectomy is:
    a. 0.1%.
    b. 1.0%.
    c. 5.0%.
    d. 10%.
    e. 20-fold higher in patients undergoing laparoscopic radical prostatectomy.

33. Rectourethral fistula (RUF) formation following brachytherapy for prostate cancer:
    a. may require complex reconstructive surgery or urinary diversion for repair.
    b. is located at the level of the prostate.
    c. is associated with fecaluria.
    d. may be associated with recurrent malignancy.
    e. may relate to all of the above.

34. A 61-year-old otherwise healthy man returns to the office with symptoms of mild stress urinary incontinence and fecaluria 3 weeks following radical retropubic prostatectomy. A VCUG is performed and reveals a 1-mm fistula at the vesicourethral junction. The prostate-specific antigen (PSA) is immeasurable, and the final pathology reveals organ-confined disease. This patient should be counseled that:
    a. a York-Mason transsphincteric approach to this fistula is associated with a high risk of anal incontinence.
    b. a trial of indwelling catheterization may result in resolution of the fistula.
    c. immediate colostomy is indicated.
    d. the stress incontinence will become more severe following repair of the fistula.
    e. urinary and fecal diversion will be necessary to repair this fistula.

35. Pyelovascular fistulae:
    a. are usually related to percutaneous procedures in the upper urinary tract.
    b. are most often due to renal malignancy.
    c. should be treated by removal of the nephrostomy tube.
    d. usually occur following radiation therapy.
    e. are usually fatal.

36. A 74-year-old woman with a history of colon cancer and external beam radiotherapy develops ureteral obstruction and a stent is placed. Three months later, she presents with severe anemia and ongoing bright red gross hematuria for several hours. On examination she is pale, tachycardic with a thready pulse and a systolic blood pressure of 60. As resuscitation is initiated with fluids and blood transfusion, the next step in management is:

    a. a CT scan of the abdomen and pelvis.
    b. cystoscopy, removal of the stent, and retrograde pyelography.
    c. immediate laparotomy and possible nephrectomy.
    d. angiography.
    e. a tagged red blood cell scan to lateralize the bleeding.

ANSWERS

1. **d. obstructed labor.** In the industrialized world, the most common cause of VVF is surgical trauma during gynecologic surgery, specifically hysterectomy. In the developing world, untreated obstructed labor results in ischemic necrosis of the anterior vaginal wall and underlying lower urinary tract and is the most common fistula in these geographic areas.

2. **a. vesicovaginal fistula.** The vast majority of urinary fistulae involve the bladder and vagina in both the industrialized and nonindustrialized world. The other types of the fistulae listed are much less common.

3. **e. all of the above.** Causes of VVF in the industrialized world include surgical trauma during hysterectomy, locally advanced gynecologic malignancy, anterior vaginal wall prolapse, anti-incontinence surgery, and pelvic radiotherapy. Intraoperative recognition and repair of bladder injury during hysterectomy should reduce the probability of VVF formation, but it does not eliminate the possibility.

4. **c. the risk of ureterovaginal fistula is greater than the risk of VVF in this setting.** The most common injury to the urinary tract during hysterectomy is a bladder laceration. Although ureteral injuries are not uncommon, they occur with far less frequency than bladder injuries. Furthermore, ureterovaginal fistulae are much less common than VVF. The absence of blue-colored fluid in the pelvis does not exclude injury to the urinary tract. For example, a small bladder laceration may not be evident, especially if the bladder is decompressed with a Foley catheter.

5. **a. are the most common etiology of VVF in Nigeria.** VVF in the developing world occur primarily due to obstructed labor. Typically, these occur in individuals who are young primigravids with a narrow bony pelvis. These fistulae are usually large; located distally in the vagina, sometimes encompassing large segments of the trigone, posterior bladder wall, and bladder neck; and are often part of a larger complex of presenting signs and symptoms termed the "obstructed labor injury complex," which includes rectovaginal fistulae. Due to their size and extensive ischemia of the surrounding tissues, these fistulae are often difficult to repair.

6. **e. ureteroscopy.** This individual does not have diagnosis of VVF, and therefore multiple considerations are present. Nevertheless, VVF is a strong possibility given the history of radiation therapy and pelvic malignancy. A VCUG can establish the presence of a fistula. Cystoscopy and biopsy of a fistula, if present, is mandatory to rule out recurrent malignancy. A CT scan of the abdomen and pelvis can evaluate for recurrent malignancy. Urodynamics may be helpful in evaluating for other types of incontinence, as well as assessing for bladder compliance and capacity in this individual, with a risk for impaired compliance due to radiation therapy. There is no indication for ureteroscopy in this individual.

7. **c. peritoneovaginal fistula.** Clear fluid draining from the vagina following surgery should be properly characterized. A urinary fistula is a possible source; however, urinary incontinence (stress, urge, overflow, etc.) are strong considerations as well. A peritoneovaginal fistula is a rare complication of hysterectomy in which peritoneal fluid leaks through the vaginal cuff. The fluid may be collected and analyzed for creatinine level. A creatinine level similar to that found in serum excludes urinary fistula as the source of the fluid. In addition, if a pyridium pad test is negative (pads are wet but are not stained orange) then this is highly suggestive of a peritoneal vaginal cuff fistula.

8. **c. 10% of cases.** Approximately 10% to 12% of individuals with VVF are found to have an associated ureteral injury.

9. **a. the optimal timing for repair of this fistula may be in 5 to 6 months.** This patient has a VVF due to radiation therapy. It is recent in onset, suggesting that the fistula is immature and has a possibility of enlarging because the radiation injury has not yet completely demarcated. The optimal timing for repair of this fistula may be in 5 to 6 months. A reevaluation at that time will be needed to assess whether the VVF is now mature and amenable to repair. Radiation-induced fistulae can be repaired vaginally, and adjuvant flaps are used to bolster the repair. The success rates for radiation-induced VVF are less than those associated with non–radiation-induced VVF, whether they are approached vaginally or abdominally.

10. **c. is suitable for the use of an omental interpositional flap.** The choice of approach for VVF repair is generally individualized based on the patient's anatomy, clinical circumstances, and the experience of the operating surgeon. In experienced hands, success rates are similar between the two approaches. Advantages of the vaginal approach include a shorter hospital stay and less postoperative morbidity compared with the abdominal approach; however, vaginal shortening may be an issue with some types of vaginal VVF repairs, including the Latzko operation.

11. **b. may be accomplished with a three- or four-layer closure.** The vaginal approach to VVF repair uses a three- or four-layer closure. Absorbable suture is preferred to avoid complications related to foreign bodies in the urinary tract, including stone formation and infection. Gracilis flaps are rarely necessary as peritoneal flaps or Martius labial fat flaps are much more convenient and local. The vaginal approach is not contraindicated in obstetric fistula, nor if the ureter is near the fistula tract.

12. **a. excision of the fistula tract.** Although some authors have suggested that excision of the epithelialized portion of the fistula tract is beneficial, it is not required in all cases.

13. **e. None of the above.** There is no evidence-based medicine to support any of these statements. Although both topical estrogens and intravenous antibiotics are commonly used, this is on the basis of expert opinion. There is no preferred method for postoperative bladder drainage following VVF repair, although unobstructed drainage is critical in preventing disruption of the suture line.

14. **e. none of the above.** The transvaginal approach to VVF repair can be used in most patients with uncomplicated VVF. There are few absolute contraindications to the vaginal approach. Nulliparous individuals with VVF located at the vaginal cuff in a high narrow vagina can be challenging to repair vaginally due to anatomic considerations, but this approach is not contraindicated.

15. **a. stress urinary incontinence.** Stress urinary incontinence may coexist with VVF; however, it is usually not related to the repair. One exception is the fistula located at the bladder neck or with involvement of the proximal urethra such as obstetric fistulae. These individuals may have new onset stress incontinence following repair due to destruction of the sphincter from the original injury.

16. **b. decreased rate of intraoperative ureteral injury.** The transabdominal approach to VVF repair has several distinct advantages compared with the transvaginal approach. However, there are no studies to suggest that ureteral injury is less common using a transabdominal approach than a transvaginal approach.

17. **c. is nondiagnostic, because there are no voiding images or postvoid images.** A postoperative cystogram should include voiding or postvoiding images to ensure that the VVF has been adequately repaired. Voiding may marginally increase the intravesical pressure, thereby providing opacification of some VVF that otherwise would be missed on simple filling cystograms. There is no standard filling volume for cystography. Generally, 2 to 3 weeks from surgery is an adequate time period for postoperative imaging. There is no indication for cystoscopy in this patient.

18. **b. external pudendal artery.** The blood supply to the Martius flap is provided from three sources: the internal and external pudendal arteries as well as the obturator artery. Generally, the small branches from the obturator artery, supplying the flap from a lateral direction, are sacrificed during mobilization. Furthermore, either the anterior (external pudendal) or posterior (internal pudendal) blood supply is divided in order to tunnel and then position the flap over the fistula.

19. **a. may be able to reach the deep pelvis without any mobilization in some patients.** The greater omentum has several favorable properties that support its use during transabdominal VVF repair. It is based on the right and left gastroepiploic arteries. Due to its rich blood supply and lymphatic properties, it can be a useful adjunctive measure in the setting of infection or inflammation. The blood supply enters the omentum perpendicular to its origin off the greater curvature of the stomach, enabling vertical incisions and mobilization into the deep pelvis. Wide mobilization may be necessary to permit the omentum to reach the deep pelvis in some cases; however, in many individuals the flap will reach into the deep pelvis without mobilization and without tension.

20. **a. ureterovaginal fistula.** This patient has at least a ureterovaginal fistula, based on the yellow-orange staining at the proximal portion of the gauze pad. This would be consistent with the normal voiding pattern. The distal blue staining would be consistent with stress incontinence as noted by the patient preoperatively. Hysterectomy is not associated with formation of urethrovaginal fistula. Vesicovaginal fistula is less likely because the staining would tend to be green (a combination of blue and yellow) and located in the midportion of the pad. A VCUG would be most helpful in definitively ruling out a vesicovaginal fistula.

21. **b. usually associated with normal voiding patterns.** Ureterovaginal fistulae involve the distal one third of the ureter. They most commonly occur in the setting of hysterectomy: Laparoscopic, abdominal, and vaginal hysterectomy may all result in ureterovaginal fistulae. Most ureterovaginal fistulae occur following hysterectomy for benign indications. Patients often do not complain of voiding dysfunction because the contralateral upper urinary tract provides filling of the bladder. VCUG is used primarily to exclude a concomitant VVF.

22. **d. vesicouterine fistula.** The most common cause of vesicouterine fistula is low-segment cesarean section. The normal physical examination suggests a lack of surgical trauma to the vagina, which most likely excludes a vaginal fistula. In the postpartum period, urine from a vesicouterine fistula will leak out of the incompetent cervical os, resulting in constant urinary leakage. A VCUG will confirm the diagnosis.

23. **a. low-segment cesarean section.** The vast majority of vesicouterine fistulae occur following low-segment cesarean section. Rarely, these may occur due to uterine rupture at the time of vaginal delivery.

24. **e. all of the above.** All of the listed options may preserve long-term fertility in patients with vesicouterine fistula. In those not desiring preservation of fertility, hysterectomy is indicated.

25. **e. vesicouterine fistula.** It is very unlikely that a vesicouterine fistula can result from such a clinical circumstance. Stress incontinence, VVF, urethrovaginal fistula, and a recurrent diverticulum may all result in the described symptoms.

26. **a. are often asymptomatic.** Distal urethrovaginal fistulae are often asymptomatic, because they originate beyond the sphincter. Vaginal voiding and pseudoincontinence may be present in some patients. A vaginal flap technique is an effective method of repair.

27. **e. diverticulitis.** Diverticulitis is the most common cause of colovesical fistula in most series. Colon cancer is the second most common cause, followed by Crohn disease.

28. **c. air in the bladder, bladder wall thickening adjacent to a loop of thickened bowel wall, and the presence of colonic diverticula.** The classic triad found on CT scan, which is suggestive of a colovesical fistula, includes: air in the bladder, bladder wall thickening adjacent to a loop of thickened bowel, and the presence of colonic diverticula.

29. **b. has a high yield in identifying potential fistulae.** The finding of bullous edema during cystoscopy is nonspecific; although, in the appropriate clinical setting, this can be very suggestive of a colovesical fistula. Eighty to 100 percent of cases of colovesical fistulae have an abnormality noted on cystoscopy. Cystoscopy and biopsy is useful to rule out a malignant fistula when this is a consideration.

30. **e. all of the above.** Air can be introduced into the bladder from instrumentation (i.e., cystoscopy or catheterization), or may be present due to infection with a gas-forming organism. Less commonly, air in the bladder results from a colovesical fistula.

31. **d. Crohn disease.** Most ureterocolic fistulae occur on the right side and occur in patients with Crohn disease. Left-sided fistulae in Crohn disease are much less common.

32. **b. 1.0%.** Most large series report a 1.0% to 1.5% incidence of rectal injury during radical retropubic prostatectomy. When recognized and repaired intraoperatively, very few of these injuries result in a rectourethral fistula. The incidence of rectal injury during laparoscopic radical prostatectomy, when performed by experienced surgeons, is similar to that reported in most open series.

33. **e. may relate to all of the above.** RUF commonly present with fecaluria, regardless of the etiology. RUF in the setting of prostatic malignancy should be biopsied to evaluate for the possibility of recurrent disease.

34. **b. a trial of indwelling catheterization may result in resolution of the fistula.** This is a small fistula and, as such, a trial of conservative therapy is warranted. Because this fistula is not associated with signs of local infection or sepsis, immediate colostomy is not indicated. A York-Mason operation is not associated with a high rate of anal incontinence. Furthermore, a single-stage approach may be attempted (without fecal diversion) in this uncomplicated fistula, if conservative measures fail. Finally, urinary incontinence may not worsen following surgical repair of the fistula.

35. **a. are usually related to percutaneous procedures in the upper urinary tract.** Pyelovascular fistulae are most often related to interventional procedures in the upper urinary tract, especially percutaneous procedures. Renal neoplasms and radiation therapy are not usually causative of these fistulae. Initial treatment consists of tamponade of the bleeding vessel. If this is unsuccessful, angiographic embolization may be necessary.

36. **d. angiography.** This individual is at high risk for a ureteroarterial fistula at the level of the stent. A CT scan, and retrograde pyelography will both most likely be nondiagnostic. Removal of stent could result in an increase in bleeding and be rapidly fatal. Angiography in the setting of active bleeding will provide both the diagnosis of a ureteroarterial fistula, if present, and a possible therapeutic intervention in the form of embolization or stent graft placement. Nephrectomy will not stop the acute hemorrhage. A red blood cell scan will be too time consuming, and although it may lateralize the side of the bleeding, it will delay a potentially lifesaving intervention.

Additional Study Points

1. Vesicovaginal fistulae may occur many years after completion of radiation therapy.
2. Clear vaginal discharge may not invariably represent a urinary fistula but may be a sign of a peritoneovaginal fistula, lymphatic fistula, vaginitis, or fallopian tube fluid.
3. Twelve percent of postsurgical vesicovaginal fistulae have an associated ureteral injury.
4. In the repair of fistulae, multiple layers should be used, and there should be no overlapping suture lines.
5. Long-term complications of vesicovaginal fistula repair include vaginal shortening and stenosis.
6. For open repair of a vesicovaginal fistula, it is essential to mobilize the bladder caudal to the fistula. Cholinergic agents are used liberally in the postoperative period following repair of a vesicovaginal fistula.
7. A Martius flap may be divided either at its superior or its inferior margin, because the vascular supply is provided at both ends of the graft.
8. A peritoneal flap is mobilized without opening the peritoneum, advancing it and securing it in a tension-free manner between the bladder and the vagina.
9. Following a ureteral injury, decompression of the upper tracks is essential.
10. Vesicouterine fistula do not always present with urinary incontinence.
11. Soft tissue flaps are an important component of successful urethrovaginal fistula repair.

chapter 78

Bladder and Female Urethral Diverticula

Eric S. Rovner, MD

QUESTIONS

1. A 68-year-old man presents with hematuria. Cystoscopy reveals a 15-cm bladder diverticulum with a 3-mm papillary lesion at the base of the diverticulum. The next step is:
   a. biopsy of the papillary lesion.
   b. transurethral resection of the papillary lesion with deep muscle resection.
   c. urodynamics and transurethral prostatectomy (TURP) if bladder outlet obstruction is noted.
   d. bladder diverticulectomy.
   e. radical cystectomy and urinary diversion.

2. Acquired bladder diverticula are commonly found in association with:
   a. prostatic obstruction.
   b. calyceal diverticula.
   c. nephrogenic adenoma.
   d. infection of perivesical glands.
   e. erectile dysfunction.

3. Congenital bladder diverticula:
   a. are associated with cellule and saccule formation.
   b. are uniformly larger and more numerous than acquired bladder diverticula.
   c. usually are located at the dome or anterior wall of the bladder.
   d. can be repaired by a transvesical approach.
   e. are associated with a high risk of malignant transformation.

4. The most common malignant tumor found in bladder diverticula is:
   a. adenocarcinoma.
   b. transitional cell carcinoma.
   c. carcinosarcoma.
   d. squamous cell carcinoma.
   e. leiomyoma.

5. A 65-year-old man with bladder outlet obstruction and a 5-cm bladder diverticulum undergoes uneventful TURP. Postoperatively, the patient's symptoms are resolved, and a voiding cystourethrogram (VCUG) demonstrates satisfactory emptying of the bladder and the bladder diverticulum. The next step is:
   a. annual surveillance with cystoscopy and urine cytology.
   b. discharge from urologic care.
   c. transvesical bladder diverticulectomy.
   d. repeat urodynamics.
   e. CT cystogram.

6. Ten years following TURP, a 71-year-old man with congestive heart failure (CHF) and atrial fibrillation who is on Coumadin has recurrent urinary tract infections (UTIs), and an American Urological Association (AUA) symptom score of 25. A videourodynamic study shows a 14-cm poorly emptying bladder diverticulum. The peak subtracted detrusor pressure (Pdet) during micturition is 15 cm H_2O with a Qmax of 3 cc/sec. Renal ultrasonography is normal. The next best step is:
   a. repeat TURP.
   b. clean intermittent self-catheterization (CIC).
   c. laser prostatectomy.
   d. bethanecol.
   e. CT urography.

7. Examination of the upper urinary tract in a patient with a right-sided 15-cm bladder diverticula and urodynamic bladder outlet obstruction will most likely show:
   a. no abnormalities.
   b. right hydroureteronephrosis.
   c. bilateral hydroureteronephrosis.
   d. right reflux nephropathy.
   e. lateral deviation of the right ureter.

8. Endoscopic examination of the lower urinary tract in the setting of bladder diverticula:
   a. is best performed with a rigid cystoscope.
   b. is associated with a high risk of perforation.
   c. should include examination of the entire interior of the diverticulum.
   d. is not indicated if an elective submucosal bladder diverticulectomy is planned.
   e. includes all of the above.

9. Pathologic examination of bladder diverticulectomy specimens usually reveals:
   a. transitional cell epithelium, muscularis mucosa, and lamina propria.
   b. cuboidal epithelium, muscularis mucosa, and lamina propria.
   c. denuded epithelium, submucosa, lamina propria, and muscularis propria.
   d. transitional cell epithelium and scattered bundles of smooth muscle.
   e. squamous cell epithelium surrounded by lamina propria.

10. Bladder diverticula:
   a. often do not produce specific symptoms.
   b. can be associated with urinary tract infections.
   c. are commonly diagnosed incidentally during the evaluation of other symptoms or conditions.
   d. may be associated with persistent pyuria.
   e. include all of the above.

11. Bladder diverticula associated with bladder outlet obstruction:
   a. are usually found in the absence of cellules and saccules.
   b. are associated with a greater than 95% prevalence of ipsilateral vesicoureteral reflux.
   c. cannot be imaged by CT.
   d. are associated with medial deviation of the pelvic ureter.
   e. are never found in the setting of hydronephrosis.

12. Common symptoms associated with urethral diverticula include all of the following EXCEPT:
   a. vaginal pruritus.
   b. dysuria.
   c. dyspareunia.
   d. postvoid dribbling.
   e. urinary frequency.

13. The prevalence of urethral diverticula is estimated to be:
   a. approximately 1% to 5% in the general population.
   b. up to 25% in autopsy studies.
   c. less than 1.5% in selected highly symptomatic patients.
   d. 25-fold more common in whites than in nonwhites.
   e. none of the above.

14. Appropriate evaluation of a patient with a suspected urethral diverticulum may include all of the following EXCEPT:
   a. endoluminal MRI of the urethra.
   b. videourodynamics.
   c. 99m–dimercaptosuccinic acid (DMSA) renal scan.
   d. transvaginal ultrasonography.
   e. voiding cystourethrography.

15. A 1.5-cm anterior vaginal wall mass is noted in a 35-year-old woman approximately 2 cm proximal to the urethral meatus without distorting the meatus. It is nontender, and stripping of the mass reveals no discharge per urethra. Urine analysis is unremarkable. This mass may represent all of the following EXCEPT a:
   a. vaginal wall cyst.
   b. Skene gland abscess.
   c. urethral diverticulum.
   d. vaginal leiomyoma.
   e. Gartner duct cyst.

16. The ostium of a urethral diverticulum is:
   a. most commonly found in the proximal one third of the urethra.
   b. most commonly found at the 10- and 2-o'clock position in the urethral lumen.
   c. usually seen on transvaginal ultrasound imaging.
   d. lined by secretory cells.
   e. often seen endoscopically as a discreet opening in the posterolateral urethra.

17. Two weeks following removal of a 5-cm proximal urethral diverticulum extending beneath the trigone of the bladder, a 48-year-old woman returns to the office with complaints of urine staining her undergarments. Possible etiologies include:
   a. urethrovaginal fistula.
   b. ureterovaginal fistula.
   c. vesicovaginal fistula.
   d. stress urinary incontinence.
   e. all of the above.

18. During performance of a urethral diverticulectomy, the Foley catheter is suddenly noted through a 0.5-cm surgically induced defect in the urethral wall as the specimen is removed from the operative field. The most appropriate next step is:
   a. mobilization of a Martius flap to buttress the urethral closure.
   b. placement of a midurethral polypropylene sling to prevent postoperative stress incontinence.
   c. primary closure of the urethra with fine absorbable suture.
   d. interposition of a biologically compatible graft, such as autologous fascia to close the gap in the urethral wall.
   e. excision and use of a portion of the urethral diverticulectomy specimen as a free graft to close the urethra.

19. The most common malignant tumor found in urethral diverticula is:
   a. adenocarcinoma.
   b. transitional cell carcinoma.
   c. carcinosarcoma.
   d. squamous cell carcinoma.
   e. none of the above.

20. Principles of surgical urethral diverticulectomy include all of the following EXCEPT:
   a. preservation or creation of urinary continence.
   b. excision of all identifiable periurethral fascia.
   c. identification of the ostium of the urethral diverticulum.
   d. closure of periurethral fascia following removal of the urethral diverticulum.
   e. watertight closure of the urethra.

21. The most likely initial event implicated in the formation of urethral diverticula is:
    a. congenital lack of fusion of the urethral crest.
    b. infection of vaginal cysts.
    c. traumatic vaginal delivery.
    d. infection of the periurethral glands.
    e. dysfunctional voiding.

22. All of the following may be associated with the postoperative course following urethral diverticulectomy surgery EXCEPT:
    a. apical vaginal prolapse.
    b. urethrovaginal fistula.
    c. recurrent urethral diverticula.
    d. UTI.
    e. persistent pelvic pain.

Imaging

1. A 47-year-old woman presents with dribbling and recurrent urinary tract infections. See Figure 78–1.

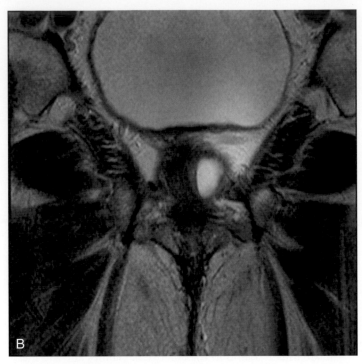

Figure 78–1, cont'd.

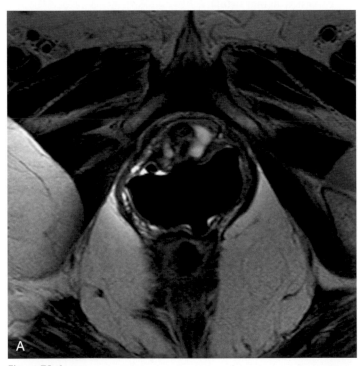

Figure 78–1.

The most likely diagnosis on this axial and coronal T2-weighted MRI done with an endovaginal coil is:
a. bladder prolapse.
b. urethral diverticulum.
c. bladder diverticulum.
d. ureteral duplication.
e. ectopic ureter.

ANSWERS

1. **a. biopsy of the papillary lesion.** Although the lesion may prove to be ultimately benign, a biopsy is necessary to exclude malignancy. Transurethral resection of a bladder tumor (TURBT) is not necessary until and unless a diagnosis of malignancy is established. TURBT of a lesion in a bladder diverticulum should be done only if absolutely necessary due to the thin wall of the diverticulum and the likelihood of perforation. The decision to proceed with definitive therapy following confirmation of a malignancy depends on several factors, including the histology, grade and stage of the tumor, and the patient's willingness and suitability for additional surgery. Transurethral resection of the prostate would not be indicated in this patient until a biopsy is

performed, the final pathology on the papillary lesion is known, and a diagnosis of benign prostatic obstruction or other indication for TURP is established. Radical cystectomy is not indicated in this case without an established diagnosis of malignancy.

2. **a. prostatic obstruction.** Acquired bladder diverticula are often associated with bladder outlet obstruction. There is no well-recognized association between bladder diverticula and the other listed entities.

3. **d. can be repaired by a transvesical approach.** When indicated, these lesions can be resected by a simple transvesical approach. The majority of congenital bladder diverticula are not associated with lower urinary tract voiding dysfunction. The pathogenesis of this lesion is felt to be a result of an anatomical weakness at the level of the ureterovesical junction. Congenital bladder diverticula are not associated with neurogenic vesicourethral dysfunction, are usually small and solitary, and are found in smooth-walled bladders without significant cellule or saccule formation.

4. **b. transitional cell carcinoma.** The most common malignant tumor found in over 70% of cases of bladder diverticula is transitional cell carcinoma. The remaining histologic types are much less common.

5. **a. annual surveillance with cystoscopy and urine cytology.** Both ongoing surveillance and operative intervention are possible treatment options in this individual; however, given the satisfactory bladder emptying, there is no indication for operative intervention at this time. Because the diverticulum empties satisfactorily, and the patient has had significant improvement in symptomatology, ongoing surveillance is the best option. However, the potential risk of malignant transformation remains and therefore, discharge from urologic care would not be appropriate. There is no indication for additional imaging or urodynamics in this asymptomatic patient.

6. **b. clean intermittent self-catheterization (CIC).** CIC will likely result in complete emptying of the lower urinary tract and reduce both the patient's symptoms and his propensity for UTIs. The diagnosis of recurrent obstruction has not been established in this patient with relatively poor contractility and therefore TURP is not indicated. Bethanechol is unlikely to significantly improve emptying of the bladder diverticulum. There is no indication for additional upper urinary tract imaging in this individual using normal renal ultrasonography.

7. **a. no abnormalities.** Bladder diverticula are most commonly associated with no changes to the upper urinary tract. Vesicoureteral reflux is not commonly associated with acquired bladder diverticula. Even in the setting of bladder outlet obstruction (BOO), the upper urinary tract is not dilated in patients with bladder diverticula.

8. **c. should include examination of the entire interior of the diverticulum.** Endoscopic examination should include visualization of the entire surface of the diverticulum. If this is not possible with rigid instrumentation, then a flexible cystoscope can be used. Biopsy of the interior of a bladder diverticulum is associated with an increased risk of perforation due to the relatively thin wall; however, simple endoscopic examination is not necessarily associated with an increased risk of perforation.

9. **d. transitional cell epithelium and scattered bundles of smooth muscle.** The adventitial layer of an excised bladder diverticulum may show scattered disorganized bundles of smooth muscle. In a true bladder diverticulum, there is usually a lack of the muscularis propria layer. The lining of a bladder diverticulum is usually transitional cell epithelium.

10. **e. include all of the above.**

11. **d. are associated with medial deviation of pelvic ureter.** Cellules and saccules are commonly found in patients with long-standing bladder outlet obstruction and are considered by some authors to be on a continuum with bladder diverticula. Although ipsilateral reflux may be present in patients with bladder diverticula, this is not a common finding. CT is an excellent modality for visualization and characterization of bladder diverticula, especially those with a narrow or obstructed neck. Medial deviation of the ureter is more common than lateral deviation of the ureter in the setting of bladder diverticula.

12. **a. vaginal pruritus.** Urethral diverticula may present with a variety of symptoms. Vaginal pruritus is not commonly reported in the setting of urethral diverticula.

13. **a. approximately 1% to 5% in the general population.** Although it is difficult to accurately quantitate the prevalence of urethral diverticula due to several factors, it is generally estimated to be 1% to 5% in the general population. The reported prevalence in autopsy studies is much lower than 25%, and the reported prevalence in highly symptomatic patients is much higher than 1.5%. Historically, the prevalence of urethral diverticula (UD) in African-Americans has been reportedly higher than that in whites, but this may be inaccurate due to reporting bias at urban academic medical centers.

14. **c. 99m–dimercaptosuccinic acid (DMSA) renal scan.** Radiographic imaging of the urethra in the setting of a suspected urethral diverticulum can be helpful in confirming the diagnosis, as well as providing information regarding relevant anatomy. The ultimate choice of imaging depends on many factors, including availability, cost, and expertise. DMSA renal scan is not indicated in the evaluation of suspected urethral diverticula.

15. **b. Skene gland abscess.** It is unlikely that this mass represents a Skene gland abscess because it is nontender and is not located distally in the region of the urethral meatus. The remaining choices are all possible. Urethral diverticula do not always result in a discharge per urethra upon stripping of the anterior vaginal wall, because the ostium of the diverticulum may be obstructed. Some diverticula are asymptomatic and are found incidentally on imaging or physical examination.

16. **e. often seen endoscopically as a discreet opening in the posterolateral urethra.** The ostium, or neck of a urethral diverticulum, is usually found posterolaterally in the middle third of the urethra. The ostium is often very difficult to visualize on any type of imaging, including ultrasonography, but can be seen endoscopically.

17. **e. all of the above.** Proximal urethral diverticula may extend beneath the bladder neck and trigone of the bladder. Therefore surgical excision of these lesions can risk stress urinary incontinence (SUI) but also injury to not only the urethra but also the bladder and distal ureter. Fortunately, these occurrences are quite rare.

18. **c. primary closure of the urethra with fine absorbable suture.** The Foley catheter is almost always seen during excision of a urethral diverticulum, especially as

the ostium is identified. The urethral defect can be closed primarily over as small as a 14-Fr Foley catheter. The other choices are either not indicated or unnecessary in the setting of an uncomplicated urethral diverticulectomy.

19. **a. adenocarcinoma.** As opposed to bladder diverticula, the most common tumor found in association with urethral diverticula is adenocarcinoma. Transitional cell carcinoma and squamous cell carcinoma are less common.

20. **b. excision of all identifiable periurethral fascia.** The periurethral fascia should be preserved during dissection of the urethral diverticulum. This tissue is used to buttress the urethral closure and close dead space remaining from a urethral diverticulectomy.

21. **d. infection of the periurethral glands.** The most likely etiology of urethral diverticula in the female is infection of the periurethral glands.

22. **a. apical vaginal prolapse.** Apical vaginal prolapse is not associated with urethral diverticulectomy. Persistent pelvic pain and/or UTI may occur despite a technically successful operation; however, a recurrent UD should be considered in the setting of these symptoms. Urethrovaginal fistula is a potential complication of urethral diverticulectomy.

Imaging

1. **b. urethral diverticulum.** The images demonstrate a fluid collection surrounding the urethra, compatible with a saddlebag urethral diverticulum. The coronal image clearly shows that the collection is separate from the bladder (options a and c are incorrect). Ectopic ureter will not have this saddlebag configuration.

Additional Study Points

1. When the diverticulum encompasses the ureteral orifice in the setting of neurogenic bladder and vesicle ureteral reflux, it is termed a Hutch diverticulum.

2. Congenital diverticula generally occur lateral and posterior to the ureteral orifice and often are associated with vesicoureteral reflux.

3. Acquired bladder diverticula usually occur in the setting of obstruction or neurogenic vesicle dysfunction.

4. The major complications of diverticula include recurrent urinary tract infections, stones, carcinoma or premalignant change in the diverticulum, and upper tract deterioration as a consequence of obstruction or reflux.

5. Many diverticula are located adjacent to the ureter and may be very adherent to it. This has implications in surgical resection.

6. The urethropelvic ligament in the female is composed of two parts: (1) endopelvic fascia and (2) periurethral fascia.

Within these two leaves of fascia lie the urethra, and this is the location of most urethral diverticula in woman.

7. The etiology of urethral diverticula in women has been attributed to recurrent urinary tract infection of periurethral glands with obstruction, suburethral abscess formation, and subsequent rupture of the infected gland into the urethra.

8. Skene glands do not communicate with the urethra.

9. Gartner duct cysts are located on the anterior lateral vaginal wall from cervix to introitus.

10. Urethral mucosa prolapse occurs in postmenopausal women and prepubertal girls.

11. A distinct layer of periurethral fascia should be preserved in managing excision of urethral diverticula for reconstruction.

Surgical Procedures for Sphincteric Incontinence in the Male: The Artificial Genitourinary Sphincter and Perineal Sling Procedures

Hunter Wessells, MD, FACS ● Andrew C. Peterson, MD, FACS

QUESTIONS

1. Which of the following is associated with a reduction in risk of artificial urinary sphincter (AUS) erosion?

   a. Transscrotal approach

   b. Proximal bulbar location

   c. Narrow-back modification

   d. InhibiZone treatment

   e. Cuff placement over bulbospongiosus muscle

2. The most significant contraindication to sling surgery for sphincteric incontinence is:

   a. impaired cognitive function.

   b. a pad weight test result of 125 mg/24 hr.

   c. prior AUS surgery.

   d. detrusor overactivity.

   e. arteriogenic erectile dysfunction.

3. The most likely cause of recurrent urinary incontinence 2 years after an AUS is:

   a. mechanical failure.

   b. atrophy.

   c. pressure-regulating balloon (PRB) aneurysm.

   d. new-onset detrusor overactivity.

   e. tubing kink.

4. A 34-year-old man with sphincteric incontinence has a history of pelvic fracture urethral disruption and closed head injury. Urodynamics show mild detrusor overactivity. The best surgical treatment is:

   a. bulbar AUS.

   b. bladder neck AUS.

   c. transobturator male sling.

   d. bone-anchored male sling.

   e. catheterizable continent stoma.

5. A 57-year-old man underwent AUS for postprostatectomy urinary incontinence 2 years ago. The expected rate of device revision over the next 3 years is:

   a. 8%.

   b. 12%.

   c. 16%.

   d. 20%.

   e. 24%.

6. In a man with a history of recurrent noninvasive bladder cancer and sphincteric urinary incontinence (UI) post-transurethral prostatectomy (TURP), the best solution for his incontinence is:

   a. bulbar AUS.

   b. bladder neck AUS.

   c. a Cunningham clamp.

   d. bone-anchored male sling.

   e. catheterizable continent stoma.

7. During urethral dissection for a first-time perineal AUS, inadvertant injury to the urethra is noted. After closing the urethral defect, the next step is:

   a. catheter drainage for 7 days and delayed replantation.

   b. placement of the cuff at a more distal location.

   c. bone-anchored sling placement at distal location.

   d. irrigation with antibiotic solution and transcorporeal cuff placement.

   e. tunica vaginalis flap coverage and bulbar cuff placement.

8. Efficacy of the male bone-anchored sling postradical prostatectomy (RP) is reduced by prior:

   a. collagen injection.

   b. adjuvant radiation therapy.

   c. transurethral resection of the prostate.

d. incision of bladder neck contracture.

e. penile prosthesis.

9. The most likely urodynamic finding in men with incontinence after RP is:

a. detrusor hyperreflexia.

b. detrusor overactivity.

c. intrinsic sphincter deficiency.

d. sensory urgency.

e. detrusor hypocontractility.

10. A 59-year-old man develops a dense vesicourethral anastomotic stricture 2 years after bulbar AUS placement for post-RP UI. The best approach for treatment is:

a. Collins knife transurethral incision.

b. laser incision.

c. open surgical reconstruction.

d. dilation with sounds.

e. antegrade transurethral incision by suprapubic cystostomy.

11. A 43-year-old man with myelomeningocele has persistent incontinence after placement of a 4.0-cm bulbar AUS. Urodynamics show a Valsalva leak point pressure (VLPP) of 55 cm H_2O and normal bladder capacity. The next step is:

a. to add a tandem cuff.

b. to reposition the cuff transcorporeally.

c. to increase PRB to 61 to 70 cm H_2O.

d. to remove and place bladder neck AUS.

e. to close the bladder neck and create a Mitrofanoff stoma.

12. The most important technical difference in implantation of a bladder neck versus bulbar AUS is the:

a. cuff measurement.

b. location of a pressure-regulating balloon.

c. preperitoneal connections.

d. choice of the pressure-regulating balloon.

e. fluid volume in device.

ANSWERS

1. **c. Narrow-back modification.** The narrow-back modification is associated with a reduced risk of erosion. The transscrotal approach may not allow the surgeon to place the cuff in a very proximal location; this is associated with potential risk of worse incontinence not erosion. There is no literature to support the value of InhibiZone treatment. Preservation of the bulbospongiosus muscle has not been shown to affect erosion rates.

2. **c. prior AUS surgery.** Radiation therapy and prior urethral surgery are relative contraindications to sling surgery due to reduced efficacy, perhaps due to poor tissue coaptation or association with more severe incontinence. Because slings do not require deliberate activation, they are more suitable for cognitively impaired patients compared with AUS. Although detrusor overactivity may reduce the efficacy of all devices, medical management can address many of these problems. Ischemic damage of the corpus spongiosum may impede proper function of slings, but no relationship has been found between cavernosal blood flow and outcomes.

3. **b. atrophy.** The narrow-backed AUS model 800 has improved mechanical reliability such that now atrophy is a more common cause of recurrent UI. New-onset detrusor overactivity is rare after AUS but may complicate any surgical treatment.

4. **d. bone-anchored male sling.** This patient has a complex history. Cognitive impairment due to closed head injury precludes either AUS implantation. After urethral disruption due to pelvic fracture, transobturator slings are not likely to provide effective elevation and elongation due to fibrosis and rhabdosphincter damage. The bone-anchored sling should be appropriate, while continent diversion should be a last resort.

5. **b. 12%.** Two- and 5-year revision rates for AUS were 16% and 28%. Thus an additional 12% failure rate is expected between years 2 and 5.

6. **b. bladder neck AUS.** The problem of urinary tract access is central to this case. Bulbar urethral procedures will not allow appropriate instrumentation and transurethral resection of recurrent tumors. A bladder neck AUS, with diameters in the 8- to 9-cm range should allow passage of a 24-Fr resectoscope.

7. **a. catheter drainage for 7 days and delayed replantation.** Urethral injury during any implant surgery places the patient at risk for device infection due to bacterial colonization of the urethra. The risk of devastating device infection outweighs any benefit, and thus the procedure should be aborted.

8. **b. adjuvant radiation therapy.** Radiotherapy is associated with a lower success rate of bone-anchored male slings, while the other conditions have not been associated with poor outcomes.

9. **c. intrinsic sphincter deficiency.** The sine qua non of UI post-RP is intrinsic sphincteric deficiency (ISD). Detrusor dysfunction may be present in up to 40% of these men, but is the primary cause of UI in less than 5%.

10. **b. laser incision.** Bulbar cuffs do not allow insertion of standard resectoscopes, making a Collins knife incision impossible. The safest approach for an initial stricture would be a laser incision through a smaller-caliber endoscope, with open surgical reconstruction being reserved for refractory cases. Dilation with sounds would be potentially risky at the bladder neck location; antegrade incision could be feasible but offers less control than the retrograde approach.

11. **d. to remove and place bladder neck AUS.** Although a tandem cuff or transcorporeal cuff could provide improved coaptation; the ultimate risk of long-term erosion makes these less desirable in a 43-year-old man. Similarly, increasing the pressure in the PRB will also increase the risk of erosion. Long-term complications of bladder neck cuffs in men with normal vesicourethral junctions are low and should be considered prior to closing the bladder neck in an otherwise adequate bladder.

12. **d. choice of pressure-regulating balloon.** Bladder neck AUS require higher pressures to ensure coaptation. Cuff measurement and PRB location require no modification; connections can be made intra-abdominally or in the subcutaneous space above the fascia, and usually the differences in fluid volume are nominal.

Additional Study Points

1. Endoscopic evaluation should precede surgical correction of urinary incontinence following radical prostatectomy or a TURP to evaluate the anatomy and eliminate bladder neck contracture.
2. An assessment of bladder capacity, compliance, and contractility is required prior to considering surgical correction of urinary incontinence.
3. Submucosal bulking agents are of limited efficacy in treating incontinence following radical prostatectomy.
4. After artificial sphincter placement, prolonged urinary retention requires suprapubic cystostomy drainage.
5. Determining the appropriate tension of the sling is the most critical portion of the operation.
6. Cuff atrophy requires downsizing, repositioning, tandem cuff placement, or transcorporeal surgery.

Benign and Malignant Bladder Disorders

chapter 80

Urothelial Tumors of the Bladder

David P. Wood, Jr., MD

QUESTIONS

1. What percentage of women will have squamous metaplasia of the bladder?
   a. 5%
   b. 15%
   c. 25%
   d. 40%
   e. 60%

2. Inverted papillomas are:
   a. a benign tumor of the bladder.
   b. a precursor to low-grade papillary cancer.
   c. chemotherapy resistant.
   d. an invasive tumor.
   e. best treated with antibiotics.

3. The incidence rate of urothelial cancer:
   a. has been decreasing recently because of less smoking.
   b. is higher in women than in men.
   c. is highest in developed countries.
   d. peaks in the 5th decade of life.
   e. is higher in Asia than Europe.

4. The mortality rate of urothelial cancer:
   a. is primarily related to lack of health care access.
   b. has been decreasing since 1990.
   c. is highest in underdeveloped countries.
   d. is proportionally higher in women than in men.
   e. is proportionally higher in white men than in African-American men.

5. What is the risk of a white male developing urothelial cancer in his lifetime?
   a. Less than 5%
   b. 20%
   c. 40%
   d. 60%
   e. 80%

6. The most common histologic bladder cancer cell type is:
   a. squamous.
   b. adeno.
   c. urothelial.
   d. small cell.
   e. leiomyosarcoma.

7. The mortality rate from bladder cancer is highest in:
   a. the United States.
   b. England.
   c. South America.
   d. China.
   e. Egypt.

8. Recent evidence suggests that physician practice may be related to bladder cancer deaths in the elderly. What percentage of deaths could be avoided?
   a. Less than 5%
   b. 30%
   c. 50%
   d. 70%
   e. 90%

9. Which gene is most commonly mutated in high-grade muscle invasive urothelial cancer?
   a. *Cyclin A*
   b. *TP53*
   c. *FGFR-3*
   d. *HRAS*
   e. *PTEN*

10. Which gene is most commonly mutated in carcinoma in situ (CIS)?
    a. *PI3K*
    b. *RB*
    c. *FGFR-3*
    d. *HRAS*
    e. *CD-44*

11. Globally, what is the relative risk of developing bladder cancer for men with chronic urinary tract infections?
    a. Less than 5 times
    b. 15 times
    c. 30 times
    d. 50 times
    e. 70 times

12. The chemotherapy proven to cause urothelial cancer is:
    a. Adriamycin.
    b. bleomycin.
    c. ifosphamide.
    d. etoposide.
    e. cyclophosphamide.

13. The increased risk of developing bladder cancer for a man who has a sister with bladder cancer is:
    a. 2 fold.
    b. 10 fold.
    c. 20 fold.
    d. 40 fold.
    e. 60 fold.

14. The risk of a family member developing bladder cancer if a first-degree relative has the disease is:
    a. related to secondhand smoke.
    b. higher in men.
    c. higher in smokers.
    d. related to inheritance of low-penetrance genes.
    e. most common in high-grade cancer.

15. The percent of patients presenting with non–muscle-invasive disease is:
    a. Less than 5%.
    b. 20%.
    c. 40%.
    d. 60%.
    e. 80%.

16. A 30-year-old man has gross hematuria and cystoscopy finds a papillary tumor. Transurethral resection of the tumor reveals a noninvasive 2-cm papillary low-malignant potential urothelial tumor. Muscle is present in the resected specimen. All of the tumor is resected. The best treatment is:
    a. intravesical BCG.
    b. repeat cystoscopy with random bladder biopsies.
    c. radical cystectomy secondary to young age.
    d. immediate mitomycin C intravesical therapy.
    e. observation.

17. The external agent most implicated in causing urothelial cancer is:
    a. β-naphthylamine.
    b. 4,4′-methylene bis(2-methylaniline).
    c. perchloroethylene.
    d. trichloroethylene.
    e. 4,4′-methylene bis(2-methylaniline).

18. If a woman stops smoking for 10 years after 30-pack-years of smoking, her risk of developing bladder cancer:
    a. is the same as if she still smoked.
    b. is the same as if she never smoked.
    c. is unrelated to the intensity of smoking.
    d. is very low because of her gender.
    e. gradually decreases over time.

19. Which food substance is associated with a low risk of urothelial cancer?
    a. Citrus
    b. Eggs
    c. Chicken
    d. Grapes
    e. Cherries

20. A man exposed to high doses of radiation (more than 500 mSv):
    a. has the same risk of urothelial cancer formation as a nuclear plant worker.
    b. will likely develop urothelial cancer within 5 years.
    c. is more likely to develop urothelial cancer if he is less than 20 years old.
    d. is 2 times more likely to develop urothelial cancer.
    e. should be quarantined for 3 months.

21. One of the main changes from the 1973 to 1998 WHO urothelial classification system was that:
    a. there should be two grades of non–muscle-invasive bladder cancer.
    b. muscle-invasive disease should be segregated into inner and outer muscle involvement.
    c. perivesical fat involvement by tumors is stage T3.
    d. CIS can be low or high grade.
    e. Ta grade 1 tumors should be considered cancerous.

22. Genetic abnormalities associated with low-malignant potential Ta tumors include:
    a. fibroblast growth factor receptor-3 (FGFR-3).
    b. TP53.
    c. retinoblastoma (RB) gene.
    d. PTEN.
    e. loss of chromosome 17.

23. Urothelial cancer noninvasively involving the prostatic urethra:
    a. is stage T4a.
    b. is stage T4b.
    c. is not part of the 2010 TNM staging system for bladder cancer.
    d. has a worse prognosis than perivesical fat involvement.
    e. should be treated with radical cystectomy.

24. A 40-year-old man has a T1 high-grade urothelial cancer on initial presentation. Muscle was present in the biopsy specimen. The next treatment is:
    a. BCG.
    b. repeat transurethral resection of a bladder tumor (TURBT).

c. radical cystectomy.

d. immediate mitomycin C instillation.

e. neoadjuvant chemotherapy followed by radical cystectomy.

25. A 73-year-old man with a history of Ta bladder cancer is found to have a 0.5-cm papillary lesion in the prostatic urethra and undergoes extensive transurethral resection of the prostate, revealing high-grade noninvasive disease of the prostatic urethra without ductal or stromal involvement. The next best step is:

a. perioperative mitomycin C.

b. surveillance cystoscopy every 3 months.

c. mitomycin C therapy.

d. induction of and maintenance with BCG therapy.

e. radical cystectomy.

26. A 62-year-old man undergoes a transurethral biopsy of a bladder tumor at the dome. Final pathology reveals muscle-invasive urothelial and small cell carcinoma. Metastatic workup is negative. The next step is:

a. intravesical gemcitabine therapy.

b. partial cystectomy.

c. radical cystoprostatectomy.

d. external beam radiotherapy.

e. chemoradiation therapy.

27. When cisplatin-based chemotherapy is used, which of the following genetic mutations is associated with the worst prognosis?

a. *FGFR-3* mutations

b. *PTEN*

c. *TP53*

d. *RB*

e. *PTEN, TP53,* and *RB*

28. Tumor suppressor genes are activated by:

a. gene amplification.

b. translocation.

c. point mutations.

d. DNA methylation.

e. microsatellite instability.

29. The risk of urologic malignancy in a man with recurrent gross hematuria, but who had a previous negative evaluation, is:

a. less than 5%.

b. 20%.

c. 40%.

d. 60%.

e. 80%.

30. Which of the following is not a high-risk factor in urothelial cancer formation in patients with microscopic hematuria?

a. Age less than 40 years

b. Smoking

c. History of pelvic radiation

d. Urinary tract infections

e. Previous urologic surgery

31. Commercially available fluorescence in-situ hybridization kits test for abnormalities in which of the following chromosomes?

a. 3, 7, 9, 17

b. 2, 5, 8

c. 4, 6, 9

d. 1, 10, 12

e. 13, 14, 16

32. Microsatellite analysis:

a. detects telomeric repeats.

b. amplifies DNA repeats in the genome.

c. evaluates abnormalities on chromosome 9.

d. detects DNA methylation.

e. identifies hereditary urothelial cancer.

33. Smoking is responsible for what percent of bladder cancer in males?

a. 5%

b. 20%

c. 40%

d. 60%

e. 80%

34. Which of the following is not sensitive to cisplatin chemotherapy?

a. High-grade urothelial cancer

b. Micropapillary cancer

c. Squamous cell cancer

d. Adenocarcinoma

e. Small cell cancer

35. Nested variant of urothelial cancer can be confused with:

a. cystitis cystica.

b. micropapillary cancer.

c. squamous cell cancer.

d. Small cell cancer.

e. high-grade urothelial cancer.

36. The most common sarcoma involving the bladder is:

a. angiosarcoma.

b. chondrosarcoma.

c. leiomyosarcoma.

d. rhabdomyosarcoma.

e. osteosarcoma.

37. Signet ring cell cancers:

a. have a good prognosis.

b. are sensitive to Adriamycin chemotherapy.

c. usually present in advanced stage.

d. are responsive to radiation therapy.

e. are low-grade at initial presentation.

38. The risk of bladder cancer formation in a spinal cord–injured patient is:

a. less than 5%.

b. 20%.

c. 40%.

d. 60%.

e. 80%.

39. For patients undergoing radical cystectomy for urothelial cancer, the risk of identifying prostatic urethral disease is:
    a. less than 5%.
    b. 20%.
    c. 40%.
    d. 60%.
    e. 80%.

40. Which of the following is not a risk factor for prostatic urethral cancer?
    a. Previous intravesical therapy
    b. CIS of the trigone
    c. CIS of the distal ureters
    d. Low-grade urothelial cancer
    e. Recurrent bladder tumors

Pathology

1. A 70-year-old man has microscopic hematuria. Cytology and CT scan are negative. Cystoscopy shows a raised 3-mm lesion on the trigone. The lesion is biopsied and depicted in Figure 80–1A and B.

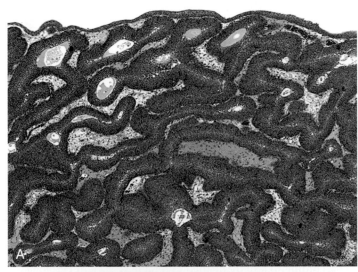

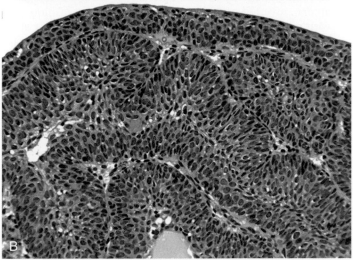

Figure 80–1. (From Bostwick DG, Cheng L. Urologic surgical pathology. 2nd edition. Edinburgh: Mosby; 2008.)

The diagnosis is:
a. inverted papilloma.
b. adenocarcinoma.
c. endometriosis.
d. cystitis glandularis.
e. transitional cell carcinoma.

2. A 65-year-old man has gross hematuria. He has a history of having had tuberculosis. Cytology is suspicious, CT scan is normal, and cystoscopy reveals a papillary lesion cephalad to the trigone. The lesion is visually completely resected and depicted in Figure 80–2.

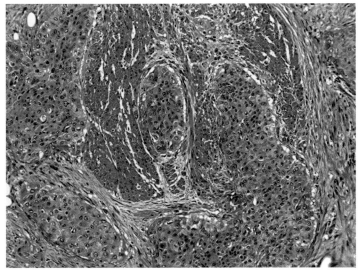

Figure 80–2. (From Bostwick DG, Cheng L. Urologic surgical pathology. 2nd edition. Edinburgh: Mosby; 2008.)

The patient should be advised to have:
a. intravesical BCG.
b. intravesical mitomycin C.
c. isoniazid (INH), rifampin, and ethambutol.
d. a cystectomy.
e. a follow-up cystoscopy in 3 months.

Imaging

1. See Figure 80–3.

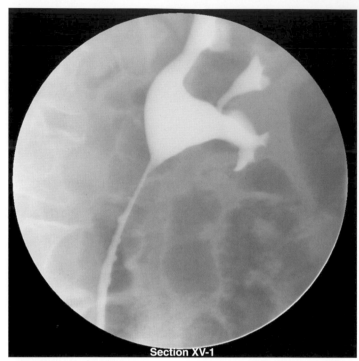

Figure 80–3.

The depicted findings have an association with:

a. bladder carcinoma.

b. previous trauma.

c. recurrent urinary tract infections.

d. urolithiasis.

e. ureteral spasm.

2. A 68-year-old man with history of smoking and hematuria undergoes a CT scan. See Figure 80–4A and B.

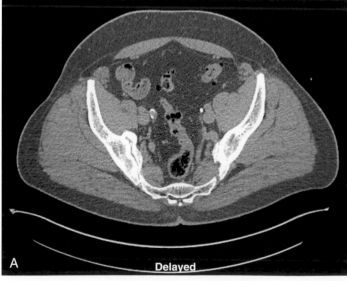

Figure 80–4.

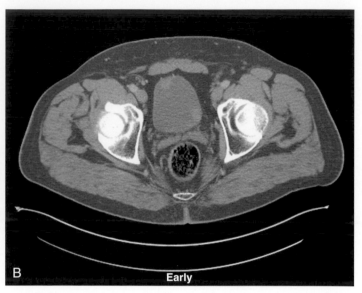

Figure 80–4, cont'd.

Figure 80–4A is an early contrast-enhanced image through the bladder, and Figure 80–4B is a delayed image through the pelvic ureters. The next step in management is:

a. shock-wave lithotripsy.

b. percutaneous nephrostolithotomy.

c. cystoscopy.

d. cystoscopy with ureteroscopy.

e. follow-up with imaging in 6 months.

ANSWERS

1. **d. 40%.** Approximately 40% of women and 5% of men have squamous metaplasia of the bladder that is usually related to infection, trauma, and surgery (Ozbey et al, 1999).* There are no racial differences, and squamous metaplasia is more common in women of childbearing age.

2. **a. a benign tumor of the bladder.** When diagnosed according to strictly defined criteria (e.g., lack of cytologic atypia), inverted papillomas behave in a benign fashion with only a 1% incidence of tumor recurrence (Sung et al, 2006; Kilciler et al, 2008). Occasionally, inverted papillomas are present with coexistent urothelial cancer elsewhere in the urinary system, occurring more commonly in the upper tract than the bladder (Asano et al, 2003). The use of fluorescent in-situ hybridization to evaluate chromosomal changes can distinguish between an inverted papilloma and a urothelial cancer with an inverted growth pattern (Jones et al, 2007).

3. **c. is highest in developed countries.** Sixty-three percent of all bladder cancer cases occur in developed countries with 55% from North America and Europe. There is a geographic difference in bladder cancer incidence rates across the world with the highest in Southern and Eastern Europe, parts of Africa, Middle East, and North America and

*Sources referenced can be found in *Campbell-Walsh Urology,* *10th Edition,* on the Expert Consult website.

the lowest in Asia and underdeveloped areas in Africa (Ferlay et al, 2007). The incidence of urothelial cancer peaks in the 7th decade of life.

4. **b. has been decreasing since 1990.** The mortality rate of urothelial cancer has decreased by 5% since 1990 primarily because of smoking cessation, changes in environmental carcinogens, and a healthier lifestyle (Jemal et al, 2008).

5. **a. Less than 5%.** A white male has a 3.7% chance of developing urothelial cancer in his lifetime, which is roughly 3 times the probability in white females or African-American males and more than 4.5 times the probability of an African-American female (Hayat et al, 2007; Jemal et al, 2008).

6. **c. urothelial.** Histologically, 90% of bladder cancers are of urothelial origin, 5% squamous cell, and less than 2% adenocarcinoma or other variants (Lopez-Beltran, 2008). Urothelial carcinoma is the most common malignancy of the urinary tract and is the second most common cause of death among genitourinary tumors.

7. **e. Egypt.** The mortality rate from bladder cancer in Egypt is 3 times higher than in Europe and 8 times more than in North America because squamous cell carcinoma is highly prevalent in Egypt (Parekh et al, 2002).

8. **b. 30%.** Mortality from bladder cancer is highest in elderly persons, particularly those greater than the age of 80, accounting for the third most common cause of cancer deaths in men over the age of 80 (Jemal et al, 2008). Whether this increase in mortality rate is related to tumor biology or changes in physician practice with the elderly is unclear. Recent evidence suggests that physician practice may be related to bladder cancer deaths in the elderly (Morris et al, 2009). These authors estimated that 31% of all bladder cancer deaths were avoidable, more commonly in noninvasive than invasive disease.

9. **b. TP53.** High-malignant potential, non-muscle invasive bladder cancer is more likely associated with deletions of tumor suppressor genes such as *TP53* and *RB*. (Chatterjee et al, 2004a; George et al, 2007; Sanchez-Carbayo et al, 2007).

10. **b. RB.** All CIS is high grade by definition. The genetic abnormalities associated with CIS include alterations to the *RB, TP53,* and *PTEN* genes (Cordon-Cardo et al, 2000; Lopez-Beltran et al, 2002; Cordon-Cardo, 2008).

11. **b. 15 times.** A retrospective review of published literature suggests that chronic urinary tract infections are associated with bladder cancer, reporting a 14 to 16 relative risk of developing bladder cancer for any history of urinary tract infection versus none (Abol-Enein, 2008).

12. **e. cyclophosphamide.** The only chemotherapeutic agent that has been proven to cause bladder cancer is cyclophosphamide (Travis et al, 1995; Nilsson and Ullen, 2008). The risk of bladder cancer formation is linearly related to the duration and intensity of cyclophosphamide treatment, supporting a causative role. Phosphoramide mustard is the primary mutagenic metabolite that causes bladder cancer in patients exposed to cyclophosphamide.

13. **a. 2 fold.** First-degree relatives of patients with bladder cancer have a twofold increased risk of developing urothelial cancer themselves, but high-risk urothelial cancer families are relatively rare (Aben et al, 2002; Murta-Nascimento et al, 2007; Kiemeney, 2008).

14. **d. related to inheritance of low-penetrance genes.** The hereditary risk seems to be higher for women and nonsmokers, but it is not related to secondhand exposure to smoking in families. Most likely, there are a variety of low-penetrance genes that can be inherited to make a person more susceptible to carcinogenic exposure, thus increasing the risk of bladder cancer formation.

15. **e. 80%.** At initial presentation, 80% of urothelial tumors are non–muscle-invasive. There are multiple growth patterns of urothelial cancer, including flat carcinoma in-situ (CIS), papillary tumors that can be low or high grade, and sessile tumors with a solid growth pattern. Non–muscle-invasive cancers can be very large because of lack of the genetic alterations required for invasion.

16. **d. immediate mitomycin C intravesical therapy.** PUNLMP is a papillary growth with minimal cytological atypia that is more than seven cells thick and is generally solitary and located on the trigone (see Fig. 80–9 in *Campbell-Walsh Urology, 10th Edition*) (Holmang et al, 2001; Sauter et al, 2004). PUNLMP is composed of thin papillary stalks where the polarity of the cells is maintained and the nuclei are minimally enlarged. PUNLMP has a low proliferation rate and is not associated with invasion or metastases. Tumor recurrence is common, and thus perioperative treatment with mitomycin C is warranted.

17. **a. β-naphthylamine.** One of the first and most common chemical agents implicated in the formation of bladder cancer in dye and rubber workers is β-naphthylamine (Case and Hosker, 1954). Activation of aromatic amines allows DNA binding by enzymes that are selectively expressed in the population, making some subjects more susceptible for cancer formation as described above related to the *NAT-2* and the *GSTM1* polymorphisms.

18. **e. gradually decreases over time.** Smoking cessation does make a difference in urothelial cancer formation. Smokers who have stopped for 1 to 3 years have a 2.6 relative risk, and those stopping for more than 15 years a 1.1 relative risk of bladder cancer formation (Wynder and Goldsmith, 1977; Smoke IAfRoCT, 2004).

19. **a. Citrus.** In general, a Mediterranean diet has the lowest urothelial cancer risk. In a case-controlled study, there were fewer cases of urothelial cancer in the group given a Mediterranean diet versus a standard Western diet probably due to the increased ingestion of fruits and vegetables (de Lorgeril et al, 1998). Both fruits and vegetables, specifically citrus, apples, berries, tomatoes, carrots, and cruciferous vegetables, contain several active compounds that are important in detoxification.

20. **d. is 2 times more likely to develop urothelial cancer.** There is a significant increased risk of dying from any cancer if a person is exposed to greater than 50 mSv. The relative risk of urothelial cancer formation is 1.63 in men and 1.74 in women. Interestingly, urothelial cancer formation after radiation is not age related, but the latency period is 15 to 30 years. However, there is no association with low-dose or industrial exposure of radiation therapy and bladder cancer formation. Importantly, urologic technicians or nuclear radiation workers do not have an increased risk of urothelial cancer formation.

21. **a. there should be two grades of non–muscle-invasive bladder cancer.** The two main changes were recognition that papillary Ta grade 1 urothelial cancers should not be considered cancers because of their indolent

growth and lack of invasion, and the second was elimination of "grade 2" cancers that became a grey zone encompassing grade 1 and grade 3 cancers causing interobserver variation.

22. **a. fibroblast growth factor receptor-3 (*FGFR-3*).** Genetic abnormalities associated with low-grade cancer include deletion of 9q and alterations of *FGFR-3*, *HRAS*, and *PI3K* (Holmang et al, 2001; Cordon-Cardo, 2008). Low-grade carcinomas are immunoreactive for cytokeratin-20 and CD-44. The *TP53*, retinoblastoma *(RB)*, and *PTEN* genes and loss of chromosome 17 are all associated with high-grade cancer.

23. **c. is not part of the 2010 TNM staging system for bladder cancer.** Extension of the tumor into the prostatic urethra without stromal invasion is currently classified under the prostatic urethral section and does not carry an adverse prognosis for patients with known bladder cancer (Pagano et al, 1996).

24. **b. repeat TURBT.** Because of this understaging, the American Urological Association (AUA) guidelines call for a repeat transurethral resection in patients with T1 tumors to assess for muscle-invasive disease even if muscle was present in the specimen (Hall et al, 2007).

25. **d. induction of and maintenance with BCG therapy.** For patients with noninvasive prostatic urethral cancer, transurethral resection of the prostate with BCG therapy is appropriate (Palou et al, 2007). For patients with prostatic ductal disease, a complete TURP is warranted, plus BCG therapy. Although a radical cystectomy could be performed, a more conservative organ-sparing treatment is recommended.

26. **e. chemoradiation therapy.** Small cell carcinoma of the bladder should be considered and treated as metastatic disease, even if there is no radiologic evidence of disease outside the bladder. Small cell carcinoma of the bladder accounts for well less than 1% of all primary bladder tumors. In general, small cell carcinoma of the bladder is very chemosensitive and the primary mode of therapy is chemoradiation therapy.

27. **e. *PTEN, TP53*, and *RB*.** Overall genetic instability is the hallmark of invasive urothelial cancer, but, specifically, alterations of *TP53*, *RB*, and *PTEN* carry a very poor prognosis (Chatterjee et al, 2004a). *FGFR-3* mutations are associated with noninvasive bladder cancer.

28. **c. point mutations.** Tumor suppressor genes are mainly activated by allelic deletion of one allele followed by point mutations of the remaining allele. Tumor suppressor genes are recessive or have a negative effect, resulting in unregulated cellular growth. Proto-oncogenes are generally activated by point mutations in the genetic code, gene amplification, and gene translocation. The activated proto-oncogenes become oncogenes that can cause cancer and is considered a positive or dominant growth effect (Lengauer et al, 1998; Wolff et al, 2005; Cordon-Cardo, 2008).

29. **a. less than 5%.** Gross, painless hematuria is the primary symptom in 85% of patients with a newly diagnosed bladder tumor (Khadra et al, 2000; Alishahi et al, 2002; Edwards et al, 2006). The gross hematuria is usually intermittent and can be related to Valsalva maneuvers; therefore any episode of gross hematuria should be evaluated even if subsequent urinalysis is negative. Fifty percent of patients with gross hematuria will have a demonstrable cause, 20% will have a urological malignancy, and 12% will have a bladder tumor (Khadra et al, 2000). The risk of malignancy in patients with recurrent gross or microscopic hematuria that had a full, negative evaluation is near zero within the first 6 years (Khadra et al, 2000).

30. **a. Age less than 40 years.** The guidelines recommend consideration for re-evaluation of low-risk individuals with microscopic hematuria, but repeat evaluation every 6 months with a urinalysis, cytology, and blood pressure (to detect renal disease) is recommended for high-risk patients. Age less than 40 is the only factor that is not associated with an increased risk of malignancy.

31. **a. 3, 7, 9, 17.** Fluorescence in-situ hybridization (FISH) identifies fluorescently labeled DNA probes that bind to intranuclear chromosomes. The current commercially available probes evaluate aneuploidy for chromosomes 3, 7, 17, and homozygous loss of 9p 21 (Zwarthoff, 2008). The median sensitivity and specificity of FISH analysis is 79% and 70%, respectively (van Rhijn et al, 2005).

32. **b. amplifies DNA repeats in the genome.** There are multiple markers available to identify short DNA repeats present throughout the chromosomes that are lost in some tumor cells. Microsatellite analysis amplifies these repeats in the genome that are highly polymorphic, and PCR amplification can detect tumor-associated loss of heterozygosity by comparing the peak ratio of the two alleles in tumor DNA in a urine sample with that ratio in a blood sample from the same individual (Steiner et al, 1997; Wang et al, 1997). The sensitivity and specificity of microsatellite analysis for the detection of urothelial carcinoma range from 72% to 97% and 80% to 100%, respectively. (Steiner et al, 1997; Wang et al, 1997). Microsatellite analysis evaluates abnormalities on all chromosomes.

33. **c. 40%.** Smoking is responsible for 30% to 50% of all bladder cancers in males, and smokers have a 2- to 6-fold greater risk of getting bladder cancer (Brennan et al, 2000; Boffetta, 2008). Smoking cessation will decrease the risk of eventual urothelial cancer formation in a linear fashion. After 15 years of not smoking, the risk of cancer formation is the same as for a person who never smoked (Smoke IAfRoCT, 2004). The strong influence of smoking in bladder cancer formation prevents accurate determination of other less significant dietary, micronutrient, or lifestyle changes that may alter bladder cancer formation.

34. **b. Micropapillary cancer.** The most effective treatment for all stages of micropapillary urothelial carcinoma is surgical resection. Treatment with transurethral resection and BCG therapy is ineffective unless the tumor is completely resected (Kamat et al, 2007). Neoadjuvant chemotherapy does not appear effective in micropapillary urothelial carcinoma, similar to ovarian cancer (Bristow et al, 2002; Kamat et al, 2007). Neoadjuvant chemotherapy may actually worsen survival by delaying therapy when compared to immediate cystectomy. Cisplatin is effective against urothelial cancer and the associated variants of squamous cell, adenocarcinoma, and small cell cancer.

35. **a. cystitis cystica.** The nested variant of urothelial cancer is a rare, but aggressive cancer that has a male to female ratio of 6:1 and can be confused with benign lesions, such as Von Brunn nests that are in the lamina propria, cystitis cystica, and inverted papillomas (Holmang and Johansson,

2001). There is little nuclear atypia in nested variant urothelial carcinoma, but the tumor cells will often contain areas with large nuclei and mitotic figures (see Fig. 80–16 in *Campbell-Walsh Urology, 10th Edition*). The mortality rate from nested variant urothelial carcinoma, despite aggressive therapy, is significant, with 70% dying of their disease within 3 years (Paik and Park, 1996).

36. **c. leiomyosarcoma.** Leiomyosarcoma is the most common histologic subtype, followed by rhabdomyosarcoma and then, rarely, angiosarcomas, osteosarcomas and carcinosarcomas. The male to female ratio is 2:1, and the average age at presentation is in the 6th decade of life. There are no clear agents that cause bladder sarcomas, although there is an association with pelvic radiation and systemic chemotherapy for other malignancies (Spiess et al, 2007). Importantly, bladder sarcomas are not smoking related.

37. **c. usually present in advanced stage.** Primary signet ring cell carcinoma of the bladder is extremely rare occupying less than 1% of all epithelial bladder neoplasms (Morelli et al, 2006). Signet ring cell carcinoma can be of urachal origin and directly extend into the bladder. These tumors generally present as high-grade, high-stage tumors, and have a uniformly poor prognosis. The primary treatment is radical cystectomy; however, in the majority of cases there are regional or distant metastases at the time of presentation, and the mean survival time is less than 20 months (Torenbeek et al, 1996). There are reports of elevated carcinoembryonic antigen (CEA) in patients with signet ring cell carcinoma. The prognostic significance of this elevated serum marker is unclear (Morelli et al, 2006). Understaging is very common in signet ring cell carcinoma, with peritoneal studding common at the time of surgical exploration.

38. **a. less than 5%.** Spinal cord–injured patients are at risk for developing squamous cell carcinoma, most likely due to chronic catheter irritation and infection. Older studies have suggested a 2.5% to 10% incidence of squamous cell carcinoma in the spinal cord–injured population, with a mean delay of 17 years after the spinal cord injury (Kaufman et al, 1977). More recent analysis of the association of spinal cord–injury and bladder cancer formation has shown a remarkably lower risk of bladder cancer formation of 0.38%, most likely because of better catheter care (Bickel et al, 1991). This supports the concept that chronic infection and foreign bodies can lead to bladder cancer formation.

39. **c. 40%.** Prostatic urethral cancer is associated with urothelial cancer of the bladder in 90% of cases, primarily CIS, and most will have multifocal bladder tumors. However, the incidence of prostatic urethral disease in patients with primary urothelial cancer is only 3% (Rikken et al, 1987; Millan-Rodriguez et al, 2000). Secondary prostatic urethral involvement in patients with a history of urothelial cancer is approximately 15% at 5 years and 30% at 15 years, almost uniformly associated with extensive intravesical therapy (Herr and Donat, 1999). For patients undergoing radical cystectomy for urothelial cancer, the risk of identifying prostatic urethral disease is 40%.

40. **d. Low-grade urothelial cancer.** Risk factors for prostatic urethral involvement are CIS of the trigone, bladder neck, distal ureters, recurrent bladder tumors, and a history of intravesical chemotherapy (Wood et al, 1989b). Low-grade tumors rarely involve the prostatic urethra.

Pathology

1. **a. Inverted papilloma.** These lesions are benign, usually occur in older men, and are often located near or on the trigone.
2. **d. a cystectomy.** The tumor invades the muscularis propria; notice the muscle bundles. Therefore the patient has at least a T2 tumor.

Imaging

1. **a. bladder carcinoma.** Pseudodiverticulosis of the ureter is associated with bladder carcinoma in 30% of cases. This association has led many to recommend that patients with this diagnosis undergo surveillance of their bladder for the development of urothelial neoplasms. The etiology is unknown.
2. **d. cystoscopy with ureteroscopy.** There are multiple enhancing masses in the fluid-filled urinary bladder on the early image. On the delayed image, the ureters are opacified with contrast, and there is a filling defect seen in the mildly dilated right ureter, suspicious for a synchronous ureteral lesion.

Additional Study Points

1. Inverted papillomas are associated with chronic inflammation.
2. Cystitis glandularis may be associated with pelvic lipomatosis.
3. Bladder cancers in adolescents and young adults generally are well differentiated and noninvasive.
4. The intensity and duration of smoking is linearly related to the risk of developing bladder cancer with no plateau; cessation of smoking reduces the risk.
5. There is a clear association between a healthy diet and a decreased risk of urothelial cancer.
6. There is no convincing evidence that alteration in fluid intake, alcohol consumption, ingestion of artificial sweeteners, or analgesic abuse increase the risk of bladder cancer; however, chronic irritation, bacterial infection, and radiation have all been associated with the development of bladder cancer.
7. Eighty percent of the time, low-grade, low-stage urothelial neoplasia (papillary urothelial neoplasia of low malignant potential) is associated with loss of chromosome 9.
8. With low-grade, low-stage urothelial neoplasia (PUNLMP), the terms low grade and high grade replace the old system of grade 1, 2, and 3.
9. Prostatic urethral involvement by transitional cell carcinoma without invasion carries a relatively good prognosis; when it invades the prostatic stroma, the prognosis is less good, and when it directly invades the substance of the prostate from the bladder, the prognosis is poor.
10. Low-grade papillary lesions have a 60% recurrence rate but less than a 10% rate of progression to muscularis propria

invasion, whereas high-grade lesions, particularly T1 may have a stage progression in up to 50% of cases. Moreover, high-grade non–muscularis propria invasive tumors have an 80% incidence of recurrence.

11. Angiolymphatic invasion is a poor prognostic sign.

12. In muscularis propria invasive urothelial cancer, alterations in *TP53, RB,* and *PTEN* are poor prognostic indicators.

13. Genetic alterations in low-grade non–muscularis propria invasive disease include alterations in *FGFR-3* and deletions in chromosome 9.

14. Porphyrin-induced fluorescent cystoscopy and narrow-band imaging cystoscopy have been used to increase the sensitivity of cystoscopy.

15. To date, none of the urinary markers are sensitive or specific enough to replace cystoscopy for monitoring bladder cancer.

16. Sarcomas of the bladder, in decreasing order of frequency, include leiomyosarcoma, rhabdomyosarcoma, angiosarcoma, osteosarcoma, and carcinosarcoma.

17. *Schistosoma haematobium* is the causative agent of squamous cell carcinoma in endemic regions.

18. Altered growth patterns such as micropapillary and nested patterns carry a poor prognosis.

chapter 81

Non–Muscle-Invasive Bladder Cancer (Ta, T1, and CIS)

J. Stephen Jones, MD, MBA ● William A. Larchian, MD

QUESTIONS

1. Postoperative intravesical chemotherapy (administered in the recovery room) is appropriate for which of the following patients?
   a. Solitary, 3-cm, low-grade-appearing tumor on posterior bladder wall
   b. Multifocal ($n = 4$), low-grade, low-stage bladder tumors, all 4 to 10 mm in diameter
   c. 6.5-cm, high-grade, broad-based tumor on lateral wall with deep resection
   d. a and b
   e. a to c

2. Which of the following agents is contraindicated for postoperative intravesical chemotherapy (administered in the recovery room)?
   a. Thiotepa
   b. Bacille Calmette-Guérin (BCG)
   c. Mitomycin C
   d. Epirubicin
   e. b and c

3. Potential advantage(s) of tumor markers such as BTA, stat NMP-22, and UroVysion (FISH) when compared with urinary cytology for monitoring patients with bladder cancer are improved:
   a. sensitivity.
   b. specificity.
   c. positive predictive value.
   d. a and c.
   e. a to c.

4. Progression rates for low-grade Ta tumors:
   a. range from 0% to 3%.
   b. range from 3% to 10%.
   c. range from 10% to 17%.
   d. range from 17% to 25%.
   e. are greater than 25%.

5. General anesthesia is most important when resecting a bladder tumor in which setting?
   a. Large, mobile papillary tumor
   b. Tumor in a posterior wall diverticulum
   c. Lateral location, at about 4 or 8 o'clock
   d. Extensive CIS
   e. Tumor at dome and along anterior bladder wall

6. A healthy 55-year-old man undergoes resection of a 2-cm bladder tumor in a posterior wall bladder diverticulum. Pathology demonstrates a pT1G3 bladder tumor with associated areas of carcinoma in situ (CIS). Muscularis mucosa is involved, but there is no definite muscularis propria in the specimen. Optimal management includes:
   a. repeat resection to stage the cancer.
   b. intravesical BCG therapy.
   c. partial cystectomy with excision of the diverticulum.
   d. radical cystectomy and neobladder urinary diversion.
   e. chemotherapy and radiation therapy.

7. The most important principle to follow when resecting tumor near or overlying a ureteral orifice is:
   a. stent frequently.
   b. avoid resection in most cases.
   c. avoid cautery in this area.
   d. resect at will; a stent or nephrostomy tube can be placed later.
   e. obtain an ultrasound preoperatively and place a nephrostomy tube if hydronephrosis is found.

8. A restaging transurethral resection of bladder tumor (TURBT) with possible postoperative intravesical chemotherapy (administered in the recovery room) is indicated in which of the following situations?
   a. pT1, G2 tumor with no muscularis propria identified
   b. pTa, G1 tumor that is multifocal ($n = 5$), for which resection appeared to be complete, but postoperative intravesical therapy was not administered
   c. pT1, G3 tumor with muscularis propria identified and negative

d. a and c

e. a to c

9. The optimal laser for fulguration of bladder tumors is:

   a. CO_2.

   b. Nd:YAG.

   c. holmium.

   d. potassium titanyl phosphate (KTP).

   e. argon.

10. Intravesical mitomycin C chemotherapy for high-risk superficial bladder cancer:

    a. reduces the risk of progression.

    b. reduces the risk of recurrence.

    c. is preferred over BCG, particularly for CIS.

    d. is virtually free of side effects.

    e. is less expensive than BCG.

11. Contraindications to intravesical BCG therapy include all of the following EXCEPT:

    a. cirrhosis.

    b. history of tuberculosis.

    c. total incontinence.

    d. immunosuppression.

    e. all of the above.

12. The combination of reduced-dose BCG and interferon-α for intravesical therapy is:

    a. more effective than BCG alone.

    b. more toxic than BCG alone.

    c. preferred first-line therapy for patients with multifocal CIS.

    d. less expensive than BCG alone.

    e. a reasonable option for BCG failures after one course of therapy.

13. Common side effects of thiotepa include:

    a. irritative voiding symptoms and fever.

    b. hematuria and irritative voiding symptoms.

    c. bladder contraction and myelosuppression.

    d. irritative voiding symptoms and myelosuppression.

    e. flulike symptoms and fever.

14. Long-term (15 years) outcome after intravesical BCG therapy for patients with high-risk non–muscle-invasive bladder cancer include which of the following?

    a. Approximately 50% progression rate

    b. Approximately 25% alive and with bladder intact

    c. A high incidence of recurrence in extravesical sites (prostatic urothelium and upper tracts)

    d. Approximately 33% cancer-related mortality rates

    e. All of the above

15. Understaging for patients with pT1G3 bladder cancer is approximately:

    a. 5% to 10%.

    b. 10% to 20%.

    c. 20% to 30%.

    d. 30% to 50%.

    e. 50% to 70%.

16. A patient is diagnosed with a 1-cm pTaG1 bladder cancer. Imaging of the upper tracts:

    a. is not indicated.

    b. should be performed only at diagnosis.

    c. should be performed at diagnosis and 5 years later.

    d. should be performed at diagnosis and every other year thereafter.

    e. should be performed at diagnosis and every year thereafter.

17. For patients with stage pTaG1 bladder tumor and a negative cytology, random bladder biopsies:

    a. are more likely to be positive in the prostatic fossa than the bladder.

    b. must be done in a systematic manner.

    c. should include sampling of the muscularis mucosa and preferably the muscularis propria as well.

    d. are indicated at initial diagnosis and need not be repeated if negative.

    e. are not indicated in most cases.

18. The risk of progression to muscle invasive disease for patients with untreated CIS of the bladder is approximately:

    a. 5% to 15%.

    b. 15% to 25%.

    c. 25% to 35%.

    d. 35% to 45%.

    e. greater than 45%.

19. Current consensus about p53 as a prognostic marker for bladder cancer is that it is:

    a. an established predictive factor for response to BCG therapy.

    b. an independent predictor of tumor progression for patients with pT1G3 disease.

    c. a stronger predictor than grade for pTa tumors.

    d. of no clinical value at present.

    e. not prospectively validated.

20. Which of the following disease entities is least common?

    a. pTaG1

    b. pTaG3

    c. pT1G3

    d. CIS of any form

    e. pT2-3

ANSWERS

1. **d. a and b.** Postoperative intravesical chemotherapy should be considered for most cases of new or recurrent non–muscle-invasive bladder cancer because it has been shown to reduce recurrence rates and improve outcomes for this disease. One exception is the patient in whom an extensive resection has been performed or whenever there is a possible perforation. In these patients intravesical chemotherapy should be withheld due to concern about local extravasation and absorption.

2. **b. Bacille Calmette-Guérin (BCG).** BCG should never be given in association with known trauma to the urinary tract such as after TURBT due to concern over systemic

absorption and sepsis. All of the other agents have shown efficacy in this setting with a favorable morbidity profile.

3. **a. sensitivity.** Tumor markers such as BTA stat, NMP-22, and UroVysion (FISH) provide improved sensitivity, particularly for low-grade tumors. High specificity is the strength of urinary cytology. This approaches 90% to 100% in many series and cannot be improved on with these other markers. Positive predictive value is highest for urinary cytology because the number of false-positives is low. Put another way, if the cytology is positive, the patient usually has active disease.

4. **b. range from 3% to 10%.** Recurrence is common (50% to 70%) for patients with low-grade, pTa tumors, but progression to higher tumor stage is uncommon, occurring in about 5% to 10% of patients.

5. **c. Lateral location, at about 4 or 8 o'clock.** Resection along the lateral bladder wall posterolaterally places one in proximity to the obturator nerve, and this can lead to an obturator reflex. This can predispose to bladder wall perforation. In this situation, general anesthesia with complete paralysis is often indicated to allow the procedure to be performed in a safe and facile manner.

6. **d. radical cystectomy and neobladder urinary diversion.** This patient should be strongly considered for radical cystectomy. Partial cystectomy is not a good option due to the presence of CIS, which indicates a high risk of field effect disease and subsequent recurrence. Deeper biopsies would risk perforation and would be unlikely to influence management. Understaging is common with tumors in diverticuli, and high-grade invasive tumors like this are best managed with radical cystectomy to ensure local disease control and optimize outcomes on a long-term basis.

7. **c. avoid cautery in this area.** A stent should be avoided if possible to prevent reflux of tumor cells into the upper tracts. In most cases this area can be resected, and most ureters will remain unobstructed as long as the orifice is identified and cautery is not used in this area. Preoperative placement of a nephrostomy tube is often unnecessary as long as renal function is stable. Many patients with hydronephrosis will have invasive disease and will be undergoing urinary diversion in the near future, and this will relieve the obstruction. Hence temporary nephrostomy tube placement is usually not required.

8. **d. a and c.** Patients with pT1 tumor for whom the muscularis propria was not identified are understaged about 50% of the time, and a repeat resection is clearly indicated. Repeat resection of patients with a pT1G3 tumor with muscularis propria present and negative reveals residual or invasive disease 30% of the time. A repeat TURBT is thus indicated in both of these patient populations to accurately stage the tumor and optimize patient management.

9. **b. Nd:YAG.** The Nd:YAG laser has the best properties (e.g., depth of penetration, intensity of energy for effective tumor ablation) for coagulation of bladder tumors and the greatest clinical experience demonstrating safety and efficacy in appropriately selected patients.

10. **b. reduces the risk of recurrence.** Mitomycin C (MMC) is expensive, especially when compared with BCG. It can reduce the risk of recurrence, but there is no convincing evidence that it can reduce progression rates, which is true for all forms of intravesical chemotherapy. Most comparative studies and meta-analyses suggest an advantage

to BCG, particularly for CIS. MMC can lead to local bladder irritation and dermatitis and is thus far from risk free.

11. **e. all of the above.** BCG is contraindicated in patients with liver disease (isoniazid cannot be given if they develop BCG sepsis), a personal history of TB, total incontinence (they cannot retain the BCG, so efficacy would be poor), and immunosuppression (BCG's mechanism of action is to stimulate an immune response). Other contraindications included disrupted urothelium, gross hematuria, or active or persistent urinary tract infection.

12. **e. a reasonable option for BCG failures after one course of therapy.** Combined therapy with BCG and interferon-α has shown activity in BCG failures and is one viable option for this challenging patient population. However, it is more expensive and there are no data to suggest that it is more effective than BCG alone. BCG remains the treatment of choice for CIS. BCG and interferon-α is well tolerated with a side effect profile that is better on average than BCG alone because most of the side effects are related to the BCG and its dose is reduced in this regimen.

13. **d. irritative voiding symptoms and myelosuppression.** Irritative voiding symptoms are reported by 12% to 69% of patients receiving intravesical thiotepa. The low molecular weight of this agent (189 kD) predisposes to systemic absorption and myelosuppression. These are the two most common side effects of this agent.

14. **e. All of the above.** Data about long-term outcomes for patients with high-risk superficial bladder cancer treated with intravesical BCG therapy are derived primarily from the experience of Memorial Sloan-Kettering (Cookson et al, 1997).* In this series 50% of patients progressed, and one third died of cancer progression. Approximately one third developed disease in the prostatic fossa or upper tracts and only 27% survived with an intact bladder. Such data should be considered when counseling patients about treatment options for high-risk disease.

15. **d. 30% to 50%.** The risk of understaging of a pT1G3 bladder tumor is about 30%, but it is even higher if there is no muscularis propria in the specimen. Altogether, the risk is about 30% to 50% in this high-risk patient population.

16. **a. is not indicated.** The incidence of upper tract tumor associated with pTaG1 bladder cancer is extremely low (0.3% to 2.3%), and current consensus is that upper tract imaging is not indicated in this patient population (Oosterlinck et al, 2005).

17. **e. are not indicated in most cases.** The yield of random bladder biopsy in patients with low-grade, low-stage bladder tumors and a negative cytology is low and is not indicated unless high-risk features are present.

18. **e. greater than 45%.** Untreated CIS is very high risk (>50%) for progressing to muscle-invasive disease. Even patients with a complete response to intravesical BCG will experience progression in 30% to 40% of cases on longitudinal follow-up (Sylvester et al, 2005).

19. **e. not prospectively validated.** Almost all studies of p53 as a prognostic marker have been retrospective to date. Although promising, this marker will require prospective validation before it can be generally used for clinical decision making. However, the balance of available data has

---

*Sources referenced can be found in *Campbell-Walsh Urology, 10th Edition,* on the Expert Consult website.

been promising, and the use of this marker for decision making in challenging cases has been advocated by many in this field. Most studies suggest that p53 is not a good predictor of response to BCG therapy, and it is clearly not better than grade for predicting outcomes for pTa disease. Its ultimate role for predicting progression for pT1G3 tumors is not well defined at present.

20. **b. pTaG3.** pTaG1 represents 50% to 70% of all non–muscle-invasive bladder tumors and is the most common of these entities. CIS is commonly associated with high-grade tumors and, overall, is found in about 10% to 20% of non–muscle-invasive bladder tumors. pT1G3 is found in about 20% of patients with non–muscle-invasive bladder tumors. pT2-3 represents about 20% of all bladder cancer patients. pTaG3 is often misclassified and in reality only represents about 5% to 10% of all non–muscle-invasive tumors (Sylvester et al, 2005).

Additional Study Points

1. Low-grade Ta bladder cancer recurs at a rate of 50% to 70% and progresses in approximately 5%.
2. High-grade T1 lesions recur in more than 80% of cases and progress in 30% to 50%.
3. The most important risk factor for progression is grade.
4. A nodular or sessile appearance suggests deeper invasion.
5. Lymphovascular invasion increases the risk of muscularis propria invasion.
6. Hydronephrosis is often but not always associated with muscularis propria invasion.
7. Papillary low-grade tumors can often be removed with the resectoscope loop without the use of electrocautery.
8. A separate biopsy of the base of the tumor should be obtained after initial resection.
9. Tumors about the ureteral orifice should be resected with pure cutting current.
10. Mitomycin C is the most effective adjuvant intravesicle therapy and, when used, should be administered within 6 hours of tumor resection.
11. All chemotherapy should be withheld when there is an extensive resection or when there is a concern that a perforation may have occurred.
12. BCG should never be administered immediately following a tumor resection.
13. The mechanism of action of BCG is initially binding to fibronectin and then the production of multiple cytokines.
14. After induction therapy, patients receiving maintenance BCG have a statistically significant decrease in recurrence rate compared with those receiving induction therapy alone.
15. BCG may delay the progression of high-risk bladder cancer; however, ultimately there may be no difference in long-term survival. Indeed, if the patient is followed long enough, there may be no effect on progression.
16. Quinolones should not be administered with BCG.
17. BCG plus interferon-α has a potential role regardless of prior BCG experience.
18. Risk factors for progression in patients with non–muscularis propria–invasive bladder cancer include high grade, tumors invading deeply into the lamina propria, lymphovascular invasion, associated CIS, and disease that is refractory to initial therapy.
19. Although upper tract disease occurs in 4% to 6% of patients, when it does occur the mortality rate is 40% to 70%.

Management of Metastatic and Invasive Bladder Cancer

Seth P. Lerner, MD, FACS ● Cora N. Sternberg, MD, FACP

QUESTIONS

1. A 52-year-old woman with a remote history of carcinoma in situ (CIS) for which she received bacille Calmette-Guérin (BCG) treatment has a new T1G3 tumor completely resected. There is scant muscularis propria in the transurethral resection of the bladder tumor (TURBT) specimen. The next step is:
   a. reinduce with BCG plus maintenance BCG.
   b. administer BCG treatment plus interferon-α.
   c. have the patient receive intravesical chemotherapy with valrubicin or gemcitabine.
   d. re-resect with muscularis propria in the specimen.
   e. have the patient undergo a radical cystectomy.

2. A 55-year-old woman is found to have a 3-cm nodular lesion in the bladder dome, which on histology is determined to be small cell carcinoma, deeply invasive into the lamina propria but with negative muscularis propria involvement. Random biopsies and urine cytology are negative. CT scans of the thorax, abdomen, and pelvis are normal. The best initial treatment is:
   a. intravesical BCG with later maintenance.
   b. repeat TURBT within 6 weeks to assess for residual disease or understaging.
   c. partial cystectomy.
   d. radical cystectomy.
   e. neoadjuvant systemic chemotherapy.

3. A 57-year-old man undergoes a TURBT of a sessile bladder tumor. The pathology reveals a T1TCC. Before deciding on additional treatment, a repeat resection must be done if the pathology has:
   a. lymphovascular invasion.
   b. CIS.
   c. G3 disease.
   d. no muscularis propria.
   e. no muscularis mucosa.

4. A 42-year-old potent man is diagnosed with a 4-cm micropapillary transitional cell carcinoma (TCC) that extensively invades the lamina propria. Muscularis propria is present and not involved. Lymphovascular invasion is identified. The next step is:

   a. restaging TURBT and intravesical BCG if muscle invasion is absent.
   b. partial cystectomy followed by radiation therapy.
   c. neoadjuvant cisplatin-based chemotherapy followed by radical cystectomy.
   d. nerve-sparing radical cystectomy.
   e. cisplatin-based chemotherapy and radiation therapy.

5. An orthotopic neobladder in a woman undergoing anterior pelvic exenteration for muscle invasive bladder cancer is contraindicated in the setting of:
   a. age older than 75.
   b. nodal metastases.
   c. recurrent urinary tract infection (UTI).
   d. bilateral hydronephrosis.
   e. posterior tumor invading the anterior vaginal wall.

6. A 65-year-old man undergoes three cycles of neoadjuvant M-VAC chemotherapy for T3bNXM0 TCC. After completing chemotherapy, there is no tumor on TURBT. The next step should be:
   a. observation with cystoscopy in 3 months.
   b. BCG weekly for 6 weeks.
   c. bladder biopsies.
   d. radiation therapy.
   e. radical cystectomy.

7. Which of the following immunohistochemistry profiles in bladder cancer is associated with the most aggressive tendencies?
   a. High p53 and Rb staining, low Ki67 and E-cadherin
   b. High p53 and Ki67 staining, absent Rb and E-cadherin
   c. High Rb and E-cadherin, low p53 and Ki67
   d. High Ki67 and Rb, low p53 and E-cadherin
   e. Low p53, Rb, E-cadherin and Ki-67

8. A 53-year-old woman with a T2NXM0 bladder TCC undergoes a radical cystectomy and continent diversion. Final pathology shows pT3a N1 with a single microscopic positive lymph node in the perivesical fat. The next step is to undergo:
   a. a PET/CT scan.
   b. adjuvant chemotherapy.
   c. adjuvant radiotherapy.

d. combined radiotherapy and chemotherapy.

e. more extensive lymphadenectomy.

9. A 48-year-old otherwise healthy man has a CT scan and TURBT, which reveal a T4aNXM0 TCC of the bladder. The next step is:

   a. neoadjuvant chemotherapy followed by radical cystectomy.

   b. radical cystectomy followed by adjuvant chemotherapy.

   c. radical cystectomy and then check tumor p53 status (if altered, give chemotherapy).

   d. preoperative radiotherapy followed by radical cystectomy.

   e. neoadjuvant chemotherapy with restaging bladder biopsies and surveillance if no clinical evidence of cancer.

10. A 62-year-old man has T3b invasive bladder TCC. Transurethral resection biopsy of the prostatic urethra shows a single focus of CIS. He does not want an external appliance. At the time of cystectomy he should have:

    a. frozen section of apical urethra margin and, if negative, an orthotopic neobladder.

    b. urethrectomy and continent cutaneous diversion.

    c. urethrectomy and ileal conduit.

    d. preoperative radiation therapy followed by cystectomy.

    e. bladder salvage with chemoradiation therapy.

11. A 58-year-old male former smoker with a past history of cystectomy for a T3bN1 invasive bladder cancer has a CT scan 5 years later that reveals one pulmonary lesion. The next step is:

    a. cisplatin chemotherapy.

    b. systemic cisplatin-based combination chemotherapy.

    c. preoperative radiotherapy followed by removal of the lung lesion.

    d. radiation therapy to the lung lesion alone.

    e. evaluation for possible lung primary carcinoma.

12. A 65-year-old patient, who has had neoadjuvant M-VAC chemotherapy and cystectomy 6 months ago for a T3bN1 invasive bladder cancer, presents with multiple lung lesions. The next treatment that should be considered is:

    a. cisplatin single-agent chemotherapy.

    b. repeat M-VAC chemotherapy.

    c. pemetrexed and gemcitabine combination chemotherapy.

    d. gemcitabine and paclitaxel combination chemotherapy.

    e. radiotherapy to the lung lesions.

ANSWERS

1. **d. re-resect with muscularis propria in the specimen.** Re-resection into muscularis propria is required for accurate staging of T1 cancers. European Association of Urology (EAU) and American Urological Association (AUA) guidelines are consistent regarding the need for routine re-resection of all T1G3 tumors. The understaging rate of T1 tumors is as high as 40% and is highest when there is no muscularis propria in the specimen (Dutta, 2001).* Treating with intravesical immunotherapy or chemotherapy before accurate staging risks missing T2 disease for which

intravesical treatment is inadequate therapy and survival probabilities are significantly reduced compared with cystectomy for less than T2 disease (Schrier et al, 2004).

2. **e. neoadjuvant systemic chemotherapy.** Small cell carcinoma is a rare variant of urothelial cancer that can comprise 100% or a fraction of the tumor. Its biologic behavior appears similar to small cell lung carcinoma with a high propensity for metastatic disease. Consensus opinion favors neoadjuvant chemotherapy with etoposide and cisplatin or enrollment in a clinical trial testing novel agents followed by either radical cystectomy or radiotherapy (Siefker-Radtke et al, 2004; Bex et al, 2009).

3. **d. no muscularis propria.** The understaging risk is up to 60% when there is no muscularis propria in the TUR specimen (Dutta, 2001). AUA and EAU guidelines are consistent in recommending this in all patients with T1G3 urothelial bladder cancer (www.uroweb.org; www.auanet.org). Upstaging to T2 is associated with a significant increased risk for cancer specific mortality (Dalbagni et al, 2009).

4. **d. nerve-sparing radical cystectomy.** Kamat and colleagues (2006) reported 44 patients with micropapillary non–muscle-invasive bladder cancer. Of 27 patients treated with BCG, 67% progressed to muscle invasive cancer including 22% with metastatic disease. Thirty patients underwent cystectomy, and only 19% remained alive with their bladder in place. On this basis, the current recommendation is to proceed directly to cystectomy. This patient should be offered nerve-sparing surgery, which is not associated with an increased risk of local pelvic recurrence.

5. **e. posterior tumor invading the anterior vaginal wall.** The distal two thirds of the female urethra may serve as an adequate sphincter mechanism provided the risk of cancer in the retained urethra is low (Schilling et al, 2008). Anterior vaginal wall involvement by a posterior-based bladder tumor or bladder neck or urethra involvement is a contraindication to urethra sparing and orthotopic bladder replacement because one cannot get an adequate distal vaginal margin and urethra margin (Stein et al, 1998). Age is not a contraindication as long as there is good pelvic support minimizing the risk of stress incontinence and the patient is capable of intermittent catheterization should the need arise. Nodal metastasis is associated with a 15% local recurrence rate with only a modest risk of invasion of the neobladder, and a thorough node dissection minimizes this risk (Lerner, 2009). Bilateral hydronephrosis while indicating a deeply invasive cancer is not a de facto contraindication (Stimson et al, 2010). UTI should be controlled before surgery, and any structural upper tract anomalies that may contribute to the risk of UTI should be resolved.

6. **e. radical cystectomy.** On average, 50% of patients with a clinical complete response have residual cancer in the radical cystectomy specimen (Sternberg et al, 2003). Failure to consolidate chemotherapy with surgery to remove the bladder or partial cystectomy in the case of a small (<3 cm) tumor in an area suitable for this approach exposes the patient to the risk of progression and lower survival probability.

7. **b. High p53 and Ki67 staining, absent Rb and E-cadherin.** High p53 nuclear immunoreactivity reflects the prolonged half-life of the altered p53 protein and is associated with a higher probability of recurrence following

---

*Sources referenced can be found in *Campbell-Walsh Urology, 10th Edition*, on the Expert Consult website.

cystectomy. Loss of Rb (retinoblastoma) immunoreactivity is associated with altered RB gene function and worse prognosis, and the combination of p53 and Rb alterations combined confers a worse prognosis than when only one or the other biomarker is altered (Chaterjee et al, 2003; Shariat et al, 2004). Increased Ki-67 staining reflects increased proliferation. E-cadherin is a cell adhesion molecule, and loss of E-cadherin has been associated with more advanced disease and worse prognosis in several studies (Byrne et al, 2001; Margulis et al, 2009).

8. **b. adjuvant chemotherapy.** Adjuvant cisplatin-based combination chemotherapy should be considered. Randomized trials have thus far not been definitive in overall survival on this subject. A meta-analysis suggests a 9% absolute benefit in overall survival, but the trials represent small numbers of patients, often closed early or due to poor accrual, and not all of the patients in adjuvant chemotherapy trials are represented (Advanced Bladder Cancer Meta-analysis Collaboration, 2005a).

9. **a. neoadjuvant chemotherapy followed by radical cystectomy.** Neoadjuvant chemotherapy with cisplatin-based combination chemotherapy has demonstrated a 5% absolute benefit in overall survival in a meta-analysis using individual patient data on 3005 patients from 11 randomized trials treated with neoadjuvant chemotherapy (Advanced Bladder Cancer Meta-analysis Collaboration, 2005b).

10. **a. frozen section of apical urethra margin and, if negative, an orthotopic neobladder.** CIS of the prostatic urethra is a risk factor for developing a second primary urothelial cancer of the retained urethra. However, in the setting of an orthotopic neobladder the risk of a second primary tumor of the retained urethra is less than 5% (Stein et al, 2005). The only contraindication to performing an orthotopic neobladder is a positive apical urethra margin and inability to achieve a negative margin of the retained urethra (Lerner et al, 2008b). Urethrectomy is never indicated solely on the basis of focal CIS of the prostatic urethra.

11. **e. evaluation for possible lung primary carcinoma.** Patients with a history of smoking may also develop second tumors such as lung cancer. In this case a single lesion may represent a primary tumor, which could be completely resected (El-Hakim et al, 2004).

12. **d. gemcitabine and paclitaxel combination chemotherapy.** After cisplatin-based combination chemotherapy with M-VAC, good results have been obtained in the second-line setting with a combination of gemcitabine and paclitaxel combination chemotherapy (Sternberg et al, 2001).

Additional Study Points

1. Among those with muscularis propria–invasive bladder cancer, 80% present with it at initial presentation.
2. Deaths due to bladder cancer invariably occur as a result of distant metastases present at the time of local regional therapy and usually occur within the first 2 years following treatment. Therefore muscularis propria–invasive bladder cancer should be considered a systemic disease.
3. The micropapillary variant is an aggressive disease and does not respond particularly well to chemotherapy.
4. T-1 grade 3 bladder tumors should routinely be re-resected because understaging is not an uncommon event.
5. Fat can be observed in the bladder wall and should not be confused with perivesical fat.
6. Lymphatic and vascular invasion is a risk factor for metastases.
7. Following chemotherapy, metastases may occur in unusual locations such as the central nervous system.
8. The incidence of pelvic node metastases is directly related to the depth of invasion and the presence of lymphovascular invasion.
9. Up to 50% of patients with muscularis propria–invasive bladder cancer succumb to their disease.
10. Of the randomized trials evaluating neoadjuvant therapy, none have shown a definite survival advantage.
11. Appropriate candidates for bladder preservation (transurethral tumor resection, chemotherapy and radiation therapy thereby preserving the bladder) are those who have solitary T-2 lesions of small diameter with no associated hydronephrosis and a visibly complete resection. The patient should have normal renal function.
12. Up to 15% of patients with muscularis propria invasive tumors have no residual disease following transurethral tumor resection.
13. Factors that affect outcome include stage, performance, status, lymphovascular invasion, age, gender, and histology.
14. Predictors of a poor prognosis include poor performance status and the presence of visceral metastases.

Surgery for Bladder Cancer

Ryan Kent Berglund, MD ● Harry W. Herr, MD

QUESTIONS

1. Which of the following statements regarding the arterial supply to the bladder is TRUE?
   a. The inferior vesical artery arises from the posterior trunk of the internal iliac artery.
   b. The superior vesical artery arises from the anterior trunk of the internal iliac artery.
   c. The majority of the blood supply to the bladder is derived from the obturator artery.
   d. The inferior gluteal artery sends no branches to the bladder.
   e. The bladder cannot be mobilized substantially because of its tenuous blood supply.

2. Which of the following statements regarding cold-cup biopsy of bladder lesions is TRUE?
   a. It is useful for biopsy of large bladder tumors.
   b. It is most amenable to lesions on the inside of the bladder neck.
   c. It is difficult to perform through a standard cystoscope.
   d. It requires suprapubic pressure if the lesion is located on the trigone.
   e. It allows for better tissue procurement without coagulation defects when compared with standard loop resection.

3. Tumor characteristics that would allow for transurethral resection as the sole treatment for muscle-invasive disease include which of the following?
   a. High grade
   b. Multifocal
   c. Papillary
   d. Tumor base larger than 2 cm
   e. Sessile

4. A suitable bowel preparation for a radical cystectomy should include all of the following EXCEPT:
   a. a cathartic such as GoLYTELY.
   b. metronidazole.
   c. gentamicin.
   d. neomycin.
   e. a clear liquid diet.

5. What is the cephalad limit to a standard pelvic lymphadenectomy?
   a. Peritoneal reflection
   b. Bifurcation of the common iliac artery
   c. Vas deferens
   d. Median umbilical ligament
   e. Node of Cloquet

6. What is the mortality rate associated with radical cystectomy?
   a. 0.1% to 0.2%
   b. 1% to 3%
   c. 5% to 7%
   d. 9% to 11%
   e. 15% to 17%

7. What is the incidence of urethral recurrence after radical cystoprostatectomy?
   a. 0.5% to 4%
   b. 4% to 18%
   c. 19% to 28%
   d. 29% to 37%
   e. 38% to 48%

8. Which of the following statements regarding urethrectomy in the male is TRUE?
   a. The dissection is much easier if carried out several weeks after radical cystectomy.
   b. Drainage is not recommended after urethrectomy.
   c. The bulbar urethral arteries should be preserved throughout the dissection.
   d. When a urethrectomy is performed, the best position for the patient is the exaggerated lithotomy.
   e. It is necessary to split the glans to remove all of the transitional cell epithelium at the meatus.

9. Which of the following statements regarding urethral involvement in bladder cancer in the female patient is TRUE?
   a. Female patients have a much higher incidence of urethral involvement than do male patients.
   b. Orthotopic bladder substitution can rarely be used in the female patient because of the risk of urethral recurrence.

c. Intraoperative frozen section is the best way to determine whether the urethra is suitable for orthotopic reconstruction.

d. Tumor involvement at the bladder neck always signifies urethral involvement.

e. Incidence of urethral involvement in female patients has been shown to be consistently above 15%.

10. A complete anterior exenteration in the female includes all of the following procedures EXCEPT:

a. cystectomy.

b. hysterectomy.

c. bilateral pelvic lymphadenectomy.

d. pubovaginal sling.

e. partial vaginectomy.

11. All of the following can be considered indications for simple cystectomy EXCEPT:

a. pyocystis in a neurogenic bladder.

b. colovesical fistula after urinary diversion.

c. urachal adenocarcinoma.

d. hemorrhagic cystitis resulting from cyclophosphamide.

e. pain and incomplete emptying in patients with prior supravesical diversions.

12. What is the advantage of partial cystectomy over total cystectomy in the management of bladder cancer?

a. More accurate staging

b. Improved survival

c. Preservation of bladder and sexual function

d. Possibility of using surveillance cystoscopy

e. Lower recurrence rates of tumor

13. Which of the following is a contraindication to partial cystectomy?

a. Tumor location at the dome of the bladder

b. Grade 1 transitional cell carcinoma

c. Tumor within a bladder diverticulum

d. Multifocal tumor associated with multifocal carcinoma in situ (CIS)

e. Urachal adenocarcinoma

14. Which of the following statements about pelvic lymphadenectomy is NOT correct?

a. Extended dissection to the aortic bifurcation is associated with increased incidence of lymphocele.

b. En bloc resection yields fewer lymph nodes than dissecting separate packets.

c. Extended lymphadenectomy improves survival in N0 patients.

d. Extended lymphadenectomy improves survival in patients with limited lymph node metastases.

e. The lateral extent of the dissection is the genitofemoral nerve.

15. All of the following are vascular branches off of the internal iliac artery EXCEPT:

a. obturator artery.

b. internal pudendal artery.

c. inferior epigastric artery.

d. medial umbilical ligament.

e. superior gluteal artery.

16. The cavernous nerves that facilitate erection originate from the:

a. nervi erigentes.

b. superior hypogastric plexus.

c. obturator nerve.

d. pudendal nerve.

e. genitofemoral nerve.

17. Vascular control during radical cystoprostatectomy in the male patient is essential at each of the following locations EXCEPT:

a. dorsal venous complex of the penis.

b. superior vesical artery.

c. lateral vesical pedicles.

d. posterior vascular pedicle between rectum and Denonvilliers fascia.

e. prostatic pedicles.

18. Which of the following is a contraindication to vagina-preserving cystectomy?

a. CIS of the distal right ureter

b. Clinical stage T3 cancer noted on examination under anesthesia

c. Multifocal high-grade Ta transitional cell carcinoma

d. Having received neoadjuvant chemotherapy

e. History of urge urinary incontinence

19. Restaging transurethral resection of the bladder is indicated to rule out:

a. tentacular spread of the primary tumor.

b. multifocal CIS.

c. prostatic involvement.

d. incomplete initial resection.

e. all of the above.

20. Elements unique to radical surgery for cancer include all of the following EXCEPT:

a. wide local excision.

b. lymphadenectomy.

c. removal of contiguous nonessential organs.

d. avoidance of tumor violation and spillage.

e. copious irrigation of the surgical field after en bloc specimen removal.

21. The cavernous nerves lie in close proximity to all of the following structures that are encountered during radical cystoprostatectomy EXCEPT the:

a. superior vesical artery.

b. seminal vesicles.

c. lateral prostatic fascia.

d. dorsal venous complex of the penis.

e. prostatic pedicles.

22. Urethrectomy should be performed at the time of radical cystoprostatectomy when there is/are:

a. CIS in the prostate.

b. pathologic T3 disease in the bladder trigone.

c. planned ileal conduit urinary diversion.

d. frozen section positive deep obturator lymph nodes.

e. grossly positive urethral frozen section margin.

23. Lymph nodes that should be included in a standard lymphadenectomy include all of the following EXCEPT:

a. Cloquet node.

b. presacral.

c. deep obturator.

d. external iliac.

e. common iliac.

24. Urachal adenocarcinoma:

a. is often treated with partial cystectomy.

b. is histologically similar to adenocarcinoma of the colon.

c. requires concurrent en bloc umbilectomy at partial cystectomy.

d. frequently metastasizes.

e. is all of the above.

ANSWERS

1. **b. The superior vesical artery arises from the anterior trunk of the internal iliac artery.** The urinary bladder has a rich blood supply derived from the superior and inferior vesical branches that arise from the anterior trunk of the internal iliac artery and by smaller branches from the obturator and internal gluteal arteries.

2. **e. It allows for better tissue procurement without coagulation defects when compared with standard loop resection.** If the bladder lesion is small, it may be amenable to cold-cup biopsy and fulguration. This technique has the advantage of tissue procurement without coagulation defects from the resectoscope.

3. **c. Papillary.** No randomized studies have compared transurethral resection alone with cystectomy. However, there is probably a small subset of patients with stage T2 transitional cell carcinoma who may be candidates for resection therapy alone. These patients are likely to have tumors that are small, solitary, papillary, moderately differentiated, less than 2 cm in diameter at the tumor base, and stage T2 or minimal stage T3a.

4. **c. gentamicin.** Clear liquids are recommended for the 2 days before surgery. Polyethylene glycol-electrolyte solution (GoLYTELY) is given on the day before surgery, and oral antibiotics containing either neomycin or erythromycin base and metronidazole are administered on the day before surgery.

5. **b. Bifurcation of the common iliac artery.** The bifurcation of the common iliac artery is the cephalad limit of the dissection.

6. **b. 1% to 3%.** The operative mortality rate for radical cystectomy has been shown to be between 1% and 3% in most modern series.

7. **b. 4% to 18%.** The incidence of urethral recurrence has been documented in prior studies to be between 4% and 18%.

8. **d. When a urethrectomy is performed, the best position for the patient is the exaggerated lithotomy.** The urethrectomy from the perineal approach is most easily performed with the patient in the exaggerated lithotomy position.

9. **c. Intraoperative frozen section is the best way to determine whether the urethra is suitable for orthotopic reconstruction.** An intraoperative frozen section of the proximal urethra should now be considered the best way to determine whether a female patient is a suitable candidate for orthotopic neobladder.

10. **d. pubovaginal sling.** The anterior approach has advantages in that it allows for simultaneous pelvic lymphadenectomy, cystectomy, urethrectomy, hysterectomy, salpingo-oophorectomy, and partial vaginectomy if clinically indicated for extensive carcinomatous involvement.

11. **c. urachal adenocarcinoma.** Various benign conditions that may warrant simple cystectomy include pyocystis, neurogenic bladder, severe urinary incontinence, severe urethral trauma, large vesical fistula, cyclophosphamide cystitis, and radiation cystitis after treatment of other pelvic malignancies.

12. **c. Preservation of bladder and sexual function.** The benefits of partial cystectomy include complete pathologic staging of the tumor and pelvic lymph nodes, as well as preservation of both bladder and sexual function.

13. **d. Multifocal tumor associated with multifocal carcinoma in situ (CIS).** Absolute contraindications to partial cystectomy would include multifocal CIS.

14. **a. Extended dissection to the aortic bifurcation is associated with increased incidence of lymphocele.** An extended pelvic lymphadenectomy does increase operating time but has not been associated with increased complications such as lymphocele, bleeding, or deep venous thrombosis. Submitting separate node packets significantly increases the yield of nodes compared with an en bloc resection. The increased number of lymph nodes resected has improved survival in patients with both negative nodes and limited lymph node metastases.

15. **c. inferior epigastric artery.** The inferior epigastric artery originates from the external iliac artery and anastomoses with the superior epigastric artery along the rectus abdominis muscle. The obturator artery leaves the pelvis via the obturator foramen, where it supplies muscular and bony structures outside the pelvis. The internal pudendal artery supplies the blood supply to the external genitalia. The medial umbilical ligament is a paired structure that is the obliterated remnant of the paired fetal umbilical arteries. The superior gluteal artery is the first and largest branch of the internal iliac artery posteriorly that supplies much of the blood supply to the gluteus maximus muscle. When ligating the internal iliac for bleeding, the ligation should be applied distal to this branch to prevent claudication.

16. **a. nervi erigentes.** The nervi erigentes or pelvic splanchnic nerves arise from the spinal sacral nerves (S2-S4) to provide parasympathetic innervation to facilitate erection. The superior hypogastric plexus contains postganglionic nerves, which stimulate emission and ejaculation. The obturator nerve supplies motor innervation for thigh adduction. The pudendal nerve provides sensory input from the external genitalia and motor output from the urinary and rectal sphincters. The genitofemoral nerve provides sensory input from the anterior thigh and scrotal and labial skin and motor input to the cremasteric muscle.

17. **d. posterior vascular pedicle between rectum and Denonvilliers fascia.** The plane between Denonvilliers fascia and the anterior rectal wall represents an avascular

plane with limited blood supply. The superior vesical artery is a major branch of the internal iliac and contributes to the majority of the superior pedicle blood supply to the bladder. The lateral vesical pedicles are a clustering of arteries and veins supplied laterally via the internal iliac artery and vein. Control of the dorsal vein of the penis is an essential step in prostatic apical dissection. The prostatic pedicles are the distal-most blood supply originating from the lateral major blood vessels.

18. **b. Clinical stage T3 cancer noted on examination under anesthesia.** Clinical stage T3 cancer is at high risk of local invasion of the bladder wall, and anterior pelvic exenteration should be performed. CIS of the ureter plays no role in vaginal-sparing surgery. Multifocal high-grade Ta TCC in and of itself is not a contraindication to vaginal preservation if confirmed on restaging TUR. TUR should be performed after neoadjuvant chemotherapy for restaging, and if organ confined disease is confirmed, vaginal sparing is acceptable. Urge urinary incontinence is a local symptom in the bladder and does not necessarily represent locally advanced disease.

19. **e. all of the above.** Microscopic tentacular spread of the primary tumor is a common source of early recurrence of tumor. Multifocal CIS can be ruled out by sampling several distinct areas of the bladder. Noting prostatic involvement is necessary for both staging and surgical planning if a neobladder is being considered. Initial resection is often not complete due to poor visualization with bleeding and cautery artifact.

20. **c. removal of contiguous nonessential organs.** Although indicated in certain radical surgeries, not all contiguous nonessential organs must be removed. Wide local excision with a buffering zone of normal adjacent tissue is necessary to prevent positive surgical margins. Lymphadenectomy is both a diagnostic and therapeutic procedure in radical surgery for bladder cancer. Tumor violation and spillage contribute to local recurrence. Copious irrigation can help reduce local recurrence from inadvertently spilled tumor cells.

21. **a. superior vesical artery.** The nervi erigentes originate in the sacral plexus and travel laterally along the rectal wall, providing branches to the genital organs via the cavernous nerves. The superior vesical artery is not located near these delicate structures. The nerve enters the prostatic fascia on the posterolateral surface of the prostate distal to the prostatic pedicles. The nerves course along to the apex of the prostate below the dorsal venous complex of the penis, and from there they innervate the cavernosal bodies.

22. **e. grossly positive urethral frozen section margin.** A grossly positive urethral frozen section margin indicates urethral involvement of disease, and formal urethrectomy should be performed at that time to prevent a positive surgical margin and prevent future recurrence. CIS in the prostate does not necessitate urethrectomy unless there is urethral involvement at the margin. Otherwise, routine urethrectomy is unnecessary in cases of locally confined, locally advanced, and metastatic disease.

23. **a. Cloquet node.** This is the superior-most deep inguinal lymph node and is rarely involved in metastatic bladder cancer. All of the other nodes are in the drainage distribution of the bladder and should be included in a standard lymph node dissection.

24. **e. is all of the above.** Urachal adenocarcinoma is an aggressive disease that frequently metastasizes. Due to its occurrence in the bladder dome in areas of colonic metaplasia, its location is conducive to partial cystectomy. En bloc umbilectomy is necessary at the time of surgery, though, due to the urachus being embryologically continuous with the umbilicus. Microscopically, urachal adenocarcinoma resembles colorectal cancers.

Additional Study Points

1. Before endoscopic treatment of bladder cancer, the patient should have upper tract imaging.
2. Initial transurethral resection of a bladder tumor should routinely be performed to include muscle. There should be a 2- to 3-cm visibly negative margin on the surface.
3. Immediately following transurethral resection of bladder tumors, intravesical installation of doxorubicin or mitomycin-C modestly reduces recurrences but has little effect on progression.
4. Bacille Calmette-Guérin should never be instilled immediately following bladder tumor resection.
5. Before a cystectomy, the sight of the abdominal stoma should be marked by an enterostomal therapist with the patient awake so that the proper location may be ascertained.
6. If prostate- or prostate capsule-sparing techniques are to be used in orthotopic bladder construction, preoperative evaluation to rule out occult cancer—either transitional cell or prostate adenocarcinoma—should be performed.
7. A radical cystectomy in the female includes complete removal of the urethra including the meatus.
8. Patients amenable to partial cystectomy should have a solitary lesion without associated CIS in which a 2-cm margin may be obtained, which is far enough away from the ureteral orifices and bladder neck so that closure can be accomplished without compromising these structures.
9. Sixty-four percent of patients undergoing radical cystectomy have at least one perioperative complication in the first 3 months postoperative; 13% experience high-grade complications. The majority of complications are gastrointestinal.
10. The boundaries of a standard lymph node dissection are the genitofemoral nerve laterally, internal iliac artery medially, Cooper ligament caudally, and crossing of the ureter at the common iliac artery cranially.

Robotic and Laparoscopic Bladder Surgery

Lee Richstone, MD ● Douglas S. Scherr, MD

QUESTIONS

1. Laparoscopic ureteral reimplantation can be performed:
   a. with a cross-trigonal approach.
   b. with a Boari flap or bladder advancement flap.
   c. with a psoas hitch.
   d. via a traditional laparoscopic or robotic approach.
   e. with all of the above.

2. All of the following are essential surgical aspects of the Boari flap or bladder advancement flap EXCEPT:
   a. An adequate-size bladder must be present (>300 mL).
   b. The contralateral vesical pedicle may be transected if necessary.
   c. The bladder flap should be slightly shorter than anticipated because bladder tissue can be easily stretched.
   d. A tension-free anastomosis is important.
   e. Typically, a refluxing ureteral anastomosis is created.

3. Principles of open, laparoscopic, or robotic vesicovaginal fistula repair include all of the following EXCEPT:
   a. good exposure of the fistulous tract.
   b. wide excision of the fibrous and scar tissue.
   c. tension-free repair of the vagina and bladder.
   d. interposition of a flap of peritoneum or omentum.
   e. adequate drainage.

4. Contraindications for laparoscopic enterocystoplasty include all of the following EXCEPT:
   a. diverticulosis.
   b. inflammatory bowel disease.
   c. renal failure.
   d. noncompliance.
   e. ulcerative colitis.

5. Which of the following statements is NOT correct regarding laparoscopic enterocystoplasty?
   a. Subtotal cystectomy may be necessary.
   b. The mesenteric pedicle of the selected bowel segment is wide and broad based.

   c. The mesenteric window is closed.
   d. Reestablishment of bowel continuity is a critical step of the operation and may be performed extracorporeally for added security, if necessary.
   e. Bowel-to-bladder anastomosis is optimally performed with interrupted serosa-to-serosa sutures.

6. Partial cystectomy may be performed in all of the following circumstances EXCEPT:
   a. tumor at the bladder dome.
   b. tumor in the bladder diverticulum.
   c. solitary invasive bladder tumor located at a distance from the ureteric orifices.
   d. history of multiple tumors or carcinoma in situ (CIS).
   e. good bladder capacity.

7. Which of the following statements is TRUE regarding partial cystectomy?
   a. Thirty to 40 percent of patients with bladder cancer are candidates for a partial cystectomy.
   b. Five-year survival rates range from 80% to 90%.
   c. Laparoscopic partial cystectomy is now an established procedure.
   d. All of the above
   e. None of the above

8. Which of the following is a contraindication for laparoscopic radical cystectomy today?
   a. Multiple bladder tumors
   b. Nonbulky, invasive bladder cancer
   c. T4 disease
   d. Moderate obesity
   e. Previous open pelvic surgery

9. Regarding radical cystectomy, all of the following have been performed laparoscopically EXCEPT:
   a. extended pelvic lymph node dissection.
   b. uterus- and vagina-sparing radical cystectomy.
   c. anterior pelvic exenteration in the female.
   d. orthotopic neobladder.
   e. Indiana pouch, constructed intracorporeally.

10. Anatomic boundaries of extended pelvic lymph node dissection include all of the following EXCEPT the:
    a. external iliac artery (lateral).
    b. obturator nerve (posterior).
    c. aortic bifurcation area (proximal).
    d. Cooper ligament.
    e. bladder (medial).

11. Future directions for laparoscopic radical cystectomy are likely to include which of the following?
    a. Careful, prospective, long-term evaluation of oncologic and functional outcomes
    b. Intracorporeal performance of radical cystectomy and extracorporeal performance of bowel work
    c. Elimination of bowel through use of novel bladder substitutes
    d. International collaboration
    e. All of the above

ANSWERS

1. **e. with all of the above.** All of the included answers are correct regarding laparoscopic ureteral reimplantation. Minimally invasive ureteral reimplantation can be performed in a refluxing or nonrefluxing fashion and with a cross-trigonal or tunneled approach if so desired. In cases with larger ureteral loss a Boari flap or bladder advancement flap can be used, or a psoas hitch can be performed replicating open techniques. Lastly, both laparoscopic and robotic approaches to ureteral reimplantation have been described.

2. **c. The bladder flap should be slightly shorter than anticipated because bladder tissue can be easily stretched.** A tension-free anastomosis of the anterolateral bladder flap based on the ipsilateral vesical pedicle is critical. The bladder flap should be somewhat longer and wider than anticipated because the nondistended bladder shrinks in size, thus placing tension on the anastomosis. Ideally, a flap length-to-breadth ratio of 3:1 ensures good vascularity of its apex.

3. **b. wide excision of the fibrous and scar tissue.** Wide circumferential excision of the fistula and associated scar tissue is not necessary and may not even be feasible. Only the fibrotic VVF tract and its edges need to be excised. Adequate mobilization of the anterior vaginal wall and posterior bladder wall is performed to achieve a tension-free repair. Care is taken not to compromise the ureteral orifices. An interposition graft of omentum is anchored between the vagina and the bladder with a stitch.

4. **a. diverticulosis.** The presence of bowel pathology such as diverticulitis or ulcerative colitis requires the use of alternative, nondiseased bowel segments. Similar to open surgery, laparoscopic enterocystoplasty should not be performed in the presence of advanced renal or liver failure, inflammatory bowel disease, or short gut syndrome or in a patient who is unable or noncompliant in performing intermittent catheterization reliably. Diverticulosis is not a contraindication for performing enterocystoplasty.

5. **e. Bowel-to-bladder anastomosis is optimally performed with interrupted serosa-to-serosa sutures.** The technical principles of enterocystoplasty are identical between open surgical and laparoscopic techniques. Generous mobilization of the bladder allows creation of an adequate anteroposterior cystotomy. Subtotal cystectomy is necessary only in patients with severely symptomatic interstitial cystitis. An optimal segment of bowel based on a broad, well-vascularized mesenteric pedicle that will reach the pelvis without tension is selected. The bowel segment is isolated, bowel continuity is reestablished by either intracorporeal or extracorporeal techniques, and the mesenteric window is closed. The isolated bowel segment is detubularized, and a bowel plate is created appropriately. A tension-free, watertight, full-thickness, circumferential, running anastomosis of the bowel segment to the bladder is created. Adequate urinary drainage is established.

6. **d. history of multiple tumors or carcinoma in situ (CIS).** Contraindications to partial cystectomy include multiple bladder tumors, tumors involving the bladder neck or posterior urethra or trigone, and concomitant carcinoma in situ. History or current evidence of multifocal transitional cell carcinoma with or without CIS is a contraindication for partial cystectomy. The ideal patient for partial cystectomy is one who has a solitary, organ-confined invasive bladder tumor located at the dome of a good-capacity bladder, without any concomitant multifocality or CIS.

7. **e. None of the above.** In large series of patients with bladder cancer, less than 10% of the patients are candidates for a partial cystectomy. In the properly selected patient, 5-year survival ranges from 50% to 70%. Laparoscopic partial cystectomy has only been performed in a few selected cases and is currently a controversial procedure.

8. **c. T4 disease.** Laparoscopic radical cystectomy is an emerging procedure performed at centers of laparoscopic expertise. At this writing, laparoscopic radical cystectomy should be offered to nonobese patients with nonbulky, organ-confined bladder cancer without pelvic lymphadenopathy on preoperative CT. Various conditions such as morbid obesity, prior radiotherapy, or pelvic surgery are relative contraindications because of the increase in laparoscopic technical complexity. Locally advanced T4 disease should not be approached laparoscopically.

9. **e. Indiana pouch, constructed intracorporeally.** Since the initial report of laparoscopic cystectomy in 1992 by Parra and colleagues, more than 300 laparoscopic radical cystectomies have been performed worldwide. In the female, laparoscopic anterior pelvic exenteration and uterus, fallopian tube, and vagina-sparing radical cystectomy have been performed. In the male, conventional radical cystectomy and prostate-sparing radical cystectomy have been performed. Bilateral extended pelvic lymph node dissection with mean nodal yields of 21 lymph nodes has been reported. With regard to urinary drainage, ileal conduit, Mainz pouch, Indiana pouch (extracorporeally constructed), and orthotopic neobladder have all been performed laparoscopically. However, long-term follow-up outcomes are still lacking.

10. **a. external iliac artery (lateral).** Laterally, the dissection is extended up to the genitofemoral nerve. At the conclusion of an extended bilateral pelvic lymph node dissection, the external and internal iliac artery and vein, common iliac artery, obturator nerve, pelvic side wall, and perivesical area should be bilaterally devoid of lymphatic fatty tissue.

11. **e. All of the above.** Laparoscopic radical cystectomy is an evolving treatment modality with increasing experience being reported from multiple centers worldwide. With earlier detection of bladder cancer, careful application of laparoscopic techniques, and meticulous long-term follow-up, laparoscopic radical cystectomy is likely to emerge as a viable treatment option for the selected patient with bladder cancer.

Additional Study Points

1. Bladder surgery and the associated urinary diversion are associated with some of the highest rates of complications in urologic surgery.
2. Bladder diverticulectomy may be indicated in those of considerable size in which there is incomplete emptying, chronic or repeated urinary tract infection, bladder calculi, pain, or malignancy.
3. Any outlet obstruction must be addressed before the time of diverticulectomy.
4. In constructing a Boari flap, it is critical to ensure that the base of the flap is wide enough to provide for adequate vascularity. The base should be at least twice as wide as the apex to prevent contracture.
5. Any patient considered for augmentation cystoplasty should be capable of self-intermittent catheterization.
6. In a partial cystectomy, a 2-cm margin should be outlined endoscopically with the electrocautery before opening the bladder because a decompressed bladder may distort the adequacy of the resection margin.

Use of Intestinal Segments in Urinary Diversion

Douglas M. Dahl, MD ● W. Scott McDougal, MD, MA (Hon)

QUESTIONS

1. When a portion of stomach is to be used for augmentation, it should:
   a. always be based on the right gastroepiploic artery.
   b. include only the antrum.
   c. never extend to the pylorus.
   d. include a significant portion of the lesser curve.
   e. be mobilized with the omentum.

2. The ileum differs from the jejunum in that:
   a. it has a larger diameter.
   b. the mesentery is thinner.
   c. it has multiple arcades.
   d. the vessels in the mesentery are larger.
   e. the mesentery is longer.

3. When stomach is used for urinary diversion, the electrolyte abnormality that may occur is most commonly what type of metabolic alkalosis?
   a. Hyperchloremic
   b. Hypochloremic
   c. Hyperkalemic
   d. Hypernatremic
   e. Hypocalcemic

4. Postoperative bowel obstruction is most common when which of the following segments is used for diversion?
   a. Right colon
   b. Stomach
   c. Sigmoid
   d. Ileum
   e. Transverse colon

5. Mechanical bowel preparation results in a reduction in:
   a. bacterial counts per gram of enteric contents.
   b. bacterial count in the jejunum.
   c. total number of bacteria in the bowel.
   d. bacterial counts in the stomach.
   e. bacterial counts in the ileum.

6. Systemic antibiotics in elective surgery should be given:
   a. before the patient is anesthetized.
   b. before the skin incision is made.
   c. intraoperatively before closure commences.
   d. any time in the perioperative period.
   e. for 3 to 5 days postoperative.

7. The most common cause of a lethal bowel complication is:
   a. use of prior irradiated bowel.
   b. lack of mechanical bowel prep.
   c. lack of antibiotic bowel prep.
   d. placement of a drain adjacent to the anastomosis.
   e. failure to give preoperative antibiotics.

8. When stapled anastomoses are compared to sutured anastomoses, there is/are:
   a. fewer leaks.
   b. less compatibility with urine.
   c. reduced overall operative time.
   d. lesser incidence of bowel obstruction.
   e. earlier return of bowel function.

9. The use of a nasogastric tube in the postoperative period:
   a. hastens the return of intestinal motility.
   b. reduces the incidence of bowel leak.
   c. reduces postoperative vomiting.
   d. increases the risk of aspiration.
   e. reduces the incidence of anastomotic leak.

10. The abdominal stoma for a conduit should be:
    a. flush with the skin.
    b. placed through the belly of the rectus muscle.
    c. made as a loop to reduce parastomal hernia.
    d. made with the colon for the least complication rate.
    e. placed in the right lower quadrant.

11. The loop end ileostomy is best used in:
    a. the obese patient.
    b. the thin patient.
    c. when a stoma is revised.

    d. in female patients.

    e. in spinal cord injury patients.

12. Ureteral strictures occurring after an ileal conduit not associated with the ureteral intestinal anastomosis most frequently occur:

    a. at the ureteral pelvic junction.

    b. in the right ureter several centimeters proximal to the ureteral intestinal anastomosis.

    c. on the left side where the ureter crosses the aorta.

    d. in the mid ureter.

    e. in either ureter within several centimeters proximal to the anastomosis.

13. Renal deterioration after a conduit diversion with normal kidneys occurs in what percent of renal units?

    a. 20%

    b. 40%

    c. 50%

    d. 70%

    e. 80%

14. The most common cause of death in patients with ureterosigmoidostomies over the long term is:

    a. cancer.

    b. renal failure.

    c. acid base abnormalities.

    d. the primary disease.

    e. ammonium intoxication.

15. The minimal glomerular filtration rate (GFR) in mL/min necessary for a continent diversion is:

    a. 70.

    b. 60.

    c. 35.

    d. 25.

    e. 20.

16. The urinary diversion with the least number of intraoperative and immediate postoperative complications is:

    a. ileal conduit.

    b. colon conduit.

    c. Koch pouch.

    d. Indiana pouch.

    e. neobladder.

17. The jejunal conduit syndrome is manifested by:

    a. hyperchloremic metabolic acidosis.

    b. hypochloremic metabolic alkalosis.

    c. hyperkalemic, hyponatremic metabolic acidosis.

    d. hypokalemic, hyponatremic metabolic alkalosis.

    e. hyperkalemic metabolic alkalosis.

18. The primary advantage of a transverse colon conduit is:

    a. its ease of construction.

    b. the ability to perform a nonrefluxing anastomosis.

    c. less likely to be injured by radiation.

    d. reduced electrolyte problems.

    e. equidistant from each kidney, allowing for short ureteral length on both sides.

19. Total body potassium depletion is most common in:

    a. ureterosigmoidostomy.

    b. ileal conduit.

    c. colon conduit.

    d. sigmoid conduit.

    e. gastrocystoplasty.

20. In urinary intestinal diversion serum creatinine may not be an accurate reflection of renal function because of:

    a. interfering substances.

    b. tubule secretion.

    c. tubule reabsorption.

    d. bowel reabsorption.

    e. decreased renal elimination.

21. Patients with urinary diversions who have a hyperchloremic metabolic acidosis over time:

    a. retain the ability to maintain the acidosis.

    b. lose the ability for electrolyte transport in the intestinal segments.

    c. compensate for the metabolic acidosis, thus eliminating risk.

    d. intermittently absorb ammonia when infection is present.

    e. tend to retain potassium.

22. Bone density abnormalities:

    a. are unlikely to occur with ileum.

    b. are most likely to occur with colon.

    c. are more common in patients with persistent hyperchloremic metabolic acidosis.

    d. are common in patients with total body potassium depletion.

    e. are unlikely to occur in patients with conduits.

23. Urinary intestinal diversion in children:

    a. increases the need for vitamin D.

    b. increases the need for calcium.

    c. limits linear growth.

    d. decreases epiphyseal growth.

    e. results in premature epiphyseal closure.

24. Cancer occurring in urinary intestinal diversion is most likely to occur in:

    a. augmentations.

    b. colon conduits.

    c. ileal conduits.

    d. ureterosigmoidostomies.

    e. sigmoid conduits.

25. Reconfiguring the bowel over the long term results in:

    a. decreased motor activity.

    b. increased volume.

    c. decreased metabolic complications.

    d. decreased absorption of solutes.

    e. increased absorption of solutes.

26. The syndrome of severe metabolic alkalosis in patients who have had a gastrocystoplasty is most likely to occur in patients who have:

a. decreased aldosterone levels.

b. jejunum interposed in the urinary tract.

c. total body potassium depletion.

d. elevated gastrin levels.

e. decreased renin levels.

Imaging

1. See Figure 85–1.

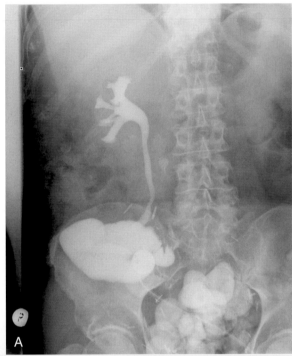

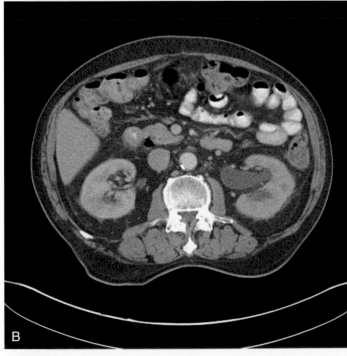

Figure 85–1.

A 72-year-old man who had a cystectomy and ileal conduit urinary diversion for high-grade, T3 transitional cell carcinoma undergoes a loopogram (*A*) and a contrast-enhanced CT scan (*B*). The most likely diagnosis is:

a. normal studies.

b. stricture at the left uretero-ileal anastomosis.

c. recurrent urothelial tumor.

d. technically poor-quality loopogram.

e. abnormal reflux into the right ureter and collecting system.

ANSWERS

1. **c. never extend to the pylorus.** When a wedge of fundus is employed, it should not include a significant portion of the antrum and should never extend to the pylorus or all the way to the lesser curve of the stomach.

2. **c. it has multiple arcades.** The ileum, being more distal in location, has a smaller diameter. It has multiple arterial arcades, and the vessels in the arcades are smaller than those in the jejunum.

3. **b. Hypochloremic.** Complications specific to the use of stomach include the hematuria-dysuria syndrome and uncontrollable metabolic alkalosis in some patients. When stomach is used, a hypochloremic, hypokalemic metabolic alkalosis may ensue.

4. **d. Ileum.** The incidence of postoperative bowel obstruction is 4% to 10%. Colon, stomach, and sigmoid obstruction result in a 4% incidence, less than that occurring with ileum.

5. **c. total number of bacteria in the bowel.** The mechanical preparation reduces the amount of feces, whereas the antibiotic preparation reduces the bacterial count. A mechanical bowel preparation reduces the total number of bacteria but not their concentration.

6. **a. before the patient is anesthetized.** Systemic antibiotics must be given before the operative event if they are to be effective.

7. **a. use of prior irradiated bowel.** In one study of urinary intestinal diversion, 75% of the lethal complications that occurred in the postoperative period were related to the bowel. Eighty percent of these patients had received radiation before the intestinal surgery.

8. **b. less compatibility with urine.** In general, anastomoses using reabsorbable sutures or reabsorbable staples are preferable for intestinal segments that are exposed to urine.

9. **c. reduces postoperative vomiting.** In several studies there was no significant difference in major intestinal complications between those who had postoperative nasogastric tubes and those who did not; however, those who did not have gastric decompression showed a much greater incidence of abdominal distention, nausea, and vomiting.

10. **b. placed through the belly of the rectus muscle.** All stomas should be placed through the belly of the rectus muscle and be located at the peak of the infraumbilical fat roll.

11. **a. the obese patient.** The loop end ileostomy is usually easier to perform than the ileal end stoma in the patient who is obese.

12. **c. on the left side where the ureter crosses the aorta.** Of importance is that ureteral strictures also occur

away from the ureterointestinal anastomosis. This stricture is most common in the left ureter and is usually found as the ureter crosses over the aorta beneath the inferior mesenteric artery.

13. **a. 20%.** Patients who are studied over the long term show a significant degree of renal deterioration. Indeed, 20% of renal units have shown significant anatomic deterioration.

14. **b. renal failure.** The most common cause of death in patients who have had a ureterosigmoidostomy for more than 15 years is acquired renal disease (i.e., sepsis or renal failure).

15. **b. 60.** If the patient is able to achieve a urine pH of 5.8 or less, can establish a urine osmolality of 600 mOsm/kg or greater in response to water deprivation, has a GFR that exceeds 60 mL/min, and has minimal protein in the urine, he or she may be considered for a retentive diversion.

16. **a. ileal conduit.** It is the simplest type of conduit diversion to perform and is associated with the fewest number of intraoperative and immediate postoperative complications.

17. **c. hyperkalemic, hyponatremic metabolic acidosis.** The early and long-term complications are similar to those listed for ileal conduit except that the electrolyte abnormality that occurs is hyperkalemic, hyponatremic metabolic acidosis instead of the hyperchloremic metabolic acidosis of ileal diversion.

18. **c. less likely to be injured by radiation.** The transverse colon is used when one wants to be sure that the segment of conduit employed has not been irradiated in individuals who have received extensive pelvic irradiation.

19. **a. ureterosigmoidostomy.** Hypokalemia and total body depletion of potassium may occur in patients with urinary intestinal diversion. This is more common in patients with ureterosigmoidostomies than it is in patients who have other types of urinary intestinal diversion.

20. **d. bowel reabsorption.** Because urea and creatinine are reabsorbed by both the ileum and the colon, serum concentrations of urea and creatinine do not necessarily accurately reflect renal function.

21. **a. retain the ability to maintain the acidosis.** The ability to establish a hyperchloremic metabolic acidosis appears to be retained by most segments of ileum and colon over time.

22. **c. are more common in persistent hyperchloremic metabolic acidosis.** Osteomalacia in urinary intestinal diversion may be due to persistent acidosis, vitamin D resistance, and excessive calcium loss by the kidney. It appears that the degree to which each of these contributes to the syndrome may vary from patient to patient.

23. **c. limits linear growth.** There is considerable evidence to suggest that urinary intestinal diversion has a detrimental effect on growth and development.

24. **d. ureterosigmoidostomies.** The highest incidence of cancer occurs when the transitional epithelium is juxtaposed to the colonic epithelium and both are bathed by feces.

25. **b. increased volume.** Reconfiguring bowel usually increases the volume, but its effect on motor activity and wall tension over the long term is unclear at this time.

26. **d. elevated gastrin levels.** The syndrome of severe metabolic alkalosis is most likely to occur in patients with high resting gastrin levels who are dehydrated and fail to empty their pouch in a timely manner.

Imaging

1. **b. stricture at the left uretero-ileal anastomosis.** The loopogram study is of good quality and demonstrates good opacification of the right ureter and collecting system, an expected finding (options d and e are incorrect). The lack of reflux into the left ureter and collecting system may be indicative of a stricture at the left uretero-ileal anastomosis, substantiated by the hydronephrotic left collecting system on the CT. Urothelial tumor recurrence is not a common cause for absence of reflux into the ureters on a loopogram (option c is less likely).

Additional Study Points

1. Perioperative care. The use of a preoperative mechanical bowel prep, oral antibiotic bowel prep, and postoperative nasogastric tube decompression in patients undergoing bowel surgery is controversial. Intravenous antibiotics administered 1 hour before the surgical incision is not controversial and is supported by many studies. Indeed, patients undergoing elective intestinal surgery in the studies that show no advantage to a mechanical and/or antibiotic bowel prep received preoperative intravenous antibiotics. It should be appreciated that these studies involve isolated anastomoses—not large segments of bowel that are opened, as is the case in urologic procedures.

2. Ureteral intestinal anastomotic strictures. Antirefluxing anastomoses have a 10% to 20% stricture rate; refluxing anastomoses have a 3% to 10% stricture rate. The Wallace ureteral intestinal anastomosis has the lowest stricture rate.

3. Renal function and urinary diversion. Serum creatinine and blood urea nitrogen do not accurately reflect renal function in patients with intestine in the urinary track because these substances when excreted by the kidney are reabsorbed by the bowel. This is more likely to be a problem in continent diversions. A GFR of at least 60 mL/min and an ability to acidify the urine are necessary prerequisites for a continent diversion.

4. The electrolyte abnormality that occurs when ileum or colon are used for the diversion is a hyperchloremic metabolic acidosis. These patients may have a potassium deficiency as well.

Cutaneous Continent Urinary Diversion

James M. McKiernan, MD ● G. Joel DeCastro, MD, MPH ● Mitchell C. Benson, MD

QUESTIONS

1. A 45-year-old man had an ileal conduit diversion as a child for bladder exstrophy. He requests a continent diversion. Serum creatinine is 2 mg/dL. Loopogram shows bilaterally thin ureters with small kidneys. Which is the best procedure?

   a. Ureterosigmoidostomy

   b. T-pouch using the ileal conduit

   c. Abandon continent diversion

   d. Penn pouch using the ileal conduit

   e. Indiana pouch

2. A 45-year-old man underwent ileal conduit urinary diversion as a child for bladder exstrophy. He presents requesting continent diversion. Serum creatinine is 2 mg/dL. Loopogram shows bilateral hydronephrosis and a pipe-stem conduit. What is the best course of action?

   a. Mainz II to avoid problems with dilated ureters

   b. T pouch abandoning the disease conduit

   c. No continent diversion

   d. Drain the upper tracts and reassess renal function

   e. Proceed to neobladder construction

3. A patient undergoing a cystectomy and planned continent cutaneous diversion has positive ureteral margin biopsies up to 2 cm above each iliac artery, at which point negative biopsies are obtained. What is the best course of action?

   a. Use the terminal ileum for ureteral implantation and a Mitrofanoff continence mechanism

   b. No continent diversion

   c. Mobilize the kidneys and stretch the ureters to the reservoir

   d. Use a T pouch with a long chimney

   e. Cutaneous ureterostomies

4. Preservation of the ileocecal valve can be maintained with which catheterizable pouch?

   a. T pouch or Kock pouch

   b. Le Bag

   c. Indiana pouch

   d. Mainz I or II

   e. Penn Pouch

5. In which procedure to repair a nipple valve would resection of additional bowel be routinely required?

   a. Stones on exposed staples

   b. Nipple valve slippage

   c. Nipple valve atrophy

   d. Pin-hole leak

   e. Anastomotic leak

6. A 10-year-old child has an ileal conduit for myelomeningocele. The conduit was replaced on two occasions for pipe-stem conduit development. The conduit is again affected by the same process. The patient's family wants a continent diversion. Which is the best procedure?

   a. Ureterosigmoidostomy

   b. Revise the conduit

   c. T pouch using the ileal conduit

   d. Penn pouch using the ileal conduit

   e. Indiana pouch using the ileal conduit

7. A patient with chronic active hepatitis and invasive bladder cancer associated with intravesical carcinoma in situ is scheduled for a cystoprostatectomy. The serum creatinine concentration is 1 mg/dL. Prostatic urethral biopsy shows mild atypia. What is the best diversion?

   a. T pouch

   b. Ileal conduit

   c. Right colon reservoir

   d. Mainz II

   e. Cutaneous ureterostomies

8. The highest reoperation rate in catheterizable pouches occurs with what type of sphincter?

   a. In situ appendix

   b. Imbricated terminal ileum

   c. Plicated terminal ileum

d. Nipple valves

e. Transposed appendix

9. Which of the Mitrofanoff sphincter deficiencies can be corrected surgically?

a. Length of the appendix

b. Absence of the appendix

c. Stenosis of the appendix

d. All of the above

10. Hematuria and skin breakdown may occur with what type of pouch?

a. T

b. Gastric

c. Mainz

d. Right colon

e. All of the above

11. Preoperative colonoscopy is indicated in candidates for which reservoir procedures?

a. Ileal

b. Jejunal

c. Rectal

d. Gastric

e. All of the above

12. What condition is more common in absorbable stapled ileal pouches?

a. Urine leaks

b. Valve failure

c. Hydronephrosis

d. Ischemic pouch contraction

e. Ureteral stricture

13. Anastomotic transitional cell carcinoma develops in a patient who has undergone cystectomy and continent cutaneous urinary diversion. What is the best treatment?

a. Distal ureterectomy and reimplantation

b. Conversion to ileal conduit

c. Ileal ureter interposition

d. Nephroureterectomy

e. Cutaneous ureterostomies

14. Drainage of mucus is most difficult with which sphincteric mechanism?

a. Kock valve

b. In-situ appendix

c. Imbricated ileum

d. Plicated ileum

e. Transposed appendix

15. Which continent cutaneous diversion allows for a refluxing ureteroenteric anastomosis?

a. Mitrofanoff with implantation of the ureters into terminal ileum

b. Mitrofanoff with implantation of the ureters into the colon

c. T pouch

d. Kock pouch

e. Indiana pouch

16. Three years after radical cystectomy and construction of a Kock pouch, a patient presents with right lower quadrant discomfort and associated spurts of urinary leakage. The test most likely to diagnose the condition is:

a. CT.

b. intravenous pyelogram (IVP).

c. urine culture and sensitivity.

d. cystogram of pouch.

e. urodynamics.

17. Three years after cystectomy and Kock pouch for bladder cancer, a patient presents with recurrent episodes of bilateral pyelonephritis. The test most likely to provide the correct diagnosis is:

a. CT.

b. IVP.

c. urine culture and sensitivity.

d. cystogram of the pouch.

e. MRI.

18. What is the most important feature in preventing nipple valve slippage?

a. Absorbable staples

b. Length of the intussusception

c. Resecting adequate mesentery

d. Attaching the nipple valve to the side wall of the reservoir

e. Length of staple line

19. In a patient with pipe-stem conduit and bilateral hydronephrosis requesting conversion to continent urinary diversion, nephrostomy drainage results in clearance values of 40 mL/min on the right and 10 mL/min on the left. Serum creatinine is 1.8 mg/dL. The next step in management is:

a. Mainz II to avoid problems with the dilated ureters.

b. T pouch abandoning the disease conduit.

c. no continent diversion.

d. ureterosigmoidostomy.

e. neobladder.

20. A patient with squamous cell cancer of the bladder desires cystectomy and continent diversion. He has lost 20 pounds in the month before surgery. The next step in management is:

a. increase oral intake.

b. conduct preoperative hyperalimentation.

c. conduct postoperative hyperalimentation.

d. proceed directly with surgery.

e. count calories.

21. Preoperative evaluation with an oatmeal enema is required in which procedure?

a. Right colon reservoir

b. Mainz I pouch

c. Mainz II procedure

d. Le Bag pouch

e. Indiana pouch

22. Follow-up urinary cytology and colonoscopy should be employed in which type of continent diversion?
    a. Ureterosigmoidostomy
    b. Mainz II procedure
    c. Right colon reservoir
    d. All of the above

23. Nocturnal emptying of the patient's reservoir is required in which type of diversion?
    a. Ureterosigmoidostomy
    b. T pouch
    c. Right colon reservoir
    d. Penn pouch
    e. Ileal conduit

24. The appendix is sacrificed in patients undergoing which pouch construction?
    a. Indiana
    b. Le Bag
    c. Mainz I
    d. All of the above

25. Pouch stone development occurs most commonly with which pouch?
    a. T pouch
    b. Kock pouch
    c. Penn pouch
    d. Gastric-ileal composite pouch
    e. Le Bag

26. What is the typical catheter used for appendiceal sphincters?
    a. 22-Fr straight-tipped
    b. 22-Fr coudé-tipped
    c. 14-Fr straight-tipped
    d. 14-Fr coudé-tipped
    e. 20-Fr coudé-tipped

27. Urinary retention resulting from continent diversion occurs most commonly with what type of sphincter?
    a. Appendiceal stoma
    b. Benchekroun hydraulic valve
    c. Nipple valve sphincter
    d. Imbricated Indiana mechanism

28. Immediate postoperative initial pouch capacity is least in which pouch?
    a. T or Kock ileal
    b. Right colon
    c. Gastric
    d. Mainz I
    e. Transverse colon

29. Elevated pouch pressures would potentially facilitate the continence mechanism seen with which valve or sphincter?
    a. Benchekroun ileal valve
    b. Kock valve
    c. Appendiceal tunnel
    d. Imbricated Indiana mechanism
    e. All of the above

30. The long-term failure rate of continence mechanisms is greatest with which mechanism?
    a. T pouch valve
    b. Appendiceal tunnel
    c. Benchekroun hydraulic valve
    d. Imbricated terminal ileum

31. Absorbable staples in continent urinary diversion are best suited to what type of reservoir pouch?
    a. Ileal
    b. Right colon reservoir
    c. Gastric-ileal composite
    d. Gastric
    e. None of the above

32. When creating a large intestinal reservoir from absorbable staples, why is bowel eversion necessary?
    a. Because staples should not be used in reservoir construction
    b. To inspect the inside of the reservoir
    c. To avoid injury to the mesenteric blood supply
    d. To allow application of the second row of staples
    e. None of the above

33. Which of the following conditions make patients unsuitable candidates for continent urinary diversion?
    a. Multiple sclerosis
    b. Quadriplegia
    c. Mental impairment
    d. Severe physical impairment
    e. All of the above

34. Which of the following sutures should not be used in the construction of a reservoir?
    a. Chromic catgut
    b. Plain catgut
    c. Silk
    d. Polyglycolic acid (Dexon)
    e. Polyglactin (Vicryl)

35. Which of the following diversions place the patient at risk for the development of a late malignancy?
    a. Ureterosigmoidostomy
    b. T pouch
    c. Mainz II
    d. Indiana pouch
    e. All of the above

36. Which of the following diversions places the patient at greatest risk for the development of a late malignancy?
    a. Ureterosigmoidostomy
    b. T pouch
    c. Mainz II
    d. Indiana reservoir
    e. Le Bag

37. Continent urinary diversion has which of the following effects?
    a. Results in a psychotic depression
    b. Results in an improved psychosocial adjustment

c. Results in violent behavior

d. Bipolar behavior

e. None of the above

38. According to most randomized studies, which type of urinary diversion is associated with the highest reported quality of life?

a. Uretero-sigmoidostomy

b. Continent ileal reservoir (Kock pouch)

c. Ileal conduit

d. Orthotopic neobladder

e. None—no conclusive studies have established higher satisfaction or quality of life with any one specific continent diversion

39. Which of the following is NOT true of continent urinary diversion?

a. It is the gold standard of urinary diversion.

b. It is a safe and reliable urinary diversion.

c. It is associated with an increased complication rate.

d. It is appropriate for selected individuals.

e. It requires stricter selection criteria than incontinent diversion.

40. Which of the following circumstances would contraindicate a rectal bladder?

a. Prior pelvic irradiation

b. Unilateral ureteral dilation

c. Bilateral ureteral dilation

d. Lax anal sphincter tone

e. All of the above

41. During the construction of a continent cutaneous urinary diversion, the surgeon should:

a. not be concerned about the continence mechanism because the mechanism will mold to the catheter.

b. not test the continence mechanism for ease of catheterization.

c. not be concerned about pouch integrity because the pouch will seal itself.

d. do none of the above.

e. do all of the above.

42. If the urine in a continent cutaneous reservoir is found to be infected, what should be done?

a. Nothing needs to be done in the absence of symptoms.

b. The urine should always be sterilized with appropriate antibiotics.

c. The infection should be eradicated and prophylactic antibiotics prescribed.

d. Administer an intravenous pyelogram to check for upper tract damage.

e. Perform a pouch-o-gram.

43. The most appropriate and conservative care for pouch rupture is:

a. broad-spectrum antibiotic therapy.

b. careful radiologic imaging and antibiotic therapy.

c. surgical exploration for repair of the rupture and broad-spectrum antibiotic therapy.

d. pouch drainage and broad-spectrum antibiotic therapy.

e. bilateral percutaneous nephrostomies.

44. The first pouch to employ the Mitrofanoff principle was the:

a. Mainz I.

b. Penn.

c. Kock.

d. Indiana.

e. Le Bag.

45. Which of the following represents the advantage of the gastric pouch?

a. Electrolyte reabsorption is reduced.

b. Absorptive malabsorption is avoided.

c. Acid urine may reduce the risk of infection.

d. All of the above

e. None of the above

46. When converting from an ileal conduit to a continent diversion, the conduit should be:

a. discarded because it is older and subject to higher complications.

b. preserved for the ureteroileal anastomosis.

c. incorporated into the continent diversion when possible.

d. discarded because it is a potential nidus of infection.

e. None of the above

47. Which of the following is TRUE of absorbable staples?

a. Their use has been shown to shorten operative time.

b. They are safe and reliable.

c. Unlike nonabsorbable staples, they must not be overlapped.

d. All of the above

e. None of the above

ANSWERS

1. **c. Abandon continent diversion.** A creatinine level greater than 1.8 mg/dL indicates a level of renal function insufficient for continent diversion.

2. **d. Drain the upper tracts and reassess renal function.** The best course of action is to place ureteral cutaneous stents bilaterally (bypassing the pipe-stem segment) and reassess urinary function. In evaluating the hydronephrotic patient with impaired renal function for continent diversion, upper tract drainage is advised. If necessary, bilateral nephrostomy tubes can be employed.

3. **a. Use the terminal ileum for ureteral implantation and a Mitrofanoff continence mechanism.** The best course of action is to perform a right colon reservoir with anastomosis of the ureters to the terminal ileum. The appendix or other pseudo-appendiceal (Mitrofanoff) mechanisms can be used for continence. The terminal ileum can accommodate short ureters.

4. **a. T pouch or Kock pouch.** Preservation of the ileocecal valve can be maintained with the T or Kock pouch. All other pouches employ right colon, so that the ileocecal valve is sacrificed.

5. **c. Nipple valve atrophy.** Nipple valve atrophy requires that a new nipple valve be made of additional bowel.

6. **b. Revise the conduit.** With significant small bowel compromise, as well as loss of the ileocecal valve in a neurogenic bladder patient, severe diarrhea may ensue.

7. **b. Ileal conduit.** The best approach is cystoprostatectomy and a conduit. Normal hepatic function is mandated in any patient undergoing continent diversion.

8. **d. Nipple valves.** The highest reoperation rate is associated with nipple valve sphincter failure.

9. **d. All of the above.** The caliber of Mitrofanoff mechanisms, the length of the appendix, stenosis, and even absence of the appendix can be resolved by surgical variations.

10. **b. Gastric pouch.** Hematuria and cutaneous skin erosion may occur with a gastric pouch. With gastric reservoirs or composite reservoirs, the low pH of the urine may lead to hematuria and cutaneous breakdown.

11. **c. Rectal reservoirs.** Preoperative colonoscopy is relatively indicated in candidates for any pouch. Any pouch using colon mandates preoperative colonic evaluation.

12. **d. Ischemic pouch contraction.** Because of the overlap of staple lines in absorbable stapled ileal pouches, ischemic pouch contraction may occur.

13. **a. Distal ureterectomy and reimplantation.** An additional segment of ileum can serve as a proximal limb to the reservoir. If nephrectomy is necessary, careful attention must be paid to the residual renal function.

14. **b. In-situ appendix.** The small-diameter catheter used in draining appendiceal sphincter pouches allows for less effective mucus drainage.

15. **a. Mitrofanoff with implantation of the ureters into terminal ileum.** The implantation of the ureters into the terminal ileum may allow for reflux. The ileal cecal valve and the isoperistaltic ileal segment may either prevent or diminish reflux.

16. **c. urine culture and sensitivity.** The most important diagnostic test is urine culture. The symptoms described are those of pouchitis. This is treated by appropriate antibiotic therapy.

17. **d. cystogram of the pouch.** The proximal nipple valve may have failed, leading to reflux and pyelonephritis. This is tested by the pouch-o-gram.

18. **d. Attaching the nipple valve to the side wall of the reservoir.** This results in a relative lengthening of the valve rather than a foreshortening of the valve with pouch filling.

19. **c. no continent diversion.** In this case, although the serum creatinine level returns to 1.8 mg/dL, the clearance value measured is less than the 60 mL/min required for continent diversion. Continent diversion should be abandoned, and simple replacement of the conduit considered.

20. **b. conduct preoperative hyperalimentation.** The 10-pound weight loss indicates a potential for nutritional depletion or metastatic disease. A careful search for metastatic disease should be undertaken. For the patient with nutritional depletion, preoperative hyperalimentation is suggested to be of value.

21. **c. Mainz II procedure.** Any procedure that relies on the intact anal sphincter for continence (i.e., the Mainz II pouch) requires an assessment of the sphincter before carrying out the operation. This can be assessed by an oatmeal enema, which mimics the constitution of a combination of the urinary and fecal streams.

22. **d. All of the above.** Follow-up urinary cytology and colonoscopy is mandatory with any procedure that combines urinary and fecal streams. Because of an increased risk of malignancy even in the absence of admixture of urine and stool, all large intestinal pouches should be subjected to annual investigation by pouchoscopy and cytology.

23. **a. Ureterosigmoidostomy.** Nocturnal reservoir emptying may be required with any of the continent cutaneous reservoirs to prevent overdistention and possible rupture but is mandatory with ureterosigmoidostomy owing to the additional risk of fecal incontinence and metabolic acidosis.

24. **d. All of the above.** The appendix is sacrificed in patients undergoing Indiana, Le Bag, and Mainz I pouch reconstruction because it can serve as a nidus for infection and abscess formation.

25. **b. Kock pouch.** Pouch stone development occurs most commonly with the Kock pouch. Despite the exclusion of distal staples, the stapling techniques used to secure nipple valves will lead to a higher potential for stone development than in pouches not requiring nipple valves.

26. **d. 14-Fr coudé-tipped.** Larger catheters will not fit into the appendix. A straight catheter is more difficult to pass.

27. **c. Nipple valve sphincter.** Urinary retention occurs most commonly with nipple valve sphincters. If the chimney of the nipple valve is not near the surface of the abdomen, the catheter can be misdirected into folds of bowel rather than through the nipple valve.

28. **a. T or Kock ileal.** Immediate postoperative initial pouch capacity is least in ileal reservoirs (i.e., the T or Kock pouch). Small bowel pouches have initial capacities that are much lower than right colon pouches.

29. **a. Benchekroun ileal valve.** Because the Benchekroun ileal valve is hydraulic, higher pouch pressures would facilitate continence, whereas lower pouch pressures might lead to incontinence.

30. **c. Benchekroun hydraulic valve.** The long-term outcome of Benchekroun hydraulic ileal valve mechanisms is possibly the worst of all reported sphincteric mechanisms.

31. **b. Right colon reservoir.** The use of absorbable staples is best suited to large bowel pouches. With large bowel pouches there is no problem with staple lines causing subsequent bowel ischemia.

32. **d. To allow application of the second row of staples.** In an absorbable-stapled right colon pouch, bowel eversion is required to allow for the application of the second row of staples. Staple lines must not cross because this will prevent the bulky, absorbable staples from seating properly. The bowel is everted, a cut is made beyond the end of the staple line, and the next line of staples is applied.

33. **e. All of the above.** Patients with multiple sclerosis, quadriplegic individuals, frailty, and mental impairment will at some point in their lives require the care of family members or visiting nurses, so they are poor candidates for any form of continent diversion.

34. **c. Silk.** All sutures used in the urinary tract should be absorbable.

35. **e. All of the above.** Late malignancy has been reported in all bowel segments exposed to the urinary stream, whether or not there is a commingling with feces.

36. **a. Ureterosigmoidostomy.** Although late malignancy has been reported in all bowel segments exposed to the urinary stream, whether or not there is a commingling with feces, the mixture of urothelium, urine, and feces poses the greatest risk.

37. **b. Results in an improved psychosocial adjustment.** Many studies from throughout the world have suggested an improved psychosocial adjustment of the patient undergoing continent urinary and fecal diversion compared with those patients with diversions requiring collecting appliances.

38. **e. None—no conclusive studies have established higher satisfaction or quality of life with any one specific continent diversion.** There is insufficient quality of life data from randomized studies comparing continent and incontinent urinary diversions to establish the superiority of any one technique.

39. **a. It is the gold standard of urinary diversion.** Ileal conduit should be considered the "gold standard" of urinary diversion.

40. **e. All of the above.** Dilated ureters, pelvic irradiation, and lax anal sphincteric tone are all contraindications to the procedure.

41. **d. do none of the above.** The continence mechanism must be catheterized to ensure ease of catheter passage. This is an extremely important and crucial maneuver because the inability to catheterize is a serious complication that will often result in the need for reoperation.

42. **a. Nothing needs to be done in the absence of symptoms.** Most authors would suggest that bacteriuria in the absence of symptomatology does not warrant antibiotic treatment.

43. **c. surgical exploration for repair of the rupture and broad-spectrum antibiotic therapy.** In general, these patients require immediate pouch decompression, radiologic pouch studies, and surgical exploration with pouch repair. If the amount of urinary extravasation is small and the patient does not have a surgical abdomen, catheter drainage and antibiotic administration may suffice in treating intraperitoneal rupture of a pouch. Patients managed with this conservative approach require careful monitoring.

44. **b. Penn.** The Penn pouch was the first continent diversion employing the Mitrofanoff principle, wherein the appendix served as the continence mechanism.

45. **d. All of the above.** Electrolyte reabsorption is greatly diminished, shortening of the absorptive bowel does not occur, and the acid urine may decrease the likelihood of reservoir colonization.

46. **c. incorporated into the continent diversion when possible.** The authors prefer to use the conduit in some form whenever possible. The use of an existing bowel segment has the potential to diminish metabolic sequelae and may result in a lower complication rate.

47. **d. All of the above.** The use of absorbable staplers has substantially reduced the time required to fashion bowel reservoirs and has demonstrated short-term and long-term reliability with respect to reservoir integrity and volume. They must not be overlapped because overlapping will prevent the proper close of the staple.

Additional Study Points

1. The ability to self-catheterize is essential in patients who are to be considered for a continent cutaneous diversion.

2. All patients should be prepared for the possibility of a traditional ileal conduit if intraoperative circumstances warrant it.

3. A patient should have a minimum creatinine clearance of 60 mL/min to undergo a continent urinary diversion.

4. Single J ureteral stents are used in all continent diversions. The stents are brought out through a separate abdominal stab wound, and a Malecot catheter should be placed into the reservoir and brought out through a separate stab wound as well.

5. In continent diversions it is not clear at this time whether antirefluxing ureteral intestinal anastomoses are necessary to preserve the upper tracts.

6. Most patients are satisfied with the type of urinary diversion irrespective of whether it is continent or not.

7. It is often useful to secure the reservoir to the anterior abdominal wall to prevent the reservoir from migrating. This is conveniently done where the Malecot exits the reservoir onto the anterior abdominal wall.

8. Renal and hepatic function must be carefully evaluated before a continent diversion is performed. Significant abnormalities in either are a contraindication to continent diversion.

Orthotopic Urinary Diversion

Eila C. Skinner, MD ● Donald G. Skinner, MD ● John P. Stein, MD

QUESTIONS

1. Which of the following patients should NOT be offered an orthotopic neobladder?
   a. An 82-year-old healthy man
   b. A 65-year-old woman with a creatinine of 1.8 and marked right hydronephrosis
   c. A 50-year-old man 2 years following low anterior colon resection with adjuvant chemotherapy and external beam radiation to the pelvis
   d. A 60-year-old woman with diabetes and hypertension
   e. A 58-year-old woman with palpable induration of the anterior vaginal apex

2. The risk factor most predictive for urethra recurrence following cystectomy for urothelial carcinoma is:
   a. prostatic stromal invasion.
   b. node-positive disease.
   c. carcinoma in situ in females.
   d. pathologic stage pT3b tumor at the trigone.
   e. history of multiple prior tumors.

3. All currently recommended types of orthotopic diversion:
   a. use less than 50 cm of bowel.
   b. preserve the ileocecal valve.
   c. use detubularized bowel for the reservoir.
   d. incorporate some form of antireflux technique.
   e. use ileum or ileum plus right colon.

4. Before considering a continent orthotopic diversion, what evaluation is mandatory?
   a. Prostatic urethral biopsy
   b. Evaluation of renal function
   c. Colonoscopy to rule out colon polyps
   d. Biopsy of the bladder neck in a female
   e. Video urodynamics to test the integrity of the external sphincter

5. The primary innervation of the rhabdosphincter that is responsible for continence following an orthotopic diversion is:
   a. parasympathetics from S2-S4.
   b. the sciatic nerve.
   c. sympathetic nerves from the hypogastric plexus.
   d. the pudendal nerve.
   e. the femoral nerve.

6. In performing a cystectomy and orthotopic ileal neobladder in a male, the most important step in preserving subsequent continence is to:
   a. construct a large-capacity reservoir.
   b. avoid excess dissection below the levator fascia.
   c. perform a nerve-sparing procedure in all cases.
   d. avoid removal of the presacral lymph nodes.
   e. place a suprapubic catheter during the early postoperative period.

7. Asymptomatic bacteriuria in patients with orthotopic diversion:
   a. carries a high risk of subsequent pyelonephritis.
   b. leads to an increase in urethral recurrence.
   c. does not generally require treatment.
   d. is rare in most reported series.
   e. suggests probable outlet obstruction.

8. Use of metallic surgical staples should be avoided in construction of a continent diversion because:
   a. it is less secure than a hand-sewn closure.
   b. they tend to be buried in the bowel mucosa.
   c. the staples increase the risk of subsequent infection.
   d. the staples become a nidus for stone formation.
   e. they increase the risk of cancer developing in the segment.

9. A 71-year-old man is found on routine follow-up to have a pelvic recurrence 13 months after cystectomy and Studer pouch ileal neobladder. The mass is 2.5 cm in the obturator fossa, abutting the pouch. He has good daytime continence but occasionally leaks at night. The next step is:
   a. resection of the mass with removal of the pouch and conversion to an ileal conduit.
   b. placement of bilateral nephrostomy tubes to divert the urine.

c. placement of a permanent suprapubic tube.

d. resection of the mass.

e. systemic chemotherapy with or without external beam radiation.

10. A 58-year-old man with clinical T3 bladder cancer is to undergo systemic chemotherapy followed by radical cystectomy. He wants to have an orthotopic diversion performed with a robotic-assisted minimally invasive technique. What should he be advised of when comparing his preference with open techniques?

a. The most difficult part of this surgery is performing an adequate extended lymphadenectomy.

b. Minimally invasive cystectomy has been proven to be less effective from an oncologic perspective.

c. It is straightforward to perform this entire surgery using pure laparoscopic techniques.

d. Robotic-assisted cystectomy has markedly reduced the early and late complications of the surgery.

e. The surgery tends to be faster with less blood loss.

11. A 66-year-old man 2 years after a cystectomy and Hautmann ileal neobladder for pathologic stage T2N0M0 bladder cancer is found on routine CT scan to have a distended neobladder. He has a postvoid residual of more than 800 mL. Cystoscopy and digital rectal examination are normal. The next step is to:

a. teach the patient intermittent catheterization.

b. dilate the urethra with van Buren sounds.

c. instruct the patient to perform both Credé and Valsalva maneuvers while voiding.

d. Convert the diversion to an ileal conduit.

e. Decompress the neobladder with a catheter for 2 weeks and then resume regular voiding.

12. Quality of life studies of patients with orthotopic diversion:

a. are best done by the physician asking the patient about the function of his or her neobladder.

b. have uniformly shown that patients with continent diversions have a better quality of life than those with ileal conduits.

c. can be easily done with questionnaires used for other populations.

d. have often been underpowered or affected by selection bias.

e. have shown that most patients with any urinary diversion have poor quality of life.

ANSWERS

1. **e. A 58-year-old woman with palpable induration of the anterior vaginal apex.** Invasion of the anterior vaginal wall is a contraindication for orthotopic diversion in women. In retrospective studies vaginal invasion was associated with a high risk of urethral involvement with the cancer. In women, when the bladder neck is involved, approximately 50% have urethra involvement.

2. **a. prostatic stromal invasion.** The risk of urethra carcinoma developing in patients with bladder cancer is approximately 5% to 7%. The most important risk factor for urethra involvement in males is prostatic involvement with transitional cell carcinoma. In many studies when only the

mucosa of the prostate is involved, few patients develop urethra carcinoma. When there is ductal involvement, approximately 5% to 10% develop urethra cancer, and when there is stromal invasion 11% to 18% develop urethra cancer.

3. **c. use detubularized bowel for the reservoir.** Splitting the bowel down its long axis and folding it to form a spherical shape is a key maneuver in all successful types of orthotopic diversion. This disrupts high-pressure contractions and results in a low-pressure reservoir with the maximum volume for a given surface area.

4. **b. Evaluation of renal function.** Patients with significantly decreased renal function are at increased risk of developing chronic acidosis and metabolic abnormalities with a continent diversion. This is due to the reabsorption of electrolytes by the bowel mucosa. A creatinine clearance of at least 35 mL/min is a prerequisite for considering continent diversion.

5. **d. the pudendal nerve.** The rhabdosphincter is primarily innervated by the pudendal somatic nerve fibers.

6. **b. avoid excess dissection below the levator fascia.** The nerve fibers from the pudendal nerve course within the levator muscles to innervate the rhabdosphincter. Thus one should avoid overdissection around the urethra or using deep suture bites to control the dorsal venous complex.

7. **c. does not generally require treatment.** Although there is some controversy about the need to treat asymptomatic bacteruria in these patients, most authors agree that it can be left untreated with a low incidence of pyelonephritis or other serious sequelae.

8. **d. the staples become a nidus for stone formation.** Metal staples that do not become covered by mucosa will be a nidus for stone formation. The experience with the hemi-Kock neobladder (the nipple valve is fixed with metal staples) has shown a high incidence of stones in these patients.

9. **e. systemic chemotherapy with or without external beam radiation.** Pelvic recurrence after cystectomy is almost always incurable and is best treated with systemic chemotherapy. Heroic surgical re-resection is usually not successful. The neobladder is not usually involved or disrupted by the recurrent disease. Surgery should be reserved for an otherwise healthy patient with outlet obstruction, recurrent hematuria, or upper tract obstruction.

10. **a. The most difficult part of this surgery is performing an adequate extended lymphadenectomy.** Robot-assisted laparoscopic cystectomy is becoming increasingly popular. The cystectomy itself is straightforward using these techniques, but accomplishing a complete extended bilateral node dissection can be difficult. Generally the neobladder has been constructed extracorporeally through a small incision.

11. **a. teach the patient intermittent catheterization.** Chronic urinary retention can occur with all types of orthotopic diversion and appears to be more common in women than men. Cystoscopy and cytology should be done to rule out cancer recurrence or a true stricture. Thereafter the patient should be taught self-catheterization, and many patients are satisfied with this treatment (which usually significantly improves continence). Some authors have advocated incision of mucosal folds at the urethral anastomosis, but care must be taken to avoid injury to the sphincter. There is no role for pharmacologic intervention

in patients with urinary retention who have had an orthotopic bladder.

12. **d. have often been underpowered or affected by selection bias.** Most quality of life studies in patients with continent urinary diversion suffer from major methodological problems. The gold standard of a randomized prospective trial is of course not practical. Most reviews of the literature have concluded that a clear advantage of one type of diversion over another has not been demonstrated.

Additional Study Points

1. The volume of the reservoir generally increases over time. Reservoirs constructed from ileum generally have a greater increase in volume over time than pouches constructed with colon.

2. The risk factors in women most predictive of urethra cancer developing are vaginal wall invasion or bladder neck involvement of the transitional cell carcinoma.

3. The majority of patients who have a urethra recurrence are symptomatic on presentation. A urinary cytology has a variable rate of yield but is generally low in this group of patients.

4. When orthotopic bladders are constructed in elderly patients, there is a slower time to achieve continence, an increased rate of stress incontinence, and an increased incidence of nighttime incontinence when compared with younger patients.

5. In order to consider a patient a candidate for a continent diversion, he or she must have a glomerular filtration rate in excess of 35 mL/min and the kidneys must be capable of concentrating and acidifying the urine.

6. All patients who are considered for a continent diversion should be willing and capable of doing self-catheterization, although for selected patients this may not be necessary.

7. In preserving the urethra for an orthotopic bladder in males, one should be careful of the dorsal venous complex, preserve the puboprostatic ligaments, and avoid deep bites into the pelvic floor. In females the endopelvic fascia and levator muscles should be preserved.

8. In patients with orthotopic bladders approximately one quarter have asymptomatic bacteruria.

9. The need to perform an antireflux mechanism for the ureters in an orthotopic urinary diversion is unproved.

10. If there is any suggestion that a nerve-sparing technique might result in a positive surgical margin, the nerve should be sacrificed. This does not mean that the diversion cannot be successfully performed and that the patient will not be continent.

11. Nighttime incontinence occurs in approximately 25% to 75% of patients.

12. Urinary retention following orthotopic urinary diversion occurs in 10% to 25% of patients and is more common in women than in men.

13. It may take 3 to 6 months in many patients to develop daytime continence. Nocturnal continence may take more than a year after surgery.

14. If a patient has an undrained urine leak postoperative, percutaneous drainage and/or nephrostomy is preferable to open surgical repair because the latter is extremely difficult and the complication rate is high.

15. Obstruction from an antireflux valve may be clinically silent, and patients may present with hydronephrosis and/or renal failure.

16. A pouch vaginal fistula is a morbid complication in female patients and is most likely to occur when the anterior vagina is removed along with the bladder. It is best prevented by interposition of an omental pedicle.

17. Quality of life surveys have not shown one type of urinary diversion to be superior over another. Most patients are reasonably well adapted socially, physically, and psychologically to their diversion. The key to this adaptation is appropriate and realistic preoperative education.

Genital and Lower Urinary Tract Trauma

Allen F. Morey, MD, FACS ● Daniel D. Dugi III, MD

QUESTIONS

1. Which of the following is an absolute indication for open repair of blunt bladder rupture injury?
   a. Significant extraperitoneal bladder rupture with extravasation of contrast agent into the scrotum
   b. Significant extraperitoneal bladder rupture with gross hematuria
   c. Significant extraperitoneal bladder rupture that has not healed after 3 weeks of Foley catheter drainage
   d. Intraperitoneal bladder rupture
   e. Significant extraperitoneal bladder rupture associated with pelvic fracture requiring treatment by external fixation

2. Which of the following is TRUE regarding cystography for diagnosis of bladder injury?
   a. If the patient is already undergoing computed tomography (CT) for evaluation of associated injuries, CT cystography should be performed via antegrade filling of the bladder after intravenous administration of radiographic contrast material and clamping the Foley catheter.
   b. If plain film cystograms are obtained, the study is considered negative and complete if there is no extravasation of contrast agent seen on the filling film.
   c. CT cystography is best performed with undiluted contrast medium.
   d. An absolute indication for immediate cystography is the presence of pelvic fracture and microhematuria.
   e. None of the above

3. Which of the following is TRUE about blunt bladder rupture injuries?
   a. They are present in 90% of patients presenting with pelvic fractures.
   b. They coexist with urethral disruption in 50% of cases.
   c. Extraperitoneal ruptures are always amenable to nonoperative treatment.
   d. High mortality rate is primarily related to nonurologic comorbidities.
   e. They are associated with microhematuria or no hematuria in 40% of cases.

4. The risk of complications from nonoperative treatment of extraperitoneal bladder rupture is increased by:
   a. associated orthopedic injury.
   b. associated vaginal injury.
   c. associated urethral injury.
   d. associated rectal injury.
   e. all of the above.

5. Three months after a urethral distraction injury a patient is found to have a 2-cm obliterative posterior urethral defect. Which of the following is TRUE about the repair?
   a. One-stage, open, perineal anastomotic urethroplasty is preferred.
   b. Orthopedic hardware in the pubic symphysis area is a contraindication to open posterior urethroplasty.
   c. Buccal mucosa graft urethroplasty is recommended.
   d. UroLume stent placement is recommended.
   e. The patient is at high risk for incontinence after posterior urethral reconstruction surgery.

6. In a patient with a pelvic fracture from blunt trauma in whom no urine is returned after catheter placement, what is the best initial method to evaluate urethral injury?
   a. Retrograde urethrography
   b. CT of abdomen and pelvis
   c. Filiforms and followers
   d. Bladder ultrasonography
   e. None of the above

7. What is the best method to evaluate suspected penile rupture?
   a. Exploration of the penile corpora through a circumcision incision
   b. Ultrasonography of the penis
   c. Exploration of the penile corpora through a midline scrotal incision
   d. Magnetic resonance imaging of the penis
   e. Cavernosography

8. During exploration after a scrotal gunshot wound, 20% of the left testicular capsule is found to be disrupted. What should be done?

    a. Left orchiectomy

    b. Application of wet dressings and delayed testicular surgery

    c. Left testicular reconstruction with synthetic graft

    d. Closure of the scrotal laceration followed by ultrasonography

    e. Immediate primary repair of the left testis

9. A 23-year-old man is found to have an 80% transection of the proximal bulbar urethra after a gunshot wound with a 22-caliber pistol. A 1-cm urethral defect is visualized during cystoscopy. What is the most appropriate therapy?

    a. Buccal mucosa graft urethroplasty

    b. Spatulated, stented, tension-free, watertight repair of the urethra with absorbable sutures

    c. Suprapubic tube placement

    d. Urethral catheterization alone

    e. Perineal urethrostomy

10. Which of the following statements regarding penile fracture is FALSE?

    a. Most injuries occur ventrolaterally.

    b. Rupture of a superficial vein can sometimes mimic the presentation of a corporeal tear.

    c. Retrograde urethrography should be uniformly performed to assess for urethral injury.

    d. Patients with penile fracture who are treated nonoperatively are more likely to have longer hospital stays, a higher risk of infection, and penile curvature than those whose fracture is repaired surgically.

    e. Physical examination is usually sufficient in making the diagnosis or for deciding on surgical exploration.

11. The blood in a hematocele is contained in which of the following?

    a. Tunica albuginea

    b. Tunica vaginalis

    c. Dartos muscle

    d. Camper fascia

    e. Spermatic cord

12. Blunt scrotal trauma that results in testis rupture:

    a. is usually a bilateral process.

    b. is often diagnosed by the presence of intratesticular hypoechoic areas on ultrasonography.

    c. has a degree of hematoma that correlates with the extent of injury.

    d. requires conservative management that results in acceptable viability and function.

    e. is definitively diagnosed during physical examination alone in most cases.

13. Which of the following is TRUE regarding penile amputation injury?

    a. Microscopic reanastomosis of the corporeal arteries is recommended.

    b. The severed phallus should be placed directly on ice during transport.

    c. Microscopic dorsal vascular and neural reanastomosis is the best method of repair.

    d. Primary macroscopic reanastomosis invariably results in erectile dysfunction.

    e. Skin loss is rarely a problem after macroscopic repair.

14. What is the best option for coverage of acute penile skin loss?

    a. Foreskin flap for small distal lesions

    b. Meshed skin graft in a young child

    c. Wet-to-dry dressings

    d. Thigh flaps

    e. Burying the penile shaft in a scrotal skin tunnel

15. Advantages of open suprapubic tube placement after posterior urethral disruption injuries include:

    a. inspection of bladder.

    b. an opportunity for controlled antegrade urethral realignment.

    c. allowance for large-bore catheter insertion.

    d. not jeopardizing continence or potency rates.

    e. all of the above.

Imaging

1. See Figure 88–1.

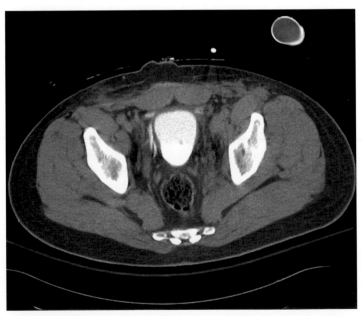

Figure 88–1.

This CT scan in a 22-year-old man involved in an motor vehicle accident indicates that the most likely diagnosis is:

a. extraperitoneal bladder injury.

b. intraperitoneal bladder injury.

c. bladder contusion.

d. combined intra peritoneal and extraperitoneal bladder injury.

e. ureteral injury.

ANSWERS

1. **d. Intraperitoneal bladder rupture.** When intraperitoneal bladder laceration occurs after blunt trauma a large laceration of the bladder dome is usually produced that predisposes to urinary ascites and/or peritonitis if it is not repaired promptly.

2. **e. None of the above.** The CT cystogram must be performed via retrograde distention of the bladder with a diluted contrast medium. Most bladder lacerations are associated with gross hematuria not microhematuria. A drainage film is required to complete a plain film cystogram.

3. **d. High mortality rate is primarily related to nonurologic comorbidities.** Bladder lacerations occur in roughly 10% of pelvic fractures and often occur in the context of multisystemic trauma.

4. **e. all of the above.** All of the listed concomitant injuries increase the risk of complications such as abscess, fistula, or incontinence.

5. **a. One-stage, open, perineal anastomotic urethroplasty is preferred.** Posterior urethral reconstruction including excision of the fibrotic segment with distal urethral mobilization and primary anastomosis is associated with the best long-term outcomes after urethral disruption. Incontinence occurs in less than 5% of patients.

6. **a. Retrograde urethrography.** Retrograde urethrography is the most reliable imaging study for urethral evaluation.

7. **a. Exploration of the penile corpora through a circumcision incision.** Penile exploration through a circumcision incision should be performed when a clinical diagnosis of penile rupture is suspected. Although MRI has been found to provide accurate images, its routine use is not justified in this setting owing to cost and availability constraints.

8. **e. Immediate primary repair of the left testis.** Immediate primary repair should be attempted in the setting of subtotal injury to an otherwise viable testis. Even extensive testicular injuries often can be safely salvaged, and tunica vaginalis grafts provide better outcomes than do synthetic grafts for complex repair.

9. **b. Spatulated, stented, tension-free, watertight repair of the urethra with absorbable sutures.** Immediate urethral repair with fine absorbable suture over a Foley catheter is associated with superior outcomes after penetrating injury. A proximal bulbar urethral pathologic process in a young man is uniquely amenable to primary anastomotic repair.

10. **c. Retrograde urethrography should be uniformly performed to assess for urethral injury.** Flexible cystoscopy performed at the time of surgical exploration is the simplest and most sensitive means to assess for urethral injury. Urethrography is of low yield in men with no hematuria, no blood at the meatus, and no voiding symptoms; and intraoperative flexible cystoscopy is an appropriate alternative method of urethral evaluation.

11. **b. Tunica vaginalis.** Blood fills the space between the visceral and parietal layers of the tunica vaginalis.

12. **b. is often diagnosed by the presence of intratesticular hypoechoic areas on ultrasonography.** Testicular rupture is often difficult to detect clinically. Ultrasound evaluation usually shows intratesticular heterogeneity as a sentinel finding; detection of a defect of the tunica albuginea is less common.

13. **c. Microscopic dorsal vascular and neural reanastomosis is the best method of repair.** Microvascular reanastomosis of the dorsal neurovascular structures is suggested as the preferred treatment modality whenever possible. Reanastomosis of the corporeal arteries is not recommended.

14. **a. Foreskin flap for small distal lesions.** Redundant foreskin provides excellent closure when ample viable tissue exists.

15. **e. all of the above.** Antegrade urethral realignment may simplify treatment of the defect, and a large-bore suprapubic catheter placed near the midline will promote subsequent identification of the prostatic apex during delayed reconstruction while preventing tube encrustation or obstruction.

Imaging

1. **a. extraperitoneal bladder injury.** There is stranding in the soft tissues around the urinary bladder, and extraluminal contrast medium is seen in the space of Retzius anterior to the bladder, as well as in the right perivesical space. With intraperitoneal injuries, contrast medium would outline the bowel and not be confined to the perivesical space. Ureteral injuries are unusual with blunt abdominal trauma and would not have this appearance.

Additional Study Points

1. Penile fracture generally occurs at the base of the penis in a ventrolateral location where the tunica albuginea is thinnest.

2. Dog bites of the penis are treated with copious irrigation, debridement, and primary closure. Human bites should be irrigated, debrided, treated with antibiotics, and left open.

3. A fractured testis should be explored and repaired because the salvage rate is higher than when conservative non-operative therapy is employed.

4. Noncomplicated extraperitoneal bladder ruptures may be treated with urethral catheter drainage alone.

5. The bulbomembranous junction is more vulnerable to injury during pelvic fracture than is the prostatomembranous junction; thus, the external sphincter is often intact. In children, urethral disruptions generally occur at the bladder neck. In females the urethral avulsion usually occurs proximally.

6. In females, urethral disruptions should be primarily repaired and vaginal lacerations should be closed.

7. Initial suprapubic cystostomy is the standard of care for major straddle injuries involving the urethra with primary anterior urethral realignment.

Lower Urinary Tract Calculi

Brian M. Benway, MD • Sam B. Bhayani, MD

QUESTIONS

1. Vesical calculus disease is usually associated with what condition in the United States?
   a. Foreign bodies
   b. Urinary tract infections
   c. Catheterization
   d. Bladder outlet obstruction
   e. None of the above

2. Magnesium ammonium phosphate stones are most often formed in association with infection with which bacteria?
   a. *Pseudomonas*
   b. *Providencia*
   c. *Klebsiella*
   d. *Staphylococcus*
   e. *Proteus*

3. Urease-producing bacteria hydrolyze urea into:
   a. uric acid.
   b. carbon monoxide.
   c. carbon dioxide.
   d. ammonium.
   e. carbon dioxide and ammonium.

4. Which continent diversion has the highest risk of stone formation?
   a. Mainz pouch
   b. Kock pouch
   c. Orthotopic hemi-Kock pouch
   d. Indiana pouch
   e. Cecal reservoir

5. Risk factors for the formation of stones in patients with urinary diversions include all of the following EXCEPT:
   a. hypocitruria.
   b. hyperchloremic metabolic acidosis.
   c. hypercalciuria.
   d. hyperoxaluria.
   e. urinary tract infection.

6. What is the most accurate examination to document the presence of a bladder stone?
   a. Ultrasonography
   b. Excretory urography
   c. Computed tomography
   d. Cystoscopy
   e. Plain (kidney/ureter/bladder) radiography

7. Appropriate treatment options for bladder calculi include all of the following EXCEPT:
   a. irrigation with Suby solution G.
   b. shockwave lithotripsy.
   c. electrohydraulic lithotripsy.
   d. ultrasonic lithotripsy.
   e. holmium laser lithotripsy.

8. Urethral calculi in women are associated with which of the following?
   a. Metabolic disturbances
   b. Urethral stricture
   c. Urethral diverticulum
   d. Foreign bodies
   e. None of the above

9. All of the following regarding primary bladder calculi in children are true EXCEPT:
   a. the peak incidence is between the ages of 2 and 4.
   b. patients usually present with multiple calculi.
   c. the incidence is much higher in males than females.
   d. formation is associated with low-phosphate diets.
   e. formation is generally not associated with urinary tract infection.

10. Endoscopic management of bladder calculi is considered an acceptable intervention in:
    a. a 26-year-old man with a history of neurogenic bladder who underwent augmentation cystoplasty at the age of 12 and performs transurethral clean intermittent catheterization.
    b. a 12-year-old girl with myelomeningocele who underwent bladder neck closure and creation of a Mitrofanoff catheterizable stoma at the age of 8.

c. a 76-year-old man with a history of bladder cancer who underwent cystectomy with Indiana pouch diversion.

d. a 65-year-old woman with a history of bladder cancer who underwent cystectomy with Kock pouch diversion.

e. a and d.

11. All of the following are true about bladder calculi in augmented bladders EXCEPT:

a. mean time to first stone formation is 2 to 6 years after augmentation.

b. catheterization through a Mitrofanoff stoma is associated with an increased risk of stone formation.

c. males are 3 to 10 times more likely to develop stones than females.

d. autoaugmentation is associated with a comparatively low risk of bladder stone formation.

e. All of the above are true.

12. Bladder stone formation in patients who have undergone kidney or pancreatic transplantation have been associated with:

a. nonabsorbable suture material used for the anastomosis.

b. incomplete bladder emptying due to diabetic cystopathy.

c. bacteriuria associated with included duodenal segments.

d. metabolic acidosis due to bicarbonate leak.

e. all of the above.

13. Which of the following is(are) typically associated with preputial calculi?

a. Stranguria

b. Phimosis

c. Voided urine culture positive for enterococcus or *Escherichia coli*

d. a and b.

e. b and c.

14. Which of the following statements about prostatic calculi is(are) TRUE?

a. Most prostatic calculi are asymptomatic.

b. Large prostatic calculi most commonly involve the central zone of the prostate.

c. Serum prostate-specific antigen and intraprostatic stone volume are directly correlated.

d. Uric acid is the predominant component of prostatic calculi.

e. All of the above

ANSWERS

1. **d. Bladder outlet obstruction.** Bladder outlet obstruction may be an etiologic factor in over 75% of bladder calculi cases and is most often related to benign prostatic hyperplasia.

2. **e. *Proteus*.** Whereas all these organisms produce urease, infection with *Proteus* species is most commonly associated with bladder calculi.

3. **e. carbon dioxide and ammonium.** Urease hydrolyzes urea, forming ammonium and carbon dioxide, which increases urinary pH. Alkaline urine promotes supersaturation and precipitation of crystals of magnesium ammonium phosphate and carbonate apatite.

4. **b. Kock pouch.** The Kock pouch has a 4% to 43% incidence of stone formation. The predominant location of calculi in the Kock pouch is along staple lines of the afferent nipple valve. Substituting polyglycolic mesh for Marlex mesh in collar construction and limiting the number of staples has reduced the incidence of pouch calculi.

5. **d. Hyperoxaluria.** Patients with augments and diversions often have reabsorption of urinary solutes, especially sulfate and ammonium, through the intestinal segment with resultant metabolic disturbances. Chronic hyperchloremic metabolic acidosis may develop that, in turn, can result in hypercalciuria, hyperphosphaturia, hypermagnesuria, and hypocitraturia, predisposing the patient to urinary tract calculi.

6. **d. Cystoscopy.** Cystoscopy is the single most accurate examination to document the presence of a bladder calculus. Cystoscopy also assists in surgical planning by identifying prostatic enlargement, bladder diverticulum, or urethral stricture that may need correction before or in conjunction with the treatment of the stone.

7. **a. Irrigation with Suby solution G.** Dissolution as primary treatment for bladder calculi can be protracted and is, now, rarely employed.

8. **c. Urethral diverticulum.** Urethral calculi in females are exceptionally rare due to low rates of bladder calculi and a short urethra that permits passage of many smaller calculi. Calculi in the female urethra are typically associated with urethral diverticulum or urethrocele.

9. **b. patients usually present with multiple calculi.** Primary bladder calculi in children are generally solitary and, once removed, recurrence is rare. Primary bladder calculi are 9 to 33 times more common in boys, and are generally not associated with anatomic, functional, or infectious abnormalities. Cereal diets low in phosphate and animal protein are considered an important risk factor. Dietary modification results in a sharp decrease in stone formation.

10. **e. a and d.** Endoscopic instrumentation is not advised in patients who have undergone continent diversion with Indiana or Penn pouches, or for those with Mitrofanoff catheterizable stomas, because there is a significant risk of injury to the continence mechanisms and the narrow limbs themselves. Although percutaneous intervention is generally advised for the treatment of stones in patients with pouch diversions, the large caliber of the catheterizable limb and the nipple valve of the Kock pouch will tolerate endoscopic instrumentation. Transurethral endoscopic management is generally considered safe in augmented bladders, regardless of the type of substitution performed.

11. **c. males are 3 to 10 times more likely to develop stones than females.** Unlike the nonaugmented population, females who have undergone augmentation cystoplasty are more likely to develop bladder calculi than males, likely owing to the higher incidence of cloacal abnormalities, which require additional procedures to establish continence. Bladder stone formation is more common in patients who have undergone intestinal substitution, as opposed to gastric and ureteric substitution or autoaugmentation, although the role of intestinal mucus in stone formation remains a matter of debate.

12. **e. all of the above.** All of the above have been found to be associated with bladder stone formation after renal

transplantation, as well as pancreatic allografts, which are drained via the bladder. Although scant reports have noted stone formation on absorbable suture, the overwhelming majority of stone formation occurs in the presence of nonabsorbable suture or clip material.

13. **e. b and c.** Stranguria is a common presenting complaint in patients with migratory urethral calculi but is rarely associated with preputial calculi. Rather, progressive voiding complaints are the norm, with rare progression to urinary retention.

14. **a. Most prostatic calculi are asymptomatic.** The vast majority of prostatic calculi are asymptomatic and are an infrequent cause of lower urinary tract symptomatology. The majority of stones are found in the posterior and posterolateral zones of the prostate, and large stones are rarely found within the central zone. Serum prostate-specific antigen levels are unaffected by the presence of prostate calculi. Prostatic calculi are generally composed of calcium phosphate and calcium carbonate, which form on nidi of inspissated prostatic secretions.

Additional Study Point

1. Clean intermittent catheterization is associated with a significant reduction in risk of bladder stone formation compared with an indwelling catheter.

Prostate

Development, Molecular Biology, and Physiology of the Prostate

David M. Berman, MD, PhD ● Ronald Rodriguez, MD, PhD ● Robert W. Veltri, PhD

QUESTIONS

1. Which of the following is not considered a sex accessory tissue?
   a. Prostate gland
   b. Seminal vesicles
   c. Tunica albuginea
   d. Ampullae
   e. Bulbourethral gland

2. Which one of the following statements about the seminal vesicles is TRUE?
   a. All placental mammals have seminal vesicles.
   b. Dogs have seminal vesicles but rats do not.
   c. Seminal vesicle carcinoma is a significant veterinary health problem in dogs.
   d. Dogs have seminal vesicles but not vasa deferentia.
   e. Rats have seminal vesicles but dogs do not.

3. Which one of the following statements about seminal vesicle and prostate epithelium is FALSE?
   a. Seminal vesicle epithelial nuclei are more similar to each other in size and shape than prostate nuclei.
   b. Seminal vesicle epithelial cells are more likely to contain intracytoplasmic pigment than prostate epithelial cells.
   c. Prostate and seminal vesicle epithelia both have distinct basal and luminal compartments.
   d. Prostate epithelium has a basal cell compartment but seminal vesicle does not.
   e. Epithelium has a basal cell compartment but seminal vesicle does not.

4. All of the following proteins are abundantly present in seminal plasma EXCEPT:
   a. tyrosine kinase.
   b. fructose.
   c. citric acid.
   d. spermine.
   e. prostaglandins.

5. Which fetal hormone stimulates the development of the wolffian ducts?
   a. Estradiol
   b. Dihydrotestosterone (DHT)
   c. Estrone
   d. Testosterone
   e. Inhibin

6. Which one of the following statements about fetal development of the lower urogenital tract is FALSE?
   a. The urogenital sinus derives from the cloaca.
   b. The cloaca gets its name (L. "sewer") because it receives input from the gastrointestinal and urinary tracts.
   c. The seminal vesicles derive from the posterior portion of the wolffian ducts, whereas the prostate derives from the anterior portion.
   d. Nkx3.1 is the earliest molecular marker of prostate development.
   e. The urogenital sinus is a primordial structure that contributes to bladder *and* prostate development.

7. Which fetal hormone is most important in stimulating the growth of the prostate during development?
   a. Estradiol
   b. DHT
   c. Estrone
   d. Testosterone
   e. Inhibin

8. Which one of the following statements is TRUE regarding the role of androgens in prostate development?
   a. Males will develop prostates in the presence of sufficiently high levels of androgens but females will not.
   b. Females will develop prostates in the presence of sufficiently high levels of androgens but males will not.
   c. Both males and females will develop prostates in the presence of sufficiently high levels of androgens.
   d. Prostate tissue rudiments with a normal androgen receptor in the epithelium but mutant androgen receptor

in the mesenchyme will develop into normal prostates in the presence of sufficiently high levels of androgen.

   e. Prostate tissue rudiments with androgen receptor overexpression in the epithelium but mutant androgen receptor in the mesenchyme will develop into normal prostates in the absence of androgen.

9. An andromedin is:

   a. a cofactor that binds to androgens.

   b. any virilizing hormone (any hormone that facilitates male sexual maturation).

   c. a virilizing paracrine hormone that is secreted by a cell in response to androgen and does not require androgen receptor for its reception.

   d. a receptor for a virilizing hormone.

   e. a specific receptor for androstenedione.

10. Which molecular pathway is incorrectly paired with its proposed function in prostate development?

   a. TGF-β: Growth inhibitor

   b. DHT: Activates transcription of androgen receptor target genes in the mesenchyme

   c. Nkx3.1: Activates genes that drive septation of the cloaca

   d. Cre: Viral gene used to engineer excision of genes of interest in transgenic mice

   e. Noggin: Antagonizes binding of bone morphogenetic proteins at their receptors

11. Which of the following is TRUE regarding neuroendocrine cells found within the prostate?

   a. The major secretory product is serotonin.

   b. A minor component of the secretory products is bombesin.

   c. Another name for them is AFUD.

   d. A major secretory product of the neuroendocrine cells is thyroid-stimulating hormone (TSH).

   e. Insulin is the major stimulator of secretion in the neuroendocrine cell system within the prostate.

12. Which of the following secretory products is not known to be expressed by mature terminally differentiated prostate epithelial cells?

   a. Prostate-specific antigen (PSA)

   b. Prostate acid phosphatase

   c. Androgen receptor

   d. Synaptophysin

   e. 15-Lipoxygenase

13. Which of the following biomarkers is not characteristic of prostate stem cells?

   a. CD49f

   b. Sca1

   c. Keratins 5/14

   d. Enrichment in proximal prostatic ducts

   e. PSA

   f. Trop2

14. Which α_1-adrenergic receptor subtype is linked to smooth muscle contraction in the prostate?

   a. α_D

   b. α_{1A}

   c. α_{1B}

   d. α_2

   e. α_{2B}

15. Which of the following is TRUE regarding testosterone?

   a. Testosterone is synthesized by the Sertoli cells of the testes.

   b. Testosterone is synthesized by the Leydig cells of the testes.

   c. Testosterone is a direct precursor of pregnenolone.

   d. 5α-Reductase is an enzyme that converts DHT into testosterone.

   e. Aromatase converts estrogens into testosterone.

16. The normal concentration of DHT in the plasma of normal males is:

   a. 100 ng/dL.

   b. 300 ng/dL.

   c. 400 ng/dL.

   d. 50 ng/dL.

   e. 20 ng/dL.

17. Dehydroepiandrosterone (DHEA) has been suggested as a major source of testosterone within the plasma. What percentage of total testosterone has been determined to be derived from DHEA?

   a. 1%

   b. 2%

   c. 5%

   d. 15%

   e. 20%

18. To what is the majority of testosterone in the plasma bound?

   a. Insulin

   b. Cholesterol

   c. Prostaglandins

   d. TP53

   e. Sex hormone–binding globulin (SHBG)

19. Which of the following is not a well-recognized type of growth control regulating the prostate?

   a. Endocrine factors

   b. Neuroendocrine factors

   c. Anabolic factors

   d. Autocrine factors

   e. Extracellular matrix factors

20. Which of the following is TRUE regarding androgen receptor intracellular events?

   a. DHT or testosterone binding to specific nucleotide receptors in the cytoplasm

   b. Dimerization and activation of the steroid receptor

   c. Endocytosis of native androgen

   d. Transport of the active receptor and androgen from the nucleus to the cell membrane

   e. Release of coactivators from the androgen receptor elements

21. How many isoforms of 5α-reductase exist?
    a. 1
    b. 4
    c. 2
    d. 7
    e. 3

22. Which 5α-reductase isoform predominates in the prostate gland?
    a. Type 1
    b. Type 2
    c. Type 3
    d. Type 4
    e. Type 5

23. All of the following characteristics have been found to be characteristic of a prostate intermediate epithelial cell EXCEPT:
    a. keratin 5/14.
    b. keratin 8/18.
    c. c-kit.
    d. proliferative activity.
    e. contact with basal cells.

24. Which of the following biologic functions is not regulated by the laminins?
    a. Cell adhesion
    b. Proliferation
    c. Differentiation
    d. Chromatin remodeling
    e. Migration

25. What proportion of the total human ejaculate comes from the prostate?
    a. 1/2
    b. 1/6
    c. 1/4
    d. 1/8
    e. 1/16

26. Seminal plasma has unusually high concentrations of all of the following EXCEPT:
    a. zinc.
    b. insulin.
    c. fructose.
    d. spermine.
    e. PSA.

27. What is the source of fructose in seminal plasma?
    a. Prostate gland
    b. Bulbourethral gland
    c. Vas deferens
    d. Seminal vesicles
    e. Basal cells

28. All of the following are secretory products of the prostate EXCEPT:
    a. hK17.
    b. prostate-specific transglutaminase 4.

    c. KLK-L11.
    d. prostatic acid phosphatase (PAP).
    e. PSP-94.

29. For chromatin remodeling and activation of transcription all but which one of these molecular components is required?
    a. CPB/p300
    b. SWI-SNF
    c. Histone 1A (H1A)
    d. Androgen receptor
    e. TRAP/DRIP

30. TRUE or FALSE: The androgen receptor is activated only by DHT, which is the active form of androgen after conversion from testosterone by 5α-reductase.
    a. True
    b. False

31. Transcriptional regulation by the androgen receptor is directed by all of the following EXCEPT:
    a. occupancy of the ligand binding domain by an active androgen.
    b. pioneer factors, such as Fox A1, which organize the target regions of the genome to which the androgen receptor will regulate.
    c. androgen response elements, which are binding sequences in the DNA to which the zinc fingers of the androgen receptor bind directly.
    d. intracellular calcium levels.

32. Compartmentalization of the androgen receptor from the cytosol to the nucleus is dependent on:
    a. dimerization.
    b. adenosine triphosphate (ATP).
    c. RAN-mediated transport.
    d. nuclear localization and nuclear export signals.
    e. all of the above.

33. Which feature of the androgen receptor polymorphisms is thought to impact on the overall activity of androgen target gene induction?
    a. Zinc finger motifs
    b. Poly CAG repeats
    c. Nuclear export signals
    d. Ligand binding domain

34. Which of the following is TRUE with regard to the effects of estrogens in prostate development?
    a. Estrogens are not required for the development of a prostate because ER-α and ER-β knockout mice have phenotypically normal prostates.
    b. ER-α regulates ductal formation.
    c. ER-β is required for prostates to allow sperm to mature to an active form.
    d. b and c

35. When the androgen receptor binds to an androgen response element, which of the following is(are) true?
    a. The dimerization of the receptor is always head to head, regardless of whether the sequence is a direct repeat or an inverted repeat.

b. The dimerization occurs head to head for an inverted repeat and head to tail for a direct repeat.

c. The dimerization of the androgen receptor occurs on the DNA template in a process that requires ATP and heat shock proteins.

d. The androgen receptor can bind to a target androgen response element in either a head-to-head or a head-to-tail orientation, depending on the orientation of the structural gene.

ANSWERS

1. **c. Tunica albuginea.** Sex accessory tissues include the prostate gland, seminal vesicles, ampullae, and bulbourethral glands. They are believed to play a major, but unknown, role in the reproductive process.

2. **e. Rats have seminal vesicles but dogs do not.** All placental mammals have prostates, but some, including the dog, lack seminal vesicles. Rats and mice do have seminal vesicles.

3. **c. Prostate and seminal vesicle epithelia both have distinct basal and luminal compartments.** Seminal vesicle epithelium has variably sized and shaped nuclei and intracytoplasmic pigment. Both features are absent in normal prostate epithelium.

4. **a. tyrosine kinase.** In the human, the sex accessory tissues produce extremely high concentrations of many important and potent biologic substances that appear in the seminal plasma, such as fructose (2 mg/mL), citric acid (4 mg/mL), spermine (3 mg/mL), and prostaglandins (200 mg/mL); extremely high concentrations of zinc (150 mg/mL); proteins (40 mg/mL); and specific proteins such as immunoglobulins, proteases, esterases, and phosphatases.

5. **d. Testosterone.** The wolffian ducts develop into the seminal vesicles, epididymis, vas deferens, ampulla, and ejaculatory duct; and the developmental growth of this group of glands is stimulated by fetal testosterone and not DHT.

6. **c.** The seminal vesicles derive from the posterior portion of the wolffian ducts, whereas the prostate derives from the anterior portion. The prostate develops from the urogenital sinus not the wolffian duct.

7. **b. DHT.** In contrast, the prostate first appears and starts its development from the urogenital sinus during the third month of fetal growth and development is directed primarily by DHT, not testosterone.

8. **c. Both males and females will develop prostates in the presence of sufficiently high levels of androgens.** If androgen (testosterone or DHT) levels are sufficiently high at the right time in fetal development, prostate development will proceed in the urogenital sinus regardless of whether the embryo is male or female. For prostate development to proceed, androgen receptor is required to be functional in the mesenchyme.

9. **c. a virilizing paracrine hormone that is secreted by a cell in response to androgen and does not require androgen receptor for its reception.** An andromedin is a hypothetical paracrine hormone that is made by the prostatic mesenchyme in response to androgen receptor activation. It acts on prostate epithelium to induce prostate development and growth.

10. **c. Nkx3.1: Activates genes that drive septation of the cloaca.** Nkx3.1 is a homeobox family transcription factor that participates in gene regulation, but Nkx3.1 knockout mice have a higher incidence of neoplasia and mild branching defects in the prostate. They do not show cloacal defects. Cloacal defects are seen in compound mutations of paralogous homeobox (Hox) genes *Hoxa13* and *Hoxd13*.

11. **d. A major secretory product of the neuroendocrine cells is thyroid-stimulating hormone (TSH).** There are three types of prostate neuroendocrine cells, with the major type containing both serotonin and TSH. The two minor cell types contain calcitonin and somatostatin. Neuroendocrine cells are also termed APUD, for amine precursor uptake decarboxylase cells, and bring about their regulatory activity by the secretion of hormonal polypeptides or biogenic amines such as serotonin (5-hydroxytryptamine), which is a common marker for these cells.

12. **d. Synaptophysin.** Numerous proteins have been identified as being expressed in terminally differentiated epithelial cells. Secretory cells stain abundantly with PSA, acid phosphatase, androgen receptor, leucine amino peptidase, and 15-lipoxygenase. They are also rich in keratins (subtypes 8 and 18). Synaptophysin is made by the neuroendocrine cells.

13. **e. PSA.** PSA is made by prostate luminal cells; keratin 8/18 is made by intermediate cells; chromogranin-A is made by neuroendocrine cells.

14. **b. α_{1A}.** Research work has demonstrated three subtypes of the α_1-adrenergic receptor (α_{1A}, α_{1B}, and α_{1D}), of which the α_{1A} receptor appears to be linked to contraction.

15. **b. Testosterone is synthesized by the Leydig cells of the testes.** Foremost among the hormones and growth factors that stimulate the prostate is the prohormone testosterone, which must be converted within the prostate into the active androgen DHT. Testosterone is synthesized in the Leydig cells of the testes from pregnenolone by a series of reversible reactions; however, once testosterone is reduced by 5α-reductase into DHT or to estrogens by aromatase, the process is irreversible. In other words, whereas testosterone can be converted into DHT and into estrogens, estrogens and DHT cannot be converted into testosterone.

16. **d. 50 ng/dL.** The concentration of DHT in the plasma of normal men is very low, 50 ng/dL, in comparison to testosterone.

17. **a. 1%.** Less than 1% of the total testosterone in the plasma is derived from DHEA.

18. **e. sex hormone–binding globulin (SHBG).** The majority of testosterone bound to plasma protein is associated with SHBG.

19. **c. Anabolic factors.** These interactive types of growth control are usually accomplished by several generalized systems (see Fig. 90–6 in *Campbell-Walsh Urology, 10th Edition*) and include (1) endocrine factors or long-range signals arriving at the prostate by serum transport of hormone originating from the secretions of distant organs (this would include serum hormone-like steroids such as testosterone, estrogens, and serum endocrine polypeptide hormones such as prolactin and gonadotropins); (2) neuroendocrine signals originating from neural stimulation such as serotonin (5-hydroxytryptamine), acetylcholine, and

norepinephrine; (3) paracrine factors or soluble tissue growth factors that stimulate or inhibit growth and are elaborated over short ranges between neighboring cells within the prostate tissue compartment such as basic fibroblast growth factor and epidermal growth factor; (4) autocrine factors or growth factors such as autocrine motility factor, produced and released by a cell and then fed back on the same cell's external membrane receptors to regulate its own growth or function; (5) intracrine factors, factors that share structural and regulatory features with autocrine factors but that work inside the cell; (6) extracellular matrix factors, insoluble tissue matrix systems that make direct and coupled contact by being attached through integrins and adhesion molecules of the basal membrane to couple cytoskeleton organization with the extracellular matrix components that include the glycosaminoglycans such as heparin sulfate; and (7) cell-cell interactions.

20. **b. Dimerization and activation of the steroid receptor.** A simplified schematic of the temporal sequence of intracellular events is depicted in Figures 90–10 and 90–11 in *Campbell-Walsh Urology, 10th Edition* and includes (1) cellular uptake of testosterone; (2) testosterone converted to DHT by metabolism of 5α-reductase; (3) DHT or testosterone binding to a specific androgen receptor in the cytoplasm; (4) dimerization and activation of the steroid receptor by a variety of post-translational steps, including, for instance, phosphorylation; (5) active nuclear transportation of the activated androgen receptor in an ATP-dependent manner; (6) chromatin remodeling via interaction with coregulatory molecules; (7) transactivation or transrepression via interactions with other coactivators or corepressor, in a histone acetyl transferase-dependent process; (8) binding of the activated receptor/coactivator complex to androgen receptor elements that are short, specific sequences of DNA recognized by androgen receptor dimers; and (9) gene regulation, in which the receptor acts as a transcription factor and, when bound to the DNA and matrix in proximity to androgen target genes, increases the RNA polymerase (Pol II) transcription of the DNA into messenger RNA.

21. **c. 2.** In the human, rat, and monkey there are two isoforms of 5α-reductase.

22. **b. Type 2.** The type 2 isoform is mutated in 5α-reductase deficiency and is the dominant isoform present in the prostate gland.

23. **c. c-kit.** The following molecules have not been demonstrated to be indicative of intermediate cells; high levels of androgen receptor, Sca-1, c-kit, and c-Met. Intermediate cells reside between and contact both basal and luminal/secretory cells.

24. **d. Chromatin remodeling.** The key functional properties of the laminins include cell adhesion, proliferation, differentiation, growth, and migration. Laminin surrounds the basement membrane of prostate acinar epithelial cells, capillaries, smooth muscle, and nerve fibers but not lymphatics, lymphocytes, or fibroblasts; and the laminin's structure and its distribution is disrupted in benign prostatic hyperplasia and higher-grade prostatic intraepithelial neoplasia and higher-grade prostate neoplasms.

25. **b. 1/6.** The major contribution to the volume of seminal plasma (average 3 mL) comes from the seminal vesicles (1.5 to 2 mL); from the prostate (0.5 mL); and from the Cowper gland and glands of Littre (0.1 to 0.2 mL).

26. **b. insulin.** In relation to other body fluids, the seminal plasma is unusual because of its very high concentrations of potassium, zinc, citric acid, fructose, phosphorylcholine, spermine, free amino acids, prostaglandins, and enzymes, most notably acid phosphatase, diamine oxidase, β-glucuronidase, lactate dehydrogenase, α-amylase, prostate-specific antigen, and seminal proteinase.

27. **d. Seminal vesicles.** The source of fructose in human seminal plasma is the seminal vesicles. Patients with congenital absence of the seminal vesicles also have an associated absence of fructose in their ejaculates.

28. **a. hK17.** Major secretory protein markers that are found in abundance and have clinical significance include (1) prostate-specific antigen (human kallikrein 3 [hK3 (protein) or KLK3 (gene)]; (2) human kallikrein 2 (hK2 or *KLK2*); (3) prostate KLK-L1; (4) prostatic acid phosphatase (PAP); and (5) prostate-specific protein (PSP-94), also termed β-microseminoprotein.

29. **c. Histone 1A (H1A).** To achieve such coordinate regulation, the protective packaging of DNA is engineered through an elegant system of tightly wound DNA around an eight-component histone core called a nucleosome. This core consists of dimers of H2A, H2B, H3, and H4, whose ability to compact DNA is directly regulated by post-translational modifications. The selective regulation of such post-translational histone modification constitutes a major regulatory mechanism for gene expression and is referred to as the "histone code" (see Fig. 90–11 in *Campbell-Walsh Urology, 10th Edition*). Histone modifications include acetylation, phosphorylation, ubiquinization, and methylation.

30. **b. False.** The androgen receptor is activated by weak adrenal androgens, testosterone, or DHT, although DHT is clearly the most potent of all the known androgens. It is estimated that DHT is between 2.5- to 10-fold more active at target gene activation than testosterone.

31. **d. intracellular calcium levels.** Although intracellular calcium is known to regulate a large number of physiologic processes, it does not have a known role in regulating androgen receptor function.

32. **e. all of the above.** After binding ligand, the androgen receptor dissociates from chaperonins, dimerizes, and then is transported to the nucleus via a nuclear localization motif, which activates Ran-dependent active transport, a process that is ATP dependent.

33. **b. Poly CAG repeats.** The shorter the length, the more active the androgen receptor is thought to function.

34. **a. Estrogens are not required for the development of a prostate because ER-α and ER-β knockout mice have phenotypically normal prostates.**

35. **a. The dimerization of the receptor is always head to head, regardless of whether the sequence is a direct repeat or an inverted repeat.** Although most models predicted that inverted repeats and direct repeats androgen response elements would have dimers that bind with opposite polarity, this prediction was not observed in x-ray crystallography studies.

Additional Study Points

1. The seminal vesicles are extremely resistant to disease.
2. There are two major cellular compartments in the prostate: epithelial and stromal.
3. The stromal compartment consists of connective tissue, smooth muscle cells, and fibroblasts.
4. Because the plasma half-life of testosterone is 10 to 20 minutes, patients who undergo a bilateral orchiectomy are functionally castrate within 1 to 2 hours after surgery.
5. The androgen receptor is transported to the nucleus and then back to the cytoplasm.
6. The longer the CAG glutamine repeats in the androgen receptor, the lower its activity in activating target genes.
7. The source of prostaglandins is the seminal vesicles.
8. Complexed PSA is irreversibly bound to α_1-antichymotrypsin and α_2-macroglobulin.
9. Semenogelin is degraded by PSA and gives rise to the coagulum of the semen.
10. Kallikrein 14 exerts an effect on seminal liquefaction. The biologic function of semenogelin involves capacitation.
11. Few drugs reach concentrations in the prostatic secretions that approach or surpass their concentrations in the blood. The exceptions include erythromycin, sulfonamides, tetracycline, clindamycin, trimethoprim, and the fluoroquinolones.
12. Prostatic fluid is more acidic than is serum.

Benign Prostatic Hyperplasia: Etiology, Pathophysiology, Epidemiology, and Natural History

Claus G. Roehrborn, MD

QUESTIONS

1. Which statement is correct regarding the role of androgenic hormones in the etiology of BPH?
   a. Testosterone and dihydrotestosterone are the sole causes of the hyperplasia taking place in the prostate after the age of 40 years.
   b. The volume of androgen receptors in the prostate decreases with aging, leading to a lesser response to androgenic stimuli.
   c. Dihydrotestosterone is considered the more potent of the androgenic steroid hormones by a factor of approximately 10:1.
   d. Of the two 5α-reductase isoforms, type 1 is most commonly found in the prostate.
   e. Only testosterone produced in the testis and not in the adrenal gland enters into the prostate gland.

2. Regarding genetic and familial factors in the etiology of BPH, which statement is TRUE?
   a. There is no evidence that BPH is a familial disease.
   b. Any man who underwent TURP should alert his sons that their chance of having to have TURP is three times greater than age-matched controls.
   c. Cases of familial BPH tend to occur in men with smaller prostates than the sporadic cases of BPH.
   d. Approximately 50% of cases of BPH in men who undergo surgery when younger than the age of 60 are estimated to be inheritable.
   e. The most likely inheritance pattern is autosomal recessive.

3. The prevalence of a disease is defined as the number of:
   a. diseased people per 100,000 population per year.
   b. existing cases per 100,000 population at a distinct target date.
   c. deaths per 100,000 population per year.
   d. deaths per number of diseased.
   e. cumulative cases of a disease over a specified time period.

4. Concerning the autopsy prevalence of BPH or stromoglandular hyperplasia:
   a. no adequate studies have been done to date.
   b. it is commonly found in men of all ages.
   c. it is very uncommon in men younger than the age of 30 years.
   d. it is found in 100% of men beginning at the age of 40 years.
   e. international comparisons are impossible owing to a lack of its definition.

5. Which of the following statements regarding the International Prostate Symptom Score (IPSS) is TRUE?
   a. Moderate symptom severity is defined as a score from 10 to 20 points.
   b. The IPSS score addresses irritative and obstructive symptoms and issues of incontinence.
   c. Quantitative symptom scores in BPH are not as important as are objective measures such as a flow rate recording.
   d. The IPSS score has been translated and validated in many languages.
   e. Physicians and nurses may fill out the IPSS score for their patients after consultation.

6. Which statement is TRUE regarding prostate volume?
   a. International studies show significant similarity in prostate volume in white, age-stratified men.
   b. Prostate volume assessment by digital rectal examination (DRE) is reproducible across examiners.
   c. Although there is a steady increase in total prostate volume with age, the transition zone volume increases only marginally.
   d. Magnetic resonance imaging measurements are, in general, smaller compared with transrectal ultrasound measurements.
   e. DRE estimation of prostate volume is fairly accurate when done by an experienced urologist.

7. Concerning liver disease and BPH, which of the following statements is TRUE?

   a. Ethanol consumption increases circulating levels of estrogens.

   b. The risk of having surgery for BPH is increased in heavy drinkers.

   c. The intake of ethanol can decrease serum testosterone levels by a variety of mechanisms.

   d. Most autopsy studies find a higher prevalence of BPH in men with liver cirrhosis.

   e. In men with liver disease histologic specimens of the prostate show a similar influence of estrogen such as seen in hormonally treated prostate cancer.

8. How do medications influence symptoms and flow rate?

   a. There is no documented influence of any medication on symptoms or flow rate.

   b. Antihistamines and bronchodilators significantly decrease urinary flow rates.

   c. Calcium channel blockers and β-adrenergic blockers reduce urinary flow rates significantly.

   d. Antidepressants, antihistamines, and bronchodilators increase the symptom score by several points.

   e. Anticholinergic agents decrease the peak urinary flow rate markedly.

9. Concerning correlations between baseline parameters, which statement is TRUE?

   a. A clinically useful correlation exists between prostate volume and serum prostate antigen (PSA) level.

   b. Many studies have shown a significant correlation between the transition zone volume and symptom severity.

   c. Correlation of symptoms, bother, interference, and quality of life are poor.

   d. Urinary flow rate and prostate volume correlate highly with serum PSA level.

   e. Serum PSA level shows a strong correlation with symptom frequency and bother.

10. Which statement is correct regarding the study of the natural history of BPH?

    a. Placebo groups from treatment trials are useful because they do not have treatment biases.

    b. A longitudinal population-based study has the fewest biases and is the most useful type of study.

    c. Control groups from intervention or medical therapy trials reflect the natural history of the disease in unselected community-dwelling men.

    d. Placebo groups have fewer selection biases compared with population-based studies.

    e. No such studies have been conducted.

11. Regarding the magnitude of the placebo response and its perception, which of the following statements is TRUE?

    a. Placebo response is not dependent on the baseline severity score.

    b. Most patients report subjective improvement when the drop from baseline is 30%.

    c. The higher the baseline score, the more of a drop is required for patients to subjectively feel improved.

    d. Perception of improvement is independent of baseline score.

    e. There are convincing data to demonstrate that the final score after treatment is more important than the baseline score or the drop from baseline.

12. Descriptive studies of the incidence rates of acute urinary retention (AUR) have demonstrated that:

    a. depending on the population studied, incidence rates less than 5 to more than 130 cases/1000 man-years have been reported.

    b. the incidence rates reported do not differ significantly between various studies and populations.

    c. AUR has been poorly defined, and therefore no incidence rate can be calculated.

    d. incidence rates of approximately 10/1000 man-years have been reported in all watchful waiting studies.

    e. incidence rates of AUR have not been reported in the urologic literature, only prevalence rates.

13. What is the most significant finding regarding analytical epidemiology of AUR?

    a. Serum PSA level is a more powerful predictor of AUR than is age.

    b. Serum PSA level and prostate volume have limited ability to predict episodes of AUR.

    c. Urinary flow rates in placebo control groups are strong predictors of AUR episodes.

    d. Age has been found to be the most significant risk factor for AUR in population-based studies.

    e. There is virtually no relationship between symptom frequency and bother and AUR episodes.

14. Which statement regarding surgery for BPH is TRUE?

    a. The incidence rates of surgery are similar across wide geographic regions and ethnic backgrounds.

    b. Compared with AUR, surgery is a less traumatic end point.

    c. Surgery is a less common end point compared with AUR.

    d. Most patients with BPH eventually require surgery for their condition.

    e. Surgery rates for BPH have remained stable since about 1990.

ANSWERS

1. **c. Dihydrotestosterone is considered the more potent of the androgenic steroid hormones by a factor of approximately 10:1.** The androgenic steroid hormones testosterone and dihydrotestosterone (DHT) have a permissive role in the development of BPH but are not the sole cause. The androgen receptor remains at high levels in the prostate in aging men and specifically in BPH tissues, maintaining responsiveness to androgenic stimuli. The most common of the two 5α-reductase isoforms is type 2 in the benignly enlarged prostate gland. DHT is considered more potent than testosterone by a factor of approximately 10:1.

2. **d. Approximately 50% of cases of BPH in men who undergo surgery when younger than the age of 60 are estimated to be inheritable.** There is significant evidence to suggest that some cases of BPH are familial,

with autosomal dominant being the most likely inheritance pattern. An increased risk for BPH surgery exists mostly for men who come to BPH surgery when younger than the age of 60, and men with familial cases of BPH have larger glands than men with sporadic cases.

3. **b. existing cases per 100,000 population at a distinct target date.** When studying diseases by descriptive or analytical epidemiologic methods it is important to have a good understanding of the definitions that apply. Most epidemiologic terms are expressed as rates, which are the number of cases for persons expressed over the population. The definitions that are of relevance are incidence rates = the number of diseased people/100,000 population/year; prevalence = the number of existing cases of the disease of interest/100,000 at a distinct target date; mortality rate, which is the number of deaths/100,000 population/year; and fatality, which equals the number of deaths due to the disease/number of diseased people.

4. **c. it is very uncommon in men younger than the age of 30 years.** The autopsy prevalence of BPH has been studied as early as 1984 by Berry and colleagues.* Since then, many studies have been done on virtually all continents in many ethnic groups. It is astonishing that these studies find a very significant agreement in terms of the actual prevalence of histologic BPH or stromoglandular hyperplasia around the world. Stromoglandular hyperplasia or BPH is very uncommon in men younger than the age of 30 but then increases steadily in an almost linear manner. In fact, approximately 90% of men in their 80s have evidence of stromoglandular hyperplasia.

5. **d. The IPSS score has been translated and validated in many languages.** The IPSS symptom score is a seven-question self-administered questionnaire that yields a total score ranging from 0 to 35 points. Men who score 0 to 7 points are classified as mildly symptomatic, those scoring from 8 to 19 points as moderately symptomatic, and those from 20 to 35 points as severely symptomatic. The IPSS score addresses irritative and obstructive but no incontinence symptomatology. It is widely accepted that quantitative symptom scores are far more important than, for example, urinary flow rate recordings. Fortunately, the IPSS score, the most widely utilized instrument, has been translated and culturally validated in many languages.

6. **a. International studies show significant similarity in prostate volume between white age-stratified men.** Prostate volume can relatively easily be assessed by transrectal ultrasonography (TRUS). TRUS has been found to be a reliable measure that is reproducible across examiners in contrast to digital rectal examination (DRE), which is only poorly reproducible. MRI is very expensive and it yields in general a larger volume compared with TRUS measurements. Of note is the fact that international studies show significant similarity in regard to total and transitional zone prostate volume in white, age-stratified men.

7. **c. The intake of ethanol can decrease serum testosterone levels by a variety of mechanisms.** It is known that alcohol intake may decrease plasma testosterone levels by reducing production of and increasing clearance of testosterone. However, despite this hypothetical reason for a

lower incidence, an inverse relationship has been described. The age-adjusted multivariant relative risks for undergoing surgery for BPH in men drinking more than three or four glasses of alcohol per day is lower than in age-matched controls. Of course, this could be due to a bias against surgery in patients who are heavy drinkers and therefore in poor health. It is interesting to note, however, that in the majority of studies, namely, four of five, a lower prevalence of BPH is found in men with cirrhosis compared with those without cirrhosis.

8. **d. Antidepressants, antihistamines, and bronchodilators increase the symptom score by several points.** There is only one study that systematically assessed the effect of medications on urinary symptoms and flow rate. Cold medications containing α-sympathomimetics tend to exacerbate lower urinary tract symptoms by the expected effect on the smooth muscle of the bladder outlet. Data from the Olmsted County Study of Urinary Symptoms and Health Status Among Men show that daily use of antidepressants, antihistamines, or bronchodilators is associated with a 2- to 3-point increase in the symptom score. However, only the daily use of antidepressants is associated with a decrease in the age-adjusted urinary flow rate.

9. **a. A clinical useful correlation exists between prostate volume and serum PSA level.** In general there is an absence of useful baseline correlations between subjective and objective parameters such as symptoms, frequency, quality of life, and urinary flow rate measures of obstruction and prostate volume. However, symptom, bother, and interference with quality of life show excellent correlation with each other, and a clinically useful correlation exists between total and transition zone prostate volume and serum PSA in men with BPH.

10. **b. A longitudinal population-based study has the fewest biases and is the most useful type of study.** There are several ways to study the natural history of BPH. One can look at watchful waiting cohorts or placebo-controlled groups of medication trials or study population-based groups of men longitudinally over time. The latter is clearly the best way of studying the natural history of the disease because it incurs the fewest biases. However, it is also the most tedious and most expensive method. Placebo groups in medication trials clearly suffer from enrollment biases but do provide useful information.

11. **c. The higher the baseline score, the more of a drop is required for patients to subjectively feel improved.** The placebo response is partially a regression to the mean and partially an effect induced by the interaction between patient and doctor. The response is clearly dependent on the baseline severity score with patients' higher scores having a larger decrease from baseline. The perception of subjective improvement has been shown to be dependent on the drop from baseline as well as on the baseline itself. For example, the higher the baseline score, the more of a drop from baseline is required for patients to have a subjective perception of improvement. Overall, a 3-point decrease is associated with a subjective perception of improvement.

12. **a. depending on the population studied, incidence rates less than 5 to more than 130 cases/1000 man-years have been reported.** AUR has been studied over the past few years in population-based studies as well

---

*Sources referenced can be found in *Campbell-Walsh Urology, 10th Edition,* on the Expert Consult website.

as in placebo-control groups from long-term treatment trials. The incidence rates differ significantly between different studies owing to the inclusion and exclusion criteria and selection biases. Fortunately, AUR is a very clearly defined outcome and, thus, incidence rates can easily be calculated and compared.

13. **d. Age has been found to be the most significant risk factor for AUR in population-based studies.** In population-based studies such as the Olmsted County Study of Urinary Symptoms and Health Status Among Men, age is the most significant predictor of AUR. Data from placebo groups of long-term medical treatment trials demonstrate that serum PSA is the most powerful predictor of AUR together with prostate volume. Although this appears to be on the surface a contradiction, it can be relatively easily explained by the fact that in BPH treatment trials, elderly men with already an existing diagnosis of BPH are enrolled. Thus, age plays a lesser factor in terms of predicting AUR. In population-based studies in which men stratified by age are followed over long periods of time, age plays a more significant factor compared with PSA.

14. **b. Compared with AUR, surgery is a less traumatic end point.** Incidence rates of surgery vary significantly across geographic regions and patients with different ethnic backgrounds. Depending on the interaction between patient and physician, the physician can convince the patient to undergo surgery or, based on the patient's comorbidities, talk him out of surgery. The same cannot be said for urinary retention. It is clear that a vast majority of patients do not require surgery in the course of their disease but, rather, can be treated effectively with reassurance alone or medication.

Additional Study Points

1. BPH is characterized by an increased number of epithelial and stromal cells, not an increase in their size.
2. Androgens are required for normal cell proliferation and differentiation and actively inhibit cell death.
3. Serum estrogen levels increase in men with age.
4. Early periurethral nodules are stromal; transition cell zone proliferation is glandular.
5. Prostatic stroma represents 40% of the gland. Smooth muscle is a prominent component of the stroma.
6. Autonomic system overactivity may contribute to lower urinary tract symptoms in men with BPH.
7. Symptoms using the AUA Symptom Index are classified as mild if the score is 0 to 7, moderate if it is 8 to 19, and severe if it is 20 to 35.
8. Men and women experience a decrease in maximum urinary flow rate as they age.
9. Bladder fibrosis is seen in both sexes with advancing age.
10. After spontaneous AUR, 15% of patients will have another episode and three fourths will undergo surgery; after precipitated AUR, 9% will have another episode and 26% will undergo surgery.

Evaluation and Nonsurgical Management of Benign Prostatic Hyperplasia

Thomas Anthony McNicholas, MBBS, FRCS, FEBU ●
Roger Sinclair Kirby, MD, MA, FRCS ● Herbert Lepor, MD

QUESTIONS

1. Benign prostatic hyperplasia (BPH) originates in the:
   a. transition zone.
   b. peripheral zone.
   c. periurethral glands.
   d. transition zone and periurethral zone.
   e. anterior zone.

2. A strong correlation exists between prostate volume and:
   a. serum prostate-specific antigen (PSA).
   b. International Prostate Symptom Score (IPSS).
   c. peak urinary flow rate (PFR).
   d. postvoid residual (PVR) urine volume.
   e. sexual activity.

3. Medications that may exacerbate lower urinary tract symptoms (LUTS) include (multiple answers are possible):
   a. α-adrenergic antagonists.
   b. α-adrenergic agonists.
   c. β-adrenergic agonists.
   d. muscarinic agonists.
   e. phosphodiesterase inhibitors.

4. The primary objective of the digital rectal examination (DRE) in the evaluation of men with LUTS is to:
   a. estimate prostate volume.
   b. obtain prostatic secretions.
   c. identify prostate nodules.
   d. determine rectal tone.
   e. determine pelvic sensation.

5. In older men with LUTS, which test should be routinely performed?
   a. Urinalysis
   b. Peak flow rate
   c. Serum creatinine assay
   d. Renal ultrasonography
   e. Urodynamics

6. It is advisable in a man with BPH and a slightly elevated creatinine concentration to perform:
   a. transurethral resection of the prostate (TURP).
   b. intravenous pyelography.
   c. renal ultrasonography.
   d. urodynamic study.
   e. computed tomography.

7. What percentage of men have histologically proven BPH with a serum PSA value of 4.0 ng/mL or greater?
   a. 5%
   b. 15%
   c. 30%
   d. 50%
   e. 70%

8. An IPSS of 20 indicates severe:
   a. LUTS.
   b. BPH.
   c. bladder outlet obstruction.
   d. bladder dysfunction.
   e. erectile dysfunction.

9. An absolute indication for surgery (TURP or open prostatectomy) is:
   a. severe symptoms.
   b. PVR urine volume of 300 mL or more.
   c. single episode of acute urinary retention (AUR).
   d. refractory gross hematuria secondary to BPH.
   e. discovery of prostate cancer.

10. A low PFR suggests:
    a. severe symptoms.
    b. bladder outlet obstruction.
    c. impaired detrusor contractility.
    d. b or c.
    e. poor testing methodology.

11. What is the next step for a man with a PVR urine volume of 300 mL?
    a. Repeat the PVR
    b. Upper urinary tract imaging
    c. Urodynamic testing
    d. TURP
    e. Drug therapy

12. The probability that a urodynamic study helps to decrease the failure rate of TURP in men with a PFR of 15 mL/sec is approximately:
    a. 10%.
    b. 25%.
    c. 50%.
    d. 75%.
    e. 100%.

13. What is the percentage of men with LUTS who have uninhibited contractions?
    a. 10%
    b. 30%
    c. 60%
    d. 80%
    e. 100%

14. What is the likelihood that uninhibited detrusor contractions in men with BPH will resolve after TURP?
    a. Never
    b. Unlikely
    c. Likely
    d. Always
    e. Unpredictable

15. The finding of bladder trabeculation suggests:
    a. high-grade obstruction.
    b. high success rate after TURP.
    c. high PVR urine volume.
    d. none of the above.
    e. all of the above.

16. Imaging of the upper tract is indicated for:
    a. prostate glands weighing more than 50 g.
    b. urinalysis demonstrating hematuria.
    c. bladder trabeculation.
    d. severe LUTS.
    e. a family history of prostate cancer.

17. An improvement in the IPSS of 5 units correlates with a symptom improvement that is:
    a. marked.
    b. moderate.
    c. slight.
    d. none.
    e. poor.

18. Urodynamic testing reliably predicts response after:
    a. TURP.
    b. α-adrenergic blockers.
    c. 5α-reductase inhibitors.
    d. laser vaporization.
    e. none of the above.

19. There is compelling evidence that PVR urine volume is:
    a. related to symptom severity.
    b. associated with the risk for urinary tract infection (UTI).
    c. both a and b.
    d. neither a nor b.
    e. predictable.

20. The definition of detrusor instability is bladder pressure greater than which level at a bladder volume of 300 mL or less?
    a. 5 cm H_2O
    b. 15 cm H_2O
    c. 40 cm H_2O
    d. 60 cm H_2O
    e. 70 cm H_2O

21. The likelihood that a man with acute urinary retention will develop a subsequent episode of urinary retention within 1 week is approximately:
    a. 20%.
    b. 40%.
    c. 60%.
    d. 80%.
    e. 100%.

22. The incidence of developing acute urinary retention is related to:
    a. prostate size.
    b. age.
    c. severity of symptoms.
    d. age and size of the prostate.
    e. all of the above.

23. The best way to eliminate bias in a clinical study is to use:
    a. honest investigators.
    b. a placebo-controlled, double-blind design.
    c. randomization.
    d. large sample size.
    e. paid investigators.

24. The larger the sample size, the:
    a. less treatment effect required to achieve statistical significance.
    b. better the study.
    c. greater the treatment effect required to achieve statistical significance.
    d. worse the study is.
    e. none of the above.

25. Which of the following is the attractive feature of medical therapy relative to TURP?
    a. Fewer side effects
    b. Reversible side effects
    c. Less serious side effects
    d. Oral therapy
    e. All of the above

26. During the past decade the incidence of TURP in the United States has decreased by approximately:
    a. 10%.
    b. 50%.
    c. 100%.
    d. 200%.
    e. 300%.

27. Which of the following percentages of men older than 50 years of age have moderate or severe LUTS?
    a. 2%
    b. 5%
    c. 30%
    d. 50%
    e. 75%

28. The ideal candidate for medical therapy should have symptoms that are:
    a. severe.
    b. moderate.
    c. minimal.
    d. bothersome.
    e. acceptable or not bothersome.

29. Smooth muscle accounts for what percentage of the area density of the prostate?
    a. 5%
    b. 10%
    c. 20%
    d. 40%
    e. 60%

30. The tension of prostate smooth muscle is mediated by the:
    a. α_1 receptor.
    b. α_2 receptor.
    c. β_2 receptor.
    d. muscarinic cholinergic receptor.
    e. androgen receptor.

31. What is the advantage of terazosin over prazosin?
    a. Its longer half-life
    b. Its better absorption
    c. Its greater α_1-receptor selectivity
    d. Its lesser expense
    e. None of the above

32. Which α_1 receptor subtype mediates prostate smooth muscle tension?
    a. α_{1A}
    b. α_{1B}
    c. α_{1C}
    d. α_{1D}
    e. α_{1E}

33. The improvement in IPSS after terazosin administration depends on baseline:
    a. age.
    b. prostate size.
    c. PVR urine volume.
    d. total symptom score.
    e. None of the above

34. The mean treatment-related improvement in response to terazosin in IPSS units is approximately:
    a. 2.
    b. 4.
    c. 6.
    d. 8.
    e. 10.

35. The durability of the improvement in symptom scores and PFRs for α_1-adrenergic blockers has been reported to be up to how many months?
    a. 12
    b. 42
    c. 60
    d. 92
    e. 120

36. Which of the following α-adrenergic blockers does not lower blood pressure in men with uncontrolled hypertension?
    a. Terazosin
    b. Doxazosin
    c. Tamsulosin
    d. Prazosin
    e. Indoramin

37. Retrograde ejaculation is most commonly seen with:
    a. terazosin.
    b. prazosin.
    c. finasteride.
    d. alfuzosin
    e. tamsulosin.

38. Approximately what percentage of men have both BPH and hypertension?
    a. 5%
    b. 15%
    c. 30%
    d. 50%
    e. 70%

39. What is the likely mechanism for dizziness with α_1-adrenergic blocker therapy?
    a. Vascular
    b. Central nervous system
    c. Carotid baroreceptor
    d. Psychological factors
    e. None of the above

40. The major advantage of tamsulosin 0.4 mg over terazosin 10 mg is:
    a. greater efficiency.
    b. less retrograde ejaculation.
    c. no dose titration.
    d. greater lowering of blood pressure.
    e. it is less expensive.

41. The embryologic development of the prostate is mediated primarily by:
    a. testosterone.
    b. dihydrotestosterone.
    c. androstenedione.
    d. estradiol.
    e. progesterone.

42. Finasteride and dutasteride significantly decrease the long-term risk of:
    a. acute urinary retention.
    b. surgical intervention.
    c. both a and b.
    d. neither a nor b.
    e. erectile dysfunction.

43. Finasteride is most effective at relieving hematuria in men with:
    a. prostatitis.
    b. enlarged prostate.
    c. transurethral prostatectomy.
    d. obstructing prostate.
    e. anticoagulant therapy.

44. Dutasteride:
    a. is a dual inhibitor of type 1 and type 2 5α-reductase.
    b. is more effective than finasteride.
    c. results in a 95% reduction in PSA after 6 months of therapy.
    d. is less likely than finasteride to result in loss of libido.
    e. improves erectile function.

45. The adverse event that limits the use of flutamide as a primary treatment of BPH is:
    a. breast tenderness.
    b. diarrhea.
    c. erectile dysfunction.
    d. loss of libido.
    e. hypertension.

46. A potential advantage of cetrorelix, a gonadotropin-releasing hormone antagonist, for the treatment of BPH is:
    a. lower cost.
    b. ability to titrate the level of androgen suppression.
    c. ease of administration.
    d. rapid response.
    e. less erectile dysfunction.

47. A Veterans Affairs study demonstrated that terazosin is more effective than finasteride at rapidly relieving symptoms in men with:
    a. small prostates.
    b. intermediate-size prostates.
    c. large prostates.
    d. severe symptoms.
    e. all of the above.

48. In the Veterans Affairs study, over 12 months, finasteride was no better than placebo at:
    a. improving symptoms.
    b. lowering micturition voiding pressure.
    c. decreasing prostate size.
    d. improving PFRs.
    e. all of the above.

49. The MTOPS study confirmed that:
    a. α-adrenergic blockers and 5α-reductase inhibitors are equivalent in relieving symptoms.
    b. α-adrenergic blockers reduce the risk of AUR over 7 years of treatment.
    c. finasteride reduces the risk of adenocarcinoma of the prostate.
    d. a combination of an α-adrenergic blocker and a 5α-reductase inhibitor is the most effective way of preventing BPH progression.
    e. finasteride improved sexual function.

50. The CombAT study showed that in men with larger prostates:
    a. the combination of dutasteride and tamsulosin was more effective than either agent alone.
    b. over time, the symptomatic response to dutasteride exceeded that to tamsulosin.
    c. both a and b.
    d. neither a nor b.
    e. tamsulosin did not affect ejaculation.

51. Antimuscarinic therapy is contraindicated in men with LUTS/BPH.
    a. Yes, in all such men.
    b. No, only in men with large and persistent residual urine volumes.
    c. No, not if combined with α-adrenergic blockers.
    d. Only in those with an enlarged prostate.
    e. No, it can be used in all men with symptoms of overactive bladder.

52. Men with significant obstruction, large residual urine volumes, and overactive bladder who fail first-line treatment with α-adrenergic blockers should be considered for:
    a. the addition of an antimuscarinic drug.
    b. surgical therapy.
    c. the addition of phosphodiesterase inhibitors.
    d. upper tract imaging.
    e. none of the above.

53. If a man with LUTS, stabilized on doxazosin, complains of erectile dysfunction he should NOT be given:
    a. low-dose sildenafil.
    b. low-dose vardenafil.
    c. low-dose tadalafil.
    d. alprostadil.
    e. a vacuum pump.

54. The amount spent on phytotherapy for the treatment of BPH is estimated to be:
    a. $10 million.
    b. $100 million.

c. $1 billion.

d. $10 billion.

e. $15 billion.

55. The definitive mechanism of action for *Serenoa repens* is:

a. inhibition of 5α-reductase.

b. inhibition of cyclooxygenase.

c. inhibition of lipoxygenase.

d. downregulation of androgen receptor.

e. inconclusive.

56. Potential future therapeutic avenues in BPH pharmacotherapy include:

a. nitric oxide donors.

b. α-adrenoceptor agonists.

c. HMG coenzyme A inhibitors.

d. endothelin antagonists.

e. selective estrogen receptor modulators.

57. The next major step in the treatment of LUTS will require:

a. unraveling the pathophysiology of LUTS.

b. more selective α_1 blockers.

c. dual inhibitors of dihydrotestosterone.

d. new strategies for relaxing prostate smooth muscle.

e. more selective 5α-reductase inhibitors.

ANSWERS

1. **d. transition zone and periurethral zone.** The proliferative process originates in the transition zone and the periurethral glands.

2. **a. serum prostate-specific antigen (PSA).** A strong correlation exists between serum PSA levels and prostate volume.

3. **b *and* d.** Current prescription and over-the-counter medications should be examined to determine whether the patient is taking drugs that impair bladder contractility (anticholinergics) or that increase outflow resistance (α-sympathomimetics).

4. **c. identify prostate nodules.** The DRE and neurologic examination are done to detect prostate or rectal malignancy, to evaluate anal sphincter tone, and to rule out any neurologic problems that may cause the presenting symptoms.

5. **a. Urinalysis.** In older men with BPH and a higher prevalence of serious urinary tract disorders, the benefits of an innocuous test such as urinalysis clearly outweigh the harm involved.

6. **c. renal ultrasonography.** An elevated serum creatinine level in a patient with BPH is an indication for imaging studies (ultrasonography) to evaluate the upper urinary tract.

7. **c. 30%.** Twenty-eight percent of men with histologically proven BPH have a serum PSA level greater than 4.0 ng/mL.

8. **a. LUTS.** The International Prostate Symptom Score (IPSS), which is identical to the American Urological Association Symptom Index (AUASI), is recommended as the symptom scoring instrument to be used for the baseline assessment of symptom severity in men presenting with LUTS. When the IPSS system is used, symptoms can be classified as mild (0 to 7), moderate (8 to 19), or severe (20 to 35). The IPSS cannot be used to establish the diagnosis of BPH.

9. **d. refractory gross hematuria secondary to BPH.** Surgery is recommended if the patient has refractory urinary retention (at least one failed attempt at catheter removal) or any of the following conditions, clearly secondary to BPH: recurrent urinary tract infection, recurrent gross hematuria, bladder stones, renal insufficiency, or large bladder diverticula.

10. **d. b or c.** One study found that flow rate recording cannot distinguish between bladder outlet obstruction and impaired detrusor contractility as the cause for a low PFR.

11. **a. Repeat the PVR.** Residual urine volume measurement has significant intraindividual variability that limits its clinical usefulness.

12. **a. 10%.** One study recommended invasive urodynamic testing for patients with a PFR higher than 15 mL/sec. For the population in their study this would have resulted in an additional 9% of patients being excluded from surgery and a decrease in failure rate to 8.3%.

13. **c. 60%.** Overactive contractions are present in about 60% of men with LUTS and correlate strongly with irritative voiding symptoms.

14. **c. Likely.** Uninhibited detrusor contractions resolve in most patients after surgery.

15. **d. none of the above.** Bladder trabeculation may predict a slightly higher failure rate in patients managed by watchful waiting but does not predict the success or failure of surgery.

16. **b. urinalysis demonstrating hematuria.** Upper urinary tract imaging is not recommended for routine evaluation of men with LUTS unless they also have one or more of the following: hematuria, urinary tract infection, renal insufficiency (ultrasonography recommended), history of urolithiasis, and history of urinary tract surgery.

17. **b. moderate.** The group mean changes in IPSS for subjects rating their improvement as markedly, moderately, or slightly improved, unchanged, or worse were −8.8, −5.1, −3.0, −0.7, and +2.7, respectively.

18. **e. none of the above.** Urodynamic testing does not predict symptom improvement after α-adrenergic blockade, transurethral microwave thermotherapy, or prostatectomy.

19. **d. neither a nor b.** One study reported no correlation between the IPSS and PVR urine volume. There are also no data documenting that the incidence of UTI is related to PVR urine volume.

20. **b. 15 cm H₂O.** The definition of detrusor instability is the development of a detrusor contraction exceeding 15 cm H_2O at a bladder volume less than or equal to 300 mL.

21. **d. 80%.** Of 59 Danish patients presenting to an emergency department with acute retention, 73% had recurrent urinary retention within 1 week after removal of the catheter.

22. **e. all of the above.** The incidence of AUR was related to age, severity of symptoms, and size of the prostate gland.

23. **b. a placebo-controlled, double-blind design.** The only mechanism to ensure that the potential bias of the subject and the investigator does not influence the outcome is a randomized, double-blind, placebo-controlled design.

24. **a. less treatment effect required to achieve statistical significance.** The larger the number of subjects enrolled in a study, the smaller the change required to achieve statistical significance.

25. **e. All of the above.** The attractive feature of medical therapy relative to prostatectomy is that clinically significant outcomes are obtained with fewer, less serious, and reversible side effects.

26. **b. 50%.** A 55% reduction in transurethral prostatectomy has occurred despite the progressively increasing number of men enrolled in the Medicare program.

27. **c. 30%.** Approximately 30% of American men older than 50 years of age have moderate to severe symptoms.

28. **d. bothersome.** The ideal candidate for medical therapy should have symptoms that are bothersome and have a negative impact on the quality of life.

29. **d. 40%.** Smooth muscle is one of the dominant cellular constituents of BPH, accounting for 40% of the area density of the hyperplastic prostate.

30. **a. α_1 receptor.** The tension of prostate smooth muscle is mediated by the α_1-adrenergic receptor.

31. **a. Its longer half-life.** Terazosin and doxazosin are long-acting α-adrenergic blockers that have been shown to be safe and effective for the treatment of BPH.

32. **a. α_{1A}.** Prostate smooth muscle tension has been shown to be mediated by the α_{1A}-adrenergic receptor.

33. **e. None of the above.** The relationships between percent change in total symptom score and PFR versus baseline age, prostate size, PFR, PVR urine volume, and total symptom score were examined to identify clinical or urodynamic factors that predicted response to terazosin therapy. No significant association was observed between treatment effect and any of these baseline factors.

34. **b. 4.** The treatment-related improvement (terazosin minus placebo) in the IPSS and urinary PFR was 3.9 symptom units and 1.4 mL/sec, respectively.

35. **b. 42.** The initial improvements in symptom scores and PFR in 450 subjects were maintained for up to 42 months.

36. **c. Tamsulosin.** The advantage of not lowering blood pressure in men who are hypertensive at baseline is open to debate.

37. **e. tamsulosin.** The treatment-related incidences of asthenia, dizziness, rhinitis, and abnormal ejaculation observed for 0.4 mg of tamsulosin were 2%, 5%, 3%, and 11%, respectively, and for 0.8 mg of tamsulosin were 3%, 8%, 9%, and 18%, respectively.

38. **c. 30%.** Approximately 30% of men treated for BPH have coexisting hypertension.

39. **b. Central nervous system.** The α_1-adrenergic receptor–mediated dizziness and asthenia are likely due to effects at the level of the central nervous system.

40. **c. no dose titration.** The major advantage of 0.4 mg tamsulosin and slow-release alfuzosin is the lack of requirement for dose titration.

41. **b. dihydrotestosterone.** The embryonic development of the prostate is dependent on the androgen dihydrotestosterone.

42. **c. both a and b.** The Proscar Long-Term Efficacy and Safety Study (PLESS) represents one of the longest duration multicenter randomized, double-blind, placebo-controlled studies reported in the literature on medical therapy for BPH. The unique findings of PLESS were related to incidences of both AUR and surgical intervention for BPH. The risk reduction of AUR and BPH-related surgery was clinically relevant, especially in men with very large prostates. Dutasteride studies showed a risk reduction of AUR of 57% and the risk reduction of BPH-related surgery of

48% compared with placebo (Roehrborn et al, 2002).* Pooled results of a 2-year open-label extension study indicate that the risk reduction of AUR and BPH-related surgery was durable over 4 years (Debruyne et al, 2004).

43. **c. transurethral prostatectomy.** These preliminary observations have been confirmed by a randomized, double-blind, placebo-controlled study demonstrating that finasteride prevents recurrent gross hematuria secondary to BPH after prostatectomy.

44. **a. is a dual inhibitor of type 1 and type 2 5α-reductase.** This is unlike finasteride, which only inhibits the type 2 isoform.

45. **a. breast tenderness.** The incidences of breast tenderness and diarrhea in the flutamide group were 53% and 11%, respectively.

46. **b. ability to titrate the level of androgen suppression.** A potential advantage of a gonadotropin-releasing hormone antagonist over the luteinizing hormone–releasing hormone agonists in the treatment of BPH is the ability to titrate the level of androgen suppression.

47. **e. all of the above.** In the study the mean group differences between terazosin versus placebo and terazosin versus finasteride for all of the outcome measures other than prostate volume were highly statistically significant. Terazosin was more effective than finasteride in those subjects with large prostates.

48. **a. improving symptoms.** The mean group differences between finasteride and placebo were not statistically significant for IPSS, Symptom Problem Index, BPH Impact Index, and PFR.

49. **d. a combination of an α-adrenergic blocker and a 5α-reductase inhibitor is the most effective way of preventing BPH progression.** This was the key conclusion of the important MTOPS study that looked at finasteride versus doxazosin versus a combination of both and placebo in men with symptomatic BPH.

50. **c. Both a and b.**

51. **b. No, only in men with large and persistent residual urine volumes.** Antimuscarinics are only contraindicated if there is a large residual urine because such men have a higher risk of retention.

52. **b. surgical therapy.**

53. **c. low-dose tadalafil.** The manufacturers of tadalafil recommend avoiding using it with doxazosin. However, care should be taken with the addition of any phosphodiesterase inhibitor to men already optimized on an α-adrenergic blocker because there is an increased risk of symptomatic hypotension in all men being considered for this combination.

54. **c. $1 billion.** Usage of these agents in the United States and throughout the world has escalated. It has been estimated that more than $1 billion was spent in the United States alone for these products.

55. **d. inconclusive.** Although experimental data have suggested numerous possible mechanisms of actions for the phytotherapeutic agents, it is uncertain which, if any, of these proposed mechanisms is responsible for the clinical responses.

---

*Sources referenced can be found in *Campbell-Walsh Urology*, *10th Edition*, on the Expert Consult website.

56. **e. Endothelin antagonists.** Although currently untested, endothelin antagonists represent a possible therapeutic avenue in BPH.

57. **a. unraveling the pathophysiology of LUTS.** Our current understanding of the pathophysiology of clinical BPH is rudimentary. It is, therefore, imperative to develop a more comprehensive understanding of the pathophysiology of symptoms.

Additional Study Points

1. In patients with severe irritable symptoms and dysuria, urine cytology should be performed.
2. Surgery is generally recommended for patients with refractory urinary retention, recurrent urinary tract infections, recurrent gross hematuria, bladder stones, renal insufficiency, and large bladder diverticula.
3. Flow rates are inaccurate if the voided volume is less than 150 mL. A PFR is better than an average flow rate.
4. Patients with a PFR greater than 15 mL/sec are less likely to have good treatment outcomes after prostatectomy than are patients with a PFR below 15 mL/sec.
5. It takes at least a 3-point change in the IPSS for the patient to perceive a difference.
6. Conservative therapy to reduce the severity and bother of symptoms involves decreasing fluid intake especially before bedtime, moderating alcohol and caffeine intake, and maintaining timed voiding schedules.
7. α-Adrenergic blockers may influence smooth muscle growth in the prostate. They may induce apoptosis.
8. α-Adrenergic blockers may induce the floppy iris syndrome, and patients should be warned of this if they are to have cataract surgery.
9. The maximal reduction in prostate volume requires 6 months after initiation of androgen suppressive therapy.
10. The rationale for aromatase inhibition is that estrogens may be involved in the pathogenesis of BPH.
11. Finasteride reduces prostate volume by about 20%.
12. Anticholinergic receptor blockers may be safely administered in patients with bladder outlet obstruction to reduce frequent voiding if they have PVR urine volumes less than 200 mL and do not report increasing hesitancy and show signs of increasing PVR urine volume when placed on such therapy.
13. Phosphodiesterase inhibitors have been known to improve IPSS scores. Phosphodiesterase inhibitors do not improve flow rate.
14. Concomitant use of α-adrenergic blockers and phosphodiesterase inhibitors may lead to hypotension.

Minimally Invasive and Endoscopic Management of Benign Prostatic Hyperplasia

John M. Fitzpatrick, MCh, FRCSI

QUESTIONS

1. Intraprostatic stents were developed after first being used to treat which of the following conditions?
   a. Peripheral vascular disease
   b. Coronary artery disease
   c. Urethral strictures
   d. Bronchial obstruction
   e. Lacrimal duct obstruction

2. The recognized role for the use of intraprostatic stents is:
   a. to replace transurethral resection of the prostate (TURP).
   b. in preoperative patients likely to develop retention.
   c. in patients unfit for TURP.
   d. in patients receiving anticoagulants.
   e. for temporary relief of obstruction.

3. The most common complication associated with temporary stents is:
   a. urinary retention.
   b. stent migration.
   c. clot retention.
   d. urinary incontinence.
   e. encrustation.

4. Which of the following statements is TRUE of transurethral needle ablation (TUNA)?
   a. It causes necrosis at 15 days.
   b. It induces fibrosis at 7 days.
   c. It causes damage to α-adrenergic receptors at 1 week.
   d. It affects nitric oxide synthase receptors, which are least vulnerable to damage.
   e. It does not affect prostate-specific antigen (PSA) staining.

5. The complication most commonly reported after TUNA is:
   a. hemorrhage.
   b. urinary retention.
   c. irritative voiding symptoms.
   d. urinary tract infection.
   e. urethral strictures.

6. Transurethral microwave therapy (TUMT) has been shown to:
   a. damage nerve fibers, with necrosis possible.
   b. induce apoptosis of prostatic cells.
   c. be superior to TURP in terms of clinical efficacy.
   d. cause retrograde ejaculation.
   e. induce post-treatment voiding difficulties with low-energy treatment.

7. Treating symptomatic benign prostatic hyperplasia with the laser:
   a. causes the greatest degree of tissue vaporization with the holmium:yttrium-aluminum-garnet laser.
   b. is most appropriate for large prostates.
   c. is associated with a low incidence of postoperative urinary infection.
   d. has a hemorrhage rate of 8%.
   e. causes erectile dysfunction in 46% of patients.

8. An absolute indication for TURP is:
   a. postvoid residual urine volume of 250 mL.
   b. recurrent urinary infections.
   c. American Urological Association Symptom Index score of 20 or greater.
   d. detrusor pressure at a maximum flow of 65 cm H_2O.
   e. inability to use medical treatment because of side effects.

9. Postoperative complications have been related to preoperative measurement of:
   a. urinary flow rate.
   b. detrusor pressure at a maximum urinary flow rate.
   c. postvoid residual urine volume.
   d. prostatic size.
   e. serum creatinine value.

10. Outflow obstruction can be predicted by:
    a. serum creatinine value.
    b. urine culture results.
    c. maximum urinary flow rate.
    d. cystoscopy.
    e. pressure-flow studies.

11. TURP should begin with:
    a. incision of the bladder neck.
    b. resection of the middle lobe.
    c. resection of the bladder neck.
    d. resection of prostatic tissue at the 12-o'clock position.
    e. resection of prostatic tissue at the 3- or 9-o'clock position.

12. The most common complication after TURP is:
    a. failure to void.
    b. hemorrhage requiring transfusion.
    c. clot retention.
    d. urinary tract infection.
    e. transurethral resection syndrome.

13. Transurethral vaporization of the prostate (TUVP) results in:
    a. vaporization.
    b. coagulation.
    c. desiccation.
    d. vaporization and desiccation.
    e. cauterization.

14. In short-term studies, TUVP has been shown to be comparable to TURP in what area?
    a. Urinary flow rate improvement
    b. Incidence of postoperative hemorrhage
    c. Postoperative urinary infection
    d. Sexual complications
    e. Improvement in postvoid residual urine volume

15. Which of the following statements is TRUE of transurethral incision of the prostate (TUIP)?
    a. It is appropriate for large prostates.
    b. It has a high complication rate.
    c. It causes retrograde ejaculation in up to 37% of cases.
    d. It commonly results in TURP syndrome.
    e. It was described by Bottini in 1900.

ANSWERS

1. **b. Coronary artery disease.** Stents were first introduced as a method of treating certain cardiovascular conditions.

2. **c. in patients unfit for TURP.** Eventually it became clear that the major role for stents was likely to be found in the management of patients who were unfit for surgery, either in the short or in the long term, in whom the alternative would have been months or indeed a lifetime of indwelling urethral catheterization.

3. **d. urinary incontinence.** In the largest number of patients (318) reported from one center, complications were divided into none, moderate, and severe. In the patients who were described as having severe complications, stress or urgency incontinence occurred in 63, emptying problems in 8, and frequency and/or nocturia (>3 episodes) in 57.

4. **c. It causes damage to α-adrenergic receptors at 1 week.** In studies with the TUNA system, necrosis was maximal at 7 days, with fibrosis developing by 15 days. In treated areas there was an absence of staining for PSA, smooth muscle actin, and α-adrenergic neural tissue. Nitric oxide synthase receptors were found to be most vulnerable

to thermal damage and occurred earliest, with damage to the α-adrenergic receptors maximal at 1 to 2 weeks.

5. **b. urinary retention.** By far the most common complication reported, however, is post-treatment urinary retention, occurring at a rate of 13.3% to 41.6%. It can be expected that within the first 24 hours about 40% of patients will experience urinary retention.

6. **b. induce apoptosis of prostatic cells.** In one study, apoptosis was verified by the terminal deoxynucleotidyl nick-end labeling (TUNEL) technique in sections showing histologic changes suggestive of apoptosis, such as pyknotic nuclei and chromatin segregation. Necrotic areas were frequently seen in the prostate to a depth of 4 to 5 cm. Outside these necrotic areas, normal and apoptotic areas were interspersed, the latter confirmed by TUNEL. The area of tissue damage seen after TUMT was relatively small compared with the volume of the prostates. The heat was implicated as the cause of the apoptosis, but there was no speculation as to the exact mechanism whereby heat brought about this effect.

7. **a. causes the greatest degree of tissue vaporization with the holmium-yttrium-aluminum-garnet laser.** The vaporization techniques using the neodymium:yttrium-aluminum-garnet (Nd:YAG) laser with high-energy density beams at high power (60 to 100 W) at a wavelength of 1064 nm have been effective for removing small amounts of tissue immediately during the procedure. However, this is a relatively inefficient technique because of the high power required. The holmium:yttrium-aluminum-garnet (Ho:YAG) laser energy is absorbed by water (unlike the Nd:YAG) at a wavelength of 2140 nm and causes considerable tissue vaporization. The methods of using the Ho:YAG laser have evolved because of several modifications in both the technology and the methodology. The technique has passed through simple vaporization to combined endoscopic laser ablation of the prostate and is now used to resect large pieces of prostatic tissue.

8. **b. recurrent urinary infections.** Although symptoms constitute the primary reason for recommending intervention, in patients with an obstructing prostate there are some absolute indications. These are acute urinary retention, recurrent infection, recurrent hematuria, and azotemia.

9. **e. serum creatinine value.** Patients with a serum creatinine level greater than 1.5 mg/dL had a 25% incidence of postoperative complications, versus an incidence of 17% in those who had a normal creatinine level.

10. **e. pressure-flow studies.** Pressure-flow studies are recommended as an optional test. This is one of the best ways to evaluate a patient's degree of obstruction and detrusor function, particularly when the diagnosis is unclear.

11. **d. resection of tissue at the 12-o'clock position.** The resection begins at the bladder neck, starting at the 12-o'clock position and is carried down to the 9-o'clock position, in a stepwise manner.

12. **a. failure to void.** The most common complications in the immediate postoperative period were, in one study, failing to void (6.5%), bleeding requiring transfusion (3.9%), and clot retention (3.3%).

13. **d. vaporization and desiccation.** With TUVP, two electrosurgical effects are combined: vaporization and desiccation. Vaporization steams tissue away using high heat, and coagulation uses lower heat to dry out tissue.

14. **a. Urinary flow rate improvement.** One study showed that in a relatively small number of cases, TUVP was as effective as TURP in relieving urodynamically proven outflow obstruction but the overall complication rate for TUVP was 17.5%.

15. **c. It causes retrograde ejaculation in up to 37% of cases.** TUIP causes a decrease in retrograde ejaculation compared with TURP. The incidence of retrograde ejaculation after TURP ranges from 50% to 95%, but after TUIP it has been reported as occurring in 0% to 37% of cases.

Additional Study Points

1. Complications of urethral stent placement include hematuria, migration, infections, incrustation, epithelial hyperplasia, irritative urinary symptoms, and painful ejaculation.

2. With the use of TUNA there is a 14% requirement for re-operation in less than 2 years. Thus long-term efficacy has not been clearly demonstrated.

3. TUMP offers less morbidity than TURP but is not as effective in relieving outlet obstruction or improving symptoms.

4. A peak urinary flow rate of less than 15 mL/sec does not differentiate between outflow obstruction and detrusor impairment.

5. Venous bleeding after TURP can be controlled by filling the bladder with 100 mL of irrigating fluid and placing the catheter on traction for 5 to 10 minutes.

6. The TUR syndrome is secondary to dilutional hyponatremia and may present as mental confusion, nausea, vomiting, hypertension, bradycardia, and visual disturbances.

7. Intraoperative priapism is managed by injecting an α-adrenergic agent into the corpora.

8. Outcomes of a TURP are best for men who are most bothered by their symptoms.

9. TUIP is particularly effective for those with bladder neck occlusion in patients with small prostates and in those who are young.

Retropubic and Suprapubic Open Prostatectomy

Misop Han, MD, MS ● Alan W. Partin, MD, PhD

QUESTIONS

1. The major advantage of open prostatectomy over transurethral resection of the prostate (TURP) in the management of a prostatic adenoma includes:
   a. removal of the prostatic adenoma under direct vision.
   b. decreased risk of hypernatremia.
   c. shortened convalescence period.
   d. decreased perioperative hemorrhage.
   e. enhanced preservation of erectile function.

2. The suprapubic prostatectomy, in comparison to the retropubic prostatectomy, allows:
   a. direct visualization of the prostatic adenoma during enucleation.
   b. better visualization of the prostatic fossa after enucleation to obtain hemostasis.
   c. easier management of a large median lobe and/or bladder calculi.
   d. an extraperitoneal approach.
   e. possible management of concomitant ureteral calculi.

3. The suprapubic approach for a prostatectomy is ideal for the patient with a large prostatic adenoma and:
   a. multiple small bladder calculi.
   b. total prostate-specific antigen level (PSA) greater than 10.0 ng/mL.
   c. erectile dysfunction.
   d. symptomatic bladder diverticulum.
   e. presence of dilated renal pelvis.

4. The most appropriate definitive treatment options for the patient with a 120-g prostatic adenoma and a symptomatic bladder diverticulum are:
   a. retropubic open prostatectomy with fulguration of the bladder diverticulum.
   b. administration of a long-acting α-adrenergic antagonist and prophylactic antibiotics.
   c. TURP followed by bladder diverticulectomy in 3 months.
   d. TURP and partial cystectomy.
   e. suprapubic prostatectomy with bladder diverticulectomy.

5. The contraindications to open prostatectomy include:
   a. biopsy-proven prostate cancer.
   b. bladder diverticulum.
   c. large bladder calculi secondary to obstruction.
   d. recurrent urinary tract infection.
   e. acute urinary retention.

6. Both retropubic and suprapubic prostatectomies:
   a. are performed in the space of Retzius.
   b. are ideal for patients with a large, obstructive prostatic adenoma and a concomitant, small bladder tumor.
   c. allow direct visualization of prostatic adenoma during enucleation.
   d. cause no trauma to the urinary bladder.
   e. require the control of dorsal vein complex before enucleation of an obstructive prostatic adenoma.

7. The most common adverse event of the open prostatectomy is:
   a. erectile dysfunction.
   b. bladder neck contracture.
   c. retrograde ejaculation.
   d. deep vein thrombosis.
   e. stress urinary incontinence.

ANSWERS

1. **a. removal of the prostatic adenoma under direct vision.** When compared with TURP, open prostatectomy offers the advantages of lower re-treatment rate and more complete removal of the prostatic adenoma under direct vision and avoids the risk of dilutional hyponatremia that occurs in approximately 2% of patients undergoing TURP.

2. **c. easier management of a large median lobe and/or bladder calculi.** The major advantage of the suprapubic procedure over the retropubic approach is that it allows direct visualization of the bladder neck and bladder mucosa. As a result, this operation is ideally suited for patients with (1) a large median lobe protruding into the bladder, (2) a clinically significant bladder diverticulum, or (3) large bladder calculi. It also may be preferable

for obese men, in whom it is difficult to gain direct access to the prostatic capsule and dorsal vein complex.

3. **d. symptomatic bladder diverticulum.** The primary indication for a suprapubic prostatectomy is the need to perform simultaneous bladder surgery such as a diverticulectomy.

4. **e. suprapubic prostatectomy with bladder diverticulectomy.** Open prostatectomy should be considered when the obstructive tissue is estimated to weigh more than 75 g. If sizable bladder diverticula justify removal, suprapubic prostatectomy and diverticulectomy should be performed concurrently.

5. **a. biopsy-proven prostate cancer.** Contraindications to open prostatectomy include a small fibrous gland, the presence of prostate cancer, and previous prostatectomy or pelvic surgery that may obliterate access to the prostate gland.

6. **a. are performed in the space of Retzius.** The advantages of a retropubic over a suprapubic approach for an open prostatectomy are clear visualization of the prostatic fossa after enucleation of the adenoma for better control of the bleeding and minimal trauma to the bladder, thus lessening postoperative bladder spasms. A suprapubic prostatectomy causes trauma to the urinary bladder. Both retropubic and suprapubic prostatectomies are performed in the space of Retzius.

7. **c. retrograde ejaculation.** Erectile dysfunction occurs in 3% to 5% of patients undergoing an open prostatectomy; it is more common in older men than in younger men. Retrograde ejaculation occurs in 80% to 90% of patients after surgery. The risk of this adverse effect is reduced if the bladder neck is preserved at the time of surgery. Also, 2% to 5% of patients will develop a bladder neck contracture 6 to 12 weeks after an open prostatectomy.

Additional Study Points

1. Of the indications for prostatectomy—(a) acute urinary retention, (b) recurrent or persistent urinary tract infections, (c) significant symptoms of bladder outlet obstruction not responsive to medical therapy, (d) persistent gross hematuria from the prostate, (e) pathologic changes of the kidneys secondary to prostatic obstruction, and (f) bladder calculi—the only absolute indication among these for prostatectomy is pathologic changes of the kidneys secondary to prostatic obstruction. All the others are relative indications because they on occasion may be corrected without the need for prostatectomy.

2. One should not consider doing an open prostatectomy for glands of less than 75 g. If an open prostatectomy is planned and it is discovered intraoperatively that the prostate is less than 50 g, it is prudent to close the patient and perform a transurethral resection of the prostate, because performing an open prostatectomy on small glands carries an extremely high complication rate.

3. Open prostatectomy should be considered in patients who cannot be placed in the lithotomy position and who have a sufficiently large gland that can be enucleated. Small fibrous glands, the presence of prostate cancer, previous prostatectomy, and pelvic surgery are contraindications to open prostatectomy.

4. Although a cystoscopic examination is not indicated for routine evaluation of obstructive voiding symptoms, one must estimate the size of the prostate adenoma preoperatively to schedule the patient appropriately. Cystoscopy may be a crucial component of that estimation. Moreover, in patients who have hematuria or a urethral stricture or in whom one needs to evaluate a known bladder calculus or diverticulum, cystoscopy is indicated.

5. More than 10% of patients undergoing open prostatectomy will require one or more units of blood either intraoperatively or postoperatively.

6. The risks of open prostatectomy include urinary incontinence, erectile dysfunction, retrograde ejaculation, urinary tract infections, bladder neck contracture, urethral stricture, and the need for a blood transfusion.

7. Nonurologic complications include pulmonary embolus, myocardial infarction, and stroke.

8. A chromic suture placed at the 5- and 7-o'clock positions at the level of the bladder neck in the prostatic fossa secures the major arterial supply to the prostate and aids in hemostasis. If the bladder neck appears obstructive, a wedge is excised dorsally and the bladder mucosa advanced into the prostatic fossa and secured with 4-0 chromic suture.

9. A method of controlling persistent hemorrhage from the prostatic fossa that cannot be controlled by the hemostatic sutures or fulguration may be accomplished with the Malament suture. A nylon suture is placed in a purse-string fashion around the bladder neck, brought out through the skin, and secured over the urethral catheter with the balloon inflated in the bladder, thus effectively tamponading the prostatic fossa. After several days the suture may be removed when hemostasis is adequate.

10. After a suprapubic prostatectomy a Malecot suprapubic tube is placed. The proper flow of continuous irrigation is entering through the urethral catheter and exiting from the suprapubic tube.

11. Erectile dysfunction occurs in 5% and retrograde ejaculation in over 90%; 5% of patients develop bladder neck contractures.

Epidemiology, Etiology, and Prevention of Prostate Cancer

Robert Abouassaly, MD, MSc ● Ian M. Thompson, Jr., MD ●
Elizabeth A. Platz, ScD, MPH ● Eric A. Klein, MD

QUESTIONS

1. Following the prostate-specific antigen (PSA) "cull effect," the incidence of prostate cancer in the United States:
   a. is decreasing.
   b. is stable.
   c. is increasing.
   d. increased initially, then decreased.
   e. is fluctuating.

2. In the United States, the highest prostate cancer incidence rates are seen in:
   a. whites.
   b. African-Americans.
   c. Hispanic/Latinos.
   d. Asian Americans
   e. American Indians.

3. Worldwide, prostate cancer:
   a. is the leading cancer diagnosis in men.
   b. is the leading cause of cancer-related mortality.
   c. is more common in northern European countries than in southern European ones.
   d. is entirely genetic in origin.
   e. has higher 5-year rates in Denmark, Poland, and Algeria compared with the United States, Canada, and Australia.

4. Regarding two large randomized trials assessing the effect of PSA screening on prostate cancer mortality:
   a. the European Randomized Study of Screening for Prostate Cancer (ERSPC) had a shorter median follow-up than the Prostate, Lung, Colorectal, and Ovarian (PLCO) cancer screening trial.
   b. the ERSPC showed no significant difference in survival between screened and unscreened men.
   c. the PLCO cancer screening trial demonstrated a 20% risk reduction in prostate cancer mortality in screened men compared with unscreened men.
   d. contamination of the control arm with PSA screening is a criticism of the PLCO cancer screening trial.
   e. both studies clearly show no benefit to PSA screening for prostate cancer.

5. Compared with a man with no family history of prostate cancer, the risk of developing prostate cancer in a man with one affected first-degree relative is:
   a. unchanged.
   b. 1.5 times higher.
   c. 2 to 3 times higher.
   d. 5 times higher.
   e. 100%.

6. HPC1-associated prostate cancers are:
   a. histologically similar to sporadic prostate cancer.
   b. caused by defects in the *BRCA2* gene.
   c. deficient in DNA repair.
   d. inherited in X-linked fashion.
   e. inherited in an autosomal-recessive fashion.

7. Biologic functions of known prostate cancer susceptibility genes include:
   a. control of the inflammatory response.
   b. antioxidant enzymes.
   c. DNA repair mechanisms.
   d. genes involved in susceptibility to infection.
   e. all of the above.

8. All of the following statements regarding gene fusions in prostate cancer are correct, EXCEPT:
   a. it results from the fusion of the 5′ untranslated end of the *TMPRSS2* serine protease gene to members of the *ETS* family of oncogenic transcription factors.
   b. the most common fusion in screen-detected prostate cancer involves *TMPRSS2* fused to *ETV1*.
   c. the *TMPRSS2* gene is expressed in malignant but not benign prostatic epithelium.
   d. *TMPRSS2* expression has been shown to be induced by estrogens.
   e. *TRMPSS*-related gene fusions are not specific for the presence of prostate cancer.

9. All of the following statements regarding estrogens and prostate cancer are correct EXCEPT:
   a. estrogen's treatment effect is primarily related to a negative feedback on the hypothalamo-pituitary-gonadal axis.

b. estrogen's treatment effect is partly through a direct inhibitory effect of estrogens on prostate epithelial cell growth.

c. aromatase-knockout mice all develop prostate cancer in their lifetime.

d. stromal estrogen receptor (ER) α expression is silenced in early prostate cancers and re-emerges with disease progression.

e. prostate epithelial ERβ may play an important role in initiation of prostate cancer.

10. Elevated serum levels of insulin-like growth factor-1 (IGF-1) have been associated with:

a. higher serum PSA levels.

b. lower body mass index.

c. reduced intraprostatic inflammation.

d. higher risk of developing prostate cancer.

e. lower serum testosterone levels.

11. Evidence suggesting that vitamin D affects the risk of prostate cancer includes the fact that:

a. men living in areas with less ultraviolet (UV) exposure have lower prostate cancer mortality rates.

b. vitamin D levels are higher in older men.

c. a calcium-poor diet predisposes men to prostate cancer.

d. native Japanese, whose diet is rich in vitamin D derived from fish, have a high incidence of prostate cancer.

e. polymorphisms conferring lower vitamin D receptor activity are associated with increased risk for prostate cancer.

12. High body mass index is associated with:

a. protection against oxidative stress.

b. higher circulating androgens.

c. lower serum PSA levels.

d. better cancer-specific survival after radical prostatectomy.

e. lower free IGF-1.

13. Hypermethylation of the following genes may play a role in prostate cancer etiology:

a. DNA repair genes (GSTP1, GPX3, and GSTM1).

b. hormonal response genes (ERα, ERβ, and RARβ).

c. genes controlling the cell cycle (CyclinD2 and 14-3-3σ).

d. tumor suppressor genes (APC, RASSF1α, DKK3, TP16INK4α, E-cadherin, and TP57WAF1).

e. all of the above.

14. Which of the following statements regarding genes involved in prostate cancer is correct?

a. Mutations of proto-oncogenes are usually associated with advanced disease.

b. There is evidence that telomere lengthening plays a role in prostate cancer.

c. The enzyme glutathione-S-transferase–1 (GST-1) is always active in prostate cancer.

d. Drugs that increase vascular endothelial growth factor (VEGF) activity are being investigated in the treatment of prostate cancer.

e. Absent expression of prostate membrane-specific antigen (PSMA) is observed after androgen withdrawal and in hormone refractory disease.

15. The major goal of a chemoprevention strategy is reduction in:

a. disease incidence and morbidity.

b. cost associated with treatment.

c. disease-promoting lifestyle habits.

d. disease-related mortality.

e. the placebo effect.

16. The major finding of the Prostate Cancer Prevention Trial (PCPT) was that:

a. finasteride reduced the 7-year period prevalence of prostate cancer by 25%.

b. more men who took finasteride died of prostate cancer than those who did not.

c. finasteride biased the interpretation of the prostate biopsies.

d. finasteride worked best in men with a positive family history.

e. finasteride improved sexual function but not voiding symptoms.

17. In the interpretation of the PCPT, "overdetection bias" refers to:

a. more men taking finasteride were sampled.

b. the histologic effect of finasteride on tumor grade.

c. more men on placebo had high-grade cancers.

d. the effect of volume reduction on tumor detection.

e. the effect of volume increase on tumor detection.

18. Findings of the Selenium and Vitamin E Cancer Prevention Trial (SELECT) include:

a. a significant reduction in the incidence of prostate cancer in the combination arm.

b. a significant increased incidence of prostate cancer in the vitamin E arm.

c. a significant increased incidence of diabetes mellitus in the selenium arm.

d. all of the above.

e. no significant difference in prostate cancer incidence in all four arms.

19. The protective effect of lycopene against prostate cancer may best be achieved by consuming:

a. cooked foods.

b. the pure form as oral capsules.

c. the pure form with other antioxidants.

d. raw vegetables.

e. fresh fruit.

20. In the PCPT, compared with placebo, finasteride use was associated with a higher incidence of:

a. prostatitis.

b. urinary tract infection.

c. surgical intervention for lower urinary tract symptoms.

d. erectile dysfunction.

e. low-grade prostate cancer.

21. The HPC1 gene (coding for the enzyme ribonuclease L [RNaseL]):

a. causes apoptosis.

b. is mutated in most men with prostate cancer.

c. is inhibited by selenium and vitamin E.

d. is regulated by androgens.

e. is inactive in men with benign prostatic hyperplasia.

22. The existence of multiple prostate cancer susceptibility genes suggests:

   a. a dominant inheritance pattern.

   b. common clinical features associated with all identified genes.

   c. genetic heterogeneity in the cause of prostate cancer.

   d. a need for yearly screening in those with a family history.

   e. multifocal tumors in affected individuals.

23. Which of the following statements regarding statins and prostate cancer is CORRECT?

   a. They elevate serum PSA.

   b. They inhibit 3-hydroxy-3-methylglutaryl coenzyme A (HMG-CoA), the rate-limiting enzyme in cholesterol biosynthesis.

   c. A recent meta-analysis found a significant association with reduced prostate cancer incidence.

   d. Statin users tend to be less healthy and medically compliant than nonusers.

   e. Prostate cancer detected in statin users has worse prognosis when stage-matched to controls.

24. A 62-year-old man with a PSA of 5.7 and a family history of prostate cancer undergoes a radical prostatectomy for clinical stage T1c prostate cancer. Pathology reveals an organ-confined Gleason 6 (3 + 3) tumor with negative margins. Molecular analysis of this tumor reveals an inactivating mutation in *HPC1*. He should be advised:

   a. to begin immediate hormonal therapy.

   b. to undergo adjuvant radiation therapy.

   c. that he is at risk of developing a central nervous system tumor.

   d. that his mother was an *HPC1* carrier.

   e. to begin serial PSA levels.

25. Hereditary prostate cancer is defined as:

   a. family history of prostate cancer.

   b. prostate cancer in a father or brother.

   c. prostate cancer in a man under age 55.

   d. prostate cancer in three successive generations.

   e. family with two affected members.

ANSWERS

1. **d. increased initially, then decreased.** According to Surveillance, Epidemiology, and End Results (SEER) program estimates, the incidence of prostate cancer peaked in 1992, approximately 5 years after introduction of PSA as a screening test, fell precipitously until 1995, increased slowly at a slope similar to that observed prior to the PSA era until 2001, and has decreased again in recent years (see Fig. 95–1 in *Campbell-Walsh Urology, 10th Edition*).

2. **b. African-Americans.** African-American men have the highest reported incidence of prostate cancer in the world, with an incidence of 255.5 per 100,000 person-years and a relative incidence of 1.6 compared with white men in the United States (American Cancer Society, 2008).* Although African-Americans have experienced a greater decline in mortality than white men since the early 1990s, their death rates remain more than 2.4 times higher than whites. Many biologic, environmental, and social hypotheses have been advanced to explain these differences, ranging from postulated differences in genetic predisposition; differences in mechanisms of tumor initiation, promotion and/or progression; higher fat in diets, higher serum testosterone levels, or higher body mass index; structural, financial, and cultural barriers to screening, early detection and aggressive therapy; and physician bias. There are currently no data that clearly indicate any of these hypotheses are the determinants of the observed differences in incidence or mortality, and it seems likely that the source of the disparity is multifactorial.

3. **c. is more common in northern European countries than in southern European ones.** Prostate cancer is the fourth most common male malignancy worldwide. Scandinavian countries have a particularly high rate of prostate cancer diagnosis and death when compared with southern European countries. In a recent study, age-standardized 5-year survival rates were found to vary greatly worldwide, ranging from 80% or higher in the United States, Australia, and Canada to less than 40% in Denmark, Poland, and Algeria.

4. **d. contamination of the control arm with PSA screening is a criticism of the PLCO cancer screening trial.** The European Randomized Study of Screening for Prostate Cancer (ERSPC) had longer median follow-up than the Prostate, Lung, Colorectal, and Ovarian (PLCO) cancer screening trial. The ERSPC had a median follow-up of 9 years, compared with 7 years in the PLCO trial. A risk reduction of 20% in prostate cancer death was observed in the ERSPC, whereas the PLCO trial failed to demonstrate a benefit to screening. The PLCO trial has been criticized for its relatively short follow-up given prostate cancer's long natural history, and for the fact that more than half the men in the control arm actually had a PSA test done outside of the trial.

5. **c. 2 to 3 times higher.** In someone with a positive family history of prostate cancer, the relative risk increases according to the number of affected family members, their degree of relatedness, and the age at which they were affected (see Table 95–2 in *Campbell-Walsh Urology, 10th Edition*).

6. **a. histologically similar to sporadic prostate cancer.** HPC1-associated cancers are caused by defects in the *RNaseL* gene, which has antiviral and pro-apoptotic functions but does not affect DNA repair mechanisms. These tumors have autosomal-dominant inheritance and are histologically indistinguishable from sporadic cancers.

7. **d. all of the above.** All of these biologic functions are represented in genes shown to predispose men with variant gene structure to prostate cancer.

8. **a. it results from the fusion of the 5′ untranslated end of the *TMPRSS2* serine protease gene to members of the *ETS* family of oncogenic transcription factors.** The most common fusion identified in localized prostate cancer involves TMPRSS2

---

*Sources referenced can be found in *Campbell-Walsh Urology, 10th Edition*, on the Expert Consult website.

fused to *ERG* (*ETS*-related gene, 21q22.3) in approximately 50% of patients (Kumar-Sinha et al, 2008). The *TMPRSS2* gene is prostate specific, and is expressed in both benign and malignant prostatic epithelium. *TMPRSS2* expression has been shown to be induced by androgens. *TRMPSS*-related gene fusions are highly specific for the presence of prostate cancer.

9. **c. aromatase-knockout mice all develop prostate cancer in their lifetime.** Aromatase-knockout mice cannot produce 17β-estradiol locally in the prostate, and despite elevated testosterone and dihydrotestosterone, they do not develop prostate cancer (McPherson et al, 2001).

10. **d. higher risk of developing prostate cancer.** A recent combined analysis found a positive correlation between serum concentration of IGF-1 and subsequent prostate cancer risk. The odds ratio in the highest versus lowest quintile was 1.38 (95% CI = 1.19 to 1.60) (Roddam et al, 2008).

11. **e. polymorphisms conferring lower vitamin D receptor activity are associated with increased risk for prostate cancer.** Interest in vitamin D as a determinant of prostate cancer risk comes from several epidemiologic observations: (1) men living in northern latitudes with less exposure to sunlight-derived UV exposure have a higher mortality rate from prostate cancer; (2) prostate cancer occurs more frequently in older men in whom vitamin D deficiency is more common both because of less UV exposure and age-related declines in the hydroxylases responsible for synthesis of active vitamin D; (3) African-Americans, whose skin melanin blocks UV radiation and inhibits activation of vitamin D, have the highest worldwide incidence and mortality rates for prostate cancer; (4) dietary intake of dairy products rich in calcium, which depresses serum levels of vitamin D, are associated with a higher risk of prostate cancer; and (5) native Japanese, whose diet is rich in vitamin D derived from fish, have a low incidence of prostate cancer. Finally, polymorphisms resulting in vitamin D receptors with lower activity have been associated with increased risk for prostate cancer.

12. **c. lower serum PSA levels.** Higher body mass index has been associated with increased biologic measures of oxidative stress, lower circulating androgen levels, lower serum PSA (perhaps as a consequence of lower circulating androgens), higher serum-free IGF-1 levels, and worse cancer specific survival after radical prostatectomy.

13. **e. all of the above.** A variety of genes implicated in prostate cancer initiation and progression are affected by these processes, including hypermethylation of hormonal response genes (*ERα*, *ERβ*, and *RARβ*), genes controlling the cell cycle (*CyclinD2* and *14-3-3σ*), tumor cell invasion/tumor architecture genes (*CD44*), DNA repair genes (*GSTP1*, *GPX3*, and *GSTM1*), tumor suppressor genes (*APC*, *RASSF1α*, *DKK3*, *TP16INK4α*, *E-cadherin*, and *TP57WAF1*), signal transduction genes (*EDNRB* and *SFRP1*), and inflammatory response genes (*PTGS/COX2*); hypomethylation of *CAGE*, *HPSE*, and *PLAU*; histone hypoacetylation of *CAR*, *CPA3*, *RARB*, and *VDR*; and histone methylation of *GSTP1* and *PSA*.

14. **a. Mutations of proto-oncogenes are usually associated with advanced disease.** There is increasing evidence that telomere shortening during cell division and oxidative cell damage, possibly as a result of chronic inflammation, may play a role in prostate carcinogenesis.

The expression of *GSTP1* is absent in approximately 70% of prostatic intraepithelial neoplasia (PIN) and virtually all cases of prostate cancer, making it the most common genetic alteration in this malignancy. Therapeutic inhibition of the VEGF receptor signaling pathway is currently being investigated in the treatment of prostate cancer. Overexpression of *PSMA* is observed after androgen withdrawal and in hormone refractory disease, and is the basis of clinical imaging studies using anti-PSMA monoclonal antibodies.

15. **a. disease incidence and morbidity.** As observed by Thomas Adams, "Prevention is so much better than cure, because it saves the labor of being sick." Thus the major goal of chemoprevention is reduction in disease incidence and its attendant morbidity, with reduced cost and mortality being secondary advantages.

16. **a. finasteride reduced the 7-year period prevalence of prostate cancer by 25%.** The main findings of the PCPT were: (1) the prevalence of prostate cancer was reduced by 24.8% (HR = 0.75, 95% CI = 18.6 to 30.6), from 24.4% to 18.4% in those randomized to finasteride compared with placebo; (2) the prevalence of Gleason grade 7 to 10 tumors was higher in the finasteride group than placebo (6.4 vs. 5.1%, HR = 1.27, 95% CI = 1.07 to 1.50); (3) the risk reduction associated with finasteride among risk groups defined by age, family history, race, and PSA were of the same general magnitude; (4) sexual side effects were more common with finasteride, whereas urinary symptoms were more common with placebo; and (5) there were an equal number of deaths due to prostate cancer in each study arm, and finasteride worked equally well in men with and without a family history of prostate cancer.

17. **d. the effect of volume reduction on tumor detection.** A similar number of tissue cores were taken on end-of-study biopsy in both arms of the PCPT, and because the finasteride-treated glands were on average 25% smaller than those on the placebo arm, a relatively larger proportion of the gland was sampled and evaluated histologically, leading to an increased chance of detecting cancer ("overdetection bias"). This suggests the possibility that the risk reduction associated with finasteride may in fact be larger than observed.

18. **e. no significant difference in prostate cancer incidence in all four arms.** There were statistically nonsignificant increased risks of prostate cancer in the vitamin E group (HR = 1.13, 99% CI = 0.95 to 1.35, P = .06) and type 2 diabetes mellitus in the selenium group (RR = 1.07, 95% CI = 0.94 to 1.22, P = .16) (Lippman et al, 2009).

19. **a. cooked foods.** Lycopene is a red-orange carotenoid found primarily in tomatoes and tomato-derived products, including tomato sauce, tomato paste, and ketchup, and other red fruits and vegetables. In an in-vivo model in which male rats were treated with *N*-methyl-*N*-nitrosourea and testosterone to induce prostate cancer, a protective effect was observed both for calorie restriction and tomato powder but not pure lycopene. This observation suggests that tomato products contain compounds in addition to lycopene that modify prostate carcinogenesis and that reduced caloric consumption, and a diet rich in tomato-based foods may be more beneficial than taking oral lycopene supplements in reducing the risk of prostate cancer.

20. **d. erectile dysfunction.** The incidence of erectile dysfunction and other sexually related side effects was more

frequent in the finasteride arm, whereas the incidence of prostatitis, urinary tract infection, benign prostatic hyperplasia, urinary retention, and surgical intervention for lower urinary tract symptoms or retention was lower.

21. **a. causes apoptosis.** RNase L is the terminal enzyme of the 2-5A system, an RNA degradation pathway that plays an important role in mediating the biologic effects of interferons, especially in response to viral infection. Type I interferons induce a family of 2-5A synthetases that are activated by double-stranded RNA (dsRNA) resulting in the conversion of adenosine triphosphate to a series of short 2′- to 5′-linked oligoadenylates (2-5A). 2-5A binds with high affinity to RNase L, converting it from its inactive form as a monomer to a potent dimer that degrades single-stranded RNA, preventing viral replication, interfering with protein synthesis, and causing caspase-mediated apoptosis (see Fig. 95–5 in *Campbell-Walsh Urology, 10th Edition*).

22. **c. genetic heterogeneity in the cause of prostate cancer.** Current evidence suggests that most prostate cancer is polygenic in origin.

23. **b. They inhibit 3-hydroxy-3-methylglutaryl coenzyme A (HMG-CoA), the rate-limiting enzyme in cholesterol biosynthesis.** Statin users have been shown to have lower serum PSA levels than nonusers. A meta-analysis of six randomized clinical trials, six cohort, and seven case-control studies found no association between statin use and overall prostate cancer incidence, but did find a protective association with advanced prostate cancer (RR = 0.77, 95% CI = 0.64 to 0.93) (Bonovas et al, 2008). Statin users tend to be healthier and more medically compliant than nonusers, making them more likely to undergo PSA screening, and possibly resulting in earlier cancer detection.

24. **e. to begin serial PSA levels.** The presence of a mutation in *HPC1* has not been shown to be associated with adverse outcome after curative treatment so that this patient's management should be dictated by his pathologic stage. Gleason stage 6 disease that is organ confined has a very favorable prognosis, and the appropriate management is serial monitoring of PSA.

25. **d. prostate cancer in three successive generations.** Hereditary prostate cancer is a subset of the familial form and has been defined as nuclear families with more than three affected members, prostate cancer in three successive generations, or two affected individuals diagnosed with cancer before age 55.

Additional Study Points

1. The median age for diagnosis of prostate cancer is 68 years. Men with prostate cancer younger than 50 years account for 2% of all cases.
2. Prostate cancer is an indolent disease with a very low cause-specific death rate and will only impact life expectancy in a minority of men.
3. The risk of developing prostate cancer increases with the number of family members with prostate cancer, their degree of relatedness, and the age at which they were affected.
4. Approximately 15% of patients with prostate cancer have the familial or hereditary form.
5. Carriers of the *BRCA2* gene have an increased risk for developing prostate cancer.
6. Chronic inflammation and infections may play a role in the genesis of prostate cancer.
7. Estrogens may act as procarcinogens in the prostate.
8. It is likely that the androgen receptor is biologically important even after androgen deprivation therapy.
9. Finasteride improves the sensitivity of PSA and the digital rectal exam.

Pathology of Prostatic Neoplasia

Jonathan I. Epstein, MD

QUESTIONS

1. Which of the following statements regarding prostatic intraepithelial neoplasia (PIN) is FALSE?
   a. Low-grade PIN should not be commented on in diagnostic reports.
   b. PIN by itself does not give rise to an elevated serum prostate-specific antigen (PSA).
   c. High-grade PIN predominates in the transition zone.
   d. The incidence of high-grade PIN on needle biopsy averages 5% to 10%.
   e. High-grade PIN is thought to be a precursor to many prostate cancers.

2. According to the largest studies, when high-grade PIN is found by needle biopsy, what is the approximate probability of finding carcinoma on subsequent biopsy?
   a. 0% to 5%
   b. 5% to 10%
   c. 20% to 30%
   d. 40% to 50%
   e. 70% to 80%

3. What percentage of stage T1c cancers are located predominantly in the transition zone?
   a. 5%
   b. 15%
   c. 30%
   d. 50%
   e. 70%

4. What percentage of prostate cancer is multifocal?
   a. 15%
   b. 25%
   c. 40%
   d. 60%
   e. 85%

5. The Gleason grade in a radical prostatectomy factors in the:
   a. two highest-grade architectural patterns.
   b. most prevalent, second most prevalent architectural patterns, and a tertiary grade if present.
   c. highest- and lowest-grade architectural patterns.
   d. highest architectural pattern, highest cytologic grade, and tertiary grade if present.
   e. most prevalent architectural pattern, cytologic grade, and tertiary grade if present.

6. Which of the following statements is FALSE regarding a needle biopsy showing a small focus of atypical glands?
   a. The average incidence of atypical glands on biopsy is less than 10%.
   b. Cases diagnosed as atypical have a relatively high likelihood of being changed upon expert review.
   c. Repeat biopsy should increase the sampling of the initial atypical site.
   d. The risk of cancer on subsequent biopsy is 40% to 50%.
   e. The level of serum PSA correlates with the risk of cancer on subsequent biopsy.

7. What percentage of tumors with positive margins progress after radical prostatectomy?
   a. 10%
   b. 30%
   c. 50%
   d. 70%
   e. 90%

8. Which of the following is least crucial to note in every radical prostatectomy pathology report?
   a. Margin status
   b. Gleason score
   c. Organ-confined status
   d. Perineural invasion
   e. Seminal vesicle invasion status

9. Which of the following subtypes of prostate cancer is associated with a worse prognosis compared with ordinary acinar carcinoma?
   a. Sarcomatoid carcinoma
   b. Ductal adenocarcinomas
   c. Small cell carcinomas
   d. Squamous cell carcinoma
   e. All of the above

10. Which of the following immunohistochemical markers is least useful in distinguishing between prostate adenocarcinoma and transitional cell carcinoma?
    a. Prostate-specific antigen (PSA)
    b. Prostate serum acid phosphatase (PSAP)
    c. Thrombomodulin

d. 34BE12

e. Cytokeratin 20

Pathology

1. See Figure 96–1.

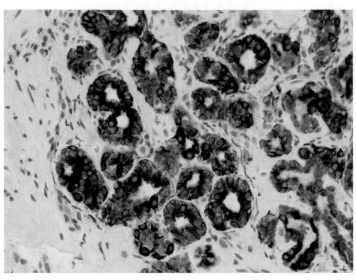

Figure 96–1. (From Bostwick DG, Cheng L. Urologic surgical pathology. 2nd ed. Edinburgh: Mosby; 2008.)

A 68-year-old man with an abnormal digital rectal exam and a PSA of 2.0 ng/mL has a needle biopsy of the prostate. The figure depicts the tissue stained with high–molecular weight cytokeratin. The diagnosis is:

a. adenocarcinoma of the prostate.

b. squamous cell carcinoma of the prostate.

c. benign prostatic hyperplasia.

d. prostatic intraepithelial neoplasia.

e. normal seminal vesicle.

2. See Figure 96–2.

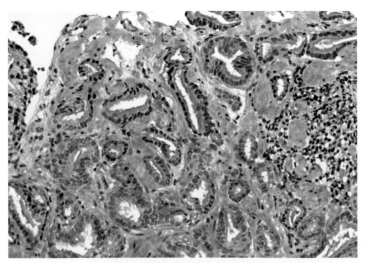

Figure 96–2. (From Bostwick DG, Cheng L. Urologic surgical pathology. 2nd ed. Edinburgh: Mosby; 2008.)

A 55-year-old man has a prostate biopsy for a PSA of 4.5 ng/mL. The diagnosis is:

a. benign prostatic hyperplasia (BPH).

b. adenocarcinoma of the prostate.

c. prostatitis.

d. lymphoma of the prostate.

e. hormonal effect on the prostate.

ANSWERS

1. **c. High-grade PIN predominates in the transition zone.** Several studies have noted an increase of high-grade PIN in the peripheral zone of the prostate, corresponding to the site of origin for most adenocarcinomas of the prostate.

2. **c. 20% to 30%.** The largest studies published to date on this issue report a 23% to 35% probability of cancer found on subsequent biopsy.

3. **b. 15%.** In clinical stage T2 carcinomas and in 85% of nonpalpable tumors diagnosed on needle biopsy (stage T1c), the major tumor mass is peripherally located.

4. **e. 85%.** Adenocarcinoma of the prostate is multifocal in more than 85% of cases.

5. **b. most prevalent, second most prevalent architectural patterns, and a tertiary grade if present.** It is recommended that in radical prostatectomy specimens, the routine Gleason score, consisting of the most prevalent and second most prevalent architectural patterns, should be recorded along with a note stating that there is a tertiary high-grade pattern (Pan et al, 2000).*

6. **e. The level of serum PSA correlates with the risk of cancer on subsequent biopsy.** Surprisingly, in men with a prior atypical biopsy, the level of serum PSA elevation or results of digital rectal examination do not correlate with the risk of a subsequent biopsy showing carcinoma.

7. **c. 50%.** In only approximately 50% of men with positive margins does the disease progress after radical prostatectomy.

8. **d. Perineural invasion.** Perineural invasion by itself in radical prostatectomy specimens does not worsen prognosis, because perineural invasion merely represents extension of tumor along a plane of decreased resistance and not invasion into lymphatics (Hassan and Maksem, 1980; Ng et al, 2004).

9. **e. All of the above.** Mucinous adenocarcinoma of the prostate gland is one of the least common morphologic variants of prostatic carcinoma. It has an aggressive biologic behavior and, like nonmucinous prostate carcinoma, has a propensity to produce bone metastases and increased serum acid phosphatase and PSA levels with advanced disease. The average survival time of patients with small cell carcinoma of the prostate is less than 1 year. Most prostatic duct adenocarcinomas are of advanced stage at presentation and have an aggressive course. Pure primary squamous carcinoma of the prostate is rare and is associated with a poor survival.

10. **e. Cytokeratin 20.** CK7 and CK20 positivities in transitional cell carcinoma are 70% to 100% and 15% to 71%, respectively. The problem with these markers is that they are not specific.

*Sources referenced can be found in *Campbell-Walsh Urology,* 10th *Edition,* on the Expert Consult website.

Pathology

1. **c. benign prostatic hyperplasia.** High–molecular weight cytokeratin stains the basal cell layer. Because the immunohistochemical stain is positive (brown color), the basal layer is present, and therefore the glands are benign.

2. **b. adenocarcinoma of the prostate.** Note the absence of the basal layer and prominent nucleoli, both hallmarks of adenocarcinoma of the prostate. This is a Gleason 6 adenocarcinoma of the prostate.

Additional Study Points

1. Prostatic intraepithelial neoplasia (PIN) is classified into low and high grade.
2. Low-grade PIN does not increase the risk of prostate cancer. Many believe that high-grade PIN is a precursor of prostate cancer; however, the evidence for this is indirect.
3. Rebiopsying patients with PIN is unnecessary unless there are multiple cores involved with high-grade PIN or there are other clinical indications.
4. Eighty-five percent of prostate adenocarcinomas are located in the peripheral zone, and 85% are multifocal.
5. Peripherally located cancers tend to extend outside the prostate through the perineural space. The presence of perineural invasion within the prostate does not worsen the prognosis. By contrast, vascular invasion increases the risk of metastatic disease.
6. Prostate cancer metastasizes, in descending order, to lymph nodes, bone, lung, bladder, liver, and adrenal glands.
7. In general, tumor volume correlates with stage and extraprostatic extension.
8. Transition zone tumors require larger volumes than do peripheral zone tumors for comparable rates of extraprostatic extension and/or distant metastases.
9. For needle biopsy specimens, the primary pattern (dominant pattern) and the highest grade (irrespective of volume) should be reported as the Gleason sum.
10. Adverse findings on needle biopsy generally accurately predict adverse findings in radical prostatectomy specimens. However, favorable findings on needle biopsy do not necessarily predict favorable findings in the radical prostatectomy specimen.
11. Benign glands are differentiated from malignant glands in that the former contain basal cells. These can be labeled, if necessary, with high–molecular weight cytokeratin and TP63. Patients with atypical glands (atypical hyperplasia, atypical small acinar proliferation) reported on biopsy specimens have a high likelihood of cancer on rebiopsy. Such findings should prompt a rebiopsy.
12. Adenosis (atypical adenomatous hyperplasia) is characteristically found in the transition zone, and although it may mimic carcinoma histologically, there is no increased risk of developing adenocarcinoma in patients with this diagnosis.
13. Only 25% of men with seminal vesicle invasion and few with lymph node metastases are biochemically free of disease following radical prostatectomy 10 years postoperatively.
14. Tumor volume correlates well with pathologic stage and Gleason grade in clinical T2 cancers; however, it is not an independent predictor of cancer progression once grade, stage, and margins are accounted for.
15. Endocrine therapy results in atrophic changes with squamous metaplasia in the prostate. Carcinomas in patients who have had endocrine therapy may appear artifactually higher in grade.
16. Primary urothelial carcinomas of the prostate show a propensity to infiltrate the bladder neck and surrounding tissue such that more than 50% of the patients are stage T3 or T4, and 20% have distant metastases at the time of presentation.

Ultrasonography and Biopsy of the Prostate

Edouard J. Trabulsi, MD, FACS ● Ethan J. Halpern, MD, MSCE ●
Leonard G. Gomella, MD, FACS

QUESTIONS

1. Prostatic corpora amylacea are:
   a. always associated with prostate infection.
   b. most commonly seen between the transition and peripheral zone of the prostate.
   c. pathognomonic for acute prostatitis.
   d. associated with hypoechoic lesions and prostate cancer.
   e. are calcifications in the peripheral zone exclusively and are located in blood vessels.

2. Which of the following statements is TRUE about transrectal ultrasonography of the seminal vesicles?
   a. Masses in the seminal vesicles are the most common lesion seen on transrectal ultrasonography (TRUS) of the prostate.
   b. The seminal vesicles are usually asymmetrical and normally measure less than 2 cm in length in the adult.
   c. Most cystic masses in the seminal vesicle are malignant and related to prostate cancer.
   d. A solid mass in the seminal vesicle is always associated with malignancy.
   e. Solid masses in the seminal vesicle can be caused by schistosomiasis in endemic regions.

3. Which of the following statements about transrectal ultrasonography after radical prostatectomy is FALSE?
   a. It should show a smooth tapering of the bladder neck to the urethra.
   b. It often reveals a hypoechoic mass anterior to the anastomosis, which usually represents recurrent cancer.
   c. It should have an intact fat plane between the bladder neck/urethra and the rectum.
   d. It should always be accompanied by biopsies of the perianastomotic area and bladder neck in patients with prostate-specific antigen (PSA) recurrence.
   e. It is contraindicated because of potential disruption of the anastomosis.

4. Which of the following statements concerning ultrasonographic estimates of prostate size/volume is TRUE?
   a. Only one formula (prolate ellipse) is acceptable to determine prostate volume.

   b. There is a poor correlation between radical prostatectomy specimen weights and volume as measured by TRUS.
   c. The mature average prostate is between 20 and 25 g and remains relatively constant until about age 50, when the gland enlarges in many men.
   d. Prostate cancer is always associated with an increase in overall volume of the prostate.
   e. Planimetry with a stepping device should be used for routine prostate volume determinations.

5. A hypoechoic lesion of the prostate can be caused by all of the following EXCEPT:
   a. hematologic malignancies.
   b. prostate cancer.
   c. transition zone, benign prostatic hyperplasia nodules.
   d. granulomatous prostatitis.
   e. normal urethra.

6. Which one of the following is NOT considered to be a commonly agreed upon indication for transrectal prostate biopsy?
   a. PSA velocity greater than 0.75 to 1.0 ng/dL/year
   b. Nodule on digital rectal examination regardless of PSA level
   c. Routine evaluation of male infertility
   d. Free PSA of less than 10% with a total PSA less than 10 ng/dL
   e. Diagnosis of recurrence after radiation therapy in a rising PSA

7. Which of the following statements is TRUE about anesthesia for TRUS prostate biopsy?
   a. Intrarectal lidocaine gel is as effective as the injection of lidocaine.
   b. It is not necessary even with extended-core biopsies owing to the small size of the needle.
   c. It is best performed using direct injection of lidocaine into the prostate gland.
   d. It is typically performed using lidocaine, a long 22-gauge spinal needle, and the biopsy channel of the ultrasound probe.
   e. It is typically performed using digital guidance to ensure that the base of the prostate near the seminal vesicles is infiltrated.

8. When performing TRUS prostate biopsy:

   a. the left lateral decubitus position is most commonly used.

   b. color and power Doppler should be available to localize the malignant foci.

   c. enemas should not be used before the procedure and may increase the risk of bleeding.

   d. intravenous antibiotic prophylaxis is necessary in all patients to prevent urosepsis.

   e. the dorsal lithotomy position increases the diagnostic accuracy of the prostate biopsies.

9. When performing TRUS prostate biopsy:

   a. only hypoechoic lesions should be sampled.

   b. a minimum of 10 to 12 systematic biopsies is now most commonly used.

   c. the transition zone should be included in all initial biopsies, because of the high incidence of cancer in this area.

   d. sextant biopsy represents the standard of care for the diagnosis of prostate cancer today.

   e. isoechoic lesions are rarely cancerous and should not be sampled unless they are calcified.

10. Which of the following statements is TRUE concerning fine-needle aspiration of the prostate?

    a. Complications are greater than with TRUS needle biopsy techniques.

    b. Diagnostic accuracy in determining Gleason score is superior to that with core needle biopsy.

    c. It is more costly than other TRUS biopsy techniques commonly used.

    d. It is commonly used outside the United States and has a low morbidity.

    e. It is the most accurate way to diagnose and grade prostate cancer.

11. Which of the following statements about antibiotic prophylaxis for TRUS biopsy is TRUE?

    a. It eliminates the risk of any infection.

    b. It reduces the risk of febrile urinary tract infection requiring hospitalization.

    c. It is not necessary if the probe is sterilized and an enema is given.

    d. Epididymitis is the most common infection after TRUS biopsy even if antibiotics are used.

    e. Bacteriuria is the only indication for antibiotics after TRUS prostate biopsy.

12. Hematospermia after TRUS biopsy:

    a. usually requires hospitalization.

    b. is eliminated with the routine use of antibiotics.

    c. usually clears immediately after TRUS biopsy.

    d. can persist for up to 4 to 6 weeks after TRUS biopsy.

    e. is eliminated if the probe is held firmly against the prostate after the needle is passed.

13. Which of the following statements is TRUE in men with a negative prostate biopsy?

    a. They can be assured that no cancer is present.

    b. They will require repeated biopsy if one of the cores contains seminal vesicle.

    c. Transurethral biopsy is the next step after an initial negative biopsy.

    d. Additional biopsies demonstrate decreasing yield of detecting cancer, and the cancer tends to be of lower grade and stage.

    e. They should undergo transperineal biopsy for all future biopsies because these have been shown to be the most accurate approach in large randomized European trials.

14. Color and power Doppler examinations are being used to improve the diagnostic accuracy of TRUS needle biopsy of the prostate. Which of the following statements is FALSE?

    a. On color Doppler, red signals indicate arterial flow and blue signals indicate venous flow.

    b. These are the most accurate technologies to use to diagnose prostate cancer on TRUS-directed biopsy.

    c. Power Doppler cannot identify slow-moving blood in vessels.

    d. Ultrasound contrast media appears to enhance the utility of color and power Doppler examinations.

    e. Doppler ultrasonography may be effective in predicting Gleason grade and outcome in prostate cancer.

Pathology

1. See Figure 97–1.

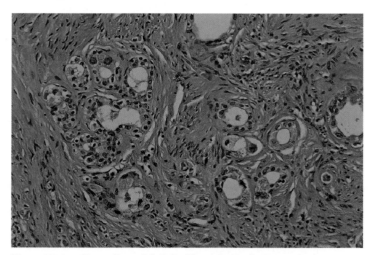

Figure 97–1.   (From Bostwick DG, Cheng L. Urologic surgical pathology. 2nd ed. Edinburgh: Mosby; 2008.)

A 65-year-old man has a needle biopsy of a palpably normal prostate for a PSA of 7.3 ng/mL. The pathology specimen depicted in the figure shows:

a. benign prostatic hyperplasia.

b. adenocarcinoma of the prostate.

c. normal seminal vesicle.

d. tuberculosis of the prostate.

e. carcinosarcoma of the prostate.

ANSWERS

1. **b. most commonly seen between the transition and peripheral zone of the prostate.** Corpora amylacea develop in the surgical capsule between the transition and peripheral zones of the prostate.

2. **e. Solid masses in the seminal vesicle can be caused by schistosomiasis in endemic regions.** Although cystic lesions of the seminal vesicle can be presumed to be benign, solid masses represent a small chance of malignancy. Schistosomiasis should be considered in the differential diagnosis of a solid seminal vesicle mass, especially in endemic regions.

3. **b. It often reveals a hypoechoic mass anterior to the anastomosis, which usually represents recurrent cancer.** Many patients will demonstrate a nodule of tissue anterior to the anastomosis, representing the ligated dorsal vein complex.

4. **c. The mature average prostate is between 20 and 25 g and remains relatively constant until about age 50, when the gland enlarges in many men.** The prostate size increases at puberty. Many men develop symptomatic enlargement of the prostate that typically begins after age 50.

5. **a. hematologic malignancies.** Many lesions can be hypoechoic, and many will prove to be malignant, reinforcing the need for biopsy of these lesions if seen. Many cancers, including hematologic malignancies of the prostate, are isoechoic.

6. **c. Routine evaluation of male infertility.** Although a TRUS of the prostate may be useful to identify anatomic abnormalities of the prostate, biopsy of the prostate is not part of routine infertility evaluation.

7. **d. It is typically performed using lidocaine, a long 22-gauge spinal needle, and the biopsy channel of the ultrasound probe.** All recent studies indicate that infiltration of lidocaine around the neurovascular bundles increases tolerability of TRUS prostate biopsy.

8. **a. the left lateral decubitus position is most commonly used.** TRUS biopsy has become the gold standard to diagnose prostate cancer. It is most commonly performed with the patient in the left lateral decubitus position. Dorsal lithotomy may also be used in certain circumstances.

9. **b. a minimum of 10 to 12 systematic biopsies is now most commonly used.** Sextant biopsy revolutionized the utility of TRUS biopsy to diagnose prostate cancer. However, significant numbers of cancers were missed based on the analysis of radical prostatectomy specimens. Increasing to a minimum of 10 to 12 systematic biopsies has increased the diagnostic yield on the first biopsy session.

10. **d. It is commonly used outside the United States and has a low morbidity.** Fine-needle aspiration is associated with a low morbidity and is used extensively outside the United States. The concern about the procedure is that it requires great skill to analyze the samples, and grading may not be as accurate as core sampling.

11. **b. It reduces the risk of febrile urinary tract infection requiring hospitalization.** Although the short-term use of prophylactic antibiotics can reduce the incidence of serious infections, it does not completely eliminate the risk of infection.

12. **d. can persist for up to 4 to 6 weeks after TRUS biopsy.** Patients should be counseled about the likelihood of hematospermia after TRUS biopsy.

13. **d. Additional biopsies demonstrate decreasing yield of detecting cancer, and the cancers tend to be of lower grade and stage.** A large European screening study suggested that as the number of biopsy sessions increased to ultimately diagnose prostate cancer, the cancers diagnosed after several biopsy sessions were generally of lower grade and stage.

14. **a. On color Doppler, red signals indicate arterial flow and blue signals indicate venous flow.** Advanced ultrasound techniques, such as color and power Doppler, are being investigated to improve the diagnostic accuracy of TRUS biopsy. The color registration on routine color Doppler refers to the direction of flow relative to the transducer and is not related to specific arterial or venous flow.

Pathology

1. **c. normal seminal vesicle.** The normal finding is not uncommonly found in prostate biopsy specimens. Note the large nuclei of some cells and the absence of nucleoli. Lipofuscin pigment, which is yellow-brown in color (not depicted here) when present in the epithelial cells, confirms the diagnosis of seminal vesicle.

Additional Study Points

1. Calcifications may be seen along the surgical capsule, which is at the junction between the transition zone and the peripheral zone. Multiple diffuse calcifications are often found incidentally and are not diagnostic of a specific pathologic entity.

2. A mass in the seminal vesicle that is cystic is usually benign, whereas a solid lesion has a small probability of being malignant. Schistosomiasis may cause solid lesions in the seminal vesicle.

3. Increasing the frequency of ultrasonography increases the resolution; decreasing the frequency increases the depth of penetration. It is important to eliminate an air interface between the ultrasound probe and the tissue being visualized.

4. A volume calculation of the prostate requires three dimensions: an anteroposterior (AP) and sagittal measurement. Formulas used to calculate volume include those for an ellipse, a sphere, or a prolate (egg shape). When a more accurate determination is required, multiple sections of the prostate must be measured using the technique of planimetry.

5. The presence of müllerian duct cysts and seminal vesicle cysts may be associated with unilateral renal agenesis.

6. Thirty-nine percent of cancers are isoechoic; 1% may be hyperechoic. A hypoechoic lesion is malignant 17% to 57% of the time. An irradiated prostate is diffusely hypoechoic.

7. There is no PSA threshold at any age that can absolutely rule out cancer.

8. The preferred antibiotic prophylaxis for a prostate biopsy is a fluoroquinolone given 1 to 2 hours prior to the procedure and for 48 hours after the procedure. For those patients at risk for endocarditis or those who have a prosthesis requiring additional coverage, intravenous ampicillin or vancomycin, if penicillin allergic, and gentamicin

followed by fluoroquinolones is the appropriate prophylaxis.

9. Proper analgesia is performed by injecting 5 mL lidocaine at the level of the seminal vesicles near the bladder base bilaterally.

10. The best visualization of the biopsy needle path is in the sagittal plane.

11. For individuals lacking a rectum, an ultrasound-directed transperineal needle biopsy or a CT-guided needle biopsy may be performed.

12. For patients who have had multiple biopsies and when there still is a high suspicion of cancer, one must be certain that the transition zone and anterior prostate have been biopsied. This may be accomplished using ultrasonography and a perineal template or by transurethral resection.

13. Complications of prostate biopsy include febrile urinary tract infections, bacteremia, acute prostatitis, bleeding, hematospermia, and acute urinary retention.

14. Investigational imaging modalities, such as contrast medium–enhanced transurethral ultrasonography and elastography, may allow more precise targeted biopsies of areas likely to contain cancer.

15. Magnetic resonance (MR) spectroscopy has the potential in the future for detecting areas of cancer and directing biopsy or treatment to these areas.

Prostate Cancer Tumor Markers

Robert H. Getzenberg, PhD ● Alan W. Partin, MD, PhD

QUESTIONS

1. Serum prostate-specific antigen (PSA) levels are specific for the presence of prostate:
   a. disease.
   b. cancer.
   c. enlargement.
   d. inflammation.
   e. none of the above.

2. Most detectable PSA in sera is bound to:
   a. albumin.
   b. α_1-antichymotrypsin (ACT).
   c. α_2-macroglobulin.
   d. human kallikrein.
   e. none of the above.

3. TRUE or FALSE: As many as 75% of men presenting with elevated PSA levels are found not to have prostate cancer after transrectal ultrasonography (TRUS) biopsy.
   a. True
   b. False

4. Compared with prostatic tissue PSA levels, prostatic tissue levels of hK2 are:
   a. elevated in well-differentiated prostate cancer tissue.
   b. elevated in poorly differentiated prostate cancer tissue.
   c. depressed in well-differentiated prostate cancer tissue.
   d. depressed in poorly differentiated prostate cancer tissue.
   e. not measurable in prostatic cancer tissue.

5. The serum urine prostate cancer biomarker PCA-3 represents a:
   a. gene on chromosome 20q13.4.
   b. noncoding gene in the *TP53* cluster.
   c. noncoding mRNA with no known protein product.
   d. glycosylated protein of molecular weight 60 kD.
   e. high–molecular weight nuclear matrix protein.

6. TRUE or FALSE: Evaluation of tissue from prostate cancer specimens has demonstrated higher mRNA expression levels compared with normal prostate tissue, suggesting that prostate cancer cells make more PSA than normal prostatic tissue.
   a. True
   b. False

7. A man with a PSA of 4 ng/mL while taking finasteride for 2 years stops this medication and begins taking saw palmetto. What should his PSA be on his next annual check-up?
   a. 2 ng/mL
   b. 4 ng/mL
   c. 6 ng/mL
   d. 8 ng/mL
   e. 10 ng/mL

8. The serum prostate cancer biomarker EPCA-2 has demonstrated value for the:
   a. detection of prostate cancer metastases.
   b. staging and localization of bone metastasis.
   c. diagnosis.
   d. staging.
   e. diagnosis and staging.

9. proPSA represents:
   a. the early form of the PSA protein in urine.
   b. PSA that has been autocleaved by another molecule several times.
   c. an early form of bound PSA found within the nucleus.
   d. an uncleaved free PSA molecule with a leader sequence.
   e. PSA that gets paid a high salary for hitting home runs.

10. Compared with men without prostate cancer, the fraction of free or unbound PSA in serum from men with prostate cancer:
    a. is equal.
    b. is lower.
    c. is greater.
    d. is undetectable by current assays.
    e. varies depending on which assay is used.

11. The value percentage of free PSA has been approved by the U.S. Food and Drug Administration (FDA) for use in improving:
    a. cancer detection in men with PSA levels less than 4 ng/mL.
    b. cancer detection in men with benign digital rectal examinations and PSA levels of 4 to 10 ng/mL.
    c. the determination of prognosis.
    d. cancer detection in men found to have atypical small acinar proliferation (ASAP).

e. cancer detection in men with a family history of prostate cancer.

12. After starting finasteride, serum PSA should _____ and the percentage of free PSA should _____.
    a. increase, not change
    b. increase, increase
    c. decrease, not change
    d. decrease, decrease
    e. not change, not change

13. Immunohistochemical studies have demonstrated different expression patterns for hK2 and PSA in benign versus cancerous tissue and may be best described as:
    a. benign: intense PSA and minimal hK2 expression.
    b. cancer: intense PSA and minimal hK2 expression.
    c. benign: minimal PSA and hK2 expression.
    d. benign: intense PSA and hK2 expression.
    e. cancer: minimal PSA and hK2 expression.

14. In which of these regions may the methylation status affect gene expression and play a role in carcinogenesis?
    a. Stop codon
    b. Glycine-cytosine–rich regions
    c. Promoter region
    d. Thymine islands
    e. All of the above

15. The products of hypermethylated genes evaluated in prostate cancer development are:
    a. UROC28 and hepsin.
    b. GSTP1, APC, and RASSF1A.
    c. DD3, PAC, and NMP 48.
    d. all of the above.

ANSWERS

1. **e. none of the above.** Although PSA is widely accepted as a prostate cancer tumor marker, it is organ specific and not disease specific. Unfortunately there is an overlap in the serum PSA levels among men with cancer and benign disease. Thus elevated serum PSA levels may reflect alterations within the prostate secondary to tissue architectural changes, such as cancer, inflammation, or benign prostatic hyperplasia (BPH).

2. **b. α₁-antichymotrypsin.** The current clinically relevant immunodetectable complexed forms of PSA are bound to ACT and, to a lesser extent, to α₁-protease inhibitor (API). The sum of these and other presently unknown PSA complexes is represented by the term complexed PSA (cPSA). The major form of cPSA in serum, PSA bound to ACT, is found in greater serum concentrations in men with cancer than in men with benign disease.

3. **a. True.** Although up to 30% of men presenting with an elevated PSA level may be diagnosed after this invasive procedure, as many as 75% to 80% will not be found to have cancer.

4. **b. elevated in poorly differentiated prostate cancer tissue.** Immunohistochemical studies reveal different tissue expression patterns for hK2 and PSA. In benign epithelium, PSA is intensely expressed compared with the minimal immunoreactivity of hK2. This is in contrast to cancerous tissue, in which more intense expression of hK2 is seen.

5. **c. noncoding mRNA with no known protein product.** Using differential display and Northern blot analysis to compare normal and prostate cancer tissue, investigators identified the *DD3/PCA3* prostate-specific gene on chromosome 9q21-22. Study of this gene has determined that it may function as noncoding mRNA, because it has been found to be alternatively spliced, contains a high density of stop codons, and lacks an open reading frame.

6. **b. False.** Although prostate cancer cells do not necessarily make more PSA than normal prostate cells, elevated serum levels are likely a result of cancer progression and destabilization of the prostate histologic architecture (Stamey et al, 1987).* Studies have demonstrated that prostate cancer cells do not make more PSA but rather less PSA than normal prostatic tissue (Meng et al, 2002). Evaluation of tissue from prostate cancer specimens have demonstrated up to 1.5-fold lower mRNA expression levels compared with normal prostate tissue (Meng et al, 2002).

7. **d. 8 ng/mL.** Finasteride (5 mg) and other 5α-reductase inhibitors for treatment of BPH have been shown to lower PSA levels by an average of 50% after 6 months of treatment (Guess et al, 1993). Thus one can multiply the PSA level by 2 to obtain the "expected" PSA level of a patient who has been on finasteride for 6 months or more. Although saw palmetto has not been shown to affect PSA levels, possible contamination of these unregulated supplements may include compounds that can alter PSA levels (i.e., PC-SPES, now off the market).

8. **e. diagnosis and staging.** Initial work with EPCA-2 for prostate cancer has demonstrated marked improvements in our ability to diagnose and stage prostate cancer.

9. **d. an uncleaved free PSA molecule with a leader sequence.** PSA originates with a 17–amino acid chain that is cleaved to yield a precursor inactive form of PSA termed proPSA (pPSA). The precursor form of PSA contains a 7–amino acid proleader peptide, in addition to the 237 constituent amino acids of mature PSA, and it is termed [–7] pPSA. Once released, the proleader amino acid chain is cleaved at the amino terminus by hK2, converting pPSA to its active 33-kD PSA form. In addition to hK2, pPSA may be activated to PSA by other prostate kallikreins, including hK4. Incomplete removal of the 7–amino acid leader chain has led to the identification of various other truncated or clipped forms of pPSA. These include pPSAs with 2-, 4-, and 5-leader amino acids ([–2]pPSA, [–4]pPSA, and [–5]pPSA). With cellular disruption, these inactive forms circulate as free PSA and may constitute the majority of the circulating free PSA in patients with prostate cancer.

10. **b. is lower.** Although prostate cancer cells do not produce more PSA than benign prostate epithelium, the PSA produced from malignant cells appears to escape proteolytic processing. Thus men with prostate cancer have a greater fraction of serum PSA complexed to ACT and a lower percentage of total PSA that is free compared with men without prostate cancer (Christensson et al, 1993; Leinonen et al, 1993; Lilja et al, 1993; Stenman et al, 1994).

---

*Sources referenced can be found in *Campbell-Walsh Urology, 10th Edition,* on the Expert Consult website.

11. **b. cancer detection in men with benign digital rectal examinations and PSA levels of 4 to 10 ng/mL.** Currently the percentage of free PSA is FDA approved for use to aid PSA testing in men with benign digital rectal examinations and minimal PSA elevations, within the diagnostic gray zone of 4 to 10 ng/mL.

12. **c. decrease, not change.** Free PSA and total PSA both decrease in men on finasteride. Because both decline, the percentage of free PSA is not altered significantly by this medication (Keetch et al, 1997; Panneck et al, 1998).

13. **a. benign: intense PSA and minimal hK2 expression.** Immunohistochemical studies reveal different tissue expression patterns for hK2 and PSA. In benign epithelium, PSA is intensely expressed compared with the minimal immunoreactivity of hK2 (Tremblay et al, 1997; Darson et al, 1999). This is in contrast to cancerous tissue, in which more intense expression of hK2 is seen. Furthermore, hK2 immunohistochemically stains the different Gleason grades of prostate cancer differently than does PSA. This inverse staining relationship of hK2 is seen as intense staining in high-grade (Gleason primary grade 4 to 5) cancers and lymph node metastasis compared with minimal staining of low-grade (Gleason primary grade 1 to 3) cancers and even weaker association in benign tissue, in which PSA exhibits intense staining (Darson et al, 1997, 1999; Tremblay et al, 1997; Kwiatkowski et al, 1998).

14. **b. Glycine-cytosine–rich regions.** Segments within the gene promoter that are composed of glycine-cytosine–rich regions are termed CpG islands. Alterations in the methylation status of these regions may affect gene expression and have been shown to play a role in carcinogenesis (Jones et al, 2002). Furthermore, cumulative effects of environmental exposures, such as diet and stress, throughout one's life may impact DNA methylation status and thus contribute to risk of cancer development (Li et al, 2004).

15. **b. GSTP1, APC, and RASSF1A.** The products of hypermethylated genes that have been evaluated in prostate cancer development are glutathione *S*-transferase P1 (GSTP1), APC, and RAS-association domain family protein isoform A (RASSF1A).

Additional Study Points

1. Prostate–specific membrane antigen (PSMA) has been identified in the central nervous system, intestine, and prostate.
2. PSA is a member of the human kallikrein gene family. PSA and human kallikrein-2 have been used in prostate cancer detection.
3. Ectopic expression of PSA occurs in breast tissue, adrenal, and renal carcinomas.
4. PSA is organ specific not disease specific; its half-life is 2 to 3 days.
5. 5α-Reductase inhibitors reduce serum PSA by 50%.
6. Prostate cancer cells make less PSA than normal prostate tissue, gram for gram. Blacks without prostate cancer have higher PSA values than whites. PSA expression is strongly influenced by androgens. Ejaculation can lead to a false increase in PSA. If it is elevated following an ejaculation, the PSA should be rechecked 48 hours following sexual abstinence.
7. Seventy percent of serum PSA is bound to three proteins: α_2-macroglobulin, α_1-protease inhibitor, and α_1-antichymotrypsin. Patients with prostate cancer have a higher fraction of circulating PSA bound to these proteins, i.e., they have a lower free PSA.
8. When PSA is released from the cell, a portion of an attached amino acid chain is cleaved, leaving a smaller amino acid chain attached, which inactivates its biologic activity. This molecule is termed proPSA. When this amino acid chain is cleaved from proPSA, PSA becomes active as a serum protease. ProPSA may be used to diagnose prostate cancer.
9. Early prostate cancer antigen 2 (EPCA-2) is a nuclear matrix protein that may have utility in prostate cancer detection and for differentiating between organ-confined and non–organ-confined disease.
10. PCA-3 is a urine-based marker used in the diagnosis of prostate cancer.
11. Identifying circulating tumor cells has great promise both for the diagnosis and staging of malignancies, including prostate cancer.
12. Prostate cancer susceptibility genes have been located on a number of chromosomes and are thought to increase the risk of developing prostate cancer.
13. Micro-RNAs are involved in the regulation of messenger RNAs and may serve as useful markers for detecting prostate cancer.
14. Metabolomics or the metabolic products of cancer cells have promise for detecting cancers in biopsy specimens.

Early Detection, Diagnosis, and Staging of Prostate Cancer

Stacy Loeb, MD ● Herbert Ballentine Carter, MD

QUESTIONS

1. What is the most useful first-line test for the diagnosis of prostate cancer?
   a. Digital rectal examination (DRE)
   b. Prostate-specific antigen (PSA) assay
   c. Prostatic acid phosphatase (PAP) assay
   d. Transrectal ultrasonography (TRUS)
   e. Combination of DRE and PSA

2. Most immunodetectable PSA in sera is bound to which of the following?
   a. Albumin
   b. α1-Antichymotrypsin (ACT)
   c. α2-Macroglobulin (MG)
   d. Human kallikrein
   e. Globulin

3. Serum PSA levels vary with which factor?
   a. Age
   b. Race
   c. Prostate volume
   d. ACT concentration
   e. Age, race, and prostate volume

4. Serum PSA elevations are specific for prostate:
   a. disease.
   b. cancer.
   c. enlargement.
   d. inflammation.
   e. none of the above.

5. A 60-year-old man taking finasteride (Proscar) for 2 years with a PSA value of 4 ng/mL would most likely, if he were not taking finasteride, have which PSA value?
   a. 2 ng/mL
   b. 6 ng/mL
   c. 8 ng/mL
   d. 12 ng/mL
   e. 4 ng/mL

6. Which of the following tests has the highest positive predictive value for prostate cancer?
   a. PSA
   b. DRE
   c. TRUS
   d. Combination of DRE and TRUS
   e. Human glandular kallikrein (hK2)

7. Which of the following statements about prostate cancer staging is FALSE?
   a. A goal of staging is to predict prognosis.
   b. Staging facilitates the selection of rational therapy on the basis of predicted extent of disease.
   c. Imaging can accurately identify all cases of pelvic lymph node metastases.
   d. PSA and DRE are components of the staging evaluation.
   e. Pelvic lymphadenectomy is the gold standard for the detection of pelvic lymph node metastases.

8. The currently available modalities for assessing disease extent in men with prostate cancer include:
   a. DRE.
   b. serum PSA.
   c. histologic grade.
   d. bone scan.
   e. all of the above.

9. Pathologic staging is superior to clinical staging because all of the following factors are confirmed in the final pathologic examination EXCEPT:
   a. PSA.
   b. surgical margin status.
   c. seminal vesicle involvement.
   d. tumor volume.
   e. capsular penetration.

10. What pathologic finding or findings at radical prostatectomy are highly predictive of the presence of occult metastatic disease?

    a. Positive surgical margins

    b. Seminal vesicle involvement

    c. Lymph node involvement

    d. Both b and c

    e. Both a and b

11. The finding of pathologic perineural invasion of cancer (PNI) on a prostate biopsy specimen suggests:

    a. organ-confined disease.

    b. low-grade disease at radical prostatectomy.

    c. a greater likelihood of capsular penetration.

    d. pelvic lymph node involvement.

    e. a bilateral nerve-sparing prostatectomy should not be considered.

12. Which staging modality provides the highest degree of understaging?

    a. Bone scan

    b. Immunoscintigraphy

    c. PSA

    d. PAP

    e. DRE

13. As general guidelines regarding PSA levels and pathologic stage, which of the following statements is TRUE?

    a. Twenty-five percent of men with a PSA value less than 4.0 ng/mL have organ-confined disease.

    b. One-hundred percent of men with a PSA value greater than 50 ng/mL have pelvic lymph node involvement.

    c. Ten percent of men with a PSA value greater than 10 ng/mL have extraprostatic extension.

    d. Serum PSA has no predictive value for staging.

    e. Seventy percent or more of men with a PSA value between 4.0 and 10.0 ng/mL have organ-confined disease.

14. With respect to the Gleason primary and secondary grade, all of the following statements are TRUE EXCEPT:

    a. primary grade ranges from 1 to 5.

    b. secondary grade ranges from 1 to 5.

    c. secondary grade and primary grade are summed to provide a Gleason score (2 to 10).

    d. the primary grade represents the second largest area of cancer on the biopsy specimen.

    e. the presence of a Gleason primary or secondary grade 4 or 5 on any biopsy specimen is predictive of poorer prognosis.

15. Which of the following variables are used to predict pathologic stage in the Partin tables?

    a. PSA

    b. Number of positive biopsy cores

    c. Gleason score

    d. Clinical stage

    e. a, c, and d are all correct

Imaging

1. See Figure 99–1.

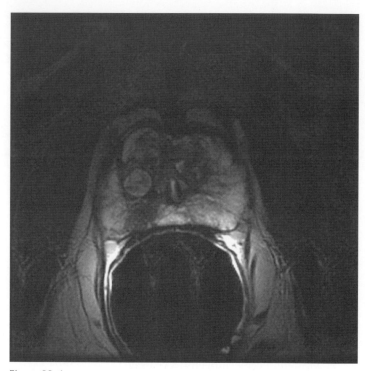

Figure 99–1.

A 59-year-old man with PSA of 5 ng/dL has this axial T2-weighted endorectal coil MRI. The most likely diagnosis is:

a. extracapsular spread of prostate cancer.

b. cancer confined to gland.

c. enlarged central gland due to benign prostatic hypertrophy.

d. neurovascular bundle involvement.

e. seminal vesicle involvement.

ANSWERS

1. **e. Combination of DRE and PSA.** The DRE and serum PSA are additive and are the most useful first-line tests for assessing the risk that prostate cancer is present in an individual.

2. **b. α1-Antichymotrypsin (ACT).** Most detectable PSA in sera (65% to 90%) is bound to ACT.

3. **e. Age, race, and prostate volume.** In the absence of prostate cancer, serum PSA levels vary with age, race, and prostate volume.

4. **e. none of the above.** Serum PSA elevations may occur as a result of disruption of the normal prostatic architecture that allows PSA to diffuse into the prostatic tissue and gain access to the circulation. This can occur in the setting of prostate disease (benign prostatic hyperplasia [BPH], prostatitis, and prostate cancer) and with prostate manipulation (prostate massage, prostate biopsy). The presence of prostate disease (prostate cancer, BPH, and prostatitis) is the most important factor affecting serum levels of PSA. PSA elevations may indicate the presence of

prostate disease, but not all men with prostate disease have elevated PSA levels. Furthermore, PSA elevations are not specific for cancer.

5. **c. 8 ng/mL.** Finasteride (a 5α-reductase inhibitor for treatment of BPH) at 5 mg has been shown to lower PSA levels by approximately 50% after 12 months of treatment. Thus one can multiply the PSA level by 2 to obtain the "true" PSA level of a patient who has been taking finasteride for 12 months or more. After 2 and 7 years of finasteride therapy, the PSA level should be multiplied by a factor of 2.3 and 2.5, respectively. Men who are to be treated with finasteride should have a baseline PSA measurement before initiation of treatment and should be followed with serial PSA measurements. If there is a rise in the PSA value when the patient is taking finasteride, these men should be suspected of having an occult prostate cancer.

6. **a. PSA.** PSA is the single test with the highest positive predictive value for cancer.

7. **c. Imaging can accurately identify all cases of pelvic lymph node metastases.** The goals in staging of prostate cancer are twofold: (1) to predict prognosis and (2) to rationally select therapy on the basis of predicted extent of disease.

8. **e. all of the above.** The currently available modalities for assessing disease extent in men with prostate cancer are DRE, serum tumor markers, histologic grade, radiographic imaging, and pelvic lymphadenectomy.

9. **a. PSA.** Pathologic staging is more useful than clinical staging in the prediction of prognosis because tumor volume, surgical margin status, extent of extracapsular spread, and involvement of seminal vesicles and pelvic lymph nodes can be determined.

10. **d. Both b and c.** The finding of seminal vesicle invasion or lymph node metastases on pathologic evaluation after radical prostatectomy is associated with a low probability of total eradication of tumor and a high probability of distant disease.

11. **c. a greater likelihood of capsular penetration.** PNI in a prostatectomy specimen has little independent prognostic staging value as initially reported by Byar and Mostofi (1972).* However, in biopsy cores, its presence is associated with a higher chance of non–organ-confined disease at prostatectomy. de la Taille and colleagues (1999) demonstrated that the presence of PNI on a biopsy specimen was closely associated with high PSA values, poorly differentiated tumor, and involvement of multiple cores with cancer, and thus a higher pathologic stage. Approximately 75% of men with PNI on a biopsy specimen will have capsular penetration on examination of the prostatectomy specimen.

12. **e. DRE.** Histologic evaluation of surgical specimens after radical prostatectomy for presumed organ-confined disease demonstrates a significant degree of understaging by DRE. Understaging of disease increases with increasing clinical stage.

13. **e. Seventy percent or more of men with a PSA value between 4.0 and 10.0 ng/mL have organ-confined disease.** As a general guideline, the majority of men (80%) with PSA values less than 4.0 ng/mL have pathologically organ-confined disease, two thirds of men with PSA levels between 4.0 and 10.0 ng/mL have organ-confined cancer, and more than 50% of men with PSA levels more than 10.0 ng/mL have disease beyond the prostate. Pelvic lymph node involvement is found in nearly 20% of men with PSA levels greater than 20 ng/mL and in most men (75%) with serum PSA levels greater than 50 ng/mL.

14. **d. the primary grade represents the second largest area of cancer on the biopsy specimen.** The Gleason grading system is based on a low-power microscopic description of the architectural pattern of the cancer. A Gleason grade (or pattern) of 1 to 5 is assigned as a primary grade (the pattern occupying the greatest area of the specimen) and a secondary grade (the pattern occupying the second largest area of the specimen). A Gleason sum (2 to 10) is determined by adding the primary grade and the secondary grade. The presence of Gleason pattern 4 or greater (primary or secondary) or a Gleason sum of 7 or greater is predictive of a poorer prognosis.

15. **e. a, c, and d are all correct.** The "Partin tables" are probability tables for the determination of pathologic stage that are based on three parameters: preoperative clinical stage, serum PSA level, and Gleason sum. In the Partin tables, numbers within the nomogram represent the percent probability of having a given final pathologic stage based on logistic regression analyses for all three variables combined; dashes represent data categories in which insufficient data existed to calculate a probability. This information is useful in counseling men with newly diagnosed prostate cancer with respect to treatment alternatives and probability of complete eradication of tumor.

Imaging

1. **b. cancer confined to gland.** The small focus of prostate cancer is seen as a well-demarcated low signal-intensity area in the right peripheral zone. The seminal vesicles are not included on this image (option e is incorrect) and cannot be assessed. The low signal-intensity capsule is well seen, bordering the tumor focus (options a and d are incorrect). Although there are a few enlarged nodules in the central gland, the gland itself is small in size (option c is incorrect).

Additional Study Points

1. PSA levels are lower in hypergonadal men; statins may reduce PSA, whereas BPH, prostatitis, prostate manipulation, and prostate cancer increase levels of PSA.
2. PSA may be elevated within 24 hours following ejaculation; DRE does not result in a significant fluctuation of PSA.
3. Surgical therapy for BPH may reduce PSA.
4. A PSA velocity of more than 0.75 ng/mL/year in patients with levels between 4 and 10 prompts a concern for prostate cancer.
5. A low noncomplexed PSA (free PSA) has a higher association with prostate cancer than does a high level of free PSA (>20%).

*Sources referenced can be found in *Campbell-Walsh Urology*, 10th *Edition*, on the Expert Consult website.

Definitive Therapy of Localized Prostate Cancer: An Overview

William J. Catalona, MD ● Misop Han, MD, MS

QUESTIONS

1. Prostate cancer is the cause of mortality in what percentage of U.S. men?
   a. 1%
   b. 3%
   c. 10%
   d. 16%
   e. 30%

2. An outcome comparison between different treatment modalities for localized prostate cancer is difficult because:
   a. most patients diagnosed with prostate cancer receive the same treatment.
   b. outcome measures are similar.
   c. the treatment outcomes in any patient series may be influenced by the malignant potential of the tumors as well as the treatment used.
   d. there are many effective treatments for clinically localized prostate cancer.
   e. randomized clinical trials eliminate selection bias.

3. The correct rationale behind watchful waiting protocols for localized prostate cancer is:
   a. a prospective, randomized clinical trial demonstrated similar local cancer progression and metastasis rates for patients with clinically localized prostate cancer managed with deferred treatment and radical prostatectomy.
   b. in most watchful waiting studies, only about 15% of patients develop objective evidence of tumor progression within 5 years.
   c. an accurate assessment of clinically insignificant or indolent cancers is determined by biopsy results.
   d. watchful waiting allows timely intervention as long as patients with localized prostate cancer are followed up semiannually with digital rectal examination and PSA levels.
   e. the potential benefits of surgery do not outweigh potential complications in men with a life expectancy of less than 10 years and a low-grade prostate cancer.

4. What is an appropriate criterion used for recommending intervention during active surveillance for prostate cancer?
   a. PSA velocity less than 0.5 ng/mL/year
   b. More than 10% of a biopsy core involvement
   c. Previous cryotherapy of the prostate gland
   d. Gleason pattern 4 or 5 present
   e. Any positive repeat biopsy

5. What recent innovation has been most responsible for the wider use of radical prostatectomy?
   a. Discovery that the pudendal nerves are responsible for urinary continence
   b. Preservation of the external sphincter muscle that yields urinary continence rates in excess of 90%
   c. Frequent use of saturation biopsy under general anesthesia
   d. Magnification provided by robotic-assisted prostatectomy
   e. Elimination of pelvic lymphadenectomy in patients with low-risk tumor features

6. What features characterize the following radical prostatectomy approach?
   a. Perineal: more blood loss and a longer operative time than the retropubic approach
   b. Retropubic: higher risk for rectal injury and postoperative fecal incontinence
   c. Laparoscopic: lowest complication rate
   d. Laparoscopic: lowest positive surgical margin rate
   e. Robotic: three-dimensional visualization

7. What outcome do the Partin tables predict?
   a. Clinical stage
   b. Gleason score
   c. Pathologic stage
   d. Biochemical recurrence-free probability
   e. Cancer-specific survival probability

8. During the nerve-sparing portion of radical retropubic prostatectomy, a surgeon should:
   a. dissect the neurovascular bundles free of the posterolateral surface of the prostate gland.

b. use bipolar electrocautery to transect the urethra.

c. perform a retrograde dissection to identify the neurovascular bundles at the bladder neck.

d. release the endopelvic fascia after the neurovascular bundle dissection.

e. use a harmonic scalpel to release neurovascular bundles.

9. Which of the following is most closely associated with urinary continence recovery following radical retropubic prostatectomy?

a. Preoperative renal function

b. Pathologic tumor stage

c. Performance of nerve-sparing surgery

d. Patient age

e. Bladder neck–sparing dissection

10. The return of erectile function following radical retropubic prostatectomy correlates best with:

a. absence of preoperative hormonal therapy.

b. absence of postoperative radiation therapy.

c. absence of antihypertensive therapy.

d. absence of a smoking history.

e. nerve-sparing status.

11. What is true of "PSA bounce"?

a. It is strongly associated with an intermittent androgen ablation therapy.

b. It usually occurs within 2 years of radiation therapy.

c. It should be treated immediately with combined androgen blockage therapy.

d. It is more commonly associated with external beam radiation therapy.

e. It does not exceed an increase of 2 ng/mL following radiation therapy.

12. What is the ASTRO (American Society of Therapeutic Radiation Oncology) definition for recurrence following radiation therapy?

a. Three consecutive rises of PSA following radiation therapy and back-dates the time of cancer progression to halfway between the second and third rise of PSA levels

b. Three consecutive rises of PSA following radiation therapy with at least one PSA bounce

c. Three PSA increases measured 12 months apart and back-dates the time of cancer progression to halfway between the first and the second rising PSA levels

d. Three consecutive PSA increases measured 6 months apart and back-dates the time of cancer progression to halfway between the PSA nadir and the first rising PSA level

e. Three consecutive PSA increases of total 2 ng/mL after reaching a PSA nadir

13. Which of the following criteria is a relative contraindication to external beam radiation therapy to the prostate?

a. Previous radical retropubic prostatectomy

b. Lower urinary tract symptoms

c. Previous transurethral resection of prostate (TURP)

d. Serum PSA less than 2 ng/mL

e. History of hematospermia

14. Which of the following parameters is most predictive of a favorable response to postoperative salvage radiation therapy?

a. Preoperative PSA less than 10 ng/mL

b. Extracapsular tumor extension

c. PSA doubling time of more than 3 months

d. Positive surgical margin

e. Preradiation PSA greater than 2 ng/mL

15. Which of the following parameters is most associated with improved prostate cancer–specific survival with salvage radiotheraphy for recurrence after surgery?

a. PSA doubling time of less than 6 months

b. Concurrent hormonal therapy

c. Lymph node metastasis

d. Initiation of salvage radiotherapy after PSA has risen above 2 ng/mL

e. Previous robot-assisted laparoscopic prostatectomy

ANSWERS

1. **b. 3%.** About 1 in 6 men are diagnosed with prostate cancer during their lifetime. Because of effective treatment of some prostate cancers and the biologic indolence relative to the life expectancy of others, only about 16% of men diagnosed with prostate cancer ultimately die of it. As a result, prostate cancer is the cause of death in about 3% of the U.S. male population.

2. **c. the treatment outcomes in any patient series may be influenced by the malignant potential of the tumors as well as the treatment used.** Patients whose tumor has a low malignant potential are predetermined to fare better with most treatments. Therefore the treatment outcomes in any patient series may be influenced by the malignant potential of the tumors and also by the treatment used. Accordingly, it is difficult to compare the results of different reports, because the patient populations usually are not strictly comparable.

3. **e. the potential benefits of surgery do not outweigh potential complications of surgery in men with a life expectancy of less than 10 years and a low-grade prostate cancer.** Traditionally, watchful waiting has been reserved for men with a life expectancy of less than 10 years and a low-grade (Gleason score 2 to 5) prostate cancer. However, active surveillance is now being studied in younger patients with low-volume, low- or intermediate-grade tumors to avoid or delay treatment that might not be immediately necessary.

4. **d. Gleason pattern 4 or 5 present.** During active surveillance, intervention is recommended if Gleason pattern 4 or 5 is present, more than two biopsy cores are involved, or more than 50% of a biopsy core is involved. Progression is more likely in patients who have cancer present on every biopsy procedure.

5. **b. Preservation of the external sphincter muscle that yields urinary continence rates in excess of 90%.** Recent innovations that have led to the wider use of radical prostatectomy include (1) the development of the anatomic radical retropubic prostatectomy that allows the dissection to be performed with good visualization and preservation of the cavernosal nerves responsible for erectile function, and preservation of the external sphincter muscle,

which yields urinary continence rates in excess of 90%; (2) the development of extended ultrasound-guided biopsy regimens, performed under local anesthesia as an office procedure; and (3) the widespread use of PSA testing, which has led to the great majority of patients being diagnosed with clinically localized disease.

6. **e. Robotic: three-dimensional visualization.** Remotely controlled, robot-assisted laparoscopic surgery recently has been popularized because of its greater technical ease for the surgeon, especially for tying sutures and performing the vesicourethral anastomosis. The availability of three-dimensional visualization is also an advantage over standard laparoscopic techniques.

7. **c. Pathologic stage.** Because imaging studies are not accurate for staging prostate cancer, preoperative clinical and pathologic parameters are used in the Partin tables to predict the pathologic stage and thus identify patients most likely to benefit from the operation.

8. **a. dissect the neurovascular bundles free of the posterolateral surface of the prostate gland.** Meticulous dissection is required to preserve the neurovascular bundles during the nerve-sparing radical retropubic prostatectomy. In performing nerve-sparing surgery, the neurovascular bundles are identified at the apex of the prostate, and the bundles are dissected free of the posterolateral surface of the prostate gland.

9. **d. Patient age.** The return of urinary continence following radical retropubic prostatectomy is strongly associated with patient age: More than 95% of men younger than age 50 are continent following surgery; 85% of men older than age 70 regain complete continence.

10. **e. nerve-sparing status.** The return of erectile function following radical retropubic prostatectomy correlates with the age of the patient, preoperative potency status, extent of nerve-sparing surgery, and the era of surgery.

11. **b. It usually occurs within 2 years of radiation therapy.** Inflammation in the prostate gland can produce transient PSA elevation, called a PSA "bounce" following radiation therapy. PSA bounce usually occurs during the first two years after treatment and is less common with external beam therapy than with brachytherapy.

12. **d. Three consecutive PSA increases measured 6 months apart and back-dates the time of cancer progression to halfway between the PSA nadir and the first rising PSA level.** Until recently, the most frequently used definition for recurrence following radiation therapy was the American Society of Therapeutic Radiation Oncology (ASTRO) definition. It requires three consecutive PSA increases measured 6 months apart and back-dates the time of cancer progression to halfway between the PSA

nadir and the first rising PSA level. Thus it usually takes years to determine whether progression has occurred after radiotherapy. In recent years, the Phoenix definition was proposed to replace the ASTRO definition. It eliminates back-dating but requires the PSA level to rise by 2 ng/mL before treatment failure is declared. Thus the time to recurrence is further prolonged after the PSA level begins to rise, and often it takes a considerably longer time for the PSA level to increase by 2 ng/mL. In some instances, adjuvant hormone therapy may be initiated before the PSA rises to 2 ng/mL. In practice, the Phoenix definition can yield results that are even more favorable than those obtained with the ASTRO definition.

13. **c. Previous transurethral resection of prostate (TURP).** A prior transurethral resection of the prostate is a relative contraindication to brachytherapy and external beam radiation therapy because the prostate does not hold the seeds well, and radiation after transurethral resection of the prostate is associated with an increased risk for urethral stricture. The presence of severe obstructive urinary symptoms is also a relative contraindication because of the risk for acute urinary retention, which is an even greater risk in patients treated with brachytherapy. Another relative contraindication is inflammatory bowel disease.

14. **d. Positive surgical margin.** Adjuvant radiotherapy is most likely to benefit patients with positive surgical margins or extracapsular tumor extension without seminal vesicle invasion or lymph node involvement. However, not all patients with extracapsular tumor extension or positive margins have tumor recurrence without radiotherapy, and most patients with highly adverse findings have treatment failure with distant metastases, despite adjuvant radiotherapy.

15. **a. PSA doubling time of less than 6 months.** Trock and associates (2008)* reported on a retrospective study of men with PSA failure after radical prostatectomy that is unique because patients received either no treatment, salvage radiation therapy, or salvage radiation therapy with androgen-deprivation therapy. They reported that salvage radiation was associated with a threefold reduction in prostate cancer mortality, and although the addition of hormone therapy provided no additional decrease in the risk for mortality, the patients who received hormone therapy had higher-risk disease. Therefore hormone therapy probably provided additional benefit for these high-risk patients. The benefit was strongest in those with the shortest PSA doubling times.

---

*Sources referenced can be found in *Campbell-Walsh Urology, 10th Edition,* on the Expert Consult website.

Additional Study Points

1. Approximately 90% of prostate cancer cases detected appear to be localized at the time of detection.
2. Patients who have greater than a 10-year life expectancy and may be considered for active surveillance should have low-volume disease, low- or intermediate-grade tumors (up to Gleason 3 + 4 = 7), nonpalpable lesions, and PSAs that are below 10. Some would suggest that any Gleason grade of 4 or 5 on biopsy makes the patient ineligible for active observation.
3. Patients who are actively observed should routinely have an interval biopsy. Follow-up biopsies in which no cancer is detected significantly decreases the risk of progression in these patients.
4. Approximately 25% to 50% of patients who choose active observation develop objective evidence of tumor progression within 5 years.
5. The median time from PSA failure to the development of metastatic disease after radical prostatectomy is 8 years,

and from the time of metastases to death is 5 years. Thus there is a total of 13 years following detectable PSA after radical prostatectomy before death due to prostate cancer usually occurs. Moreover, only one third of the patients with detectable PSAs will develop clinical metastases.

6. Neoadjuvant hormone therapy does not enhance the resectability of prostate cancer in those patients undergoing a radical prostatectomy.

7. Nerve grafting when a neurovascular bundle must be sacrificed has not been proven to be effective.

8. Ultrasensitive PSA measurements postprostatectomy may falsely classify patients as having a tumor recurrence.

9. Adverse prognostic factors following radical prostatectomy include non–organ-confined disease, seminal vesicle invasion, positive surgical margins, and lymph node metastases.

10. In those instances of high-grade adenocarcinomas and neuroendocrine tumors that do not produce much PSA, recurrent disease is diagnosed by palpation, thus indicating a role for DRE in monitoring.

11. The most common late complications of radical prostatectomy are erectile dysfunction, urinary incontinence, inguinal hernia, and urethral stricture.

12. Intensity-modulated radiation therapy (IMRT) generally delivers in excess of 75 Gy.

13. Side effects of external beam radiation therapy include 5% to 10% persistent irritable bowel symptoms and 10% to 15% intermittent rectal bleeding. About half the patients will be impotent.

14. Patients who have high-volume disease or high Gleason scores benefit from androgen-deprivation therapy prior to administering radiation therapy.

15. Brachytherapy using either iodine-125 or palladium-103 delivers 125-145 Gy to the prostate.

16. Not all patients with extracapsular tumor extension or positive surgical margins have a PSA failure. Those patients would not be expected to benefit from adjuvant radiation therapy.

Expectant Management of Prostate Cancer

James A. Eastham, MD ● Peter T. Scardino, MD, FACS

QUESTIONS

1. Watchful waiting is appropriate for men who:
   a. are 70 years of age or older.
   b. have impalpable cancer not visible on imaging studies.
   c. have a serum prostate-specific antigen (PSA) level less than 10 ng/mL.
   d. have a life expectancy approximately 10 years or less and well to moderately differentiated cancer.
   e. have no major comorbidities.

2. Which of the following is important for monitoring men on watchful waiting?
   a. Periodic PSA testing
   b. Serial transrectal ultrasound
   c. Repeat prostate biopsy
   d. Endorectal MRI
   e. None of the above

3. For men with well or moderately differentiated prostate cancer on watchful waiting, the 10-year cancer-specific mortality is approximately:
   a. 1%.
   b. 5%.
   c. 15%
   d. 30%.
   e. 50%.

4. For men with well-differentiated prostate cancer, the rate of metastases within the first 10 years of watchful waiting is approximately:
   a. 5%.
   b. 10%.
   c. 20%.
   d. 50%.
   e. 75%.

5. Compared with men treated by radical prostatectomy, men on watchful waiting have a higher risk of:
   a. bowel problems.
   b. obstructive voiding problems.
   c. metastases.
   d. death from prostate cancer.
   e. all of the above.

6. The best way to select men for active surveillance is:
   a. age at the time of cancer diagnosis.
   b. life expectancy.
   c. PSA level.
   d. results of imaging studies.
   e. assessment by multiple variables such as Epstein's risk assessment or nomogram.

7. During follow-up of men on active surveillance, how is digital rectal examination (DRE) most valuable?
   a. DRE is an indicator that a repeat biopsy is warranted.
   b. DRE is a means to assess prostate size as an indication for transurethral resection of the prostate.
   c. DRE is an indicator to order an imaging study such as transrectal ultrasound or an endorectal MRI.
   d. DRE is a predictor of cancer progression.
   e. DRE has no apparent value in this setting.

ANSWERS

1. **d. have a life expectancy approximately 10 years or less and well to moderately differentiated cancer.** Watchful waiting is a reasonable option in patients with a life expectancy of 10 years and clinically localized, well differentiated, or moderately differentiated prostate cancer.

2. **e. none of the above.** Because the goal of watchful waiting is to limit morbidity and not to administer potentially curative treatment, PSA testing, repeat biopsy, and imaging studies are unimportant.

3. **c. 15%.** According to a study by Bill-Axelson and colleagues (2008),* men who were managed conservatively had a 14% cancer-specific mortality rate at 10 years after diagnosis.

4. **c. 20%.** Chodak and colleagues (1994) found that, for men with well-differentiated, clinical stage T1 to T2 cancer managed conservatively, the risk of metastasis at 10 years was 19%.

---

*Sources referenced can be found in *Campbell-Walsh Urology, 10th Edition,* on the Expert Consult website.

5. **e. all of the above.** In a randomized comparison of watchful waiting and radical prostatectomy in Sweden, men on watchful waiting experienced significantly more obstructive voiding complaints, bowel problems, metastases, and death from prostate cancer.

6. **e. assessment by multiple variables such as Epstein's risk assessment or nomogram.** Models that incorporate multiple factors have proven to be better predictors of indolent prostate cancer than any single factor.

7. **a. DRE is an indicator that a repeat biopsy is warranted.** None of the current active surveillance studies has found DRE to be an independent predictor of cancer progression, although it can be useful in determining that a repeat biopsy should be taken.

Additional Study Points

1. Forty-two percent of American men 50 years of age or older who die of causes other than prostate cancer have prostate cancer at autopsy.

2. In the prostate cancer prevention trial it was found that 6.2% of men with a PSA less than 0.5 ng/mL had prostate cancer on biopsy.

3. It is generally accepted that organ-confined cancer less than 0.5 mL in volume with no Gleason grade 4 or 5 component is indolent and poses little if any risk to the patient.

4. Current studies suggest that 20% to 40% of prostate cancers that are detected would never have been found in a subject's lifetime without screening—in other words, will never affect the patient's life.

5. The criteria generally used for selection of individuals for active observation include (a) no Gleason grade 4 or 5 in the biopsy; (b) no more than three cores positive, none of which is more than 50% involved (some suggest that there should be <3 mm of total involvement in the biopsy cores); (c) no palpable disease (controversial); and (d) a PSA less than 10 ng/mL with a PSA density less than 0.15 ng/mL per gram of tissue.

6. In most series of patients on active observation, approximately a third over a period of 5 years will receive definitive treatment.

7. PSA kinetics are extremely complex, so it is difficult to establish specific PSA criteria that predict progression.

8. A repeat biopsy is an integral part of all active observation protocols.

9. Indications for abandonment of active observation are an increased amount of cancer on repeat biopsy, an increased Gleason sum, a rapidly rising PSA, and patient anxiety.

10. Definitive therapy for disease progression in those on active observation appears to be effective in the majority of patients, although no long-term studies are available to firmly establish this.

Radical Retropubic and Perineal Prostatectomy

Alan W. Partin, MD, PhD ● Edward M. Schaeffer, MD, PhD ●
Herbert Lepor, MD ● Patrick C. Walsh, MD

QUESTIONS

1. What is the arterial blood supply to the prostate?
   a. The pudendal artery
   b. The superior vesical artery
   c. The inferior vesical artery
   d. The external iliac artery
   e. The obturator artery

2. What vessels are located in the neurovascular bundle?
   a. Capsular arteries and veins
   b. Pudendal artery and vein
   c. Hemorrhoidal artery and vein
   d. Santorini plexus
   e. Accessory pudendal artery

3. A radical prostatectomy may compromise the arterial blood supply to the penis by injuring the aberrant blood supply from which artery?
   a. The obturator artery
   b. The inferior vesical artery
   c. The superior vesical artery
   d. The penile artery
   e. All of the above

4. The main parasympathetic efferent innervation to the pelvic plexus arises from:
   a. S1.
   b. S2-S4.
   c. T11-L2.
   d. L3-S1.
   e. T5-T8.

5. What is the relationship of the neurovascular bundle to the prostatic fascia?
   a. Inside Denonvilliers fascia
   b. Outside the lateral pelvic fascia
   c. Inside the prostatic fascia
   d. Between the layers of the prostatic fascia and the levator fascia
   e. Both inside and outside the prostatic fascia

6. Why is there less blood loss during radical perineal prostatectomy?
   a. It is easier to ligate the dorsal vein complex through the perineal approach than through the retropubic approach.
   b. There is no need to divide the puboprostatic ligaments.
   c. The dorsal vein complex is not divided because the dissection occurs beneath the lateral fascia and anterior pelvic fascia.
   d. Because the perineum is elevated, there is lower venous pressure.
   e. The arterial supply to the prostate is ligated early.

7. Which anatomic structure is responsible for the maintenance of passive urinary control after radical prostatectomy?
   a. Bladder neck
   b. Levator ani musculature
   c. Preprostatic sphincter
   d. Striated urethral sphincter
   e. Bulbar urethra

8. What is the major nerve supply to the striated sphincter and levator ani?
   a. The neurovascular bundle
   b. The sympathetic fibers from T11 to L2
   c. The pudendal nerve
   d. The obturator nerve
   e. The accessory pudendal nerve

9. What is the posterior extent of the pelvic lymph node dissection?
   a. The hypogastric vein
   b. The obturator nerve
   c. The obturator vessels
   d. The sacral foramen
   e. The pelvic side wall musculature

10. In opening the endopelvic fascia, there are often small branches traveling from the prostate to the pelvic sidewall. These branches are tributaries from the:
    a. obturator artery.
    b. external iliac artery.

c. inferior vesical artery.

d. pudendal artery and veins.

e. neurovascular bundle.

11. How extensively should the puboprostatic ligaments be divided?

a. Superficially, with just enough incised to expose the junction between the anterior apex of the prostate and the dorsal vein complex

b. Extensively, down to the pelvic floor, including the pubourethral component

c. Not at all; the puboprostatic ligaments should be left intact

d. Widely enough to permit a right angle to be placed around the dorsal vein complex

e. Not at all; the puboprostatic ligaments do not need to be divided to perform a radical prostatectomy

12. When the dorsal vein complex is divided anteriorly, what is the most common major structure that can be damaged, and what is the most common adverse outcome?

a. Aberrant pudendal arteries; impotence

b. Neurovascular bundle; impotence

c. Striated urethral sphincter; incontinence

d. Levator ani musculature; incontinence

e. Both a and b

13. What is the most common site for a positive surgical margin and when does this occur?

a. Posterolateral; during release of the neurovascular bundle

b. Posterior; when the prostate is dissected from the rectum

c. Apex; during division of the striated urethral sphincter-dorsal vein complex

d. Bladder neck; during separation of the prostate from the bladder

e. Seminal vesicles

14. How should the back-bleeders from the dorsal vein complex on the anterior surface of the prostate be oversewn and why?

a. The edges should be pulled together in the midline to avoid bleeding.

b. Bunching sutures should be used to avoid excising too much striated sphincter.

c. The edges should be oversewn in the shape of a V to avoid advancing the neurovascular bundles too far anteriorly on the prostate.

d. They should be oversewn horizontally to avoid a positive surgical margin.

e. Oversewing the proximal dorsal vein complex is not required.

15. After the dorsal vein complex has been ligated and the urethra has been divided, what posterior structure, other than the neurovascular bundles, attaches the prostate to the pelvic floor?

a. Rectourethralis

b. Denonvilliers fascia

c. Rectal fascia

d. Posterior portion of the striated sphincter complex

e. Neurovascular bundles

16. What are the advantages of releasing the levator fascia higher at the apex?

a. More soft tissue on the prostate

b. Less traction on the neurovascular bundles as they are released

c. Preservation of anterior nerve fibers

d. Less blood loss

e. Better visualization of the location of the cancer

17. Once the apex of the prostate has been released, what is the best way to retract the prostate for exposure of the neurovascular bundle?

a. Traction on the catheter, producing upward rotation of the apex of the prostate

b. Use of a sponge stick to roll the prostate on its side

c. Downward displacement of the prostate with a sponge stick

d. Use of finger dissection to release the prostate posteriorly

e. Dissection with the sucker

18. To avoid a positive surgical margin, what is the best way to release the neurovascular bundle?

a. Right-angle dissection beginning on the posterior surface of the prostate and dissecting anterolaterally

b. Using sharp dissection, laterally dissecting toward the rectum

c. Using finger dissection to fracture the neurovascular bundle from the prostate

d. Using electrocautery to separate the neurovascular bundle from the prostate

e. Elevation of the prostate with traction on the Foley catheter

19. What is the latest point at which a decision can be made regarding preservation or excision of the neurovascular bundle?

a. When perineural invasion is identified on the needle biopsy specimen

b. When the neurovascular bundle is being released from the prostate and fixation is identified

c. When the prostate has been removed and tissue covering the posterolateral surface of the prostate is thought to be inadequate

d. When the patient is found to have a positive biopsy result at the apex

e. When the Partin tables indicate a greater than 50% chance of extraprostatic extension

20. Before the lateral pedicles are divided, what is the last major branch of the neurovascular bundle that must be identified and released?

a. Apical branch

b. Posterior branch

c. Capsular branch

d. Bladder neck branch

e. Seminal branch

21. When the vesicourethral anastomosis sutures are being tied, if tension is found, what is the best way to release it?

a. Creating an anterior bladder neck flap

b. Placing the Foley catheter on traction postoperatively

c. Releasing attachments of the bladder to the peritoneum

d. Using vest sutures

e. Releasing the urethra from the pelvic floor

22. If there is excessive bleeding from the dorsal vein complex while it is being divided, what should be done?

    a. Abandon the operation and close the incision

    b. Ligate the hypogastric arteries

    c. Inflate a Foley balloon and place traction on it

    d. Divide the dorsal vein complex completely over the urethra and oversew the end

    e. Deflate the Foley catheter

23. If a rectal injury occurs during the operation, the most appropriate next step is:

    a. to create a loop colostomy.

    b. to create an end colostomy.

    c. to create a Hartman pouch.

    d. to ensure interposition of the omentum following repair of the injury.

    e. to repair the rectal injury in two layers.

24. In postoperative patients who require transfusions of blood for hypotension, the best approach is to:

    a. avoid re-exploration because it might damage the anastomosis.

    b. perform re-exploration.

    c. place the Foley catheter on traction.

    d. administer fresh frozen plasma.

    e. serially monitor the patient in an intensive care unit setting.

25. What is the best way to ensure good coaptation of the anastomotic mucosal surfaces to avoid a bladder neck contracture?

    a. Hold the catheter on traction while tying the sutures

    b. Use a sponge stick in the perineum

    c. Use a Babcock clamp to hold the bladder down

    d. Use vest sutures

    e. Evert the bladder mucosa

26. What is the most common cause of incontinence after radical prostatectomy?

    a. Intrinsic sphincter deficiency

    b. Detrusor instability

    c. Failure to reconstruct the bladder neck

    d. Injury to the neurovascular bundles

    e. Bladder neck contracture

27. Preservation of the seminal vesicles during radical prostatectomy has demonstrated:

    a. improved erectile function in the majority of men.

    b. no increase in biochemical recurrence.

    c. improved early and late urinary control.

    d. increased rate of pelvic abscess.

    e. none of the above.

28. Preservation of the bladder neck during radical prostatectomy has demonstrated:

    a. improved erectile function.

    b. improved long-term urinary control.

c. decreased surgical margins.

d. improved anastomotic stricture rate.

e. none of the above.

29. What percentage of men who had bilateral sural nerve grafting demonstrated full erections sufficient for penetration?

    a. 9%

    b. 13%

    c. 26%

    d. 38%

    e. 57%

30. Sural nerve grafts are placed:

    a. end to end on the ipsilateral side from the tumor.

    b. above the bladder neck and below the pubic arch.

    c. in reverse to the natural position (proximal to distal and distal to proximal).

    d. in a circle to enhance nerve growth factor release.

    e. next to the prostatectomy specimen in the pelvis until it is time for anastomosis.

31. Which complication has changed dramatically with experience with salvage prostatectomy?

    a. Overall urinary incontinence

    b. Potency

    c. Blood loss

    d. Rectal injury

    e. Stricture rate

32. Which of the following statements about perineal prostatectomy is FALSE?

    a. The pathologic outcomes are similar to those of radical retropubic prostatectomy and proven over considerable time.

    b. It has experienced a resurgence of interest as a result of its low morbidity and rapid convalescence.

    c. It fell out of favor as the principle technique in the 1970s secondary to high intraoperative blood loss.

    d. Nerve-sparing techniques have been applied to the approach, allowing for postoperative potency.

    e. Partin tables allow for relatively accurate predictions of pathologic stage, forfeiting the need for staging lymphadenectomy in many patients.

33. With regard to postoperative neurapraxia, which of the following statements is TRUE?

    a. The literature supports that it is almost always transient.

    b. It usually results in a motor deficit that is transient.

    c. Most studies show that a self-limited neurapraxia occurs in approximately 25% of patients.

    d. The same rates of neurapraxia tend to occur in retropubic prostatectomy as well.

    e. This is a major source of morbidity and the reason many surgeons do not use this approach.

34. Which of the following statements with regard to rectal injury associated with perineal prostatectomy is FALSE?

    a. If unrecognized it may result in the occurrence of a rectocutaneous or urethrocutaneous fistula.

b. Despite the close proximity of the rectum in the initial dissection, the incidence is fairly low.

c. It can be avoided when an assistant places gentle downward pressure on the Lowsley tractor while the rectourethralis muscle is divided.

d. If repaired with a two-layer closure, most clinical sequelae are avoided.

e. After repair with a two-layer closure, the operation can continue without a problem.

35. When selecting a patient for radical perineal prostatectomy, which of the following must always be considered?

a. Gleason score of biopsy specimen

b. Preoperative serum prostatic-specific antigen (PSA)

c. Mild degenerative lumbar disk disease

d. a and b only

e. All of the above

36. Which of the following is TRUE regarding the radical perineal prostatectomy?

a. Patients who require lymph node sampling for staging purposes should undergo a radical retropubic prostatectomy because the radical perineal prostatectomy, when combined with a laparoscopic lymph node dissection, yields much higher morbidity and is not cost effective.

b. Patients with ankylosis of the hips or spine may not tolerate a radical perineal prostatectomy.

c. Patients with a prior history of renal transplant surgery with the allograft in the right iliac fossa are not candidates for a radical perineal prostatectomy.

d. Morbid obesity is becoming a common contraindication to a radical perineal prostatectomy.

e. None of the above.

37. Which of the following statements regarding blood loss during radical perineal prostatectomy is TRUE?

a. Because transfusion rates are low, a blood type and crossmatch are not recommended before starting the case.

b. Unlike a radical retropubic prostatectomy, the dorsal venous complex is not usually encountered and blood loss is significantly reduced.

c. Transfusion rate in most reports is approximately 15%.

d. The dorsal venous complex is ligated early, resulting in reduced blood loss.

e. Rates of transfusion are generally greater than those in the retropubic literature.

38. Which of the following statements concerning postoperative care is TRUE?

a. The diet is rapidly advanced to a regular diet.

b. Most patients are discharged from the hospital by postoperative day 2.

c. A rectal suppository is administered on a scheduled basis while in the hospital to minimize Foley catheter discomfort except in cases of intraoperative rectal injury.

d. a and b only

e. All of the above

39. Which of the following statements is TRUE with regard to potency outcomes of the radical perineal prostatectomy?

a. Using a nerve-sparing technique, potency is shown to return in up to 70% of men.

b. Older patients are as likely to be as potent as younger patients if a nerve-sparing technique is employed.

c. Pharmacotherapy is demonstrated to improve postoperative potency status.

d. All of the above

e. a and c only

40. In a perineal prostatectomy, exposure of the urethra is facilitated by:

a. encircling the urethra with umbilical tape.

b. the Lowsley retractor.

c. division of the puboprostatic ligaments.

d. division of the dorsal venous complex.

e. retraction of the neurovascular bundles medially.

41. Which of the following statements concerning the technique of urethral anastomosis is TRUE?

a. The presence of the Lowsley retractor assists in identifying the membranous urethral stump for the initial placement of interrupted sutures.

b. A running suture technique is advocated for a watertight anastomosis.

c. The visualization of the anastomosis is difficult, one of the few disadvantages of the radical perineal prostatectomy.

d. The sutures are interrupted in a tennis racquet fashion.

e. The indwelling Foley catheter is not passed until after the anterior vesicourethral anastomotic sutures are placed and tied down.

ANSWERS

1. **c. The inferior vesical artery.** The prostate receives arterial blood supply from the inferior vesical artery.

2. **a. Capsular arteries and veins.** The capsular branches run along the pelvic sidewall in the lateral pelvic fascia posterolateral to the prostate, providing branches that course ventrally and dorsally to supply the outer portion of the prostate. Histologically, the capsular arteries and veins are surrounded by an extensive network of nerves. These capsular vessels provide the macroscopic landmark that aids in the identification of the microscopic branches of the pelvic plexus that innervate the corpora cavernosa.

3. **e. All of the above.** The major arterial supply to the corpora cavernosa is derived from the internal pudendal artery. However, pudendal arteries can arise from the obturator, inferior vesical, and superior vesical arteries. Because these aberrant branches travel along the lower part of the bladder and anterolateral surface of the prostate, they are divided during radical prostatectomy. This may compromise arterial supply to the penis, especially in older patients with borderline penile blood flow.

4. **b. S2-S4.** The autonomic innervation of the pelvic organs and external genitalia arises from the pelvic plexus, which is formed by parasympathetic visceral efferent preganglionic fibers that arise from the sacral center (S2 to S4).

5. **d. Between the layers of the prostatic fascia and the levator fascia.** The neurovascular bundles are located in the lateral pelvic fascia between the prostatic and levator fasciae (see Fig. 102–4 in *Campbell-Walsh Urology, 10th Edition*).

6. **c. The dorsal vein complex is not divided because the dissection occurs beneath the lateral fascia and anterior pelvic fascia.** In an effort to avoid injury to the dorsal vein of the penis and Santorini plexus during radical perineal prostatectomy, the lateral fascia and anterior pelvic fascia are reflected off the prostate. This accounts for the reduced blood loss associated with radical perineal prostatectomy.

7. **d. Striated urethral sphincter.** The striated sphincter contains fatigue-resistant, slow-twitch fibers that are responsible for passive urinary control.

8. **c. The pudendal nerve.** The pudendal nerve provides the major nerve supply to the striated sphincter and levator ani.

9. **a. The hypogastric vein.** The obturator artery and vein are skeletonized but are usually left undisturbed and are not ligated unless excessive bleeding occurs. The dissection then continues down to the pelvic floor, exposing the hypogastric veins.

10. **d. pudendal artery and veins.** The incision in the endopelvic fascia is carefully extended in an anteromedial direction toward the puboprostatic ligaments. At this point, one often encounters small arterial and venous branches from the pudendal vessels, which perforate the pelvic musculature to supply the prostate. These vessels should be ligated with clips to avoid coagulation injury to the pudendal artery and nerve, which are located just deep to this muscle as they travel along the pubic ramus.

11. **a. Superficially, with just enough incised to expose the junction between the anterior apex of the prostate and the dorsal vein complex.** The dissection should continue down far enough to expose the juncture between the apex of the prostate and the anterior surface of the dorsal vein complex at the point where it will be divided. The pubourethral component of the complex must remain intact to preserve the anterior fixation of the striated urethral sphincter to the pubis.

12. **c. Striated urethral sphincter; incontinence.** The goal is to divide the complex with minimal blood loss while avoiding damage to the striated sphincter.

13. **c. Apex; during division of the striated urethral sphincter-dorsal vein complex.** The exact plane on the anterior surface of the prostate can be visualized, avoiding inadvertent entry into the anterior prostate and ensuring minimal excision of the striated sphincter musculature. This is the most common site for positive surgical margins because it can be difficult to identify the anterior apical surface of the prostate.

14. **c. The edges should be oversewn in the shape of a V to avoid advancing the neurovascular bundles too far anteriorly on the prostate.** To avoid back-bleeding from the anterior surface of the prostate, the edges of the proximal dorsal vein complex on the anterior surface of the prostate are sewn in the shape of a V with a running 2-0 absorbable suture. If one tries to pull these edges together in the midline, the neurovascular bundles can be advanced too far anteriorly on the prostate.

15. **d. Posterior portion of the striated sphincter complex.** The posterior band of urethra is now divided to expose the posterior portion of the striated urethral sphincter complex. The posterior sphincter complex is composed of skeletal muscle and fibrous tissue.

16. **b. Less traction on the neurovascular bundles as they are released and c. Preservation of anterior nerve fibers.** The purpose of this technique is to speed up recovery of sexual function by reducing traction on the branches of the nerves to the cavernous bodies and striated sphincter and/or avoiding inadvertent transection of the small branches that travel anteriorly. However, because there is less soft tissue at the apex, the risk of positive margins may be increased.

17. **b. Use of a sponge stick to roll the prostate on its side.** When the surgeon releases the neurovascular bundle, there should be no upward traction on the prostate. Rather, the prostate should be rolled from side to side.

18. **a. Right-angle dissection beginning on the posterior surface of the prostate and dissecting anterolaterally.** After the plane between the rectum and prostate in the midline has been developed, it is possible to release the neurovascular bundle from the prostate, beginning at the apex and moving toward the base, by using the sponge stick to roll the prostate over on its side. Beginning on the rectal surface, the bundle is released from the prostate by spreading a right angle gently. With use of this plane, Denonvilliers fascia and the prostatic fascia remain on the prostate; only the residual fragments of the levator fascia are released from the prostate laterally.

19. **c. When the prostate has been removed and tissue covering the posterolateral surface of the prostate is thought to be inadequate.** Clues that indicate that wide excision of the neurovascular bundle is necessary include inadequate tissue covering the posterolateral surface of the prostate once the prostate had been removed, leading to secondary wide excision of the neurovascular bundle. This last point is important to understand. The surgeon does not have to make the decision about whether to excise or preserve the neurovascular bundle until the prostate is removed, and, if there is not enough soft tissue covering the prostate, one can excise the neurovascular bundle then.

20. **b. Posterior branch.** The surgeon should look for a prominent arterial branch traveling from the neurovascular bundle over the seminal vesicles to supply the base of the prostate. This posterior vessel should be ligated on each side and divided. By this method, the neurovascular bundles are no longer tethered to the prostate and fall posteriorly.

21. **c. Releasing attachments of the bladder to the peritoneum.** The anterior suture is tied initially. There should be no tension. If there is, the bladder should be released from the peritoneum.

22. **d. Divide the dorsal vein complex completely over the urethra and oversew the end.** If there is troublesome bleeding from the dorsal vein complex at any point, the surgeon should completely divide the dorsal vein complex over the urethra and oversew the end. This is the single best means to control bleeding from the dorsal vein complex. Any maneuver short of this will only worsen the bleeding. To gain exposure for the prostatectomy, one must put traction on the prostate. If the dorsal vein is not

completely divided, traction opens the partially transected veins and usually worsens the bleeding.

23. **d. to ensure interposition of the omentum following repair of the injury.** It is wise to interpose omentum between the rectal closure and the vesicourethral anastomosis to reduce the possibility of a rectourethral fistula.

24. **b. perform re-exploration.** Our findings suggest that patients requiring acute transfusions for hypotension after radical prostatectomy should undergo exploration to evacuate the pelvic hematoma in an effort to decrease the likelihood of bladder neck contracture and incontinence.

25. **c. Use a Babcock clamp to hold the bladder down.** We have found that the use of a Babcock clamp to approximate the bladder neck and urethra while the anastomotic sutures are tied has virtually eliminated bladder neck contractures in our practice.

26. **a. Intrinsic sphincter deficiency.** After radical prostatectomy, incontinence is usually secondary to intrinsic sphincter deficiency.

27. **e. none of the above.** Sparing of the seminal vesicles has not improved incontinence, potency, nor margin status; and there have been no reported cases of pelvic abscess.

28. **e. none of the above.** Sparing of the bladder neck has not improved incontinence, potency, margin status, or stricture rates.

29. **c. 26%.** The percentage of men who had bilateral sural nerve grafting and demonstrated full erections (sufficient for penetration) was 26%.

30. **c. in reverse to the natural position (proximal to distal and distal to proximal).** Sural nerve grafts are placed in reverse to the natural position (proximal to distal and distal to proximal).

31. **d. Rectal injury.** Only rectal injury rates have dramatically changed.

32. **c. It fell out of favor as the principle technique in the 1970s secondary to high intraoperative blood loss.** In the 1970s the procedure fell out of favor because the importance of pelvic lymphadenectomy was understood for the purposes of staging. However, with the advent of Partin tables, surgeons could accurately predict the chances of lymph node involvement, obviating the need for staging lymphadenectomy. Furthermore, laparoscopic lymphadenectomy has gained favor and allows for radical perineal prostatectomy and lymph node dissection in one operative setting in those where it is required. Pathologic outcomes are not significantly different for either procedure. It offers shorter hospital stays and lower costs than the retropubic prostatectomy. Blood loss is significantly lower than with the retropubic approach. A nerve-sparing technique can be accomplished through the perineal approach.

33. **a. The literature supports that it is almost always transient.** Sensory neurapraxia of the lower extremity is reported to occur in approximately 2% of radical perineal prostatectomy cases. However, one study did report an incidence of 25%. This is reported significantly more often than with retropubic prostatectomy. True motor deficits are rare. Because of the transient nature, this is not a major source of morbidity.

34. **c. It can be avoided when an assistant places gentle downward pressure on the Lowsley tractor while the rectourethralis muscle is divided.** Traction on the Lowsley tractor during division of the rectourethralis muscle tents the rectum upward and increases the likelihood of injury. Traction should not be placed until after the rectourethralis muscle is divided. When unrecognized, a fistula may ensue. Although one report showed an incidence of rectal injury in 11% of cases, most series recognize an incidence of 1% to 5%. When recognized and repaired at the time of injury, the operation can continue without a problem.

35. **d. a and b only.** The patient's Gleason score and PSA value help determine the likelihood of organ-confined disease and, thus, the candidacy for a radical perineal prostatectomy. A history of degenerative disk disease is not a contraindication to surgery.

36. **b. Patients with ankylosis of the hips or spine may not tolerate a radical perineal prostatectomy.** Because of the necessity of either an exaggerated lithotomy or modified exaggerated lithotomy position, ankylosis of the hips or spine may be a contraindication to the procedure. Concomitant radical perineal prostatectomy and laparoscopic lymph node dissection results in little increased morbidity and remains cost effective when compared with radical retropubic prostatectomy. Patients with prior renal transplantation or morbid obesity are often better candidates for a perineal approach than the retropubic approach.

37. **b. Unlike a radical retropubic prostatectomy, the dorsal venous complex is not usually encountered and blood loss is significantly reduced.** The dorsal venous complex is usually not encountered, resulting in relatively lower blood loss when compared with the retropubic approach. A blood type and antibody screen are performed in the days or hours before surgery, but a crossmatch is generally unnecessary. Transfusion rates are generally around 5%.

38. **d. a and b only.** Postoperatively, the diet is advanced rapidly as tolerated, patients ambulate early, and the overwhelming majority of patients are discharged by the second postoperative day. However, rectal stimulation or manipulation is prohibited in the postoperative period.

39. **e. a and c only.** In a series by Weldon and colleagues (1997),* up to 70% of the patients were potent postoperatively. Furthermore, pharmacotherapy has been demonstrated to improve potency outcomes. However, older age has been demonstrated to be a risk factor for postoperative impotence.

40. **b. the Lowsley retractor.** The apex of the prostate and adjacent urethra can be palpated easily due to the presence of the Lowsley retractor.

41. **e. The indwelling Foley catheter is not passed until after the anterior vesicourethral anastomotic sutures are placed and tied down.** During placement of the anterior vesicourethral anastomotic sutures, a red rubber catheter is placed transurethrally and used to identify the membranous urethral stump and also provide traction on the urethra to assist in placement of the sutures. The red rubber catheter is then removed, and the indwelling Foley catheter is then placed retrograde into the bladder. Simple interrupted sutures are placed for the anastomosis. A tennis racquet technique is used for bladder neck reconstruction if necessary.

---

*Sources referenced can be found in *Campbell-Walsh Urology*, 10th *Edition*, on the Expert Consult website.

Additional Study Points

1. The dorsal vein has three major branches: a superficial branch in the midline and two lateral branches that span over the lateral aspects of the prostate.

2. The prostate is covered with three distinct fascial layers: Denonvilliers fascia, prostatic fascia, and levator fascia.

3. Denonvilliers fascia is most prominent and dense near the base of the prostate and overlying the seminal vesicles and thins dramatically more caudad at its termination at the striated sphincter.

4. Laterally the prostatic fascia fuses with the levator fascia.

5. Following radical prostatectomy, 15% to 20% of men develop an inguinal hernia. It is usually an indirect inguinal hernia.

6. The final decision whether to preserve the neurovascular bundles is made at surgery.

7. Findings that would indicate a neurovascular bundle should be resected include palpable induration in the lateral pelvic fascia and a neurovascular bundle that appears fixed to the prostate.

8. Thermal energy should never be used on or near the neurovascular bundles.

9. Bladder neck contractures occur in less than 10% of patients.

10. Factors important for recovery of erectile function include patient age, preoperative potency status, and preservation of the neurovascular bundles.

11. Potency improves with time such that in one study 42% of patients were potent at 3 months and 73% at a year.

12. In a randomized study using sural nerve grafting to preserve potency in patients in whom a neurovascular bundle needed to be sacrificed, there was no difference in those grafted versus those who were not.

13. Salvage radical prostatectomy should only be considered in men who have unequivocally clinically localized prostate cancer.

14. Complications following salvage radical prostatectomy include 50% incontinence, 24% anastomotic stricture, and nearly universal erectile dysfunction with approximately a 45% recurrence rate at 5 years.

15. Complete excision of the seminal vesicle during radical prostatectomy is recommended for cancer control.

Laparoscopic and Robotic-Assisted Laparoscopic Radical Prostatectomy and Pelvic Lymphadenectomy

Li-Ming Su, MD ● Joseph A. Smith, Jr., MD

QUESTIONS

1. With laparoscopic/robotic prostatectomy a continuous suture for the vesicourethral anastomosis:
   a. avoids incontinence.
   b. has a high rate of bladder neck contracture.
   c. can be performed with the need for only a single knot.
   d. requires an indwelling catheter for at least 2 weeks.
   e. eliminates the need for a pelvic drain.

2. With laparoscopic/robotic radical prostatectomy, positive margin rates are not influenced by:
   a. surgical technique.
   b. patient selection.
   c. the method of pathologic analysis.
   d. transperitoneal versus extraperitoneal exposure.
   e. tumor grade and stage.

3. Compared with open surgical approaches, laparoscopic/robotic prostatectomy has been consistently shown to decrease:
   a. postoperative pain.
   b. urinary incontinence.
   c. bleeding.
   d. erectile dysfunction.
   e. positive margins.

4. Positive surgical margins with laparoscopic/robotic prostatectomy:
   a. decrease as technical experience is gained.
   b. are rare at the prostatic apex.
   c. occur only when extracapsular disease is present.
   d. are seen most commonly at the prostate base.
   e. can be avoided by using a robotic-assisted approach.

5. An advantage of extraperitoneal versus transperitoneal approach to laparoscopic/robotic prostatectomy is:
   a. faster operating room time.
   b. shorter hospitalization.
   c. increased working space.
   d. avoidance of bowel manipulation.
   e. fewer positive margins.

6. Laparoscopic pelvic lymph node dissection:
   a. is difficult to perform along with robotic radical prostatectomy.
   b. should always be performed transperitoneally.
   c. has an increased risk of thromboembolic complication compared with open approaches.
   d. should only be performed for tumors lower than or equal to Gleason grade 7.
   e. can allow lymph node removal comparable with open surgery.

7. Rectal injury with laparoscopic/robotic radical prostatectomy:
   a. is best avoided by antegrade release of the rectum from the posterior prostate.
   b. is usually from trocar placement.
   c. can be avoided by bluntly dividing Denonvilliers fascia.
   d. should be treated with an immediate diverting colostomy.
   e. is often unrecognized and heals spontaneously.

8. Bleeding during laparoscopic/robotic radical prostatectomy is usually minimal because:
   a. the plane of periprostatic tissue dissection is different than with open surgery.
   b. the dorsal vein complex does not have to be divided.
   c. the pneumoperitoneum tamponades venous bleeding.
   d. suturing is easier than with open surgery.
   e. the Trendelenburg position decreases venous pressure.

9. Robotic assistance with laparoscopy is most useful in:
   a. trocar insertion and removal.
   b. maintaining a steady insufflation pressure.
   c. decreasing operating room costs.

d. facilitating suturing.

e. eliminating the need for a table side assistant.

10. The neurovascular bundle lies within which two periprostatic fascial planes?

a. Prostate capsule and prostatic fascia

b. Prostate capsule and levator fascia

c. Prostatic fascia and levator fascia

d. Denonvilliers fascia and prostate capsule

e. Denonvilliers fascia and endopelvic fascia

11. Antegrade laparoscopic dissection of the prostate results in less blood loss as compared with the retrograde approach due in part to:

a. early division of the dorsal venous complex and prostatic pedicles.

b. early division of the prostatic pedicles and late division of the dorsal venous complex.

c. less tissue manipulation.

d. better visualization.

e. late division of the dorsal venous complex and prostatic pedicles.

12. The higher cost of laparoscopic/robotic-assisted as compared with open radical prostatectomy is mostly a consequence of:

a. higher blood loss and transfusion rates.

b. a higher complication rate.

c. a longer operative time and disposable equipment.

d. longer hospital stays.

e. higher surgical and anesthesia charges.

13. As a consequence of the CO_2 pneumoperitoneum used during minimally invasive prostatectomy, the anesthesia team must be most aware of the potential for:

a. bleeding and hypotension.

b. hypoxia and acidosis.

c. tachycardia and hypertension.

d. bradycardia and hypotension.

e. hypercarbia and oliguria.

14. Positive margins at the prostatic apex:

a. are more common with the robotic-assisted technique as compared with open surgery.

b. can occur due to protrusion of the posterior prostatic apex beneath the urethra.

c. can occur more commonly with retrograde versus antegrade dissection of the prostate.

d. are less common in laparoscopic versus open surgery.

e. are less common than at the prostatic base.

15. Men who are not candidates for laparoscopic/robotic-assisted laparoscopic radical prostatectomy include those with:

a. palpable tumors.

b. history of prior pelvic surgery.

c. morbid obesity.

d. uncorrectable bleeding diatheses.

e. prior neoadjuvant hormonal therapy.

ANSWERS

1. **c. can be performed with the need for only a single knot.** The vesicourethral anastomosis may be accomplished using either an interrupted closure or a running continuous suture with a single knot (van Velthoven et al, 2003).*

2. **d. transperitoneal versus extraperitoneal exposure.** Comparison of margin status between high-volume centers with the operations performed by experienced surgeons has shown no definitive advantage for one surgical approach over the other in achieving negative surgical margins (Brown et al, 2003; Khan and Partin, 2005).

3. **c. bleeding.** Because most of the blood loss that occurs during radical prostatectomy is from venous sinuses, the tamponade effect from the pneumoperitoneum helps diminish ongoing blood loss during laparoscopic robotic prostatectomy (LRP)/robot-assisted laparoscopic prostatectomy (RALP). Blood loss of less than a few hundred milliliters is routinely reported (Guillonneau et al, 2001; Hoznek et al, 2002).

4. **a. decrease as technical experience is gained.** In most series of LRP and RALP, positive margin percentages decrease as greater familiarity with the procedure is obtained (Ahlering et al, 2004b; Salomon et al, 2004; Rassweiler et al, 2005).

5. **d. avoidance of bowel manipulation.** As the extraperitoneal technique avoids violation of the peritoneal envelope, bowel manipulation is avoided. It is for this reason that patients with extensive prior abdominal surgery can undergo successful laparoscopic and robotic prostatectomy by the extraperitoneal route.

6. **e. can allow lymph node removal comparable with open surgery.** Pelvic lymphadenectomy can be performed by open or laparoscopic techniques with no significant difference in nodal yield.

7. **a. is best avoided by antegrade release of the rectum from the posterior prostate.** Thorough dissection of the rectum off of the posterior prostate is critical to minimize the risk of rectal injury during subsequent steps such as division of the urethra and dissection of the prostatic apex. With LRP and RALP, sharp and complete incision of the posterior layer of Denonvilliers fascia is necessary after seminal vesicle dissection to allow adequate mobilization of the rectum.

8. **c. pneumoperitoneum tamponades venous bleeding.** Because most of the blood loss that occurs during radical prostatectomy is from venous sinuses, the tamponade effect from the pneumoperitoneum helps diminish ongoing blood loss during LRP/RALP. Blood loss of less than a few hundred milliliters is routinely reported (Guillonneau et al, 2001; Hoznek et al, 2002).

9. **d. facilitating suturing.** Most surgeons, however, believe that the robotic technology significantly facilitates suturing (especially for the vesicourethral anastomosis) and other aspects of the surgical dissection (Dasgupta, 2005).

10. **c. prostatic fascia and levator fascia.** The neurovascular bundle travels between two distinct fascial planes that surround the prostate, namely, the prostatic fascia and levator fascia.

*Sources referenced can be found in *Campbell-Walsh Urology, 10th Edition,* on the Expert Consult website.

11. **b. early division of the prostatic pedicles and late division of the dorsal venous complex.** Because the dorsal venous complex is divided early in the operation and the prostatic pedicles late, there is potentially a greater risk of ongoing bleeding with the retrograde technique (Rassweiler et al, 2001). In contrast, during the antegrade neurovascular bundle dissection, the arterial blood supply to the prostate (via the prostatic pedicles) is divided early and the dorsal venous complex is divided near the end of the operation, thus reducing blood loss during the operation.

12. **c. a longer operative time and disposable equipment.** In the study by Link and colleagues (2004), the factors that most influenced overall cost in order of importance included operative time, length of hospital stay, and consumable items (e.g., disposable laparoscopic equipment and trocars).

13. **e. hypercarbia and oliguria.** The anesthesiologist must be aware of the potential consequences of CO_2 insufflation and pneumoperitoneum including oliguria and hypercarbia.

14. **b. can occur due to protrusion of the posterior prostatic apex beneath the urethra.** Before division of the posterior urethra, great care must be taken to inspect the contour of the posterior prostatic apex. In some patients, the posterior prostatic apex can protrude beneath the urethra, resulting in an iatrogenic positive margin if not identified.

15. **d. uncorrectable bleeding diatheses.** Contraindications to minimally invasive laparoscopic prostatectomy include uncorrectable bleeding diatheses or the inability to undergo general anesthesia due to severe cardiopulmonary compromise.

Additional Study Points

1. Accessory pudendal arteries traveling longitudinally along the anteromedial aspect of the prostate should be preserved because they may be important in preserving blood flow for erectile function.
2. When dissecting at the tip of the seminal vesicles, care should be taken not to use electrocautery because damage to the cavernosal nerves that travel adjacent to this area may be incurred.
3. The apical dissection is the most common sight of positive margins following radical prostatectomy. It is important to note that at the apex there may be an anterior and posterior overlying lip of prostate tissue that needs to be recognized and included with the specimen before transecting the urethra.
4. A transperitoneal approach is not totally protective against the formation of a lymphocele. Clips should be used if lymphatics are identified to reduce the incidence of lymphocele formation.

Radiation Therapy for Prostate Cancer

Anthony V. D'Amico, MD, PhD ● Juanita M. Crook, MD, FRCPC ● Clair J. Beard, MD ●
Theodore L. DeWeese, MD ● Mark Hurwitz, MD ● Irving D. Kaplan, MD

QUESTIONS

1. An advance in the radiotherapeutic management of prostate cancer includes which of the following?
   a. Three-dimensional conformal technique and image guidance for radioactive source placement in the prostate gland
   b. The ability to remove all uncertainty related to patient setup
   c. The ability to deliver three-dimensional conformal radiation therapy with no risk of side effects
   d. The ability to cure all patients with prostate cancer
   e. The ability to identify who has clinically significant prostate cancer

2. What are four important predictors of prostate cancer–specific mortality after external beam radiation therapy?
   a. Patient's age, performance status, height, and weight
   b. Biopsy Gleason score, age, weight, and height
   c. Biopsy Gleason score, age, height, and weight
   d. Biopsy Gleason score, prostate-specific antigen (PSA) level, percentage of prostate biopsies, and clinical stage
   e. Biopsy Gleason score, PSA level, clinical stage, and height

3. The percentage of positive prostate biopsies is:
   a. not an important predictor of PSA failure-free survival after external beam radiation therapy.
   b. equal to the number of cores sampled divided by 100.
   c. not an important predictor of prostate cancer–specific mortality after external beam radiation therapy in low-risk patients.
   d. able to identify the patients at higher risk of prostate cancer–specific mortality despite having low-risk disease.
   e. equal to the PSA value divided by the biopsy Gleason score.

4. Which of the following statements is TRUE regarding local control after radiation therapy for prostate cancer?
   a. It is an unimportant end point because it does not predict for survival.
   b. Local control improves with higher radiation doses.
   c. Local control is associated with a longer time to PSA nadir and lower nadir.
   d. a and b
   e. b and c

5. Which of the following statements is TRUE regarding the PSA bounce phenomenon after prostate brachytherapy?
   a. It is seen in 25% to 30% of prostate brachytherapy cases using permanent seed implant monotherapy.
   b. It may occur anytime between 8 and 30 months after implant.
   c. The patient may be asymptomatic.
   d. It may be associated with a positive biopsy showing treatment effect.
   e. All of the above

6. What are the three most important predictors of PSA failure-free survival after external beam radiation therapy?
   a. Patient's age, performance status, and weight
   b. Patient's age, PSA level, and weight
   c. PSA value, biopsy Gleason score, and clinical T stage
   d. PSA value, biopsy Gleason score, and age
   e. Biopsy Gleason score, age, and weight

7. Two years after definitive radiotherapy for prostate cancer, what should the serum PSA level be?
   a. Undetectable
   b. Less than 0.5 ng/mL
   c. Stable and not rising
   d. Normal
   e. None of the above

8. One year after radiotherapy, the serum PSA value has fallen to within the "normal range" (2.5 ng/mL) but then starts to rise, with subsequent readings of 3.5 and 5.1 ng/mL over a 6-month period. The most appropriate management is:
   a. Tell the patient that radiation therapy has not worked and discuss salvage prostatectomy and cryosurgery.
   b. Tell the patient that the PSA value is still normal and not to worry.

c. Tell the patient that he likely has a recurrence and that rising PSA may indicate a distant component to the failure.

d. None of the above

e. Both a and b

9. With regard to the PSA nadir after radiation therapy, which of the following statements is TRUE?

a. An early nadir is good.

b. Patients showing distant failure reach a nadir later.

c. Patients who are cured may take 24 to 30 months to reach a nadir.

d. A nadir greater than 0.5 ng/mL means that treatment has failed.

e. None of the above

10. Prostate biopsy samples should be negative for disease by what time after radiation therapy?

a. 6 months

b. 12 months

c. 18 months

d. 30 months

e. None of the above

11. Which of the following statements is TRUE regarding local control after radiation therapy for prostate cancer?

a. It is an unimportant end point because it does not predict for survival.

b. It is lower in patients with early disease because they receive lower doses of radiation.

c. It is equal for all types of radiation treatment.

d. It is associated with treatment technique and dose of radiation.

e. None of the above

12. Which of the following statements is TRUE regarding conformal radiation therapy?

a. It is available in almost all radiation centers.

b. It is more accurate than conventional radiation.

c. It is unassociated with improved outcomes in prostate cancer patients.

d. It is a form of particle therapy.

e. None of the above

13. Which of the following statements is TRUE regarding complications after radiation therapy?

a. They are related to treatment technique, type of radiation used, and total dose given.

b. They are identifiable in the majority of treated patients.

c. They are higher with dose escalation protocols.

d. They are lower with particle beam therapy.

e. None of the above

14. Dose escalation trials using conformal radiation show improved outcomes at which of the following doses?

a. 60 Gy

b. 66 Gy

c. 70 Gy

d. Greater than 75 Gy

e. None of the above

15. Dose escalation trials show a benefit for all of the following groups EXCEPT:

a. patients with favorable tumors (T1 or T2, Gleason score of <7) and PSA levels less than 10.

b. patients with favorable tumors (T1 or T2, Gleason score of <7) and PSA levels greater than 20.

c. patients with unfavorable tumors (T2b or T3, Gleason score of >7) and PSA levels less than 10.

d. patients with unfavorable tumors (T2b or T3, Gleason score of ≥7) and PSA levels greater than 4.

e. None of the above

16. Which of the following statements is TRUE regarding particle beam therapy?

a. It has a theoretical advantage over photon therapy.

b. It has been shown to be more effective than photon therapy.

c. It is less expensive than photon therapy.

d. It is less toxic than photon therapy.

e. None of the above

17. Which of the following statements is TRUE regarding intensity-modulated radiation therapy?

a. It is a form of particle therapy.

b. It has been proved to improve treatment outcome.

c. It gives equal emphasis to the target tissue (prostate) and normal tissue (bladder and rectum) during treatment planning.

d. It can be delivered inexpensively because of software improvements.

e. None of the above

18. With regard to complications of permanent implant brachytherapy, which of the following statements is TRUE?

a. There is a higher rate of urinary toxicity than with external beam irradiation.

b. There is a higher rate of rectal toxicity than with external beam irradiation.

c. There is a higher rate of impotence than in radical prostatectomy.

d. There is a higher rate of impotence than in external beam irradiation.

e. None of the above

19. Which of the following statements is TRUE regarding high-dose-rate brachytherapy?

a. It is usually delivered as monotherapy for advanced prostate cancer.

b. It uses high-activity iodine-103 or paladium-103 (^{103}Pd) as the source.

c. It does not require a surgical procedure.

d. It is generally delivered in several fractions as a boost to external beam irradiation.

e. None of the above

20. When comparing iodine-125 (^{125}I) to ^{103}Pd, which of the following statements is TRUE?

a. ^{125}I has a shorter half-life than ^{103}Pd.

b. ^{125}I delivers a significantly higher dose to the rectum when compared with 103Pd.

c. ^{125}I delivers a significantly higher dose to the urethra when compared with 103Pd.

d. The dose prescribed for a ^{125}I implant is higher than the dose for a ^{103}Pd implant.

e. None of the above

21. When prostate brachytherapy monotherapy is compared with a brachytherapy boost, which of the following statements is TRUE?

   a. A higher implant dose is used with monotherapy than with the boost.

   b. Brachytherapy monotherapy is associated with a higher rate of rectal complications than is brachytherapy boost.

   c. Brachytherapy monotherapy is preferred for patients with preexisting urinary outlet obstruction.

   d. Brachytherapy monotherapy is preferred for larger glands.

   e. None of the above

22. Prostate brachytherapy monotherapy is appropriate for which group of patients?

   a. Patients with T3 cancer

   b. Patients with T1c prostate cancer

   c. Patients with a high probability of organ-confined disease

   d. Patients with a high probability of organ-confined disease, prostates weighing less than 60 g, and low American Urological Association (AUA) symptom scores

   e. None of the above

23. MRI-guided prostate brachytherapy is able to provide optimal placement of the radioactive sources within the prostate gland for what reason?

   a. A real-time imaging mechanism permits the physician to verify that the trajectory of the catheter containing the radioactive sources is in the ideal location when compared with the preplan.

   b. The magnetic field aligns the sources perfectly.

   c. The procedure can be done under local anesthesia.

   d. A Foley catheter is not necessary.

   e. a and b

24. With MRI-guided prostate brachytherapy, patients with large prostate glands (>60 g) can have implants and still have low acute urinary retention rates (4%) for what reason?

   a. MRI guidance allows for urethral sparing.

   b. MRI guidance allows for fewer sources.

   c. A Foley catheter is not necessary with MRI-guided brachytherapy.

   d. A cystoscopy is not performed with MRI-guided brachytherapy.

   e. The procedure can be performed using local anesthesia.

25. What is the principal reason for neoadjuvant androgen suppression before initiation of radiation therapy?

   a. To prevent early development of metastatic disease

   b. To reduce prostate size, thus minimizing the field size and side effects of external beam treatment

   c. To reduce the tumor burden requiring eradication with radiation

   d. To delay the need for radiation

   e. To improve overall survival

26. For a patient with a Gleason 8 prostate cancer, which of the following statements is best supported by the findings of phase 3 studies? Androgen suppression:

   a. is always used with radiation.

   b. improves overall survival when used with radiation.

   c. improves biochemical freedom from failure (bNED) survival when given in addition to standard dose radiation.

   d. has no role in treatment on the basis of this factor alone.

   e. is given for 4 months before radiation.

27. What do the findings of RTOG 92-02 indicate when androgen suppression is given in combination with radiation for T3 Gleason score 7 disease?

   a. Prolonged adjuvant androgen deprivation provides added benefit as compared with neoadjuvant therapy alone.

   b. The optimal duration of androgen suppression with radiation is now defined.

   c. Prolonged androgen deprivation results in improved overall survival.

   d. Neoadjuvant androgen deprivation is sufficient.

   e. Radiation alone is suboptimal therapy.

28. A patient has a history of hormone-refractory metastatic prostate cancer. He now has a new painful lesion of his upper femoral shaft. What is a typical course of palliative radiation therapy for this man?

   a. One fraction of radiation at 3000 cGy

   b. 7 weeks of daily radiation to 7000 cGy

   c. 10 fractions of daily radiation to 3000 cGy

   d. One fraction of daily radiation to 7000 cGy

   e. None of the above

29. A patient with a history of metastatic prostate cancer, under treatment with a luteinizing hormone-releasing hormone agonist and a nonsteroidal antiandrogen, presents with a 3-week history of increasing middle to low back pain and 2 days of leg weakness. The next step is:

   a. increasing the dose of nonsteroidal antiandrogen.

   b. MRI of the thoracic and lumbar spine.

   c. radiation therapy with a systemic radionuclide such as strontium-89.

   d. treatment with a selective cyclooxygenase-2 inhibitor for 5 to 7 days and reevaluation.

   e. None of the above

30. What is the most common toxicity of systemic radionuclide therapy with strontium-89 and samarium-153?

   a. Hematologic toxicity, particularly with a decrement in the platelet count

   b. Neurologic toxicity including tinnitus

   c. Genitourinary toxicity, particularly azotemia

   d. Hepatic toxicity associated with an elevation of transaminase levels

   e. None of the above

31. What would be an attractive gene therapy approach that could be combined with radiation for the treatment of prostate cancer?

   a. One that requires prolonged transgene expression

   b. One that kills cells by a mechanism that complements and does not overlap with radiation-induced cell death

c. One that requires all prostate cancer cells to be transduced

d. a and c

e. None of the above

Imaging

1. A voiding cystourethrogram on a 72-year-old man who presents with urinary tract infections 2 years after combination external beam radiation therapy and brachytherapy for prostate cancer is depicted in Figure 104–1.

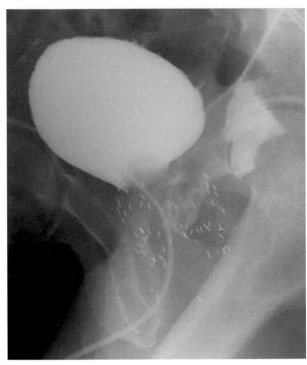

Figure 104–1.

The most likely diagnosis is:

a. brachytherapy seed migration.

b. urethra rectal fistula.

c. vesico sigmoid fistula.

d. vesico rectal fistula.

e. urethro cutaneous fistula.

ANSWERS

1. **a. Three-dimensional conformal technique and image guidance for radioactive source placement in the prostate gland.** The first advance has been the generation of linear accelerators and conformal techniques capable of delivering high doses of radiation deep within the pelvis while simultaneously respecting the normal tissue tolerance of the anterior rectal wall, prostatic urethra, femoral heads, and bladder neck. The second advance was made when image-guided techniques were introduced for use during the insertion of radioactive sources directly into the prostate gland.

2. **d. Biopsy Gleason score, prostate-specific antigen (PSA) level, percentage of prostate biopsies, and clinical stage.** The pretreatment prognostic factors that have established roles in predicting recurrence include the PSA value, biopsy Gleason score, and the 1992 American Joint Committee on Cancer Staging (AJCCS) clinical stage.

3. **d. able to identify the patients at higher risk of prostate cancer-specific mortality despite having low-risk disease.** Of particular importance is that the majority of patients (158/207 [76%]) in the intermediate-risk group could be classified into either a 30% or an 85% 5-year PSA control high- or low-risk cohort, respectively, by using the preoperative prostate biopsy data.

4. **e. b and c.**

5. **e. All of the above.**

6. **c. PSA value, biopsy Gleason score, and clinical T stage.** The pretreatment prognostic factors that have established roles in predicting recurrence include the PSA value, biopsy Gleason score, and the 1992 AJCCS clinical stage.

7. **c. Stable and not rising.** It is clear that there is no distinct PSA threshold that defines successful treatment but that PSA stability after the nadir is important.

8. **c. Tell the patient that he likely has a recurrence and that rising PSA may indicate a distant component to the failure.** The level of PSA nadir achieved to some extent reflects the type of failure. The median PSA nadir for patients exhibiting local failure is 2 to 3 ng/mL, and for those exhibiting distant failure it is 5 to 10 ng/mL. The postnadir doubling time of the PSA value also correlates with the type of failure, with distant failures having shorter PSA doubling times of 3 to 6 months and local failures having longer PSA doubling times of 11 to 13 months.

9. **c. Patients who are cured may take 24 to 30 months to reach a nadir.** The time to nadir has been shown to be inversely proportional to disease-free survival. The median time to nadir in patients who remain free from failure is 22 to 33 months, with 92% of men whose PSA value reached a nadir at 36 months or longer remaining disease free.

10. **d. 30 months.** In a series of 498 men followed with sequential systematic postirradiation biopsies, biopsy samples cleared at a mean time of 30 months after radiation therapy.

11. **d. It is associated with treatment technique and dose of radiation.** Tumor control was better in patients who received higher doses of radiation to larger fields, at the expense of increased complications.

12. **b. It is more accurate than conventional radiation.** The result is loosely described as conformal radiation therapy because the radiation beams conform to the shape of the treatment target.

13. **a. They are related to treatment technique, type of radiation used, and total dose given.** The percentage of patients who experience side effects and the severity of the side effects differ somewhat from series to series depending on the morbidity scale used and also on whether the assessment is physician or patient based.

14. **d. Greater than 75 Gy.** Dose escalation therapy, to doses greater than 75 Gy, is still experimental, but the early data appear to be highly favorable.

15. **a. patients with favorable tumors (T1 or T2, Gleason score of <7) and PSA levels of less than 10.** Patients with favorable tumors (Gleason score of <6, T1 or

T2a) who also had a PSA level of less than 10 ng/mL derived no benefit from dose escalation because all patients in this group did well. Patients with unfavorable tumors (Gleason score of 7 to 10 and T2b or T3) who also had a PSA level of greater than 20 ng/mL also derived no benefit from dose escalation.

16. **a. It has a theoretical advantage over photon therapy.** The heavy particle beams are difficult to produce and to control but have certain theoretical advantages over conventional x-ray and electron beams.

17. **c. It gives equal emphasis to the target tissue (prostate) and normal tissue (bladder and rectum) during treatment planning.** The goal of this method of treatment planning and delivery is to maximize treatment to the target (e.g., prostate) while minimizing treatment to the surrounding tissues to a degree that is not possible with conformal therapy.

18. **a. There is a higher rate of urinary toxicity than with external beam irradiation.** One study showed that 37% of patients report grade 1 urinary toxicity (symptoms not requiring medical intervention) within the first 60 days after implantation. Grade 2 urinary toxicity (requiring medical intervention), with a mean duration of 19 months after implantation and with a likelihood of resolution of 68% at 36 months, has been reported. Significant continued obstruction requiring self-catheterization occurs in 1% to 5% of patients.

19. **d. It is generally delivered in several fractions as a boost to external beam irradiation.** This therapy is delivered as a boost in two to four applications, either before or after external beam irradiation.

20. **d. The dose prescribed for a ^{125}I implant is higher than the dose for a ^{103}Pd implant.** Higher-activity seeds are required for ^{103}Pd versus ^{125}I to deliver a similar tumoricidal dose (i.e., 1.3 mCi per palladium seed vs. 0.4 mCi per iodine seed).

21. **a. A higher implant dose is used with monotherapy than with the boost.** There is relatively little radiation delivered to the rectum with brachytherapy alone. However, the prostatic urethra receives a full dose. When an implant is combined with external-beam therapy, the dosage to the urethra is less but increased radiation is received by the rectum. Glands exceeding 60 g do not lend themselves to monotherapy because it is difficult to treat the entire gland with this modality alone.

22. **d. Patients with a high probability of organ-confined disease, prostates weighing less than 60 g, and low American Urological Association (AUA) symptom scores.** Larger prostatic volumes—specifically glands greater than 60 g—were associated with urinary toxicities. Other investigators reported that transurethral prostatic resection in the distant past is not a contraindication to implantation. Patients with a pretreatment AUA score greater than 20 demonstrated a 29% risk of developing urinary retention, whereas a pretreatment score of less than 10 was associated with a 2% risk.

23. **a. A real-time imaging mechanism permits the physician to verify that the trajectory of the catheter containing the radioactive sources is in the ideal location when compared with the preplan.** By using this technique, the three-dimensional trajectory that the catheter containing the radioactive sources traverses can be checked intraoperatively and compared, within a few seconds, with the ideal location based on the preplan using real-time MRI.

24. **a. MRI guidance allows for urethral sparing.** Therefore despite implanting 45 men with glands greater than 60 g, the acute urinary retention rate was 4% and the need for prolonged use of oral α_{1a}-adrenergic blockers was 5%, consistent with a urethral-sparing technique.

25. **c. To reduce the tumor burden requiring eradication with radiation.** Short-duration neoadjuvant androgen suppression therapy may be used with the goal of reducing the local tumor burden, requiring eradication by subsequent radiation.

26. **c. improves biochemical freedom from failure (bNED) survival when given in addition to standard dose radiation.** Among strategies to improve outcome for patients with locally advanced prostate cancer, hormonal manipulation in combination with radiation therapy has consistently demonstrated improvement in treatment outcome as compared with standard-dose radiation alone. A meta-analysis of both retrospective and prospective trials of androgen deprivation in combination with radiation therapy demonstrated near-universal benefit in regard to local/regional control, disease-free survival, and bNED survival.

27. **a. Prolonged adjuvant androgen deprivation provides added benefit as compared with neoadjuvant therapy alone.** The optimal type, timing, and duration of androgen suppression in combination with radiation therapy remains to be defined. In RTOG 92-02, patients with T2c-T4, N0-1, M0 disease were randomized to receive a total of 4 months of total androgen suppression with radiation administered after 2 months or the same regimen followed by an additional 2 years of goserelin. Subgroup analysis revealed significant improvement in overall survival for patients with Gleason scores 8 to 10.

28. **c. 10 fractions of daily radiation to 3000 cGy.** A frequently used regimen in the United States is to give 3000 cGy in 10 divided fractions.

29. **b. MRI of the thoracic and lumbar spine.** The diagnostic tool of choice to evaluate a spinal cord compression is MRI.

30. **a. Hematologic toxicity, particularly with a decrement in the platelet count.** Toxicity of strontium-89 is mainly hematologic. Platelet depression is dose dependent.

31. **b. One that kills cells by a mechanism that complements and does not overlap with radiation-induced cell death.** A rational combination of one of these approaches with a more standard cytotoxic therapy such as radiation may provide superior cell killing as a result of nonoverlapping modes of cell death.

Imaging

1. **b. urethra rectal fistula.** There is partial opacification of the irregular prostatic urethra with immediate filling of the rectum. The bladder is normal in appearance, making option d incorrect. Colonic diverticulitis is an important cause of colovesical fistulae but does not usually cause urethrorectal fistulae. The contrast is in the rectum—thus a urethrocutaneous fistula is not likely. The seeds are located in the area one would expect following brachytherapy.

Additional Study Points

1. The advantage of brachytherapy is that there is a rapid falloff of dose within a few millimeters of the seed implant.

2. A pretreatment PSA velocity of greater than 2 ng/mL/yr is associated with an increased risk of biochemical failure following radiation therapy.

3. The definition of failure following radiation therapy is three consecutive rises in PSA following the nadir. It is recommended that these determinations be obtained 3 to 4 months apart.

4. A PSA nadir of less than 0.5 ng/mL is correlated with successful treatment.

5. PSA nadir is the strongest predictor of outcome.

6. Approximately 50% of potent men are impotent at 5 years following conformal external beam radiation therapy.

7. Conformal radiation therapy (CRT) uses a computerized algorithm to conform the dose of radiation to the contours of the prostate.

8. Intensity-modulated radiation therapy (IMRT) uses a set of radiation beams with changing intensities distributed across the field.

9. When IMRT is compared with CRT, lower doses are delivered to critical tissues such as rectum, bladder, and small bowel.

10. Heavy particle beams such as neutrons and protons exhibit a Bragg effect. This is manifested by a sharp falloff beyond the particle's tissue range, thus delivering little radiation beyond that point.

11. 125 Iodine has a half-life of approximately 60 days; palladium 103 has a half-life of 17 days.

12. Steroid administration along with radiation therapy is an integral part of the treatment for spinal cord compression due to prostate cancer.

Cryotherapy for Prostate Cancer

David C. Miller, MD, MPH ● Louis Leon Pisters, MD ● Arie S. Belldegrun, MD

QUESTIONS

1. Technical innovations improving cryotherapy for prostate cancer include all EXCEPT the use of:
   a. transrectal ultrasound.
   b. urethral warming catheters.
   c. warming of neurovascular bundles.
   d. thermocouples placed in critical areas of the prostate.
   e. smaller-diameter cryoprobes allowing percutaneous insertion.

2. Which of the following statements concerning contemporary cryogenic systems is FALSE?
   a. They are based on employing pressurized gas rather than liquid cryogens.
   b. Multipoint sensors allow cryosurgeons to monitor temperatures along an entire tissue plane.
   c. Argon gas is employed for tissue freezing.
   d. They rely on retropubic cryoneedle placement.
   e. Helium gas is employed for active tissue thawing.

3. What is the most clinically important parameter of tissue ablation other than lowest temperature achieved by cryotherapy?
   a. The diameter of the cryoprobe
   b. The number of freeze/thaw cycles
   c. The velocity of tissue thawing
   d. The velocity of tissue freezing
   e. The duration of freezing

4. Typically, the cryoprobes that are activated first in cryotherapy for prostate cancer are located:
   a. medially.
   b. posteriorly.
   c. laterally.
   d. anteriorly.
   e. periurethrally.

5. What is the characteristic appearance of frozen tissue on ultrasound?
   a. Mixed echogenicity
   b. Hyperechogenicity
   c. Anechogenicity
   d. Hypoechogenicity
   e. None of the above

6. Prostate cell death is likely to occur completely in a single freeze cycle when tissue temperature reaches:
   a. 20° C.
   b. 0° C.
   c. −20° C.
   d. −40° C.
   e. none of the above.

7. A patient with Gleason grade 3+4, clinical stage T1c prostate cancer associated with a serum prostate-specific antigen (PSA) value of 8.6 ng/mL is noted to have a prostate gland volume of 70 mL and an American Urological Association (AUA) Symptom Score of 18. Which of the following statements is TRUE?
   a. This patient is best treated with cryotherapy.
   b. This patient requires microwave therapy of the prostate before cryotherapy.
   c. This patient will likely develop urinary tract obstruction after cryotherapy.
   d. This patient should undergo neoadjuvant hormone therapy to reduce the gland before cryotherapy.
   e. This patient cannot undergo cryotherapy.

8. Failure after prostate cryotherapy may be defined as:
   a. failure to reach PSA nadir by 2 months.
   b. PSA cutoff greater than 0.1 ng/mL.
   c. three consecutive elevations in PSA after nadir.
   d. PSA rise of 2 ng/mL above post-treatment nadir.
   e. c and d.

9. Two years after cryosurgery for clinical stage T2a, PSA 7.0, Gleason grade 3 + 4 cancer, a patient is found to have benign glands on a prostate biopsy specimen from the right apex. No malignancy is detected. The PSA level is detectable at 0.2 ng/mL. What is the next step in management?
   a. Repeat cryoablation of the left lobe
   b. Radiation therapy
   c. Surveillance
   d. Androgen deprivation
   e. Repeat biopsy

10. Which clinical parameter most accurately predicts for cancer control after cryotherapy?

    a. PSA nadir less than 0.1 ng/mL

    b. Preoperative Gleason score less than 6

    c. Preoperative serum PSA level less than 15 ng/mL

    d. A prostate volume less than 40 mL

    e. Preoperative T stage

11. Potential advantages of primary cryotherapy for prostate cancer over other local therapies include all EXCEPT:

    a. It is capable of destroying a biologically heterogeneous population of cancer cells including cell populations that are resistant to radiation therapy and hormonal therapy.

    b. The freezing process can extend beyond the capsule of the prostate, potentially eradicating extracapsular disease.

    c. It is proven to be beneficial with adjuvant therapies.

    d. It can be repeated with minimal morbidity.

    e. It can treat high Gleason score prostate cancer.

12. Salvage cryotherapy for radiorecurrent prostate cancer:

    a. will not reduce the PSA below 0.4 ng/mL.

    b. may be useful in the control of local spread in the face of distant metastases.

    c. has the same incidence of incontinence and fistula rates as primary cryotherapy.

    d. may be performed on all patients for whom irradiation fails.

    e. is unlikely to cure high-risk disease (PSA >10 ng/nL and Gleason score >7).

13. Clinical pretreatment factors associated with early treatment failure after salvage cryotherapy include:

    a. postradiation PSA greater than 10 ng/mL.

    b. recurrent cancer with Gleason score 9 or greater.

    c. postradiation PSA doubling time 16 months or less.

    d. all of the above.

    e. none of the above.

14. The most common complication after cryotherapy for prostate cancer is:

    a. rectourethral fistula.

    b. incontinence.

    c. erectile dysfunction.

    d. urethral sloughing.

    e. pelvic pain.

15. Two months after cryotherapy, a patient complains of urinary frequency and dysuria. Urinalysis reveals pyuria. What is the most likely diagnosis?

    a. Pelvic abscess

    b. Urethral sloughing

    c. Extravasation of urine

    d. Rectourethral fistula

    e. Bladder neck contracture

ANSWERS

1. **c. warming of neurovascular bundles.** Use of transrectal ultrasonography (TRUS) for real-time monitoring of the freezing process, use of a urethral warming catheter, use of thermocouples placed in critical areas of the prostate, and improved cryoprobes allowing percutaneous insertion are technical innovations that have all contributed to improving cryotherapy for prostate cancer.

2. **d. They rely on retropubic cryoneedle placement.** With contemporary cryogenic systems, the transition from liquid to gas allowed for the development of ultrathin 17-gauge (1.47-mm) cryoprobes, which permitted direct transperineal (not retropubic) needle placement through a template without making incisions or using tract dilatation and insertion kits. Each of the remaining responses is correct.

3. **b. The number of freeze/thaw cycles.** In a clinical setting, the number of freezing cycles, the lowest temperature achieved, and the existence of any regional "heat sinks" may be more important factors relating to cancer destruction. Repeating a freeze/thaw cycle results in more extensive tissue damage compared with a single cycle.

4. **d. anteriorly.** To maintain TRUS visibility, the freezing is started at the anterior probe layer and continued posteriorly. Uncovered areas may be visualized, and a correcting maneuver may be used. If the freezing is started posteriorly, the acoustic shadowing would prevent visualization of tissue beyond the ice.

5. **d. Hypoechogenicity.** Frozen tissue is significantly different from unfrozen tissue in sound impedance, resulting in strong echo reflection at the interface of frozen and normal tissue. The frozen area can be seen as a well-marginated hyperechoic rim with acoustic shadowing by ultrasonography. Sonography provides no information about the temperature distribution within the ice, nor does it show the extent of freezing at the lateral or anterior aspects of the prostate.

6. **d. –40° C.** Complete cell death is unlikely to occur at temperatures higher than –20° C, and temperatures lower than –40° C are required to completely destroy cells.

7. **d. This patient should undergo neoadjuvant hormone therapy to reduce the gland before cryotherapy.** A gland in excess of 50 mL may be treated best with neoadjuvant androgen deprivation to reduce target volume and allow for more effective cryoablation.

8. **e. c and d.** There is no established definition of biochemical failure after cryotherapy, and different PSA cutoff levels of 0.3, 0.4, 0.5, and 1.0 ng/mL have been used in numerous studies. The American Society for Therapeutic Radiology and Oncology (ASTRO) definitions of failure based on three consecutive rises in the PSA level or PSA nadir plus 2 (Phoenix definition) have also been used.

9. **c. Surveillance.** Benign epithelium, often very focal, has been seen in up to 71% of patients after cryotherapy. The significance of benign epithelium is unknown, and such findings may represent areas of the prostate not frozen to low temperatures, perhaps in the area of the urethral warmer.

10. **a. PSA nadir less than 0.1 ng/mL.** Biochemical failure is lowest among patients who achieve a PSA nadir less than 0.1 ng/mL. Biopsy failure is also lowest in those patients with PSA nadirs less than 0.1 ng/mL.

11. **It is proven to be beneficial with adjuvant therapies.** Potential advantages that primary cryotherapy for prostate cancer offers over other local therapies include the capability of destroying a biologically heterogeneous population of cancer cells including cell populations that are resistant to radiation therapy and hormonal therapy, extension of the freezing process beyond the capsule of the prostate, potentially eradicating extracapsular disease, repeat of treatment with minimal morbidity, and treatment of high Gleason score prostate cancer.

12. **e. is unlikely to cure high-risk disease (PSA >10 ng/mL and Gleason score >7).** In patients who have experienced radiation therapy failure for prostate cancer, those with a PSA greater than 10 ng/mL and Gleason score of the recurrent cancer greater than or equal to 9 are unlikely to be successfully salvaged. The incidence of incontinence and fistulas is higher in salvage cryotherapy.

13. **d. all of the above.** Clinical factors associated with early treatment failure after salvage cryotherapy for radiorecurrent prostate cancer include a PSA level greater than 10 ng/mL, Gleason score greater than or equal to 9, and a postradiation PSA doubling time of 16 months or less.

14. **c. erectile dysfunction.** The most common complication after cryotherapy for prostate cancer is erectile dysfunction. Rectourethral fistula, incontinence, urethral sloughing, and pelvic pain are complications that can occur after cryotherapy. More contemporary series report higher impotence rates of 80% or more. This is probably because of the use of multiple freeze/thaw cycles and extension of the ice ball beyond the prostate into the area of the neurovascular bundles.

15. **b. Urethral sloughing.** Tissue sloughing is manifested by irritative and obstructive voiding symptoms. Pyuria is noted as well. Urinary retention is not uncommon. This condition typically occurs 3 to 8 weeks after the procedure. Initial management consists of antibiotics.

Additional Study Points

1. The mechanisms of injury for cryotherapy involve dehydration of the cell with rupture of the cell membrane, toxic concentration of cellular constituents, and vascular injury.
2. Cell destruction is determined by the cooling rate, warming rate, and lowest temperature achieved.
3. Slow thawing is more effective than rapid thawing in terms of tissue destruction.
4. Contraindications to prostate cryotherapy include a prior transurethral resection of the prostate, symptoms of significant urinary obstruction, large prostate size, and rectal pathology.
5. Salvage radiation following failure of cryotherapy appears to be effective and safe.
6. Complications of cryotherapy include erectile dysfunction, which is common; long-term incontinence in 1% to 10% of patients; symptomatic urethral sloughing in 5% to 15% of patients; pelvic, rectal, or perineal pain; rectal urethral fistula; and osteitis pubis in a minority of patients.

High-Intensity Focused Ultrasound for the Treatment of Prostate Cancer

Michael O. Koch, MD

QUESTIONS

1. High-intensity focused ultrasound (HIFU) exerts what effect on prostate tissue?
   a. Tissue fragmentation with disruption of vascular architecture
   b. Coagulative necrosis
   c. Nuclear injury
   d. Cavitation
   e. Disruption of protein synthesis

2. The revised ASTRO-Phoenix criteria of prostate-specific antigen (PSA) nadir + 2 ng/mL were designed to:
   a. allow comparison of different modalities for localized prostate cancer.
   b. determine the curative potential of HIFU.
   c. allow the comparison of different radiation modalities in preventing progressive prostate cancer.
   d. determine the curative potential of radiation modalities.
   e. allow comparison of surgical and radiation-based treatments.

3. The most common side effect of HIFU for localized prostate cancer is:
   a. impotence.
   b. urinary retention.
   c. bladder neck stricture.
   d. urethrorectal fistulae.
   e. incontinence.

4. The determination of true efficacy of HIFU for localized prostate cancer is limited by:
   a. short follow-up.
   b. invalid PSA end points.
   c. false-negative biopsies.
   d. changing technology.
   e. all of the above.

ANSWERS

1. **b. Coagulative necrosis.** Highly focused sound energy results in mechanical and thermal effects on tissue. In the case of HIFU, the primary mechanism of tissue ablation is by raising the temperature in the tissue above the level needed to create coagulative necrosis.

2. **c. allow the comparison of different radiation modalities in preventing progressive prostate cancer.** The Astro-Phoenix criterion was developed to allow comparisons among various forms of radiation therapy with or without the concomitant use of hormonal therapy. The recommendations of the task force that developed these criteria specifically stated that it would be inappropriate to use this end point for surgery or for thermal-based therapies.

3. **b. urinary retention.** HIFU results in acute swelling of the prostate gland, resulting in temporary urinary retention that usually lasts 1 to 2 weeks. This occurs in the majority of patients with the other complications listed occurring much less frequently.

4. **e. all of the above.** HIFU may become a highly effective and widely used technology for the treatment for early prostate cancer. However, the current published literature is limited by short follow-up and lack of end points, which are proven to be predictive of disease specific morbidity or mortality in the context of this technology.

Additional Study Points

1. HIFU provides an energy source 10,000 times stronger than diagnostic ultrasound, producing a focal area of heat with temperatures that can exceed 80° C.
2. Complications following HIFU therapy include transient urinary retention in almost all, prolonged urinary retention in 9%, urethral stricture in 3.6%, and rectal urethral fistula in 1% to 3%.

chapter
107

Treatment of Locally Advanced Prostate Cancer

Maxwell V. Meng, MD • Peter R. Carroll, MD, MPH

QUESTIONS

1. Identification of patients with high-risk prostate cancer is best achieved by:
   a. transrectal ultrasonography.
   b. serum prostate-specific antigen (PSA).
   c. digital rectal examination.
   d. serum PSA, biopsy grade, and clinical stage.
   e. PSA kinetics.

2. Using the Kattan postoperative nomogram, which of the following contributes most to the risk of biochemical recurrence after radical prostatectomy?
   a. Positive surgical margin
   b. Pretreatment serum PSA of 17 ng/mL
   c. Gleason 4 + 3 disease
   d. Established capsular penetration
   e. Seminal vesicle invasion

3. Neoadjuvant androgen deprivation before radical prostatectomy leads to:
   a. improved biochemical-free survival.
   b. improved overall survival.
   c. reduced positive surgical margins.
   d. reduced local recurrence.
   e. increased operative morbidity.

4. In men with locally advanced prostate cancer undergoing prostatectomy, clinical overstaging (i.e., pathologically organ-confined disease) occurs in:
   a. less than 10%.
   b. 15% to 30%.
   c. 40% to 60%.
   d. 70% to 80%.
   e. greater than 90%.

5. The use of high-dose antiandrogen monotherapy after prostatectomy in men with locally advanced disease:
   a. reduces disease progression.
   b. increases cardiac morbidity.
   c. does not have an impact on sexual function.
   d. improves overall survival.
   e. improves local disease control.

6. In men with locally advanced/high risk prostate cancer, the most effective treatment among the following options is:
   a. brachytherapy plus external beam radiation therapy.
   b. neoadjuvant androgen deprivation (AD) plus external beam radiation therapy.
   c. neoadjuvant AD plus external beam radiation therapy plus adjuvant AD.
   d. concurrent AD plus external-beam radiation therapy.
   e. long-term AD alone.

7. Risk assessment schemes for prostate cancer are most accurate for patients with:
   a. low-risk disease.
   b. high-risk disease.
   c. the disease.
   d. metastatic disease.
   e. locally advanced cancers.

8. The current appropriate dose for adjuvant radiation therapy after radical prostatectomy is:
   a. less than 45 Gy.
   b. 45 to 50 Gy.
   c. 51 to 55 Gy.
   d. 56 to 60 Gy.
   e. greater than 60 Gy.

9. The use of androgen deprivation in combination with radiation therapy for those with high-risk cancers is associated with all of the following EXCEPT:
   a. improved local control.
   b. improved biochemical-free survival.
   c. less gastrointestinal toxicity.
   d. worsened sexual function.
   e. more urinary frequency.

10. The benefits of early radiation therapy after radical prostatectomy in men with locally advanced disease are observed:
   a. for improved local control.
   b. for improved overall survival.
   c. in men with positive surgical margins.
   d. in none of the above.
   e. in all of the above.

ANSWERS

1. **d. serum PSA, biopsy grade, and clinical stage.** Although clinical stage, serum PSA, and Gleason score all individually predict pathologic stage and prognosis, the combination of these three variables increases the accuracy of this assessment.

2. **b. pretreatment serum PSA of 17 ng/mL.** Despite the trend toward lower serum PSA at the time of diagnosis, PSA remains an important predictor of treatment failure and greater elevations (>8 ng/mL) of PSA contribute significantly to calculated biochemical recurrence.

3. **c. reduced positive surgical margins.** The randomized and nonrandomized studies of neoadjuvant androgen deprivation in men with lower clinical stage (cT1-T2) clearly demonstrate a reduction in the rate of positive surgical margins; however, this advantage has not been observed in men with cT3c and has not translated into improved long-term PSA-free survival.

4. **b. 15% to 30%.** Recent data suggest that clinical overstaging occurs in approximately 27% of men with clinical stage T3 disease undergoing prostatectomy, consistent with the range in the literature of 7% to 26%.

5. **a. reduces disease progression.** Bicalutamide at greater dose (150 mg) appears to have a positive effect in those men with locally advanced disease, with 43% reduction in disease progression and potential benefit of improved survival; however, it should be remembered that high-dose bicalutamide given to men with localized prostate cancer is associated with increased risk of death (hazard ratio: 1.23).

6. **c. neoadjuvant AD plus external beam radiation therapy plus adjuvant AD.** The accumulated data from multiple RTOG and EORTC trials suggest that improved outcomes are achieved with greater duration of administration of androgen deprivation in combination with external beam radiation therapy, with apparent benefit of both neoadjuvant and adjuvant therapy.

7. **a. low-risk disease.** Validation has confirmed the general accuracy of the available risk assessment tools, but there is a tendency to overestimate the risk of cancer recurrence in men with high-risk disease features.

8. **e. greater than 60 Gy.** There is a trend to improve response to adjuvant radiation therapy, and most contemporary series report doses greater than 60 Gy, with a potential threshold of either 61.2 or 64 Gy.

9. **c. less gastrointestinal toxicity.** The longer application (>6 to 9 months) of androgen deprivation in conjunction with radiation therapy may be associated with increased rectal morbidity and sexual dysfunction.

10. **e. in all of the above.** Data from EORTC 22911 and SWOG 8794 clearly demonstrate a benefit of adjuvant RT in men with pT3 disease, after radical prostatectomy, with respect to biochemical relapse-free, metastasis-free, and overall survival, as well as improved local control. The EORTC study suggests that patients who benefit the most are those with positive surgical margins.

Additional Study Points

1. At least 10% of men with newly diagnosed prostate cancer have locally advanced disease.

2. Risk assessment for locally advanced disease is best determined by a combination of PSA, T stage, cancer grade, and extent of cancer in the biopsy.

3. PSA recurrence following radical prostatectomy is affected by extracapsular extension, seminal vesicle invasion, positive lymph nodes, and positive surgical margins.

4. Neoadjuvant androgen deprivation therapy before radical prostatectomy has no role.

5. Early androgen deprivation therapy appears to have a potential survival advantage in subsets of men with more aggressive disease at the expense of the side effects of the therapy.

6. The role of adjuvant radiation therapy following radical prostatectomy is controversial. A subset of patients apparently benefits from adjuvant radiation therapy. Unfortunately, all studies to date are flawed such that specific subsets of patients who will benefit have not been adequately defined.

Clinical State of the Rising PSA Value after Definitive Local Therapy: A Practical Approach

Michael J. Morris, MD ● Howard I. Scher, MD

QUESTIONS

1. The most important therapeutic consideration in selecting either local salvage therapy or systemic therapy for a patient with a rising PSA value after definitive local therapy is:

   a. patients with a rising PSA level after definitive local therapy should be started on hormonal therapy because they are destined to experience systemic relapse.

   b. patients with a rising PSA level should undergo salvage local procedures, such as radiation or cryotherapy or prostatectomy, before undergoing any systemic treatment.

   c. patients with a rising PSA level and no metastatic disease should be started on chemotherapy.

   d. patients with a rising PSA level should undergo neither systemic nor local treatments, because the only appropriate context in which to begin any intervention is when they have developed radiographic metastases.

   e. patients with a rising PSA level should be risk stratified and treated with a modality of therapy that matches their risk of relapse, risk of developing local versus systemic disease, and risk of dying of other causes.

2. Which of the following best describes the state of knowledge of systemic treatment for patients with a rising PSA?

   a. Randomized prospective data have demonstrated that patients with a rising PSA value live longer if they are started on hormones as soon as the PSA level is detectable rather than waiting until there are radiographic metastases.

   b. There have been no randomized trials performed in this population demonstrating that any therapy is superior to observation. Therefore the most appropriate treatment for these patients is to place them in a clinical trial, if a reasonable and appropriate study is available in the community.

   c. Patients enrolled in clinical trials have shown an improvement in survival when hormones are used for early node-positive patients and as adjuvant therapy after radiation therapy as opposed to deferred strategies. These clinical trials are clearly applicable to patients with a rising PSA level, and therefore early hormonal therapy is the standard of care.

   d. Bicalutamide, 150 mg daily, will prolong survival and preserve quality of life.

   e. Zoledronic acid has been shown to be beneficial in prolonging the time to developing bone metastases in the nonmetastatic population with a rising PSA level.

3. The PSA doubling time (PSADT) can be used as part of:

   a. prognosis for time to metastatic disease.

   b. prognosis for prostate cancer–specific survival.

   c. prognosis for likelihood of remaining free of evidence of disease after salvage radiation therapy.

   d. all of the above.

   e. a and c only.

4. The PSA value is used in clinical trials involving patients with a rising PSA level in which of the following ways?

   a. The post-treatment PSA level decline is a surrogate for survival.

   b. A post-treatment PSA decline of 50% is the only means by which experimental therapies should be judged as either a success or failure.

   c. The patient's PSA kinetics should be used to assess the patient's probability of progression-free survival, overall survival, or a clinical event such as developing metastases to help formulate eligibility criteria.

   d. A rising PSA level on therapy is a universally accepted indicator that the patient's disease has progressed.

   e. A PSADT of 15 months suggests a high risk of developing early metastatic disease.

5. Which of the following characterizes the clinical state of "rising PSA"?

   a. Postoperative patients enter it when the PSA level is detectable.

   b. Postirradiation patients enter it when the PSA is 0.1.

   c. Patients who have not received definitive therapy enter it when their PSA level rises.

d. Patients enter it when they have consistently rising PSA values in accordance with an indication of treatment failure for their primary therapy and have negative imaging studies.

e. The definition of a patient who has entered the state of "rising PSA" is independent of the previous treatment that the patient has received.

6. High-dose bicalutamide (150 mg) as monotherapy for patients with a rising PSA level:

   a. should still be considered investigational.

   b. is standard treatment for patients with a rising PSA level.

   c. is approved by the U.S. Food and Drug Administration.

   d. has a proven survival advantage over standard treatment with a gonadotropin-releasing hormone agonist.

   e. has all of the benefits of a gonadotropin-releasing hormone agonist and none of the drawbacks

ANSWERS

1. **e. patients with a rising PSA level should be risk stratified and treated with a modality of therapy that matches their risk of relapse, risk of developing local versus systemic disease, and risk of dying of other causes.** Prognostic models to predict the likelihood of developing metastatic disease versus achieving a durable remission after local salvage treatments are available. These models use such prognostic features as Gleason score, staging at the time of primary definitive local therapy, the timing of relapse relative to primary therapy, the PSA at relapse that is triggering a decision in regard to salvage, and PSA kinetics. Once the likelihood of developing metastatic disease, of benefiting from local therapy, and of dying of disease versus other causes are addressed and the need for treatment determined, consideration can be given to what options are available and the likelihood of success in controlling the disease or, preferably, eliminating it completely.

2. **b. There have been no randomized trials performed in this population demonstrating that any therapy is superior to observation. Therefore the most appropriate treatment for these patients is to place them in a clinical trial, if a reasonable and appropriate study is available in the community.** An issue that has long been debated is what is the optimal time to begin androgen-deprivation therapy, because there have been no clinical trials to compare hormones with expectant observation specifically in the rising PSA population. Indeed, the American Society of Clinical Oncology Clinical Practice Guidelines argue formally against an "early" treatment policy (Loblaw et al, 2004, 2007).* Yet, there is a significant body of literature to suggest that early hormonal therapy has the potential to confer a survival advantage in selected patients relative to an approach in which hormones are deferred to the point of having radiographically evident metastases. Most are randomized trials of androgen deprivation applied before, during, and after radiation therapy for variable amounts of time from 6 months to continuous that show improvements in disease-free and

overall survival compared with either no hormonal therapy or hormonal therapy that has been deferred until the time of metastatic disease (Lawton et al, 2001; Bolla et al, 2002; Pilepich et al, 2003, 2005; D'Amico et al, 2004, 2008; Horwitz et al, 2008). The caveat is that the patients in the state of localized disease enrolled in these trials may not be directly comparable to those in the clinical state of rising PSA value who have already failed either local or combined modality treatments and are now at risk for developing radiographic metastases as the next point in the natural history. High-dose bicalutamide has not been directly or rigorously tested in this population relative to a placebo or castrating therapy, and zoledronic acid has not been shown to prolong survival in any prostate cancer population.

3. **d. all of the above.** In general, low pretreatment PSA levels, lower-grade tumors, low clinical or pathologic staging, late time from definitive local therapy to PSA relapse, and long PSADTs generally provide a prognosis for a low likelihood of developing distant radiographically apparent metastases (Pound, 1999; Buskirk et al, 2006; Stephenson et al, 2007). High-grade disease, short time intervals to biochemical relapse (<2 years vs. >2 years), and a PSADT of less than 10 months versus more than 10 months predicted for a shorter time to radiographic progression (Pound, 1999). In an updated analysis, time to PSA failure was no longer predictive when PSADT was considered (Antonarakis et al, 2009). In numerous studies, PSADT is the dominant factor used to assess the risk of developing metastasis-free survival (Roberts et al, 2001; Valicenti et al, 2006). In one study, a PSADT of less than 6 months was associated with a 5-year progression-free survival of 64% versus 93% for patients who had a longer PSADT (Roberts, 2001). Data now exist that demonstrate an association between PSADT and disease-specific survival after radiation therapy (Lee et al, 1997; Zagars and Pollack, 1997; Sandler et al, 2000; D'Amico et al, 2002, 2003), and the post-treatment PSADT with time to prostate cancer-specific and all-cause mortality (all $P < .001$).

4. **c. The patient's PSA kinetics should be used to assess the patient's probability of progression-free survival, overall survival, or a clinical event such as developing metastases to help formulate eligibility criteria.** Patients with unfavorable PSA kinetics who are at a high risk of metastases or death from disease are a group who not only need systemic therapy but are most likely to benefit. This patient group can be divided into three categories based on prognosis: low-risk patients are unlikely to develop metastases, symptoms, or death from disease and should be managed expectantly; intermediate-risk patients can be considered for investigational approaches designed to slow the disease to the point at which the patient dies of other causes (tantamount to cure) or receives androgen deprivation; and high-risk patients (those with PSADTs of 9 months or less) can be considered for androgen deprivation or, ideally, enrolled in a clinical trial. There are several useful end points for trials in this clinical state. The most immediate of these is the post-therapy change in PSA level. The attraction of measuring serial PSA levels is that these assays can be obtained simply and frequently with minimal inconvenience to the patient. However, ease of use and mathematical objectivity should not be confused with

---

*Sources referenced can be found in *Campbell-Walsh Urology*, 10th Edition, on the Expert Consult website.

true surrogacy for clinical benefit. Time to PSA progression can be defined by an increase to a predetermined number or an increase by an absolute percentage or a change in the postintervention rate of rise. The definition must also vary for drugs that produce "no change," those that produce a decline, or those that produce an undetectable PSA. As noted previously, the demonstration of an association does not equate with surrogacy, and there remains a large proportion of the association between PSA-based metrics and clinical outcomes that is yet unexplained.

5. **d. Patients enter it when they have consistently rising PSA values in accordance with an indication of treatment failure for their primary therapy and have negative imaging studies.** When a patient has entered the clinical state of a "rising PSA" depends on the primary therapy he has received and the sensitivity of the assay used to measure PSA.

6. **a. should still be considered investigational.** Some practitioners treat patients in this clinical state with antiandrogen monotherapy based on results of the Early Prostate Cancer Trial (Iversen et al, 2004; Wirth et al, 2004; McLeod et al, 2006). Single-agent bicalutamide has also been studied in patients with either metastatic or locally advanced disease in two trials (Boccardo et al, 2002; Tyrrell et al, 2006). None of these trials directly addresses the population at hand with rigor sufficient to call high-dose bicalutamide a true standard of care. Although practitioners do use high-dose bicalutamide outside the context of a clinical trial, its value in this population over and above either castrating therapy or nothing at all is uncertain. This dose of bicalutamide,

however, is not approved in the United States and has no proven survival advantage over treatments with testosterone-lowering agents, and its risk-benefit ratio has not been definitively tested in this population (Boccardo et al, 2002; Tyrrell et al, 2006).

Additional Study Points

1. After discontinued use of ablative hormonal therapy, testosterone levels generally return to baseline within 3 to 6 months; however, some patients can have extremely prolonged recovery periods.

2. In the overwhelming majority of patients, biochemical relapse occurs far earlier than the development of radiographically observed metastases.

3. Parameters often used in predicting the significance of a rising PSA level include pretreatment PSA level, grade of tumor, pathologic stage, time to relapse, and PSADT.

4. PSADT is often used to predict the time to the development of metastatic disease; however, it is unlikely that PSA kinetics follow the model of a single exponential equation. Therefore it is extremely difficult in many patients over a long period of time to characterize the PSADT.

5. The use of adjuvant therapy after a rising PSA value should take into account its effects on cognitive function, well-being, sexual health, cardiovascular risk, and the likelihood that it would be effective in eradicating disease.

6. Patients who have demonstrable disease in the prostatic bed after radical prostatectomy should be considered for salvage radiation and/or hormonal therapy.

Hormone Therapy for Prostate Cancer

Joel B. Nelson, MD

QUESTIONS

1. The effectiveness of estrogen as a hormone therapy for prostate cancer is primarily based on:
   a. direct cytotoxic effects of estrogen on prostate cancer cells.
   b. competitive binding of estrogen to the androgen receptor.
   c. inhibition of the conversion of cholesterol to pregnenolone.
   d. desensitizing luteinizing hormone–releasing hormone (LH-RH) receptors in the anterior pituitary.
   e. negative feedback on luteinizing hormone (LH) secretion by the pituitary.

2. The expected response of a man to the administration of the nonsteroidal antiandrogens is:
   a. LH increases, testosterone decreases, and estrogen decreases.
   b. LH increases, testosterone increases, and estrogen decreases.
   c. LH increases, testosterone increases, and estrogen increases.
   d. LH decreases, testosterone decreases, and estrogen increases.
   e. LH decreases, testosterone increases, and estrogen increases.

3. All of the following therapeutic approaches for androgen axis blockade are in current clinical use EXCEPT:
   a. inhibition of androgen synthesis.
   b. blocking androgen action by binding to the androgen receptor in a competitive fashion.
   c. ablating the source of androgens.
   d. direct inhibition of androgen receptor–mediated pathways.
   e. inhibition of LH-RH and LH release.

4. Nonsteroidal antiandrogens:
   a. do not act as agonists for prostate cancer cells when used in combination with LH-RH agonists.
   b. allow long-term maintenance of erectile function and sexual activity at rates similar to men undergoing surgical castration.
   c. commonly induce gastrointestinal toxicity, manifest as constipation, leading, on occasion, to fecal impaction.
   d. cause pancreatic toxicity, ranging from reversible mild to fulminant, life-threatening suppurative pancreatitis requiring periodic monitoring of serum amylase and lipase.
   e. cause fluid retention and thromboembolism in the majority of patients.

5. Which of the following nonsteroidal antiandrogens is associated with a delayed adaptation to darkness after exposure to bright illumination and interstitial pneumonitis?
   a. Bicalutamide
   b. Flutamide
   c. Hydroxyflutamide
   d. Nilutamide
   e. Cyproterone acetate

6. Concerning LH-RH agonists:
   a. based on a review of 24 trials, involving more than 6600 patients, survival after therapy with an LH-RH agonist was significantly better than surgical castration.
   b. although depot preparations and osmotic pump devices allow dosing to extend from 28 days to 1 year, the most effective dosing regimen is daily.
   c. current LH-RH agonists are based on analogues of the native LH-RH decapeptide by amino acid substitutions, particularly position 6 of the peptide.
   d. widespread use of orally effective LH-RH agonists has been limited by severe allergic reactions in some patients, even after previously uneventful treatment.
   e. use of LH-RH agonists is limited to combined androgen blockade.

7. Each of the following has been associated with a favorable initial response to androgen-deprivation therapy (ADT) EXCEPT:
   a. magnitude of the prostate-specific antigen (PSA) level decline.
   b. rapidity of the PSA level decline.
   c. PSA doubling time before initiating ADT.
   d. Gleason score of the primary tumor.
   e. maintenance of a detectable PSA value.

8. Which of the following statements about the complications of ADT is TRUE?

   a. Most men undergoing ADT have normal bone mineral density before initiating therapy, and it usually takes at least a decade of treatment before the average man will develop osteopenia.

   b. Hot flashes occur in about one fourth of men on ADT but should always be treated because of the associated rare but life-threatening cardiovascular side effects.

   c. Erectile dysfunction after surgical castration or use of an LH-RH is common but not inevitable: although 1 in 5 men maintain some sexual activity, only 1 in 20 maintain high levels of sexual interest (libido).

   d. Because most men on ADT maintain lean muscle mass the increase in weight is due to increases in adipose tissue.

   e. Gynecomastia and mastodynia are common with estrogenic compounds and antiandrogens but are effectively treated by external-beam radiation therapy after they occur.

9. Which of the following statements about the combination of 3 months of neoadjuvant ADT before radical prostatectomy is TRUE?

   a. Positive surgical margin rates are significantly reduced with patients on ADT.

   b. There is a significant reduction in biochemical (PSA) progression with patients on ADT.

   c. The benefit of neoadjuvant ADT appears to be in men with locally advanced disease and/or those with high-grade disease.

   d. Antiandrogen monotherapy has not shown a significant reduction of biochemical failure, but LH-RH agonists have demonstrated this reduction.

   e. Although the results of prospective randomized studies of this combination are mixed, the overall body of evidence supports the use of ADT in this setting.

10. Combined androgen blockade:

   a. is designed to address the low levels of testicular androgens remaining after the use of LH-RH agonists or antagonists.

   b. typically uses antiandrogens at the time of PSA rise after treatment with an LH-RH agonist.

   c. has not shown a survival advantage compared with an LH-RH agonist alone.

   d. significantly benefits men with minimally metastatic disease when used in combination with surgical castration.

   e. with the use of cyproterone acetate has a slightly worse outcome.

11. Compared with deferred ADT, early ADT instituted before the development of objective metastatic disease:

   a. provides an overall survival advantage in all clinical disease states.

   b. has an equivalent quality of life.

   c. does not increase overall death rates.

   d. does not prevent the emergence of hormone-refractory prostate cancer.

   e. should be offered to men with PSA recurrence after radical prostatectomy because of the rapid disease progression in this clinical setting.

12. In men with lymph node metastatic prostate cancer discovered at the time of radical prostatectomy a significant overall survival benefit of immediate ADT:

   a. is limited to those with extrapelvic positive nodes.

   b. has been demonstrated in men who have also undergone subsequent radical prostatectomy.

   c. has been demonstrated in men who have not undergone subsequent radical prostatectomy.

   d. b and c are correct.

   e. a, b, and c are correct.

13. From a strictly financial point of view, which of the following forms of ADT is the least expensive?

   a. Scrotal orchiectomy

   b. LH-RH agonist

   c. Diethylstilbestrol

   d. Antiandrogen monotherapy

   e. LH-RH antagonist

14. Compared with continuous ADT, intermittent ADT has been shown in randomized prospective studies to:

   a. delay progression to hormone-refractory prostate cancer.

   b. improve quality of life.

   c. improve cancer-specific survival.

   d. All of the above

   e. None of the above

15. There is general consensus that ADT should always be initiated in a hormonally intact patient in which of the following clinical settings?

   a. Before radical prostatectomy with a clinical T2 tumor

   b. In all clinical stages when undergoing external-beam radiation therapy

   c. In a patient with clinically localized prostate cancer who does not want local treatment

   d. In a patient with symptomatic metastatic disease

   e. In a patient with high-grade prostatic intraepithelial neoplasia on needle biopsy who refuses a subsequent biopsy

ANSWERS

1. **e. negative feedback on luteinizing hormone (LH) secretion by the pituitary.** After the success of surgical castration in treating prostate cancer, the first central inhibition of the hypothalamic-pituitary-gonadal axis exploited the potent negative feedback of estrogen on LH secretion. Estradiol is 1000-fold more potent at suppressing LH and follicle-stimulating hormone (FSH) secretion by the pituitary compared with testosterone. Although estrogen has some direct cytotoxic effects on prostate cancer cells, this is not its primary mode of action. All antiandrogens competitively bind to the androgen receptor. Aminoglutethimide inhibits the conversion of cholesterol to pregnenolone, an early step in steroidogenesis. The LH-RH agonists desensitize LH-RH receptors in the anterior pituitary.

2. **c. LH increases, testosterone increases, and estrogen increases.** Unlike the steroidal antiandrogens, such as cyproterone acetate, which have central progestational inhibitory effects, the nonsteroidal antiandrogens simply block androgen receptors, including those in the hypothalamic-pituitary axis. Because those central androgen receptors no longer sense the normal negative feedback exerted by testosterone, both LH levels and the normal testicular response to increased LH-testosterone levels increase. Peripheral conversion of this excessive testosterone also increases estrogen levels, leading to the gynecomastia and mastodynia associated with the nonsteroidal antiandrogens.

3. **d. direct inhibition of androgen receptor–mediated pathways.** There are four therapeutic approaches for androgen axis blockade in current clinical use (see Table 109–2 in *Campbell-Walsh Urology, 10th Edition*). All current forms of ADT function by reducing the ability of androgen to activate the androgen receptor, whether through lowering levels of androgen or by blocking androgen/androgen receptor binding. Therefore, the androgen receptor is not directly affected by ADT, leading many to hypothesize that hormone-refractory prostate cancer is a reactivation of androgen receptor–mediated pathways.

4. **b. allow long-term maintenance of erectile function and sexual activity at rates similar to men undergoing surgical castration.** By blocking testosterone feedback centrally the nonsteroidal antiandrogens cause LH and testosterone levels to increase, allowing antiandrogen activity without inducing hypogonadism, and potency can be preserved. In clinical trials specifically examining erectile function and sexual activity in men on antiandrogen monotherapy, however, long-term preservation of those domains was 20% and not significantly different than men undergoing surgical castration. All antiandrogens can act agonistically on prostate cancer cells and, when used in combination with LH-RH agonists, withdrawal of the antiandrogen can lead to declines in the level of PSA and even objective responses. The common gastrointestinal toxicity is diarrhea, most often seen with flutamide. Liver toxicity, ranging from reversible hepatitis to fulminate hepatic failure, is associated with all nonsteroidal antiandrogens and requires periodic monitoring of liver function tests. The steroidal antiandrogen cyproterone acetate is associated with fluid retention and thromboembolism.

5. **d. Nilutamide.** About one fourth of men on nilutamide therapy will note a delayed adaptation to darkness after exposure to bright illumination, and nilutamide is also associated with interstitial pneumonitis in approximately 1% of patients that can progress to pulmonary fibrosis. Hydroxyflutamide is the active metabolite of flutamide. Cyproterone acetate is a steroidal antiandrogen.

6. **c. current LH-RH agonists are based on analogues of the native LH-RH decapeptide by amino acid substitutions, particularly position 6 of the peptide.** The LH-RH agonists exploit the desensitization of LH-RH receptors in the anterior pituitary after chronic exposure to LH-RH, thereby shutting down the production of LH and, ultimately, testosterone. Analogues of native LH-RH increase their potency and half-lives (see Table 109–3 in *Campbell-Walsh Urology, 10th Edition*). The initial flare in LH and testosterone may last 10 to 20 days, and coadministration of an antiandrogen is required for only 21 to 28 days. Survival after therapy with an LH-RH agonist was equivalent to that of orchiectomy. The clinical utility of the first LH-RH agonists was hampered by their short-half lives, requiring daily dosing. The LH-RH antagonist abarelix has been associated with severe allergic reactions: all LH-RH agonists are administered either intramuscularly or subcutaneously. LH-RH can be used without combination with an antiandrogen.

7. **e. the maintenance of a detectable PSA value.** The odds ratio of progressing to androgen-refractory progression at 24 months of starting ADT was 15-fold higher in those who did not achieve an undetectable PSA value. The magnitude and rapidity of the level of PSA decline, the pre-ADT PSA doubling time, and pretreatment testosterone levels are all associated with the response to ADT. For each unit increase in Gleason score the cumulative hazard of androgen-refractory progression was nearly 70%.

8. **c. Erectile dysfunction after surgical castration or use of an LH-RH is common but not inevitable: although 1 in 5 men maintain some sexual activity, only 1 in 20 maintain high levels of sexual interest (libido).** The loss of sexual functioning is not inevitable with surgical or chemical castration, with up to 20% of men able to maintain some sexual activity. Libido is more severely compromised, with approximately 5% maintaining a high level of sexual interest. More than half of men undergoing ADT meet the bone mineral density criteria for osteopenia or osteoporosis; it is estimated that osteopenia will develop in the average man within 4 years of initiating ADT. Hot flashes are among the most common side effects of ADT, affecting between 50% and 80% of patients. Hot flashes should be treated only in those who find them bothersome. Loss of muscle mass and increase in percent fat body mass are common in men undergoing ADT. Prophylactic radiation therapy (10 Gy) has been used to prevent or reduce gynecomastia and mastodynia, but it has no benefit once these side effects have already occurred.

9. **a. Positive surgical margin rates are significantly reduced in patients on ADT.** In both nonrandomized and randomized clinical trials, the pathologic positive surgical margin rate is significantly reduced. In one study the positive surgical margin rate fell from nearly 50% in hormonally intact patients to 15% in patients on ADT. Despite this improvement there has not been a corresponding significant reduction in biochemical (PSA) progression in patients on ADT, a finding in four separate prospective randomized studies. The benefit of ADT in men with locally advanced disease and/or high-grade disease has been in combination with external-beam radiation therapy. There is no evidence any form of 3-month neoadjuvant ADT before radical prostatectomy reduces biochemical failure rates.

10. **e. using cyproterone acetate has a slightly worse outcome.** In studies of combined androgen blockade using the steroidal antiandrogen cyproterone acetate compared with LH-RH agonists alone, the outcomes were slightly worse with the combination, suggesting increased non–prostate cancer deaths with this agent. Combined androgen blockade is designed to block the possible contribution of adrenal androgens to prostate cancer progression. Combined androgen blockade uses an antiandrogen along with an LH-RH agonist: addition of an antiandrogen at the time of

PSA rise (evidence of hormone-refractory disease) is considered secondary hormonal manipulation. There are several clinical trials that have shown a slight but significant survival advantage for combined androgen blockade. A landmark randomized clinical trial comparing surgical castration alone to surgical castration combined with flutamide did not show a significant benefit in men with minimal metastatic disease.

11. **d. does not prevent the emergence of hormone-refractory prostate cancer.** The timing of the initiation of ADT has not prevented the development of hormone-refractory prostate cancer. Although early ADT may provide an overall survival advantage in certain clinical disease states, in most studies there is no significant overall survival advantage. Indeed, in localized, low-risk prostate cancer, early ADT is associated with an increase in overall death rates. The natural history of disease progression after biochemical failure after radical prostatectomy is protracted: median time to bone metastases is 8 years.

12. **b. has been demonstrated in men who have also undergone subsequent radical prostatectomy.** A randomized prospective study of men with positive regional, pelvic lymph nodes discovered at the time of radical prostatectomy showed an overall survival advantage to immediate ADT. In that study all men also underwent the radical prostatectomy. A similar study, performed by the European Organization for the Research and Treatment of Cancer, in men who did not undergo radical prostatectomy if positive nodes were discovered did not show a significant survival advantage to immediate ADT.

13. **c. Diethylstilbestrol.** At a dose of 1 to 3 mg/day with no prophylactic breast irradiation, this drug is the least expensive form of ADT. LH-RH agonists would be less expensive than scrotal orchiectomy only if the patient lived a few months after the administration of ADT. Combined androgen blockade is the most expensive form of ADT.

14. **e. none of the above.** Randomized prospective studies of intermittent ADT are ongoing and no results are yet available. The possible benefits of intermittent ADT listed have not been demonstrated.

15. **d. In a patient with symptomatic metastatic disease.** In hormonally intact men with symptomatic metastatic prostate cancer, ADT is always indicated. There is no significant biochemical (PSA) disease-free advantage in men treated with neoadjuvant ADT. The benefits of ADT in combination with external-beam radiation therapy are in men with locally advanced and/or high-grade disease. The use of ADT in men with low-risk, localized prostate cancer is associated with a significantly lower overall survival. There is no indication for ADT in the management of prostatic intraepithelial neoplasia.

Additional Study Points

1. Antiandrogens bind to the androgen receptor in a competitive fashion. They are either steroidal or nonsteroidal.
2. Steroidal antiandrogens suppress LH release. Thus the steroidal antiandrogens block the effects of testosterone on the receptor as well as lower testosterone through their progestational central inhibition effect.
3. When performing an orchiectomy, double ligating the transected segments of the cord with one being a trans-fixion suture is advised.
4. Initial exposure to LH-RH agonists results in a flare of testosterone; the clinical effects of the flare may be blocked by the simultaneous administration of an anti-androgen. The two drugs should be administered together, and the antiandrogen therapy should be continued for 3 weeks.
5. After 4 years of androgen deprivation, the average man is osteopenic.
6. Hot flashes may be treated with megestrol, 20 mg twice daily.
7. Androgen deprivation therapy results in bone loss, sexual dysfunction, hot flashes, decreased cognitive function, changes in muscle mass, anemia, and gynecomastia.
8. Twenty percent of individuals with metastatic prostate cancer die of non–prostate cancer causes.
9. Bilateral orchiectomy reduces testosterone by 90% within 24 hours.

Treatment of Castration-Resistant Prostate Cancer

Emmanuel S. Antonarakis, MD ● Michael A. Carducci, MD ●
Mario A. Eisenberger, MD

QUESTIONS

1. All of the following represent appropriate management in a patient with evidence of prostate cancer progression after initial hormonal therapy EXCEPT:

    a. obtain a serum testosterone level to evaluate adequate gonadal suppression, restage the disease with radiographs and scans, maintain gonadal suppression, and plan the next therapeutic step.

    b. if the patient is on an antiandrogen in addition to a luteinizing hormone–releasing hormone (LH-RH) analogue, discontinue this for 4 weeks in the case of flutamide/nilutamide and for 8 weeks in the case of bicalutamide.

    c. if the patient has no symptoms, the workup shows that he has adequate gonadal suppression (serum testosterone <50 ng/mL), and the only evidence of disease progression is a rising prostate-specific antigen (PSA) and scans are unchanged, try a second-line hormonal therapy before chemotherapy is offered.

    d. if the patient experiences severe focal bone pain that requires regular use of narcotic analgesics, consider palliative radiation therapy.

    e. restage with radiographs and scans, evaluate serum testosterone level if less than 50 ng/mL, and discontinue all hormonal therapy (LH-RH analogue and antiandrogen) for 4 to 8 weeks before planning the next therapeutic step.

2. A patient has a rising PSA value after 24 months of treatment with an LH-RH analogue; the workup shows no evidence of metastasis (as prior to initiation of hormonal therapy). Which of the following constitutes the most reasonable approach?

    a. Send the patient to an oncologist for initiation of chemotherapy.

    b. Continue follow-up with regular PSA tests and restage when the patient becomes symptomatic.

    c. Radiate the prostatic bed and the pelvis.

    d. Assess the PSA doubling time (PSADT): if less than 6 months, consider treatment as soon as possible; otherwise, observation may be reasonable.

    e. Evaluate the adequacy of gonadal suppression (check serum testosterone level) and plan for second-line endocrine manipulations.

3. A patient with bone metastases shows evidence of rising serum PSA levels while on second-line hormonal agents and continued LH-RH agonist. Bone scintiscan indicates slow progression, and he has no symptoms. Which of the following constitutes the most appropriate management?

    a. Plan for next endocrine treatment approach, including the infusion of zoledronate given 3 times yearly.

    b. Administer docetaxel, 75 mg/m^2 every 3 weeks, and zoledronate, 4 mg monthly.

    c. Administer a radiopharmaceutical.

    d. Treat aggressively with high-dose bicalutamide, calcium, and vitamin D.

    e. Wait until he becomes symptomatic.

4. A patient with diffuse bone metastases develops severe back pain. The PSA level is stable. The next step is:

    a. give analgesics as needed and consider a workup when the PSA value rises.

    b. add zoledronate to management.

    c. consider radiation therapy.

    d. order radiation therapy followed by docetaxel.

    e. order magnetic resonance imaging (MRI) of the spine to rule out cord compression.

5. A patient who is stable on hormonal therapy for many years develops a rapid deterioration with perirectal pain, liver metastasis, and weight loss. The PSA level is undetectable. Computed tomography of the pelvis shows a large pelvic mass. The next step is:

    a. begin docetaxel because he has castration-resistant prostate cancer (CRPC).

    b. administer radiation to the pelvis followed by docetaxel.

    c. treat with bicalutamide because the PSA level is still low.

    d. perform a biopsy of the pelvic mass to rule out the neuroendocrine/anaplastic subtype.

    e. send him for a colonoscopy because he probably has another cancer because the PSA value is negative.

6. The previous patient's pelvic mass is sampled, and the pathology report shows a small cell carcinoma. The best approach is:
   a. radiation therapy followed by second-line hormonal therapy until progression; then offer chemotherapy.
   b. docetaxel combined with zoledronate.
   c. chemotherapy with carboplatin and etoposide preceded or followed by irradiation.
   d. a bronchoscopy, because of the histology (small cell carcinoma).
   e. radiation to the pelvis followed by ketoconazole and hydrocortisone.

7. Results of the phase 3 TAX-327 trial showed significant improvements in which of the following outcomes in patients with CRPC treated with docetaxel versus mitoxantrone?
   a. Overall survival
   b. PSA response
   c. Pain response
   d. Quality of life
   e. All of the above

8. Which of the following is TRUE for estramustine phosphate?
   a. It is critical to use it combined with docetaxel.
   b. It has significant single-agent activity in CRPC.
   c. It has no activity at all in CRPC.
   d. Thromboembolic events are usually prevented by prophylactic anticoagulation.
   e. It adds significant toxicity to docetaxel without an apparent survival benefit.

9. The following are all TRUE regarding toxicity of docetaxel chemotherapy EXCEPT:
   a. it may cause myelosuppression.
   b. it may cause fatigue and neurotoxicity.
   c. it may cause edema.
   d. it may cause modest elevation of liver function test results.
   e. toxicity overrides quality of life benefits.

10. Bone loss associated with androgen-deprivation therapy is characterized by:
    a. proliferation of osteoblasts.
    b. hypocalcemia.
    c. depletion of osteoclasts.
    d. increased osteoclastic activity.
    e. hypercalcemia

11. In prostate cancer, which of the following is TRUE about bone metastases?
    a. They are always osteoblastic, because of growth factor effects.
    b. Pathologic fractures are common.
    c. Hypercalcemia is common.
    d. They are mostly lytic, associated with a predominant osteoclastic effect associated with treatment.
    e. There is increasing evidence that growth factors, cytokines, and other proteins may play a role in the development of bone metastases.

12. Which of the following is TRUE about zoledronate?
    a. Side effects include anemia and renal dysfunction.
    b. It rarely may cause osteonecrosis of the jaw in patients who are undergoing dental work.
    c. It reduces the increase in osteoclastic activity associated with androgen deprivation.
    d. It is approved for the treatment of hypercalcemia.
    e. All of the above

13. A decline in serum PSA level associated with administration of chemotherapy for metastatic CRPC:
    a. represents evidence of therapeutic benefit but not necessarily longer survival.
    b. is seen in about 50% of patients receiving docetaxel treatment.
    c. is usually seen in the first 3 months of treatment.
    d. All of the above
    e. None of the above

14. Which of the following is TRUE about brain metastasis in prostate cancer?
    a. It is seen in about 25% of patients with CRPC.
    b. It is common in patients progressing rapidly on hormonal therapy.
    c. Routine MRI of the brain should be considered in all CRPC patients.
    d. It is seen in less than 1% of patients, except when they demonstrate the neuroendocrine phenotype.
    e. Brain metastasis associated with small cell histology should be treated surgically.

15. Taxanes, including docetaxel, have which of the following clinical and biologic properties?
    a. They are antimitotic agents.
    b. They induce BCL2 phosphorylation.
    c. They are associated with an increased accumulation of cells in the G_2M phase of the cell cycle.
    d. They cause radiosensitization in vitro.
    e. All of the above

16. Which of the following is a target for the development of novel treatments in CRPC?
    a. CYP17 enzyme
    b. *PTEN*-associated signaling pathways
    c. Endothelin axis
    d. RANKL overexpression in bone metastasis
    e. All of the above

17. All of the following are TRUE about the androgen receptor (AR) in prostate cancer progression to the castration-resistant phenotype EXCEPT:
    a. AR can never be found in the castration-resistant state.
    b. aberrant function is not an uncommon feature as the disease progresses toward the castration-resistant state; this is clinically manifested by responses to withdrawal of antiandrogens.
    c. transcriptional activity of AR can be seen without ligand activation.
    d. ligand-independent activation can be seen via growth factors pathways.

e. wild-type AR remains active after testosterone suppression.

18. Which of the following is TRUE regarding immunologic therapy for prostate cancer?
    a. Sipuleucel-T (Provenge) has demonstrated improved median overall survival compared with placebo in a multicenter phase 3 trial (IMPACT) involving men with metastatic CRPC.
    b. A phase 3 trial (VITAL-1) of GVAX versus docetaxel/prednisone in asymptomatic men with chemotherapy-naive CRPC showed an overall survival advantage in the GVAX study arm.
    c. A phase 3 trial (VITAL-2) of docetaxel/prednisone versus docetaxel/GVAX in patients with symptomatic metastatic CRPC showed an overall survival advantage in the docetaxel/GVAX study arm.
    d. Inhibition of cytotoxic T lymphocyte–associated antigen 4 (CTLA-4) with the monoclonal antibody ipilimumab has never been associated with autoimmune toxicities.
    e. None of the above

ANSWERS

1. **e. Restage with radiographs and scans, evaluate serum testosterone level if less than 50 ng/mL, and discontinue all hormonal therapy (LH-RH analogue and antiandrogen) for 4 to 8 weeks before planning the next therapeutic step.** This is false because the LH-RH analogue should be continued indefinitely in all patients. Discontinuation of antiandrogens (both steroidal and nonsteroidal) can result in short-term clinical responses expressed by decreases in PSA levels, symptomatic benefits, and, less frequently, objective improvements in soft tissue and bone metastasis in a small proportion of these patients. Because of this, it is recommended that in patients treated with antiandrogens in combination with other forms of androgen deprivation the first step should involve the discontinuation of these agents and provide careful observation, including serial monitoring of PSA levels for a period 4 to 8 weeks before embarking on the next therapeutic maneuver.

2. **e. Evaluate adequacy of gonadal suppression (check serum testosterone level) and plan for second-line endocrine manipulations.** Patients with evidence of inadequate suppression of testosterone may respond with readjustment of gonadal suppressive treatment. Second-line endocrine maneuvers are effective in 20% to 60% of these patients and are certainly much less toxic. Furthermore, the benefits of chemotherapy in this setting (castration-resistant, nonmetastatic disease) have not been demonstrated. Given the major difference in terms of incidence and type of toxicities seen with sequential hormonal therapy versus cytotoxic chemotherapy, in the absence of data, it is recommended to implement the least toxic approach first. Clinical trials are clearly recommended for such patients.

3. **b. Administer docetaxel, 75 mg/m² every 3 weeks, and zoledronate, 4 mg monthly.** Docetaxel has become the agent of choice in this setting as of 2004, based on a large phase 3 randomized trial, TAX-327 (see Figs. 110–3 to 110–5 and Tables 110–3 to 110–5 in *Campbell-Walsh Urology, 10th Edition*), which demonstrated its superiority to the previous standard, mitoxantrone and prednisone (Tannock

et al, 2004).* TAX-327 enrolled 1006 patients with no prior chemotherapy and stable pain scores to one of three arms, all with concomitant prednisone at 5 mg PO twice daily: mitoxantrone, 12 mg/m² IV every 3 weeks; docetaxel, 75 mg/m² IV every 3 weeks; and docetaxel, 30 mg/m² IV weekly. Patients remained on gonadal suppression (LH-RH agonist) but had all other hormonal agents discontinued within 4 to 6 weeks. Treatment duration was 30 weeks in all arms, or a maximum of 10 cycles in the every-3-week arms, with more patients completing treatment in the every-3-week docetaxel group than the mitoxantrone group owing mostly to differences in disease progression (46% vs. 25%). After a median 20.7-month follow-up, overall survival in the every-3-week docetaxel group was 18.9 months with a pain response rate of 35% and a PSA response of 45%, contrasted to weekly docetaxel at 17.3 months, 31%, and 48%, respectively. This translated into a 24% relative risk reduction in death (95% CI 6% to 48%, $P = .0005$) with every-3-week docetaxel (see Fig. 110–4 in *Campbell-Walsh Urology, 10th Edition*). Patients on the mitoxantrone study arm had a median survival of 16.4 months, a pain response of 22%, and a PSA response of 32%.

Bisphosphonates have become an integral part in the management of metastatic prostate cancer to the bones. These compounds reduce bone resorption by inhibiting osteoclastic activity and proliferation. Zoledronate is a potent intravenous bisphosphonate approved for the treatment of hypercalcemia and the treatment of decreased bone mineral density in postmenopausal women (Green and Rogers, 2002). Recent experience in patients with progressive CRPC with bone metastasis showed zoledronate reduced the incidence of skeletal-related events compared with placebo in a prospective randomized trial. In addition, it has also been shown to increase mineral bone density in patients with prostate cancer receiving long-term androgen deprivation (Smith at al, 2003; Saad et al, 2004). At the present time this compound is indicated for the treatment of patients with progressive prostate cancer with evidence of bone metastasis at doses of 4 mg given by short intravenous infusion repeated at intervals of 3 to 4 weeks for several months. Side effects include fatigue, myalgias, fever, anemia, and mild elevations of serum creatinine concentration.

4. **e. order magnetic resonance imaging (MRI) of the spine to rule out cord compression.** Spinal MRI is routinely used to exclude the possibility of significant epidural disease, and it has almost entirely replaced other methodology such as CT myelography and conventional myelograms. Cancer-related pain is undoubtedly the most debilitating symptom associated with metastatic prostatic carcinoma. Prompt recognition of the various pain syndromes associated with this disease is critical to accomplish effective control of this devastating symptom. The most common pain syndromes and their respective therapeutic considerations are described in Table 110–6 in *Campbell-Walsh Urology, 10th Edition*.

5. **d. perform a biopsy of the pelvic mass to rule out the neuroendocrine/anaplastic subtype.** Laboratory and clinical evidence indicate that alterations in the differentiation pathway (neuroendocrine transformation) of

---

*Sources referenced can be found in *Campbell-Walsh Urology, 10th Edition,* on the Expert Consult website.

prostate cancer can be seen in a variable proportion of patients with primarily advanced disease (diSant'Agnese, 1995). The therapeutic implications of this finding are of significance because tumors demonstrating the neuroendocrine phenotype usually represent an inherently endocrine-resistant disease, and in view of their different clinical and biologic properties compared with the usual adenocarcinoma of the prostate, these tumors usually require separate therapeutic considerations.

6. **c. chemotherapy with carboplatin and etoposide preceded or followed by irradiation.** Treatment is usually similar to that in patients with other neuroendocrine tumors, such as small cell carcinoma of the lung, and include combinations of cisplatin/carboplatin and etoposide (Frank et al, 1995), paclitaxel/docetaxel, and topotecan. Radiation is very effective and should be considered in cases with bulky disease and brain metastasis and when local disease control in critical areas will have a positive impact in quality of life (pain, potential pathologic fractures, and bladder outlet obstruction). A combined chemoradiation approach is frequently necessary to accomplish maximal control of disease.

7. **e. All of the above.** TAX-327 and SWOG-9916 are the two seminal studies that both demonstrated a survival advantage in men with CRPC for docetaxel over mitoxantrone-prednisone, establishing docetaxel as the standard chemotherapy treatment for this disease.

8. **e. It adds significant toxicity to docetaxel without an apparent survival benefit.** This was demonstrated in the SWOG-9916 study, a large phase 3 trial in which 770 patients with progressive CRPC were randomly assigned to oral estramustine (280 mg three times daily) plus docetaxel (60 mg/m^2 every 3 weeks) versus mitoxantrone (12 mg/m^2 every 3 weeks) plus prednisone (see Figs. 110–6 to 110–8 in *Campbell-Walsh Urology, 10th Edition*) (Petrylak et al, 2004). In this study, median overall survival was longer in the docetaxel-estramustine group than in the mitoxantrone-prednisone group (17.5 vs. 15.6 months, $P = .02$), with a corresponding hazard ratio for death of 0.80 (95% CI, 0.67 to 0.97). Because of the high rate of thromboembolic events with estramustine, prophylactic low-dose warfarin and aspirin were given to patients in that study arm, but this did not reduce the incidence of thromboembolism. Although comparisons between the docetaxel arms across the two pivotal trials may not be appropriate because of differences in schedule, patient populations, and docetaxel dosing (60 mg/m^2 in SWOG-9916 and 75 mg/m^2 in TAX-327), it may be concluded that estramustine is unlikely to add significantly to the activity of docetaxel.

9. **e. toxicity overrides quality of life benefits.** Toxicity in the every-3-week versus weekly docetaxel arms was notable for more hematologic toxicity in the every-3-week arm (3% neutropenic fever versus 0%, and 32% grade 3/4 neutropenia versus 1.5%) (see Table 110–5 in *Campbell-Walsh Urology, 10th Edition*) but slightly lower rates of nausea and vomiting, fatigue, nail changes, hyperlacrimation, and diarrhea. Neuropathy was slightly more common in the every-3-week arm (grade 3/4 in 1.8% vs. 0.9%). Quality of life as measured by the FACT-P scores did not differ significantly among the docetaxel schedules but was more favorable than in the mitoxantrone arm.

10. **d. increased osteoclastic activity.** Bone loss associated with prostate cancer can result from an enhanced osteoclastic activity associated with long-term androgen suppression, which in turn will cause excessive resorption of bone mineral and organic matrix.

11. **e. There is increasing evidence that growth factors, cytokines, and other proteins may play a role in the development of bone metastasis.** Bone loss associated with prostate cancer can result from an enhanced osteoclastic activity associated with long-term androgen suppression, which in turn will cause excessive resorption of bone mineral and organic matrix. Tumor cells may also cause mineral release and matrix resorption in the areas involved by metastatic disease (Galasko, 1986). In addition to various cytokines, growth factors, tumor necrosis factors, and bone morphogenic proteins have been shown in preclinical studies to play a major role in the induction of both osteoclastic and osteoblastic activity (Reddi and Cunningham, 1990). In prostate cancer, bone metastases are predominantly but not always blastic, which reflects a predominance of osteoblastic activity in the process of bone remodeling.

12. **e. All of the above.** Zoledronate is a potent intravenous bisphosphonate approved for the treatment of hypercalcemia and the treatment of decreased bone mineral density in postmenopausal women (Green and Rogers, 2002). At the present time this compound is indicated for the treatment of patients with progressive prostate cancer with evidence of bone metastasis at doses of 4 mg given by short intravenous infusion repeated at intervals of 3 to 4 weeks for several months. Side effects include fatigue, myalgias, fever, anemia, and mild elevations of the serum creatinine concentration. Hypocalcemia has been described, and concomitant use of oral calcium supplements (1500 mg/day) and vitamin D (400 units/day) is recommended. An unusual but important complication is the development of severe jaw pain associated with osteonecrosis of the mandibular bone.

13. **d. All of the above.** In addition to a falling PSA value, several other parameters can be used to predict response to chemotherapy, and a number of prognostic models evaluating baseline and post-treatment characteristics have been developed (Smaletz et al, 2002; Halabi et al, 2003). Among various parameters with consistent prognostic significance are baseline performance status, presence of pain, and pretreatment hemoglobin level. Other possible parameters include baseline PSA level, extent of bone scintiscan involvement (number and pattern/distribution of bone lesions), and presence of visceral disease. Semi-quantitative methods to evaluate PSA mRNA expression in circulating tumor cells (using reverse transcription/polymerase chain reaction) and various PSA constructs (e.g., PSA doubling time, PSA velocity) are among the post-treatment parameters most likely to be of prognostic significance (Kantoff et al, 2001; Scher et al, 2004; Armstrong et al, 2007).

14. **d. It is seen in less than 1% of patients, except when they demonstrate the neuroendocrine phenotype.** In these cases, brain metastases should be treated with a combination of chemotherapy and brain irradiation.

15. **e. All of the above.** Docetaxel is a cytotoxic agent and member of the taxoid family. It induces apoptosis in cancer cells through TP53-independent mechanisms that are believed to be due to its inhibition of microtubule

depolymerization and inhibition of antiapoptotic signaling. The induction of microtubule stabilization intracellularly through β-tubulin interactions causes guanosine triphosphate (GTP)-independent polymerization and cell cycle arrest at G_2M, and some have reported a twofold greater microtubule affinity compared with paclitaxel. Additionally, docetaxel has been found to induce BCL2 phosphorylation in vitro, a process that has been correlated with caspase activation and loss of its normal antiapoptotic activity. Unable to inhibit the proapoptotic molecule BAX, phosphorylated BCL2 may also induce apoptosis through this independent mechanism. However, additional mechanisms may be important, such as CDKN1Bkip1 induction and repression of BCL-XL.

16. **e. All of the above.** Table 110–7 in *Campbell-Walsh Urology, 10ᵗʰ Edition,* summarizes ongoing clinical trials evaluating novel targeted therapies for men with CRPC. New drug development for metastatic prostate cancer has been reviewed by Armstrong and George (2008).

17. **a. AR can never be found in the castration-resistant state.** In prostate cancer, various molecular changes in the AR have been shown to parallel disease progression in castrate patients and in some situations may provide the explanation for the responses associated with some therapeutic maneuvers (antiandrogen withdrawal effect, responses to secondary endocrine manipulations with compounds that bind to AR). Despite this, a precise role of the AR in the pathogenesis of disease progression remains to be better elucidated. A novel AR-modulating agent, MDV3100, is thought to act by inhibiting AR translocation into the nucleus and has entered phase 1/2 human clinical trials.

18. **a. Sipuleucel-T (Provenge) has demonstrated improved median overall survival compared with placebo in a multicenter phase 3 trial (IMPACT) involving men with metastatic CRPC.** In this trial, which accrued a total of 512 patients, sipuleucel-T demonstrated a modest survival advantage compared with placebo in this patient population (median survival 25.8 vs. 21.7 months, hazard ratio 0.78; $P = .03$) (Dendreon Inc., 2009). Three-year survival was also improved by 38% with sipuleucel-T compared with placebo (31.7% vs. 23.0%). None of the GVAX trials has ever shown an improvement in survival, and both VITAL-1 and VITAL-2 were terminated early because of data observed at the time of interim analyses suggesting that the survival improvements initially hypothesized were unlikely to be observed if the trials were to be continued (Higano et al, 2009). Alarmingly, in the VITAL-2 study, mortality was higher in patients on the docetaxel/GVAX arm (Small et al, 2009).

Additional Study Points

1. The average survival of the prostate cancer patient is 24 to 36 months after the documentation of metastatic disease.
2. It is the general consensus that patients should be maintained on ablative hormonal therapy during the course of subsequent chemotherapy indefinitely even though they are resistant to it.
3. After the development of the castration-resistant state a sequential hormonal approach is usually used; the drugs employed include aminoglutethimide and ketoconazole.
4. Obstructive uropathy is not an uncommon complication of metastatic prostate cancer.
5. Docetaxel is the standard treatment for metastatic castration-resistant prostate cancer.
6. Mitoxantrone is used to palliate symptoms.
7. Any patient with back pain and a history of bone metastases should be aggressively evaluated for epidural cord compression. The treatment of this is high-dose intravenous corticosteroids, radiation therapy, and/or surgical decompression.
8. Bone metastases in prostate cancer are usually blastic; hypercalcemia is rare.

Pediatric Urology

Normal Development of the Genitourinary Tract

John M. Park, MD

QUESTIONS

1. The fetal kidneys develop from which of the following embryonic structures?
   a. Paraxial (somite) mesoderm
   b. Intermediate mesoderm
   c. Neural tube
   d. Lateral mesoderm
   e. Urogenital sinus

2. Which of the following statements regarding the mesonephros is FALSE?
   a. It serves as a transient excretory organ during the development of the definitive kidneys metanephros.
   b. Certain elements of the mesonephros persist as part of the reproductive tract.
   c. The excretory portion of the mesonephros begins to degenerate during the first year of life.
   d. Development of the nephric ducts (also called wolffian ducts) precedes that of the mesonephric tubules.
   e. During the early development, the mesonephros lies medial to the developing mullerian ducts.

3. At what gestational time point does the metanephros development begin?
   a. 20th day
   b. 24th day
   c. 28th day
   d. 32nd day
   e. 36th day

4. Which of the following statements is TRUE regarding metanephric development?
   a. It requires the reciprocal inductive interaction between müllerian duct and metanephric mesenchyme.
   b. The calyces, pelvis, and ureter derive from the differentiation of the metanephric mesenchyme.
   c. Older, more differentiated nephrons are located at the periphery of the developing kidney, whereas newer, less differentiated nephrons are found near the juxtamedullary region.
   d. In humans, although renal maturation continues postnatally, nephrogenesis is completed by birth.
   e. The metanephric development requires the inductive effect of the urogenital sinus.

5. The fused lower pole of the horseshoe kidney is trapped by which of the following structures during the ascent?
   a. Inferior mesenteric artery
   b. Superior mesenteric artery
   c. Celiac artery
   d. Common iliac artery
   e. Aorta

6. The homozygous gene disruption (gene knockout) in which of the following does *NOT* lead to a significant renal maldevelopment in mice?
   a. *Wt1*
   b. *Pax2*
   c. Glial cell line–derived neurotrophic factor (GDNF)
   d. *Tp53*
   e. *Ret*

7. Which of the following statements is FALSE regarding GDNF?
   a. It is a ligand for the RET receptor tyrosine kinase.
   b. *GDNF* gene knockout mice demonstrate an abnormal renal development.
   c. It is expressed in the metanephric mesenchyme but not in the ureteric bud.
   d. GDNF arrests the ureteric bud growth in vitro.
   e. GDNF expression is restricted by FoxC1 and FoxC2 transcription factors.

8. Which of the following statements is FALSE regarding the renin-angiotensin system during renal and ureteral development?
   a. The embryonic kidney is able to produce all components of the renin-angiotensin system.
   b. Both subtypes of angiotensin II receptor, AT1 and AT2, are expressed in the developing metanephros.
   c. *At1* knockout mice demonstrate a spectrum of congenital urinary tract abnormalities, including ureteropelvic junction obstruction and vesicoureteral reflux.
   d. Infants born to mothers treated with angiotensin-converting enzyme inhibitors during pregnancy have

increased rates of oligohydramnios, hypotension, and anuria.

e. Pharmacologic inhibition of angiotensin-converting enzyme in the neonatal rat produces irreversible abnormalities in renal function and morphology.

9. The urachus involutes to become:

a. verumontanum.

b. median umbilical ligament.

c. appendix testis.

d. epoöphoron.

e. prostatic utricle.

10. Which of the following statements is FALSE regarding bladder development?

a. The bladder body is derived from the urogenital sinus whereas the trigone develops from the terminal portion of the mesonephric ducts.

b. Bladder compliance seems to be low during early gestation, and it gradually increases thereafter.

c. Epithelial-mesenchymal inductive interactions appear to be necessary for proper bladder development.

d. Histologic evidence of smooth muscle differentiation begins near the bladder neck and proceeds toward the bladder dome.

e. By the 12th week the urachus involutes to become a fibrous cord, which becomes the median umbilical ligament.

11. The primordial germ cell migration and the formation of the genital ridges begin at which time point during gestation?

a. Third week

b. Fifth week

c. Seventh week

d. Ninth week

e. 12th week

12. Which of the following statements is FALSE regarding the paramesonephric (müllerian) ducts?

a. Both male and female embryos form paramesonephric (müllerian) ducts.

b. In male embryos the paramesonephric ducts degenerate under the influence of the müllerian-inhibiting substance (MIS) produced by the Leydig cells.

c. In male embryos the paramesonephric ducts become the appendix testis and the prostatic utricle.

d. In female embryos the paramesonephric ducts form the female reproductive tract, including fallopian tubes, uterus, and upper vagina.

e. The paramesonephric duct derivatives are absent in patients with complete androgen insensitivity syndrome.

13. Which of the following structures in the male reproductive tract develops from the urogenital sinus?

a. Vas deferens

b. Seminal vesicles

c. Prostate

d. Appendix epididymis

e. Prostatic utricle

14. Which of the following statements is FALSE regarding normal prostate development?

a. It requires the conversion of testosterone into dihydrotestosterone by 5α-reductase.

b. It is dependent on epithelial-mesenchymal interactions under the influence of androgens.

c. It is first seen at the 10th to 12th week of gestation.

d. It requires the effects of müllerian-inhibiting substance.

e. Androgen receptors in the urogenital sinus mesenchyme are required for prostate specification and differentiation.

15. In female embryos the remnants of the mesonephric ducts persist as the following structures EXCEPT:

a. epoöphoron.

b. paroöphoron.

c. hymen.

d. Gartner duct cysts.

e. ectopic ureter.

16. Which of the following statements is FALSE regarding the external genitalia development?

a. The appearance of the external genitalia is similar in male and female embryos until the 12th week.

b. The external genital appearance of males who are deficient in 5α-reductase is similar to that of females.

c. In males, the formation of distal glandular urethra may occur by the fusion of urethral folds proximally and the ingrowth of ectodermal cells distally.

d. In females, the urethral folds become the labia majora, and the labioscrotal folds become the labia minora.

e. Mice and humans with functional loss of androgen receptors demonstrate a complete feminization of the external genitalia.

17. The testes descend to the level of the internal inguinal ring by which time point during gestation?

a. Sixth week

b. Third month

c. Sixth month

d. Ninth month

e. At birth

18. Which of the following statements is FALSE regarding the SRY (the Sex-determining Region of the Y chromosome)?

a. Its expression triggers the primitive sex cord cells to differentiate into the Sertoli cells.

b. Approximately 25% of sex reversal conditions in humans are attributable to SRY mutations.

c. It is located on the short arm of the Y chromosome.

d. It causes the regression of mesonephric ducts.

e. The identity of protein encoded by the SRY has not been determined.

ANSWERS

1. **b. Intermediate mesoderm.** Mammals develop three kidneys in the course of intrauterine life. The embryonic kidneys are, in order of their appearance: the pronephros, the mesonephros, and the metanephros. The first two kidneys regress in utero, and the third becomes the

permanent kidney. In terms of embryology, all three kidneys develop from the intermediate mesoderm.

2. **c. The excretory portion of the mesonephros begins to degenerate during the first year of life.** Like the pronephros, the mesonephros is also transient, but in mammals it serves as an excretory organ for the embryo while the definitive kidney, the metanephros, begins its development. Development of the nephric ducts (also called wolffian ducts) precedes the development of the mesonephric tubules. Soon after the appearance of the nephric ducts during the fourth week, mesonephric vesicles begin to form. Initially, several spherical masses of cells are found along the medial side of the nephrogenic cords at the cranial end. This differentiation progresses caudally and results in the formation of 40 to 42 pairs of mesonephric tubules, but only about 30 pairs are seen at any one time because the cranially located tubules start to degenerate starting at about the fifth week. By the fourth month the human mesonephros has almost completely disappeared, except for a few elements that persist into maturity. Certain elements of the mesonephros are retained in the mature urogenital system as part of the reproductive tract.

3. **c. 28th day.** The definitive kidney, the metanephros, forms in the sacral region as a pair of new structures, called the ureteric buds, sprout from the distal portion of the nephric duct and come in contact with the blastema of metanephric mesenchyme at about the 28th day.

4. **d. In humans, although renal maturation continues postnatally, nephrogenesis is completed by birth.** It requires the inductive interaction between the ureteric bud and metanephric mesenchyme. The calyces, pelvis, and ureter derive from the ureteric bud. Older, more differentiated nephrons are located in the inner part of the kidney near the juxtamedullary region. In humans, although renal maturation continues to take place postnatally, nephrogenesis is completed before birth.

5. **a. Inferior mesenteric artery.** The inferior poles of the kidneys may fuse, forming a horseshoe kidney that crosses over the ventral side of the aorta. During ascent, the fused lower pole becomes trapped under the inferior mesenteric artery and thus does not reach its normal position.

6. **d. *Tp53*.** Mutant *Wt1* mice do not form ureteric buds, and in *Pax2* knockout mice no nephric ducts, müllerian ducts, ureteric buds, or metanephric mesenchyme form and the animals die within 1 day of birth because of renal failure. Ureteric bud formation is impaired in GDNF and *Ret* knockout mice, but *Tp53* knockout mice do not demonstrate significant renal developmental anomaly.

7. **d. GDNF arrests the ureteric bud growth in vitro.** GDNF promotes ureteric bud growth in vitro. Although the importance of RET in kidney development was clearly demonstrated, it is only recently that its ligand, GDNF, has been identified. GDNF is a secreted glycoprotein that possesses a cystine-knot motif. GDNF is expressed within the metanephric mesenchyme prior to ureteric bud invasion, and ureteric bud formation is impaired in GDNF knockout mice.

8. **c. *At1* knockout mice demonstrate a spectrum of congenital urinary tract abnormalities, including ureteropelvic junction obstruction and vesicoureteral reflux.** *At2* knockout mice demonstrate a spectrum of congenital urinary tract abnormalities, including ureteropelvic junction obstruction, multicystic dysplastic kidney, megaureter, vesicoureteral reflux, and renal hypoplasia.

9. **b. median umbilical ligament.** By the 12th week the urachus involutes to become a fibrous cord, which becomes the median umbilical ligament.

10. **d. Histologic evidence of smooth muscle differentiation begins near the bladder neck and proceeds toward the bladder dome.** Between the 7th and 12th weeks the surrounding connective tissues condense and smooth muscle fibers begin to appear, first at the region of the bladder dome and later proceeding toward the bladder neck.

11. **b. Fifth week.** During the fifth week, primordial germ cells migrate from the yolk sac along the dorsal mesentery to populate the mesenchyme of the posterior body wall near the 10th thoracic level. In both sexes the arrival of primordial germ cells in the area of future gonads serves as the signal for the existing cells of the mesonephros and the adjacent coelomic epithelium to proliferate and form a pair of genital ridges just medial to the developing mesonephros.

12. **b. In male embryos the paramesonephric ducts degenerate under the influence of the müllerian-inhibiting substance (MIS) produced by the Leydig cells.** A new pair of ducts, called the paramesonephric (müllerian) ducts, begins to form just lateral to the mesonephric ducts in both male and female embryos. These ducts arise by the craniocaudal invagination of thickened coelomic epithelium, extending all the way from the third thoracic segment to the posterior wall of the developing urogenital sinus. The caudal tips of the paramesonephric ducts adhere to each other as they connect with the urogenital sinus between the openings of the right and left mesonephric ducts. The cranial ends of the paramesonephric ducts form funnel-shaped openings into the coelomic cavity (the future peritoneum). As developing Sertoli cells begin their differentiation in response to the *SRY* (Sex-determining Region of the Y chromosome), they begin to secrete MIS, which causes the paramesonephric (müllerian) ducts to regress rapidly between the 8th and 10th weeks. Small müllerian duct remnants can be detected in the developed male as a small tissue protrusion at the superior pole of the testis, called the appendix testis, and as a posterior expansion of the prostatic urethra, called the prostatic utricle. In female embryos, MIS is absent, so the müllerian ducts do not regress and instead give rise to fallopian tubes, uterus, and vagina.

13. **c. Prostate.** Vas deferens, seminal vesicles, and appendix epididymis all develop from the mesonephric ducts. The prostate and bulbourethral glands develop from the urogenital sinus.

14. **d. It requires the effects of müllerian-inhibiting substance.** The prostate gland begins to develop during the 10th to 12th weeks as a cluster of endodermal evaginations budding from the pelvic urethra (derived from the urogenital sinus). These presumptive prostatic outgrowths are induced by the surrounding mesenchyme, and this process depends on the conversion of testosterone into dihydrotestosterone by 5α-reductase. Similar to renal and bladder development, prostatic development depends on mesenchymal-epithelial interactions but is under the influence of androgens. There is no evidence that MIS plays a direct role in prostate development.

15. **c. Hymen.** In the absence of MIS and androgens, the mesonephric (wolffian) ducts degenerate and the paramesonephric (müllerian) ducts give rise to the fallopian tubes, uterus, and upper two thirds of the vagina. The remnants of mesonephric ducts are found in the mesentery of the ovary as the epoöphoron and paroöphoron and near the vaginal introitus and anterolateral vaginal wall as Gartner duct cysts. The hymen develops from the endodermal membrane located at the junction between the vaginal plate and the definitive urogenital sinus, which is the future vestibule of the vagina.

16. **d. In females, the urethral folds become the labia majora and the labioscrotal folds become the labia minora.** The early development of the external genital organ is similar in both sexes until the 12th week. Early in the 5th week, a pair of swellings called cloacal folds develops on either side of the cloacal membrane. These folds meet just anterior to the cloacal membrane to form a midline swelling called the genital tubercle. During the cloacal division into the anterior urogenital sinus and the posterior anorectal canal, the portion of the cloacal folds flanking the opening of the urogenital sinus becomes the urogenital folds and the portion flanking the opening of the anorectal canal becomes the anal folds. A new pair of swellings, called the labioscrotal folds, then appears on either side of the urogenital folds. In the absence of dihydrotestosterone, the primitive perineum does not lengthen and the labioscrotal and urethral folds do not fuse across the midline in the female embryos. The phallus bends inferiorly, becoming the clitoris, and the definitive urogenital sinus becomes the vestibule of the vagina. The urethral folds become the labia minora, and the labioscrotal folds become the labia majora. The external genital organ develops in a similar manner in genetic males who are deficient in 5α-reductase and therefore lack dihydrotestosterone.

17. **b. Third month.** The testis reaches the level of internal inguinal ring by the third month and passes through the inguinal canal to reach the scrotum between the seventh and ninth months.

18. **d. It causes the regression of mesonephric ducts.** When the Y-linked master regulatory gene, called *SRY,* is expressed in the male, the epithelial cells of the primitive sex cords differentiate into Sertoli cells and this critical morphogenetic event triggers subsequent testicular development. Analysis of DNA narrowed the location of the *SRY* to a relatively small region within the short arm of the chromosome. It is now clear that only about 25% of sex reversals in humans can be attributed to disabling mutations of the *SRY.*

Additional Study Points

1. The glomerulus, proximal tubule, loop of Henle, and distal tubule are derived from the metanephric mesenchyme.
2. The remainder of the collecting system is formed from the ureteric bud (wolffian duct).
3. The Weigert-Meyer rule states that the most lateral and cephalad ureteric orifice arises from the lower pole and may demonstrate reflux whereas the most medial and caudad orifice drains the upper pole and may be associated with a ureterocele.
4. Sertoli cells produce mullerian-inhibiting substance, which causes regression of the mullerian ducts.
5. Testosterone is secreted by the Leydig cells and stimulates the wolffian ducts to form the vas deferens and seminal vesicles.
6. The prostate and bulbourethral glands develop from the urogenital sinus.
7. Circulating androgens play a critical role in the development of the prostate.
8. When 5α-reductase is deficient, prostatic growth and development is severely compromised.
9. In the absence of müllerian-inhibiting substance and androgens, the wolffian ducts degenerate and the müllerian ducts give rise to the fallopian tubes, uterus, and upper two thirds of the vagina.
10. Boys with spina bifida have a 23% incidence of cryptorchidism.
11. If the *SRY* gene complex is translocated to an X chromosome, an XX female will have male characteristics.

Renal Functional Development and Diseases in Children

Lane S. Palmer, MD, FAAP, FACS ● Howard Trachtman, MD

QUESTIONS

1. In the human, nephrogenesis is completed by:
   a. 20 weeks.
   b. 24 to 28 weeks.
   c. 30 to 32 weeks.
   d. 34 to 36 weeks.
   e. the postnatal period.

2. A 4-year-old boy presents with swelling and decreased urine output. He has had eyelid edema on awakening for the past week. His blood pressure is 90/50 mm Hg, and he has marked eyelid edema, distended abdomen, and pitting edema of the legs and feet. Urinalysis showed a specific gravity of 1.030, pH 5, 3+ protein, and trace amount of blood. Serum studies show a sodium level of 131 mEq/L, blood urea nitrogen value of 30 mg/dL, creatinine level of 0.3 mg/dL, and albumin level of 1.6 g/dL. The appropriate next step in management is:
   a. admission to inpatient unit for quantitation of urinary protein excretion.
   b. renal imaging.
   c. initiation of oral diuretics and asking parents to collect a timed urine specimen for protein at home, with outpatient follow-up.
   d. workup for occult malignancy.
   e. serum cholesterol evaluation.

3. A 6-year-old healthy girl undergoes a routine physical examination. Urinalysis reveals a specific gravity of 1.020, pH 6, trace protein, and moderate amount of blood on dipstick testing. The microscopic test shows 5 to 6 red blood cells per high-powered field. An inappropriate next step is:
   a. renal ultrasonography.
   b. random urine calcium and creatinine determinations.
   c. clean-catch urine culture.
   d. an empirical 10-day course of antibiotics.
   e. a repeat urinalysis in 2 weeks.

4. A urinalysis in an 8-year-old boy shows a specific gravity of 1.030, pH 5, trace protein, and moderate amount of blood. He has a normal physical examination including blood pressure of 96/56 mm Hg. On further history he was hospitalized 2 months ago with poststreptococcal glomerulonephritis. The most appropriate course of action is:
   a. cystoscopy.
   b. renal ultrasonography.
   c. a course of antibiotics after obtaining a urine culture.
   d. to reassure his family and obtain records from the outside institution.
   e. computed tomography.

5. A 6-year-old boy presents to the emergency department with the new onset of left-sided flank pain, gross hematuria, and vomiting. His blood pressure is 120/70 mm Hg, and the physical examination reveals right costovertebral angle tenderness. The urinalysis shows brown urine with a specific gravity of 1.030, pH 7, large amount of blood, and 2+ protein. The next step in diagnostic evaluation should NOT include:
   a. high-resolution computed tomography of abdomen/pelvis without contrast.
   b. microscopic examination of the urine.
   c. cystoscopy.
   d. renal ultrasonography.
   e. serum electrolyte determination.

6. A 9-year-old girl presents after passing a 3-mm stone. On analysis, the stone is composed 100% of calcium oxalate. The next step is to:
   a. start a thiazide diuretic.
   b. obtain a 24-hour urine collection to test for calcium, creatinine, oxalate, and citrate.
   c. start potassium citrate.
   d. restrict dietary calcium.
   e. restrict dietary oxalate.

7. A 6-year-old boy presents to the emergency department with new onset of headache and gross hematuria. He has no dysuria or fever but has vomited three times. He had a sore throat the week before, but it has resolved. His blood pressure is 140/90 mm Hg, and physical examination reveals a heart murmur. The urinalysis shows brown

urine with a specific gravity of 1.030, pH 7, large amount of blood, and 2+ protein. The next step in the diagnostic evaluation should include all of the following EXCEPT:

a. computed tomography of the abdomen and pelvis.

b. comprehensive metabolic panel.

c. C3 determination.

d. antistreptolysin O titer.

e. microscopic examination of the urine.

8. A 3-year-old boy presents to the emergency department with a respiratory problem and gross hematuria. He has no dysuria or abdominal pain but has fever, rhinorrhea, and cough. His blood pressure is 120/70 mm Hg, and physical examination shows rhinorrhea, mild pharyngeal erythema, and no peripheral edema or abdominal tenderness. The urinalysis shows brown urine with a specific gravity of 1.030, pH 7, large amount of blood, and 2+ protein. (His mother also has had hematuria in the past, and his maternal uncle is deaf and on hemodialysis.) The next step in diagnostic evaluation includes all of the following EXCEPT:

a. computed tomography of the abdomen and pelvis.

b. comprehensive metabolic panel.

c. renal biopsy.

d. antistreptolysin O titer and C3.

e. microscopic examination of the urine.

9. A 16-year-old boy with end-stage renal disease is managed with peritoneal dialysis (PD). He develops a fever of 102° F, abdominal pain, and vomiting. The next step in management is to:

a. obtain blood and urine cultures.

b. start broad-spectrum antibiotics.

c. collect a specimen of dialysate for white blood cell count and culture.

d. change to hemodialysis.

e. administer intraperitoneal antibiotics.

10. An 8-year-old boy is found to have a blood urea nitrogen level of 60 mg/dL and a creatinine of 2.7 mg/dL. His urinary sodium level is 13 mEq/L, fractional excretion of sodium (FE_{Na}) is 0.8%, and urinary osmolality is 410 mOsm/Kg. The most likely cause of his renal failure is:

a. posterior urethral valves.

b. gastroenteritis with diarrhea.

c. gentamicin administration.

d. contrast nephropathy.

e. hepatorenal syndrome.

11. A 9-year-old boy is found during routine examination to have a blood pressure of 120/90 mm Hg. The child was calm, and a properly sized blood pressure cuff was used for the measurement. The best next step in management is to:

a. repeat the measurement next week in the office.

b. obtain a fasting lipid profile.

c. perform renal ultrasonography.

d. obtain selective renin levels.

e. perform ambulatory blood pressure monitoring (ABPM).

ANSWERS

1. **d. 34 to 36 weeks.** The metanephros begins its inductive phase after 5 weeks of gestation; and, in the human, nephrogenesis follows a sigmoidal curve, with most rapid increase in midgestation, and is completed by 34 to 36 weeks.

2. **a. admission to inpatient unit for quantitation of urinary protein excretion.** The patient has hypoalbuminemia, edema, and proteinuria and most likely has nephrotic syndrome. The initial illness is best treated with inpatient admission to complete the diagnostic studies (quantitate urinary protein, measure plasma lipids) and provide education of the family, including institution of a low-salt diet. Oral prednisone is started because a renal biopsy is rarely indicated. Oral diuretics are not commonly prescribed unless careful observation is possible due to poor response and the potential for thromboses. Malignancy is rarely associated with nephrotic syndrome in children, and therefore a workup is not indicated. Imaging of the urinary tract is rarely indicated in children with nephrotic syndrome. Fortunately, most children with primary nephrotic syndrome respond to corticosteroids within 14 days and have spontaneous diuresis with loss of edema and proteinuria.

3. **d. an empirical 10-day course of antibiotics.** Although asymptomatic hematuria may be caused by occult urinary tract infection, empirical treatment without culture is never the correct approach. Unfortunately, this scenario happens far too often in the primary care world. It is reasonable to repeat the urinalysis before proceeding with diagnostic evaluation. If the hematuria persists, then imaging the kidneys and urinary tract and screening for hypercalciuria is a reasonable approach.

4. **d. to reassure the family and obtain records from the outside institution.** Given the previous history of postinfectious glomerulonephritis (in his case due to a preceding streptococcal infection), the most likely cause of microscopic hematuria is resolving nephritis. The microhematuria may persist for up to 1 year, while the proteinuria and macroscopic hematuria usually resolve within the 2-week acute phase. It would be helpful to confirm the diagnosis by review of medical records.

5. **c. cystoscopy.** The clinical picture is that of a child presenting with a renal calculus. Cystoscopy is rarely indicated in the diagnostic evaluation, although it might be included during the treatment phase of nephrolithiasis in children. High-resolution computed tomography without administration of a contrast agent is the test of choice, but one cannot argue with ultrasonography as a first test. Examination of the urine is also a viable first step because children with nephritis occasionally complain of flank pain.

6. **b. obtain a 24-hour urine collection to test for calcium, creatinine, oxalate, and citrate.** A metabolic evaluation for the cause of calcium oxalate nephrolithiasis should be initiated because the differential diagnosis includes hyperoxaluria, hypercalciuria, renal tubular acidosis, or idiopathic calcium stones. In children, preventative treatment is rarely initiated without attempts to diagnose the underlying metabolic disturbance. Dietary calcium restriction is never a treatment for children with calcium stones with or without hypercalciuria.

7. **a. computed tomography of the abdomen and pelvis.** With symptomatic hypertension and gross hematuria, one must entertain the possibility of acute glomerulonephritis. The prior history of pharyngitis is consistent with poststreptococcal-associated disease. Examination of the urine sediment for signs of glomerulonephritis (cellular casts) and documentation of renal function and electrolytes as well as elevated antistreptolysin O titer and decreased C3 are the usual steps taken to confirm the diagnosis. Hypertension is treated aggressively with salt restriction, loop diuretics, and antihypertensive agents. Resolution of the hypertension parallels resolution of the acute phase.

8. **a. computed tomography of the abdomen and pelvis.** The presentation of gross hematuria during a respiratory infection is not characteristic of postinfectious glomerulonephritis because the onset of nephritis usually follows the infection. The positive family history is important because the onset of macroscopic hematuria during a respiratory infection is characteristic of two forms of chronic glomerulonephritis: IgA nephropathy and Alport hereditary nephritis. Imaging is usually not indicated if glomerulonephritis can be confirmed by microscopic examination of the urine. Patients with both IgA and hereditary nephritis would be expected to have normal C3. A renal biopsy is needed for diagnosis of IgA and is usually needed for diagnosis of hereditary nephritis except in the case in which the affected relative has already undergone biopsy.

9. **c. collect a specimen of dialysate for white blood cell count and culture.** Peritonitis is the most common complication of PD. Although the patient should undergo a full fever workup including urine and blood cultures, the diagnosis is secured by collecting a sample of dialysate, which is often cloudy, and finding 100 WBCs/mm^3 of which 50% are neutrophils. Antibiotics will be administered after the cultures are collected. PD can continue while treating the peritonitis.

10. **b. gastroenteritis with diarrhea.** The biochemical analysis that was provided indicates a prerenal cause of acute renal injury. Both gastroenteritis and hepatorenal syndrome are categorized as prerenal whereas contrast nephropathy and aminoglycoside toxicity cause intrinsic renal damage. Of the two prerenal causes, gastroenteritis with diarrhea is much more common.

11. **a. repeat the measurement next week in the office.** This child's blood pressure is elevated and should be repeated and hypertension confirmed. ABPM would be the ideal method for confirmation but is recommended in children older than 10 years old. Therefore the blood pressure should be re-measured in the office. If hypertension is confirmed, then the workup will include a complete metabolic panel, lipid profile, an echocardiogram, and renal ultrasonography. Angiography and selective renin levels would be performed in the case of severe or recalcitrant hypertension.

Additional Study Points

1. The glomerular filtration rate at birth is 10% to 15% of the adult value owing to a decreased number of perfused cortical nephrons.
2. Renal function is impaired in the fetus and infant: FE_{Na} is increased, acidification is limited, potassium secretion is compromised, and the ability to concentrate the urine is impaired.
3. Normal FE_{Na} for an infant is 1% to 3% (for an adult it is less than 1%).
4. Normal serum bicarbonate in an infant is 15 to 18 mM/L because of the physiologic limitations for acidification.
5. Glomerular filtration rate is dependent on gestational age and doubles in the first 2 weeks of life.
6. Water makes up 80% of the body weight of a newborn.
7. Isolated asymptomatic microscopic hematuria is generally benign.
8. Hematuria in the presence of significant proteinuria indicates glomerular disease.
9. Fanconi syndrome is a generalized dysfunction of the proximal renal tubule.
10. Renal tubular acidosis has three basic types: type I or distal, type II or proximal, and type IV due to aldosterone deficiency.
11. Aldosterone plays a pivotal role in increasing Na$^+$,K$^+$-ATPase and enhancing the activity of H$^+$ pumps.
12. Patients with renal tubular acidosis generally present with failure to thrive.
13. The most common cause of acquired nephrogenic diabetes insipidus is obstructive uropathy. Other causes include lithium and amphotericin administration.
14. Polyuria, polydipsia, and poor growth are common presenting symptoms in children with renal tubular diseases.
15. Hypercalciuria and hypocitraturia are the two most common causes of urolithiasis in children.
16. Converting a patient with acute kidney injury from oliguria to nonoliguria does not increase glomerular filtration rate or alter the course.
17. Substantial nephron loss during acute kidney injury warrants life-long monitoring for progression to chronic renal failure.
18. A native nephrectomy before renal transplantation should be considered in patients with severe uncontrollable hypertension, significant proteinuria, recurrent pyelonephritis, severe hydronephrosis, infected or symptomatic polycystic kidneys, or persistent anti–glomerular basement membrane antibody levels.

Congenital Urinary Obstruction: Pathophysiology and Clinical Evaluation

Craig A. Peters, MD, FACS, FAAP ● Robert L. Chevalier, MD

QUESTIONS

1. After relief of a unilateral ureteral obstructing lesion, decreased relative uptake compared with the contralateral kidney on radionuclide renal imaging is most likely due to:
   a. glomerular hyperfiltration.
   b. asymmetrical renal growth.
   c. established renal tubular fibrosis.
   d. neural imbalance.
   e. compensatory hypertrophy.

2. Congenital obstruction differs from acquired obstruction in that it:
   a. affects glomerular development.
   b. induces interstitial fibrosis.
   c. affects tubular function.
   d. causes renal atrophy.
   e. alters renal homeostasis.

3. Renal dysplasia associated with obstruction is characterized by:
   a. renal atrophy.
   b. glomerular cysts.
   c. fibromuscular collars.
   d. heterotopic bone formation.
   e. excess production of afferent arteriole renin.

4. In a unilaterally hydronephrotic kidney, supranormal function on a renal scan is indicative of:
   a. renal hyperplasia.
   b. vascular recruitment due to obstruction.
   c. artifactual increased tubular uptake.
   d. uncertain prognosis.
   e. significant obstructive effect.

5. In the obstructed kidney, epidermal growth factor (EGF) has been shown to:
   a. reduce glomerular sclerosis.
   b. accelerate interstitial fibrosis.
   c. reduce renin recruitment in the afferent arteriole.

d. improve collecting duct function.
   e. reduce renal apoptosis.

6. Epithelial-mesenchymal transformation in the developing kidney is:
   a. seen only in the setting of obstruction.
   b. integral to glomerular development.
   c. the basis for glomerular sclerosis.
   d. reflected in the presence of α-smooth muscle actin.
   e. a one-way process.

7. Regulation of the extracellular matrix in the kidney:
   a. depends on normal expression of EGF.
   b. depends on balanced activity of tissue inhibitors of metalloproteinases (TIMPs) and matrix metalloproteinases (MMPs).
   c. depends entirely on collagen synthesis.
   d. is not related to angiotensin expression.
   e. is independent of transforming growth factor-β activity.

8. The principal effects of congenital renal obstruction are:
   a. hypoplasia and increased epithelial-mesenchymal transformation.
   b. glomerulosclerosis, interstitial fibrosis, and atrophy.
   c. glomerulosclerosis, renin downregulation, and tubular hypertrophy.
   d. increased growth, fibrosis, and tubular atrophy.
   e. altered growth regulation, renal differentiation, and functional integration.

9. Inflammatory changes in the congenitally obstructed kidney:
   a. are similar to that seen in postnatally obstructed kidneys.
   b. are mediated by the renin-angiotensin system.
   c. are minimal in the absence of overt infection.
   d. are the key element in glomerular damage.
   e. affect renal interstitial fibrosis.

10. In the fetal kidney, angiotensin activity:
    a. is tightly regulated by EGF.
    b. acts predominantly through the angiotensin AT1 receptor.

c. affects epithelial-mesenchymal transformations.

d. is an important regulator of renal growth.

e. is unaffected by renal obstruction.

ANSWERS

1. **b. asymmetrical renal growth.** When renal function appears to decline after relief of obstruction it is often due to different growth and functional development rates of the two kidneys, when the affected kidney cannot increase its absolute function as rapidly as the other intact kidney. This produces a progressive differential functional uptake on nuclear imaging that gives the impression of functional loss that is relative and not absolute.

2. **a. affects glomerular development.** Only congenital obstruction will change glomerular development, whereas acquired obstruction can produce all of the other changes indicated. As it occurs during development, congenital obstruction can produce an altered developmental pattern whereas acquired obstruction does not change an already established pattern but only damages or distorts it.

3. **c. fibromuscular collars.** One of the histologic hallmarks of dysplasia are fibromuscular collars, so-called primitive ducts reflecting abnormal differentiation of the peritubular mesenchyme. Renal growth impairment is common with dysplasia, however this is not atrophy but growth failure. Glomerular cysts are not characteristic of dysplasia. Heterotopic cartilage may be seen but not bone. Excess renin expression may be seen in obstruction without dysplasia.

4. **d. uncertain prognosis.** It remains controversial as to the basis for supranormal function on renal scan in the setting of hydronephrosis. In some cases it is thought to be artifactual but may also reflect a compensatory mechanism that reflects obstructive effects. There is no evidence that it reflects vascular recruitment, but it may be mediated by vascular factors.

5. **e. reduce renal apoptosis.** Administration of EGF to the congenitally obstructed kidney can reduce renal apoptosis and reduce the effects of growth impairment. The other effects have not been reported.

6. **d. reflected in the presence of α-smooth muscle actin.** Epithelial-mesenchymal transformations are an important part of renal development but have not been shown to be part of normal glomerular development. It is the presumed basis for the presence of α-smooth muscle actin in the obstructed kidney. It is bidirectional.

7. **b. depends on balanced activity of tissue inhibitors of metalloproteinases (TIMPs) and matrix metalloproteinases (MMPs).** Extracellular membrane (ECM) regulation is due to collagen synthesis rates as well as to the rate of ECM breakdown. The latter is determined by the balanced activities of the TIMPs and MMPs; these are regulated in part by transforming growth factor-β and the renin-angiotensin system.

8. **e. altered growth regulation, renal differentiation, and functional integration.** The key patterns defining congenital renal obstruction are altered growth regulation, renal differentiation, and functional integration, although interstitial fibrosis, tubular hypotrophy, and increased epithelial-mesenchymal transformation are components of these changes.

9. **c. are minimal in the absence of overt infection.** In contrast to acquired obstruction, congenital obstruction is not characterized by a significant inflammatory infiltrate, except when complicated by infection.

10. **d. is an important regulator of renal growth.** In the developing kidney, angiotensin is an important growth regulator, as well as mediator of fibrosis, and is altered significantly by obstruction. Fetal angiotensin acts predominantly through the angiotensin AT2 receptor until late in gestation when the AT1 receptor begins to exert a greater role.

Additional Study Points

1. A damaged kidney does not have the functional reserve to maintain normal renal function over time as the child grows. Thus, over time, the creatinine concentration will rise in patients who have no functional reserve in their nephron mass.

2. Obstructive processes may produce dysplasia.

3. In some cases, congenitally obstructed kidneys are smaller. This is not a result of atrophy but of hypoplasia.

4. A critical determinant of dysplasia in the kidney is complete obstruction early in gestation.

5. A universal characteristic of obstruction is renal fibrosis with infiltration of the interstitium with extracellular matrix.

6. It appears that nitric oxide regulates obstructive fibrosis and that increased amounts of nitric oxide reduce the degree of interstitial fibrosis.

7. Measures of urinary sodium, chloride, osmolality, and calcium correlate with fetal renal function. When these measures approach serum levels, irreversible damage is suggested.

8. The distinctness of the calyx is helpful in determining the functionality of the obstruction. Thus, no caliectasis suggests a mild to minimal degree of functional obstruction.

9. ^{99m}Tc-Mercaptoacetyltriglycine is generally used for diuretic renography. It is taken up and excreted by the renal tubules relatively rapidly with little glomerular filtration.

10. If the diuretic renogram shows a $t_{1/2}$ greater than 20 minutes, the kidney is presumed to be obstructed; if it is less than 10 minutes it is presumed normal; if it is between 10 and 20 minutes it is considered indeterminate.

11. Obstruction can be very harmful to the developing kidney far beyond that seen in the mature kidney. The effects of obstruction may be not be reversible owing to alterations in structure and function in the developing kidney that does not occur in the mature kidney.

12. When obstruction results in a growth impairment, the results are fewer nephron units and delayed nephron maturation.

13. Angiotensin appears to be a key modulator of the inflammatory response in ureteral obstruction.

14. Renal renin is increased in the obstructed kidney.

Perinatal Urology

Richard S. Lee, MD ● Joseph G. Borer, MD

QUESTIONS

1. A 34-week female fetus has normal amniotic fluid and unilateral upper pole hydroureteronephrosis with no evidence of an intravesical ureterocele. What does this most likely represent?
   a. Vesicoureteral reflux (VUR)
   b. Ureteropelvic junction obstruction
   c. Obstructed ectopic ureter
   d. Cloacal malformation
   e. None of the above

2. Which of the following statements are TRUE?
   a. Intermittent or varying degrees of hydronephrosis or a hydroureter is pathognomonic of VUR.
   b. VUR cannot be definitively diagnosed on prenatal ultrasound evaluation.
   c. Increasing degrees of hydronephrosis increase the risk of VUR.
   d. Decreasing degrees of hydronephrosis decrease the risk of VUR.
   e. None of the above

3. A 37-week-old fetus with a previously normal ultrasound examination has a newly diagnosed enlarged left kidney with loss of corticomedullary differentiation, echogenic streaks, branching hyperechoic vessels, and a calcified intramural inferior vena caval plaque. What is the most likely diagnosis?
   a. Renal artery thrombosis
   b. Renal vein thrombosis
   c. Congenital mesoblastic nephroma
   d. Autosomal-recessive polycystic kidney disease
   e. Wilms tumor

4. A 31-week male fetus has a thick-walled dilated bladder, dilated posterior urethra, unilateral severe hydroureteronephrosis, and late-onset oligohydramnios (>29 weeks). There are no other ultrasound findings. Serial bladder taps have been performed with the latest indices: sodium 90 mEq/L (previous 115 mEq/L), chloride 100 mEq/L (previous 120 mEq/L), and osmolality 190 mOsm/kg (previous 225 mOsm/kg). The next step is:
   a. early delivery at 31 weeks.
   b. early delivery after 32 weeks.

   c. in-utero urinary tract decompression with shunt.
   d. amnioinfusion with concomitant in-utero shunt placement.
   e. observation with delivery at term.

5. In which scenario is in-utero decompression by shunt most reasonable?
   a. Single male fetus with decreasing amniotic fluid after 28 weeks
   b. Single male fetus with severe bilateral renal cystic disease at 24 weeks
   c. Female fetus with bilateral echogenic kidneys, decompressed bladder volume, and oligohydramnios
   d. Single male fetus with severe hydronephrosis and oligohydramnios at 21 weeks
   e. A twin male fetus with severe hydronephrosis and oligohydramnios at 21 weeks and a normal twin

6. To best distinguish between severe unilateral hydronephrosis and a multicystic dysplastic kidney (MCDK), which of the following best represents an MCDK?
   a. Minimal or absent renal parenchyma
   b. Absence of a central large cyst
   c. Appearance of multiple noncommunicating cysts
   d. a, b, and c
   e. a and c

7. A 28-week fetus has bilaterally enlarged echogenic kidneys without renal cysts, hepatobiliary dilatation, and severe oligohydramnios. These findings suggest which diagnosis?
   a. Autosomal-recessive polycystic kidney disease
   b. Posterior urethral valves
   c. Bilateral MCDK
   d. Autosomal-dominant polycystic kidney disease
   e. Bilateral multilocular cystic nephroma

8. A 2-month-old male infant with an antenatal history of left moderate to severe hydronephrosis has a postnatal ultrasound evaluation at 24 hours of life demonstrating mild hydronephrosis. Follow-up ultrasonography at 2 months demonstrates left severe hydronephrosis. This can be explained by:
   a. intermittent changing hydronephrosis consistent with VUR.
   b. physiologic oliguria.

c. worsening obstruction.

d. ureterocele disproportion.

e. none of the above.

9. Prenatal imaging findings that are consistent with bladder exstrophy include all of the following EXCEPT:

a. absence of bladder filling documented on repetitive fetal imaging.

b. volume of amniotic fluid appropriate for fetal gestational age.

c. lower abdominal wall mass.

d. spinal cord or spinal column abnormality.

e. low-set umbilicus and inability to clearly visualize genitalia.

10. Cloacal exstrophy is most likely in the differential diagnosis when fetal ultrasonography and/or magnetic resonance imaging identify:

a. normal number, location, and anatomy of the kidneys.

b. omphalocele.

c. lower abdominal wall mass, absence of bladder filling on serial imaging, ectopic kidney, and spinal cord tethering.

d. 46,XY karyotype on amniocentesis and diminutive genitalia.

e. renal agenesis and contralateral hydronephrosis.

11. A 46,XX karyotype, cystic pelvic mass, bilateral hydroureteronephrosis, and the presence of ascites in a fetus are findings and characteristics most consistent with the diagnosis of:

a. cloacal exstrophy.

b. cloaca.

c. bladder exstrophy.

d. imperforate anus.

e. prune-belly syndrome.

12. Which of the following statement(s) regarding the identification of a solid renal mass on fetal imaging is/are FALSE?

a. When possible, delivery should be planned at a pediatric tertiary care center to avoid a potentially life-threatening condition in early neonatal life.

b. A solid renal mass identified in the fetus is most often consistent with a malignant tumor.

c. Prenatal identification of a renal mass warrants careful immediate postnatal monitoring of the neonate.

d. A solid renal mass in the fetus is a relatively common finding.

e. Both b and d

ANSWERS

1. **c. Obstructed ectopic ureter.** A duplication anomaly with upper pole hydroureteronephrosis is typically associated with a ureterocele, ectopic ureterocele, or an ectopic ureter causing obstruction. A dilated ureter is typically identified.

2. **b. VUR cannot be definitively diagnosed on prenatal ultrasound evaluation.** Previous studies have demonstrated that the degree of hydronephrosis does not correlate with the incidence of VUR.

3. **b. Renal vein thrombosis.** The ultrasound appearance of the kidney during renal vein thrombosis can be renal enlargement, loss of the corticomedullary differentiation, echogenic streaks, lack of definition of renal sinus echoes, and loss of venous flow in the affected kidney evident on Doppler imaging.

4. **e. observation with delivery at term.** Serial bladder sampling over 3 days has been used to help determine if the fetus is a viable candidate. The serial nature of the procedure allows one to see the subsequent trend of urine osmolality and electrolyte composition as a reflection of fetal kidney response. This fetus has encouraging urine electrolytes and only unilateral hydroureteronephrosis.

5. **d. Single male fetus with severe hydronephrosis and oligohydramnios at 21 weeks.** In-utero intervention is currently indicated when the fetus's life is at risk. In-utero decompression by shunting is only indicated in instances of presumed bladder obstruction in the setting of oligohydramnios. In-utero intervention in the case of a twin gestation may place the other fetus at risk and therefore is not recommended.

6. **d. a, b, and c.** The findings of multiple noncommunicating cysts, minimal or absent renal parenchyma, and the absence of a central large cyst are diagnostic of a multicystic dysplastic kidney.

7. **a. Autosomal-recessive polycystic kidney disease.** Bilaterally enlarged echogenic kidneys without renal cystic disease, particularly if associated with hepatobiliary dilatation or oligohydramnios, are suggestive of autosomal-recessive polycystic kidney disease.

8. **b. physiologic oliguria.** It is important to keep in mind that a postnatal ultrasound examination performed within the first 48 hours of life may not yet demonstrate hydronephrosis or may underestimate the degree of hydronephrosis secondary to physiologic oliguria.

9. **d. spinal cord or spinal column abnormality.** Ultrasound findings in a fetus with bladder exstrophy include nonvisualization of the fetal bladder, lower abdominal wall mass immediately inferior to a low-lying umbilicus, and diminutive genitalia. Other findings that may be evident to the experienced observer include normal kidneys in orthotopic position, normal vertebrae and spinal cord, abnormal symphyseal diastasis, and anteriorly displaced anus.

10. **c. lower abdominal wall mass, absence of bladder filling on serial imaging, ectopic kidney, and spinal cord tethering.** The prenatal diagnosis of cloacal exstrophy should be suspected with findings of nonvisualization of the bladder in association with a low-lying umbilicus, lower abdominal wall mass—typically omphalocele—and kidney (number, location, and/or appearance) and lumbosacral spine abnormalities.

11. **b. cloaca.** Persistent cloaca should be considered in any female fetus presenting with hydronephrosis and a large cystic mass arising from the pelvis.

12. **e. Both b and d.** Congenital mesoblastic nephroma is a rare benign congenital renal tumor and is the most common solid renal tumor in the neonatal period. Malignant tumors are rare. Delivery at a pediatric tertiary care center should be planned to avoid a potentially life-threatening condition in early neonatal life.

Additional Study Points

1. Oligohydramnios may be the result of urinary tract obstruction or poor renal function.
2. Inability to identify the bladder on repeat prenatal ultrasound studies should suggest the diagnosis of exstrophy.
3. Dilatation of the posterior urethra (keyhole sign) suggests posterior urethral valves.
4. Neural tube defects are diagnosed prenatally by α-fetoprotein and screening with ultrasonography.
5. Adrenal hemorrhage may appear as eggshell calcifications in contrast to the fine stippled calcifications of neuroblastoma.
6. An indication that renal function is salvageable is suggested by a fetal urine specimen in which the urinary sodium value is less than 100 mEq/L, the chloride value is less than 110 mEq/L, and the osmolality is less than 200 mOsm/kg.
7. Postnatal ultrasonography performed within the first 48 hours of life may not demonstrate hydronephrosis owing to decreased urine formation.
8. A dimercaptosuccinic acid scan is used for confirmation of the diagnosis when the ultrasound findings are not classic for multicystic dysplastic kidney—to differentiate it from cystic nephroma.

Evaluation of the Pediatric Urology Patient

Douglas A. Canning, MD ● Sarah M. Lambert, MD

QUESTIONS

1. Which one of the following patients does NOT need to be seen emergently?
   a. A newborn with hydronephrosis in a solitary kidney
   b. A 4-year-old boy with acute right scrotal pain
   c. A 12-year-old girl with microscopic hematuria during a routine examination
   d. An 8-year-old boy with sickle-cell anemia and a 5-hour history of priapism
   e. A male newborn with a distended bladder, bilateral hydronephrosis, and respiratory insufficiency

2. Which of the following is a potential complication of neonatal circumcision?
   a. Wound infection
   b. Meatal stenosis
   c. Death
   d. Penile curvature
   e. All of the above

3. The pediatric kidney is particularly susceptible to trauma due to:
   a. relatively increased renal size.
   b. limited visceral adipose tissue.
   c. limited chest wall protection.
   d. increased mobility.
   e. All of the above

4. The optimal timing of spinal ultrasonography during screening for occult spinal dysraphism is:
   a. after puberty.
   b. before 6 months of age.
   c. between 1 year and 6 years.
   d. none of the above.
   e. all of the above.

5. What is the most commonly detected etiology for asymptomatic microscopic hematuria in children?
   a. Fibroepithelial polyp
   b. Hypercalciuria
   c. Poststreptococcal glomerulonephritis
   d. Uncomplicated urinary tract infection
   e. Hyperuricosuria

6. Findings associated with the Beckwith-Wiedemann syndrome include:
   a. macroglossia.
   b. hepatosplenomegaly.
   c. nephromegaly.
   d. all of the above.
   e. only a and b.

7. A voiding cystourethrogram is essential in the diagnosis of which clinical conditions?
   a. Ureteropelvic junction obstruction
   b. Primary obstructive megaureter
   c. Posterior urethral valve
   d. Nephrolithiasis
   e. All of the above

8. When should a newborn with suspected congenital adrenal hyperplasia be tested?
   a. At the first well-baby visit
   b. Before discharge from the nursery
   c. No testing is required
   d. None of the above
   e. Both a and b

9. All of the following statements about the pediatric abdominal examination are true EXCEPT:
   a. renal pathology is the source of up to two thirds of neonatal abdominal masses.
   b. abdominal distention at birth or shortly afterward suggests either obstruction or perforation of the gastrointestinal tract.
   c. the abdominal wall is normally strong, especially in infants with hydronephrosis.
   d. a solid flank mass may be due to renal vein thrombosis.
   e. All of the above

10. Which of the following statements is TRUE about cutaneous markers of occult spinal dysraphism?
    a. Forty percent of patients with atypical presacral dimples have associated occult spinal dysraphism.

b. A combination of two or more congenital midline skin lesions is the strongest marker of occult spinal dysraphism.

c. An "atypical" presacral dimple, as defined, may indicate spina bifida or cord tethering, if the dimple is in the midline, less than 2.5 cm from the anal verge at birth, or shallower than 0.5 cm.

d. All of the above are true.

e. Both a and b are true.

11. Sexual abuse can be associated with which of the following physical examination findings?

a. Bruised vaginal mucosa in a prepubertal child

b. Penile discharge

c. A normal genital and perineal examination

d. a and c

e. a, b, and c

12. Urethral meatal stenosis occurs in the newborn:

a. as a result of birth trauma.

b. after urinary tract infection.

c. after a newborn physical examination.

d. after healing of the inflamed, denuded glans after circumcision.

e. from undergarment irritation.

13. In newborns with ambiguous genitalia, what does a symmetrical gonadal examination suggest?

a. Congenital adrenal hyperplasia or true hermaphroditism

b. Mixed gonadal dysgenesis or androgen insensitivity syndrome

c. Congenital adrenal hyperplasia or mixed gonadal dysgenesis

d. Congenital adrenal hyperplasia or androgen insensitivity syndrome

e. True hermaphroditism or mixed gonadal dysgenesis

14. Secondary urinary incontinence is defined as:

a. diurnal and nocturnal enuresis.

b. incontinence associated with urinary tract infection.

c. urinary incontinence associated with constipation.

d. urinary incontinence after a dry interval greater than 6 months.

e. urinary incontinence associated with a neurologic condition.

15. A newborn should have a hydrocele surgically corrected in the newborn period if:

a. it is large.

b. it is changing in volume.

c. it accompanies a symptomatic hernia.

d. a, b, and c.

e. b and c.

ANSWERS

1. **c. A 12-year-old girl with microscopic hematuria during a routine examination.** In the absence of other symptoms, microscopic hematuria in children is not an emergency. Bilateral hydronephrosis or hydronephrosis in a solitary kidney both represent emergencies and should be evaluated as soon as possible. Acute scrotal pain should always be considered testicular torsion until proven otherwise. Boys with sickle cell anemia are at increased risk for priapism and should always be treated immediately to decrease the long-term sequela associated with priapism.

2. **e. All of the above.** Wound infections, meatal stenosis, death, and removal of insufficient foreskin are all potential complications of neonatal circumcision.

3. **e. All of the above.** The pediatric kidney is particularly susceptible to trauma due to limited visceral adipose tissue, limited chest wall protection, relatively increased renal size, and increased mobility of the kidney.

4. **b. before 6 months of age.** Ossification of the posterior elements after 6 months of age prevents an acoustic ultrasound window. After 6 months, a spinal MRI is recommended when an occult spinal dysraphism is suspected.

5. **b. Hypercalciuria.** Most microscopic hematuria in children is transient and the source is not identified. The most commonly identified etiology of asymptomatic microhematuria in children is hypercalciuria.

6. **d. all of the above.** Beckwith-Wiedemann syndrome is caused by a mutation on chromosome 11p15.5. Clinical features include exomphalos, macroglossia, and gigantism in the neonate. Many of the affected infants have hypoglycemia in the first few days of life. Patients are at increased risk of developing specific tumors (e.g., adrenal carcinoma, Wilms tumors, hepatoblastoma, and rhabdomyosarcoma).

7. **c. Posterior urethral valve.** The diagnosis of posterior urethral valves requires visualization of the urethra during voiding. Bladder diverticula, a pronounced bladder neck, dilated posterior urethral, vesicoureteral reflux, and valve leaflets can all be associated with posterior urethral valves and are visible on voiding cystourethrogram. Ureteropelvic junction obstruction and primary obstructive megaureter are both obstructions above the level of the urethra and are usually evaluated with ultrasonography and a MAG3 renal scan or magnetic resonance urogram. Nephrolithiasis is typically evaluated using ultrasonography and CT scan when necessary.

8. **b. Before discharge from the nursery.** Congenital adrenal hyperplasia may result in salt wasting; therefore infants with ambiguous genitalia must be quickly evaluated and stabilized.

9. **c. the abdominal wall is normally strong, especially in infants with hydronephrosis.** Renal pathology accounts for approximately two thirds of abdominal masses found in the neonate. Solid masses include neuroblastoma, congenital mesoblastic nephroma, teratoma, and renal enlargement due to renal vein thrombosis. The abdominal wall is normally weak in premature infants and on occasion in those with hydronephrosis.

10. **e. Both a *and* b are true.** The lower back should be examined for any evidence of cutaneous markers of occult spinal dysraphisms that may account for abnormal bladder function. In a series of 207 neonates with sacral and presacral cutaneous stigmata, 40% of patients with atypical dimples were found to have occult spinal dysraphism. An "atypical" presacral dimple is defined as a dimple that is off center, more than 2.5 cm from the anal verge at birth, or deeper than 0.5 cm.

11. **e. a, b, *and* c.** Although penile discharge and bruised vaginal mucosa can reflect sexual abuse, the possibility of sexual abuse should not be dismissed in the absence of physical examination findings. Only 11% of girls evaluated in a sexual abuse clinic demonstrated suggestive physical examination findings.

12. **d. after healing of the inflamed, denuded glans after circumcision.** Meatal stenosis is common after circumcision. It may result from contraction of the meatus after healing of the inflamed, denuded glans tissue that occurs after retraction of the foreskin or from damage to the frenular artery at the time of circumcision.

13. **d. Congenital adrenal hyperplasia or androgen insensitivity syndrome.** Particular attention to the symmetry of the examination is important if a disorder of sexual differentiation is thought to exist. A symmetrical gonadal examination (gonads palpable on each side or impalpable on both sides) suggests a global disorder, such as congenital adrenal hyperplasia or androgen insensitivity.

14. **d. urinary incontinence after a dry interval greater than 6 months.** Although urinary incontinence can be associated with infection, constipation, and neurologic disease, secondary urinary incontinence is defined as occurring after a dry interval greater than 6 months.

15. **e. b *and* c.** A hydrocele that changes in volume suggests a patent processus vaginalis. These infants are at risk for an inguinal hernia. The processus vaginalis is not likely to close after birth. If a hernia has been symptomatic, it should be corrected in the newborn period.

Additional Study Points

1. The most common malignant abdominal tumor in infants is a neuroblastoma, followed by Wilms tumor.

2. Very few undescended testes will descend after 3 months of age.

3. The most common prepubertal testicular tumor is teratoma, followed by rhabdomyosarcoma, epidermoid cyst, yoke sac tumor, and germ cell tumor, in that order.

4. Very few children hold the urine and not the stool. Conversely, children who retain stool nearly always retain urine.

5. Gross hematuria in the newborn is an emergency, because it may indicate renal vein thrombosis or renal artery thrombosis.

6. In general, blunt renal trauma is treated nonoperatively, except when there is a major vascular avulsion or extensive urinary extravasation.

7. In the newborn, the foreskin is adherent to the glans, and adhesions should not be separated unless a circumcision is performed.

8. A positive dip stick for blood requires a microscopic examination. Absence of red blood cells in the microscopic examination indicates hemoglobinuria or myoglobinuria.

Infection and Inflammation of the Pediatric Genitourinary Tract

Linda Marie Dairiki Shortliffe, MD

QUESTIONS

1. Boys have more urinary tract infections (UTIs) than girls:
   a. during the first year of life.
   b. when they become sexually active.
   c. during elementary school years.
   d. if they are uncircumcised toddlers.
   e. at puberty.

2. Characteristics of bacteria more likely to infect the kidney include:
   a. growth in mannose.
   b. hemolysis.
   c. P fimbriae.
   d. KOH staining.
   e. urease production.

3. Intracellular bacterial pods may allow microbial adaptation and protection through:
   a. uroplakins.
   b. bacterial clonal genes.
   c. Toll-like receptors.
   d. the Tamm-Horsfall protein.
   e. biofilms.

4. Risk factors for recurrent UTI in young women include:
   a. age at first UTI and UTI in mother.
   b. other congenital abnormalities.
   c. vesicoureteral reflux.
   d. recent antimicrobial usage.
   e. encopresis and voiding history.

5. Incidence of vesicoureteral reflux differs by:
   a. circumcision status.
   b. ethnicity or race.
   c. gene polymorphisms.
   d. bacterial colonization.
   e. blood group antigen.

6. The best urinary indicators of infection on urinalysis are positive:
   a. pyuria, leukocyte esterase, and catalase.
   b. nitrite, microscopic red blood cell (RBC) and white blood cell (WBC) casts.
   c. glitter cells in spun urine.
   d. microscopic bacteria, leukocyte esterase, and nitrite.
   e. Gram stain and nitrite.

7. A source of bacterial persistence is:
   a. sexual activity.
   b. prepuce.
   c. struvite calculus.
   d. fecal colonization.
   e. increased postvoid residual.

8. A radiologic finding of pyelonephritis is:
   a. a hot spot on a ^{99m}Tc-dimercaptosuccinic acid (DMSA) nuclear renogram.
   b. a focal renal wedge lesion on intravenous pyelogram.
   c. hypoechogenicity on renal ultrasonography.
   d. ureteral dilation.
   e. renal pelvic debris.

9. Renal scarring in association with vesicoureteral reflux is caused by:
   a. the "water hammer" effect of vesicoureteral reflux.
   b. intrarenal reflux with pyelotubular backflow.
   c. bacteriuria and vesicoureteral reflux.
   d. compound calyces.
   e. elevated bladder pressure.

10. In children, the likelihood of renal scarring correlates with:
    a. the number of occurrences of UTI.
    b. the severity of fever.
    c. intrapelvic pressure.
    d. renal dysplasia.
    e. the duration of vesicoureteral reflux.

11. Nocturnal enuresis accompanies recurrent UTIs in children, and:
    a. treatment is associated with decreased UTIs.
    b. these are independent findings.
    c. vesicoureteral reflux may be involved.
    d. both findings are likely to resolve spontaneously by puberty.
    e. dysfunctional voiding is likely.

12. Increased periurethral bacterial colonization is present:
    a. in children who experience recurrent UTIs.
    b. on the foreskin of boys age 5 and older.
    c. when children are constipated.
    d. during antimicrobial therapy.
    e. in children with vesicoureteral reflux.

13. During pregnancy what is more likely to occur?
    a. UTIs
    b. Renal scarring
    c. Bacteriuria progressing to pyelonephritis
    d. Vesicoureteral reflux
    e. Asymptomatic bacteriuria

14. During pregnancy, females who have had surgically corrected vesicoureteral reflux for breakthrough UTIs:
    a. will be protected from UTIs.
    b. do not need urinary tract antimicrobial prophylaxis.
    c. do not have accelerated renal insufficiency.
    d. do need the urine screened for bacteriuria.
    e. risk increased fetal complications.

15. Evaluation and management of the first UTI in a 2-year-old child should include:
    a. a DMSA scan.
    b. parenteral antimicrobial agents.
    c. a WBC count and nitrite test.
    d. an erythrocyte sedimentation rate (ESR) and creatinine test.
    e. prophylactic antimicrobial agents until imaging is performed.

16. When a child does not appear to improve after 2 to 3 days of appropriate antimicrobial therapy for the first UTI, one should:
    a. perform a DMSA scan.
    b. obtain a complete blood count (CBC) and blood cultures.
    c. perform renal and bladder ultrasonography.
    d. perform voiding cystourethrography.
    e. change antimicrobial therapy.

17. A characteristic sign of mature renal scarring on a DMSA renogram is:
    a. focal circular area of diminished uptake.
    b. diffuse renal enlargement.
    c. wedged-shaped areas of increased uptake.
    d. polar areas of diminished uptake.
    e. areas of increased focal cortical activity.

18. When an asymptomatic UTI is diagnosed:
    a. it should be treated to prevent recurrence.
    b. about a third clear spontaneously.
    c. the infecting bacteria commonly have P pili.
    d. imaging evaluation is not needed unless it is the second UTI.
    e. monthly urinary specimens are needed to check for UTI.

19. Appropriate treatment of children with UTI includes:
    a. follow-up culture after 48 hours.
    b. hospitalization of all infants younger than age 6 months.
    c. single-dose oral treatment for most school-age children.
    d. "switch" therapy for febrile children with UTI.
    e. radiologic evaluation after the second febrile UTI.

20. In a 6-year-old girl with recurrent UTIs, occasional diurnal incontinence, and normal genitourinary tract by renal and bladder ultrasonography and voiding cystourethrogram:
    a. monthly screening cultures should be performed.
    b. annual renal and bladder ultrasonography is warranted.
    c. urodynamics should be performed.
    d. constipation should be suspected.
    e. daily perineal hygiene should be initiated.

21. Good practice to lower incidence of surgical site infections includes all of the following EXCEPT:
    a. short hospitalization.
    b. preoperative antimicrobial agents 3 hours before all open operations.
    c. bowel preparation before bowel surgery with mechanical preparation and nonabsorbable oral and intravenous antibiotics.
    d. clipping hair in the operating room if hair needs removal.
    e. vancomycin 120 minutes before surgery when required because of allergies.

22. An 8-year-old boy recovering from a bone marrow transplant has frequency, urgency, and dysuria with hematuria and is treated for a UTI. The cultures return in 48 hours and show no growth, so the antimicrobial treatment is stopped, but the symptoms continue. The next step should be to:
    a. perform renal arteriography.
    b. perform cystoscopy.
    c. give interferon and acyclovir.
    d. reculture urine.
    e. perform renal and bladder ultrasonography and voiding cystourethrography.

23. A 12-year-old boy is explored for possible testicular torsion, but epididymitis is found, and urine cultures show no growth. The next step should be:
    a. antimicrobial treatment, renal and bladder ultrasonography, and voiding cystourethrogram.
    b. antimicrobial treatment and testicular color flow Doppler ultrasonography in 3 months.
    c. no further treatment.
    d. an intravenous pyelogram.
    e. a testicular biopsy, special cultures, and ultrasonography of the testes.

24. After 10 days of urethral catheter drainage, the urine from a 5-year-old child with multiple traumatic injuries grows 10,000 CFU/mL of *Candida glabrata*. The next step is to:
    a. give parenteral amphotericin before catheter removal.
    b. change the catheter.
    c. give intravesical amphotericin irrigation before catheter removal.
    d. change the indwelling catheter and alkalinize the urine.
    e. perform renal and bladder ultrasonography.

25. After an acute UTI, when selecting a drug for low-dose urinary tract antimicrobial prophylaxis:
    a. the same drug that was used for treatment should be optimal.
    b. serum concentrations of drug should be high.
    c. urinary excretion should be rapid.
    d. there should be minimal effect on the fecal flora.
    e. drug dosage should be higher for the first few weeks.

26. Nitrofurantoin is useful for treating recurrent UTIs because it:
    a. has high serum and tissue concentrating levels.
    b. has a hemolytic effect.
    c. affects the bacterial biofilm.
    d. diffuses into the vagina and decreases bacterial colonization.
    e. has lower systemic absorption and may generate less microbial resistance.

27. In CT evaluation of a possible renal abscess:
    a. cortical attenuation is diagnostic.
    b. striations are characteristic.
    c. delayed renal views 2 to 3 hours later may be needed.
    d. wedge defects are helpful.
    e. vascular phase is most important.

ANSWERS

1. **a. during the first year of life.** Only during the first year of life do males get more UTIs than females, and during that period, uncircumcised boys have up to 10 times the risk of circumcised boys of having a UTI.

2. **c. P fimbriae.** Two important markers for *Escherichia coli* virulence are mannose-resistant hemagglutination (MRHA) characteristics and P blood group–specific adhesins (P fimbriae or P pili).

3. **e. biofilms.** Biofilms appear to allow microbial adaptation to variable environments and then allow aggregate detachment that will cause systemic infection, antimicrobial resistance by plasmid exchange, endotoxin production, and overall increased resistance to host immune systems.

4. **a. age at first UTI and UTI in mother.** Two distinct risks for recurrent UTI in young women (age 18 to 30 years) are age at first UTI (<age 15; odds ratio [OR] = 3.9) and UTI in the mother (OR = 2.3).

5. **b. ethnicity or race.** Several studies show that African Americans have fewer UTIs, lower incidence of vesicoureteral reflux, and perhaps less likelihood of reflux nephropathy than Hispanics or whites.

6. **d. microscopic bacteria, leukocyte esterase, and nitrite.** The combination of positive leukocyte esterase and nitrite testing and microscopic confirmation of bacteria has almost 100% sensitivity for detection of UTI, and when all (or leukocyte esterase and nitrite tests) are negative, the negative predictive value approaches 100%.

7. **c. struvite calculus.** Sources of urinary tract bacterial persistence are usually found early in children, because imaging is performed after the first UTI. The discovery of surgically correctable sources of bacterial persistence is obviously important. The majority of recurrent UTI is, however, reinfection with the same or a different organism that ascends from the bowel and is not surgically correctable.

8. **d. ureteral dilation.** Focal or general renal enlargement or swollen kidneys may be found in acute pyelonephritis; other findings on ultrasonography include thickening of the renal pelvis, hypoechogenicity, focal or diffuse hyperechogenicity, and ureteral dilation.

9. **c. bacteriuria and vesicoureteral reflux.** Renal scarring in association with vesicoureteral reflux occurs when bacteriuria is present.

10. **a. the number of occurrences of UTI.** The likelihood of renal scarring directly correlates, moreover, with the number of UTI occurrences.

11. **b. these are independent findings.** Epidemiologic investigations show monosymptomatic nocturnal enuresis is unassociated with UTI, but diurnal enuresis or a combination of diurnal and nocturnal enuresis, even if as infrequent as once a week, may be associated with pediatric UTI.

12. **a. in children who experience recurrent UTIs.** Women and children who suffer repeated UTIs remain more colonized by periurethral gram-negative bacteria than those who do not. Times and conditions of increased periurethral colonization are, therefore, associated with increased risk of UTI.

13. **c. bacteriuria progressing to pyelonephritis.** The likelihood that the bacteriuria may progress to pyelonephritis is greatly increased. Thirteen and a half to 65% of pregnant women who are bacteriuric on a screening urinary culture will develop subsequent pyelonephritis during pregnancy if untreated, whereas pyelonephritis is rarely the consequence of uncomplicated cystitis in a nonpregnant woman.

14. **d. do need the urine screened for bacteriuria.** If vesicoureteral reflux is surgically corrected, these patients should not be assured that pyelonephritis during pregnancy is impossible or even unlikely. The urine of these pregnant women must still be screened routinely for bacteriuria.

15. **e. prophylactic antimicrobial agents until imaging is performed.** After the therapeutic regimen for acute UTI, the child should be started on a daily prophylactic antimicrobial agent until full radiologic evaluation of the urinary tract may be conveniently performed in the next days to weeks.

16. **c. perform renal and bladder ultrasonography.** Early urinary tract imaging is important in a seriously ill and/or febrile child in whom the site of infection is unclear or who has unusual circumstances. Circumstances include newly diagnosed azotemia or a poor response to appropriate antimicrobial drugs after 3 to 4 days.

17. **d. polar areas of diminished uptake.** Later, after the acute episode heals, scans will show (1) a normal pattern, (2) generally diminished uptake and small kidney volume, (3) diminished uptake in the medial kidney, or (4) polar defects with diminished uptake in the renal poles.

18. **b. about a third clear spontaneously.** A majority of infants who have covert bacteriuria may clear their bacteriuria without treatment; others state that only about 30% of asymptomatic school-age girls with asymptomatic UTI clear spontaneously without treatment.

19. **d. "switch" therapy for febrile children with UTI.** A large series of children from 3 months to 5 years had successful treatment of febrile UTI with intravenous gentamicin (5 mg/kg/day once daily) until afebrile (2 to 4 days), given in a day treatment center of a tertiary-care

hospital, followed by an oral antibiotic for a total of 10 days.

20. **d. constipation should be suspected.** Girls with recurrent UTI are more likely to have a family history of UTI, infrequent voiding, poor fluid intake, and stool retention.

21. **b. preoperative antimicrobial agents 3 hours before open operations.** The most recent published Centers for Disease Control and Prevention (CDC) guidelines that are related to surgical-site infections were published in 1999 and summarized by Nichols (2001).* None of the guidelines is specific for children or includes genitourinary operations. The CDC recommends (1) not removing hair unless it will interfere with the operation and, if removed, clipping immediately before operation; (2) identifying and treating all remote infections; (3) maintaining as short a hospitalization as possible; (4) administering antimicrobial agents only when indicated, based on published recommendations for a specific operation; (5) administering antimicrobial agents intravenously to ensure bactericidal serum and tissue levels when the incision is made (60 minutes beforehand with most agents and 120 minutes beforehand with vancomycin) and maintaining these levels for a few hours after closure, with discontinuation no later than 24 hours after surgery, even if drainage catheters are left in place; (6) preparing bowel for elective operations with mechanical bowel preparation, including enemas and cathartic agents and nonabsorbable oral antimicrobial agents the day before surgery in addition to the intravenous drugs; and (7) withholding routine vancomycin usage.

22. **c. give interferon and acyclovir.** The BK virus, a DNA virus of the polyomavirus genus, has been found in the urine of bone marrow transplantation, and other immunosuppressed patients having hemorrhagic cystitis (2 weeks to 5 months after transplantation), causing both

symptomatic (hematuria and dysuria) and asymptomatic infections.

23. **a. antimicrobial treatment, renal and bladder ultrasonography, and voiding cystourethrogram.** During or after treatment of the acute bacterial urinary and epididymal infections, radiologic evaluation of the urinary tract should be performed, as with any UTI. In young boys and infants, epididymitis is more likely to be related to genitourinary abnormalities (abnormal connections) or systemic hematogenous dissemination than in older males. Urethral and urinary cultures from the prepubertal male are likely to show either nothing or gram-negative organisms and thus be referred to as "nonspecific epididymitis," whereas in the postpubertal sexually active boys, the cause may involve sexually transmitted organisms (*Neisseria gonorrhoeae, Chlamydia trachomatis*).

24. **c. give intravesical amphotericin irrigation before catheter removal.** Although stopping unnecessary antimicrobial agents, changing or removing the indwelling catheter, and urinary alkalinization may be helpful, these means do not clear many cases of funguria. Recent prospective studies with intravesical amphotericin B bladder irrigation and oral fluconazole appear to show that both may clear funguria, although fungal recurrences are common.

25. **d. there should be minimal effect on the fecal flora.** The ideal prophylactic agent should have low serum and high urinary concentrations, have minimal effect on the normal fecal flora, be easily administered and tolerated, and be cost effective.

26. **e. has lower systemic absorption and may generate less microbial resistance.** Nitrofurantoin is an effective urinary prophylactic agent because its serum levels are low, its urinary levels are high, and it produces minimal effect on the fecal flora.

27. **c. delayed renal views 2 to 3 hours later may be needed.** Scans delayed 3 or more hours may help in differentiating renal abscess from hypofunctioning parenchyma in severe pyelonephritis.

---

*Sources referenced can be found in *Campbell-Walsh Urology, 10th Edition,* on the Expert Consult website.

Additional Study Points

1. Urinary tract infections cause abnormally elevated renal pelvic pressures.
2. Clinical symptoms correlate poorly with bacterial localization in the urinary tract.
3. Microbial lipopolysaccharides trigger urothelial receptors (Toll-like receptors) to activate the innate local immune system, activating cytokines, chemokines, and neutrophils.
4. For children, when performing intermittent catheterization, neither sterile nor single-use lubricated catheters, or antimicrobial prophylaxis, are recommended.
5. In teenage females, sexually transmitted infections may progress to pelvic inflammatory disease, infertility, and result in chronic pelvic pain.
6. Suprapubic bladder aspiration is the most reliable method of determining whether a urinary tract infection is present.
7. Elevated C-reactive protein has been associated with serious bacterial infections in children.
8. Children with glucose-6-phosphate dehydrogenase deficiency should not be given nitrofurantoin.
9. Children with gross polynephritic nephropathy (reflux nephropathy) have a 10% to 20% risk of hypertension.
10. Significant proteinuria is a routine finding in patients with vesicoureteral reflux who have progressive deterioration of renal function.
11. Adenovirus is the most common cause of acute viral hemorrhagic cystitis in children.
12. Any catheter that has been left in place for more than 4 days will result in infected urine.

Anomalies of the Upper Urinary Tract

Ellen Shapiro, MD ● Stuart B. Bauer, MD ● Jeanne S. Chow, MD

QUESTIONS

1. During a left inguinal herniorrhaphy, the vas was absent, and a 3-mm golden yellow nodule was found along the spermatic cord. This boy may also have:
   a. a left appendage epididymis.
   b. left renal agenesis.
   c. a malpositioned left adrenal gland.
   d. an absent left head of epididymis.
   e. an absent left testis.

2. A 14-year-old girl with abdominal pain undergoes abdominal and pelvic ultrasonography. A solitary right kidney is seen. Her abdominal pain is most likely associated with:
   a. skeletal anomalies.
   b. a unicornuate uterus.
   c. an imperforate hymen.
   d. a didelphic uterus.
   e. an absent left ovary.

3. A 27-year-old man has infertility. Pelvic ultrasonography reveals a right pelvic kidney and a left orthotopic kidney. The most likely cause of his infertility is:
   a. an absence of the right vas.
   b. a history of bilateral cryptorchidism.
   a. an absence of the mid and lower pole of the right epididymis.
   b. dysplasia of the right testis.
   e. a subcornonal hypospadias.

4. The renal segment with the most variable blood supply is the:
   a. apex.
   b. upper.
   c. middle.
   d. lower.
   e. posterior.

5. A 29-year-old hypertensive woman was found to have a 2.7 cm renal artery aneurysm. Excision is recommended:
   a. if the aneurysm increases in size to 3 cm.
   b. when the woman is no longer of child-bearing age.
   c. at this time.

   d. if there is no arteriovenous (A-V) fistula.
   e. when the hypertension is well controlled.

6. A 5-year-old girl with a pelvic kidney has hydronephrosis most commonly due to:
   a. vesicoureteral reflux.
   b. malrotation.
   c. ureterovesical junction obstruction.
   d. ureteropelvic junction obstruction.
   e. ectopic ureter.

7. A newborn girl was noted prenatally to have coarctation of the aorta and a horseshoe kidney. The next step is:
   a. a voiding cystourethrogram.
   b. magnetic resonance urography (MRU) with gadolinium.
   c. an echocardiogram.
   d. to obtain a karyotype.
   e. a skeletal series.

8. Unilateral renal agenesis is commonly associated with the:
   a. normal position of the splenic flexure.
   b. normal position of the adrenal gland.
   c. ipsilateral undescended testis.
   d. normal position of the hepatic flexure.
   e. rudimentary uterus.

9. Bilateral renal agenesis is associated with mutations of:
   a. *GFRα1*.
   b. *GDNF*.
   c. *RET*.
   d. *WNT*.
   e. *Pax2*.

10. Unilateral renal agenesis can be reliably diagnosed by finding:
    a. a single umbilical artery.
    b. preauricular skin tag(s).
    c. an imperforate hymen.
    d. absence of renal artery at L1-L2.
    e. specific radiographic evidence.

11. Male predominance of occurrence is most striking in:
    a. unilateral renal agenesis.
    b. bilateral renal agenesis.

c. crossed fused ectopia.

d. ectopic kidney.

e. calyceal diverticulum.

12. The incidence of unilateral renal agenesis is:

   a. 1 : 2500.

   b. 1 : 4000.

   c. 1 : 1100.

   d. 1 : 5000.

   e. 1 : 500.

13. Unilateral renal agenesis and a unicornuate uterus will form when the embryologic insult occurs at which gestational time?

   a. Before the 4th week

   b. At the start of the 4th week

   c. At the end of the 4th week

   d. At the start of the 5th week

   e. At the end of the 5th week

14. In autopsy studies, unilateral renal agenesis was found in association with:

   a. an absence of the gonad.

   b. a normally developed ureter.

   c. an ectopic ureteral orifice.

   d. adrenal agenesis.

   e. an absence of the head of the epididymis.

15. Most ectopic kidneys are clinically asymptomatic EXCEPT:

   a. pelvic kidneys.

   b. thoracic kidneys.

   c. kidneys with ectopic ureters.

   d. lumbar kidneys.

   e. abdominal kidneys.

16. The isthmus of a horseshoe kidney is located adjacent to which vertebrae?

   a. T12 and L1

   b. L1 and L2

   c. L3 and L4

   d. L5 and S1

   e. S1 and S2

17. Between the 6th and 9th week, normal rotation of the kidney toward the midline to attain its orthotopic position involves:

   a. 60 degrees of lateral rotation.

   b. 90 degrees of lateral rotation.

   c. 180 degrees of lateral rotation.

   d. 90 degrees of medial rotation.

   e. 180 degrees of medial rotation.

18. Congenital renal arteriovenous fistulas are:

   a. usually bilateral.

   b. cirsoid in configuration.

   c. symptomatic before the 3rd decade.

   d. more common in males.

   e. usually located in the lower pole.

19. Bilateral megacalycosis:

   a. occurs more frequently in females.

   b. has an increased number of dilated calyces.

   c. is associated with ureteral dilation.

   d. is autosomal recessive in inheritance pattern.

   e. shows an obstructive pattern on renal scan.

ANSWERS

1. **b. left renal agenesis.** The finding of a 3-mm golden yellow nodule is indicative of ectopic adrenal tissue. The absent vas should raise a red flag for possible ipsilateral renal agenesis, because the ureteral bud and vas are both derived from the wolffian duct. In one study, 79% of adult males with an absence of the vas deferens have an absent ipsilateral kidney with left-sided lesions predominating. The lower pole and midpole of the epididymis are wolffian duct derivatives. The head of the epididymis is derived from the mesonephric tubules that link the mesonephric or wolffian duct with the gonad.

2. **d. didelphic uterus.** Unilateral renal agenesis can be associated with didelphic uterus and obstruction of the ipsilateral vagina, resulting in hydrocolpos. This would likely explain this girl's abdominal pain.

3. **b. a history of bilateral cryptorchidism.** This man's infertility is most likely due to a history of bilateral cryptorchidism. An ipsilateral absent vas, abnormal epididymis, or a unilateral dysplastic gonad would not lead to infertility because a normal contralateral testis is present in those situations. Bilateral cryptorchidism has been associated with infertility.

4. **a. apex.** The vessel to the apical segment has the greatest variation in origin; it arises from (1) the anterior division (43%), (2) the junction of the anterior and posterior divisions (23%), (3) the main stem renal artery or aorta (23%), or (4) the posterior division of the main renal artery (10%).

5. **c. at this time.** Generally, excision is recommended if (1) the hypertension cannot be easily controlled; (2) incomplete ringlike calcification is present; (3) the aneurysm is larger than 2.5 cm; (4) the patient is female and of child-bearing age, because rupture during pregnancy is a possibility; (5) the aneurysm increases in size on serial angiograms; or (6) an arteriovenous fistula is present.

6. **d. ureteropelvic junction obstruction.** The renal pelvis is usually anterior (instead of medial) to the parenchyma, because the kidney has incompletely rotated. As a result, 56% of ectopic kidneys have a hydronephrotic collecting system. Half of these cases are due to obstruction of the ureteropelvic or the ureterovesical junction (70% and 30%, respectively), 25% from reflux grade III or greater, and 25% from the malrotation alone.

7. **d. to obtain a karyotype.** Horseshoe kidney and coarctation of the aorta are seen in patients with Turner syndrome (45,X). Therefore a karyotype should be obtained. Other stigmata may include lymphedema, shield chest, low hairline, and webbed neck.

8. **b. normal position of the adrenal gland.** Unilateral renal agenesis is commonly associated with an adrenal gland that is in a normal position, although it may be flattened. Regardless of sex, both gonads are usually normal. The most common müllerian duct anomalies are a true unicornuate uterus with complete absence of the ipsilateral

horn and fallopian tube or a bicornuate uterus with rudimentary development of the horn on the affected side. A plain film of the abdomen showing the gas pattern of the splenic flexure in the left renal fossa suggests left renal agenesis, ectopia, or crossed ectopia, whereas the gas pattern of the hepatic flexure positioned in the right renal fossa suggests congenital absence of the right kidney.

9. **c. *RET*.** The association between abnormal kidney development and mutations of *RET*, *GDNF*, and *GFRα1* in 29 stillborn fetuses with bilateral renal agenesis (BRA) or unilateral renal agenesis (URA). Mutations in *RET* were found in 7 of 19 fetuses with BRA and 2 of 10 fetuses with URA. A mutation in *GDNF* was found in only 1 fetus with URA who also had mutations in *RET*. No *GFRα1* mutations were observed. These data suggest that congenital renal agenesis results from *RET* mutations that prevent or impede the embryonic development of RET-dependent structures.

10. **e. specific radiographic evidence.** Unilateral renal agenesis can be diagnosed reliably with a combination of radiographic examinations, including a plain film of the abdomen, abdominal and pelvic ultrasonography, dimercaptosuccinic acid (DMSA) scan, and/or magnetic resonance angiography (MRA).

11. **b. bilateral renal agenesis.** Male predominance is most striking in bilateral renal agenesis, with almost 75% of individuals being male. For unilateral renal agenesis, there is a male to female ratio of 1.8:1. Crossed fused ectopia has a slight male predominance (3:2), while ectopic kidneys have no significant difference between the sexes in incidence.

12. **c. 1:1100.** The incidence of unilateral renal agenesis is 1:1100.

13. **a. Before the 4th week.** Unilateral renal agenesis and a unicornuate uterus will form when the embryologic insult occurs before the 4th week. If the insult occurs early in the 4th week of gestation and affects both the wolffian duct and the ureteral bud, maldevelopment of the wolffian duct affects renal development, müllerian duct elongation, contact with the urogenital sinus, and subsequent fusion. Therefore a didelphic uterus will form with obstruction of the horn and vagina on the side of the unilateral renal agenesis. If the insult occurs after the 4th week and the wolffian duct and müllerian duct elongation and differentiation proceed normally, and only the ureteral bud

and metanephric blastema are affected, thereby resulting in isolated unilateral renal agenesis.

14. **d. adrenal agenesis.** In autopsy studies of unilateral renal agenesis, adrenal agenesis occurs in fewer than 10%, although the ipsilateral adrenal gland may be flattened. The ureter is not normally developed, and the ipsilateral ureter is completely absent in about 60% of the cases. The gonad is usually normal in both sexes. The head of the epididymis is normally formed, because it is derived from the mesonephric tubules that link the mesonephric duct to the gonad.

15. **c. kidneys with ectopic ureters.** Most ectopic kidneys are clinically asymptomatic, except for the unusual cases of an ectopic kidney with an ectopic ureter.

16. **c. L3 and L4.** The isthmus of a horseshoe kidney is located adjacent to the L3 and L4 vertebrae.

17. **d. 90 degrees of medial rotation.** Between the 6th and 9th week, normal rotation of the kidney toward the midline to attain its orthotopic position involves 90 degrees of medial rotation.

18. **b. cirsoid in configuration.** Fewer than 25% of all renal arteriovenous fistulas (AVFs) are congenital. They are identifiable by their cirsoid configuration and multiple communications between the main or segmental renal arteries and venous channels. Although congenital, they rarely present clinically before the third or fourth decade. Women are affected three times as often as men, and the right kidney is involved slightly more often than the left. The lesion is usually located in the upper pole (45% of cases), but, not infrequently, it may be found in the midportion (30%) or in the lower pole (25%) of the kidney.

19. **b. has an increased number of dilated calyces.** Megacalycosis is defined as a nonobstructive enlargement of calyces resulting from malformation of the renal papillae. The calyces are generally dilated and malformed and may be increased in number. The renal pelvis is not dilated, nor is its wall thickened, and the ureteropelvic junction (UPJ) is normally funneled without evidence of obstruction. The ureter is usually normal. It occurs predominantly in males in a ratio of 6:1. Bilateral disease has been seen almost exclusively in males, whereas segmental unilateral involvement occurs only in females.

Additional Study Points

1. In bilateral renal agenesis, 40% of the affected infants are stillborn. The ureters are almost always absent, and the bladder is either absent or hypoplastic. The adrenal glands, however, are usually in their normal anatomic position.

2. In patients with bilateral renal agenesis associated with oligohydramnios, Potter fascies are pathognomonic of the process. Pulmonary hypoplasia is frequently present.

3. A single umbilical artery has been associated with renal anomalies.

4. In unilateral renal agenesis, the ipsilateral ureter is completely absent in 60% of the cases. Abnormalities of the contralateral ureter are not uncommon; reproductive tract anomalies in females are also common.

5. With unilateral renal agenesis, one quarter of the contralateral ureters reflux.

6. There is an association of genital anomalies with renal ectopia. The upper pole of the ectopic kidney usually joins with the lower pole of the normal kidney.

7. In all types of fusion anomalies, the ureter from each kidney is usually orthotopic.

8. The highest incidence of associated anomalies occurs with solitary renal ectopia. Associated anomalies in the male include cryptorchidism and vaginal atresia or unilateral uterine anomalies in the female.

9. In a horseshoe kidney, the isthmus is bulky and consists of parenchymatous tissue with its own blood supply.

10. The blood supply to a horseshoe kidney is variable.
11. UPJ obstruction in horseshoe kidneys occurs one third of the time.
12. The incidence of Wilms tumors in horseshoe kidneys is higher than would be expected in the general population.
13. Renal arteries are end arteries and, as such, have no collaterals.
14. Arteriovenous fistulas may result in hypertension in 50% of cases, due to relative ischemia beyond the fistula. It is renin-mediated hypertension.
15. Infundibulopelvic stenosis is usually bilateral and commonly associated with vesicoureteral reflux.

chapter 118

Renal Dysgenesis and Cystic Disease of the Kidney

John C. Pope IV, MD

QUESTIONS

1. Which of the following is a correct match?
   a. von Hippel-Lindau disease and adenoma sebaceum
   b. Tuberous sclerosis and angiomyolipoma
   c. Autosomal dominant polycystic kidney disease (ADPKD) and salt-losing nephropathy
   d. Congenital nephrosis (Finnish type) and medullary cysts
   e. Autosomal recessive polycystic kidney disease (ARPKD) and colonic diverticulosis

2. The primary feature(s) associated with Ask-Upmark Kidney (segmental hypoplasia) is/are:
   a. hypertension.
   b. renal artery intimal disease.
   c. found in young men and boys.
   d. b and c.
   e. a and c.

3. The development of acquired renal cystic disease (ARCD) is most related to which factor?
   a. Age of the patient
   b. Duration of renal failure
   c. Recent initiation of hemodialysis
   d. *Escherichia coli* infection
   e. Genetic defect on chromosome 16

4. Which statement(s) about ARPKD is/are TRUE?
   a. The most severe forms develop later in childhood or adolescence.
   b. No matter the severity of the renal disease, all patients will have liver involvement in the form of congenital hepatic fibrosis.
   c. In newborns, ultrasound findings include very enlarged kidneys with increased parenchymal echogenicity.
   d. a and b
   e. b and c

5. Which of the following statements accurately describes a fundamental process essential for the development of renal cysts?
   a. Proliferation of epithelial cells in segments of the renal collecting system

   b. Accumulation of fluid within an expanding segment of the glomerulus
   c. An imbalance of the secretory and absorptive properties in proliferating tubular epithelial cells
   d. Hypertrophy of the basement membrane within the ascending loop of Henle
   e. Glomerular outpouching resulting from elevated glomerular hydrostatic pressure

6. Which of the following statement(s) is/are correct about ADPKD?
   a. The genetic defect is located on the short arm of chromosome 16.
   b. Most affected infants have congenital hepatic fibrosis.
   c. Renal cysts are infrequently seen on ultrasonographic scans of affected patients before 30 years of age.
   d. Glomerular cysts are never found in the kidneys of newborns diagnosed with ADPKD.
   e. The incidence of renal cell carcinoma in ADPKD is twice that in the normal population.

7. The following are extrarenal manifestations of ADPKD EXCEPT:
   a. hepatic cysts.
   b. intracranial (berry) aneurysms.
   c. cerebellar hemangioblastomas.
   d. colonic diverticulosis.
   e. mitral valve prolapse.

8. Which of the following statements is FALSE regarding unilateral multicystic dysplastic kidneys?
   a. The majority of multicystic dysplastic kidneys become smaller or ultrasonographically undetectable with time.
   b. There is an absence of communication between cysts on ultrasonographic scans.
   c. Cysts are usually found in communication with each other when injected intracystically with contrast material.
   d. The sine qua non for diagnosis of a multicystic dysplastic kidney is the presence of primitive ducts.
   e. Multicystic dysplastic kidneys appear more often in females and more often on the right side.

9. Flank pain is one of the most common presenting symptoms of ADPKD in adult patients. This is often caused by:
   a. bleeding into a cyst.
   b. renal cell carcinoma.
   c. cyst rupture.
   d. b and c.
   e. a and c.

10. Which gene is associated with a multiple malformation syndrome and clear cell renal cell carcinoma?
    a. *PDK1*
    b. *PDK2*
    c. *TG737*
    d. *Wnt-2*
    e. *VHL*

11. A benign multilocular cyst is seen most often:
    a. in males younger than 4 years of age and in females older than 30 years of age.
    b. in females younger than 4 years of age and in males older than 30 years of age.
    c. in males between 4 and 30 years of age.
    d. equally in both sexes before 4 years of age and in females after 30 years of age.
    e. equally in both sexes before 4 years of age and in males after 30 years of age.

12. What is the primary distinguishing factor between juvenile nephronophthisis (NPH) and medullary cystic kidney disease (MCKD)?
    a. NPH presents with polyuria and polydipsia, while MCKD does not.
    b. NPH is an autosomal recessive disorder, while MCKD is an autosomal dominant disease.
    c. NPH is diagnosed histologically with severe interstitial fibrosis, while MCKD is diagnosed by the presence of glomerulosclerosis.
    d. Most patients with MCKD have extrarenal manifestations of the disease, while patients with NPH are usually affected only in the kidneys.
    e. In patients with NPH, renal failure occurs in the third to fourth decade, while in patients with MCKD, renal failure typically occurs in adolescence.

13. A patient with which of the following entities has the highest likelihood of having a renal cell carcinoma develop?
    a. ADPKD
    b. Tuberous sclerosis
    c. von Hippel-Lindau disease
    d. Acquired renal cystic disease
    e. Medullary sponge kidney

14. Which of the following is FALSE pertaining to multicystic dysplastic kidneys (MCDK)?
    a. MCDK is one of the most common causes of an abdominal mass in the newborn.
    b. In patients with MCDK, the contralateral renal moiety is frequently affected by urologic disease.

    c. MCDK is often difficult to differentiate from severe ureteropelvic junction obstruction.
    d. Data from large series show that MCDK is associated with an increased risk for hypertension.
    e. Roughly 40% of MCDKs will spontaneously involute over time.

15. Which of the following would confirm the diagnosis of tuberous sclerosis?
    a. Renal angiomyolipoma and multiple renal cysts
    b. Hamartomatous rectal polyps and facial adenoma sebaceum
    c. Renal angiomyolipoma and cardiac rhabdomyoma
    d. Multiple renal cysts, hepatic fibrosis, and pheochromocytoma
    e. Mitral valve prolapse, renal angiolipoma, and gingival fibromas

16. The following are TRUE of von Hippel-Lindau (VHL) disease EXCEPT:
    a. VHL disease is an autosomal dominant syndrome.
    b. VHL disease is caused by a mutation in the tumor suppressor gene, *VHL*, located on chromosome 3.
    c. epididymal cysts are not infrequent in patients with VHL disease.
    d. pheochromocytomas, cerebellar hemangioblastomas, and retinal angiomas are common extrarenal manifestations of VHL disease.
    e. renal cell carcinomas, the most common manifestation, are seen in the vast majority of patients.

17. Renal sinus cysts are most likely derived from:
    a. vascular elements.
    b. renal parenchyma.
    c. renal pelvis.
    d. lymphatic system.
    e. nephrogenic rests.

18. Most simple renal cysts identified in utero represent:
    a. the first sign of a multicystic kidney.
    b. the first sign of ARPKD.
    c. the first sign of ADPKD.
    d. a calyceal diverticulum.
    e. resolve before birth.

19. Approximately what percentage of individuals older than 60 years will have an identifiable renal cyst on computed tomography (CT)?
    a. 1% to 5%
    b. 10%
    c. 33%
    d. 75%
    e. 90%

20. Which of the following group of antibiotics includes the best choice for treating an infected renal cyst in a patient with ADPKD?
    a. Trimethoprim-sulfamethoxazole, chloramphenicol, fluoroquinolones
    b. Cephalosporins, trimethoprim-sulfamethoxazole, doxycycline

   c. Gentamicin, cephalosporins, vancomycin

   d. Fluoroquinolones, metronidazole (Flagyl), vancomycin

   e. Doxycycline, amoxicillin, gentamicin

21. All of the following are reasonable treatment strategies for patients with ADPKD EXCEPT:

   a. management of hypertension.

   b. avoidance of surgical treatment for large or multiple cysts in patients with chronic flank pain.

   c. surgical treatment of symptomatic urinary stone disease.

   d. use of lipophilic antibiotics for treatment of a suspected renal cyst infection.

   e. screening with magnetic resonance imaging (MRI) or CT for berry aneurysms in patients with a family history of subarachnoid hemorrhage.

22. In neonates with a unilateral multicystic kidney, what is the incidence of contralateral vesicoureteral reflux?

   a. 0% to 7%

   b. 18% to 43%

   c. 50% to 67%

   d. 75%

   e. 7% to 15%

23. What is the most likely cause of flank pain and hematuria in a 50-year-old patient with end-stage renal disease who has been undergoing dialysis for 5 years?

   a. Acute renal vein thrombosis

   b. Acute renal artery thrombosis

   c. Renal cell carcinoma

   d. ARCD

   e. Uric acid stones

24. Which group of three findings best describes the typical ultrasonographic image of a multicystic dysplastic kidney?

   a. The cysts are organized around a central large cyst; there is no identifiable renal sinus; and there are communications between the cysts.

   b. The cysts have a haphazard distribution; there is absence of a central or medial large cyst; and there are no obvious communications between the cysts.

   c. The cysts have a haphazard distribution; there is no obvious renal sinus; and there is a large central cyst.

   d. Connections exist between the cysts; a medial cyst is present; and a renal sinus is usually present.

   e. The cysts are organized at the periphery; the largest is the central one; and there is an identifiable renal sinus.

25. The Mayer-Rokitansky-Küster-Hauser syndrome refers to which group of associated findings?

   a. Wilms tumor, nephrotic syndrome, ambiguous genitalia

   b. Caudad ureteric budding, lateral orifice position, lower pole dysplasia

   c. Hypertension, vesicoureteral reflux, deep cortical depression over an area of the kidney with "thyroidization" of tubules

   d. Bilateral renal agenesis, respiratory failure, oligohydramnios

   e. Unilateral renal agenesis or renal ectopia, ipsilateral müllerian defects, vaginal agenesis

26. Which one of the following conditions is most representative of a neoplastic growth?

   a. Benign multilocular cyst

   b. Oligomeganephronia

   c. Multicystic dysplastic kidney

   d. Calyceal diverticulum

   e. Ask-Upmark kidney

27. Which of the following is the best match?

   a. ARPKD and congenital hepatic fibrosis

   b. Medullary sponge kidney and predominance of glomerular cysts

   c. Juvenile nephronophthisis and cortical cysts

   d. Ask-Upmark kidney and hypotension

   e. von Hippel-Lindau disease and adenoma sebaceum

28. Which of the following matches is correct?

   a. ARPKD and chromosome 2

   b. ADPKD and chromosomes 4 and 16

   c. Tuberous sclerosis and chromosomes 9 and 15

   d. von Hippel-Lindau disease and chromosome 4

   e. Juvenile nephronophthisis and chromosome 6

29. A renal cyst with increased number of septa and prominent calcification in a nonenhancing cyst wall does not require exploration. According to the Bosniak grading system this cyst would be categorized as:

   a. I.

   b. II.

   c. II F.

   d. III.

   e. IV.

30. Ultrasonography in neonates with ARPKD reveals kidneys that are hyperechogenic or "bright" in appearance. This finding is due to:

   a. the presence of many small punctate calcifications within the renal papillae.

   b. dysplastic, diseased renal parenchyma.

   c. a vast increase in small fat deposits within the renal sinuses.

   d. the presence of numerous microcysts created by tightly compacted, dilated collecting ducts that result in innumerable ultrasonographic interfaces.

   e. the presence of renal hamartomas with increased cortical vascularity.

31. Ultrasound and/or CT criteria for the diagnosis of a simple renal cyst include all the following EXCEPT:

   a. sharp, thin, distinct smooth walls and margins.

   b. Thickness of cyst wall less than or equal to 3 mm.

   c. acoustic enhancement behind cyst (ultrasound).

   d. spherical or ovoid shape.

   e. homogeneous with absence of internal echoes.

32. A 50-year-old man with known von Hippel-Lindau disease presents with a single episode of gross hematuria. CT scan reveals a 3-cm enhancing mass in the upper pole of each kidney. Metastatic evaluation is negative. He is

otherwise healthy. Appropriate treatment at this point would be:

a. bilateral radical nephrectomy with the placement of a peritoneal dialysis catheter.

b. bilateral upper pole partial nephrectomy.

c. right radical nephrectomy with left upper pole partial nephrectomy.

d. observation with serial CT every 4 months.

e. CT-guided needle biopsy of each lesion with surgical removal if diagnosis confirms renal cell carcinoma.

ANSWERS

1. **b. Tuberous sclerosis and angiomyolipoma.** Angiomyolipomas occur in 40% to 80% of patients with tuberous sclerosis.

2. **a. Hypertension.** Hypertension and its sequelae (headache, hypertensive encephalopathy, retinopathy, etc.) are the hallmarks of Ask-Upmark kidney. Segmental vascular anomalies have been cited as a possible cause of the hypertension, but there is no evidence that renal artery intimal disease is associated. This disease is primarily found in young women and girls.

3. **b. Duration of renal failure.** At first, ARCD was thought to be confined to patients receiving hemodialysis. However, it shortly became apparent that the disorder is almost as common in patients receiving peritoneal dialysis and that it may develop in patients with chronic renal failure who are being managed medically without any type of dialysis. Thus ARCD appears to be a feature of end-stage kidney disease rather than a response to dialysis.

4. **e. b *and* c.** The most severe form of ARPKD appears earliest in life, i.e., newborn period. All patients with ARPKD have liver involvement in the form of hepatic fibrosis and vary in the degree of biliary ectasia and periportal fibrosis. In both fetus and newborn, ultrasonography identifies bilateral, very enlarged, diffusely echogenic kidneys, especially when compared with the echogenicity of the liver. The increased echogenicity is due to the presence of numerous microcysts (created by tightly compacted, dilated collecting ducts) that result in innumerable interfaces. Compared with normal newborn kidneys, in ARPKD the pyramids are hyperechogenic because they blend in with the rest of the kidney, and the kidneys typically have a homogeneous appearance.

5. **c. An imbalance of the secretory and absorptive properties in proliferating tubular epithelial cells.** The fundamental processes that are essential for the development and progressive enlargement of renal cysts include (1) proliferation of epithelial cells in segments of renal tubule, (2) accumulation of fluid within the expanding tubule segment, and (3) disturbed organization and metabolism of the extracellular matrix. An imbalance of the secretory and absorptive properties in proliferating epithelial cells leads to a net accumulation of fluid in otherwise normal renal tubules. Recent evidence indicates that, beyond the loop of Henle, tubule cells have the capacity to secrete solutes and fluid on stimulation with $3',5'$-cyclic adenosine monophosphate (cAMP). This secretory flux operates in competition with the more powerful mechanism by which sodium (Na^+) is reabsorbed through apical epithelial Na^+ channels (ENaC). Under conditions in which

Na^+ reabsorption is diminished, the net secretion of sodium chloride (NaCl) and fluid occurs.

6. **a. The genetic defect is located on the short arm of chromosome 16.** Infants with ARPKD have hepatic fibrosis, and infants with ADPKD rarely have hepatic fibrosis but commonly have cysts in the liver. Renal cysts are frequently seen on ultrasonography by the age of 20 years. Glomerular cysts are sometimes found in the kidneys of newborns diagnosed with ADPKD. The risk of renal cell carcinoma in patients with ADPKD is no higher than that in the general population.

7. **c. cerebellar hemangioblastomas.** All are extrarenal manifestations of ADPKD except cerebellar hemangioblastomas, which are seen in patients with von Hippel-Lindau disease.

8. **e. Multicystic dysplastic kidneys appear more often in females and more often on the right side.** At any age, the condition is more likely to be found on the left. Males are more likely to have unilateral multicystic dysplastic kidneys (2.4 : 1).

9. **a. bleeding into a cyst.** Pain (flank and/or abdominal) is the most common presenting symptom in adults. This results from a number of possible factors: mass effect (cysts impinging on abdominal wall or neighboring organs), bleeding into the cysts, urinary tract infection (including infected cysts), and nephrolithiasis.

10. **e. *VHL*.** The gene associated with the transmission of von Hippel-Lindau disease is located on chromosome 3. In non–von Hippel-Lindau patients with sporadic clear cell renal cell carcinoma, 50% of cell lines are associated with a mutational form of the *VHL* gene.

11. **a. in males younger than 4 years of age and in females older than 30 years of age.** The great majority of patients present before the age of 4 years or after the age of 30 years. Five percent present between 4 and 30 years of age. The patient is 2 times as likely to be male if younger than 4 years and 8 times as likely to be female if older than 30 years of age.

12. **b. NPH is an autosomal recessive disorder, while MCKD is an autosomal dominant disease.** Although either condition can occur sporadically, juvenile nephronophthisis usually is inherited as an autosomal recessive trait, while medullary cystic disease usually is inherited in an autosomal dominant fashion. Juvenile nephronophthisis and medullary cystic disease both cause polydipsia and polyuria in more than 80% of cases, but not to the extent observed in patients with diabetes insipidus. Pathologically, NPH and MCKD are similar. Histologically, there is a characteristic triad present that includes (1) irregular thickening and disintegration of the tubular basement membrane, (2) marked tubular atrophy with cyst development, and (3) interstitial cell infiltration with fibrosis. Twenty percent of juvenile nephronophthisis families have extrarenal manifestations, while MCKD usually affects only the kidneys. Another important difference between the two entities is that renal failure develops in patients with NPH at a mean age of 13 years and almost always before 25 years. MCKD is a milder disease when it presents in early adulthood but it will manifest in all patients by 50 years of age (Bernstein and Gardner,

1979).* End-stage renal disease (ESRD) in patients with MCKD most often develops in the third or fourth decade.

13. **c. von Hippel-Lindau disease.** Tuberous sclerosis and von Hippel-Lindau disease are associated with epithelial hyperplasia (and adenomas as well) and have an increased incidence of renal cell carcinoma (tuberous sclerosis, 2%, and von Hippel-Lindau disease, 35% to 38%).

14. **d. Data from large series show that MCDK is associated with an increased risk for hypertension.** All statements are true of MCDK except that large series indicate MCDK is NOT associated with an increased risk of hypertension.

15. **c. Renal angiomyolipoma and cardiac rhabdomyoma.** Definitive diagnosis of tuberous sclerosis (TSC) is dependent on the presence of certain major and minor clinical features. The diagnosis of TSC requires two major features (renal angiomyolipoma, facial angiofibromas or forehead plaques, nontraumatic ungual or periungual fibroma, three or more hypomelanotic macules, shagreen patch, multiple retinal nodular hamartomas, cortical tuber, subependymal nodule, subependymal giant cell astrocytoma, cardiac rhabdomyoma, lymphangioleiomyomatosis) or one major plus two minor features (multiple renal cysts, nonrenal hamartoma, hamartomatous rectal polyps, retinal achromic patch, cerebral white matter radial migration tracts, bone cysts, gingival fibromas, "confetti" skin lesions, multiple enamel pits).

16. **e. renal cell carcinomas, the most common manifestation, are seen in the vast majority of patients.** All statements are true of VHL disease except that renal cysts, NOT *renal cell carcinoma*, are the most common and often earliest manifestation as seen in 76% of patients.

17. **d. lymphatic system.** The predominant type of renal sinus cyst appears to be one derived from the lymphatics.

18. **e. resolve before birth.** In 28 of 11,000 fetuses with renal cysts, 25 fetuses had the cysts resolve before birth. Of two cysts that remained postnatally, in one it was the first sign of a multicystic kidney.

19. **c. 33%.** In adults, the frequency of renal cyst occurrence increases with age. Using CT, one group demonstrated a 20% incidence of cysts by 40 years of age and approximately 33% incidence of cysts after 60 years of age.

20. **a. Trimethoprim-sulfamethoxazole, chloramphenicol, fluoroquinolones.** In the experience of one group of researchers, the only dependable antibiotics were those that were lipid soluble, namely, trimethoprim-sulfamethoxazole and chloramphenicol. Chloramphenicol produced better results. The fluoroquinolones, which are also lipid soluble, are proving useful. If a patient with suspected pyelonephritis does not respond to an antibiotic, and if the antibiotic used is not lipid soluble, one must consider whether the infection may be present in a noncommunicating cyst.

21. **b. avoidance of surgical treatment for large or multiple cysts in patients with chronic flank pain.** All are reasonable treatment strategies for a patient with ADPKD, except when conservative measures of chronic pain treatment fail, surgical management must be considered.

Ultrasonography- or CT-guided cyst aspiration is a straightforward procedure and may be both diagnostic and therapeutic. Surgical unroofing of multiple or very large cysts can potentially alleviate symptoms of pain and can be performed either laparoscopically or through open flank or dorsal lumbotomy incisions. Surgical intervention appears to only improve symptomatology and does not appear to either accelerate the decline of renal function or preserve declining renal function.

22. **b. 18% to 43%.** Contralateral vesicoureteral reflux is seen even more often than contralateral ureteropelvic junction obstruction, being identified in 18% to 43% of infants.

23. **d. ARCD.** The most common presentation of ARCD is loin pain, hematuria, or both. Bleeding occurs in as many as 50% of patients.

24. **b. The cysts have a haphazard distribution; there is absence of a central or medial large cyst; and there are no obvious communications between the cysts.** Renal masses in infants most often represent either multicystic kidney disease or hydronephrosis, and it is important to distinguish the two, especially if the surgeon wishes to remove a nonfunctioning hydronephrotic kidney or repair a ureteropelvic junction obstruction while leaving a multicystic organ in situ. In newborns, ultrasonography is generally the first study performed. In a few cases, it is difficult to distinguish multicystic kidney disease from severe hydronephrosis. In general, however, the multicystic kidney has a haphazard distribution of cysts of various sizes without a larger central or medial cyst and without visible communications between the cysts. Frequently, very small cysts appear in between the large cysts. By comparison, in ureteropelvic junction obstruction, the cysts or calyces are organized around the periphery of the kidney, connections can usually be demonstrated between the peripheral cysts and a central or medial cyst that represents the renal pelvis, and there is an absence of small cysts between the larger cysts (see Fig. 114–20 in *Campbell-Walsh Urology, 9th Edition*). When there is an identifiable renal sinus, the diagnosis is more likely to be hydronephrosis than multicystic kidney.

25. **e. Unilateral renal agenesis or renal ectopia, ipsilateral müllerian defects, vaginal agenesis.** The term Mayer-Rokitansky-Küster-Hauser syndrome refers to a group of associated findings that include unilateral renal agenesis or renal ectopia, ipsilateral müllerian defects, and vaginal agenesis. Drash syndrome includes Wilms tumor, nephrotic syndrome, and ambiguous genitalia; the findings of caudad ureteric budding, lateral orifice position, and lower pole dysplasia follow the bud theory; the grouping of hypertension, vesicoureteral reflux, and deep cortical depression over an area of the kidney with "thyroidization" of tubules defines the Ask-Upmark kidney; and the grouping of bilateral renal agenesis, respiratory failure, and oligohydramnios can lead the fetus to be born with Potter syndrome and Potter facies.

26. **a. Benign multilocular cyst.** For the benign multilocular cystic lesion, certain authors prefer the term cystic nephroma, because this term implies a benign but neoplastic lesion.

27. **a. ARPKD and congenital hepatic fibrosis.** All patients with ARPKD have varying degrees of congenital hepatic fibrosis.

---

*Sources referenced can be found in *Campbell-Walsh Urology, 10th Edition*, on the Expert Consult website.

28. **b. ADPKD and chromosomes 4 and 16.** For the genetic cystic disease ADPKD, the chromosomal defect is on chromosome 16 for *PKD1* and 4 for *PKD2; PKD3* has not been mapped. Autosomal recessive polycystic kidney disease involves chromosome 6; tuberous sclerosis involves chromosomes 9 and 16; von Hippel-Lindau disease involves chromosome 3; and juvenile nephronophthisis involves chromosome 2.

29. **c. II F.** The Bosniak classification has recently been updated to include category II F as defined in the answer.

30. **d. the presence of numerous microcysts created by tightly compacted, dilated collecting ducts that result in innumerable ultrasonographic interfaces.** In both fetus and newborn with ARPKD, ultrasonography identifies bilateral, very enlarged, diffusely echogenic kidneys, especially when compared with the echogenicity of the liver. The increased echogenicity is due to the presence of numerous microcysts (created by tightly compacted, dilated collecting ducts) that result in innumerable interfaces. Compared with normal newborn kidneys, in ARPKD the pyramids are hyperechogenic because they blend in with the rest of the kidney, and the kidneys typically have a homogeneous appearance.

31. **b. Thickness of cyst wall less than or equal to 3 mm.** One can safely make the diagnosis of a classic benign simple cyst by ultrasonography when the following criteria are met: (1) absence of internal echoes; (2) sharply defined, thin, distinct wall with a smooth and distinct margin; (3) good transmission of sound waves through the cyst with consequent acoustic enhancement behind the cyst; and (4) spherical or slightly ovoid shape. The CT criteria for a simple cyst are similar to those used in ultrasonography: (1) sharp, thin, distinct, smooth walls and margins; (2) spherical or ovoid shape; and (3) homogeneous content.

32. **b. bilateral upper pole partial nephrectomy.** Because the tumors that characterize VHL disease are frequently multiple, bilateral, and recurrent, close surveillance and minimization of surgical procedures constitute the mainstay of treatment. For patients who have VHL disease and all patients who have hereditary cancer syndromes, the goal of treatment is cancer control, not cancer cure, and preservation of functional parenchyma to avoid the morbidity associated with renal loss. In patients who have VHL disease, surgical resection is performed with the understanding that microscopic disease probably is left behind. Currently, nephron-sparing surgery should be considered the standard of care for treating low-grade RCC in the setting of VHL disease. Patients with high-grade disease are still probably best served with bilateral nephrectomy. Although having the objective of sparing as much renal parenchyma as possible and preventing metastasis of the lesions already present, it is not curative surgery (Reed, 2009). Although this approach does not reduce the risk of recurrence, reported to be 75% to 85%, the 10-year disease-specific survival rates are quite high (81% to 94%) (Malek, 1987; Steinbach, 1995; Roupret, 2003; Ploussard, 2007). Classically, the survival rate after nephrectomy has been only 50%. Because most of these tumors are low grade, a nephron-sparing approach provides very good survival rates while avoiding the diminished quality of life that comes with bilateral nephrectomy and subsequent dialysis/transplantation. Laparoscopic and percutaneous image-guided ablative techniques, such as radiofrequency ablation and cryoablation, have also been used and are currently under investigation.

Additional Study Points

1. Potter facies is manifested by hypertelorism, prominent inner canthal folds, and a recessive chin.
2. Dysplasia is histologically manifested by embryonic, immature mesenchyme, and primitive renal components.
3. Renal hypoplasia is manifested by less than the normal number of calyces and nephrons with absence of dysplasia.
4. Oligomeganephronia is a reduced number of nephrons with hypertrophy of the remaining nephrons. Many patients with the disorder develop renal failure.
5. The Ask-Upmark kidney (segmental hypoplasia) is often associated with reflux and patients develop severe hypertension.
6. Autosomal dominant polycystic kidney disease is associated with cysts of the liver, pancreas, spleen and lungs, berry aneurysms, colonic diverticula, aortic aneurysms, and mitral valve prolapse.
7. Benign multilocular cyst and cystic nephroma fall into a spectrum of disease, with multilocular cyst on the one end being benign and, on the other end of the spectrum, cystic Wilms tumors being malignant. Multilocular cyst with nodules of Wilms tumor lies in the middle.
8. In the adult, there is a multilocular cystic renal cell carcinoma. Multilocular cystic lesions should therefore be removed.
9. One third of patients with medullary sponge kidneys have hypercalciuria.

Core Principles of Perioperative Management in Children

Carlos R. Estrada, Jr., MD ● Lynne R. Ferrari, MD

QUESTIONS

1. Prematurity and intrauterine growth restriction are defined as born before:
   a. 38 weeks and weighing less than 1500 g, respectively.
   b. 37 weeks and weighing less than 2500 g, respectively.
   c. 36 weeks and weighing less than 2500 g, respectively.
   d. 37 weeks and weighing less than 1500 g, respectively.
   e. 36 weeks and weighing less than 1500 g, respectively.

2. During the fetal stage of lung development, all branching resulting in the terminal bronchial airways occurs by:
   a. 12 weeks gestation.
   b. 10 weeks gestation.
   c. 16 weeks gestation.
   d. 20 weeks gestation.
   e. 24 weeks gestation.

3. Compared with the adult heart, the neonatal and pediatric myocardium are:
   a. stiffer and less compliant.
   b. less stiff and less compliant.
   c. stiffer and more compliant.
   d. less stiff and more compliant.
   e. identical.

4. Following the relatively rapid rise in glomerular filtration rate (GFR) over the first few months of life, adult GFR is reached by:
   a. 3 to 4 years.
   b. 4 to 5 years.
   c. 6 months.
   d. 12 to 24 months.
   e. 10 years.

5. For a 7-month-old infant in the postoperative period who weighs 9 kg, the most appropriate maintenance fluid is:
   a. D5 ¼ NS + 20 mEq/L KCl at 36 mL/hr.
   b. D5 ½ NS + 20 mEq/L KCl at 45 mL/hr.
   c. D5 ½ NS + 20 mEq/L KCl at 18 mL/hr.

   d. D5 ¼ NS at 36 mL/hr.
   e. D5 ½ NS + 20 mEq/L KCl at 36 mL/hr.

6. The school-aged child typically most fears:
   a. death.
   b. that they may not meet the expectations of adults.
   c. loss of control.
   d. injury.
   e. separation from their primary caregivers.

7. For a healthy child undergoing uncomplicated surgery, the risk of an adverse event is approximately:
   a. 1 in 10,000.
   b. 1 in 200.
   c. 1 in 2,000,000.
   d. 1 in 100,000.
   e. 1 in 200,000.

8. Routine diagnostic testing for surgery in a healthy 12-month-old child includes:
   a. a chest x-ray and complete blood count.
   b. a complete blood count, electrolytes, and prothrombin time (PT)/partial thromboplastin time (PTT).
   c. a chest x-ray, complete blood count, and PT/PTT.
   d. hemoglobin/hematocrit determination.
   e. no studies.

9. In preparation for surgery, children should fast from clear liquids:
   a. for 2 hours prior to surgery.
   b. for 3 hours prior to surgery.
   c. for 4 hours prior to surgery.
   d. for 6 hours prior to surgery.
   e. being NPO after midnight.

10. For a child 6 years of age, assessment of postoperative pain is best done by:
   a. simply asking him or her about the pain.
   b. relying on appearance, because children cannot hide their pain well.

c. using a visual analog scale.

d. using a faces scale.

e. asking the child's parents.

11. Poor and rapid metabolizers of codeine can be expected to:

a. have good and poor pain relief, respectively.

b. have little effect and have dangerously high plasma morphine levels, respectively.

c. have dangerously high plasma morphine levels and little effect, respectively.

d. have identical CYP2D6 enzyme genotypes.

e. most likely be of North African and white descent, respectively.

12. Surgical antibiotic prophylaxis for a major class II operation is best:

a. administered the night before surgery.

b. administered following incision.

c. administered immediately after surgery is complete.

d. administered 1 hour prior to incision.

e. not recommended/administered.

13. Blood volume in children can be most closely estimated as:

a. 55 mL/kg.

b. 25 to 50 mL/kg.

c. 70 to 80 mL/kg.

d. 100 mL/kg.

e. 65 to 70 mL/kg.

14. Fever (>38.5° C rectal temperature) in children within 24 hours of surgery is most likely due to:

a. urinary tract infection.

b. surgical-site infection.

c. deep vein thrombosis.

d. atelectasis.

e. dehydration.

ANSWERS

1. **b. Born before 37 weeks and weighing less than 2500 g, respectively.** A baby born before 37 weeks gestation is considered premature. The severity of prematurity may be indicated by the birth weight, although these two factors are not necessarily related. Infants weighing 2500 g or less at birth are considered low birth weight (LBW) in prematurity, but in an infant born full term, this weight would indicate intrauterine growth restriction (IUGR). This is an important distinction, because full term neonates with IUGR usually have different problems than premature infants.

2. **c. 16 weeks gestation.** Proper intrauterine growth and development are dependent on presence of normal amniotic fluid volume. Of particular relevance to urologists is lung development, which is dependent on amniotic fluid. The fetal stage of lung development begins at 7 weeks gestation and proceeds to term. By the end of the 16th week gestation, all lung branching occurs, resulting in the terminal bronchial airways. After this time, the only further growth that occurs is elongation and widening of existing airways.

3. **a. stiffer and less compliant.** The neonatal and pediatric myocardium is stiffer and less compliant compared with the adult heart. This results in diminished preload capacity so that increases in end-diastolic ventricular volume and increases in right ventricular pressure result in decreased cardiac output at lower levels than in adult patients. In addition, infants and children have relatively higher resting heart rates. As a result, cardiac output in children is heart rate dependent, because the stroke volume is relatively fixed. Decreases in heart rate in infants and children will result in decreases in cardiac output to a greater extent than a similar decrease in heart rate in an adult patient. A reduction of a child's heart rate to that of a typical adult would result in marked decrease in cardiac output.

4. **d. 12 to 24 months.** In utero, renovascular resistance is high, limiting renal blood flow. Immediately following birth, the distribution of renal cortical blood flow changes, with increased perfusion of the outer cortex and increased reactivity of the renal vascular bed. Consequently, the glomerular filtration rate (GFR) rises quickly despite renal blood flow remaining unchanged. In addition, water and electrolyte homeostasis is difficult to predict. GFR and tubular function double by 1 month of age (Kaskel),* and over the first 3 months of life, renovascular resistance continues to decrease, which results in further rises in GFR. Following this relatively rapid rise, GFR continues to increase more slowly toward adult levels, which are reached by 12 to 24 months of life. The maturation of renal tubular function lags behind the maturation of glomerular function, and therefore the neonate can concentrate urine to only approximately 50% of adult capability.

5. **e. D5 1/2 NS + 20 mEq/L KCl at 36 mL/hr.** The total requirements for maintenance fluids can be calculated using the Holliday-Segar formula. After calculating the fluid requirement, children usually receive either D5 ¼ NS + 20 mEq/L KCl or D5 ½ NS 20 mEq/L KCl. Children who are less than 6 months old are generally given the solution with ¼ NS, because of their high water needs per kilogram. Children 6 months and older, however, should receive the solution with ½ NS.

6. **b. that they may not meet the expectations of adults.** Age-appropriate treatment of children is essential to provide the best possible perioperative experience. Infants fear separation from their primary caregivers and exhibit stranger anxiety. Toddlers fear loss of control, so enabling a child to make choices, such as asking if the child has a color preference for his or her hospital gown, will diminish anxiety. Preschool-age children fear injury; they may fear, for example, that a blood draw may result in not enough blood being left in their bodies. The school-age child typically fears that he or she may not meet the expectations of adults. They are reluctant to ask questions for fear that they should already know the answer. Adolescents fear death and usually do not understand bodily functions.

7. **e. 1 in 200,000.** Most parents will express that they experience more anxiety about the anesthetic than the risks of the surgery. For a healthy child undergoing uncomplicated surgery, the risk of an adverse event is approximately 1 in 200,000. The risk of death under anesthesia is the most feared complication. This risk is 1 in

---

*Sources referenced can be found in *Campbell-Walsh Urology, 10th Edition,* on the Expert Consult website.

10,000 for all patients of any age undergoing any surgical procedure. However, the risk of death directly attributable to the anesthetic approaches zero, although the risk of cardiac arrests due to anesthesia remains approximately 4.5 in 10,000. The incidence of anesthetic-related complications and death is highest during the first year of life at 43:10,000, but this decreases dramatically during the second year of life to 5:10,000. Anesthetic risks increase by a factor of six during emergency procedures in all age groups.

8. **e. no studies.** Routine diagnostic testing in preparation for surgery is rarely indicated in healthy children, and studies that are ordered should be selected based on the general medical health of the patient and the procedure being performed. In general, measurement of hemoglobin/hematocrit in a healthy child undergoing elective surgery is unnecessary. A hemoglobin/hematocrit should be measured if significant blood loss is anticipated or if the child is younger than 6 months old or was born prematurely.

9. **a. 2 hours prior to surgery.** It is no longer advisable or safe to restrict children to "NPO after midnight." The American Society of Anesthesiologists recommends fasting from clear fluids for 2 hours prior to anesthesia. Clear liquids consist of water, nonparticulate juices (e.g., apple, white grape), Pedialyte, and Popsicles. Fasting from breast milk for 4 hours and formula for 6 hours is recommended. The suggested fasting period for solid food is 6 hours for regular meals and 8 hours for fat-containing meals. However, individual institutions may have specific practice guidelines.

10. **d. using a faces scale.** In general, children 8 years and older can reliably report pain on the visual analog scale used in adults. Children between the ages of 3 and 7 years can better report pain using a faces scale that uses a series of drawings depicting increasing levels of distress.

11. **b. have little effect and have dangerously high plasma morphine levels, respectively.** Codeine is a relatively weak opioid given its extremely low affinity for opioid receptors, and most of its analgesic effect is due to the 10% that is metabolized to morphine. The metabolism to morphine is predominantly by *O*-demethylation by the cytochrome P450 enzyme CYP2D6, which is known to show genetic polymorphism. Therefore variations in CYP2D6 will result in variable abilities to metabolize codeine. In this way, individuals may be classified as poor metabolizers or ultrarapid metabolizers, depending on the phenotype of their CYP2D6 enzyme.

12. **d. administered 1 hour prior to incision.** The timing of surgical antimicrobial prophylaxis is critically important, and the first dose should be given 30 minutes to 3 hours prior to incision to achieve bactericidal levels of the antibiotic at the site of incision.

13. **c. 70 to 80 mL/kg.** Blood volume in children varies with age, but can be estimated as 70 to 80 mL/kg.

14. **d. atelectasis.** Postoperative fever is a very common early surgical problem, and its etiology is taught in the first days of medical school surgery clerkships as the four Ws: wind, wound, water, and walking. "Wind" refers to atelectasis, "wound" to a surgical-site infection (SSI), "water" to a urinary tract infection (UTI), and "walking" to fever caused by deep vein thrombosis (DVT) in the lower extremities. Fever, defined as greater than 38.5° C rectal temperature, is common within 24 hours of surgery and is usually caused by atelectasis.

Additional Study Points

1. Please see Table 119–2 in *Campbell-Walsh Urology, 10th Edition* for more information on fluid calculations in children.
2. Lung development is dependent on an adequate amount of amniotic fluid.
3. A fetus with severe oligohydramnios may suffer pulmonary fibrosis.
4. Cardiac output in children is heart rate dependant; the stroke volume is relatively fixed.
5. Neonates have an increased susceptibility to infection due to impaired T-lymphocyte function and deficiency of immunoglobulins.
6. The immune system does not become fully competent until about 8 years of age.
7. Anesthesia is most risky in the first year of life.
8. A family history of anesthesia-related events, liver problems, and malignant hyperthermia is part of the preoperative assessment.
9. Children should take clear liquids up to 2 hours prior to anesthesia; and solid foods should not be consumed for 8 hours prior to anesthesia.
10. In premature infants who undergo anesthesia, the major risk postoperatively is apnea; similarly, in full-term infants younger than 4 weeks of age, apnea is the major postoperative risk.
11. Children with spina bifida have a high incidence of latex sensitivity.

chapter 120

Anomalies and Surgery of the Ureter in Children

Michael C. Carr, MD, PhD ● Pasquale Casale, MD

QUESTIONS

1. Which of the following is NOT correct concerning laparoscopic pyeloplasty?
   a. Discounted early as unacceptable due to degree of difficulty
   b. Can be performed after a failed previous pyeloplasty
   c. Has an overall higher success rate than endopyelotomy
   d. Can be performed in patients of all ages
   e. Many different techniques for laparoscopic approach have been described

2. In regard to closure of trocar sites:
   a. closing fascial wounds more than 3 mm is recommended.
   b. fascial closure devices facilitate closure in the obese patient.
   c. omentum is the most common herniated intra-abdominal structure.
   d. trocar hernias may be closed at the bedside with local anesthesia.
   e. all of the above are true.

3. Which is NOT true for transperitoneal procedures?
   a. Sutures may be passed through the anterior abdominal wall.
   b. For lower abdominal procedures, infants are best positioned across the foot of the bed.
   c. Laxity of the infant abdominal wall can limit exposure due to compression.
   d. Cannula fixation is a common problem in pediatric laparoscopy.
   e. Visibility is usually a problem.

4. A recognized dangerous complication of laparoscopy in all infants is:
   a. hypothermia.
   b. ventilatory compromise.
   c. abdominal adhesions.
   d. decreased renal perfusion.
   e. compartmental syndrome.

5. Which of the following is a contraindication to laparoscopic surgery in the pediatric population?
   a. Septic shock
   b. Spinal deformity
   c. Previous abdominal surgery
   d. Weight
   e. Intestinal malrotation

6. Hypothermia during laparoscopy in all infants is caused by:
   a. abdominal irrigation.
   b. high-frequency ventilation.
   c. room temperature insufflation.
   d. evaporation.
   e. cold room temperature.

7. Regarding pediatric minimally invasive surgery in obese patients:
   a. a suture can be placed from the skin at the entry site to the cannula to keep the cannula from sliding off if rapid desufflation is encountered.
   b. hitch stitches are helpful.
   c. an insufflation needle works well in most children, because the abdominal wall is thin.
   d. bladeless optical trocars for the camera port might be helpful.
   e. higher insufflation pressures are needed.

8. Which of the following is TRUE regarding primary obstructive megaureters?
   a. It is caused by an aperistaltic juxtavesical segment that is unable to propagate urine at acceptable rates of flow.
   b. It most commonly occurs with neurogenic and non-neurogenic voiding dysfunction or infravesical obstructions such as posterior urethral valves.
   c. It may be due to acute infections, nephropathies, and other medical conditions that cause significant increases in urinary output that overwhelm maximal peristalsis.
   d. It is diagnosed when reflux, obstruction, and secondary causes of dilatation are ruled out.
   e. None of the above

9. Which of the following is TRUE regarding secondary obstructive megaureters?
   a. It is caused by an aperistaltic juxtavesical segment that is unable to propagate urine at acceptable rates of flow.
   b. It most commonly occurs with neurogenic and non-neurogenic voiding dysfunction or infravesical obstructions such as posterior urethral valves.

c. It may be due to acute infections, nephropathies, and other medical conditions that cause significant increases in urinary output that overwhelm maximal peristalsis.

d. It is diagnosed once reflux, obstruction, and secondary causes of dilatation are ruled out.

e. None of the above

10. Which of the following is TRUE regarding secondary nonobstructive, nonrefluxing megaureters?

a. It is caused by an aperistaltic juxtavesical segment that is unable to propagate urine at acceptable rates of flow.

b. It most commonly occurs with neurogenic and non-neurogenic voiding dysfunction or infravesical obstructions such as posterior urethral valves.

c. It may be due to acute infections, nephropathies, and other medical conditions that cause significant increases in urinary output that overwhelm maximal peristalsis.

d. It is diagnosed once reflux, obstruction, and secondary causes of dilatation are ruled out.

e. None of the above

11. Which of the following is TRUE regarding primary nonobstructive, nonrefluxing megaureters?

a. It is caused by an aperistaltic juxtavesical segment that is unable to propagate urine at acceptable rates of flow.

b. It most commonly occurs with neurogenic and non-neurogenic voiding dysfunction or infravesical obstructions such as posterior urethral valves.

c. It may be due to acute infections, nephropathies, and other medical conditions that cause significant increases in urinary output that overwhelm maximal peristalsis.

d. It is diagnosed once reflux, obstruction, and secondary causes of dilatation are ruled out.

e. None of the above.

12. Which of the following is TRUE regarding primary obstructive, nonrefluxing megaureters?

a. As long as renal function is not significantly affected and urinary infections do not become a problem, expectant management is preferred.

b. Antibiotic suppression is appropriate in most cases.

c. Close radiographic surveillance is appropriate in most cases.

d. All of the above

e. None of the above

13. Which of the following is TRUE regarding the surgical management of megaureters?

a. Ureteral tailoring is usually necessary to achieve the proper length-to-diameter ratio required of successful reimplants.

b. Plication or infolding is useful for the more severely dilated ureter.

c. Excisional tapering is preferred for the moderately dilated ureter.

d. Narrowing the ureter may theoretically lead to less effective peristalsis.

e. Patients usually have such massively dilated and tortuous ureters that straightening with removal of excess length and proximal revision becomes necessary.

ANSWERS

1. **d. Can be performed in patients of all ages.** Caution should be taken with children younger than 6 months. Although work has been done in infants, it appears that the success rates are less in the newborn to 6-month range. Some authors believe it is due to the limited working space (Tan, 1999; Kutikov, 2006).*

2. **e. all of the above are true.** It appears that opinions vary as to whether or not sites less than 10 mm should be closed. The authors' personal experience has led them to close any trocar site where the fascia can be visualized. (Tonouchi H, Ohmori Y, Kobayashi M, Kusunoki M. Trocar site hernia. Arch Surg 2004;139:1248–56.)

3. **e. Visibility is usually a problem.** Visibility is typically not a problem, because the expanded, pliable abdominal wall in children is proportionally larger than even in adult patients. (Casale P, Kojima Y. Robotic-assisted laparoscopic surgery in pediatric urology: an update. Scand J Surg 2009;98:110–9.)

4. **a. hypothermia.** If warmed insufflation gases are not used, hypothermia may ensue. Also, there is a steady increase in oxygen consumption during laparoscopy. The increase in oxygen consumption was more marked in younger children and was associated with a significant rise in core temperature. Open surgery was not associated with significant changes in core temperature or oxygen consumption. (McHoney MC, Corizia L, Eaton S, et al. Laparoscopic surgery in children is associated with an intraoperative hypermetabolic response. Surg Endosc 2006;20(3):452–7.)

5. **a. Septic shock.** Sepsis appears to be the only absolute contraindication to laparoscopy in this patient cohort due to the profound metabolic effects of the septic state. The other answers are only relative contraindications and should be addressed on an individual basis. (Casale P. Robotic pediatric urology. Expert Rev Med Devices 2008;5(1):59–64.)

6. **d. evaporation.** Evaporation is the key element in neonatal cooling during laparoscopic procedures. Bessell and colleagues found that core temperatures after insufflation with heated humidified gas were no different than that of controls in an animal model. After insufflation with cool dry gas, core temperature dropped by 1.8° C, which was significantly more than the 0.6° C drop experienced by control animals and those insufflated with heated humidified gas (P < .01). (Bessell JR, Ludbrook G, Millard SH, et al. Humidified gas prevents hypothermia induced by laparoscopic insufflation. Surg Endosc 1999;13(2):101–5.)

7. **d. bladeless optical trocars for the camera port might be helpful.** Bladeless trocars can be helpful in obese patients to ensure the peritoneal cavity is penetrated and the extraperitoneal space is traversed. (String A, Berber E, Foroutani A, et al. Use of the optical access trocar for safe and rapid entry in various laparoscopic procedures. Surg Endosc 2001;15(6):570–3.)

8. **a. It is caused by an aperistaltic juxtavesical segment that is unable to propagate urine at acceptable rates of flow.** It is generally agreed that the cause of primary obstructive megaureter is an aperistaltic

*Sources referenced can be found in *Campbell-Walsh Urology, 10th Edition,* on the Expert Consult website, unless given in full below.

juxtavesical segment 3 to 4 cm long that is unable to propagate urine at acceptable rates of flow.

9. **b. It most commonly occurs with neurogenic and non-neurogenic voiding dysfunction or infravesical obstructions such as posterior urethral valves.** This form of megaureter most commonly occurs with neurogenic and non-neurogenic voiding dysfunction or infravesical obstructions such as posterior urethral valves.

10. **c. It may be due to acute infections, nephropathies, and other medical conditions that cause significant increases in urinary output that overwhelm maximal peristalsis.** Significant ureteral dilatation can result from acute urinary tract infections (UTIs) accompanied by bacterial endotoxins that inhibit peristalsis. Resolution is expected with appropriate antibiotic therapy. Nephropathies and other medical conditions that cause significant increases in urinary output that overwhelm maximal peristalsis can also lead to progressive ureteral dilatation as collecting systems comply to handle the output from above. These conditions include lithium toxicity, diabetes insipidus or mellitus, sickle cell nephropathy, and psychogenic polydipsia.

11. **d. It is diagnosed once reflux, obstruction, and secondary causes of dilatation are ruled out.** Once reflux, obstruction, and secondary causes of dilatation are ruled out, the designation of primary nonrefluxing, nonobstructed megaureter is appropriate.

12. **d. All of the above.** Most clinicians now believe that as long as renal function is not significantly affected and urinary infections do not become a problem, expectant management is preferred. Antibiotic suppression and close radiologic surveillance are appropriate in most cases.

13. **a. Ureteral tailoring is usually necessary to achieve the proper length-to-diameter ratio required of successful reimplants.** Ureteral tailoring (excision or plication) is usually necessary. Narrowing the ureter also theoretically enables its walls to coapt properly, leading to more effective peristalsis. Revising the distal segment intended for reimplantation is all that is usually required.

Additional Study Points

1. Ureteropelvic junction (UPJ) obstruction occurs more commonly in boys and on the left side.
2. UPJ obstruction may be seen with severe vesicoureteral reflux.
3. Megaureters may be caused by vesicoureteral reflux, obstruction, or intrinsic abnormalities of the ureter.
4. Dismembered pyeloplasty for the repair of UPJ obstruction is preferred by many because of its broad applicability, ability to remove the pathologic UPJ, and the ability to incorporate a reduction pyeloplasty with the repair.
5. When performing a ureterocalicostomy, the lower pole of the kidney should be amputated, all periureteral tissue should be preserved, and a tension-free mucosal anastomosis should be performed over a stent.
6. In repairing a megaureter, it must be remembered that to preserve the blood supply to the lower ureter, which courses to it medially, tailoring of the ureter should occur laterally.

Ectopic Ureter, Ureterocele, and Ureteral Anomalies

Craig A. Peters, MD, FACS, FAAP ● Richard N. Schlussel, MD ● Cathy Mendelsohn, PhD

QUESTIONS

1. All of the following are possible drainage sites for an ectopic ureter in a female EXCEPT the:
   a. fallopian tube.
   b. uterus.
   c. ovary.
   d. vagina.
   e. urethra.

2. Inadequate interaction between the ureteral bud and metanephric blastema will most likely lead to which of the following conditions?
   a. Dysplasia
   b. Hydronephrosis
   c. Reflux
   d. Ureteral ectopia
   e. Multicystic dysplasia

3. How is the relationship between the upper and lower pole orifices in a complete ureteral duplication best described? The upper pole:
   a. orifice is cephalad and lateral to the lower orifice.
   b. ureter joins the lower pole ureter just before entry into the bladder.
   c. orifice is caudal and medial to the lower pole orifice.
   d. orifice and lower pole orifice sit transversely side by side.
   e. ureter joins the bladder neck caudal to the lower pole orifice.

4. All of the following contribute to vesicoureteral reflux EXCEPT:
   a. lateral ureteral insertion.
   b. lax bladder neck.
   c. poorly developed trigone.
   d. gaping ureteral orifice.
   e. short intramural tunnel.

5. The most common site of drainage of an ectopic ureter in a male is the:
   a. vas deferens.
   b. anterior urethra.
   c. seminal vesicle.
   d. posterior urethra.
   e. ampulla of the vas.

6. The voiding pattern most often seen in a girl with an ectopic ureter is:
   a. urge incontinence.
   b. stress incontinence.
   c. continuous incontinence.
   d. interrupted urinary stream.
   e. overflow incontinence.

7. Which of the following findings is most likely present on an ultrasound in a patient with an ectopic ureter in a duplicated system?
   a. Echogenic parenchyma of the lower pole of the kidney
   b. Medially displaced lower pole of the kidney
   c. Cystic structure in the bladder
   d. Tortuous lower pole ureter
   e. Cystic changes in the upper pole of the kidney

8. Which of the following anatomic derangements will NOT be seen in a patient with bilateral single-system ectopic ureters?
   a. Poorly developed bladder neck
   b. Decreased bladder capacity
   c. Hutch diverticulum
   d. Trigone underdevelopment
   e. Dysplastic renal parenchyma

9. Ureteroceles can be associated with all of the following EXCEPT:
   a. smoking during pregnancy.
   b. vesicoureteral reflux.
   c. white race.
   d. female gender.
   e. duplicated kidneys.

10. All of the following can be caused by a ureterocele. Which is the least likely?
    a. Bladder outlet obstruction
    b. Upper pole obstruction

c. Ipsilateral lower pole reflux

d. Urinary incontinence

e. Contralateral reflux

11. A child known to have a ureterocele based on ultrasound imaging undergoes cystography, but no filling defect is noted. The most likely explanation is:

a. ureterocele eversion.

b. lower pole reflux.

c. ureterocele effacement.

d. ureterocele prolapse.

e. ureterocele disproportion.

12. A girl undergoes open resection of a large ectopic ureterocele. After removal of the catheter, she has high postvoid residuals demonstrated on a sonogram. Which complication is most likely responsible?

a. Persistent reflux

b. Prolapsing residual ureterocele tissue

c. Neuropraxia secondary to bladder retraction

d. Excessive buttressing of deficient detrusor at the bladder neck

e. Residual flap of the ureterocele in the urethra

13. What is the preferred method of endoscopic treatment of a ureterocele?

a. Resection of the roof of the ureterocele

b. Puncture of the ureterocele's urethral extension

c. Puncture of the roof of the ureterocele

d. Transverse incision at the base of the ureterocele

e. Resection of the base of the ureterocele only

14. An adult is evaluated as a possible kidney donor. An excretory urogram demonstrates a round contrast-filled area at the bladder base with a thin radiolucent rim around it. What is the most likely diagnosis?

a. Single-system kidney with a ureterocele

b. Marked opacification delay of the kidney

c. Radiopaque stone filling the ureterocele

d. Extension of a ureterocele to the bladder neck and urethra

e. Reflux

15. A white infant is found to have a smooth interlabial mass on the posterior aspect of the urethra. What would be the most appropriate initial management?

a. Chemotherapy

b. Puncture of the mass

c. Topical estrogen cream

d. Observation

e. Resection of the mass

16. An 11-year-old child presents with flank pain and hematuria. There is left hydronephrosis to the ureteropelvic junction. There is no ureteral dilation. Diuretic renography shows symmetric uptake in both kidneys and a $t_{1/2}$ of 40 minutes. At the time of surgery a retrograde pyelogram shows a proximal ureteral filling defect. What is the best course of action?

a. Abandon the procedure and obtain CT imaging with contrast

b. Perform ureteroscopic biopsy

c. Perform radical nephroureterectomy

d. Perform ureteroscopic excision of the presumed fibroepithelial polyp

e. Proceed with dismembered pyeloplasty and resect the fibroepithelial polyp

17. Which of the following statements regarding duplex kidneys is TRUE?

a. Duplex kidneys are the same size as single-system kidneys.

b. The upper pole moiety is the more likely of the two to have a ureteropelvic junction obstruction.

c. The duplex kidney arises as a consequence of two separate ureteric buds.

d. A duplex kidney results from two separate metanephric blastemal entities arising near the mesonephric duct.

e. The lower pole ureter is less likely to have vesicoureteral reflux.

18. In a child with a functioning nondilated upper pole segment associated with an ectopic ureter, which of the following therapeutic options are most appropriate? (More than one answer may be correct.)

a. Common sheath ureteral reimplantation

b. Upper to lower uretero-pyelostomy

c. Upper to lower distal ureteroureterostomy

d. Upper pole partial nephrectomy

e. Upper pole ureteral reimplantation

19. Initial endoscopic incision of a ureterocele offers all of the following advantages EXCEPT:

a. early relief of bladder outlet obstruction.

b. potential for definitive therapy.

c. possible improvement in trigonal deficiency.

d. potential for improved function of the affected renal segment.

e. decompression of a dilated upper pole ureter.

20. What is the most common form of ureteral triplication?

a. All three ureters joining to terminate in a single bladder orifice

b. Three ureters joining to form two ureteral orifices

c. Three ureters draining as three separate orifices

d. One of the three ureters terminating ectopically, the other two draining orthotopically

e. Two ureters draining into three orifices

21. Failure of atrophy of which vessel leads to the formation of a preureteral vena cava?

a. Posterior cardinal vein

b. Subcardinal vein

c. Supracardinal vein

d. Umbilical artery

e. Inferior vitelline vein

22. Which of the following types of ureterocele is associated with the lowest incidence of secondary procedures after endoscopic treatment?

a. Ectopic ureterocele

b. Ureterocele in a female patient

c. Intravesical ureterocele

d. Ureterocele associated with a duplicated system

e. Cecoureterocele

23. After the perinatal period, what is the most common method of presentation of a ureterocele?

a. Incontinence

b. Abdominal mass

c. Failure to thrive

d. Stranguria

e. Urinary tract infection

24. A patient with a suspected ectopic ureter without hydronephrosis has a renal moiety that is difficult to define on an ultrasonographic study. Which of the following tests is a sensitive method of detecting this moiety?

a. Diethylenetriaminepentaacetic acid (DTPA) renal scanning

b. MRI of the abdomen and pelvis

c. Nuclear voiding cystourethrography

d. Positron emission tomography

e. Intravenous pyelography

ANSWERS

1. **c. ovary.** An ectopic ureter may drain into any of the structures related to the Wolffian duct and can rupture into the adjoining fallopian tube, uterus, upper vagina, or urethra.

2. **a. Dysplasia.** Clinical and experimental observations combine to support the commonly held notion that dysplasia is the product of inadequate ureteric bud-to-blastema interaction. The other conditions may include an abnormal interaction but are not specifically the result of that interaction.

3. **c. orifice is caudal and medial to the lower pole orifice.** This is due to its later incorporaton and migration into the trigonal structure. The lower pole orifice is more cranial and lateral to the caudad medial upper pole orifice.

4. **b. lax bladder neck.** It is owing to the combined effects of the lateral ureteral orifice position, the ureter's shortened submucosal course, the poorly developed trigone, and the abnormal morphology of the ureteral orifice that primary vesicoureteral reflux develops.

5. **d. posterior urethra.** In the male the posterior urethra is the most common site of the termination of the ectopic ureter. All other sites except the anterior urethra are possible sites of ectopic ureteral insertion.

6. **c. continuous incontinence.** Continuous incontinence in a girl with an otherwise normal voiding pattern after toilet training is the classic symptom of an ectopic ureteral orifice. This may not be obvious in the pre-toilet-trained girl but can occasionally be seen as slow, steady dribbling of urine on direct observation.

7. **d. Tortuous lower pole ureter.** The most obvious imaging sign on ultrasonography of an ectopic ureter is a tortuous dilated ureter due to distal obstruction. This is not always present but, when seen, should direct further attention to the distal ureter and bladder to also assess for the presence of a ureterocele, which would appear as a cystic structure in the bladder. The upper pole may be dysplastic, but cystic changes are uncommon. The lower pole is usually normal but may be hydronephrotic yet uncommonly echogenic. The lower pole is displaced laterally, not medially.

8. **c. Hutch diverticulum.** Because there is no formation of the trigone and base plate, a wide, poorly defined, incompetent vesical neck results. In rare instances, bilateral single ectopic ureters are associated with agenesis of the bladder and urethra. Commonly, the involved kidneys are dysplastic or display varying degrees of hydronephrosis. The ureters are usually dilated, and reflux is often present. The bladder neck is incompetent; therefore the child dribbles continuously. Because there is poor resistance, the bladder does not have the opportunity to distend with urine and therefore has a small capacity.

9. **a. smoking during pregnancy.** They occur most frequently in females (4:1 ratio) and almost exclusively in whites. Approximately 10% are bilateral. Eighty percent of all ureteroceles arise from the upper poles of duplicated systems, and approximately 50% will have associated vesicoureteral reflux.

10. **a. Bladder outlet obstruction.** Ultrasonographic study shows a dilated ureter emanating from a hydronephrotic upper pole (see Fig. 121–11 in *Campbell-Walsh Urology, 10th Edition*). This finding should signal the examiner to image the bladder to determine whether a ureterocele is present. If the lower pole is associated with reflux or if the ureterocele has caused delayed emptying from the ipsilateral lower pole, the lower pole may likewise be hydronephrotic. Similarly, the ureterocele may impinge on the contralateral ureteral orifice or obstruct the bladder neck and cause hydronephrosis in the opposite kidney, but the latter is uncommon. The upper pole parenchyma drained by the ureterocele will exhibit varying degrees of thickness and echogenicity. Increased echogenicity correlates with dysplastic changes. Reflux may also be seen in the contralateral system if the ureterocele is large enough to distort the trigone and the opposite ureteral submucosal tunnel. In one series, 28% of patients had reflux in the contralateral unit.

11. **c. ureterocele effacement.** Voiding cystourethrography can usually demonstrate the size and laterality of the ureterocele, as well as the presence or absence of vesicoureteral reflux. If early filling views are not obtained, the ureterocele may efface and the filling defect may not be visible. In some cases the ureterocele will evert and appear as a diverticulum.

12. **e. Residual flap of the ureterocele in the urethra.** The authors of one study emphasized the need for passing a large catheter antegrade through the bladder neck to ascertain that all mucosal lips that might act as obstructing valves have been removed. In some large ureteroceles, if repair of the maldeveloped trigone is not adequate, a posterior defect at the bladder neck can act as an obstructive valve during voiding.

13. **d. Transverse incision at the base of the ureterocele.** Our preferred method of incising the ureterocele is similar to that described by Rich and colleagues (1990),* a transverse incision through the full thickness of the ureterocele wall using the cutting current. Making the incision as distally on the ureterocele and as close to the

---

*Sources referenced can be found in *Campbell-Walsh Urology, 10th Edition,* on the Expert Consult website.

bladder floor as possible lessens the chance of postoperative reflux into the ureterocele.

14. **a. Single-system kidney.** Excretory urography often demonstrates the characteristic cobra-head (or spring-onion) deformity: an area of increased density similar to the head of a cobra with a halo or less dense shadow around it. The halo represents a filling defect, which is the ureterocele wall, and the oval density is contrast material excreted into the ureterocele from the functioning kidney.

15. **b. Puncture of the mass.** A ureterocele that extends through the bladder neck and the urethra and presents as a vaginal mass in girls is termed a *prolapsing ureterocele.* This mass can be distinguished from other interlabial masses (e.g., rhabdomyosarcoma, urethral prolapse, hydrometrocolpos, periurethral cysts) by virtue of its appearance and location. The prolapsed ureterocele has a smooth, round wall, as compared with the grapelike cluster that typifies rhabdomyosarcoma (see Fig. 121–8 in *Campbell-Walsh Urology, 10th Edition*). The color may vary from pink to bright red to the necrotic shades of blue, purple, or brown. The ureterocele usually slides down the posterior wall of the urethra and, hence, the urethra can be demonstrated anterior to the mass and catheterized. The short-term goal is to decompress the ureterocele. The prolapsing ureterocele may be manually reduced back into the bladder; however, even if this is successful, the prolapse is likely to recur. Subsequent management is determined by further functional evaluation.

16. **e. Proceed with dismembered pyeloplasty and resect the fibroepithelial polyp.** This scenario most likely represents a fibroepithelial polyp of the ureteropelvic junction creating or associated with obstruction. The best approach is to proceed with the planned pyeloplasty, identify and resect the polyp thoroughly, and perform a conventional dismembered pyeloplasty. At times polyps may be multiple and complex, so this possibility should be looked for.

17. **c. The duplex kidney arises as a consequence of two separate ureteric buds.** Duplication anomalies arise as a consequence of two ureteral buds forming and inducing separate segments of the metanephric blastema. The duplex kidney may be completely normal, although it tends to be longer than normal, but if there is abnormal development, reflux and ureteropelvic junction obstruction occurs, most often in the lower pole, while ectopic ureteral insertion with or without a ureterocele is nearly always associated with the upper pole.

18. **b *and* c.** When the upper pole of a duplex system associated with an ectopic ureter demonstrates function, preservation is typically recommended. Two reasonable options exist for this including proximal ureteropyelostomy, which excises most of the usually dilated upper pole ureter, and distal ureteroureterostomy, which permits drainage without any manipulation of the perirenal tissues. There are no data to support one over the other, and both are reasonable options. There is no evidence to indicate that the so-called "yo-yo" phenomenon of urine refluxing into more dilated segments of ureter is a clinically significant concern.

19. **c. Possible improvement in trigonal deficiency.** Transurethral puncture of a ureterocele does not improve trigonal deficiency, which can be associated with a severe ureterocele. This deficiency, which may lead to persisting reflux and bladder outlet obstruction, may require corrective surgery.

20. **a. All three ureters joining to terminate in a single bladder orifice.** In the classification used by most investigators, there are four varieties of triplicate ureter. In one variety, all three ureters unite and drain through a single orifice. This appears to be the most common form encountered, while all others have been reported.

21. **b. Subcardinal vein.** If the subcardinal vein in the lumbar portion fails to atrophy and becomes the primary right-sided vein, the ureter is trapped dorsal to it.

22. **c. Intravesical ureterocele.** Several studies have indicated that intravesical ureteroceles fared better than extravesical ureteroceles with regard to decompression, preservation of upper pole function, newly created reflux, and need for secondary procedures. Nonetheless, the clinical scenario will be the most important indicator of the appropriateness of endoscopic incision for a ureterocele in a particular patient.

23. **e. Urinary tract infection.** Many ureteroceles are still diagnosed clinically. The most common presentation is that of an infant who has a urinary tract infection or urosepsis. In the early perinatal period, prenatal identification of hydronephrosis is currently the most common means of diagnosis.

24. **b. MRI of the abdomen and pelvis.** Occasionally, the renal parenchyma associated with an ectopic ureter is difficult to locate on ultrasound and may be identified only by alternative imaging studies. In such cases in which an ectopic ureter is strongly suspected because of incontinence yet no definite evidence of the upper pole renal segment is found, CT or MRI has demonstrated the small, poorly functioning upper pole segment (see Fig. 121–16 in *Campbell-Walsh Urology, 10th Edition*).

Additional Study Points

1. An ectopic ureter in a duplex system inevitably drains the upper pole.
2. In females the ectopic ureter may enter from the bladder neck to the perineum or into the vagina, uterus, or rectum.
3. In males the ectopic ureter always enters the urogenital system above the external sphincter and may enter wolffian duct structures such as the vas deferens, seminal vesicles, and ejaculatory duct.
4. The orifice of a cecoureterocele is within the bladder; however, the ureterocele may extend beyond the bladder neck into the urethra.
5. The ectopic ureter inserts into the wolffian duct structure and not directly into a müllerian structure. Therefore in the female, in order for an ectopic ureter to enter the vagina, cervix, or uterus, it requires a rupture into those structures.
6. The Weigert-Meyer rule states that an ectopic ureter or ureterocele is associated with the upper pole and is located caudal to the lower pole ureteral orifice.
7. A young boy presenting with epididymitis might have an ectopic ureter.
8. A toilet-trained girl with verified continuous urinary leakage should be evaluated for an ectopic ureter.

9. A ureterocele or ectopic ureter associated with a patulous bladder neck may be complicated by incontinence. Cecoureteroceles are at particular risk for this.

10. On endoscopy, ureteroceles vary in their appearance with bladder filling.

11. In a transurethral incision of the ureterocele, the incision is made transversely as close to the bladder floor as possible.

12. In patients who have an ectopic ureter who present with sepsis and have massive ureteral dilatation, a temporary end ureterostomy may be the best management.

13. When the upper pole of the kidney is removed for an ectopic ureter, the residual stump is rarely problematic.

14. The separation of ureters distally in the intravesicle dissection should be discouraged because it may injure the common blood supply.

15. Conditions that routinely affect the single-system kidney generally affect the lower pole of a duplex system such as ureteropelvic junction obstruction and vesicle ureteral reflux. Conditions that affect the upper pole are more likely due to abnormal ureteral formation such as ectopia and ureterocele.

16. Fibroepithelial polyps most commonly occur at the ureteral pelvic junction but may occur anywhere in the ureter.

17. Correction of the circumcaval ureter requires ureteral division and excision or bypass of the retrocaval segment.

Vesicoureteral Reflux

Antoine E. Khoury, MD, FRCSC, FAAP ● Darius J. Bägli, MDCM, FRCSC, FAAP, FACS

QUESTIONS

1. The estimated prevalence of vesicoureteral reflux in children with a urinary tract infection (UTI) is:
   a. 1%.
   b. 3%.
   c. 5%.
   d. 10%.
   e. 30%.

2. Which of the following statements regarding reflux is FALSE?
   a. Antenatally detected reflux is associated with a male preponderance.
   b. Antenatally detected reflux is usually low grade in boys when compared with that in girls.
   c. Antenatally detected reflux is usually bilateral in boys when compared with that in girls.
   d. When reflux is detected antenatally, renal impairment is frequently present at birth and is likely due to congenital dysplasia.
   e. The majority of reflux detected later in life occurs in females.

3. Which one of the following statements regarding vesicoureteral reflux in regard to patient's race is TRUE?
   a. The incidence of vesicoureteral reflux is equal in children of all races.
   b. The disparity in the incidence of vesicoureteral reflux with respect to race becomes clearer in adulthood.
   c. The frequency of detected vesicoureteral reflux is lower in female children of African descent.
   d. African infants and white infants have a similar incidence of reflux diagnosed on the basis of antenatal hydronephrosis.
   e. There is a clear understanding regarding the predisposition of reflux because many of the studies have included patients from different countries around the world.

4. Which of the following statements is FALSE in regard to the diagnosis and treatment of sibling vesicoureteral reflux?

   a. On the basis of clinical judgment and the presence or absence of UTI, the patient's age should be taken into account in regard to the decision to proceed with diagnostic intervention to diagnose sibling reflux.
   b. It is reasonable to prescribe antibiotic prophylaxis while the decision to diagnose sibling reflux or not takes place.
   c. Once sibling reflux is diagnosed, the indications for correction are different from the indications for treating reflux in the general pediatric population diagnosed after UTI.
   d. Siblings who are younger than 5 years of age with normal imaging studies of the kidneys can be managed on the basis of clinical judgment, and it is not absolutely necessary to obtain a voiding cystogram.
   e. Siblings younger than 5 years of age who present with cortical renal defects have the most to lose by febrile UTIs in the presence of vesicoureteral reflux.

5. Primary reflux is a congenital anomaly of the ureterovesical junction with which of the following characteristics? A deficiency of the:
   a. longitudinal muscle of the extravesical ureter results in an inadequate valvular mechanism.
   b. longitudinal muscle of the intravesical ureter results in an inadequate valvular mechanism.
   c. circumferential muscle of the extravesical ureter results in an inadequate valvular mechanism.
   d. circumferential muscle of the intravesical ureter results in an inadequate valvular mechanism.
   e. longitudinal and circumferential muscles of the intravesical ureter results in an inadequate valvular mechanism.

6. What is the ratio of tunnel length to ureteral diameter found in normal children without reflux?
   a. 5:1
   b. 4:1
   c. 3:1
   d. 2:1
   e. 1:1

7. Which of the following is TRUE regarding children with non-neurogenic neurogenic bladders?

   a. Constriction of the urinary sphincter occurs during voiding in a voluntary form of detrusor-sphincter dyssynergia.

   b. Gradual bladder decompensation and myogenic failure result from incomplete emptying.

   c. Gradual bladder decompensation and myogenic failure result from increasing amounts of residual urine.

   d. All of the above apply.

   e. None of the above apply.

8. Which of the following statements is TRUE in regard to secondary vesicoureteral reflux?

   a. The most common cause of anatomic bladder obstruction in the pediatric population is posterior urethral valves, and vesicoureteral reflux is present in a great majority of these children.

   b. Anatomic obstruction of the bladder is a common cause of secondary vesicoureteral reflux in female patients.

   c. Patients with neurofunctional etiology for secondary vesicoureteral reflux benefit from immediate surgical intervention to try to correct vesicoureteral reflux.

   d. A sacral dimple or hairy patch on the lower back is not a significant finding in regard to evaluation and treatment of vesicoureteral reflux.

   e. The most common structural obstruction in male and female patients is the presence of a ureterocele at the bladder neck.

9. The complex anatomic relationships required of the ureterovesical junction may be gradually damaged by:

   a. decreases in bladder wall compliance.

   b. detrusor decompensation.

   c. incomplete emptying.

   d. all of the above.

   e. none of the above.

10. What does the initial management of functional causes of reflux involve?

    a. Surgical treatment

    b. Medical treatment

    c. Observation only

    d. All of the above

    e. None of the above

11. Signs or symptoms of voiding dysfunction include:

    a. dribbling.

    b. urgency.

    c. incontinence.

    d. "curtseying" behavior in girls.

    e. all of the above.

12. Treatment of bladder dysfunction and instability, regardless of its severity or cause, is directed at:

    a. damping uninhibited bladder contractions.

    b. dilating the urethral sphincter.

    c. lowering intravesical pressures.

    d. all of the above.

    e. a and c only.

13. There is a strong association between the presence of reflux in patients with neuropathic bladders and intravesical pressures of greater than:

    a. 10 cm H_2O.

    b. 20 cm H_2O.

    c. 40 cm H_2O.

    d. 60 cm H_2O.

    e. 80 cm H_2O.

14. Bladder infections and their accompanying inflammation can also cause reflux by:

    a. lessening compliance.

    b. elevating intravesical pressures.

    c. distorting and weakening the ureterovesical junction.

    d. All of the above

    e. None of the above

15. Which system provides the current standard for grading reflux on the basis of the appearance of contrast in the ureter and upper collecting system during voiding cystourethrography?

    a. The Heikel and Parkkulainen system

    b. The International Classification system

    c. The Dwoskin and Perlmutter system

    d. The National Classification system

    e. The Dwoskin and Parkkulainen system

16. Which of the following is TRUE regarding accurately grading reflux with coexistent ipsilateral obstruction?

    a. It is not possible.

    b. It is facilitated by obtaining a renal scan.

    c. It is facilitated by obtaining an ultrasonographic scan.

    d. It is facilitated by obtaining an excretory urogram.

    e. It is facilitated by obtaining a radionuclide cystogram.

17. Which of the following is TRUE regarding the presence of fever?

    a. It may be an indicator of upper urinary tract involvement.

    b. It may not always be a reliable sign of upper urinary tract involvement.

    c. It increases the likelihood of discovering vesicoureteral reflux.

    d. All of the above apply.

    e. None of the above apply.

18. Complete evaluation including a voiding cystourethrogram (VCUG) and ultrasound are required for which of the following patients?

    a. An uncircumcised male infant with a febrile illness and a positive urine culture obtained through a bagged specimen

    b. A 3-year-old girl admitted to the hospital with pneumonia and found to have *Escherichia coli* on a urine culture without pyuria detected by microscopic analysis

    c. A female patient with recurrent culture and urinalysis proven to have afebrile UTIs and later found to have scarring on a dimercaptosuccinic acid (DMSA) scan

    d. Any child older than 5 years of age with documented UTIs

    e. None of the above

19. Which of the following statements is TRUE regarding screening of older children who present with asymptomatic bacteriuria? They can be screened initially with:
    a. ultrasonography.
    b. cystography.
    c. excretory urography.
    d. renal scan.
    e. nothing because they do not require any screening studies.

20. Which of the following is TRUE regarding cystography?
    a. Cystography performed with a Foley catheter or while the patient is under anesthesia produces static studies that inaccurately screen for reflux or sometimes exaggerate its degree because of bladder overfilling.
    b. Cystography performed in the presence of excessive hydration may mask low grades of reflux because diuresis can blunt the retrograde flow of urine.
    c. Cystograms may show reflux only during active infections when cystitis weakens the ureterovesical junction with edema or by increasing intravesical pressures.
    d. Cystograms obtained during active infections can overestimate the grade of reflux because the endotoxins produced by some gram-negative organisms can paralyze ureteral smooth muscle and exaggerate ureteral dilatation.
    e. All of the above apply.

21. Which of the following statements is TRUE regarding radionuclide cystography?
    a. It provides similar anatomic detail to that obtained with fluoroscopic cystography.
    b. It is an accurate method for detecting and following reflux.
    c. It is associated with more radiation exposure than is fluoroscopic cystography.
    d. It is a less sensitive test than fluoroscopic cystography.
    e. It provides more anatomic detail than fluoroscopic cystography.

22. Which of the following statements is TRUE regarding ultrasonography?
    a. It is the diagnostic study of choice to initially evaluate the upper urinary tracts of patients with suspected or proven vesicoureteral reflux.
    b. It can effectively rule out reflux.
    c. It should be performed every 2 to 3 years in patients with reflux who are medically managed.
    d. It is the study of choice for assessing renal function.
    e. An ultrasonogram showing intermittent dilatation of the renal pelvis or ureter confirms the presence of reflux.

23. What is the best study for the detection of pyelonephritis and cortical renal scarring?
    a. Diethylenetriaminepentaacetic acid (DTPA) renal scan
    b. DMSA renal scan
    c. Mercaptoacetyltriglycine (MAG3) renal scan
    d. Pyelogram
    e. Renal ultrasonographic scan

24. Which of the following is TRUE regarding urodynamic studies?
    a. They may be indicated in any child suspected of having a secondary cause for reflux (valves, neurogenic bladder, non-neurogenic neurogenic bladder, voiding dysfunction).
    b. They should be performed without the use of prophylactic antibiotics in children with secondary reflux.
    c. They help direct therapy in patients with secondary reflux.
    d. All of the above apply.
    e. Only a and c are true.

25. Which of the following is TRUE in regard to the evaluation of vesicoureteral reflux?
    a. Routine cystoscopy is indicated in the workup of patients with vesicoureteral reflux.
    b. The radiation doses with modern digital techniques have improved the anatomic detail, but the radiation dose with VCUG remains significantly higher than that of a radionuclide cystogram.
    c. Grading of reflux by VCUG and radionuclide cystogram is similar and comparable between the two imaging modalities.
    d. Ultrasonography provides an alternative means to evaluate the presence or absence of vesicoureteral reflux.
    e. Uroflowmetry is a valuable tool in the workup of a patient with vesicoureteral reflux.

26. Which of the following accurately describes what happens during ureteral development? A ureteral bud that:
    a. is medially (caudally) positioned from a normal takeoff at the trigone offers an embryologic explanation for primary reflux.
    b. is laterally (cranially) positioned from a normal takeoff at the trigone offers an embryologic explanation for primary reflux.
    c. fails to meet with the renal blastema offers an embryologic explanation for primary reflux.
    d. is laterally (cranially) positioned is often obstructed.
    e. fails to meet with the renal blastema is often obstructed.

27. In regard to the diagnosis of renal scars based on renal scintigraphy, which of the following is TRUE?
    a. An area of photopenia detected during an acute episode of pyelonephritis always represents renal scar.
    b. Photopenic areas may result from postinfection renal scarring and some renal dysplasia.
    c. Ultrasound is a sensitive and accurate diagnostic modality for renal scarring.
    d. Areas for photopenia detected during an acute episode of pyelonephritis that later resolve on a subsequent renal scan represent resolution of renal scarring.
    e. All of the above apply.

28. Which of the following is TRUE regarding hypertension?
    a. In children and young adults it is most commonly caused by reflux nephropathy.

b. It is not related to the grade of reflux or severity of scarring.

c. It is not associated with abnormalities of Na+,K+-ATPase activity.

d. All of the above apply.

e. None of the above apply.

29. Which of the following factors might contribute to the effects of reflux on renal growth?

a. The congenital dysmorphism often associated with, but not caused by, reflux

b. The number and type of urinary infections and their resultant nephropathy

c. The quality of the contralateral kidney and its implications for compensatory hypertrophy

d. The grade of reflux in the affected kidney

e. All of the above

30. With regard to renal growth and reflux, which of the following is TRUE?

a. With the exception of those kidneys that are developmentally arrested, most studies implicate infection as the cause for altered renal growth.

b. Successful antireflux surgery can accelerate renal growth.

c. Successful antireflux surgery may not allow the affected kidneys to return to normal size.

d. All of the above apply.

e. None of the above apply.

31. The anatomy of patients with ureteral duplication typically follows the Weigert-Meyer rule, in which the upper pole ureter enters the bladder:

a. distally and medially, and the lower pole ureter enters the bladder proximally and laterally.

b. proximally and medially, and the lower pole ureter enters the bladder distally and laterally.

c. distally and laterally, and the lower pole ureter enters the bladder proximally and medially.

d. proximally and laterally, and the lower pole ureter enters the bladder distally and medially.

e. superior to the lower pole ureter.

32. Which of the following is TRUE regarding vesicoureteral reflux?

a. It is infrequently associated with complete ureteral duplications.

b. It may occur into either ureter of a duplicated system.

c. It more often involves the ureter from the upper pole in a duplicated system.

d. It resolves less frequently in patients with double ureters.

e. All of the above apply.

33. Which of the following regarding reflux is TRUE?

a. The reflux associated with small paraureteral diverticula resolves at rates similar to those of primary reflux and can be managed accordingly.

b. The reflux associated with paraureteral large diverticula is less likely to resolve and usually requires surgical correction.

c. The reflux associated with diverticula, in which the ureter enters the diverticulum, regardless of size, should be corrected surgically.

d. All of the above apply.

e. None of the above apply.

34. Which of the following accurately describes the state of the bladder during pregnancy?

a. Urine volume decreases in the upper collecting system as the physiologic dilatation of pregnancy evolves.

b. Bladder tone increases because of edema and hyperemia.

c. Bladder changes predispose the patient to bacteriuria.

d. All of the above apply.

e. None of the above apply.

35. During pregnancy, the presence of vesicoureteral reflux in a system already prone to bacteriuria may lead to increased morbidity. What is an additional risk factor?

a. Renal scarring

b. Tendency to get urinary infections

c. Hypertension

d. Renal insufficiency

e. All of the above

36. Which of the following is considered to be TRUE regarding reflux management?

a. Spontaneous resolution of vesicoureteral reflux is common.

b. Higher grades of vesicoureteral reflux are less likely to resolve than lower grades.

c. Reflux of sterile urine is a benign process that does not lead to significant renal damage.

d. Prolonged use of antibiotic prophylaxis has no known health consequences.

e. All of the above apply.

37. Regarding surgical correction of vesicoureteral reflux, which of the following is currently accepted?

a. Extravesical ureteral reimplantation

b. Intravesical ureteral reimplantation

c. Endoscopic injection of bulking agent

d. All of the above

e. None of the above

38. Common to each type of open surgical repair for reflux is the creation of:

a. a valvular mechanism that enables ureteral compression with bladder filling and contraction.

b. a mucosal tunnel for reimplantation having adequate muscular backing.

c. a tunnel length of three times the ureteral diameter.

d. all of the above.

e. none of the above.

39. Complete ureteral duplications with reflux can be best managed surgically by:

a. separating the ureters and reimplanting them separately.

b. a common sheath repair in which both ureters are mobilized with one mucosal cuff.

c. performing an upper to lower ureteroureterostomy and reimplanting the lower ureter.

d. performing a lower to upper ureteroureterostomy and reimplanting the upper ureter.

e. none of the above.

40. Early postoperative obstruction can occur after a ureteral reimplant due to:

a. edema.

b. subtrigonal bleeding.

c. mucus plugs.

d. blood clots.

e. all of the above.

41. If early postoperative obstruction occurs after a ureteral reimplant, the next step is:

a. immediate nephrostomy tube placement.

b. immediate placement of a ureteral stent.

c. initial observation and diversion for unabating symptoms.

d. placement of both a nephrostomy tube and a ureteral stent.

e. reoperation.

42. Which of the following is TRUE regarding persistent reflux after ureteral reimplantation?

a. It may be due to unrecognized secondary causes of reflux such as neuropathic bladder and severe voiding dysfunction.

b. It seldom results from a failure to provide adequate muscular backing for the ureter within its tunnel.

c. It may be repaired surgically using minor submucosal advancements.

d. All of the above apply.

e. None of the above apply.

43. Which of the following is TRUE regarding the treatment of vesicoureteral reflux?

a. Since the widespread acceptance of endoscopic treatment, the indications for surgical correction differ between open endoscopic and laparoscopic approach.

b. Long-term follow-up data support the durability of endoscopic injection therapy.

c. All injection materials provide a similar success rate and are just as easily injected under similar circumstances.

d. The accuracy of the needle entry point during endoscopic injection, as well as the needle placement, are important components for the success of the surgical procedure.

e. The learning curve for endoscopic injection is similar to the learning curve for open surgical reimplantation.

44. Which of the following is TRUE regarding the laparoscopic approach for ureteral reimplantation?

a. The advantages of this approach over open surgery include smaller incisions, less discomfort, brief hospitalizations, and quicker convalescence.

b. As with other laparoscopic procedures, experience is essential to the success of this approach.

c. Costs may be increased because of lengthier surgery and the expense of disposable equipment.

d. All of the above apply.

e. None of the above apply.

ANSWERS

1. **e. 30%.** A meta-analysis of studies of children undergoing cystography for various indications has indicated that the prevalence of vesicoureteral reflux is estimated to be 30% for children with UTIs and about 17% in children without infection.

2. **b. Antenatally detected reflux is usually low grade in boys when compared with that in girls.** The reflux is usually high grade and bilateral in boys when compared with reflux in girls.

3. **c. The frequency of detected vesicoureteral reflux is lower in female children of African descent.** One of the clear differences that has been established over several studies is the relative 10-fold lower frequency of vesicoureteral reflux in female children of African descent.

4. **c. Once sibling reflux is diagnosed, the indications for correction are different from the indications for treating reflux in the general pediatric population diagnosed after UTI.** By taking into account the imaging of the kidneys first, as well as the patient's age and history of UTI, a rational top-down approach to sibling reflux screening emerges. In any sibling, however, in which reflux is diagnosed, the indications for treatment remain the same as for general reflux in the pediatric population.

5. **b. longitudinal muscle of the intravesical ureter results in an inadequate valvular mechanism.** Primary reflux is a congenital anomaly of the ureterovesical junction in which a deficiency of the longitudinal muscle of the intravesical ureter results in an inadequate valvular mechanism.

6. **a. 5:1.** In Paquin's novel study, a 5:1 tunnel length–ureteral diameter ratio was found in normal children without reflux.

7. **d. All of the above apply.** On the far end of this spectrum are children with non-neurogenic neurogenic bladders. Here, constriction of the urinary sphincter occurs during voiding in a voluntary form of detrusor-sphincter dyssynergia. Gradual bladder decompensation and myogenic failure result from incomplete emptying and increasing amounts of residual urine.

8. **a. The most common cause of anatomic bladder obstruction in the pediatric population is posterior urethral valves, and vesicoureteral reflux is present in a great majority of these children.** This diagnosis is obviously limited to male patients; consequently, female patients have a lower incidence of anatomic bladder obstruction. The most common structural obstruction in female patients is the presence of a ureterocele that prolapses and obstructs the bladder neck. Between 48% and 70% of patients with posterior urethral valves have vesicoureteral reflux, and relief of obstruction appears to be responsible for resolution of the reflux in a good number of those patients. The presence of a neurologic disorder should prompt the clinician to treat based on the primary etiology as opposed to proceeding with immediate surgical correction. One important aspect of the physical examination in children who present with vesicoureteral reflux is detection of potential occult spinal dysraphism, and this includes a thorough physical examination looking for sacral dimples, hairy patches, or gluteal cleft abnormalities.

9. **d. all of the above.** Decreases in bladder wall compliance, detrusor decompensation, and incomplete emptying gradually damage the complex anatomic relationships required of the ureterovesical junction.

10. **b. Medical treatment.** The initial management of functional causes of reflux is medical. It is imperative that clinicians inquire about, and determine, the voiding patterns of children with reflux.

11. **e. all of the above.** In addition to a careful physical examination, signs or symptoms of voiding dysfunction include dribbling, urgency, and incontinence. Girls often exhibit curtseying behavior, and boys will squeeze the penis in an attempt to suppress bladder contractions.

12. **e. a and c only.** Treatment of bladder dysfunction and instability, regardless of its severity or cause, is directed at dampening uninhibited contractions and lowering intravesical pressures.

13. **c. 40 cm H$_2$O.** There is a strong association between intravesical pressures of greater than 40 cm H$_2$O and the presence of reflux in patients with myelodysplasia and neuropathic bladders.

14. **d. All of the above.** Bladder infections (UTIs) and their accompanying inflammation can also cause reflux by lessening compliance, elevating intravesical pressures, and distorting and weakening the ureterovesical junction.

15. **b. The International Classification System.** The Heikel and Parkkulainen system gained popularity in Europe a few years before the Dwoskin and Perlmutter system became widely accepted in the United States. The International Classification System devised in 1981 by the International Reflux Study represents a melding of the two. It provides the current standard for grading reflux on the basis of the appearance of contrast in the ureter and upper collecting system during voiding cystourethrography.

16. **a. It is not possible.** Accurately grading reflux is impossible with coexistent ipsilateral obstruction.

17. **d. All of the above apply.** The presence of fever may be an indicator of upper urinary tract involvement but is not always a reliable sign. However, if fever (and presumably pyelonephritis) is present, the likelihood of discovering vesicoureteral reflux is significantly increased.

18. **c. A female patient with recurrent culture and urinalysis proven to have afebrile UTIs and later found to have scarring on a dimercaptosuccinic acid (DMSA) scan.** The presence of culture-proven UTIs in the setting of an abnormal renal scan should raise the question of vesicoureteral reflux, and it is reasonable to proceed with a VCUG and ultrasound in those patients. The other clinical scenarios include a patient without pyuria and a clear alternative source for her fever, as well as an infant diagnosed with UTI with a specimen obtained through a bagged collection. In those children the diagnosis of UTI should be questioned before proceeding with evaluation through cystogram and renal ultrasonography. Patients older than 5 years of age should not undergo immediate VCUG just on the basis of the presence of a UTI.

19. **a. ultrasonography.** Older children who present with asymptomatic bacteriuria or UTIs that manifest solely with lower tract symptoms can be screened initially with ultrasonography alone, reserving cystography for those with abnormal upper tracts or recalcitrant infections.

20. **e. All of the above apply.** Excessive hydration may mask low grades of reflux because diuresis can blunt the retrograde flow of urine. Some reflux is demonstrated only during active infections when cystitis weakens the ureterovesical junction with edema or by increasing intravesical pressures. In addition, cystograms obtained during active infections can overestimate the grade of reflux because the endotoxins produced by some gram-negative organisms can paralyze ureteral smooth muscle and exaggerate ureteral dilatation.

21. **b. It is an accurate method for detecting and following reflux.** Nuclear cystography is the scintigraphic equivalent of conventional cystography. Although the technique does not provide the anatomic detail of fluoroscopic studies, it is an accurate method for detecting and following reflux.

22. **a. It is the diagnostic study of choice to initially evaluate the upper urinary tracts of patients with suspected or proven vesicoureteral reflux.** Ultrasonography has replaced the excretory urogram (intravenous pyelogram) as the diagnostic study of choice to initially evaluate the upper urinary tracts of patients with suspected or proven vesicoureteral reflux.

23. **b. DMSA renal scan.** Renal scintigraphy with technetium 99m-labeled DMSA is the best study for detection of pyelonephritis and the cortical renal scarring that sometimes results.

24. **e. Only a and c are true.** Urodynamic studies may be indicated in any child suspected of having a secondary cause for reflux (e.g., valves, neurogenic bladder, non-neurogenic neurogenic bladder, voiding dysfunction), and they help direct therapy.

25. **e. Uroflowmetry is a valuable tool in the workup of a patient with vesicoureteral reflux.** Evaluation of the lower urinary tract cannot solely rely on imaging studies because reflux is considered to be a dynamic phenomenon. Uroflowmetry provides valuable information in the clinical assessment of these patients. Modern management of reflux does not include the routine evaluation through cystoscopy. The radionuclide cystogram has historically been described as a technique that requires a significantly lower dose of radiation than a regular VCUG, but the requirements with modern digital techniques have significantly narrowed the difference between these two imaging modalities. Unfortunately, ultrasound cannot reliably detect between the presence or absence of vesicoureteral reflux.

26. **b. is laterally (cranially) positioned from a normal takeoff at the trigone offers an embryologic explanation for primary reflux.** As Mackie and Stevens have suggested, a ureteral bud that is laterally (cranially) positioned from a normal takeoff at the trigone offers an embryologic explanation for primary reflux, whereas those inferiorly (caudally) positioned are often obstructed.

27. **b. Photopenic areas may result from postinfection renal scarring and some renal dysplasia.** Vesicoureteral reflux, particularly reflux of higher grades, may result in renal dysplasia, which often appears scintigraphically identical to postinfection pyelonephritic scars. During an episode of active pyelonephritis, the renal scan may show an area of photopenia that later, if it persists, represents renal scarring secondary to the infection. Neither renal scan nor ultrasonography can differentiate accurately between renal dysplasia and renal scarring.

28. **a. In children and young adults it is most commonly caused by reflux nephropathy.** Reflux nephropathy is the most common cause of severe hypertension in children and young adults, although the actual incidence is unknown.

29. **e. All of the above.** Factors that might contribute to the effects of reflux on renal growth include the congenital dysmorphism often associated with (30% of cases), but not caused by, reflux; the number and type of urinary infections and their resultant nephropathy; the quality of the contralateral kidney and its implications for compensatory hypertrophy; and the grade of reflux in the affected kidney.

30. **d. All of the above apply.** With the exception of those kidneys that are developmentally arrested, most studies implicate infection as the cause for altered renal growth. Successful antireflux surgery can accelerate renal growth but may not allow affected kidneys to return to normal size.

31. **a. distally and medially, and the lower pole ureter enters the bladder proximally and laterally.** The anatomy of patients with ureteral duplication typically follows the Weigert-Meyer rule wherein the upper pole ureter enters the bladder distally and medially and the lower pole ureter enters the bladder proximally and laterally.

32. **b. It may occur into either ureter of a duplicated system.** Although urine may reflux into either ureter, it more commonly involves the ureter from the lower pole because of its lateral position and shorter submucosal tunnel.

33. **d. All of the above apply.** Reflux associated with small diverticula resolves at rates similar to those of primary reflux and can be managed accordingly. In contrast, reflux found with paraureteral large diverticula is less likely to resolve and usually requires surgical correction. In any case, when the ureter enters the diverticulum, regardless of size, surgery is recommended.

34. **c. Bladder changes predispose the patient to bacteriuria.** Bladder tone decreases because of edema and hyperemia, which are changes that predispose the patient to bacteriuria. In addition, urine volume increases in the upper collecting system as the physiologic dilatation of pregnancy evolves.

35. **e. All of the above.** It seems logical to assume that during pregnancy the presence of vesicoureteral reflux in a system already prone to bacteriuria would lead to increased morbidity. Maternal history also becomes a factor if past reflux, renal scarring, and a tendency to get urinary infections are included. Women with hypertension and an element of renal failure are particularly at risk.

36. **e. All of the above.** As summarized by Walker (1994),* vesicoureteral reflux resolves spontaneously in many cases but is less likely to resolve in patients with a higher grade of reflux. The reflux of sterile urine is considered to be benign, as well as the extended use of prophylactic antibiotics. Surgical open correction has a high success rate.

37. **d. All of the above.** Extravesical and intravesical ureteral reimplantation are all options for treatment of vesicoureteral reflux. In the past decade there has been widespread enthusiasm for endoscopic treatment, and different bulking agents have been used to correct vesicoureteral reflux using minimal invasive techniques.

38. **a. a valvular mechanism that enables ureteral compression with bladder filling and contraction.** Common to each technique is the creation of a valvular mechanism that enables ureteral compression with bladder filling and contraction, thus reenacting normal anatomy and function. A successful ureteroneocystostomy provides a submucosal tunnel for reimplantation having sufficient length and adequate muscular backing. A tunnel length of five times the ureteral diameter is cited as necessary for eliminating reflux.

39. **b. a common sheath repair in which both ureters are mobilized with one mucosal cuff.** Approximately 10% of children undergoing antireflux surgery have an element of ureteral duplication. The most common configuration is a complete duplication that results in two separate orifices. This is best managed by preserving a cuff of bladder mucosa that encompasses both orifices. Because the pair typically share blood supply along their adjoining wall, mobilization as one unit with a "common sheath" preserves vascularity and minimizes trauma.

40. **e. all of the above.** Early after surgery, various degrees of obstruction can be expected of the reimplanted ureter. Edema, subtrigonal bleeding, and bladder spasms all possibly contribute. Mucus plugs and blood clots are other causes. Most postoperative obstructions are mild and asymptomatic and resolve spontaneously. More significant obstructions are usually symptomatic. Affected children typically present 1 to 2 weeks after surgery with acute abdominal pain, nausea, and vomiting.

41. **c. initial observation and diversion for unabating symptoms.** The large majority of perioperative obstructions subside spontaneously, but placement of a nephrostomy tube or ureteral stent sometimes becomes necessary for unabating symptoms.

42. **a. It may be due to unrecognized secondary causes of reflux such as neuropathic bladder and severe voiding dysfunction.** Other than technical errors, failure to identify and treat secondary causes of reflux is a common cause of the reappearance of reflux. Foremost among these secondary causes are unrecognized neuropathic bladder and severe voiding dysfunction.

43. **d. The accuracy of the needle entry point during endoscopic injection, as well as the needle placement, are important components for the success of the surgical procedure.** The learning curve for endoscopic injection is believed to be different from that of open surgical reimplantation, but studies have not been carried out comparing these two surgical approaches for correction of vesicoureteral reflux. Treatment is currently based on the same indications, and these indications do not differ between the different types of intervention.

44. **d. All of the above apply.** The advantages of this approach over open surgery include smaller incisions, less discomfort, brief hospitalizations, and quicker convalescence. As with other laparoscopic procedures, a learning curve needs to be broached and experience is essential to the success of this approach. Laparoscopic reimplantation requires a team with at least two surgeons; the repair is converted from an extraperitoneal to an intraperitoneal approach; many of the available instruments are less than ideal for use in children; operative time is greater than with open techniques; and cost is increased because of lengthier surgery and the expense of disposable equipment.

*Sources referenced can be found in *Campbell-Walsh Urology, 10th Edition,* on the Expert Consult website.

Additional Study Points

1. In patients with reflux approximately one third of their siblings will have reflux.

2. Reflux that is inherited is thought to be due to an autosomal dominant pattern.

3. There is a frequent association of constipation and encopresis with reflux and UTIs.

4. If both the ureteropelvic junction (UPJ) and ureterovesical junction (UVJ) require operative repair, the UPJ should be repaired first.

5. There is an association of renal maldevelopment with high grades of reflux.

6. The cardinal renal anomalies associated with reflux are multicystic dysplastic kidney and renal agenesis; the presence of either condition mandates a VCUG.

7. Women with UTIs and reflux who have undergone a reimplantation will still be at significant risk for UTIs during pregnancy and should be monitored.

8. Almost 80% of low-grade and half of grade III reflux will resolve spontaneously.

9. Sterile reflux is benign.

10. Cohen's technique of uretero reimplantation is particularly well suited for small bladders and thick-walled bladders.

11. There is a 10% to 15% incidence of contralateral reflux after unilateral reflux is repaired.

12. Prophylactic bilateral reimplantation for unilateral reflux is not indicated.

Prune-Belly Syndrome

Anthony A. Caldamone, MD, MMS, FAAP, FACS ● John R. Woodard, MD

QUESTIONS

1. Common findings in the prune-belly syndrome include all of the following EXCEPT:
   a. deficiency of abdominal wall musculature.
   b. urinary tract dilatation.
   c. palpable undescended testes.
   d. urachal pseudodiverticulum.
   e. vesicoureteral reflux.

2. Which of the following statements regarding the prognosis of patients with prune-belly syndrome is FALSE?
   a. The patient will likely be infertile.
   b. A substantial risk of renal failure exists.
   c. Testicular descent will not occur spontaneously.
   d. The male "pseudo-prune" phenotype is protected from renal failure.
   e. Chronic constipation and ineffective cough may result from abdominal wall laxity.

3. Complications involving which of the following organ systems are most likely to threaten the early survival of an infant with prune-belly syndrome?
   a. Cardiac
   b. Renal
   c. Pulmonary
   d. Gastrointestinal
   e. Endocrine

4. Ureteral dysfunction in prune-belly syndrome is related to all of the following EXCEPT:
   a. ureteral dilatation with failure of luminal coaptation during peristalsis.
   b. reduced smooth muscle tissue.
   c. failure of propagation of an electrical conduction due to increased fibrous connective tissue.
   d. more severe proximal ureteral dysfunction with failure to conduct a urinary bolus from the renal pelvis.
   e. abnormal myofilament content in smooth muscle cells.

5. Urodynamic bladder evaluation in prune-belly syndrome is primarily characterized by bladder enlargement with:
   a. elevated voiding pressures and detrusor-sphincter dyssynergia.
   b. high-amplitude uninhibited contractions.
   c. poorly contractile detrusor or myogenic failure.
   d. poor compliance.
   e. absent sensation.

6. The classic findings on prenatal ultrasound on prune-belly syndrome include all of the following EXCEPT:
   a. ambiguous genitalia.
   b. hydroureteronephrosis.
   c. distended bladder.
   d. early fetal ascites.
   e. irregular abdominal wall circumferences.

7. A management strategy of observation in the prune-belly syndrome is strongly supported by which finding?
   a. That spontaneous improvement in dilatation of the urinary tract generally occurs after puberty
   b. That vesicoureteral reflux occurs at low pressures and does not represent a threat to renal parenchyma
   c. That the risk of obstruction after ureteral reimplantation always outweighs the benefit
   d. That operative risks in this patient population are excessive
   e. None of the above

8. Which statement is most accurate when considering management of the lower urinary tract in the patient with prune-belly syndrome?
   a. Reduction cystoplasty is indicated when bladder capacity becomes greater than expected for age.
   b. Internal urethrotomy improves postvoid residual urine volumes without risk of incontinence.
   c. Reduction cystoplasty permanently improves bladder dynamics.
   d. Internal urethrotomy should be specifically based on pressure-flow studies.
   e. Routine intermittent catheterization should be used to improve postvoid residual urine volumes in all patients.

9. Which statement regarding orchiopexy in the patient with prune-belly syndrome is TRUE?
   a. It requires a microvascular testicular autotransplantation because of the high intra-abdominal position.
   b. It maintains endocrine function but has no potential to preserve spermatogenesis.
   c. It can be best accomplished by transperitoneal mobilization before 1 year of age.

d. It should never involve use of the Fowler-Stephens technique because of unreliability of the collateral testicular blood supply.

e. It is performed if spontaneous descent fails to occur by 2 years of age.

10. The most appropriate indication for prenatal intervention in suspected prune-belly syndrome is:

a. oligohydramnios.

b. urinary ascites.

c. urethral atresia and progressive oligohydramnios.

d. pulmonary hypoplasia.

e. distended bladder.

11. The most appropriate initial management of the newborn with prune-belly syndrome includes:

a. percutaneous drainage of the upper urinary tract after stabilization.

b. stabilization and then vesicostomy if anesthetic risk permits.

c. stabilization and then bilateral cutaneous ureterostomy if anesthetic risk permits.

d. evaluation of pulmonary status and voiding cystourethrogram to rule out posterior urethral valves and reflux.

e. evaluation of pulmonary status, renal ultrasonographic study, and prophylactic antibiotics.

12. The prostatic urethra in prune-belly syndrome:

a. is dilated and associated with bladder neck hypertrophy on a voiding cystogram.

b. is sometimes associated with congenital urethral obstruction resulting in megalourethra.

c. is associated with a hypoplastic prostate with decreased epithelium and increased smooth muscle.

d. results in retrograde ejaculation.

e. is characterized by none of the above.

ANSWERS

1. **c. palpable undescended testes.** Bilateral cryptorchidism is a central feature of the syndrome, and in most patients both testes are intra-abdominal, overlying the ureters at the pelvic brim near the sacroiliac level.

2. **d. The male "pseudo-prune" phenotype is protected from renal failure.** Although it is exceptionally rare to encounter a normal urinary tract in association with the characteristic abdominal wall defect in a male, the converse is not unusual. Some patients (with pseudo-prune-belly syndrome) with a normal or relatively normal abdominal wall exhibit many or all of the internal urologic features. These features may include dysplastic or dysmorphic kidneys or dilated and tortuous ureters. One report noted eight boys with relatively mild external features of the syndrome, five of whom progressed to renal failure, evidence that these children remain vulnerable to renal deterioration.

3. **c. Pulmonary.** The most urgent matters are actually those concerned with cardiopulmonary function. Pulmonary complications including pulmonary hypoplasia, pneumomediastinum, pneumothorax, and cardiac abnormalities must be excluded.

4. **d. more severe proximal ureteral dysfunction with failure to conduct a urinary bolus from the renal pelvis.** The proximal ureter usually displays a more normal appearance, an important feature when considering corrective surgery.

5. **c. poorly contractile detrusor or myogenic failure.** Usually, the cystometrogram reveals excellent detrusor compliance; the end-filling pressure assumes a normal value; and the bladder functions well as a reservoir. However, bladder sensation during filling is shifted to the right with a delayed first sensation to void and bladder capacity may be more than double the normal volume. Less consistent and less favorable results are seen with the voiding profile. The compressor capabilities of the detrusor are diminished by the frequent presence of vesicoureteral reflux and reduced detrusor contractility.

6. **a. ambiguous genitalia.** The findings on prenatal ultrasound in prune-belly syndrome may not be diagnosed in all cases but would include hydronephrosis, an enlarged bladder, ascites presenting in the second trimester, and irregular abdominal wall circumference. Although external genital anomalies such as bilaterally undescended testes and megalourethra occur with prune-belly syndrome, these would not be detected on prenatal ultrasound as abnormalities of external genital development.

7. **e. None of the above.** The obvious implication of different studies was that a more aggressive approach was necessary to improve the fate of the infant with prune-belly syndrome. With the recognition that infection and progressive renal insufficiency are the factors that most often pose the greatest threat to quality of life and survival, surgical reconstruction to normalize the anatomy and function of the genitourinary tract was advocated. Early retailoring of the urinary system to reduce stasis and eliminate reflux or obstruction has included ureteral shortening, tapering and vesicoureteral reimplantation, and reduction cystoplasty. Reconstruction is best delayed until the child is approximately 3 months old, to allow for pulmonary maturation. This approach has been successful in achieving anatomic and functional improvement.

8. **d. Internal urethrotomy should be specifically based on pressure-flow studies.** Some initial improvement in voiding dynamics can be achieved by aggressive bladder remodeling. However, with long-term follow-up, there has been no evidence that this improvement is maintained and excessive bladder volumes tend to recur with time. Internal urethrotomy is indicated in the rare patient with true anatomic urethral obstruction or in patients with urodynamic evidence of urethral obstruction by pressure-flow studies.

9. **c. It can be best accomplished by transperitoneal mobilization before 1 year of age.** Orchiopexy in all patients is now generally performed during infancy in an effort to maintain the germ cell population and protect spermatogenesis. In the neonate and in patients up to at least 6 months of age, transabdominal complete mobilization of the spermatic cord almost always allows the testis to be positioned in the dependent portion of the scrotum without dividing the vascular portion of the spermatic cord. The Fowler-Stephens technique for performing orchiopexy in patients with intra-abdominal testes has become part of the standard urologic armamentarium.

10. **c. urethral atresia and progressive oligohydramnios.** Because most hydronephrosis in prune-belly syndrome is well tolerated, its presence alone is not an indication for intervention. Similarly, oligohydramnios, pulmonary hypoplasia, distended bladder, and urinary ascites do not independently warrant prenatal intervention. The only situation with prune-belly syndrome that is potentially reversible is the pulmonary hypoplasia that is seen from urethral atresia and due to progressive oligohydramnios. Oligohydramnios that occurs early in the second trimester is generally indicative of severe renal dysplasia.

11. **e. evaluation of pulmonary status, renal ultrasonographic study, and prophylactic antibiotics.** The most urgent matters are those concerned with cardiopulmonary function. After stabilization, urologic evaluation proceeds with physical examination and ultrasonography. Imaging requiring catheterization and the potential for introduction of bacteria should be avoided unless the results are necessary for immediate clinical decision making. Attention to sterile technique is crucial if invasive studies are performed. Once introduced, infection in a static system may be difficult to eradicate.

12. **d. results in retrograde ejaculation.** The characteristically wide bladder neck merges with a grossly dilated prostatic urethra, so the junction is nearly imperceptible both radiographically and by gross inspection. The prostatic urethra does, however, taper to a relatively narrow membranous urethra at the urogenital diaphragm. Retrograde ejaculation is common.

Additional Study Points

1. The three major findings in prune-belly syndrome are (1) deficiency of abdominal musculature, (2) bilateral intra-abdominal testes, (3) anomalous urinary tract usually composed of hydronephrosis and varying degrees of renal dysplasia.
2. The single most important determinant of renal function is the degree of renal dysplasia.
3. The majority (95%) of those with prune-belly syndrome are males.
4. The ureters lack smooth muscle cells and have an increased amount of fibrous connective tissue; the most normal portion of the ureter with the greatest amount of smooth muscle is in the proximal segment. This is the segment that should be preserved for reconstruction.
5. The bladder is usually massively dilated.
6. The vas and seminal vesicles are often atretic.
7. The fusiform type of mega urethra involves deficiencies of the corpus cavernosum and corpus spongiosum, whereas the scaphoid variety involves a deficiency of corpus spongiosum only.
8. The deficiency in the abdominal wall musculature is usually medial and inferior.
9. The disease is generally classified into three categories according to severity: category I—patients with marked oligohydramnios with renal dysplasia and pulmonary hypoplasia; category II—moderate renal insufficiency; category III—mild manifestations in which renal function is well maintained.
10. Infection and progressive renal insufficiency are the greatest threat to long-term survival.
11. Abdominal wall reconstruction has been demonstrated to improve bladder emptying and result in a more effective cough and improved defecation.

Exstrophy-Epispadias Complex

John P. Gearhart, MD • Ranjiv I. Mathews, MD

QUESTIONS

1. What is the live birth incidence of classic bladder exstrophy?
   a. 1 in 100,000
   b. 1 in 60,000
   c. 1 in 50,000
   d. 1 in 70,000
   e. 1 in 90,000

2. What is the live birth risk of bladder exstrophy in the offspring of individuals with bladder exstrophy and epispadias?
   a. 1 in 70
   b. 1 in 300
   c. 1 in 500
   d. 1 in 700
   e. 1 in 450

3. The main theory of embryologic maldevelopment in exstrophy is that of abnormal:
   a. underdevelopment of the cloacal membrane, preventing medial migration of the mesoderm tissue and proper lower abdominal wall development.
   b. overdevelopment of the cloacal membrane, preventing medial migration of the mesodermal tissue and proper lower abdominal wall development.
   c. infiltration of ectoderm into the cloacal membrane.
   d. infiltration of mesoderm into the cloacal membrane.
   e. invasion of endoderm into the cloacal membrane.

4. In evaluation of the skeletal defects of bladder exstrophy, Sponseller and colleagues (1995)* found that with classic bladder exstrophy, there are changes in the orientation of the pelvic bones. These include:
   a. external rotation of the posterior aspect of the pelvis of 12 degrees on each side.
   b. retroversion of the acetabulum.
   c. an 18-degree rotation of the anterior pelvis.

d. a 30% shortening of the pubic rami in addition to a significant pubic symphyseal diastasis.
   e. All of the above.

5. Which of the following statements is TRUE regarding hernias in children with exstrophy?
   a. Identification at the time of initial closure is not possible.
   b. They are usually unilateral.
   c. They are noted in 80% of boys and 10% of girls.
   d. The orientation of the pelvic bones makes them infrequent.
   e. A patent processus vaginalis is rarely noted.

6. Which of the following statements is TRUE regarding the male genital defect in exstrophy?
   a. The posterior length of the corporeal bodies was 30% shorter than normal controls.
   b. The diameter of the posterior corporeal segments was less than normal controls.
   c. The shortening of the penis was due entirely to the pubic diastasis.
   d. The anterior corporeal segments are 50% shorter than that of normal control subjects.
   e. The angle between the corpora cavernosa is markedly reduced in boys with exstrophy.

7. Which of the following statements best describes findings regarding the prostate in exstrophy?
   a. Volume weight and the cross-sectional area appeared normal compared with published results from control subjects.
   b. The prostate extended circumferentially around the urethra in all patients with exstrophy.
   c. Free PSA values were greater than in normal controls, indicating recurrent injury from infection.
   d. The vas deferens and seminal vesicles were abnormal due to the effect of the exstrophic bladder.
   e. Total PSA values were not measurable in men with exstrophy.

8. Which of the following accurately describes the vagina in the female patient with bladder exstrophy?
   a. Shorter than normal and of smaller caliber
   b. Vaginal orifice is displaced posteriorly due to the anterior exstrophic bladder

*Sources referenced can be found in *Campbell-Walsh Urology*, *10th Edition*, on the Expert Consult website.

c. Shorter than normal but of normal caliber

d. Longer than normal and of wider caliber

e. Cervix enters the posterior vaginal wall

9. Findings regarding the structure and innervation of the exstrophic bladder include:

   a. density and binding affinity of the muscarinic receptors that were similar to norms.

   b. a decreased ratio of collagen to muscle in the exstrophic bladder.

   c. increased myelinated nerve profiles, indicating a later developmental stage.

   d. a threefold increase in the amount of type I collagen.

   e. study of vasoactive intestinal polypeptide, protein gene product 9.5, and calcitonin gene-related peptide that indicated the presence of dysinnervation.

10. Which of the following statements best describes bladder function in patients with bladder exstrophy?

    a. In patients continent after reconstruction, normal cystometrograms are noted in 10% to 25%.

    b. Eighty percent of patients had compliant and stable bladders before bladder neck reconstruction.

    c. Involuntary contractions were noted infrequently after bladder neck reconstruction.

    d. After bladder neck reconstruction, 90% maintained normal bladder compliance.

    e. After successful closure, ultrastructure remains abnormal in the majority.

11. The characteristic prenatal appearance of bladder exstrophy includes which of the following?

    a. Absence of bladder filling

    b. Low-set umbilicus

    c. Widening of the pubic ramus

    d. Diminutive genitalia

    e. All of the above

12. Newborn patient selection for immediate reconstruction is based on:

    a. examination of the bladder in the nursery without anesthesia.

    b. complete lack of any surface defects on examination.

    c. indentation of the bladder using anesthesia or outward bulging when the child cries.

    d. size of the phallus at birth.

    e. extent of the pubic diastasis.

13. Fundamental steps in the modern staged reconstruction of bladder exstrophy include all of the following EXCEPT:

    a. early bladder, posterior urethral, and abdominal wall closure.

    b. early epispadias repair around age 1.

    c. conversion of the bladder exstrophy to complete epispadias.

    d. bladder neck reconstruction before the epispadias repair to provide early continence.

    e. ureteral reimplantation at the time of bladder neck reconstruction.

14. What is the best treatment option at the time of birth in a child whose bladder template is judged to be too small to undergo closure?

    a. Excision of the bladder with a nonrefluxing colon conduit

    b. Immediate closure with epispadias repair to provide resistance and allow the bladder to grow

    c. Delaying closure by 4 to 6 months with reassessment to see if the bladder will grow

    d. Bladder closure, augmentation, ureteral reimplantation, and a continence procedure

    e. Improve the potential for successful closure with an osteotomy

15. Combined osteotomy was developed for all of the following reasons EXCEPT:

    a. the approach allows placement of an external fixator device.

    b. superior cosmesis provided by this approach.

    c. the need to turn a patient to perform an osteotomy.

    d. better ease of pubic approximation.

    e. reduced risk of malunion of the iliac wing and reduction of blood loss.

16. Complications that are associated with osteotomy and immobilization techniques include all of the following EXCEPT:

    a. skin ulceration associated with use of mummy wrapping.

    b. failure of the bladder and abdominal wall closure associated with the use of spica casting.

    c. high rates of failure of reconstruction associated with the use of osteotomy and external fixation.

    d. transient femoral nerve palsy with the use of osteotomy.

    e. delayed union of the iliac wings after use of posterior osteotomy.

17. Other options have been described for reconstruction in bladder exstrophy. Which of the following statements is TRUE regarding the other described approaches?

    a. The Warsaw approach includes bladder neck reconstruction at the time of initial bladder closure.

    b. The Erlangen approach includes all of the features of reconstruction of the exstrophy in a single procedure.

    c. The Seattle approach (CPRE) includes bladder neck reconstruction as part of the complete reconstruction of exstrophy.

    d. Combined bladder closure and epispadias repair are performed in cases of primary exstrophy repair at birth.

    e. The Warsaw approach uses the Young repair as the preferred method for epispadias reconstruction.

18. After initial primary bladder closure in the newborn, what should be done if recurrent urinary tract infections occur?

    a. Voiding cystourethrogram

    b. Bladder CT

    c. Ureteral reimplantation

    d. Prophylaxis modified

    e. Cystoscopy

19. After successful bladder closure, management should include all the following EXCEPT:
    a. calibration of the urethral outlet 4 weeks after closure to ensure free drainage.
    b. ultrasound evaluation of the kidneys and bladder.
    c. intermittent antibiotics for urinary tract infections.
    d. complete bladder drainage by suprapubic tube clamping.
    e. yearly cystoscopic evaluation.

20. In a patient with bladder exstrophy who undergoes more than one closure of the bladder and urethral defect, what is the chance of having adequate bladder capacity for later bladder neck reconstruction?
    a. 60%
    b. 70%
    c. 20%
    d. 30%
    e. 10%

21. The key concepts in the reconstruction of epispadias include all of the following EXCEPT:
    a. correction of ventral chordee.
    b. urethral reconstruction.
    c. glans reconstruction.
    d. penile skin coverage.
    e. penile lengthening.

22. Information gleaned from most major series of bladder neck reconstruction indicates that the most important factor to predict success and eventual continence after bladder neck reconstruction is:
    a. age of the child.
    b. number of prior bladder infections.
    c. number of attempts at bladder closure.
    d. bladder capacity.
    e. vesicoureteral reflux.

23. After bladder neck reconstruction, within what time period do the majority of patients achieve daytime continence?
    a. 2 years
    b. 1 year
    c. 2 months
    d. 6 months
    e. 4 years

24. After a failed bladder closure in the newborn period, an appropriate time period should elapse before attempting a secondary repair. What should this time period be?
    a. 2 months
    b. 18 months
    c. 2 years
    d. 6 months
    e. 15 months

25. All of the following are TRUE regarding the results of modern staged reconstruction of exstrophy EXCEPT:
    a. The onset of eventual continence and continence rates were unchanged in those who had initial successful closure.

b. The modified Cantwell-Ransley repair has replaced the Young technique because there is less urethral tortuosity and lower fistula rates.
    c. Incidence of fistula formation was 12% at 3 months after epispadias repair.
    d. Continence is more likely in those patients undergoing initial closure before 72 hours of age or those who have closure after 72 hours of age with osteotomy.
    e. Continence rates are higher in those who have capacities of 85 mL or more at the time of bladder neck reconstruction.

26. Which of the following is TRUE regarding exstrophy failures?
    a. After successful secondary closure, 90% of patients develop dryness and voided continence.
    b. Dehiscence after complete primary repair may be associated with corporeal, urethral, and other major soft tissue loss.
    c. Bladder prolapse can be managed with minimal outlet procedures because this is considered a mild failure.
    d. Because the results of reclosure are poor, immediate resection of the bladder plate followed by neobladder construction is the preferred management.
    e. Posterior urethral stricture is usually a late complication occurring 4 to 6 years after initial closure.

27. Bladder neck reconstruction is designated as a failure if a 3-hour dry interval is not achieved within 2 years after surgery. Management of such failure is with the use of:
    a. collagen, which can lead to dryness.
    b. artificial urinary sphincter small bladder capacities.
    c. bladder neck transection, augmentation cystoplasty, and continent diversion.
    d. repeat bladder neck reconstruction in relatively tight bladder necks.
    e. repeat bladder neck reconstruction in bladder instability.

28. The risks of ureterosigmoidostomy in the exstrophy population include:
    a. pyelonephritis and hyperchloremic acidosis.
    b. pyelonephritis, hyponatremia, and rectal incontinence.
    c. low incidence for eventual development of cancer.
    d. poor outcomes with upper tract deterioration.
    e. prolapse of the abdominal stoma.

29. What is the live birth incidence of cloacal exstrophy?
    a. 1 in 400,000
    b. 1 in 20,000
    c. 1 in 750,000
    d. 1 in 1,000,000
    e. 1 in 500,000

30. Neurospinal abnormalities are noted in the majority of patients with cloacal exstrophy. All of the following are true EXCEPT:
    a. Thoracic defects may be noted in 10% of patients.
    b. The embryologic basis for the neurospinal defect has been identified as failure of neural tube closure.
    c. Autonomic bladder innervation is derived from a more medial location.

d. Innervation of the duplicated corporeal bodies arises from the sacral plexus and courses medial to the hemibladders.

e. Functional defects can include minimal lower extremity function.

31. Cloacal exstrophy is a multisystem abnormality. Which of the following is TRUE regarding cloacal exstrophy?

a. The bones in a child with cloacal exstrophy were microscopically, markedly different from normal controls.

b. In the presence of a normal bowel length, there is low probability for the development of short-gut syndrome.

c. The most common müllerian anomaly noted was partial uterine duplication.

d. Cardiovascular and pulmonary anomalies are frequently noted.

e. The most common upper urinary tract anomaly noted was multicystic dysplastic kidney.

32. What is the incidence of omphalocele associated with cloacal exstrophy?

a. 40%

b. 70%

c. 95%

d. 20%

e. 60%

33. In the patient with cloacal exstrophy, hindgut remnants should be preserved to:

a. enlarge the bladder.

b. permit vaginal reconstruction.

c. allow either bladder augmentation or vaginal reconstruction.

d. provide additional length of bowel for fluid absorption.

e. allow later anal pull-through surgery.

34. Gender assignment continues to remain a controversial aspect of cloacal exstrophy management. Current research indicates which of the following?

a. Psychosexual evaluation indicates that patients have marked female shift in development.

b. Patients have feminine childhood behavior but developed masculine gender identity.

c. Histology of the testis at birth is abnormal, and therefore removal has been recommended.

d. Most recommend that gender be assigned on the basis of the ability for functional reconstruction rather than on karyotype.

e. A functional and cosmetically acceptable phallus can now be constructed.

35. What is the live birth incidence of male epispadias?

a. 1 in 150,000

b. 1 in 200,000

c. 1 in 400,000

d. 1 in 117,000

e. 1 in 250,000

36. What is the incidence of reflux in patients with complete epispadias?

a. 10% to 20%

b. 90%

c. 70%

d. 50%

e. 30% to 40%

37. In the complete epispadias group, what is the predominant indicator of eventual continence?

a. Length of the urethral groove

b. Lack of spinal abnormalities

c. Bladder capacity at the time of bladder neck reconstruction

d. Age at bladder neck reconstruction

e. Age at epispadias repair and degree of resistance provided

38. Many variations in anatomy have been reported in the exstrophy-epispadias complex. All of the following are true regarding exstrophy variants EXCEPT:

a. The presence of musculoskeletal defects characteristic of the complex, with a normal urinary tract, is termed pseudoexstrophy.

b. The bladder is completely exstrophied in the superior vesical fissure variant.

c. With "covered" exstrophy, an isolated ectopic bowel segment has been frequently noted.

d. An isolated segment of bladder is left on the abdominal wall, with a complete urinary tract within the bladder in duplicate exstrophy.

e. A common embryologic origin has been postulated for developments of all of the variants.

39. Sexual function and libido in male and female exstrophy patients are:

a. normal in males, abnormal in females.

b. normal only in males.

c. normal in both males and females.

d. normal only in females.

e. abnormal in both males and females.

40. What is the most common complication after pregnancy in female exstrophy patients?

a. Premature labor

b. Rectal prolapse

c. Preeclampsia

d. Cervical and uterine prolapse

e. Oligohydramnios

41. Psychologic studies of male and female children with bladder exstrophy find that:

a. all have clinical psychopathology.

b. they do not have clinical psychopathology.

c. most have significant depression due to the condition.

d. many children have gender dysphoria.

e. half of males and half of females have clinical psychopathology.

42. Single-stage reconstruction using the complete primary exstrophy repair technique offers several advantages over staged reconstruction EXCEPT:

a. the possibility to correct the penile, bladder, and bladder neck abnormalities of bladder exstrophy with one operation.

b. the ability to achieve urinary continence without bladder neck reconstruction.

c. correction of vesicoureteral reflux at the time of surgery.

d. lower complication rates than previous attempts at single-stage reconstruction.

e. initiation of bladder cycling early in life.

43. Single-stage reconstruction using the complete primary exstrophy repair technique relies on which of the following to achieve continence?

a. Reestablishment of normal anatomic relationships

b. Bladder neck reconstruction at the time of primary surgery

c. Osteotomy at the time of single-stage reconstruction

d. Simultaneous epispadias repair

e. None of the above

44. The following postoperative factors have been shown to increase the success of reconstruction for bladder exstrophy EXCEPT:

a. immobilization with external fixators, Buck traction, a spica cast, or a mummy wrap.

b. antibiotic therapy.

c. prolonged non per os (NPO) status to avoid abdominal distention.

d. urinary diversion through ureteral stenting and suprapubic urinary drainage.

e. adequate nutritional support.

45. Single-stage reconstruction using the complete primary exstrophy repair technique can be safely performed because:

a. the neurovascular bundles of the corporeal bodies lie laterally rather than dorsally on the corporeal bodies.

b. the cavernosal bodies and urethral wedge are not actually separated from each other in this technique.

c. the blood supply to the corporeal bodies and that to the urethral wedge are independent of each other.

d. the blood supply is quickly reestablished once the components are "reassembled."

e. the distal vascular communications between the corpora and urethral wedge are preserved.

46. The proximal limit(s) of dissection using the complete primary exstrophy repair technique is/are:

a. the intersymphyseal band.

b. the muscles of the pelvic floor.

c. the rectum.

d. the corpora spongiosa.

e. the endopelvic fascia.

47. Factors that mitigate against using a single-stage reconstruction technique for cloacal exstrophy include the presence of:

a. a large omphalocele.

b. a wide pubic diastasis.

c. a concomitant myelomeningocele.

d. a small bladder plate.

e. all of the above.

48. Complications of the complete primary exstrophy repair technique include:

a. myogenic bladder failure.

b. testicular atrophy.

c. urethrocutaneous fistula.

d. hip dislocation.

e. epispadias.

ANSWERS

1. **c. 1 in 50,000.** The incidence of bladder exstrophy has been estimated as being between 1 in 10,000 and 1 in 50,000 live births.

2. **a. 1 in 70.** Shapiro determined that the risk of bladder exstrophy in the offspring of individuals with bladder exstrophy and epispadias is 1 in 70 live births, a 500-fold greater incidence than in the general population.

3. **b. overdevelopment of the cloacal membrane, preventing medial migration of the mesodermal tissue and proper lower abdominal wall development.** The theory of embryonic maldevelopment in exstrophy held by Marshall and Muecke is that the basic defect is an abnormal overdevelopment of the cloacal membrane, preventing medial migration of the mesenchymal tissue and proper lower abdominal wall development.

4. **e. All of the above.** Sponseller and colleagues found that patients with classic bladder exstrophy have a mean external rotation of the posterior aspect of the pelvis of 12 degrees on each side, retroversion of the acetabulum, and a mean 18-degree external rotation of the anterior pelvis, along with 30% shortening of the pubic rami.

5. **c. They are noted in 80% of boys and 10% of girls.** Connelly and colleagues, in a review of 181 children with bladder exstrophy, reported inguinal hernias in 81.8% of boys and 10.5% of girls.

6. **d. The anterior corporeal segments are 50% shorter than that of normal control subjects.** With the use of MRI to examine adult men with bladder exstrophy and comparison of this result with that from age- and race-matched control subjects, it was found that the anterior corporeal length in male patients with bladder exstrophy is almost 50% shorter than that of normal control subjects.

7. **a. Volume weight and the cross-sectional area appeared normal compared with published results from control subjects.** The volume, weight, and maximum cross-sectional area of the prostate appeared normal compared with published results from control subjects.

8. **c. Shorter than normal but of normal caliber.** The vagina is shorter than normal, hardly greater than 6 cm in depth, but of normal caliber.

9. **a. density and binding affinity of the muscarinic receptors that were similar to norms.** Muscarinic cholinergic receptor density and binding affinity were measured in control subjects and in patients with classic bladder exstrophy. The density of the muscarinic cholinergic receptors in both the control and exstrophy groups was similar, as was the binding affinity of the muscarinic receptor. Therefore it was thought by the authors that the neurophysiologic composition of the exstrophied bladder is not grossly altered during its anomalous development.

10. **b. Eighty percent of patients had compliant and stable bladders before bladder neck reconstruction.** Diamond and colleagues (1999), looking at 30 patients with bladder exstrophy at various stages of reconstruction, found that 80% of patients had compliant and stable bladders before bladder neck reconstruction.

11. **e. All of the above.** In a review of 25 prenatal ultrasonographic examinations with the resulting birth of a newborn with classic bladder exstrophy, several observations were made: (1) absence of bladder filling; (2) a low-set umbilicus; (3) widening pubis ramus; (4) diminutive genitalia; and (5) a lower abdominal mass that increases in size as the pregnancy progresses and as the intra-abdominal viscera increase in size.

12. **c. indentation of the bladder under anesthesia or outward bulging when the child cries.** In minor grades of exstrophy that approach the condition of complete epispadias with incontinence, the bladder may be small yet may demonstrate acceptable capacity, either by bulging when the baby cries or by indenting easily when touched by a sterile gloved finger in the operating room with the child under anesthesia.

13. **d. bladder neck reconstruction before the epispadias repair to provide early continence.** The most significant changes in the management of bladder exstrophy have been (1) early bladder, posterior urethral, and abdominal wall closure, usually with osteotomy; (2) early epispadias repair; (3) reconstruction of a continent bladder neck and reimplantation of the ureters; and, most importantly; (4) definition of strict criteria for the selection of patients suitable for this approach. Bladder neck repair usually occurs when the child is 4 to 5 years of age, has an adequate bladder capacity, and, most important, is ready to participate in a postoperative voiding program.

14. **c. Delaying closure by 4 to 6 months with reassessment to see if the bladder will grow.** Ideally, waiting for the bladder template to grow for 4 to 6 months in the child with a small bladder is not as risky as submitting a small bladder template to closure in an inappropriate setting, resulting in dehiscence and allowing the fate of the bladder to be sealed at that point.

15. **c. the need to turn a patient to perform an osteotomy.** Combined osteotomy was developed for three reasons: (1) osteotomy is performed with the patient in the supine position, as is the urologic repair, thereby avoiding the need to turn the patient; (2) the anterior approach to this osteotomy allows placement of an external fixator device and intrafragmentary pins under direct vision; and (3) the cosmetic appearance of this osteotomy is superior to that of the posterior iliac approach.

16. **c. high rates of failure of reconstruction associated with the use of osteotomy and external fixation.** Successful closure was noted in 97% of those immobilized with an external fixator and modified Buck traction.

17. **b. The Erlangen approach includes all of the features of reconstruction of the exstrophy in a single procedure.** This method is truly a "complete repair" because it accomplishes all of the facets of exstrophy reconstruction in a single procedure. Surgical repair is, however, performed at 8 to 10 weeks of age when the infant is larger and has had the opportunity to be medically stabilized.

18. **e. Cystoscopy.** An important caveat is that if there are recurrent urinary tract infections or if the bladder is distended on an ultrasonographic study, cystoscopy should be performed and the posterior urethra should be carefully examined anteriorly for erosion of the intrapubic stitch, which may be the cause of the recurrent infections.

19. **c. intermittent antibiotics for urinary tract infections.** Before removal of the suprapubic tube, 4 weeks after surgery, the bladder outlet is calibrated by a urethral catheter or a urethral sound to ensure free drainage. A complete ultrasound examination is obtained to ascertain the status of the renal pelves and ureters, and appropriate urinary antibiotics are administered because all patients will have reflux postclosure. Residual urine is estimated by clamping the suprapubic tube, and specimens for culture are obtained before the patient leaves the hospital and at subsequent intervals to detect infection and ensure that the bladder is empty.

20. **a. 60%.** In one study, if a patient underwent two closures, the chance of having an adequate bladder capacity for bladder neck reconstruction was 60%.

21. **a. correction of ventral chordee.** Regardless of the surgical technique chosen for reconstruction of the penis in bladder exstrophy, four key concerns must be addressed to ensure a functional and cosmetically pleasing penis: (1) correction of dorsal chordee, (2) urethral reconstruction, (3) glandular reconstruction, and (4) penile skin closure.

22. **d. bladder capacity.** The most important long-term factor gleaned from a review of all these series is the fact that bladder capacity at the time of bladder neck reconstruction is an important determinant of eventual success.

23. **b. 1 year.** The vast majority of patients achieve daytime continence in the first year after bladder neck reconstruction.

24. **d. 6 months.** Dehiscence, which may be precipitated by incomplete mobilization of the pelvic diaphragm, and inadequate pelvic immobilization postoperatively, wound infection, abdominal distention, or urinary tube malfunction necessitates a 6-month recovery period before a second attempt at closure.

25. **a. The onset of eventual continence and continence rates were unchanged in those who had initial successful closure.** The importance of a successful initial closure is emphasized by Oesterling and Jeffs (1987) and by Husmann and colleagues (1989), who found that the onset of eventual continence was quicker and the continence rate higher in those who underwent a successful initial closure with or without osteotomy.

26. **b. Dehiscence after complete primary repair may be associated with corporeal, urethral, and other major soft tissue loss.** Dehiscence and prolapse have also been reported after the "complete repair" and may be associated with glandular, corporeal, urethral plate, and other major soft tissue loss.

27. **c. bladder neck transection, augmentation cystoplasty, and continent diversion.** A majority of bladder neck failures require eventual augmentation or continent diversion. The artificial urinary sphincter has been used with some success in patients who have a good bladder capacity. However, in most of these failures the bladder capacity is small and augmentation will be required. At the time of reoperative surgery, either the bladder neck is transected proximal to the prostate with a Mitrofanoff

substitution or a continence procedure such as an artificial sphincter or collagen injection, or both, are performed. In our extensive experience with failed bladder neck reconstructions, most of the patients have had several surgeries and need to be dry. In such cases the most suitable alternative is bladder neck transection, augmentation, and a continent urinary stoma (Gearhart et al, 1995b; Hensle et al, 1995).

28. **a. pyelonephritis and hyperkalemic acidosis.** However, this form of diversion should not be offered until one is certain that anal continence is normal and after the family has been made aware of the potential serious complications including pyelonephritis, hyperkalemic acidosis, rectal incontinence, ureteral obstruction, and delayed development of malignancy.

29. **a. 1 in 400,000.** Fortunately, cloacal exstrophy is exceedingly rare, occurring in 1 in 200,000 to 400,000 live births.

30. **b. The embryologic basis for the neurospinal defect has been identified as failure of neural tube closure.** The embryologic basis for the neurospinal defects associated with cloacal exstrophy has been postulated to be secondary to problems with the disruption of the tissue of the dorsal mesenchyme rather than failure of neural tube closure (McLaughlin et al, 1995). Alternatively, it has been suggested that the defects that lead to the formation of cloacal exstrophy may lead to the developing spinal cord and vertebrae being pulled apart (Cohen, 1991).

31. **c. The most common müllerian anomaly noted was partial uterine duplication.** The most commonly reported müllerian anomaly was uterine duplication, seen in 95% of patients (Diamond, 1990). The vast majority of these patients had partial uterine duplication, predominantly a bicornate uterus.

32. **c. 95%.** In Diamond's series, the incidence of omphalocele was 88%, with a majority of all series reporting 95% or greater.

33. **d. provide additional length of bowel for fluid absorption.** With the recognition of the metabolic changes in patients with ileostomy, an attempt is always made to use the hindgut remnant to provide additional length of bowel for fluid absorption.

34. **e. A functional and cosmetically acceptable phallus can now be constructed.** Most authors recommend assigning gender that is consistent with karyotypic makeup of the individual if at all possible (see Fig. 61–26). This policy can be supported by a report indicating that the histology of the testis at birth is normal (Mathews et al, 1999a). Furthermore, with evolution of techniques for phallic reconstruction, a functional and cosmetically acceptable phallus can now be constructed (Husmann et al, 1989).

35. **d. 1 in 117,000.** Male epispadias is a rare anomaly, with a reported incidence of 1 in 117,000 males.

36. **e. 30% to 40%.** The ureterovesical junction is inherently deficient in complete epispadias, and reflux has been reported between 30% and 40% in a number of series.

37. **c. Bladder capacity at the time of bladder neck reconstruction.** In the epispadias group, much as in the exstrophy group, bladder capacity is the predominant indicator of eventual continence.

38. **b. The bladder is completely exstrophied in the superior vesical fissure variant.** In the superior vesical fissure variant of the exstrophy complex, the musculature and skeletal defects are exactly the same as those in classic exstrophy; however, the persistent cloacal membrane ruptures only at the uppermost portion, and a superior vesical fistula that actually resembles a vesicostomy results. Bladder extrusion is minimal and is present only over the normal umbilicus.

39. **c. normal in both males and females.** Sexual function and libido in exstrophy patients are normal.

40. **d. Cervical and uterine prolapse.** The main complication after pregnancy was cervical and uterine prolapse, which occurred frequently.

41. **b. they do not have clinical psychopathology.** The conclusions of this long-term study were that children with exstrophy do not have clinical psychopathology.

42. **c. correction of vesicoureteral reflux at the time of surgery.** In most applications of the primary exstrophy repair technique, correction of vesicoureteral reflux is not performed, although some have reported performing ureteral reimplantation. All of the other elements are considered advantages of the primary repair.

43. **a. Reestablishment of normal anatomic relationships.** The fundamental basis of the primary repair technique is to reposition the bladder neck and urethral complex into the normal pelvic position more posteriorly than at birth. This permits more normal function of the pelvic floor in maintenance of continence. The other factors do not contribute as significantly to continence.

44. **c. prolonged no per os (NPO) status to avoid abdominal distention.** It is not necessary to maintain an NPO status after primary repair because this will compromise nutrition. If an ileus develops, appropriate decompression and management are necessary because abdominal distention strains the repair. All other factors contribute to a successful outcome.

45. **c. the blood supply to the corporeal bodies and that to the urethral wedge are independent of each other.** Because the three elements of the penis, the two corpora and the urethral wedge, are fully separated in the penile disassembly, their vasculature must be proximal, which it is; and this is the reason this method is successful. Nevertheless, preservation of these proximal vascular supplies is essential.

46. **b. the muscles of the pelvic floor.** The limit of dissection along the penile structures is the pelvic floor, which is then split to permit repositioning of the bladder neck complex posteriorly.

47. **e. all of the above.** All of these factors would indicate that an attempt to perform a primary repair would be at high risk for failure, predominantly by dehiscence. Several of these factors may be present at one time.

48. **c. urethrocutaneous fistula.** The most common complication after primary repair is development of a urethrocutaneous fistula on the ventrum of the penis. Other complications can include corporeal devascularization, hydronephrosis, and hypospadias.

Additional Study Points

1. The male-to-female ratio for exstrophy is 2:1.
2. The risk of bladder exstrophy in family members is increased.
3. Rectal prolapse frequently occurs in untreated exstrophy patients who have widely separated symphyses. It disappears after exstrophy closure.
4. If rectal prolapse occurs after closure, bladder outlet obstruction should be suspected.
5. The autonomic nerves are displaced laterally in patients with exstrophy.
6. Reflux occurs in 100% of patients with exstrophy.
7. An ectopic isolated bowel segment may be present in the lower abdominal wall.
8. Osteotomy is rarely performed in newborns unless the diastasis is greater than 4 cm.
9. The most reliable predictors of urinary continence are the size of the bladder template at birth and successful primary closure.
10. Approximately 75% of patients with exstrophy are continent after repair. Continence is defined as 3 hours of dryness.
11. Cloacal exstrophy consists of exstrophy of the bladder; complete phallic separation; wide diastasis of the pubis; exstrophy of the terminal ileum, which lies between the two halves of the bladder; rudimentary hindgut; imperforate anus; omphalocele; and not infrequently associated spinal defects.
12. In adolescence and adults with exstrophy, concerns in the male are length, appearance, and deviation of the penis. In the female, concerns are the appearance of the external genitalia, adequacy of the vaginal opening, and uterine prolapse.
13. Women with exstrophy have delivered children; however, a frequent complication after pregnancy is cervical and uterine prolapse.

Bladder Anomalies in Children

Dominic C. Frimberger, MD ● Bradley P. Kropp, MD, FAAP

QUESTIONS

1. At which time point can the fetal bladder usually be first detected on ultrasound?
   a. At the 10th week of gestation
   b. At the 12th week of gestation
   c. At the 16th week of gestation
   d. Not before the third trimester
   e. Only when anomalies are present

2. What are important features on prenatal bladder ultrasound?
   a. Urine cycling
   b. Size of bladder
   c. Amniotic fluid levels
   d. Thickness of the bladder wall
   e. All of the above

3. Which of the following bladder dilatations is caused by obstruction?
   a. Posterior urethral valves
   b. Prune-belly syndrome
   c. Congenital megacystis
   d. a and b
   e. All of the above

4. Which of the following statements concerning the urachus is INCORRECT?
   a. The urachus is positioned intraperitoneally.
   b. The urachus is lined by the obliterated umbilical arteries.
   c. The urachal length varies from 3 to 10 cm.
   d. Four different urachal anomalies have been described.
   e. The urachus has three layers.

5. Primary paraureteral diverticula are seen in trabeculated bladders among many diverticula in the bladder and happen in children with infravesical obstruction.
   a. True
   b. False

6. Which other condition must be considered in the workup of a patent urachus?
   a. The presence of vesicoureteral reflux
   b. Association with bladder outlet obstruction
   c. The presence of a patent omphalomesenteric tract

   d. The presence of bladder diverticula
   e. All of the above

7. Which congenital syndrome is not associated with bladder diverticula?
   a. Ehlers-Danlos
   b. Klippel-Trenaunay
   c. Williams elfin facies
   d. Menkes syndrome
   e. None of the above

8. Which statement concerning bladder duplication is NOT true?
   a. Duplication anomalies of the external genitalia are present in up to 90% of patients.
   b. Duplication anomalies of the lower gastrointestinal tract are present in up to 80% of patients.
   c. Other abnormalities such as vesicoureteral reflux, renal ectopia, and dysplasia are commonly found.
   d. Duplications can occur in the coronal or sagittal plane.
   e. Duplications can present with one or two urethras.

ANSWERS

1. **a. At the 10th week of gestation.** The bladder can be visualized in about 50% of cases in the fetal pelvis at the 10th week of gestation, concurrent with the onset of urine production. The detection rate increases with fetal age to 78% at 11 weeks, 88% at 12 weeks, and almost 100% at 13 weeks.

2. **e. All of the above.** The fetal bladder empties every 15 to 20 minutes; therefore a second ultrasound in the same setting is mandatory in case of nonvisualization of the bladder. The fetal bladder can appear either dilated, hypoplastic, or absent on ultrasound and therefore give clues about maldevelopment of the urinary tract. Until 16 weeks of gestation, the amniotic fluid is mainly consistent with placental transudate, at which time it changes to predominantly fetal urine.

3. **a. Posterior urethral valves.** Prune-belly syndrome and congenital megacystis are characterized by nonobstructive dilatation of the urinary bladder. Posterior urethral valves cause obstructive dilatation of the bladder and upper urinary tract.

4. **a. The urachus is positioned intraperitoneally.** The urachus is preperitoneal in the center of a pyramid-shaped space. This space is lined by the obliterated umbilical

arteries, with its base on the anterior dome of the bladder and the tip directed toward the umbilicus.

5. **b. False.** Primary paraureteral diverticula are seen in smooth-walled bladders, occur isolated with no other diverticula, are intermittent in presentation, and happen in children with no infravesical obstruction.

6. **c. The presence of a patent omphalomesenteric tract.** It is important to differentiate a patent urachus from a patent omphalomesenteric duct. The presence of both anomalies in the same patient is rare. Urachal patency is often absent even with severely obstructed bladders in utero.

7. **b. Klippel-Trenaunay.** Congenital diverticula are often found in children with generalized connective tissue diseases such as Ehlers-Danlos, Williams elfin facies, and Menkes syndromes.

8. **b. Duplication anomalies of the lower gastrointestinal tract are present in up to 80% of patients.** Associated duplication anomalies of the external genitalia have been reported in up to 90% of cases, whereas associated duplication anomalies of the lower gastrointestinal tract occur in only up to 42% of cases. Association with other nonurologic congenital anomalies is more frequent in sagittal than coronal duplications.

Additional Study Points

1. The fetal bladder empties every 15 to 20 minutes, so if it is not visualized, repeat ultrasound 15 to 20 minutes later should be performed.
2. When obstruction is the cause of a dilated bladder in the fetus, the mother has oligohydramnios.
3. Congenital megacystis is defined as a dilated, thin-walled bladder with a wide and poorly developed trigone. These bladders generally have wide-gaping ureteral orifices that are displaced laterally, causing massive reflux. Correcting the reflux often restores normal voiding dynamics.
4. Urachal remnants often undergo spontaneous resolution if discovered in patients younger than 6 months. An infected urachal remnant should be initially drained and treated with antibiotics; once the infection has subsided, then an excision should be performed.
5. A urachal sinus must be differentiated from a persistent omphalomesenteric duct. This presents as a Meckel diverticulum connected to the umbilicus.
6. Urachal cysts do not communicate with either the bladder or umbilicus.
7. Portions of a bladder can be contained within a hernia sac.

Posterior Urethral Valves

Anthony J. Casale, MD

QUESTIONS

1. Most patients with posterior urethral valves are diagnosed:
   a. using antenatal ultrasound screening.
   b. as neonates with failure to thrive.
   c. in the first year of life with urinary tract infections.
   d. in mid childhood with voiding dysfunction.
   e. in adolescence with renal insufficiency.

2. The major cause of mortality today in boys with posterior urethral valves is:
   a. renal failure in the newborn period.
   b. renal failure in mid childhood.
   c. urinary sepsis in infancy.
   d. pulmonary insufficiency in the newborn period.
   e. renal insufficiency in adolescence.

3. The most important determining factor in long-term renal function in posterior urethral valves is the:
   a. degree of bladder damage.
   b. severity of hydronephrosis.
   c. ability to control infection.
   d. degree of renal dysplasia.
   e. ability to concentrate urine.

4. The valve bladder syndrome can cause the most damage by:
   a. resulting in incontinence.
   b. leading to recurrent infection.
   c. preventing adequate upper tract drainage.
   d. leading to hypertension.
   e. causing renal tubular damage.

5. Urinary ascites, vesicoureteral reflux and dysplasia (VURD), and bladder diverticula all offer what advantage to patients with posterior urethral valves?
   a. Promoting urinary drainage
   b. Providing a pressure pop-off valve
   c. Allowing free upper tract drainage through the ureterovesical junction
   d. Promoting bladder emptying
   e. Allowing early diagnosis

6. The most important feature in managing bladder dysfunction in patients with posterior urethral valves is that it:
   a. seldom causes persistent problems.
   b. is affected by renal function.
   c. causes intermittent incontinence.
   d. causes persistent reflux.
   e. is variable and changes during life.

7. In patients with posterior urethral valves and persistent reflux, it is most important to:
   a. document that the bladder can empty effectively.
   b. evaluate upper tract drainage.
   c. measure upper tract pressures.
   d. control incontinence.
   e. surgically correct the reflux in early childhood.

8. A 2-kg premature infant with posterior urethral valves and multiple medical problems is stable at 2 weeks of age. Infant cystoscopes are not available. The next step in management is:
   a. catheter drainage.
   b. cutaneous vesicostomy.
   c. cutaneous pyelostomies.
   d. cutaneous ureterostomies.
   e. percutaneous nephrostomies.

9. Antenatal intervention with a vesicoamniotic shunt is most likely to help the fetus by:
   a. improving early renal function.
   b. improving long-term renal function.
   c. preventing pulmonary hypoplasia.
   d. improving bladder function.
   e. allowing full-term delivery.

10. Ultrasound in infants with posterior urethral valves may help to predict long-term renal function by demonstrating:
    a. degree of hydronephrosis.
    b. bladder wall thickness.
    c. degree of renal dysplasia.
    d. grade of reflux.
    e. type of urethral valve.

11. Anterior urethral valves differ from posterior urethral valves in that they may appear as:
    a. bilateral hydronephrosis.
    b. urosepsis.
    c. failure to thrive.
    d. intermittent penis mass.
    e. voiding dysfunction.

12. The accuracy of diagnosing posterior urethral valves on antenatal ultrasound screening is affected by:
    a. amniotic fluid.
    b. fetal age.
    c. maternal age.
    d. fetal size.
    e. maternal hydration.

ANSWERS

1. **a. using antenatal ultrasound screening.** The diagnosis of patients with posterior urethral valves is most often made using antenatal ultrasound screening.

2. **d. pulmonary insufficiency in the newborn period.** The major cause of mortality today in posterior urethral valves is from pulmonary hypoplasia. Infants with renal failure can be dialyzed, but pulmonary insufficiency may still be fatal.

3. **d. degree of renal dysplasia.** The degree of renal dysplasia is the most important factor in determining long-term renal function. Renal dysplasia develops early in fetal life and cannot be reversed. It limits renal growth and development.

4. **c. preventing adequate upper tract drainage.** The valve bladder syndrome is the greatest threat in preventing adequate upper tract drainage. It may also contribute to infection and incontinence.

5. **b. Providing a pressure pop-off valve.** Urinary ascites, VURD, and bladder diverticula all offer relative protection to the valve patient by acting as pressure pop-off valves. In this way they may spare the kidney high pressures and may protect renal function.

6. **e. is variable and changes during life.** The most important feature to remember in managing bladder dysfunction in patients with posterior urethral valves is that it is variable and changes during life. Urodynamic monitoring is necessary in managing patients with posterior urethral valves.

7. **a. document that the bladder can empty effectively.** In patients with posterior urethral valves and persistent reflux, it is most important to document that the bladder can empty effectively. Both valve remnants and bladder dysfunction can contribute to persistent reflux.

8. **b. cutaneous vesicostomy.** Cutaneous vesicostomy is the best initial option to establish long-term bladder drainage in a small infant with posterior urethral valves when valve ablation may be technically difficult.

9. **c. preventing pulmonary hypoplasia.** Antenatal intervention with a vesicoamniotic shunt is most likely to help the fetus by helping prevent pulmonary hypoplasia. Evidence that antenatal intervention improves renal or bladder function is lacking.

10. **c. degree of renal dysplasia.** Ultrasound in infants with posterior urethral valves may help to predict long-term renal function by demonstrating the degree of renal dysplasia. Renal dysplasia is evident on ultrasound by increased echogenicity.

11. **d. intermittent penis mass.** Anterior urethral valves differ from posterior urethral valves in that they may present as an intermittent penile mass. Anterior urethral valves are often in the form of a diverticulum that fills with urine during voiding and may be visible along the shaft of the penis.

12. **b. fetal age.** The accuracy of diagnosing posterior urethral valves on antenatal ultrasound screening is affected by fetal age. Ultrasound done when the fetus is younger than 24 weeks' gestation may miss the diagnosis of posterior urethral valves.

Additional Study Points

1. Type I valves are the most common.
2. Type II folds, which emanate from the verumontanum to the bladder neck, are no longer considered valves.
3. A type III valve is a membrane lying transversely across the urethra.
4. In patients with posterior urethral valves, the bladder neck is rigid and hypertrophied.
5. Virtually all valve patients have hydroureteronephrosis.
6. Patients with posterior urethral valves fail to concentrate and acidify urine throughout childhood and adulthood.
7. Patients with urinary ascites have a poor prognosis.
8. The keyhole sign as seen on ultrasound or VCUG represents a dilated bladder and a dilated prostatic urethra with a hypertrophied bladder neck in between.
9. Vesicoureteral reflux is present at birth in 50% of patients with posterior urethral valves.
10. The goal in treating posterior urethral valves cystoscopically is to incise them, not remove them.
11. It is imperative to document that the valve remnants are no longer obstructive following therapy.
12. If upper tract drainage is required, a low loop ureterostomy is preferred because it provides adequate drainage, can be placed beneath the diaper, and offers the least difficult reconstruction.
13. High-grade reflux is often associated with severe renal dysplasia.
14. The valve bladder may lead to deterioration of the upper tracts and incontinence over the patient's life.
15. The majority of patients with valve bladder have delayed daytime and nighttime continence.
16. The independent risk factors for predicting end-stage renal disease in patients with posterior urethral valves are the nadir serum creatinine and severe bladder dysfunction.
17. Anterior urethral valves occur in the form of a diverticulum.
18. The treatment of congenital urethral strictures in the neonate is vesicostomy because the strictures are generally too long and dense to incise.

Non-Neuropathic Dysfunction of the Lower Urinary Tract in Children

C.K. Yeung, MD ● Jennifer D.Y. Sihoe, MD, BMBS, BMedSci(Hons), FRCSEd(Paed), FHKAM(Surg) ● Stuart B. Bauer, MD

QUESTIONS

1. Development of normal bladder function involves:
   a. decrease in urine production and increase in bladder capacity.
   b. increase in urine production and increase in voiding frequency.
   c. increase in bladder capacity and decrease in voiding frequency.
   d. decrease in voided volume and increase in voiding frequency.
   e. increase in bladder capacity and no change in voided volume.

2. Which of the following statements best describes urodynamic findings of maximum detrusor pressures with micturition (Pdetmax) in infants with normal lower urinary tracts? When compared to adults?
   a. There is no difference compared with adults.
   b. Lower Pdetmax is observed in infants compared with adults.
   c. Higher Pdetmax is observed in male infants only.
   d. Higher Pdetmax is observed in female infants only.
   e. Higher Pdetmax is observed in both male and female infants.

3. Which of the following statements on neurologic control of normal micturition is FALSE?
   a. Innervation of the bladder involves both the central somatic and the autonomic nervous system.
   b. Micturition is initiated with a full bladder by a simple spinal cord reflex.
   c. Micturition does not occur during sleep.
   d. Development of direct volitional control over the bladder-sphincter complex occurs.
   e. Neurologic control occurs at different levels of the central nervous system from spinal cord to brainstem.

4. A characteristic of children with the urge syndrome is:
   a. the Vincent curtsy sign.
   b. the hold maneuver.
   c. urgency.
   d. small bladder capacity.
   e. all of the above.

5. Involuntary leakage of urine on standing after voiding in a toilet-trained girl is suggestive of:
   a. vesicoureteral reflux (VUR).
   b. vesicovaginal reflux.
   c. stress incontinence.
   d. urge syndrome.
   e. Hinman syndrome.

6. Which of the following best characterizes a decompensated bladder?
   a. Large bladder capacity with poor bladder emptying
   b. Small bladder capacity with incontinence
   c. Hyperreflexic bladder with reduced bladder capacity
   d. Small bladder capacity with frequent voiding
   e. None of the above

7. Fecal retention and constipation are often associated with which of the following urinary tract abnormalities?
   a. Urinary tract infection (UTI)
   b. VUR
   c. Hydronephrosis
   d. Enuresis
   e. All of the above

8. A 3-year-old boy presents with symptomatic UTI. Micturating cystourethrography confirms bilateral grade 4 VUR, and prophylactic antibiotic therapy is begun. Which of the following statements is correct?
   a. There is a high rate of spontaneous resolution of the VUR.
   b. The risk of breakthrough UTI is minimal on prophylactic antibiotic therapy.
   c. Surgical intervention is a consideration when the child is older.
   d. A urodynamic study is warranted for appropriate management of any underlying bladder dysfunction.

e. Radiologic studies of the upper urinary tract are not necessary.

9. A 6-year-old girl presents with symptoms of urge syndrome. Which of the following investigations should be done first?

a. Micturating cystourethrogram

b. Voiding diary

c. Radiograph of lumbar spine

d. Urine culture

e. Ambulatory urodynamic study

10. Which of the following statements about urodynamic studies is correct?

a. Natural fill urodynamics can only be performed via a suprapubic catheter.

b. Conventional fill studies are performed during ambulatory urodynamics.

c. Detrusor response may be inhibited during conventional fill urodynamic studies.

d. During video-urodynamics the child is allowed to run freely within a private cubicle.

e. Urodynamic studies are used to describe the physiologic parameters involved in the bladder mechanics during voiding only.

11. Treatment of a child with primary nocturnal enuresis may involve all of the following modalities EXCEPT:

a. antibiotic prophylaxis.

b. acupuncture.

c. bowel management.

d. pelvic floor rehabilitation.

e. antimuscarinics.

12. Urodynamic studies in children with primary nocturnal enuresis commonly exhibit which of the following?

a. Normal findings

b. Marked reduction in bladder emptying efficiency

c. Low leak-point pressure

d. Poor bladder compliance

e. Reduced functional bladder capacity

ANSWERS

1. **c. increase in bladder capacity and decrease in voiding frequency.** Development of normal bladder function involves an increase in bladder capacity in response to an increase in urine production. The voiding frequency decreases with age, whereas the voided volume of each micturition increases.

2. **e. Higher Pdetmax is observed in both male and female infants.** Urodynamic studies of infants with normal lower urinary tracts have documented significantly higher Pdetmax in both male and female infants compared with adults, although male infants had significantly higher Pdetmax compared with female infants.

3. **b. Micturition is initiated with a full bladder by a simple spinal cord reflex.** Studies have shown that even in full-term fetuses and newborns, micturition is modulated by higher centers.

4. **e. all of the above.** Detrusor overactivity during filling causes frequent attacks of sudden and imperative sensations of urge (urgency) that are often counteracted by voluntary contraction of the pelvic floor muscles in an attempt to compress the urethra (hold maneuver) exhibited as squatting (Vincent curtsey sign). Children with urge syndrome have small bladder capacities for age.

5. **b. vesicovaginal reflux.** This best describes postvoid dribbling, which typically occurs when urine gets trapped in the vagina during voiding and dribbles out soon after standing in otherwise normal toilet-trained girls with no other associated urinary symptoms.

6. **a. Large bladder capacity with poor bladder emptying.** A decompensated bladder can result from chronic functional bladder outflow obstruction resulting in deterioration in detrusor contractility and emptying efficiency, which eventually leads to development of a large, floppy bladder.

7. **e. All of the above.** The close proximity of the rectum to the posterior wall of the bladder makes it possible that any gross distention of the rectum can result in mechanical compression of the bladder and bladder neck, leading to urinary obstruction. Fecal impaction may also induce bladder dysfunction, which may be manifested by VUR, enuresis, or UTI.

8. **d. A urodynamic study is warranted for appropriate management of any underlying bladder dysfunction.** Infants with UTI and VUR (especially boys) have a high prevalence of high maximum voiding pressures associated with detrusor overactivity. Bladder dysfunction has a powerful relationship with nonresolution of high-grade VUR. Treatment of the bladder dysfunction, however, was shown to result in a marked increase in the rate of spontaneous resolution and reduction in recurrent UTIs.

9. **b. Voiding diary.** A daily record of fluid intake and urine output at home under normal conditions would be most informative as a noninvasive first-line investigation to suggest any underlying bladder dysfunction and identify those issues that warrant further investigations.

10. **c. Detrusor response may be inhibited during conventional fill urodynamic studies.** Nonphysiologic filling of the bladder during conventional fill urodynamics, even at low filling rates, can lead to misinterpretation of true bladder activity during normal situations. Artificial filling may inhibit detrusor response and attenuate its maximum contractile potential, rendering detrusor instability less pronounced and undetectable.

11. **a. antibiotic prophylaxis.** A significant proportion of children with severe nocturnal enuresis has underlying bladder dysfunction that may respond to the different treatment modalities listed. There is no role for long-term antibiotic prophylaxis in these children because recurrent UTI is seldom a problem when other associated urologic anomalies are excluded.

12. **e. Reduced functional bladder capacity.** A significant proportion of children with severe nocturnal enuresis shows a marked reduction in functional bladder capacity when compared with age-matched normal controls. This may be related to the high prevalence of underlying bladder dysfunction, particularly of detrusor overactivity at night, in enuretic children.

Additional Study Points

1. In infants and young children, the bladder is an abdominal organ and can readily be palpated when full.
2. Immature detrusor sphincter coordination manifested as detrusor hypercontractility and interrupted voiding commonly occurs in the first 2 years of life and results in functional bladder outflow obstruction.
3. Even in newborns, micturition does not occur during sleep, suggesting modulation of micturition by higher centers.
4. The association of constipation with urologic pathology is referred to as the dysfunctional elimination syndrome. Abnormalities of bowel function are commonly present in young children with voiding dysfunction.
5. Giggle incontinence often results in complete emptying of the bladder.
6. In patients who develop acquired bladder sphincter dysfunction, a significant proportion also has bowel dysfunction.
7. There is a significant association of bladder dysfunction with nonresolution of high-grade vesicle ureteral reflux.
8. In children there is a poor correlation between maximal flow rate and outflow resistance. It is better to study the pattern of the flow curve.
9. In any evaluation of voiding dysfunction, abnormalities of the lower spine should be sought.
10. Nocturnal urine output in many enuretic children is in excess of bladder reservoir capacity during sleep.
11. Many enuretic children have a marked reduction in functional bladder capacity when compared with age-matched controls and may have detrusor instability as well.

Neuropathic Dysfunction of the Lower Urinary Tract

Dawn Lee MacLellan, MD, FRCSC • Stuart B. Bauer, MD

QUESTIONS

1. Urinary incontinence or voiding dysfunction in children without obvious neurologic disease is related to which of the following?
   a. Excessive urine production from nephrogenic diabetes insipidus
   b. Delayed maturation of the nervous system
   c. An ectopic ectopia
   d. All of the above
   e. b and c only

2. Rectal pressure monitoring during a cystometrogram allows for which of the following parameters?
   a. It provides a way of detecting an overactive detrusor.
   b. It determines true detrusor compliance.
   c. It differentiates detrusor from abdominal leak point pressure.
   d. All of the above
   e. None of the above

3. Eliciting an overactive detrusor is easiest to diagnose during a cystometrogram under which of the following conditions?
   a. Rapid infusion of warm saline
   b. Slow infusion of cold saline
   c. Slow infusion of warm saline
   d. Rapid infusion of cold saline
   e. Having the child cough during the examination

4. Which vitamin plays a major role in the prevention of neural tube defects?
   a. Niacin
   b. Riboflavin
   c. Folic acid
   d. B_{12}
   e. Carotene

5. Which statement is TRUE about children with a thoracic level myelomeningocele?
   a. Leg function is usually normal.
   b. Infants with this level lesion often have detrusor-sphincter dyssynergia.
   c. Infants with this level lesion have an underactive detrusor.
   d. Older children tend to have a normal upper urinary tract on ultrasonography.
   e. Older children tend to easily achieve urinary continence with just clean intermittent catheterization alone.

6. What percent of neonates with a myelomeningocele have a normal upper urinary appearance on ultrasonography within the first month of life?
   a. 45%
   b. 60%
   c. 75%
   d. 85%
   e. 95%

7. Secondary tethering of the spinal cord in infants who have had closure of the myelomeningocele in the first days of life occurs in what percentage of children?
   a. 5%
   b. 10%
   c. 15%
   d. 20%
   e. 25%

8. Credé voiding is best avoided in which of the following conditions?
   a. Vesicourethral reflux with a severely denervated urethral sphincter
   b. Vesicourethral reflux with a fully innervated urethral sphincter
   c. A poorly compliant bladder with a low leak point pressure
   d. An overactive detrusor with a low leak point pressure
   e. A compliant bladder with a low leak point pressure

9. When considering an antireflux operation in a child with a myelomeningocele, treating which urodynamic parameter beforehand is thought to be most important for achieving a successful result?
   a. Poor compliance
   b. Presence of detrusor overactivity
   c. a and b

d. Neither a nor b

e. A high leak point pressure

10. Which of the following anticholinergic medications is most potent in reducing detrusor overactivity?

a. Hyoscyamine

b. Propantheline bromide

c. Oxybutynin

d. Glycopyrrolate

e. Tolterodine

11. After a gastrocystoplasty to enlarge the bladder and counteract a poorly compliant bladder which metabolic derangement can occur if the patient is not monitored carefully?

a. Hyponatremic hypochloremic metabolic alkalosis

b. Hypernatremic hyperkalemic metabolic acidosis

c. Hypokalemic hyperchloremic metabolic alkalosis

d. Hypernatremic hypochloremic metabolic acidosis

e. Hyponatremic hyperchloremic metabolic acidosis

12. Which of the following statements is FALSE regarding sexual function in patients with myelodysplasia?

a. Females are unable to bear children in 50% of the cases.

b. Males may have normal sperm production but are unable to have adequate ejaculatory function.

c. Females have regular menses.

d. Pubertal changes tend to occur earlier in myelodysplastic children compared with normal children.

e. Incontinence of urine has little effect on the sexual behavior of males or females.

13. All of the following may be an outward physical sign of an occult spinal dysraphism EXCEPT:

a. a subcutaneous mass overlying the thoracic spine.

b. an asymmetrical gluteal cleft.

c. a draining pilonidal dimple.

d. one leg slightly longer than the other.

e. a spinal scoliosis.

14. The conus medullaris normally resides opposite which vertebral body at puberty?

a. T11

b. T12

c. L1

d. L2

e. L3

15. Which of the following maternal factors may be responsible for sacral agenesis in a neonate?

a. Exposure to progestational agents early in the pregnancy

b. Insulin-dependent diabetes early in the early gestational period

c. Insulin dependency later in the pregnancy

d. Exposure to progestational agents later in the pregnancy

e. None of the above

16. Which of the following statements is TRUE regarding the diagnosis of sacral agenesis?

a. Motor function in the lower extremities and sacral area is normal.

b. Motor function in the lower extremities and sacral area is impaired.

c. The abnormality can be diagnosed in the neonate due to an abnormal gluteal cleft.

d. Sensation in the lower extremities and sacral area is normal.

e. Sensation in the lower extremities and sacral area is impaired.

17. Which statement is TRUE regarding neurogenic bladder dysfunction in children with imperforate anus?

a. An injury to the pelvic nerves during the pull-through procedure leads to the lesion.

b. An injury to the pelvic floor muscles while separating the rectourethral fistula may cause the lesion.

c. Neurogenic bladder dysfunction is almost never seen in supralevator level lesions.

d. Neurogenic bladder dysfunction is fairly common in infralevator level lesion.

e. A spinal cord abnormality in association with imperforate anal lesions can be seen in 30% of imperforate anus cases.

18. Most children with cerebral palsy have what type of lower urinary tract function on urodynamic testing?

a. A hyperactive bladder with denervation in the external urethral sphincter

b. A hyperactive bladder with bladder sphincter dyssynergy during voiding

c. An underactive bladder with denervation in the external urethral sphincter

d. An underactive bladder with a normally innervated external urethral sphincter

e. A normally reflexic bladder with bladder sphincter synergy during voiding

19. The most common cause of a traumatic spinal cord injury in infants is:

a. a motor vehicle accident.

b. an accidental fall from a high place.

c. a hyperextension injury to the cervical spine during delivery.

d. spinal column surgery to correct either an intraspinal process or scoliosis.

e. a sports-related injury.

ANSWERS

1. **d. All of the above.** One has to consider multiple, other, possibly unrelated causes of urinary incontinence when the diagnosis is not evidently the result of a neurologic lesion.

2. **d. All of the above.** It is a mandatory parameter to accurately measure actual detrusor function (compliance, contractility, and leak point pressure) that is free of artifacts of movement.

3. **b. Slow infusion of cold saline.** A slow infusion allows the detrusor muscle to accommodate to the increasing volume in at best a reproducible physiologic way. The cold solution may stimulate the detrusor to elicit overactive contraction during filling in patients with an overactive detrusor.

4. **c. Folic acid.** Folic acid has been shown to reduce the incidence of neural tube defects in several large populations

of people when given to women of childbearing age before pregnancy is achieved.

5. **b. Infants with this level lesion often have detrusor-sphincter dyssynergia.** Seventy-four percent of neonates and 54% of older children have intact sacral cord function with absence of pontine micturition center coordination of the detrusor and urethral sphincter.

6. **d. 85%.** Fifteen to 20 percent of neonates have an abnormal urinary tract on radiologic examination when first evaluated consisting of hydroureteronephrosis secondary to spinal shock, probably from the spinal canal closure, or abnormalities that developed in utero as a result of abnormal lower urinary tract function in the form of outlet obstruction.

7. **e. 25%.** The neurologic lesion in myelodysplasia is a dynamic disease process in which changes take place throughout childhood. The exact number is variable, depending on the level of the original lesion, the thoroughness with which the children were followed, and the criteria used for diagnosing a change.

8. **b. Vesicourethral reflux with a fully innervated urethral sphincter.** When the sacral reflex arc is intact the Credé maneuver results in a reflex response in the external sphincter that increases urethral resistance and raises the pressure needed to expel urine from the bladder. This, in turn, leads to high-pressure "voiding" that can aggravate the degree of reflux present and its effect on the kidney.

9. **c. a and b.** Lowering detrusor pressure and reducing overactivity of the muscle ensure that the bladder remains a favorable organ for a successful antireflux operation.

10. **d. Glycopyrrolate.** Glycopyrrolate is the most potent oral anticholinergic drug available today, but it may have the typical belladonna-like side effects common to all these drugs (see Table 128–1 in *Campbell-Walsh Urology, 10th Edition*).

11. **a. Hyponatremic hypochloremic metabolic alkalosis.** A gastric segment removed from the gastrointestinal system can cause hyponatremic hypochloremic metabolic alkalosis because its secretory surface involves an active H^+ and Cl^- pump that is not regulated by endogenous hormones. There is no absorptive surface in the remaining sections of the bladder that can resorb these ions, and thus a metabolic derangement can rapidly occur.

12. **a. Females are unable to bear children in 50% of the cases.** Several studies have revealed that 70% to 80% of myelodysplastic women are able to become pregnant and have uneventful pregnancies and deliveries.

13. **a. a subcutaneous mass overlying the thoracic spine.** In more than 90% of children with an occult spinal dysraphism there is a cutaneous abnormality overlying the lower spine in the lower lumbar or upper sacral areas.

14. **c. L1.** Under normal circumstances the conus medullaris ends just above the L2 vertebra at birth and recedes upward to T12 by adulthood because the spinal cord grows at a slower rate than the increasing height of the vertebral bodies.

15. **b. Insulin-dependent diabetes early in the early gestational period.** Teratogenic factors may play a role in the pathogenesis of sacral agenesis because insulin-dependent diabetic mothers have a 1% chance of giving birth to a child with this disorder.

16. **c. The abnormality can be diagnosed in the neonate due to an abnormal gluteal cleft.** The only clue to the diagnosis of sacral agenesis, besides a high index of suspicion, is flattened buttocks and a low, short gluteal cleft, because sensation and lower extremity motor function is usually normal.

17. **e. A spinal cord abnormality in association with imperforate anal lesions can be seen in 30% of imperforate anus cases.** Spinal cord abnormalities including a tethered cord, thickened or fatty filum terminale, and a lipoma have been noted in 18% to 50% of patients with an imperforate anus, with the incidence varying proportionately in relation to the height of the rectal lesion.

18. **e. A normally reflexic bladder with bladder sphincter synergy during voiding.** Most children with cerebral palsy develop total urinary control. Detrusor overactivity is seen in 80%, but dyssynergy between the bladder and sphincter has only been noted in 5%, and 11% have evidence of lower motor neuron denervation in the sphincter.

19. **c. a hyperextension injury to the cervical spine during delivery.** Neonates are particularly prone to a hyperextension injury of the cervical spine during high forceps delivery.

Additional Study Points

1. During urodynamics, bladder filling should occur at a rate of the calculated bladder capacity divided by 10 per minute.
2. Normal voiding pressure in boys is 55 to 80 cm H_2O and in girls it is 30 to 65 cm H_2O.
3. In the myelomeningocele patient the bony vertebral level provides little or no clue as to the neurologic level.
4. Upper motor neuron lesions result in an overactive detrusor, exaggerated sacral reflexes, detrusor sphincter dyssynergia, a thickened bladder wall, and a closed bladder neck.
5. Lower motor neuron lesions result in a noncontractile detrusor, denervation of the external sphincter, diminished or absent sacral reflexes, and a small smooth-walled bladder with an open bladder neck.
6. Assessment of the neonate with myelomeningocele involves renal ultrasonography and measurement of the postvoid residual urine.
7. Resting bladder pressure should be maintained below 30 cm H_2O. Resting pressures above 40 cm H_2O result in upper tract deterioration.
8. The neurologic lesion in myelodysplasia is a dynamic process and changes throughout childhood.
9. Bowel incontinence is frequently unpredictable and not associated with the attainment of urinary continence in myelodysplasia patients.
10. Sacral agenesis may result in bladder dysfunction not detected at birth and is usually brought to the physician's attention when the child fails at toilet training.
11. Sacral agenesis may manifest as either an upper or lower motor neuron lesion.
12. In patients with cerebral palsy the presence of incontinence is usually related to the physical impairment.
13. In traumatic injuries of the spine, patients with upper thoracic and cervical lesions are likely to exhibit autonomic dysreflexia.

Urinary Tract Reconstruction in Children

Mark C. Adams, MD, FAAP ● David B. Joseph, MD, FACS, FAAP

QUESTIONS

1. Children with significant bladder or sphincter dysfunction requiring reconstructive surgery most likely have:
   a. bladder exstrophy or epispadias.
   b. posterior urethral valves.
   c. cloacal anomalies.
   d. prune-belly syndrome.
   e. spinal dysraphism.

2. The most important contribution to the field of pediatric reconstructive surgery has been:
   a. Mitrofanoff's description of a continent abdominal wall stoma using appendix.
   b. Lapides' introduction of clean intermittent catheterization (CIC).
   c. Goodwin's description of ileal reconfiguration.
   d. development of several effective means to increase bladder outlet resistance.
   e. recognition that a dilated ureter could be used for bladder augmentation.

3. Normal bladder compliance is based on:
   a. ample collagen type II.
   b. inverse relationship of bladder volume and bladder pressure.
   c. bladder unfolding, elasticity, and viscoelasticity.
   d. subepithelial matrix bridges associated with collagen.
   e. hypertrophic bladder bundles interspersed with collagen.

4. Chronically elevated bladder filling pressures may cause hydronephrosis, vesicoureteral reflux, and impaired renal function. The lowest pressure threshold most often reported to cause problems is:
   a. 20 cm H_2O.
   b. 30 cm H_2O.
   c. 40 cm H_2O.
   d. 50 cm H_2O.
   e. 60 cm H_2O.

5. Upper urinary tract changes associated with a poorly compliant, hyperreflexic bladder are initially treated by:
   a. autoaugmentation.
   b. pharmacologic management and intermittent catheterization.

   c. ileal augmentation.
   d. sigmoid augmentation.
   e. gastric augmentation.

6. Preoperative bladder capacity and compliance are best determined by urodynamics using:
   a. carbon dioxide as an irrigant at a slow fill rate (10% of capacity per minute).
   b. room temperature saline at a slow fill rate (10% of capacity per minute).
   c. body temperature saline at a fast fill rate (30% of capacity per minute).
   d. cooled saline at a slow fill rate (10% of capacity per minute).
   e. cooled saline at a fast fill rate (30% of capacity per minute).

7. Urinary tract reconstruction for urinary continence requires:
   a. confirmation of a normal upper urinary tract.
   b. identification of a highly compliant bladder.
   c. documentation of the presence or absence of vesicoureteral reflux.
   d. acceptance and compliance with intermittent catheterization.
   e. documentation of a serum creatinine value less than 1.4 mg/dL.

8. Mechanical bowel preparation is performed in patients undergoing:
   a. ileocystoplasty.
   b. sigmoid cystoplasty.
   c. gastrocystoplasty.
   d. ureterocystoplasty.
   e. all of the above.

9. A urinary stricture after transureteroureterostomy is most likely due to:
   a. mobilization of the crossing ureter with periureteral tissue.
   b. mobilization of the crossing ureter without angulation beneath the inferior mesenteric artery.
   c. mobilization of the recipient ureter to meet the crossing one.

d. wide anastomosis of the crossing ureter to the posteromedial aspect of the recipient.

e. watertight anastomosis.

10. Creating an antireflux mechanism is most difficult with anastomosis to the:

a. stomach.

b. ileum.

c. cecum.

d. transverse colon.

e. sigmoid colon.

11. The Young-Dees-Leadbetter bladder neck repair in children with neurogenic sphincter deficiency:

a. results in limited success because of a lack of muscle tone and activity of the native bladder neck.

b. can achieve successful continence results similar to those noted in children with bladder exstrophy.

c. does not often require bladder augmentation or intermittent catheterization.

d. is best performed in association with a Silastic sling.

e. limits the necessity for intermittent catheterization in children who could empty by a Valsalva maneuver preoperatively.

12. An ambulatory 15-year-old girl with lumbosacral myelomeningocele voids to completion with a low-pressure detrusor contraction and the Valsalva maneuver. She remains incontinent due to bladder neck and intrinsic sphincter deficiency refractory to pharmacologic management. To limit the risk of intermittent catheterization, the next step is:

a. Young-Dees-Leadbetter bladder neck repair.

b. artificial urinary sphincter placement.

c. fascial bladder neck sling placement.

d. Kropp bladder neck repair.

e. Pippi-Salle bladder neck repair.

13. One side effect associated with bladder neck repair that can be decreased with good preoperative evaluation is:

a. recurrent urolithiasis.

b. recurrent cystitis.

c. inability to spontaneously void.

d. associated need for augmentation cystoplasty.

e. unmasking of detrusor hostility, resulting in upper urinary tract changes.

14. Fascial slings used for increasing outlet resistance in children with neurogenic sphincteric incompetence:

a. are more effective in girls than in boys.

b. are dependent on the type of fascial or cadaveric tissue used.

c. are dependent on the configuration of the sling and wrap used.

d. rarely result in the need for bladder augmentation and intermittent catheterization.

e. frequently result in urethral erosion.

15. The least favorable indication for an artificial urinary sphincter is:

a. neurogenic bladder dysfunction.

b. bladder exstrophy or epispadias.

c. inability to empty the bladder by spontaneous voiding.

d. associated need for bladder augmentation.

e. prepubertal age.

16. The most common limitation of a Kropp urethral lengthening for continence is:

a. fistula from the urethra to the bladder, resulting in incontinence.

b. inability to spontaneously void, resulting in urinary retention.

c. difficulty with intermittent catheterization, particularly in boys.

d. new vesicoureteral reflux.

e. distal ureteral obstruction.

17. Urinary continence is most definitively achieved after:

a. Young-Dees-Leadbetter bladder repair.

b. placement of an artificial urinary sphincter.

c. placement of a circumferential fascial wrap.

d. urethral lengthening and reimplantation.

e. bladder neck division.

18. To avoid uninhibited pressure contractions during an enterocystoplasty:

a. large bowel should be used.

b. the intestinal segment should be reconfigured.

c. the majority of the diseased bladder should be excised.

d. a stellate incision into the bladder should be created to increase the circumference of the bowel anastomosis.

e. small mesenteric windows are created in the bowel segment.

19. Potential ways to prevent reflux when using ileum for continent diversion include all of the following except:

a. intussuscepted nipple valve.

b. split nipple cuff of ureter.

c. placement of the spatulated ureter into an incised mucosal trough.

d. flap valve created beneath a taenia.

e. placement of the ureter within a serosa-lined tunnel between two limbs of ileum.

20. The gastrointestinal segment that most often causes permanent gastrointestinal side effects when used in children with a neurogenic bladder is the:

a. stomach.

b. jejunum.

c. ileum.

d. ileocecal segment.

e. sigmoid colon.

21. The most likely problem after gastrointestinal bladder augmentation is:

a. early satiety.

b. hyperchloremic metabolic acidosis.

c. small bowel obstruction.

d. chronic diarrhea.

e. vitamin B_{12} deficiency with megaloblastic anemia.

22. The gastrointestinal segment resulting in the best long-term capacity and compliance after augmentation cystoplasty is the:
    a. gastric body.
    b. gastric antrum.
    c. ileum.
    d. cecum.
    e. sigmoid colon.

23. The risk of failure to achieve appropriate capacity and compliance after augmentation cystoplasty is:
    a. less than 5%.
    b. 5% to 10%.
    c. 11% to 15%.
    d. 16% to 20%.
    e. more than 20%.

24. The serum metabolic pattern that occurs most often after an ileocystoplasty or colocystoplasty is:
    a. hypochloremic metabolic acidosis.
    b. hyperchloremic metabolic acidosis.
    c. hypochloremic metabolic alkalosis.
    d. hyperchloremic metabolic alkalosis.
    e. hyponatremic metabolic acidosis.

25. The serum metabolic pattern that occurs most often after gastrocystoplasty is:
    a. hypochloremic metabolic acidosis.
    b. hyperchloremic metabolic acidosis.
    c. hypochloremic metabolic alkalosis.
    d. hyperchloremic metabolic alkalosis.
    e. hyponatremic metabolic acidosis.

26. The risk of intermittent hematuria and dysuria after gastrocystoplasty is most influenced by:
    a. the gastric segment used.
    b. persistent urinary incontinence.
    c. decreased renal function.
    d. diagnosis of bladder exstrophy.
    e. neurogenic bladder dysfunction.

27. Bacteriuria should be treated after bladder augmentation when:
    a. associated with CIC.
    b. urinalysis demonstrates microscopic hematuria.
    c. there is increased mucus production.
    d. etiology is posterior urethral valves.
    e. urine culture reveals growth of a urea-splitting organism.

28. The gastrointestinal segment associated with the lowest incidence of stone formation is:
    a. stomach.
    b. jejunum.
    c. ileum.
    d. cecum.
    e. sigmoid colon.

29. Adenocarcinoma of the bladder after augmentation cystoplasty can occur after:
    a. 2 years.
    b. 4 years.

c. 8 years.
d. 16 years.
e. 26 years.

30. The risk of perforation after bladder augmentation includes all but:
    a. high outflow resistance.
    b. persistent hyperreflexia or uninhibited bladder contractions.
    c. use of sigmoid colon.
    d. bladder exstrophy.
    e. neurogenic bladder dysfunction.

31. The initial management of a spontaneous perforation of an augmented bladder in a child with a neurogenic bladder is:
    a. placement of a large-bore urethral catheter for drainage.
    b. placement of a large-bore suprapubic cystotomy tube for drainage.
    c. immediate surgical exploration and repair.
    d. serial abdominal examinations.
    e. urine culture.

32. Pregnancy associated with urinary reconstruction:
    a. is reasonable after urinary diversion but is contraindicated after augmentation cystoplasty.
    b. results in the mesenteric pedicle positioned directly anterior to the uterus.
    c. results in the mesenteric pedicle deflected laterally without vascular compromise to the augmented segment.
    d. is avoided due to mechanical compression of the pedicle and ischemia with loss of the augmented segment.
    e. is contraindicated because of increased risk of systemic sepsis complicating the hydronephrosis.

33. Ureterocystoplasty is limited because:
    a. it requires an intraperitoneal approach.
    b. complete mobilization of the ureter may result in vascular compromise.
    c. dilated ureter is not as compliant as a similar-sized bowel segment.
    d. dilated ureter is not available in many patients.
    e. ureterocystoplasty precludes spontaneous voiding.

34. Autoaugmentation is contraindicated with:
    a. serum creatinine value greater than 1.4 ng/dL.
    b. CIC.
    c. vesicoureteral reflux.
    d. uninhibited bladder contractions.
    e. small bladder capacity.

35. A ureterosigmoidostomy should not be undertaken in a patient with a history of:
    a. dilated ureters.
    b. anteriorly placed rectum associated with bladder exstrophy.
    c. recurrent pyelonephritis.
    d. fecal incontinence.
    e. constipation.

36. The use of efferent nipple valves for continence in children:
    a. has not approached the results achieved in adults.
    b. has a higher complication and reoperation rate than a flap valve.
    c. is equivalent to any other continence mechanism.
    d. is often associated with difficulty in catheterization.
    e. often results in stomal stenosis.

37. The least important factor when creating an appendicovesicostomy is:
    a. taking a wide cecal cuff to decrease the risk of stomal stenosis.
    b. creating a tunnel of 4 cm, at least greater than a 5:1 ratio of tunnel length to diameter, to achieve continence.
    c. a small, uniform lumen allowing for easy catheterization.
    d. mobilizing the right colon to adequately free the appendix.
    e. tubularizing a small portion of the cecum in continuity with the appendix to increase length.

38. A frequent occurrence after an appendicovesicostomy is:
    a. urinary incontinence due to inadequate length of the flap valve mechanism.
    b. urinary incontinence due to persistently elevated reservoir pressure.
    c. appendiceal perforation that often occurs due to catheterization.
    d. appendiceal stricture or necrosis.
    e. stomal stenosis.

39. A 12-year-old obese girl with spina bifida undergoes appendicocecostomy, bladder neck sling, bladder augmentation, and continent catheterizable bladder channel. The upper urinary tract is normal. The best source of tissue for the bladder channel is:
    a. distal right ureter after right-to-left transureteroureterostomy.
    b. tapered segment of small bowel of adequate length.
    c. right fallopian tube.
    d. gastric tube.
    e. tubularized bladder flap.

40. In complex pediatric urinary undiversion procedures it is most difficult to:
    a. provide adequate outflow resistance.
    b. create a compliant urinary reservoir.
    c. achieve an effective antireflux mechanism without upper tract obstruction.
    d. provide a reliable access for intermittent catheterization.
    e. achieve urinary and fecal continence.

ANSWERS

1. **e. spinal dysraphism.** Most pediatric reconstructive procedures are undertaken to correct a problem of the native urinary tract causing progressive hydronephrosis, urinary incontinence unresponsive to medical management, or temporary diversion. Children with bladder and sphincteric dysfunction represent the most complex reconstructive cases seen in pediatric urology; children with the diagnoses of exstrophy, persistent cloaca and urogenital sinus, posterior urethral valves, bilateral single ectopic ureters, and prune-belly syndrome may be involved. However, children with a neurogenic bladder due to a myelomeningocele make up the vast majority of patients requiring this type of surgical intervention.

2. **b. Lapides' introduction of clean intermittent catheterization (CIC).** One of the most important contributions in the care of children with bladder dysfunction came with the acceptance of CIC described by Lapides and colleagues in 1972 and 1976, based on the work of Guttmann and Frankel. The effective use of CIC has allowed the application of augmentation and lower tract reconstruction to groups of patients who had not previously been candidates. The principle of intermittent catheterization allows the reconstructive surgeon to aggressively correct storage problems by providing an adequate reservoir and good outflow resistance. Spontaneous voiding, although a goal, is not imperative because catheterization can be used for emptying.

3. **c. bladder unfolding, elasticity, and viscoelasticity.** Multiple factors contribute to the property of compliance. Initially the bladder is in a collapsed state, which allows for the storage of urine at low pressure by simply unfolding. As it expands, detrusor properties of elasticity and viscoelasticity take effect. Elasticity allows the detrusor muscle to stretch without an increase in tension until it reaches a critical volume. When filling is slow, as in a natural state, or stops, there is a rapid decay in this pressure known as stress relaxation. Normally, stress relaxation is in balance with the filling rate and prevents an increase in detrusor pressure.

4. **c. 40 cm H_2O.** Elevated passive filling pressure becomes clinically pathogenic when a pressure greater than 40 cm H_2O is chronically reached. Pressure at this level sustained over a prolonged period of time impairs ureteral drainage and can result in acquired vesicoureteral reflux, pyelocaliceal changes, hydroureteronephrosis, and decreased glomerular filtration rate.

5. **b. pharmacologic management and intermittent catheterization.** Pharmacologic management can play a role in decreasing filling pressure, particularly when hyperreflexic detrusor contractions are present. A combination of medications and intermittent catheterization has a positive impact, particularly in children with neurogenic dysfunction.

6. **b. room temperature saline at a slow fill rate (10% of capacity per minute).** The testing medium and infusion rate can influence the results. Carbon dioxide is not as reliable as fluid infusion, particularly when evaluating bladder compliance and capacity. The most common fluids used for testing are saline and iodinated contrast material; both provide reproducible results. Use of testing media at body temperature is also appropriate, but room temperature has also been shown to be acceptable. End filling pressure, and bladder compliance, can be dramatically affected by simply changing the filling rate. The cystometrogram should be performed at a fill rate of 10% per minute of the predicted bladder capacity for age.

7. **d. acceptance and compliance with intermittent catheterization.** No test ensures that a patient will be able to void spontaneously and empty well after bladder augmentation or other reconstruction. Therefore, all patients must be prepared to perform CIC postoperatively. The

native urethra should be examined for the ease of catheterization. Ideally, the patient should learn CIC and practice it preoperatively until the patient, family, and surgeon are comfortable that catheterization can and will be performed reliably. In spite of a technically perfect operation, failure to catheterize and empty the bladder after reconstruction can result in upper tract deterioration, urinary tract infection, or bladder perforation.

8. **e. all of the above.** Each patient undergoes preoperative bowel preparation to minimize the potential risk of surgery if the use of any bowel is contemplated. Even when ureterocystoplasty or other alternatives are planned, intraoperative findings may dictate the need for use of a bowel segment.

9. **c. mobilization of the recipient ureter to meet the crossing one.** If the native urinary bladder is small and adequate for only a single ureteral tunnel, transureteroureterostomy and a single reimplant may be helpful. Typically, the better ureter should be implanted into the bladder. The contralateral ureter drains into the reimplanted ureter via a transureteroureterostomy. The crossing ureter should follow a smooth path and remain tension free. It should be carefully mobilized with all of its adventitia and as much periureteral tissue as possible to preserve blood supply. Care must be taken not to angulate the crossing ureter beneath the inferior mesenteric artery. The crossing ureter should be widely anastomosed to the posteromedial aspect of the recipient ureter. The recipient ureter should not be mobilized or brought medially to meet the contralateral ureter in order to minimize devascularization.

10. **b. ileum.** The necessity of ureteral reimplantation into an intestinal segment may occasionally determine the segment to be used for bladder augmentation or replacement. Long-term experience with ureterosigmoidostomy and colon conduit diversion has established an effective means of creating a nonrefluxing ureteral implant. If a gastric segment is used for bladder augmentation or replacement, the ureters may be implanted into the stomach in a manner remarkably similar to that used in the native bladder. Creating an effective antireflux mechanism into an ileal segment is more difficult. The split nipple technique described by Griffith may prevent reflux at least at low reservoir pressure.

11. **a. results in limited success because of a lack of muscle tone and activity of the native bladder neck.** Reports of success with the Young-Dees-Leadbetter bladder neck reconstruction in children with neurogenic sphincter dysfunction are limited, not only in the number of series but also in overall improvement of incontinence. Independent reviews of long-term results of this repair showed minimal success in individuals with neurogenic dysfunction. These authors speculated that the lack of success was due to a lack of muscle tone and activity in the wrapped muscle related to the neurogenic problem.

12. **b. artificial urinary sphincter placement.** The artificial urinary sphincter has been recognized as the only procedure that can result in prompt continence in selected children while preserving their ability to void spontaneously.

13. **e. unmasking of detrusor hostility, resulting in upper urinary tract changes.** It is now recognized that occlusion of the bladder neck in children with neurogenic sphincter incompetence can result in the unmasking or

development of detrusor hostility manifest by a decrease in bladder compliance or increase in detrusor hyperreflexia. Careful preoperative urodynamic assessment helps to identify some of the children who are at risk.

14. **a. are more effective in girls than in boys.** Fascial slings have been used more extensively and with better results in girls with neurogenic sphincter incompetence, although recently some success has been reported in boys. Overall long-term success with fascial slings in the neurogenic population has varied greatly from 40% to 100%.

15. **c. inability to empty the bladder by spontaneous voiding.** The ultimate benefits of the artificial urinary sphincter include its ability to achieve a high rate of continence while maintaining the potential for spontaneous voiding. For practical purposes, when intermittent catheterization is required along with augmentation cystoplasty, using native tissue for continence eliminates the long-term concern for infection/erosion and the risk of mechanical failure.

16. **c. difficulty with intermittent catheterization, particularly in boys.** One study examined the results in 23 children, 22 of whom had neurogenic sphincter incompetence, and noted continence in more than 90% of the children. The most common complication was difficult catheterization, particularly in boys. Less than half of the boys in this series were catheterized through the native urethra; the majority were catheterized via an abdominal wall stoma.

17. **e. bladder neck division.** The ultimate procedure to increase bladder outlet resistance is to divide the bladder neck so that it is no longer in continuity with the urethra. This must be accompanied by creation of a continent abdominal wall stoma and should be performed only in patients who will reliably be able to perform catheterization.

18. **b. the intestinal segment should be reconfigured.** Two studies demonstrated the advantages of opening a bowel segment on its antimesenteric border, which allows detubularization and reconfiguration of that intestinal segment. Reconfiguration into a spherical shape provides multiple advantages, including maximization of the volume achieved for any given surface area, blunting of bowel contractions, and improvement of overall capacity and compliance.

19. **d. flap valve created beneath a taenia.** Small bowel does not have a taenia; this method is appropriate for large bowel. The split nipple technique described by Griffith may prevent reflux at least at low reservoir pressure. LeDuc and colleagues in 1987 described a technique in which the ureter is brought through a hiatus in the ileal wall. From that hiatus the ileal mucosa is incised and the edges are mobilized so as to create a trough for the ureter. It may also be possible to create antireflux mechanism using a serosal-lined tunnel created between two limbs of ileum as described by Abol-Enein and Ghoneim in 1999. Reinforced nipple valves of ileum have been used extensively to prevent reflux with the Kock pouch. Good long-term results have been achieved by Skinner after several modifications.

20. **d. ileocecal segment.** Chronic diarrhea after bladder augmentation alone is rare. Diarrhea can occur after removal of large segments of ileum from the gastrointestinal tract, although the length of the segments typically used for augmentation is rarely problematic unless other problems

coexist. Removal of the ileum and ileocecal valve from the gastrointestinal tract may cause diarrhea. One study noted that 10% of patients with neurogenic dysfunction have significant diarrhea after such displacement.

21. **b. hyperchloremic metabolic acidosis.** Postoperative bowel obstruction is uncommon after augmentation cystoplasty, occurring in approximately 3% of patients after augmentation. The rate of obstruction is equivalent to that noted after conduit diversion or continent urinary diversion. Removal of the distal ileum from the gastrointestinal tract may result in vitamin B_{12} deficiency and megaloblastic anemia. The terminal 15 to 20 cm of ileum should not be used for augmentation, although problems may arise even if that segment is preserved. Early satiety may occur after gastrocystoplasty but usually resolves with time. Disorders of gastric emptying should be extremely rare, particularly when using the body of the stomach.

22. **c. ileum.** Ileal reservoirs have been noted to have lower basal pressures and less motor activity when created for continent urinary diversion. Problems with pressure after augmentation cystoplasty usually occur from uninhibited contractions caused by the bowel segment. It is extremely rare not to achieve an adequate capacity or flat tonus limb unless a technical error has occurred with use of the bowel segment. Rhythmic contractions have been noted postoperatively with all bowel segments, particularly the stomach, although ileum is the least likely to demonstrate a remarkable urodynamic abnormality.

23. **b. 5% to 10%.** Hollensbe and associates at Indiana University reported on one of the largest experiences with pediatric bladder augmentation and found that approximately 5% of patients had significant uninhibited contractions causing clinical problems. Another study found that 6% required secondary augmentation of a previously augmented bladder for similar problems in long-term follow-up.

24. **b. hyperchloremic metabolic acidosis.** The first recognized metabolic complication related to storage of urine within intestinal segments was the occasional development of hyperchloremic metabolic acidosis after ureterosigmoidostomy. Another study demonstrated the mechanisms by which acid is absorbed from urine in contact with intestinal mucosa. A later report noted that essentially every patient after augmentation with an intestinal segment had an increase in serum chloride and a decrease in serum bicarbonate levels, although clinically significant acidosis was rare if renal function was normal.

25. **c. hypochloremic metabolic alkalosis.** Gastric mucosa is a barrier to chloride and acid resorption and, in fact, secretes hydrochloric acid. The secretory nature of gastric mucosa may at times be detrimental to the patient and can result in two unique complications of gastrocystoplasty. Severe episodes of hypokalemic hypochloremic metabolic alkalosis after acute gastrointestinal illnesses have been noted after gastrocystoplasty.

26. **e. neurogenic bladder dysfunction.** Virtually all patients with normal sensation have occasional hematuria or dysuria with voiding or catheterization after gastrocystoplasty beyond that which is expected with other intestinal segments. All patients should be warned of this potential problem, although in most patients these symptoms are intermittent and mild and do not require treatment. The dysuria is less problematic in patients with limited sensation due to neurogenic dysfunction. Patients who are incontinent or have decreased renal function may be at increased risk. These problems occur less frequently after antral gastric cystoplasty in which there is a smaller load of parietal cells.

27. **e. urine culture reveals growth of a urea-splitting organism.** It appears that the use of CIC is a prominent factor in the development of bacteriuria in patients after augmentation cystoplasty. Every episode of asymptomatic bacteriuria does not require treatment in patients performing CIC. Bacteriuria should be treated when significant symptoms occur such as fever, suprapubic pain, incontinence, and gross hematuria. Bacteriuria should also be treated when the urine culture demonstrates growth of a urea-splitting organism that may lead to stone formation.

28. **a. stomach.** Most bladder stones in the augmented child are of a struvite composition. Bacteriuria has been thought to be an important risk factor. Stones have been noted after the use of all intestinal segments with no significant difference appreciated between small and large intestine. Struvite stones are less likely after gastrocystoplasty.

29. **b. 4 years.** Patients undergoing augmentation cystoplasty should be made aware of a potential increased risk of tumor development. Yearly surveillance of the augmented bladder with endoscopy should eventually be performed; the latency period until such procedures are necessary is not well defined. The earliest reported tumor after augmentation was found only 4 years after cystoplasty.

30. **d. bladder exstrophy.** The cause of delayed perforations after bladder augmentation is unknown. Perforations may occur in bladders with significant uninhibited contractions after augmentation. High outflow resistance may maintain bladder pressure rather than allowing urinary leakage and venting of the pressure, potentially increasing ischemia. The majority of patients suffering perforations after augmentation cystoplasty have a neurogenic etiology. At Indiana University, perforations were noted in 32 of 330 patients undergoing cystoplasty an average of 4.3 years after augmentation. Analysis of this experience suggested that the use of sigmoid colon was the only significant increased risk.

31. **c. immediate surgical exploration and repair.** The standard treatment of spontaneous perforation of the augmented bladder is surgical repair, as it is for intraperitoneal rupture of the bladder after trauma. The majority of patients with perforations have myelodysplasia and present late in the course of the disease because of impaired sensation. Increasing sepsis and death of the patient may result from a delay in diagnosis or treatment.

32. **c. results in the mesenteric pedicle deflected laterally without vascular compromise to the augmented segment.** Experience is limited regarding what is known about the changes to the pedicle of a bladder augmentation during pregnancy. It has been reported that the mesenteric pedicle to bladder augmentations is not stretched over the uterus at the time of cesarean section. The pedicle has been found to be deflected laterally. Urinary tract infections may be problematic in women who have undergone urinary reconstruction, including bladder augmentation. Ureteral dilatation, increased residual urine, and diminished tone to the upper tract may all be important risk factors.

33. **d. a dilated ureter is not available in many patients.** Several series have reported good results after

ureteral augmentation with a follow-up as long as 8 years. The upper urinary tract has remained stable or improved in virtually all patients. Complications are uncommon. The main disadvantage to ureterocystoplasty is the limited patient population with a poorly functioning kidney drained by a megaureter.

34. **e. small bladder capacity.** Although autoaugmentation can improve compliance, an increase in volume is "modest at best." In a report of 12 children who had undergone a detrusorotomy, 5 were considered to have excellent results, 2 had acceptable results, and 1 was lost to follow-up. The main disadvantage of autoaugmentation is a limited increase in bladder capacity such that adequate preoperative volume may be the most important predictor of success.

35. **d. fecal incontinence.** Before ureterosigmoidostomy is considered, anal sphincter competence must be ensured. Tests used to assess sphincter integrity include manometry, electromyography, and practical evaluation of the ability to retain an oatmeal enema in the upright position for a time period without soilage. Incontinence of a mixture of stool and urine results in foul soilage and must be avoided.

36. **b. has a higher complication and reoperation rate than a flap valve.** The greatest experience with nipple valves for achieving urinary continence has been with the Kock pouch. Skinner and associates made a series of modifications to aid in maintenance of the efferent nipple. Even with experience and these modifications, a failure rate of 15% or higher can be expected. Equivalent results with the nipple valve and a Kock pouch have been achieved in children.

37. **b. creating a tunnel of 4 cm, at least greater than a 5:1 ratio of tunnel length to diameter, to achieve continence.** The appendix is an ideal natural tubular structure that can be safely removed from the gastrointestinal tract without significant morbidity. The small caliber of the appendix facilitates creation of a short functional tunnel with the bladder wall. Experience has shown that continence can be achieved with only a 2-cm appendiceal tunnel.

38. **e. stomal stenosis.** Incontinence is rare with the Mitrofanoff principle and may result from inadequate length of the flap valve mechanism or persistently elevated reservoir pressure. The most common complication has been stomal stenosis and occurs in 10% to 20% of patients. Stenosis resulting in difficult catheterization may occur early in the postoperative course and requires formal revision.

39. **b. tapered segment of small bowel of adequate length.** When the appendix is unavailable for use, other tubular structures can provide a similar mechanism for catheterization and continence. Mitrofanoff, in 1980, described a similar technique using ureter. Woodhouse and MacNeily, in 1994, as well as others, have used the fallopian tube, which can accommodate catheterization. Monti and Yang have been credited with a novel modification of the tapered intestinal segment, which can be reimplanted according to the Mitrofanoff principle.

40. **c. achieve an effective antireflux mechanism without upper tract obstruction.** The key to urinary undiversion is understanding the original pathologic condition that led to diversion. One report described a 26-year experience with urinary undiversion in 216 patients. In that series, management of the bladder was relatively straightforward and effective with bladder augmentation as necessary. In that series, inadequate outflow resistance was usually treated with Young-Dees-Ledbetter bladder neck repair. Most complications were related to the ureters; 23 patients required reoperation for persistent reflux, whereas 10 did so for partial obstruction of the ureter. Those reoperation rates are indicative of the difficulty one faces in dealing with short, dilated, and scarred ureters, which may be present after urinary diversion.

Additional Study Points

1. Bladder volume in children is equal to 30 × (age in years + 2).
2. Intermittent catheterization must be taught and accepted by the patient and caregiver before any urinary reconstruction is performed.
3. There is no test that ensures the patient will be able to void spontaneously and empty well after bladder augmentation or reconstruction.
4. Most patients prefer to catheterize an abdominal wall stoma rather than the native urethra.
5. Bladder neck bulking agents are not particularly effective in children.
6. When placing the artificial sphincter it should be placed at the bladder neck in females and in prepubertal boys.
7. One third of patients will require further surgery after augmentation cystoplasty because of various problems.
8. Bacteriuria is common after intestinal cystoplasty. After intestinal cystoplasty, routine bladder irrigation should be performed to evacuate inspissated mucus.
9. Stomach should be reserved for patients who have short gut syndrome or who have received heavy pelvic irradiation.
10. Delayed spontaneous perforation of the bowel segment after intestinal cystoplasty occurs in approximately 5% of patients.

Hypospadias

Warren T. Snodgrass, MD

QUESTIONS

1. Histologic studies of embryos suggest ventral penile curvature results from:
   a. fibrosis of the urethral plate.
   b. fibrosis of the corpus spongiosum.
   c. scrotal tethering of the penile shaft.
   d. a short urethra.
   e. arrested development.

2. The underlying cause for hypospadias in most boys is:
   a. idiopathic.
   b. inadequate testosterone production.
   c. partial androgen receptor deficiency.
   d. chromosomal anomalies.
   e. prenatal exposure to environmental estrogens.

3. A 6-month-old infant presents for evaluation of subcoronal hypospadias. During physical examination the left testis is palpated in the groin but cannot be manipulated into the scrotum. The next step is to:
   a. examine the infant in 6 months to allow for testicular descent.
   b. perform ultrasonography to rule out testicular retraction.
   c. obtain a karyotype.
   d. schedule hypospadias repair now and orchiopexy in 6 months.
   e. schedule orchiopexy now with hypospadias repair in 6 months.

4. During a proximal penile shaft hypospadias repair a catheter cannot be passed into the bladder. The most likely cause is:
   a. a false passage in the urethra.
   b. an enlarged utricle.
   c. partial urethral duplication ending in a blind pouch.
   d. an elevated bladder neck.
   e. proximal urethral stricture.

5. A 6-month-old infant without other known medical problems is referred for scrotal hypospadias. He is also found to have ventral penile curvature, a deep scrotal cleft, and penoscrotal transposition, but both testes are in the scrotum. The next step is to:

   a. proceed with surgery.
   b. obtain a karyotype.
   c. order voiding cystourethrography to visualize the utricle.
   d. obtain renal ultrasonography.
   e. schedule testicular ultrasonography.

6. Preoperative testosterone stimulation before hypospadias repair has been demonstrated to:
   a. improve vascularity to the prepuce for flaps.
   b. permanently increase penile length.
   c. increase glans circumference.
   d. lengthen ventral shaft skin.
   e. promote epiphyseal closure.

7. A patient with penoscrotal hypospadias has ventral curvature of nearly 90 degrees preoperatively. After the penis is degloved and dartos tissues released, artificial erection shows the curvature has diminished to less than 30 degrees. The best next step is to:
   a. transect the urethral plate.
   b. perform dermal grafting of the corpora cavernosa at the point of greatest bending.
   c. proceed with urethroplasty.
   d. perform a midline dorsal plication.
   e. perform midline dorsal plication and ventral dermal corporal grafting.

8. A 6-month-old infant is referred for hypospadias. On examination he is found to have a dorsally hooded prepuce, ventral penile curvature, a glanular meatus, and a normal scrotum. The parents should be informed that straightening the penile curvature most likely will require:
   a. only skin degloving and ventral dartos dissection.
   b. multiple dorsal midline plications.
   c. ventral corporeal grafting.
   d. transection of the urethra.
   e. single dorsal plication and a ventral corporeal graft.

9. A 6-week-old infant is evaluated after neonatal circumcision. The primary care physician expresses concern for a "bad circ." On examination the meatus is coronal and the glans wings are separated. There is no redundant shaft skin after the circumcision except in the ventral midline near the meatus. The family should be counseled that:

a. these findings indicate urethral injury during circumcision.

b. urethroplasty will be performed best using a ventral preputial skin flap.

c. circumcision most likely has affected vascularity to the redundant ventral skin and so urethroplasty will be done best using the skin as a graft.

d. after circumcision, urethroplasty will require a buccal graft from the lower lip.

e. their infant has a hypospadias variant.

10. The parents of a 6-month-old with subcoronal hypospadias request foreskin reconstruction rather than circumcision. The family should be told:

a. preoperative testosterone therapy is necessary to enlarge the foreskin.

b. complication rates are significantly greater with preputioplasty.

c. not to retract the foreskin in the first 6 weeks after surgery.

d. to use a gentle compression dressing to minimize preputial edema after surgery.

e. the foreskin most likely will be needed for urethroplasty and so circumcision will likely be necessary.

11. Each of the following is thought to reduce the likelihood for fistula development after hypospadias surgery EXCEPT:

a. subepithelial suturing of the neourethra.

b. two-layer closure of the neourethra.

c. monofilament sutures.

d. approximation of the corpus spongiosum over the neourethra.

e. placement of a dartos flap over the neourethra.

12. A mother reports her 7-year-old son who had a penoscrotal tabularized incised plate (TIP) hypospadias repair took longer to void than a playmate during a sleepover. He does not strain to urinate and has had no urinary tract infections. Uroflowmetry shows a peak flow rate of 8 mL/sec with a plateau-shaped curve. The next step is to:

a. reassure that the flow rate is within the normal range.

b. recommend voiding cystourethrography to rule out stricture.

c. perform urethral dilation.

d. schedule for flap reoperative urethroplasty.

e. advise buccal inlay reoperative urethroplasty.

13. An 8-year old had distal hypospadias repair as an infant. Initially after surgery he was thought to have a normal urinary stream, although the parents only rarely observed urination since he used diapers. Over the past year the parents think his stream has slowed and notice he seems to have to "push" to empty his bladder. On examination there is a faint white discoloration around the meatus. Best management includes:

a. intraoperative biopsy with frozen section.

b. meatotomy for meatal stenosis.

c. flip-flap reoperative urethroplasty.

d. topical corticosteroids for 6 weeks.

e. excision of the distal urethra with a two-stage buccal graft urethroplasty.

14. A 1-year-old boy had a subcoronal hypospadias repair 6 months previously. He has a 2-mm fistula at the site of the original meatus. The distance from the fistula to the neomeatus is approximately 3 mm, and the glans wings still appear approximated. The best treatment of the fistula is:

a. a midline incision through the neomeatus to the fistula with reoperative distal urethroplasty.

b. rotational skin flap fistula closure.

c. fistula closure covered with a ventral dartos barrier flap.

d. inlay buccal graft urethroplasty.

e. dilation of the meatus for stenosis.

15. A 10-year-old presents with midshaft hypospadias persistent after seven operations on his penis. He appears to have ventral curvature greater than 30 degrees and has been circumcised. There is visible scarring between the meatus and the glans, and the scrotum is riding high on the penile shaft to near the meatus. The most appropriate next step is:

a. TIP reoperation.

b. flip-flap reoperative urethroplasty.

c. onlay flap reoperative urethroplasty.

d. inlay buccal graft urethroplasty.

e. two-stage buccal graft urethroplasty.

16. A 6-year-old who had a tubularized preputial flap hypospadias repair as an infant presents with a slow urinary stream and stranguria worsening over the past year. Physical examination is unremarkable, but the peak flow is 3 mL/sec with a postvoid residual volume of 75 mL. At surgery, cystoscopy shows a 5-mm stricture near the original meatus. This stricture is best corrected by:

a. urethral dilation.

b. direct vision internal urethrotomy (DIVU).

c. DIVU with urethral dilations for 3 months.

d. inlay buccal urethroplasty.

e. staged buccal graft reoperation.

17. A 9-year-old prepubertal boy has failed multiple operations for penoscrotal hypospadias. Examination shows a distal shaft meatus, persistent ventral curvature, and a flat ventral glans. During planned two-stage buccal graft reoperation it becomes apparent the entire neourethra will have to be excised back to the penoscrotal junction. The best plan for first-stage grafting is:

a. to use cheek tissue on the penile shaft and maintain the remnant prepuce in the glans.

b. to use cheek tissue to graft the entire defect.

c. to use cheek tissue on the penile shaft and lip tissue within the glans.

d. to use lip tissue on the penile shaft and cheek tissue within the glans.

e. to use ventral penile shaft skin to graft the entire defect.

18. An infant with distal shaft hypospadias has a narrow, flat appearance to the urethral plate. Artificial erection after degloving shows the penis to be straight. The best option for urethroplasty is:

a. meatoplasty and glansplasty (MAGPI).

b. TIP.

c. flip-flap with V incision meatoplasty.

d. to incise the urethra to the midshaft and perform onlay preputial flap repair.

e. to inlay buccal graft from the lip and then tubularize the urethral plate.

19. The parents report their 1-year-old boy seems to be having difficulty urinating 3 months after TIP repair for coronal hypospadias. They have observed the stream once or twice and thought it looked thin. On examination the glans looks entirely normal, except the meatus appears small. An 8-Fr sound will not pass the meatus. The most likely cause for this complication is:

a. balanitis xerotica obliterans.

b. ischemia of the neomeatus.

c. postoperative edema of the meatus.

d. suturing the urethral plate too far distally.

e. compression from the glans wings closure.

20. The parents report their 1-year-old boy seems to be voiding without any problems 6 months after TIP repair for coronal hypospadias, although they have not seen the actual urinary stream because he is still in diapers. On examination you observe the meatus appears small. The next step is to:

a. calibrate the meatus.

b. obtain voiding cystourethrography.

c. schedule examination under anesthesia and meatotomy.

d. recommend reoperative urethroplasty, using either a ventral flip-flap if possible or inlay buccal grafting from the lip.

e. begin daily urethral dilations for 6 weeks.

21. A Koyanagi flap repair for a child with scrotal hypospadias and ventral curvature who also needs rotational flap scrotoplasty for penoscrotal transposition is planned. The appropriate sequence of repair is to:

a. delay scrotoplasty for 6 months to protect skin flap vascularity.

b. perform urethroplasty and scrotoplasty in a single operation.

c. straighten the ventral curvature and perform scrotoplasty in the first operation and delay urethroplasty for 6 months.

d. straighten the ventral curvature and perform urethroplasty and scrotoplasty at a second procedure in 6 months.

e. correct ventral curvature and perform scrotoplasty simultaneously and stage the urethroplasty.

22. A 19-month-old presents for evaluation of scrotal hypospadias. The mother has noted his pupils seem enlarged, and she is concerned he might have developmental delay. He is crying during examination, hindering inspection of his eyes. He has scrotal hypospadias with a deep scrotal cleft, but both testes are in the scrotum. His evaluation before surgery should include:

a. renal ultrasonography.

b. testicular ultrasonography.

c. voiding cystourethrography.

d. determination of the testosterone-to-dihydrotestosterone ratio.

e. measurement of müllerian inhibition hormone.

23. A 10-year-old had a hypospadias reoperation 1 year ago that included a tunica vaginalis barrier flap over the neourethra harvested from the right testis. He reports no problems voiding, but with erection the penis is pulled to the right side. The next step is:

a. to reassure him the tension on his penis will resolve at puberty.

b. to make a small scrotal incision and transect the tunica vaginalis flap.

c. to make a midline penile incision and excise the tunica vaginalis flap.

d. to create a tunica vaginalis flap from the left testis to evenly distribute the tension on the penis during erection.

e. to instruct the patient to pull the penis toward the left during erection to relax contracted tissues.

24. A 14-year-old undergoes a first-stage buccal graft reoperation that involves grafting along the entire penile shaft. The next morning he has a visible hematoma under the shaft skin extending into the scrotum, which is enlarged to the size of a softball. The next step is to:

a. return immediately to the operating room to evacuate the hematoma.

b. apply a compression dressing over the penis and scrotum.

c. check coagulation profiles for bleeding diathesis.

d. observe with continued bed rest.

e. evacuate the hematoma and regraft the penile shaft.

25. The mother of a son with coronal hypospadias is pregnant again. She asks if the child is a male whether it is likely he also will have hypospadias. The correct response is:

a. only hypospadias associated with malformation syndromes has familial recurrence.

b. only if she was taking birth control pills containing progesterone shortly before she conceived.

c. only if her husband also has hypospadias.

d. yes, because hypospadias is a Y-linked disorder.

e. the odds are that another son would not have hypospadias.

ANSWERS

1. **e. arrested development.** Ventral curvature is thought to result from arrested development, which may then cause the ventral skin, dartos, corpus spongiosum, urethra or urethral plate, and/or corpora cavernosa to be relatively shortened. There is no fibrosis in the urethral plate, whereas a short urethra is a very rare cause of ventral curvature.

2. **a. idiopathic.** Although a minority of boys with hypospadias have demonstrated chromosomal anomalies or defects in the androgen pathway for virilization, in most the cause cannot currently be determined. Environmental estrogens have been implicated in hypospadias, but their role, if any, remains uncertain.

3. **c. obtain a karyotype.** The combination of a penile anomaly with undescended testis may indicate a disorder of sexual differentiation. Although more commonly found

with proximal hypospadias and a nonpalpable testis, it is still advised to obtain a karyotype in any child with hypospadias and cryptorchidism.

4. **b. an enlarged utricle.** The most common reason for difficulty with catheter placement during hypospadias repair is an enlarged utricle, which is most often encountered in boys with proximal hypospadias.

5. **a. proceed with surgery.** Neither karyotyping nor urinary tract imaging is indicated for isolated hypospadias, even in patients with proximal defects.

6. **c. increase glans circumference.** No study documents improved vascularity by hormonal stimulation, and increases in penile length are most often temporary. No evidence implicates premature epiphyseal closure from commonly used testosterone regimens before hypospadias surgery. Glans circumference reliably increases with testosterone therapy.

7. **d. perform a midline dorsal plication.** Curvature less than 30 degrees can be straightened by a single dorsal plication without clinically apparent shortening of the penis. Transection of the urethral plate and/or ventral corporal grafting are reserved for cases with curvature greater than 30 degrees after degloving and dartos dissection.

8. **a. only skin degloving and ventral dartos dissection.** Most often penile curvature noted in so-called chordee without hypospadias is due to shortened ventral skin and dartos and so corrects as the penis is degloved and ventral dartos dissected. Multiple plications should be avoided, ventral corporeal grafting is reserved for curvature greater than 30 degrees after degloving and ventral dartos dissection, and urethral transection for a shortened urethra is only rarely indicated in this condition.

9. **e. their infant has a hypospadias variant.** The patient has megameatus intact prepuce hypospadias variant, and urethroplasty is done without flaps or grafts by tubularizing the urethral plate.

10. **c. not to retract the foreskin in the first 6 weeks after surgery.** Disruption of the reconstructed prepuce may result from attempts to retract the foreskin early after surgery, before edema subsides and the wound heals. Otherwise complication rates are similar between patients with distal hypospadias undergoing foreskin reconstruction versus circumcision. Dressings do not significantly impact postoperative edema. The foreskin is nearly always adequate for reconstruction in boys with distal hypospadias, with no reports suggesting the need for preoperative testosterone therapy. Urethral plate tubularization removes the need to use foreskin for urethroplasty.

11. **c. monofilament sutures.** No study demonstrates outcomes are influenced by suture type.

12. **a. reassure that the flow rate is within the normal range.** Urethral strictures after hypospadias repair have been reported in patients with a peak flow less than two standard deviations from normal, usually less than 5 mL/sec, whereas this child has a peak flow within the normal range for age. Therefore the likelihood this patient has a stricture is small. Furthermore, TIP repair is uncommonly complicated by stricture.

13. **e. excision of the distal urethra with a two-stage buccal graft urethroplasty.** The history and physical findings suggest balanitis xerotica obliterans (BXO). Biopsy with frozen section usually is impractical in children, meaning therapy is directed by clinical suspicion. Meatotomy or skin flap repair of meatal stenosis most often fail in the presence of BXO, whereas excision of all tissues affected by BXO with staged buccal grafting is considered most likely to succeed without recurrent stenosis. Topical corticosteroids may be initially effective, but stenosis recurs when therapy ends, and BXO may extend proximally along the urethra to a level not reached by topical applications.

14. **c. fistula closure covered with a ventral dartos barrier flap.** A fistula with good glans approximation usually can be primarily corrected with fistula closure covered by a barrier flap. In contrast, when only a thin skin strip holds the glans wings together between the neomeatus and fistula then reoperative distal urethroplasty/glansplasty is needed. A rotational skin flap is not a good option in this case because it is necessary to dissect under the corona to completely free the fistula tract and advance a barrier flap. Although meatal stenosis has to be considered in any case with a fistula, appropriate therapy when it is present is reoperation not dilations.

15. **e. two-stage buccal graft urethroplasty.** Visible scarring is a relative contraindication to TIP or inlay reoperations, whereas skin flaps are more difficult to raise with adequate vascularity after multiple failed operations. The best plan is to excise scarred tissues and perform staged buccal graft urethroplasty.

16. **d. inlay buccal urethroplasty.** Direct vision internal urethrotomy has a long-term success rate less than 10% after tubularized preputial flap repairs. The best treatment in this case is inlay grafting into the stricture.

17. **c. to use cheek tissue on the penile shaft and lip tissue within the glans.** It is best to use lip tissue within the glans, because it is thinner than cheek tissue and so facilitates glansplasty. For a long graft covering the entire penile shaft, a combination of cheek tissue on the shaft and lip within the glans is recommended. Given the narrow and flat appearance of the glans and a history of multiple failed repairs, the skin with the glans is best excised to restore a deep groove that ultimately will result in a vertical meatus at the second stage. After multiple failed operations redundant shaft skin sufficient for grafting and subsequent urethroplasty is not available.

18. **b. TIP.** TIP repair results for distal hypospadias are not dependent on "characteristics" of the urethral plate. MAGPI is limited to glanular hypospadias. Attempts to create a vertical meatus in conjunction with skin flap repairs usually fail or give suboptimal appearance when the urethral plate is flat. There is no need to convert a distal shaft to more proximal hypospadias to perform onlay preputial flap repair, which has a higher complication rate than does a TIP repair in this situation. It is not necessary to graft the incised plate, and if that were considered in a primary operation then preputial graft rather than buccal mucosa would be preferred because it is thinner and more readily accessible.

19. **d. suturing the urethral plate too far distally.** The most common cause of meatal stenosis after a TIP repair is suturing the urethral plate too far distally. Balanitis xerotica obliterans is unlikely early after surgery and often presents as white discoloration at the meatus. Ischemia is possible but unlikely given the reliable vascularity of the urethral plate and glans tissues. Edema after surgery may slow the

urinary stream but at 3 months does not prevent passage of a sound. Glans closure does not create urethral obstruction.

20. **a. calibrate the meatus.** The meatus may appear small after TIP repair without indicating meatal stenosis. Passage of an 8- or 10-Fr sound would suffice to determine if the meatus is stenotic. Meatal stenosis occurs in less than 5% of patients after TIP repair and so a small-appearing meatus in an asymptomatic patient should not prompt immediate concern that examination under anesthesia or reoperation is needed.

21. **b. perform urethroplasty and scrotoplasty in a single operation.** The scrotum and penis develop from different anlagen with separate blood supplies, making simultaneous urethroplasty and scrotoplasty possible.

22. **a. renal ultrasonography.** The history suggests WAGR syndrome, and so renal ultrasonography is recommended because of the association with Wilms tumor.

23. **b. to make a small scrotal incision and transect the tunica vaginalis flap.** Failure to dissect the tunica vaginalis flap to the external ring can result in traction on the penis during erection deviating it toward the base of the flap. The best therapy is to make a small scrotal incision over the flap and transect it.

24. **d. observe with continued bed rest.** Graft quilting and the tie-over dressing prevent blood from accumulating under the graft. Hematoma under adjacent penile skin and within the scrotum as described here will resolve. It is unlikely a boy requiring a staged buccal graft repair has an undiagnosed coagulopathy after prior penile operations.

25. **e. the odds are that another son would not have hypospadias.** Sporadic and syndromic hypospadias can have familial recurrence. Although the likelihood a sibling will have hypospadias is increased, the overall risk remains small.

Additional Study Points

1. Dihydrotestosterone at the 8- to 12-week gestational phase is a key mediator in the proper development of the penis.
2. There is an increased risk of hypospadias in births resulting from assisted reproduction.
3. Physical examination in a patient with hypospadias may reveal a ventral deficient prepuce, downward glans tilt, deviation of the median penile raphe, ventral curvature, scrotal encroachment onto the penile shaft, scrotal cleft, and penile scrotal transposition.
4. Ventral curvature results from arrest during normal development and not from fibrous bands.
5. There are three types of hypospadias repairs: tubularization of the urethral plate, supplementation or substitution of the urethral plate with skin flaps, or urethral plate substitution with grafts.

Abnormalities of the External Genitalia in Boys

Jeffrey S. Palmer, MD, FACS, FAAP

QUESTIONS

1. In the male, which of the following stimulates the development of the external genitalia?
   a. Testosterone
   b. Human chorionic gonadotropin
   c. Dihydrotestosterone
   d. Luteinizing hormone and follicle-stimulating hormone
   e. Maternal progesterone

2. What percentage of uncircumcised boys will have persistent phimosis by 17 years of age?
   a. Less than 1%
   b. 5%
   c. 10%
   d. 15%
   e. 20%

3. Circumcision should not be performed in neonates with which condition of the genitalia?
   a. Phimosis
   b. Undescended testis
   c. Inguinal hernia
   d. Penile curvature
   e. Testicular atrophy

4. What is the most common complication associated with circumcision?
   a. Trauma to the glans
   b. Bleeding
   c. Meatal stenosis
   d. Skin bridges
   e. Balanitis xerotica obliterans (BXO)

5. A 4-year-old boy presents with phimosis and BXO of the prepuce. What is the preferred treatment?
   a. Observation
   b. Topical corticosteroids
   c. Excision of BXO skin without circumcision

   d. Warm baths
   e. Circumcision

6. Penile agenesis is associated with all of the following malformations EXCEPT:
   a. cryptorchidism.
   b. vesicoureteral reflux.
   c. horseshoe kidney.
   d. ureteropelvic junction obstruction.
   e. renal agenesis.

7. The etiology of the buried penis includes all of the following EXCEPT:
   a. suprapubic fat pad.
   b. small penis.
   c. poor penopubic fixation of the penis.
   d. obesity.
   e. cicatricial scarring after surgery.

8. A 9-month-old boy who was previously circumcised presents with a buried penis resulting from cicatricial scarring. What is the most appropriate initial treatment?
   a. Topical betamethasone and manual retraction
   b. Revision of circumcision
   c. Penopubic fixation of the penis
   d. Liposuction of the suprapubic fat pad
   e. Observation

9. What is the minimal normal stretched penile length of a full-term neonate?
   a. 1.2 cm
   b. 1.9 cm
   c. 2.5 cm
   d. 3.2 cm
   e. 4.5 cm

10. Which of the following statements is TRUE regarding a micropenis in a term male neonate?
    a. The testes are usually normal in size and not cryptorchid.
    b. It is best managed by gender reassignment.

c. It has an abnormal ratio of the length of the penile shaft to circumference.

d. It is unlikely to respond to testosterone stimulation until puberty.

e. It is less than 1.9 cm in stretched length.

11. What is the most common cause of micropenis?

a. Hypergonadotropic hypogonadism

b. Hypogonadotropic hypogonadism

c. Idiopathic

d. Growth hormone deficiency

e. Androgen insensitivity syndrome

12. Which of the following statements regarding penile masses is FALSE?

a. The treatment of parameatal urethral cysts is complete excision of the cyst.

b. The most common acquired cystic lesion of the penis is smegma under the unretractable prepuce.

c. Congenital penile nevi tend to be malignant.

d. The initial management of juvenile xanthogranulomas is expectant monitoring.

e. Epidermal inclusion cysts may form after penile surgery,

13. A 13-year-old African-American boy with sickle cell disease has a 6-hour painful erection. The initial management should include all of the following EXCEPT:

a. alkalization.

b. hydration.

c. intracavernous injections of β-adrenergic sympathomimetic agents.

d. analgesia.

e. transfusion to reduce hemoglobin S concentration.

14. Which is the following statements is TRUE regarding high-flow priapism?

a. It is usually a drug-induced etiology.

b. The aspirated blood is similar to venous blood on blood gas analysis.

c. Color Doppler ultrasonography commonly demonstrates the fistula.

d. Surgical intervention is the initial management.

e. Sickle cell disease is the most common cause.

15. Penoscrotal transposition is associated with all of the following anomalies EXCEPT:

a. sex chromosome abnormalities.

b. distal shaft hypospadias with chordee.

c. sex chromosome abnormalities.

d. Aarskog syndrome.

e. caudal regression.

ANSWERS

1. **c. Dihydrotestosterone.** Influence of dihydrotestosterone on the androgen receptors results in the differentiation of the genital tubercle, genital (labioscrotal) folds, and genital swelling at between 9 and 13 weeks of gestation into the male structures of the glans penis, penile shaft, and scrotum, respectively.

2. **a. Less than 1%.** Preputial retractability increases with age with 90% of uncircumcised boys 3 years of age with completely retractable prepuces; less than 1% by 17 years of age have phimosis. Therefore, primary phimosis is almost always resolvable during childhood without intervention.

3. **d. Penile curvature.** Circumcision should not be performed in neonates with other penile conditions that require surgical correction. These conditions include hypospadias, penile curvature, dorsal hood deformity, buried penis, and webbed penis.

4. **b. Bleeding.** The risk of complications after circumcision is 0.2% to 5%. The most common complication is bleeding, which occurs in 0.1% and is more common in older children.

5. **e. Circumcision.** Treatment of BXO includes medical and surgical management. The use of topical corticosteroids has had limited benefit to treat mild BXO of the prepuce with minimal scar formation. Circumcision is the preferred treatment.

6. **d. ureteropelvic junction obstruction.** Penile agenesis (aphallia) results from failure of development of the genital tubercle. The disorder is rare and has an estimated incidence of 1 in 10 to 30 million births. The karyotype almost always is 46,XY, and the usual appearance is that of a well-developed scrotum with descended testes and an absent penile shaft. The anus is usually displaced anteriorly. Associated malformations are common and include cryptorchidism, vesicoureteral reflux, horseshoe kidney, renal agenesis, imperforate anus, and musculoskeletal and cardiopulmonary abnormalities.

7. **b. small penis.** A buried penis can be classified into three categories based on etiology for the concealment: (1) poor penopubic fixation of the skin at the base of the penis; (2) obesity; and (3) a trapped penis from cicatricial scarring after penile surgery, typically a circumcision.

8. **a. Topical betamethasone and manual retraction.** Young children with secondary cicatricial scarring after penile surgery can undergo forceful dilation of the cicatrix with a fine hemostat in the office after the application or injection of analgesia. Another option is the combination of topical betamethasone and manual retraction.

9. **b. 1.9 cm.** Stretched penile length is determined by measuring the penis from its attachment to the pubic symphysis to the tip of the glans. One must be careful to depress the suprapubic fat pad completely to obtain an accurate measurement, especially in an obese infant or child. In general, the penis of a full-term neonate should be at least 1.9 cm long.

10. **e. It is less than 1.9 cm in stretched length.** Micropenis is a normally formed penis that is at least 2.5 SD below the mean size in stretched length for age. The ratio of the length of the penile shaft to its circumference is usually normal, but occasionally the corpora cavernosa are severely hypoplastic. The testes are usually small and frequently cryptorchid while the scrotum is usually fused and often diminutive. A stretched penile length less than 1.9 cm long is consistent with a micropenis.

11. **b. Hypogonadotropic hypogonadism.** The most common cause of micropenis is hypogonadotropic hypogonadism, which is the failure of the hypothalamus to produce an adequate amount of gonadotropin-releasing hormone (GnRH). This condition may result from hypothalamic dysfunction, which can occur in Prader-Willi

syndrome, Kallmann syndrome (genital-olfactory dysplasia), Laurence-Moon-Biedl syndrome, and the CHARGE association.

12. **c. Congenital penile nevi tend to be malignant.** Congenital penile nevi tend to be superficial and benign. Congenital penile nevi are pigmented lesions that can form on the glans and penile shaft. They tend to be superficial and benign and should be excised.

13. **c. intracavernous injections of β-adrenergic sympathomimetic agents.** The initial treatment of low-flow priapism resulting from sickle cell disease is conservative with hydration, oxygenation, alkalization, analgesia, and transfusion with the goal of reducing hemoglobin S concentration. Evacuation of blood and irrigation of the corpora cavernosa along with intracavernous injections of α-adrenergic sympathomimetic agents, such as phenylephrine or epinephrine solution, can be a concurrent therapy. Surgical intervention to allow corporeal drainage by shunt procedures is indicated if there is a lack of response to medical therapy.

14. **c. Color Doppler ultrasonography commonly demonstrates the fistula.** High-flow priapism is usually due to perineal trauma, such as a straddle injury. Corporeal irrigation is diagnostic and therapeutic. Typically, the aspirated blood is bright red and the aspirate is similar to arterial blood on blood gas analysis. Color Doppler ultrasonography often will demonstrate the fistula. The initial management is observation because spontaneous resolution may occur. Superselective embolization of cavernous and penile arteries is the next line of therapy. If not, angiographic embolization is indicated.

15. **b. distal shaft hypospadias with chordee.** Frequently, penoscrotal transposition occurs in conjunction with perineal, scrotal, or penoscrotal hypospadias with chordee. Penoscrotal transposition has also been associated with caudal regression, sex chromosome abnormalities, and Aarskog syndrome. As many as 75% of patients with complete penoscrotal transposition and a normal scrotum have a significant urinary tract abnormality, including renal agenesis and dysplasia, and other nongenitourinary anomalies.

Additional Study Points

1. The normal penile size of a neonate is 3.5 ± 0.7 cm in stretched length. It should be at least 1.9 cm. If it is below 1.9 cm it is classified as a micropenis.
2. The potential benefits of circumcision include prevention of penile cancer, urinary tract infections, sexually transmitted diseases including HIV infection, and phimosis.
3. Glanular adhesions and skin bridges are not uncommon complications of circumcision.
4. Meatal stenosis is a condition that occurs almost exclusively in children after infant circumcision.
5. If a meatotomy is performed, suturing the urethral mucosa to the glans with fine, resorbable sutures reduces the risk of recurrence.
6. The causes of micropenis include (a) hypogonadotropic hypogonadism, (b) hypergonadotropic hypogonadism (primary testicular failure), and (c) idiopathic causes.
7. Most men born with micropenis have male gender identity and satisfactory sexual function.
8. Priapism can be ischemic (veno-occlusive, low flow), nonischemic (arterial, high flow), and stuttering (intermittent).
9. Refer to Table 131–1 in *Campbell-Walsh Urology, 10th Edition* for a list of male genital anomalies that commonly occur in various syndromes.
10. Refer to Table 131–3 in *Campbell-Walsh Urology, 10th Edition* for the Tanner classification of sexual maturity stages in boys.

chapter 132

Abnormalities of the Testis and Scrotum and Their Surgical Management

Julia Spencer Barthold, MD

QUESTIONS

1. Most adolescent varicoceles evaluated by urologists are:
   a. painful.
   b. of cosmetic concern.
   c. asymptomatic.
   d. associated with an ipsilateral hydrocele.
   e. bilateral.

2. Significant testicular volume differential in cases of varicocele is defined as greater than:
   a. 5%.
   b. 5% to 10%.
   c. 10% to 15%.
   d. 15% to 20%.
   e. 25%.

3. Hydrocele formation after varicocele ligation is least likely to occur after which of the following procedures?
   a. Retroperitoneal ligation
   b. Subinguinal ligation
   c. Laparoscopic ligation
   d. Microscopic inguinal ligation
   e. Transvenous embolization

4. Irreversible ischemic injury of the testicular parenchyma may begin as early as how many hours after torsion of the spermatic cord?
   a. 1
   b. 2
   c. 4
   d. 6
   e. 8

5. Which of the following is most specific in diagnosing spermatic cord torsion?
   a. High-riding testis
   b. Absence of the cremasteric reflex
   c. Transverse lie of the testis
   d. Spermatic cord twist on high-resolution Doppler ultrasonography
   e. Acute severe pain

6. After manual detorsion of the spermatic cord, which of the following is appropriate management?
   a. Color Doppler ultrasonography
   b. Radionuclide scan
   c. Doppler examination of the testis and spermatic cord
   d. Discharge from the hospital and arrangement for an office reevaluation in 1 week
   e. Immediate scrotal exploration

7. An adolescent is evaluated for a history of self-limited, intermittent episodes of severe unilateral scrotal pain. Physical examination findings are normal. What is the most appropriate course of action?
   a. Color Doppler ultrasonography
   b. Reassessment in 6 months
   c. Elective scrotal exploration
   d. Radionuclide scrotal imaging
   e. Immediate scrotal exploration

8. When the diagnosis of torsion of the appendix epididymis is made, which of the following is optimal management?
   a. Observation
   b. Color Doppler ultrasonography
   c. Radionuclide scrotal imaging
   d. Immediate scrotal exploration
   e. Cord block and manual detorsion

9. Which of the following is the most likely diagnosis in an infant with sterile urine and epididymitis?
   a. Unilateral renal agenesis
   b. Large prostatic utricle
   c. Urethral stricture disease
   d. Persistent vasoureteral fusion
   e. Radiographically normal urinary tract

10. What is the most appropriate course of action in an otherwise healthy neonate with perinatal testicular torsion?
    a. Prompt surgical exploration of the affected testis
    b. Prompt surgical exploration of the affected testis with contralateral scrotal orchidopexy
    c. Color Doppler ultrasonography of the scrotum
    d. Radionuclide testicular scan
    e. Observation

11. What is the master gene responsible for male sexual differentiation?
    a. *RSPO1*
    b. *SOX9*
    c. *WT1*
    d. *SRY*
    e. *WNT4*

12. During male reproductive tract development, androgens mediate the differentiation of all of the following structures EXCEPT:
    a. seminal vesicles.
    b. ureter.
    c. epididymis.
    d. vas deferens.
    e. ejaculatory ducts.

13. Which of the following does not play a direct role in testicular descent?
    a. Testis
    b. Epididymis
    c. Genitofemoral nerve
    d. Gubernaculum
    e. Processus vaginalis

14. Peak levels of testosterone and insulin-like-3 (INSL3) occur in the male fetus at approximately what gestational week?
    a. 5
    b. 8
    c. 10
    d. 15
    e. 20

15. Cryptorchidism increases the risk of all of the following EXCEPT:
    a. spermatic cord torsion.
    b. clinical hernia.
    c. reactive hydrocele.
    d. infertility.
    e. testicular malignancy.

16. The risk of cryptorchidism is higher in all of the following syndromes EXCEPT:
    a. cerebral palsy.
    b. cystic fibrosis.
    c. arthrogryposis.
    d. prune-belly syndrome.
    e. posterior urethral valves.

17. All of the following are associated with patency of the processus vaginalis EXCEPT:
    a. transverse testicular ectopia.
    b. epididymal anomalies.
    c. cryptorchidism.
    d. spermatic cord torsion.
    e. polyorchidism.

18. Abdominoscrotal hydrocele is reported to be associated with all of the following features EXCEPT:
    a. a closed processus vaginalis.
    b. epididymal anomalies.
    c. testicular dysmorphism.
    d. hydronephrosis.
    e. increased pressure within the tunica vaginalis.

19. Histologic findings in cryptorchid testes may include all of the following EXCEPT:
    a. carcinoma in situ.
    b. absence of adult dark spermatogonia.
    c. early disappearance of gonocytes.
    d. failure of Sertoli cell maturation.
    e. reduced spermatogonia per tubule (S/T) ratio.

20. What percentage of undescended testes are nonpalpable at presentation?
    a. 1%
    b. 3%
    c. 10%
    d. 20%
    e. 30%

21. The disease most likely to be associated with diminished paternity is:
    a. monorchidism.
    b. bilateral cryptorchidism.
    c. subclinical varicocele.
    d. epididymitis.
    e. bilateral inguinal hernia repair.

22. During laparoscopy, spermatic cord structures exiting an open internal ring ipsilateral to a nonpalpable testis implies:
    a. vanishing testis, inguinal exploration unnecessary.
    b. vanishing testis, inguinal exploration necessary.
    c. intracanalicular atrophic testis, inguinal exploration unnecessary.
    d. intracanalicular testis, inguinal exploration necessary.
    e. further exploration unnecessary if contralateral testicular hypertrophy is present.

23. Advantages of laparoscopic management of an intra-abdominal testis include all of the following EXCEPT:
    a. it more accurately assesses the presence or absence, viability, and anatomy of the testis compared with radiographic imaging.
    b. it allows for laparoscopic repair of the ipsilateral inguinal hernia when present.
    c. it enhances surgical exposure, lighting, and magnification.

d. it allows a greater degree of proximal dissection of the spermatic vessels.

e. it allows diagnosis of associated müllerian ductal abnormalities if present.

24. Which statement is FALSE regarding Fowler-Stephens orchidopexy?

a. It is less commonly associated with testicular atrophy than laparoscopic orchidopexy.

b. It has a lower success rate in patients who have undergone previous inguinal surgery.

c. Blood supply is based on the deferential artery and collateral peritoneal vessels.

d. It should be performed at a similar age as a standard inguinal orchidopexy.

e. It should be considered if the testis is not near the internal ring.

25. Which of the following is NOT a relative indication for elective varicocele repair?

a. Pain

b. Oligospermia

c. Small testes

d. Continuous spermatic venous reflux

e. Testicular size discrepancy of greater than 20%

26. Which of the following is NOT consistent with a diagnosis of vanishing testis?

a. Patent processus vaginalis

b. Contralateral testicular hypertrophy

c. Palpable nubbin in scrotum

d. Increased serum follicle-stimulating hormone

e. Micropenis

ANSWERS

1. **c. asymptomatic.** Most adolescent varicoceles are asymptomatic.

2. **b. 15% to 20%.** In adults and adolescents, testicular size (volume) should be approximately equal bilaterally, with the normal differential not being more than 15% to 20% volume.

3. **e. Transvenous embolization.** Hydrocele formation is related to failure to preserve lymphatic vessels associated with the spermatic cord and its vessels. Hydrocele formation seems most common after retroperitoneal ligation, especially when a mass ligation technique is used, and is least likely to occur after transvenous embolization.

4. **c. 4 hours.** Irreversible ischemic injury to the testicular parenchyma may begin as soon as 4 hours after occlusion of the cord.

5. **d. Spermatic cord twist on high-resolution Doppler ultrasonography.** Spermatic cord twist on high-resolution Doppler imaging is the most specific finding, that is, the least likely to be false positive, in spermatic cord torsion.

6. **e. Immediate scrotal exploration.** It should be remembered that manual detorsion may not totally correct the rotation that has occurred and that prompt exploration is still indicated.

7. **c. Elective scrotal exploration.** If the suspicion is strong that episodes of intermittent torsion and spontaneous detorsion have occurred, the author's experience has been

that the finding of a bell-clapper deformity at exploration can be expected. Elective scrotal exploration should be performed, with scrotal fixation of both testes.

8. **a. Observation.** When the diagnosis of a torsed appendage is confirmed clinically or by imaging, nonoperative management will allow most cases to resolve spontaneously.

9. **e. Radiographically normal urinary tracts.** The majority of infants with epididymitis have sterile urine and apparently radiographically normal urinary tracts.

10. **b. Prompt surgical exploration of the affected testis with contralateral scrotal exploration.** Clearly, if the cause of scrotal swelling appears to be related to an acute postnatal event, all efforts should be made to pursue prompt surgical intervention. If torsion is confirmed, contralateral scrotal exploration with testicular fixation should be performed.

11. **d. SRY.** The *SRY* gene appears to be primarily responsible for male sexual differentiation through complex interactions involving both activation and repression of other male-specific genes.

12. **b. ureter.** Androgens (testosterone, dihydrotestosterone) mediate the differentiation of the paired wolffian ducts into the seminal vesicles, epididymis, vas deferens, and ejaculatory ducts.

13. **b. Epididymis.** Changes in the gubernaculum and processus vaginalis and their innervation by the genitofemoral nerve and hormone secretion by the testis are important in the process of testicular descent.

14. **d. 15.** Testosterone production peaks at 14 to 16 weeks of gestation and that of INSL3 peaks at 15 to 17 weeks.

15. **c. Reactive hydrocele.** All of the others are possible complications of cryptorchidism.

16. **b. cystic fibrosis.** All the other syndromes are associated with a higher risk of cryptorchidism; mutations of the cystic fibrosis gene are associated with congenital absence of the vas deferens.

17. **d. spermatic cord torsion.** Risk of torsion is associated with abnormal development of the tunica vaginalis but not patency of the processus vaginalis.

18. **b. epididymal anomalies.** The processus vaginalis is closed in cases of abdominoscrotal hydrocele; and an elongated dysmorphic testis, increased pressure within the tunica vaginalis, and hydronephrosis have all been reported.

19. **c. early disappearance of gonocytes.** Histologic abnormalities that may be present in cryptorchid testes include delayed disappearance of gonocytes, reduced numbers of adult dark spermatogonia, a reduced spermatogonia per tubule (S/T) ratio, and carcinoma in situ.

20. **d. 20%.** Approximately 20% of undescended testes are nonpalpable at presentation.

21. **b. bilateral cryptorchidism.** Although subfertility may occur in rare cases of monorchism, subclinical varicocele, recurrent epididymitis, and vasal obstruction after bilateral inguinal hernia repair, it is most likely to occur in males with a history of bilateral cryptorchidism.

22. **d. intracanalicular testis, inguinal exploration necessary.** Although atretic spermatic vessels seen exiting the internal ring may be associated with a distal vanishing testis, the appearance of the spermatic vessels during laparoscopy is subjective; therefore exploration (inguinal or laparoscopic) is needed to rule out an intracanalicular viable or atrophic testis. Further exploration is unnecessary if blind-ending intra-abdominal spermatic vessels are found.

Hypertrophy of a normally descended contralateral testis is suggestive of monorchism.

23. **b. it allows for laparoscopic repair of the ipsilateral inguinal hernia when present.** Repair of the inguinal hernia or patent processus vaginalis does not require formal repair at the time of laparoscopic orchidopexy.

24. **a. It is less commonly associated with testicular atrophy than laparoscopic orchidopexy.** Fowler-Stephens orchidopexy, either one- or two-stage, has a higher reported testicular atrophy rate compared with laparoscopic orchidopexy.

25. **d. Continuous spermatic venous reflux.** Significant pain associated with varicocele, bilateral small testes, and oligospermia are reasonable indications to proceed with repair in an adolescent male. The standard indication is ipsilateral testicular volume loss, or hypotrophy, of at least 15% to 20%, although this should be documented on serial yearly testicular examinations, because variable growth of the testes may occur during puberty. Continuous reflux may be documented on color Doppler imaging but is not a specific indication for surgery.

26. **a. Patent processus vaginalis.** Contralateral testicular hypertrophy and a palpable scrotal nubbin may present in boys with unilateral vanishing testis and increased serum follicle-stimulation hormone levels, and micropenis may be seen in boys with bilateral vanishing testes. The processus vaginalis is closed in most cases of vanishing testis.

Additional Study Points

1. Testicular hormones are required for testicular descent. Three fourths of undescended testes are palpable; two thirds are unilateral.

2. The etiology of a vanishing testis is most likely due to in utero torsion or a vascular accident.

3. The documentation of a vanishing testis requires identifying a blind-ending spermatic vessel.

4. Orchiopexy should be performed at 6 months of age in the full-term infant.

5. The use of human chorionic gonadotropin to distinguish retractile from cryptorchid testes is not reliable and therefore its use is not recommended.

6. Laparoscopic identification and mobilization of an abdominal testes is preferred. If the testis can be mobilized to the opposite inguinal ring, it generally can be placed in the scrotum.

7. Oligospermia and/or azoospermia occurs in approximately 75% of patients with bilateral cryptorchid testes and 43% of those with unilateral cryptorchid testes.

8. The incidence of abnormal hormonal and sperm parameters in cryptorchidism is higher than is the risk of infertility measured by paternity.

9. Patients with nonsyndromic cryptorchidism have a high incidence of epididymal anomalies and a patent processus vaginalis.

10. A varicocele may alter testicular growth, spermatogenesis, and fertility.

11. There is a progressive improvement in sperm quality that normally occurs with testicular growth in the teenage years; therefore many patients with varicocele and apparent hypotrophy of the testis experience normalization with growth with or without surgical repair.

12. Observation remains the approach of choice for the majority of adolescent children with a varicocele.

13. The prevalence of varicocele in adolescence is similar to that found in adults and is 14%.

14. In children with inguinal hernias a patent processus vaginalis occurs in 63% of patients younger than 2 months and in about 40% of patients between age 1 and 2 years. However, indiscriminant contralateral exploration during a unilateral herniorrhaphy is not indicated.

15. Most patients with acute torsion present within 6 hours of the onset of pain. There is often associated absence of the cremasteric reflex.

16. Thirty to 50 percent of patients with acute spermatic chord torsion report a previous history of intermittent scrotal pain.

17. Before birth, torsion generally occurs extravaginally, but after birth it usually occurs intravaginally.

18. Epididymitis with or without a concurrent urinary tract infection warrants urinary tract evaluation with imaging to rule out urethral and ureteral abnormalities.

Sexual Differentiation: Normal and Abnormal

David Andrew Diamond, MD ● Richard N. Yu, MD, PhD

QUESTIONS

1. Which of the following statements is TRUE about *SRY* (sex-determining region of the Y-chromosome gene)?

   a. It is synonymous with the H-Y antigen.

   b. The expressed SRY protein has a characteristic high-mobility group (HMG), DNA-binding domain.

   c. It is a zinc finger gene on the Y chromosome known as *ZFY.*

   d. It was genetically mapped by the study of patients with Klinefelter and Turner syndromes.

   e. It is synonymous with *Sry* in humans.

2. Which of the following statements is TRUE regarding müllerian-inhibiting substance (MIS)?

   a. It acts systemically to produce müllerian regression.

   b. It is secreted by the fetal Leydig cells.

   c. It functions normally in patients with hernia uteri inguinale.

   d. It is secreted at 7 to 8 weeks of gestation, representing the initial endocrine function of the fetal testis.

   e. It is secreted by the fetal testis at 10 weeks of gestation, after testosterone production has begun.

3. Which description of *WT1* is correct?

   a. Mutations in *WT1* can result in either Denys-Drash or Frasier syndrome.

   b. Mutations in *WT1* are associated with adrenocortical carcinoma.

   c. Loss of *WT1* function has not been associated with genitourinary anomalies.

   d. Duplication of *WT1* has been associated with dosage-sensitive sex reversal.

   e. The gene was originally isolated in cloning experiments and localized to the X chromosome.

4. Which of the following statements is TRUE regarding fetal testosterone?

   a. It results in regression of the müllerian ducts.

   b. It is produced primarily by the adrenal gland.

   c. It acts locally to virilize the urogenital sinus and genital tubercle.

   d. It acts locally to virilize the internal wolffian duct structures.

   e. It enters target tissue by active diffusion.

5. Which of the following statements is TRUE regarding dihydrotestosterone (DHT)?

   a. It produces virilization of wolffian duct structures.

   b. It is converted by 5α-reductase to testosterone in target tissues.

   c. It produces virilization of the urogenital sinus.

   d. It acts locally to produce regression of müllerian structures.

   e. It is secreted in large quantities by the fetal testis.

6. Which of the following statements is TRUE regarding patients with Klinefelter syndrome?

   a. They have at least one X and two Y chromosomes.

   b. They are at increased risk for development of adenocarcinoma of the breast.

   c. They undergo replacement of Leydig cells with hyaline.

   d. They are characteristically fertile.

   e. They bear little resemblance to XX males.

7. The streak gonad of Turner syndrome:

   a. can descend to the scrotum.

   b. has a reduced number of oocytes.

   c. in the presence of a Y chromosome results in increased risk for development of seminoma.

   d. is located in the round ligament.

   e. in the presence of a Y chromosome results in risk for development of gonadoblastoma.

8. Which of the following statements is TRUE regarding patients with "pure" gonadal dysgenesis?

   a. They frequently have chromosomal anomalies.

   b. They are at lesser risk for gonadal tumors than are patients with Turner syndrome.

   c. They lack the somatic defects associated with Turner syndrome.

d. They have gonadal histology different from that of patients with Turner syndrome.

e. They derive similar benefit from synthetic growth hormone as do patients with Turner syndrome.

9. What is the common denominator in all cases of Denys-Drash syndrome?

   a. Gonadoblastoma

   b. Nephropathy with early-onset proteinuria

   c. Wilms tumor

   d. Calyceal blunting

   e. Progressive renal failure

10. Which of the following statements is TRUE regarding patients with embryonic testicular regression or bilateral vanishing testes syndromes?

    a. They have normal testosterone and elevated estradiol levels.

    b. They have normal testosterone but decreased DHT levels.

    c. They have castrate testosterone and elevated gonadotropin levels.

    d. They have castrate testosterone and normal gonadotropin levels.

    e. They have normal follicle-stimulating hormone but decreased luteinizing hormone levels.

11. Which of the following statements is TRUE regarding the ovotestis in ovotesticular disorders of sexual development (DSD)?

    a. It cannot descend from the retroperitoneum.

    b. It is found in the minority of patients.

    c. It can be unilateral or bilateral.

    d. It has testicular and ovarian elements randomly distributed.

    e. It is impossible to cleave surgically.

12. An important consideration for gender assignment in the ovotesticular DSD patient is:

    a. the potential for fertility.

    b. the impossibility of precisely dividing an ovotestis surgically.

    c. that malignant degeneration of gonads does not occur.

    d. the familial pattern of inheritance of the disorder.

    e. the unresponsiveness of the external genitalia to testosterone.

13. Which of the following statements is TRUE regarding the 21-hydroxylase deficiency in congenital adrenal hyperplasia (CAH)?

    a. It accounts for 99% of CAH cases.

    b. It occurs as a result of gene inactivation in the majority of cases.

    c. It occurs with simple virilization in 75% of cases and salt wasting in 25% of cases.

    d. It occurs with a predictable phenotype.

    e. It is transmitted in an autosomal dominant pattern.

14. Prenatal treatment of patients with CAH with dexamethasone:

    a. is appropriate therapy in seven of eight at-risk fetuses.

    b. is initiated after a diagnosis of CAH is confirmed.

c. is of no risk to the fetus.

d. is demonstrated to be effective.

e. acts by suppressing maternal corticotropin.

15. Which of the following statements is TRUE regarding enzymatic disorders of testosterone biosynthesis?

    a. They are transmitted in an autosomal dominant pattern.

    b. They are associated with persistent müllerian structures.

    c. They appear clinically with a predictable phenotype.

    d. They may involve impaired glucocorticoid and mineralocorticoid synthesis.

    e. They may be associated with fertility.

16. Which of the following statements is TRUE regarding patients with complete androgen insensitivity?

    a. They are appropriately raised as female.

    b. They have normal wolffian duct structures.

    c. They have persistent müllerian duct structures.

    d. They should undergo orchiectomy as early as possible.

    e. They have a 2% incidence of inguinal hernia.

17. What is Reifenstein syndrome?

    a. The group of defects in testosterone biosynthesis that results in male pseudohermaphroditism

    b. A form of 5α-reductase deficiency

    c. Defects of MIS elaboration in utero

    d. A disorder of androgen receptor quantity or function

    e. An autosomal recessively transmitted disorder

18. Which of the following statements is TRUE regarding patients with 5α-reductase deficiency?

    a. Fertility is an important issue in gender assignment.

    b. Isoenzymes 1 and 2 are abnormal.

    c. Serum testosterone levels are normal, but there is a decreased testosterone/DHT ratio.

    d. Masculinization occurs at puberty.

    e. Prostatic enlargement occurs at puberty.

19. Which of the following statements is TRUE regarding patients with persistent müllerian duct syndrome?

    a. They have absent wolffian duct structures.

    b. They represent a homogeneous disorder of involving the MIS receptor.

    c. They should undergo routine removal of müllerian structures.

    d. They experience a high incidence of transverse testicular ectopia.

    e. They are uniformly infertile.

20. Which of the following statements is TRUE regarding Mayer-Rokitansky-Küster-Hauser syndrome?

    a. It presents most commonly as infertility.

    b. It is a homogeneous disorder entailing congenital absence of the uterus and vagina.

    c. It is associated with a spectrum of ovarian abnormalities.

    d. It has associated upper urinary tract anomalies, primarily with the atypical disorder.

    e. It is associated with persistent wolffian duct structures.

21. In an unambiguous neonate with hypospadias and a unilateral cryptorchid testis:
    a. midshaft location of the urethral meatus is an important risk factor for disorder of sexual differentiation.
    b. impalpability of the cryptorchid testis carries a 50% risk of a disorder of sexual differentiation.
    c. palpability of the cryptorchid testis effectively rules out disorder of sexual differentiation.
    d. perineal hypospadias is not a risk factor for a disorder of sexual differentiation.
    e. difference in tissue texture of the poles of the cryptorchid gonad is suggestive of tumor.

22. Gender identity:
    a. is synonymous with gender role.
    b. is primarily determined by prenatal exposure to androgens.
    c. is primarily determined by postnatal environmental influences.
    d. is defined as the identification of self as either male or female.
    e. does not play a role in gender dysphoria.

ANSWERS

1. **b. The expressed SRY protein has a high mobility group (HMG), DNA binding domain.** This domain can induce significant DNA binding when bound to the regulatory regions of target genes. The *SRY* gene is located on the short arm of the Y chromosome adjacent to the pseudoautosomal boundary. Deletion maps based on the genomes of these individuals were constructed by a number of laboratories, and *SRY* was mapped to the most distal aspect of the Y-unique region of the short arm of the Y chromosome, adjacent to the pseudoautosomal boundary.

2. **d. It is secreted at 7 to 8 weeks of gestation, representing the initial endocrine function of the fetal testis.** The initial endocrine function of the fetal testes is the secretion of MIS by the Sertoli cells at 7 to 8 weeks of gestation.

3. **a. Mutations in *WT1* can result in either Denys-Drash or Frasier syndrome.** Denys-Drash syndrome is characterized by a triad of Wilms tumor, congenital nephropathy, and disorder of sexual development (DSD), whereas Frasier syndrome is associated with gonadal dysgenesis, gonadoblastoma, and congenital nephropathy. *WT1* is located on chromosome 11 but is not associated with dosage-sensitive sex reversal.

4. **d. It acts locally to virilize the internal wolffian duct structures.** It was clearly demonstrated that androgen is essential for virilization of wolffian duct structures, the urogenital sinus, and genital tubercle. Testosterone, the major androgen secreted by the testes, enters target tissues by passive diffusion. The local source of androgen is important for wolffian duct development, which does not occur if testosterone is supplied only via the peripheral circulation.

5. **c. It produces virilization of the urogenital sinus.** In some cells, such as those in the urogenital sinus, testosterone is converted to DHT by intracellular 5α-reductase. Testosterone or DHT then binds to a high-affinity intracellular receptor protein, and this complex enters the nucleus, where it binds to acceptor sites on DNA, resulting in target gene activation and protein synthesis. Therefore, in tissues equipped with 5α-reductase at the time of sexual differentiation, such as prostate, urogenital sinus, and external genitalia, DHT is the active androgen.

6. **b. They are at increased risk for development of adenocarcinoma of the breast.** Gynecomastia, which can be quite marked, is a common pubertal development in patients with Klinefelter syndrome. As a result, these patients are at eight times the risk for developing breast carcinoma relative to normal males. Males with Klinefelter syndrome have one Y chromosome and at least two X chromosomes.

7. **e. in the presence of a Y chromosome results in risk for development of gonadoblastoma.** In patients with occult Y chromosomal material, the risk of gonadoblastoma, an in-situ germ cell cancer, is approximately 30%. The streak gonad is usually abdominal in location, is hypoplastic, and predominantly consists of fibrous tissue.

8. **c. They lack the somatic defects associated with Turner syndrome** (e.g., broad chest, neck webbing, cardiac and renal anomalies, and short stature). However, patients with 46,XX "pure" gonadal dysgenesis are closely related to those with Turner syndrome. Because these subjects exhibit none of the somatic stigmata associated with Turner syndrome and their condition entails gonadal dysgenesis only, this type has been regarded by some authors as pure.

9. **b. Nephropathy with early-onset proteinuria.** The full triad of the syndrome includes nephropathy, characterized by the early onset of proteinuria, and hypertension and progressive renal failure in the majority. Because incomplete forms of the syndrome may occur, the nephropathy has become regarded as the common denominator of the syndrome.

10. **c. They have castrate testosterone and elevated gonadotropin levels.** The diagnosis can be made on the basis of a 46,XY karyotype and castrate levels of testosterone despite persistently elevated serum luteinizing hormone and follicle-stimulating hormone levels.

11. **c. It can be unilateral or bilateral.** Ovotesticular DSD patients are individuals having both testicular tissue with well-developed seminiferous tubules and ovarian tissue with primordial follicles, which may take the form of one ovary and one testis or, more commonly, one or two ovotestes. Histopathology of the ovotestis will typically demonstrate well-developed ovarian tissue and a dysgenetic testicular component.

12. **a. the potential for fertility.** The most important aspect of management in ovotesticular DSD is gender assignment.

13. **b. It occurs as a result of gene inactivation in the majority of cases.** Mutations leading to gene conversion of the active *CYP21A* gene into the inactive gene occur in 65% to 90% of cases of the classic disorder (salt wasting and simple virilizing) and all cases of nonclassic 21-hydroxylase deficiency. 21-Hydroxylase deficiency accounts for 95% of CAH cases, with 75% presenting with salt wasting and 25% with simple virilization.

14. **d. is demonstrated to be effective.** Treatment should be initiated prior to 9 weeks after the last menstrual period, once pregnancy is confirmed. A number of series have established the effectiveness of prenatal treatment of CAH with dexamethasone, which suppresses fetal secretion of

adrenocorticotropic hormone. However, a diagnosis of CAH cannot be confirmed before therapy is initiated because the diagnosis is usually made by chorionic villus sampling or amniocentesis. Therefore, if treatment is initiated for all at-risk fetuses, seven of eight may be treated unnecessarily before confirmatory diagnosis.

15. **d. They may involve impaired glucocorticoid and mineralocorticoid synthesis.** A defect in any of the five enzymes required for the conversion of cholesterol to testosterone can cause incomplete (or absent) virilization of the male fetus during embryogenesis. The first three enzymes (cholesterol side chain cleavage enzyme, 3β-hydroxysteroid dehydrogenase, and 17α-hydroxylase) are present in both the adrenals and the testes. Therefore their deficiency results in impaired synthesis of glucocorticoids and mineralocorticoids in addition to testosterone.

16. **a. They are appropriately raised as female.** It is of great interest that, currently, all studies of patients with complete androgen insensitivity support an unequivocal female gender identity, consistent with androgen resistance of brain tissue as well. To date there has been no report of a patient raised as a female who needed gender reassignment to male. Development of wolffian duct structures is androgen dependent. Sertoli cells are present and produce MIS, which results in the regression of müllerian duct structures.

17. **d. A disorder of androgen receptor quantity or function.** Androgen receptor studies in cultured fibroblasts have demonstrated two forms of receptor defect in the partial androgen insensitivity syndrome. These include a reduced number of normally functioning androgen receptors and normal receptor number but decreased binding affinity.

18. **d. Masculinization occurs at puberty.** At puberty, partial masculinization occurs with an increase in muscle mass, development of male body habitus, increase in phallic size, and onset of erections. The type 2 isoenzyme is affected in patients with 5α-reductase deficiency, resulting in an increased testosterone/DHT ratio owing to a reduced testosterone-to-DHT conversion rate.

19. **d. They experience a high incidence of transverse testicular ectopia.** Persistent müllerian duct syndrome is thought to be etiologically important in transverse testicular ectopia, occurring in 30% to 50% of cases. Aberrant MIS function may be secondary to defects in the gene for MIS or in the gene for the MIS receptor.

20. **d. It has associated upper urinary tract anomalies, primarily with the atypical disorder.** Urinary tract anomalies occur more commonly in patients with the atypical form of the disorder than in patients with the typical syndrome. Patients with Mayer-Rokitansky-Küster-Hauser syndrome typically present with primary amenorrhea.

21. **b. impalpability of the cryptorchid testis carries a 50% risk of a disorder of sexual differentiation.** With a unilateral cryptorchid testis, the incidence of a disorder of sexual differentiation was 30% overall, 15% if the undescended testis was palpable, and 50% if it was impalpable.

22. **d. is defined as the identification of self as either male or female.** Gender role refers to aspects of behavior that distinguish males and females. The development of gender identity is poorly understood but is influenced by prenatal and postnatal factors. Individual conflicts with gender identity are central to the concept of gender dysphoria.

Additional Study Points

1. *SRY* initiates testicular organogenesis.
2. The prostate, urogenital sinus, and external genitalia are all sensitive to dihydrotestosterone.
3. Estrogens are not required for normal female differentiation.
4. Patients with Klinefelter syndrome have eunuchoidism, gynecomastia, azoospermia, and small testis and are tall for their age. Muscle development is poor.
5. Patients with Turner syndrome (XO) have sexual infantilism, web neck, and cubitus valgus, are of the female phenotype, are short in stature, and lack secondary sexual characteristics.
6. In patients with Turner syndrome, any Y-chromosome material increases the risk for the streak gonad developing a gonadoblastoma; these patients also have increased incidence of abnormalities of the kidney, including horseshoe kidney.
7. The diagnosis of congenital adrenal hyperplasia (CAH) of the salt-wasting variety is made by obtaining a serum 17-hydroxyprogesterone value 3 to 4 days after birth. If it is elevated, the patient has CAH.
8. In patients who have severe forms of CAH difficult to control medically, bilateral adrenalectomy may be the most effective approach.
9. A distinctly palpable gonad along the pathway of descent is highly suggestive of a testis or rarely of an ovotestis.
10. Patients with bilateral impalpable testes or a unilateral impalpable testis and hypospadias should be regarded as having a disorder of sexual development until proven otherwise whether or not the genitalia appear ambiguous. They should have a karyotype.

134

Surgical Management of Disorders of Sexual Differentiation, Cloacal Malformation, and Other Abnormalities of the Genitalia in Girls

Richard C. Rink, MD, FACS, FAAP ● Martin Kaefer, MD, FAAP, FACS

QUESTIONS

1. Mayer-Rokitansky-Küster-Hauser syndrome:
   a. presents most commonly as infertility.
   b. is a homogeneous disorder comprising congenital absence of the uterus and vagina.
   c. is associated with a spectrum of ovarian abnormalities.
   d. has associated upper urinary tract anomalies, primarily with the atypical disorder.
   e. is associated with persistent wolffian duct structures.

2. The crucial period in embryogenesis for the formation of the terminal bowel, kidney, paramesonephric ductal system, and lumbosacral spine is:
   a. 4 to 6 weeks.
   b. 8 to 10 weeks.
   c. 10 to 14 weeks.
   d. 14 to 18 weeks.
   e. more than 18 weeks.

3. Which of the following is FALSE regarding vaginal agenesis (müllerian aplasia)?
   a. It occurs with an incidence of approximately 1 in 5000 live female births.
   b. Serum follicle-stimulating hormone and luteinizing hormone levels can be expected to be abnormally high.
   c. Embryologically it results from a failure of the sinovaginal bulbs to develop and form the vaginal plate.
   d. It is a condition associated with renal abnormalities.
   e. It is a condition associated with skeletal abnormalities.

4. Skeletal anomalies are found in what percentage of patients with Meyer-Rokitansky-Küster-Hauser syndrome?
   a. 10% to 20%
   b. 25% to 35%
   c. 40% to 60%
   d. 70% to 90%
   e. 0% (they are not seen in association with the syndrome)

5. What is the most common cause of primary amenorrhea?
   a. Testicular feminization
   b. Vaginal agenesis
   c. Mixed gonadal dysgenesis
   d. Imperforate hymen
   e. Transverse vaginal septum

6. Which of the following statements regarding the genitalia of women with Meyer-Rokitansky-Küster-Hauser syndrome is FALSE?
   a. In approximately 10% of patients a normal but obstructed uterus or rudimentary uterus with functional endometrium is present.
   b. Normal fallopian tubes are seen in approximately 35% of patients.
   c. The ovaries are not functional in the majority of patients.
   d. The hymenal fringe is usually present along with a small vaginal pouch.
   e. The labia majora are typically normal in appearance.

7. Which of the following is FALSE regarding the construction of a vagina utilizing bowel?
   a. Failure to develop an adequate space between the rectum and bladder can result in compromised blood flow to the segment used for vaginal construction.
   b. In general, colon is preferred over ileum because of its lower incidence of associated postoperative stenosis.
   c. When compared with the McIndoe procedure, the bowel vagina suffers from a higher incidence of postoperative stenosis.
   d. An advantage of a bowel vagina over the McIndoe procedure includes the lubricating properties of mucus (which may help to facilitate intercourse).
   e. One specific indication for the use of ileum is a previous history of pelvic radiation.

8. Uterus didelphys with unilateral imperforate vagina most commonly presents as:
   a. primary amenorrhea.
   b. cyclical abdominal pain associated with normal cyclical menstruation.
   c. renal anomalies contralateral to the side of the obstruction.
   d. anomalies of the axial skeleton.
   e. constipation.

9. Urethral prolapse is most commonly seen in young females of which ethnic background?
   a. African-American
   b. White
   c. Asian
   d. Hispanic
   e. American Indian

10. In most cases of labial adhesions, which of the following is TRUE?
    a. They are believed to occur because of a relative state of hyperestrogenism.
    b. They should be treated with surgical lysis.
    c. They require no treatment.
    d. They occur secondary to sexual abuse.
    e. They have associated renal anomalies.

11. What is the mean age of a child with vaginal rhabdomyosarcoma?
    a. Younger than 2 years
    b. 2 to 4 years
    c. 4 to 8 years
    d. 8 to 12 years
    e. Older than 12 years

12. Urogenital sinus anomalies in disorders of sexual differentiation states are most commonly seen in association with:
    a. congenital adrenal hyperplasia.
    b. mixed gonadal dysgenesis.
    c. true hermaphroditism.
    d. cloacal anomalies.
    e. gonadal dysgenesis.

13. The most common finding in cloacal anomalies that have been diagnosed by antenatal ultrasonography is:
    a. ascites.
    b. distended rectum.
    c. distended bladder.
    d. distended vagina.
    e. distended bladder and rectum.

14. What is the most common vaginal anatomy in cloacal malformation?
    a. Single vagina, single uterus
    b. Single vagina, double uterus
    c. Two vaginas, two uteri
    d. Two vaginas, one uterus
    e. Single vagina, no uterus

15. Which of the following is not part of the normal evaluation of a child born with a cloacal anomaly?
    a. Genitography
    b. MRI of the head
    c. Echocardiography
    d. MRI of the spine

16. Neonatal vaginoplasty combined with clitoroplasty and labioplasty has all of the following advantages EXCEPT:
    a. it allows phallic skin for vaginal reconstruction.
    b. maternal estrogens increase vaginal thickness and vascularity.
    c. tissues are less scarred.
    d. vaginal stenosis is clearly less.

17. The cut-back vaginoplasty is appropriate for:
    a. labial fusion.
    b. low vaginal confluence.
    c. high vaginal confluence.
    d. vaginal atresia.
    e. vaginal agenesis.

18. Surgical management of cloacal malformations involves all of the following steps EXCEPT:
    a. decompression of the gastrointestinal tract.
    b. decompression of the genitourinary tract.
    c. vaginostomy.
    d. definitive repair of the cloaca.
    e. correction of nephron destructive anomalies.

19. Fecal continence after cloacal reconstruction is most closely related to:
    a. the level of rectal confluence.
    b. associated urinary anomalies.
    c. neurologic status.
    d. the type of repair.
    e. the timing of the repair.

ANSWERS

1. **d. has associated upper urinary tract anomalies, primarily with the atypical disorder.** Urinary tract anomalies occur more commonly in patients with the atypical form of the disorder than in patients with the typical syndrome.

2. **a. 4 to 6 weeks.** Laboratory data with teratogens support the concept of a key event occurring between the fourth and fifth weeks of gestation that results in an error in the simultaneous development of the terminal bowel, kidney, bladder, paramesonephric ductal system, and lumbosacral spine.

3. **b. Serum follicle-stimulating hormone and luteinizing hormone levels can be expected to be abnormally high.** Vaginal agenesis, which occurs with an incidence of approximately 1 in 5000 live female births, is the congenital absence of the proximal portion of the vagina in an otherwise phenotypically (i.e., normal secondary sexual characteristics), chromosomally (i.e., 46,XX), and hormonally (i.e., normal luteinizing hormone and follicle-stimulating hormone levels) intact female. It results from a failure of the sinovaginal bulbs to develop and form the vaginal plate. Hauser and Schreiner (1961)* brought further attention to the frequent association of renal and skeletal anomalies in these patients and stressed the differences between patients with these findings and those with testicular feminization.

4. **a. 10% to 20%.** Associated congenital abnormalities of the skeletal system have been described in 10% to 20% of cases.

5. **c. Mixed gonadal dysgenesis.** Meyer-Rokitansky-Küster-Hauser syndrome is, in fact, secondary only to gonadal dysgenesis as a cause of primary amenorrhea.

6. **c. The ovaries are not functional in the majority of patients.** Although occasionally cystic, the ovaries are almost always present and functional.

7. **c. When compared with the McIndoe procedure, the bowel vagina suffers from a higher incidence of postoperative stenosis.** A high incidence of postoperative vaginal stenosis necessitates postoperative vaginal dilatation in the McIndoe procedure.

8. **b. cyclical abdominal pain associated with normal cyclical menstruation.** As with other obstructive disorders, the patient may present with cyclical or chronic abdominal pain. However, unlike other obstructive processes, duplication anomalies with unilateral obstruction are not associated with primary amenorrhea.

9. **a. African-American.** This entity, which was first described by Solinger in 1732, occurs most often in prepubertal African-American girls and postmenopausal white women.

*Sources referenced can be found in *Campbell-Walsh Urology, 10th Edition,* on the Expert Consult website.

10. **c. They require no treatment.** Most children do not require treatment unless one of the aforementioned symptoms (urine pooling within the vagina, which may lead to postvoid dribbling; perineal irritation; physical findings of sexual abuse) occurs.

11. **a. Younger than 2 years.**

12. **a. congenital adrenal hyperplasia.** Urogenital sinus abnormalities are most often seen in disorders of sexual differentiation states, most commonly in association with congenital adrenal hyperplasia, which has been noted to have an incidence as frequent as 1 in 500 in the nonclassic mild forms.

13. **d. distended vagina.** The common finding in all reports has been a cystic pelvic mass between the bladder and rectum, representing a distended vagina.

14. **c. Two vaginas, two uteri.** In Hendren's report on 154 patients with cloacal anomalies, 66 patients had one vagina, 68 had two vaginas, and the vagina was absent in 20 (Hendren, 1998). The incidence of vaginal duplication is even higher in the authors' own patient population. The uterus anomaly generally is similar to the vaginal anomaly, that is, two vaginas with two uteri.

15. **b. MRI of the head.** The frequency of associated organ system abnormalities requires further radiographic evaluation. Echocardiography should always be done. MRI to evaluate the lumbosacral spine and to evaluate pelvic anatomy and musculature is necessary.

16. **d. Vaginal stenosis is clearly less.** Other investigators, including the authors' group, have thought that vaginoplasty, regardless of the vaginal location, is best combined with clitoroplasty in a single stage. This allows the redundant phallic skin to be used in the reconstruction, adding flexibility for the surgeon, which is compromised when the skin has been previously mobilized. Furthermore, the authors and others have noted that maternal estrogen stimulation of the child's genitalia results in thicker vaginal tissue, which is better vascularized, making vaginal mobilization more easily performed.

17. **a. labial fusion.** The cut-back vaginoplasty is rarely used and is appropriate only for simple labial fusion.

18. **c. vaginostomy.** Surgical management now involves four basic steps: decompression of the gastrointestinal tract, decompression of the genitourinary tract, correction of nephron destructive or potentially lethal urinary anomalies, and definitive repair of the cloaca.

19. **c. neurologic status.** Fecal continence is directly related to neurologic status.

Additional Study Points

1. The urorectal septum fuses with the cloacal membrane and divides it into a ventral urogenital membrane and a dorsal anal membrane.

2. The fibromuscular node that results from contact of the septum with the cloacal membrane is the insertion site for the perineal muscles.

3. Remnants of the prostatic ducts give rise to the Skene glands; remnants of the wolffian ducts give rise to the Gartner ducts.

4. The Bartholin glands are homologues of the bulbourethral glands in the male.

5. The proximal portion of the vagina forms from the fused paired müllerian ducts; the distal portion forms from the sinovaginal bulbs, which later canalize.

6. In planning treatment for a transverse vaginal septum, it is of critical importance to determine whether there is a cervix and, if present, its exact location relative to the septum.

7. Vaginal atresia differs from vaginal agenesis and testicular feminization in that the müllerian structures are not affected. As a result, the uterus, cervix, and upper portion of the vagina are normal.

8. A complication of the use of skin grafts to create a neovagina is the increased incidence of vaginal stenosis and the requirement for repeated vaginal dilatation.

9. Most anomalies of lateral fusion have no functional significance.

10. When an intralabial mass appears to be associated with the urethra, workup should always include renal pelvic ultrasonography.

11. In patients with congenital adrenal hyperplasia, the location of the confluence of the vagina and the urethra in relation to the bladder neck is a critical determinant in the surgical management.

12. When gonads in the neonatal period require biopsy, a deep biopsy is appropriate because the ovarian component of an ovotestis may be completely surrounded by testicular tissue or may be located in the poles.

13. Spinal cord abnormalities have been frequently detected in patients with cloacal abnormalities.

14. When clitoroplasty is performed, the glans and tunics and the neurovascular bundles should be preserved.

15. In reconstruction of distal vaginal abnormalities, the distal vagina is often narrow and the flap required to adequately exteriorize the vagina must be sutured to the normal-caliber vagina proximally.

16. In cloacal anomalies, it is optimal to repair all abnormalities at a single stage.

17. There is a high percentage of patients who have a neuropathic component to their incontinence in those who have had corrective surgery for cloacal abnormalities.

135

Surgical Management of Pediatric Stone Disease

Michael C. Ost, MD ● Francis X. Schneck, MD

QUESTIONS

1. Which component(s) of present day western diets is/are thought to contribute to the increasing prevalence of nephrolithiasis in the pediatric population?

   a. Protein

   b. Potassium and magnesium

   c. Saturated fats and cholesterol

   d. Sodium and carbohydrates

   e. Calcium

2. A 5-year-old boy is seen in the office with complaints of intermittent right flank pain. There have been no episodes of nausea, vomiting, or fevers. He has 3+ blood on a urine dip. His physical exam reveals some mild right costovertebral angle (CVA) tenderness. Which imaging modality should be used first?

   a. Intravenous pyelography (IVP)

   b. Plain radiograph (kidney-ureter-bladder [KUB])

   c. Ultrasonography

   d. Computed tomography (CT) scan

   e. Retrograde pyelogram

3. A 12-year-old girl is found to have a 5-mm left distal ureteral stone after an acute episode of left flank pain. She responded well to conservative therapy (IV hydration and pain medication) and her pain subsides. The next step is:

   a. observation, because the stone will most likely pass in 6 weeks.

   b. plan for an endourologic procedure, because, given the size of the stone, it will most likely not pass.

   c. a trial of oral therapies, such as α blockers and steroids to facilitate stone passage.

   d. a trial of oral therapy with a calcium channel blocker to facilitate stone passage.

   e. that no further interventions will be needed, because the stone has most likely passed.

4. A 10-year-old boy with spina bifida had an augment cystoplasty, bladder neck reconstruction, and bilateral Glenn-Anderson ureteral reimplantation for high-grade reflux

at age 7. He was found to have a 1-cm renal pelvic stone. The therapy least likely to yield an efficacious (stone-free) result is:

   a. shock wave lithotripsy (SWL).

   b. ureteroscopy with laser lithotripsy.

   c. ureteral stenting and ureteroscopy with laser lithotripsy 6 weeks later.

   d. percutaneous nephrolithotomy.

   e. open pyelolithotomy.

5. With regard to SWL in the treatment of pediatric nephrolithiasis, treatment failures are associated with:

   a. high stone burdens (i.e., 2-cm calcium oxalate monohydrate stone).

   b. sizeable infundibular length.

   c. an infundibulopelvic angle greater than 45 degrees.

   d. staghorn calculi.

   e. a, b, and c.

6. Complications that may occur during ureteroscopy while treating a ureteral stone include:

   a. hypothermia and hyponatremia.

   b. ureteral avulsion.

   c. hypertension.

   d. all of the above.

   e. a and b.

7. A 9-year-old female with cystinuria is found to have a right 2-cm renal pelvic stone. The best option for treating her stone is:

   a. extracorporeal shock wave lithotripsy (ESWL).

   b. ureteroscopy with laser lithotripsy and stone basketing.

   c. percutaneous nephrolithotomy (PCNL).

   d. medical therapy with potassium citrate and Thiola.

   e. anatrophic nephrolithotomy.

8. The most common chemical composition of a bladder stone found in a child from a developing country is:

   a. struvite.

   b. ammonium acid urate.

c. uric acid.

d. calcium oxalate monohydrate.

e. calcium oxalate dehydrate.

ANSWERS

1. **d. Sodium and carbohydrates.** It has been speculated that diets rich in sodium and carbohydrates may be contributing to the etiology of urolithiasis in this cohort of children.

2. **c. Ultrasonography.** Ultrasonography has a more limited role in the assessment of urolithiasis compared with CT but has the distinct advantage of no associated ionizing radiation. Therefore ultrasonography should be considered as a screening tool in the workup for non-emergent abdominal or flank pain.

3. **b. plan for an endourologic procedure, because, given the size of the stone, it will most likely not pass.** In managing stone disease in the pediatric population, it is important to note that renal calculi less than 3 mm are likely to spontaneously pass, and stones greater than or equal to 4 mm in the distal ureter are likely to require endourologic treatment. This information should be relayed to caregivers and parents.

4. **a. shock wave lithotripsy (SWL).** Recent data suggests that stone-free rates in children with a history of urologic conditions or urinary tract reconstruction are quite low (12.5%), and, with alternative surgical techniques available, they may be better served with ureterorenoscopy (URS) or PCNL.

5. **e. a, b, and c.** SWL failure and re-treatment rates were associated with increased mean stone burden, increased infundibular length, and infundibulopelvic angle greater than 45 degrees. Staghorn calculi are uncommon in children and represent a management challenge. Although monotherapy success rates are low in adults, acceptable stone-free rates in children have been achieved with SWL.

6. **e. a and b.** Irrigating fluid, which may be used under pressure, should be isotonic and at body temperature to avoid hypothermia and hyponatremia. Other complications of ureteroscopy include unrecognized ureteral injury, including mucosal flaps and tears, perforation, false passage, and partial to complete avulsion. Hypertension is not a recognized complication of ureteroscopy.

7. **c. percutaneous nephrolithotomy (PCNL).** This child would be best served with a PCNL due to a large stone burden. Although ureteroscopy is an option, multiple sessions would most likely be required. Cystine stones do not respond well to SWL. Medical therapy helps to prevent cystine stones, but not treat. Anatrophic nephrolithotomy is not an appropriate surgical treatment for this stone.

8. **b. ammonium acid urate.** Bladder stones are more often found in children from developing countries and are thought to be related endemically to malnutrition. It is thought that diets low in animal protein and phosphorous (breast milk as opposed to cow's milk), in addition to vitamin A deficiency, are contributory. Bladder stones from children in these developing countries are most often composed of ammonium acid urate. By contrast, among children from industrialized nations, bladder stones are most often found in those with spinal cord injuries or congenital abnormalities such as spina bifida. Very often these children have undergone augment cystoplasty and/or manage their bladders by clean intermittent catheterization.

Additional Study Points

1. The excretion of metabolites in the urine is different for a child as compared with an adult; adult values should not be used in evaluating calcium, phosphate, uric acid oxalate, and citrate excretion in children.

2. Stones less than 3 mm are likely to pass spontaneously.

3. When using shock wave lithotripsy, lower power settings are appropriate.

4. Ureteroscopy for distal ureteral stones achieves a higher stone-free rate.

5. Calculi up to 15 mm in the upper tract may be effectively treated ureteroscopically.

chapter
136

Urologic Considerations in Pediatric Renal Transplantation

Craig A. Peters, MD, FACS, FAAP

QUESTIONS

1. Indications for urodynamic evaluation of a child being prepared for renal transplant include:
   a. focal segmental glomerulosclerosis (FSGS) renal failure.
   b. prolonged anuria after FSGS renal failure.
   c. ongoing grade III vesicoureteral reflux.
   d. ESRD in a child with nocturnal enuresis.
   e. ESRD in a child with wetting but no urinary tract infections (UTIs).

2. Renal transplantation into a child with an augmented bladder is associated with:
   a. cyclosporine toxicity.
   b. no significant change in graft survival.
   c. hyperchloremic metabolic alkalosis.
   d. recurrent infection.
   e. refractory rejection.

3. In a 10-year-old boy with a 50-cc capacity bladder, a history of posterior urethral valves, end-stage renal disease (ESRD), and anuria, optimal bladder management in preparation for renal transplantation is:
   a. bladder cycling by intermittent catheterization.
   b. anticholinergic medications and proceeding with transplantation.
   c. ileocystoplasty.
   d. transplant into transverse colon loop and delayed augmentation.
   e. gastrocystoplasty and continent catheterizable stoma.

4. Indications for pretransplant native nephrectomy include all of the following EXCEPT:
   a. chronic two-drug hypertension.
   b. persisting grade III vesicoureteral reflux (VUR) in a 4-year-old child.
   c. multicystic dysplastic kidney (MDCK).
   d. age younger than 12 months.
   e. ESRD associated with Denys-Drasch syndrome.

5. An antirefluxing transplant ureteroneocystostomy should be performed:
   a. only in children on intermittent catheterization.
   b. only in children with neurogenic bladder dysfunction.
   c. in infants only.
   d. in children at risk for UTI or bladder dysfunction.
   e. in any child undergoing renal transplantation.

6. Following a cadaveric renal transplant for FSGS, a 10-year-old boy is found to have distal ureteral obstruction from a 4-cm stricture that fails balloon dilation and stenting. The best option for management is:
   a. psoas hitch transplant ureteroneocystostomy.
   b. ileal interposition.
   c. Boari flap-to-graft pelvis.
   d. transplant ureter–to–native ureteroureterostomy.
   e. transplant nephrectomy.

7. Six months following an uncomplicated living related-donor renal transplant, a 7-year-old girl develops acute pyelonephritis of the graft with a rise in creatinine. There is no hydronephrosis on ultrasonography. A VCUG demonstrates grade III reflux into the graft but none in the native ureters. She has normal voiding patterns. The best option for management is:
   a. continuous antibiotic prophylaxis and repeat studies in 18 months, anticipating spontaneous resolution.
   b. endoscopic injection of subureteral bulking agents.
   c. open redo transplant ureteroneocystostomy.
   d. transplant ureter–to–native ureteroureterostomy.
   e. 6 months of antibiotic prophylaxis and observation.

8. 18 months following an uncomplicated living related-donor renal transplant, a 5-year-old boy with a history of posterior urethral valves develops a rising creatinine level, graft hydronephrosis, and two febrile UTIs. VCUG shows grade III reflux into the graft and moderate bladder trabeculation similar to his pretransplant pattern. The best next step in his care is:
   a. urodynamic evaluation and likely anticholinergics and intermittent catheterization.

b. ileocystoplasty and appendicovesicostomy.

c. psoas hitch ureteral reimplantation.

d. transplant ureter–to–native ureteroureterostomy.

e. nontunneled ureteroneocystostomy.

ANSWERS

1. **e. ESRD in a child with wetting but no urinary tract infections (UTIs).** The child with ongoing wetting is the most likely to have treatable voiding dysfunction that may put the renal graft at risk. Simple bladder defunctionalization with no history of underlying bladder dysfunction is unlikely to need urodynamic evaluation and often may not need bladder cycling. Reflux alone, without recurrent UTI, wetting, or a neurogenic cause is not likely to benefit from urodynamics. Nocturnal enuresis is not an indication for invasive evaluation of bladder function.

2. **b. no significant change in graft survival.** Although early reports implied a high risk due to bladder augmentation in children undergoing renal transplant, modern series have demonstrated the safety and, indeed, the benefits of providing a low-pressure urinary reservoir on graft function. The incidence of positive urine cultures can be increased, but clinically significant infections are not markedly increased.

3. **a. bladder cycling by intermittent catheterization.** In the child with anuria, bladder function cannot be easily assessed until the bladder has been cycled. Although this child may require augmentation, that cannot be determined until after a trial of cycling is attempted. Transplanting into a diversion is not an acceptable alternative in a child who has the potential for adequate bladder function with medical management and intermittent catheterization.

4. **c. multicystic dysplastic kidney.** All of these clinical situations can justify native nephrectomy except for the presence of a MCDK. There is minimal to no risk of leaving the dysplastic kidney in place. Persisting reflux may be a relative indication, and some practitioners may chose to reimplant the native ureter or simply leave it alone if there is no significant history of infection. In some centers, children younger than 12 months do not routinely have native nephrectomy, although there is a slightly higher risk of graft loss without this.

5. **d. in children at risk for UTI or bladder dysfunction.** Any child with a risk for UTI or who has bladder dysfunction and may therefore develop a UTI, particularly if immunosuppressed, should have a nonrefluxing ureteroneocystostomy. Some centers perform a nonrefluxing ureteral implantation in all children; this is probably not essential. Older children, those with no history of bladder dysfunction or recurrent infections, or those with a history of structural abnormalities can be effectively transplanted with a refluxing ureteroneocystostomy.

6. **a. psoas hitch transplant ureteroneocystostomy.** Several options are available for salvage of the graft in this situation, but the most effective is a psoas hitch when there is still some graft ureter available. A transplant ureter–to–native ureteroureterostomy is effective, but requires nephrectomy in most cases. Boari flaps may be useful for cases in which the entire ureter is lost or if there is no native ureter remaining. Even with loss of the entire ureter, a renal pelvis–to–native ureter anastomosis is effective. Ileal interposition and graft nephrectomy are not viable options.

7. **c. open redo transplant ureteroneocystostomy.** The best option in this situation is a redo open reimplantation to create an effective antireflux tunnel. This can be done intravesically or extravesically, or, occasionally, both due to scarring and fibrosis. Spontaneous resolution is highly unlikely, and simply waiting for another episode of pyelonephritis risks graft injury. Transplant ureter–to–native ureteroureterostomy is an option but requires nephrectomy. Endoscopic injection has a limited success rate in published series, and the durability is undefined. In the setting where a repeat episode of pyelonephritis is associated with significant risk to the graft, such an approach does not seem prudent.

8. **a. urodynamic evaluation and likely anticholinergics and intermittent catheterization.** This boy is best served by a formal assessment of his bladder function, with likely use of anticholinergics to improve capacity and compliance and intermittent catheterization to provide for emptying. One can start this therapy empirically but having a baseline permits assessment of the treatment's effect. Moving directly to augmentation without knowing if medical management can be effective is not appropriate. Simply reimplanting the ureter or performing a ureter to native ureteroureterostomy without treating the likely bladder dysfunction is also not appropriate.

Additional Study Points

1. Children who present for renal transplantation often have a congenital obstruction, vesicoureteral reflux, or a neuropathic bladder as the etiology of their renal failure.

2. Indications for urodynamics include neuropathic bladder, posterior urethral valves, voiding dysfunction, hydronephrosis, or recurrent UTIs.

3. The bladder may be refunctionalized with bladder cycling; however, it may take considerable time to reach maximal functional capacity. The goal for refunctionalization should be to achieve 75% of capacity for the expected age and to maintain pressures less than 30 cm of water.

4. Any major urologic reconstruction should be undertaken well before anticipated transplantation, ideally allowing 3 months for healing to occur before the transplant.

5. Native nephrectomy is indicted in patients with malignant hypertension, profound protein loss due to nephrotic syndrome, recurrent upper tract infections, and massive reflux.

6. For patients on peritoneal dialysis, intraperitoneal surgery will require temporary transition to hemodialysis.

7. An extravesical ureteroneocystostomy is generally preferred for the ureteral anastomosis for the transplant. There is no data to support routine stenting of the transplanted ureter.

8. In the setting of a rising creatinine level and hydronephrosis, obstruction and rejection may be intermingled.

137

Pediatric Urologic Oncology

Michael L. Ritchey, MD, FAAP, FACS ● Robert C. Shamberger, MD

QUESTIONS

1. A chromosomal abnormality associated with an adverse prognosis in neuroblastoma is:
   a. mutation of chromosome 11p15.
   b. absence of the *MDR* gene.
   c. mutation of the *TP53* gene.
   d. deletion of the short arm of chromosome 1.
   e. loss of heterozygosity (LOH) for chromosome 11p13.

2. In situ neuroblastoma:
   a. invariably progresses to clinical neuroblastoma.
   b. usually regresses spontaneously.
   c. is associated with deletion of chromosome 11.
   d. is usually detected on newborn screening.
   e. is frequently associated with amplification of the N-*MYC* oncogene.

3. Ganglioneuroma is:
   a. a stroma-rich tumor by the Shimada classification.
   b. most commonly located in the adrenal gland.
   c. often found secondary to symptoms from metastatic disease.
   d. associated with acute myoclonic encephalopathy.
   e. associated with an unfavorable prognosis.

4. Screening for neuroblastoma:
   a. has improved survival in patients with neuroblastoma.
   b. has decreased the number of children older than 1 year of age with advanced staged disease.
   c. has identified more tumors with amplified N-*MYC* oncogene expression.
   d. discovers tumors with an improved prognosis.
   e. is widely performed in the United States.

5. A clinical feature associated with a favorable prognosis in neuroblastoma is:
   a. age greater than 2 years.
   b. thoracic location of the primary tumor.
   c. N-*MYC* amplification.
   d. chromosome 1p deletion.
   e. stroma-poor histology.

6. A 1-month-old girl is found to have a right suprarenal mass on abdominal ultrasonography. The mass measures 4 cm in diameter. Imaging evaluation detects liver metastases. A skeletal survey is normal. Physical examination reveals multiple subcutaneous skin nodules. The mass is removed and confirmed to be a neuroblastoma. Analysis of the tumor reveals no N-*MYC* amplification. The next best step is:
   a. observation.
   b. irradiation to the tumor bed.
   c. vincristine, cyclophosphamide, and doxorubicin.
   d. vincristine, cyclophosphamide, and irradiation to the tumor bed.
   e. autologous bone marrow transplantation after chemotherapy and total-body irradiation.

7. A 3-year-old girl has vaginal rhabdomyosarcoma. Her mother has a history of breast cancer. This patient most likely has:
   a. Beckwith-Wiedemann syndrome (BWS).
   b. Li-Fraumeni syndrome.
   c. Perlman syndrome.
   d. Fragile X syndrome.
   e. Sotos syndrome.

8. A 3-year-old boy has rhabdomyosarcoma of the prostate. An unfavorable prognostic feature of this tumor is:
   a. alveolar histologic type.
   b. embryonal histology.
   c. LOH for chromosome 11p15.
   d. botryoid pattern.
   e. spindle cell variant.

9. A 1-year-old girl previously had a partial cystectomy for rhabdomyosarcoma of the bladder. After completion of vincristine, dactinomycin, and cyclophosphamide (VAC) chemotherapy, biopsy of the bladder reveals rhabdomyoblasts. Abdominal and chest computed tomography (CT) are negative. The next step is:
   a. radiation therapy.
   b. continue chemotherapy.
   c. cystectomy with diversion.
   d. observation.
   e. a change in chemotherapy regimen.

10. A 4-year-old boy has paratesticular rhabdomyosarcoma noted on biopsy of the spermatic cord lesion. The next step is radical orchiectomy and:
    a. vincristine, dactinomycin, and cyclophosphamide.
    b. retroperitoneal lymph node dissection.
    c. retroperitoneal lymph node sampling.
    d. radiation therapy to the retroperitoneum.
    e. cisplatin, etoposide, and vincristine.

11. The WAGR (Wilms tumor, Aniridia, Genital abnormalities, mental Retardation) syndrome is most frequently associated with:
    a. deletion of chromosome 15.
    b. advanced-stage Wilms tumor.
    c. neonatal presentation of Wilms tumor.
    d. renal insufficiency.
    e. familial predisposition to Wilms tumor.

12. A 3-year-old boy had undergone treatment for hypospadias and an undescended testis as an infant. He develops renal insufficiency. Renal biopsy is consistent with a membranoproliferative glomerulonephritis. Appropriate management before renal transplantation is:
    a. a voiding cystourethrogram.
    b. gonadal biopsy.
    c. observation.
    d. bilateral nephrectomy.
    e. serial renal ultrasonograms.

13. A 2-year-old boy has a palpable right-sided abdominal mass. CT shows this to be a solid lesion. On physical examination, the patient's right arm and leg are noted to be slightly longer in length. His diagnosis is most probably:
    a. Wilms tumor.
    b. neuroblastoma.
    c. angiomyolipoma.
    d. nephroblastomatosis.
    e. renal cell carcinoma.

14. A newborn is identified with Beckwith-Wiedemann syndrome. A renal ultrasonogram is obtained. The clinical finding that best predicts the risk of subsequent Wilms tumor development is:
    a. hepatomegaly.
    b. hemihypertrophy.
    c. nephromegaly.
    d. mutation at chromosome 11p13.
    e. family history of Wilms tumor.

15. A 6-month-old girl is diagnosed with aniridia. Ultrasonography is done every 3 months. This will result in:
    a. increased survival.
    b. detection of lower-stage renal tumor.
    c. decreased incidence of bilateral tumors.
    d. decreased surgical morbidity.
    e. detection of tumors smaller than 3 cm in diameter.

16. A deletion of chromosome 11 has been found most frequently in Wilms tumor patients with:
    a. aniridia.
    b. bilateral tumors.

c. hemihypertrophy.
d. Denys-Drash syndrome.
e. Beckwith-Wiedemann syndrome.

17. A 5-year-old boy undergoes nephrectomy for a solid renal mass. Pathology reveals stage I favorable histology Wilms tumor. An increased risk for tumor relapse is associated with:
    a. tumor aneuploidy on flow cytometry.
    b. deletion of chromosome 11p13.
    c. duplication of chromosome 1.
    d. LOH for chromosome 16q.
    e. elevated serum ferritin level.

18. A 2-year-old girl undergoes left nephrectomy for Wilms tumor. A solitary left pulmonary lesion is noted on chest CT. The pathology shows favorable histology but with capsular penetration. The most important prognostic feature is:
    a. capsular penetration.
    b. histologic subtype.
    c. absence of lymph node involvement.
    d. age at presentation.
    e. presence of pulmonary metastasis.

19. The feature associated with worse survival in children with Wilms tumor is:
    a. diffuse anaplasia.
    b. diffuse tumor spill.
    c. incomplete tumor resection.
    d. tumor spread to periaortic lymph nodes.
    e. lung metastasis.

20. An increased risk for metachronous Wilms tumor is associated with:
    a. anaplastic histology.
    b. clear cell sarcoma.
    c. blastema-predominant pattern.
    d. renal sinus invasion.
    e. nephrogenic rests.

21. A 6-year-old boy has a solid abdominal mass noted on ultrasonography. A right-sided varicocele is present on physical examination. The next best step is:
    a. abdominal CT.
    b. magnetic resonance imaging (MRI) of the abdomen.
    c. chest CT.
    d. intravenous pyelogram.
    e. arteriogram.

22. A 1-year-old boy undergoes nephrectomy for Wilms tumor. The finding that has the most adverse impact on survival is:
    a. hilar lymph node involvement.
    b. renal sinus invasion.
    c. capsular penetration.
    d. ureteral extension of tumor.
    e. renal vein thrombus.

23. The factor associated with the lowest risk of local tumor relapse in children with Wilms tumor is:
    a. local tumor spill.
    b. unfavorable histology.

c. incomplete tumor removal.

d. absence of lymph node sampling.

e. capsular penetration.

24. A 4-year-old girl undergoes removal of a Wilms tumor of favorable histology. Imaging evaluation reveals multiple pulmonary metastases. Treatment should include vincristine, dactinomycin, and:

a. observation.

b. resection of the lesions.

c. doxorubicin and chest irradiation.

d. doxorubicin, cyclophosphamide, and irradiation.

e. doxorubicin and etoposide.

25. A 3-month-old boy undergoes removal of a 300-g Wilms tumor of the right kidney. The pathology shows diffuse anaplasia and tumor confined to the kidney. Lymph nodes are negative. The next step is:

a. observation.

b. vincristine and dactinomycin.

c. vincristine, dactinomycin, and irradiation of tumor beds.

d. doxorubicin, vincristine, dactinomycin, and irradiation of the tumor bed.

e. ifosfamide, etoposide, and doxorubicin.

26. A 5-year-old girl presents with hematuria. CT reveals a right abdominal mass with extension of tumor thrombus into the suprahepatic vena cava. The best next step is:

a. chemotherapy.

b. irradiation.

c. open biopsy followed by chemotherapy.

d. preoperative chemotherapy and radiation therapy.

e. primary surgical removal of the kidney and tumor thrombus.

27. A 2-year-old boy is found to have bilateral Wilms tumor. There is a tumor occupying more than 50% of the left kidney and a 4.0-cm tumor in the upper pole of the right kidney. The best next step is:

a. left nephrectomy and right renal biopsy.

b. bilateral partial nephrectomy.

c. right partial nephrectomy and left renal biopsy.

d. bilateral nephrectomies.

e. chemotherapy.

28. A 1-year-old girl has a stage III Wilms tumor. During the course of chemotherapy she develops an enlarged heart and evidence of congestive heart failure. The drug responsible for these findings is most likely:

a. dactinomycin.

b. etoposide.

c. vincristine.

d. cyclophosphamide.

e. doxorubicin.

29. A 2-year-old boy undergoes left orchiectomy. Pathology reveals a yolk sac tumor confined to the testis. CT findings of the chest and abdomen are negative. No preoperative tumor markers were obtained. At 4 weeks after surgery, tumor markers are negative. The next step is:

a. lymph node dissection.

b. observation.

c. chemotherapy.

d. staining of the tumor for α-fetoprotein.

e. retroperitoneal lymph node sampling.

30. A 1-year-old boy undergoes a left radical nephrectomy for a large renal mass. The pathologic features associated with the worst prognosis are:

a. diffuse anaplasia stage I.

b. focal anaplasia stage III.

c. rhabdoid tumor of the kidney stage III.

d. clear cell sarcoma of the kidney stage III.

e. favorable histology stage IV.

31. A newborn boy was noted to have a left renal mass on prenatal ultrasonography. Postnatal evaluation confirms a 5-cm solid mass in the lower pole of the left kidney. The right kidney is normal. Chest radiography and CT of the chest are negative for metastatic disease. The mass was completely removed by a radical nephrectomy. The tumor was confined to the kidney and weighed 300 grams. The next step in treatment is:

a. 1200-cGy abdominal irradiation to the left flank.

b. observation only.

c. dactinomycin and vincristine for 10 weeks.

d. dactinomycin and vincristine for 18 weeks.

e. 2000-cGy abdominal irradiation plus dactinomycin and vincristine for 18 weeks.

32. A 6-year-old, phenotypic boy with hypospadias and bilateral cryptorchism has a 3-cm lower abdominal mass. His karyotype is XO/XY. At abdominal exploration, a tumor is found in the right gonad. Right orchiectomy is performed. Frozen section reveals gonadoblastoma. The best next step is:

a. left orchiopexy.

b. retroperitoneal lymphadenectomy node sampling.

c. left orchiectomy.

d. chemotherapy.

e. observation.

33. A 2-year-old boy has a left upper pole testicular mass that is cystic on ultrasonography. Excision of the lesion is performed by an inguinal approach leaving the lower half of the testis. Frozen section demonstrates clear margins. Final pathology reveals teratoma, and the margins are negative for tumor. Serum α-fetoprotein and β-hCG are negative. Chest and abdominal CT are negative. The next step is:

a. radical orchiectomy and modified retroperitoneal lymph node dissection.

b. observation.

c. radical orchiectomy and combination chemotherapy.

d. radical orchiectomy.

e. radical orchiectomy and abdominal irradiation.

34. The tuberous sclerosis complex is associated with the development of angiomyolipoma and cystic renal disease. These patients have been found to have an abnormality of chromosome:

    a. 1.

    b. 7.

    c. 9.

    d. 12.

    e. 14.

35. A 3-month-old boy undergoes removal of a solid yolk sac tumor. The margins of resection are negative for tumor. Chest and abdominal CT results show no signs of metastatic disease. Two weeks postoperatively, the serum α-fetoprotein value is 35 ng/dL. The next step is:

    a. chemotherapy.

    b. retroperitoneal lymph node dissection.

    c. observation.

    d. retroperitoneal lymph node sampling.

    e. abdominal irradiation.

ANSWERS

1. **d. deletion of the short arm of chromosome 1.** Deletion of the short arm of chromosome 1 is found in 25% to 35% of neuroblastomas and is an adverse prognostic marker. The deletions are of different size, but, in a series of eight cases, a consensus deletion included the segment 1p36.1-2, suggesting that genetic information related to neuroblastoma tumorigenesis is located in this segment.

2. **b. usually regresses spontaneously.** In 1963, Beckwith and Perrin coined the term in-situ neuroblastoma for small nodules of neuroblastoma cells found incidentally within the adrenal gland, which are histologically indistinguishable from neuroblastoma. In infants younger than 3 months of age, undergoing postmortem examination, in-situ neuroblastoma was found in 1 of 224 infants. This represents an incidence of in-situ neuroblastoma 40 to 45 times greater than the incidence of clinical tumors, suggesting that these small tumors regress spontaneously in most cases. However, more recent studies have shown that these neuroblastic nodules are found in all fetuses studied and generally regress.

3. **a. a stroma-rich tumor by the Shimada classification.** The Shimada classification is an age-linked histopathologic classification. One of the important aspects of the Shimada classification is determining whether the tumor is stroma poor or stroma rich. Patients with stroma-poor tumors with unfavorable histopathologic features have a very poor prognosis (less than 10% survival). Stroma-rich tumors can be separated into three subgroups: nodular, intermixed, and well differentiated. Tumors in the last two categories more closely resemble ganglioneuroblastoma or immature ganglioneuroma and have a higher rate of survival.

4. **d. discovers tumors with an improved prognosis.** The goal of screening programs is to detect disease at an earlier stage and decrease the number of older children with advanced-stage disease and thus improve survival. An increased number of infants younger than 1 year of age have been diagnosed with the mass screening program, and most of these patients have lower-stage tumors. Regrettably, the number of children older than 1 year of age with advanced-stage disease has not decreased.

5. **b. thoracic location of the primary tumor.** The site of origin is of significance, with a better survival rate noted for nonadrenal primary tumors. Most children with thoracic neuroblastoma present at a younger age with localized disease and have improved survival even when corrected for age and stage.

6. **a. observation.** The generally favorable behavior of stage IV-S disease has been explained with the development of biologic markers. The vast majority of these infants have tumors with entirely favorable markers, thus explaining their nonmalignant behavior. A small percentage, however, have adverse markers, and it is these children who have progressive disease to which they often succumb. Resection of the primary tumor is not mandatory. Although excellent survival has been reported after surgery, information regarding histologic prognostic factors was not available for all of these patients. A more recent review was performed of a large cohort of 110 infants with stage IV-S disease. The entire cohort of infants had an estimated 3-year survival rate of 85% ± 4%. This survival rate was significantly decreased, however, to 68% ± 12% for infants who were diploid, 44% ± 33% for those who were N-*MYC* amplified, and 33% ± 19% for those with unfavorable histology tumors. Of note, there was no statistical difference in survival rate for infants who underwent complete resection of their primary tumor compared with those with partial resection or only biopsy. Patients with extensive metastatic disease who are N-*MYC*–positive represent a high-risk group.

    These patients should be considered for a more aggressive treatment with multimodal therapy as appropriate for the risk group classification.

7. **b. Li-Fraumeni syndrome.** Subgroups of children with a genetic predisposition to the development of rhabdomyosarcoma have been identified. The Li-Fraumeni syndrome associates childhood sarcomas with mothers who have an excess of premenopausal breast cancer and with siblings who have an increased risk of cancer. A mutation of the *TP53* tumor suppressor gene was found in the tumors in all patients with this syndrome.

8. **a. alveolar histologic type.** The second most common form is alveolar, which occurs more commonly in the trunk and extremities than in genitourinary sites and has a worse prognosis. Alveolar rhabdomyosarcoma also has a higher rate of local recurrence and spread to regional lymph nodes, bone marrow, and distant sites.

9. **d. observation.** If tumor is shrinking during chemotherapy, and another biopsy after completing radiotherapy shows maturing rhabdomyoblasts without frank tumor cells, total cystectomy can be postponed or avoided altogether.

10. **a. vincristine, dactinomycin, and cyclophosphamide.** Before effective chemotherapy, surgery alone produced a 50% 2-year relapse-free survival rate. With current multimodal treatment, survival rates of 90% are expected. Currently, the Intergroup Rhabdomyosarcoma Study Group recommends that children 10 years of age and older undergo ipsilateral retroperitoneal lymph node dissection before chemotherapy.

11. **d. renal insufficiency.** Patients with the WAGR syndrome have a germline deletion at 11p13. *WT1* mutations and deletions predispose patients to renal insufficiency. Both the

Denys-Drash and WAGR syndrome are associated with an increased risk of renal failure. This occurs later in the WAGR syndrome, often in the second decade of life after treatment of the Wilms tumor.

12. **d. bilateral nephrectomy.** One specific association of male pseudohermaphroditism, renal mesangial sclerosis, and nephroblastoma is the Denys-Drash syndrome. The majority of these patients progress to end-stage renal disease. A specific mutation of the 11p13 Wilms tumor gene has been identified in these children. Although XY individuals have been reported most often, the syndrome has been reported in genotypic/phenotypic females. One should have a high index of suspicion for the development of renal failure and Wilms tumor in patients with male pseudohermaphroditism.

13. **a. Wilms tumor.** Beckwith Wiedemann Syndrome (BWS) is characterized by excess growth at the cellular, organ (macroglossia, nephromegaly, hepatomegaly), or body segment (hemihypertrophy) levels. Most cases of BWS are sporadic, but up to 15% exhibit heritable characteristics with apparent autosomal dominant inheritance. The risk of nephroblastoma in children with BWS and hemihypertrophy is 4% to 10%.

14. **c. nephromegaly.** Children with BWS found to have nephromegaly (kidneys in the 95th percentile of age-adjusted renal length) are at the greatest risk for the development of Wilms tumor.

15. **b. detection of lower-stage renal tumor.** Screening with serial renal ultrasound scans has been recommended in children with aniridia, hemihypertrophy, and BWS. Review of most studies suggests that 3 to 4 months is the appropriate screening interval. Tumors detected by screening will generally be at a lower stage.

16. **a. aniridia.** Approximately 50% of patients with WAGR syndrome and a constitutional deletion on chromosome 11 will develop Wilms tumor.

17. **d. LOH for chromosome 16q.** LOH for a portion of chromosome 16q has been noted in 20% of Wilms tumors. A study of 232 patients registered on the National Wilms Tumor Study Group (NWTSG) found LOH for 16q in 17% of the tumors. Patients with tumor-specific LOH for chromosome 16q had a statistically significantly poorer 2-year relapse-free and overall survival rates than did those patients without LOH for chromosome 16q.

18. **b. histologic subtype.** Markers associated with unfavorable outcome include nuclear atypia (anaplasia), focal or diffuse, and sarcomatous tumors (rhabdoid and clear cell type). The latter two tumor types, however, are tumor categories distinct from Wilms tumor. These unfavorable features occurred in approximately 10% of patients but accounted for almost half of the tumor deaths in early NWTSG studies.

19. **a. diffuse anaplasia.** Anaplasia is associated with resistance to chemotherapy. This is evidenced by the similar incidence of anaplasia (5%) in the NWTSG and International Society of Paediatric Oncology studies. Although the presence of anaplasia has clearly been demonstrated to carry a poor prognosis, patients with stage I anaplastic Wilms tumor, as well as those with higher stages and focal rather than diffuse anaplasia, seem to have a more favorable outcome. This confirms the observation that anaplasia is more a marker of chemoresistance than inherent aggressiveness of the tumor.

20. **e. nephrogenic rests.** NWTSG investigators demonstrated the clinical importance of nephrogenic rests. Multiple rests in one kidney usually imply that nephrogenic rests are present in the other kidney. Children younger than 12 months of age diagnosed with Wilms tumor, who also have nephrogenic rests, in particular perilobar nephrogenic rests, have a markedly increased risk of developing contralateral disease and require frequent and regular surveillance for several years.

21. **b. magnetic resonance imaging (MRI) of the abdomen.** Compression or invasion of adjacent structures may result in an atypical presentation. Extension of Wilms tumor into the renal vein and inferior vena cava (IVC) can cause varicocele, hepatomegaly due to hepatic vein obstruction, ascites, and congestive heart failure. Such symptoms are found in less than 10% of patients with intracaval or atrial tumor extension.

22. **a. hilar lymph node involvement.** The most important determinants of outcome in children with Wilms tumor are histopathology and tumor stage. Accurate staging of Wilms tumor allows treatment results to be evaluated and enables universal comparisons of outcomes. The staging system used by the NWTSG is based primarily on the surgical and histopathologic findings. Examination for extension through the capsule, residual disease, vascular involvement, and lymph node involvement is essential to properly assess the extent of the tumor.

23. **e. capsular penetration.** One study identified risk factors for local tumor recurrence as tumor spillage, unfavorable histology, incomplete tumor removal, and absence of any lymph node sampling. The 2-year survival rate after abdominal recurrence was 43%, emphasizing the importance of the surgeon in performing careful and complete tumor resection.

24. **c. doxorubicin and chest irradiation.** Patients with stage III favorable histologic type tumors and stage II to III focal anaplasia are treated with dactinomycin, vincristine, and doxorubicin and 10.8-Gy abdominal irradiation. Patients with stage IV favorable histologic type tumors receive abdominal irradiation based on the local tumor stage and 12 Gy to both lungs.

25. **d. doxorubicin, vincristine, dactinomycin, and irradiation of the tumor bed.** Anaplasia tumors are resistant to chemotherapy. However, if the tumor is confined to the kidney and completely resected the prognosis is good. They do require more intense treatment than children with stage I, favorable-histology tumors.

26. **c. open biopsy followed by chemotherapy.** The current recommendations from the NWTSG are that preoperative chemotherapy is of benefit in patients with bilateral involvement, inoperable tumor at surgical exploration, and IVC extension above the hepatic veins. All other patients should undergo primary nephrectomy.

27. **e. chemotherapy.** Patients with bilateral Wilms tumor have an increased risk for renal failure. These patients should receive preoperative chemotherapy without attempts at initial surgery. Repeat imaging after 6 weeks of chemotherapy can assess response to treatment. Appropriate surgical resection may then be undertaken.

28. **e. doxorubicin.** In recent years, there has been increasing concern regarding the risk of congestive heart failure in children who receive treatment with anthracyclines such as

doxorubicin. In addition to the acute cardiotoxicity, cardiac failure can develop many years after treatment.

29. **b. observation.** The initial treatment for yolk sac tumor is radical inguinal orchiectomy. This treatment is curative in most children. Routine retroperitoneal lymph node dissection and adjuvant chemotherapy are not indicated.

30. **c. rhabdoid tumor of the kidney stage III.** Typical clinical features include early age at diagnosis (median age of less than 16 months), resistance to chemotherapy, and high mortality rate. Unlike Wilms tumor, which typically metastasizes to the lungs, abdomen/flank, and liver, rhabdoid tumor of the kidney, which also metastasizes to these sites, is distinguished by its propensity to metastasize to the brain.

31. **b. observation only.** The most common renal tumor in a newborn is congenital mesoblastic nephroma. The important aspect of the recognition of these tumors as a separate entity is the usually excellent outcome with radical surgery only. Wilms tumors do occur rarely in neonates, but these patients are eligible for observation only on current protocols.

32. **c. left orchiectomy.** Early gonadectomy is advocated, because tumors have been reported in children younger than 5 years of age. In patients with mixed gonadal dysgenesis who are reared as males, all streak gonads and undescended testes should be removed. Scrotal testes can be preserved, because they are less prone to tumor development.

33. **b. observation.** Prepubertal mature teratomas have a benign clinical course, which contrasts with the clinical behavior of teratomas in adults, which have the propensity to metastasize. This benign behavior has led to the consideration of testicular-sparing procedures rather than radical orchiectomy.

34. **c. 9.** Two genes have been identified in the tuberous sclerosis complex: *TSC1* on chromosome 9 and *TSC2* on chromosome 16. It has been postulated that these genes act as tumor suppressor genes and that the LOH of *TSC1* or *TSC2* may explain the progressive growth pattern of renal lesions seen in these patients.

35. **c. observation.** It is important to note that an elevated α-fetoprotein level after orchiectomy for yolk sac tumor in an infant does not always represent persistent disease. Normal adult reference laboratory values for α-fetoprotein cannot be used in young children, because α-fetoprotein synthesis continues after birth. Normal adult levels (<10 mg/mL) are not reached until 8 months of age.

Additional Study Points

1. Neuroblastoma is the most common extracranial solid tumor of childhood; 75% arise in the retroperitoneum, 50% in the adrenal, and 25% in the paravertebral ganglia.

2. N-*MYC* oncogene occurs in 20% of primary neuroblastoma tumors and is an adverse prognostic indicator.

3. Neuroblastoma, ganglioneuroblastoma, and ganglioneuroma form a histologic spectrum of differentiation from malignant to benign.

4. Symptoms of neuroblastoma include those due to catecholamine release, those due to vasoactive intestinal peptide (watery diarrhea), and myoclonic encephalopathy.

5. The finding of intratumor fine stippled calcifications with vascular encasement distinguishes neuroblastoma from Wilms tumor on imaging.

6. Stage IV-S (S meaning special) refers to a small primary tumor with metastases to the liver, skin, and/or bone marrow without radiographic evidence of bone metastases.

7. Complete surgical resection is curative for low-staged neuroblastoma.

8. Rhabdomyosarcoma has three histologic types: embryonal, alveolar, and undifferentiated.

9. For patients with rhabdomyosarcoma, generally, chemotherapy and radiation precede surgical resection unless the tumor is amenable to a partial cystectomy.

10. Radiation therapy for patients with bladder or prostate rhabdomyosarcoma results in a markedly reduced functional bladder capacity and abnormal voiding patterns.

11. In paratesticular rhabdomyosarcoma, children who are 10 years of age and older should have an ipsilateral retroperitoneal lymph node dissection.

12. In Wilms tumor, loss of heterozygosity at 1p and 16q is associated with an increased risk of tumor relapse and death.

13. There is an association between Wilms tumor and horseshoe kidney.

14. There are three histologic components of Wilms tumor: blastemal, epithelial, and stromal.

15. The anaplastic variant of Wilms tumor is associated with resistance to chemotherapy.

16. Clear cell sarcoma and rhabdoid tumors are not Wilms variants but, rather, distinct histologic types of renal malignancies.

17. There is an increased incidence of second malignant neoplasms in children treated for Wilms tumors.

18. Schiller-Duval bodies are a characteristic finding in yolk sac tumors of the testis.

19. Teratomas are classified as mature, immature, and malignant.

20. Mature teratomas have a benign course in childhood and are successfully treated with radical orchiectomy alone. This is not true in the adult.

21. Immature teratomas generally behave in a benign fashion in childhood unless they have foci of yolk sac tumor. If the latter is the case, they should be treated as one would treat a yolk sac tumor.

22. All streak gonads in patients with gonadal dysgenesis should be removed.

chapter 138

Pediatric Genitourinary Trauma

Douglas A. Husmann, MD

QUESTIONS

1. Which of the following signs or symptoms noted after a traumatic insult is suggestive of a preexisting renal abnormality?
   a. Microscopic hematuria with shock
   b. Gross hematuria with shock
   c. Gross hematuria with clot formation
   d. Hematuria disproportionate to severity of trauma
   e. Hematuria in the absence of coexisting injuries to the thorax, spine, pelvis/femur, or intra-abdominal organs

2. The radiographic study that is the most sensitive for the presence of a renal injury is:
   a. intravenous pyelography (IVP).
   b. magnetic resonance imaging (MRI) of abdomen.
   c. focused assessment with sonography for trauma (FAST) ultrasonography.
   d. triphasic abdominal computed tomography (CT).
   e. monophasic abdominal CT.

3. Following a traumatic injury, a CT of the abdomen reveals a renal laceration that extends into the collecting system with urinary extravasation. The injury is associated with a devitalized fragment; the grade of renal injury is:
   a. 1.
   b. 2.
   c. 3.
   d. 4.
   e. 5.

4. An 11-year-old boy sustained a renal laceration that extended into the collecting system 2 weeks previously. He has been at home for the past week with grossly clear urine. He is at home and has the sudden onset of gross hematuria with clots. The next step is:
   a. reassurance and continued observation.
   b. bed rest, force fluids, and follow-up the next day.
   c. continued observation and arranging for follow-up CT in the morning.
   d. bringing the patient by car to the office for evaluation.
   e. transportation to the emergency room by ambulance.

5. A 9-year-old boy sustained a renal laceration associated with a functional renal fragment that was completely dissociated from the kidney. He has a persistent symptomatic urinary fistula despite combined treatment with a nephrostomy tube, double-J stent, and urethral catheter. The next step is:
   a. angiographic embolization of the functional renal fragment.
   b. radiofrequency ablation (RFA) of functional renal fragment.
   c. cryotherapy of the functional renal fragment.
   d. laparoscopic partial nephrectomy.
   e. open partial nephrectomy.

6. An 8-year-old boy on intravenous (IV) prophylaxis with cephazolin undergoes angiographic embolization of a traumatic arteriovenous (AV) fistula associated with a grade 4 traumatic renal injury. His urine is clear, but, on postembolization day 1 and 2, he has febrile temperature spikes to 40° C. Blood pressure is stable. Acetaminophen is given for the fever, and blood and urine cultures are obtained. The next step is:
   a. continued observation.
   b. a change in antibiotic coverage to piperacillin.
   c. addition of metronidazole.
   d. CT of abdomen and aspiration of perinephric hematoma/urinoma.
   e. percutaneous nephrostomy drainage of urinoma.

7. A 2-year-old boy sustains a major renal laceration with a tear into the collecting system secondary to child abuse. He has persistent gross hematuria with clots and ileus, 5 days following his injury. CT scan reveals clot filling the renal pelvis and a significant perinephric urinoma; however, good flow of contrast is seen into the ipsilateral distal ureter. These findings are essentially unchanged from a CT scan done 48 hours earlier. Vital signs and hemoglobin are normal and stable. The next step is:
   a. continued observation.
   b. angiography.
   c. percutaneous nephrostomy.
   d. cystoscopy, retrograde pyelogram, and stent placement.
   e. surgical exploration and renorrhaphy.

8. Follow-up CT imaging for a grade 2 renal injury should be performed:
   a. only if the patient develops localized signs or symptoms.
   b. 2 to 3 days post-traumatic injury.
   c. 3 to 4 weeks post-traumatic injury.
   d. 3 months post-traumatic injury
   e. 1 year post-traumatic injury.

9. Retroperitoneal (renal) exploration is recommended when:
   a. a stab wound to the flank results in a grade 2 renal injury.
   b. a 38-caliber gunshot wound (GSW) results in a grade 2 renal injury.
   c. a motor vehicle accident (MVA) results in an isolated grade 4 renal injury.
   d. a nonhemorrhagic retroperitoneal mass is found on surgical exploration following a GSW.
   e. an MVA results in the need for emergent laparotomy due to vascular instability, and a retroperitoneal hemorrhage is found on exploration.

10. A 12-year-old girl is involved in a bicycle MVA. A CT scan taken 2 hours following trauma reveals an isolated renal injury with no perfusion and, subsequently, no function of the left kidney. The right kidney is within normal limits. Vital signs are stable and hemoglobin is normal. The next step is:
   a. observation.
   b. angiography with stenting of left renal artery.
   c. angiographic infusion of streptokinase into left renal artery.
   d. systemic heparinization.
   e. surgical exploration.

11. In a patient with a preexisting ureteropelvic junction (UPJ) obstruction, gross hematuria following trauma is usually due to:
   a. coexisting renal lithiasis.
   b. renal contusion.
   c. laceration through the thinned renal cortex.
   d. rupture of the renal pelvis.
   e. UPJ disruption.

12. The following is an absolute indication for CT cystography following blunt trauma:
   a. gross hematuria.
   b. abdominal wall bruising.
   c. pelvic fracture.
   d. lumbar spinal fracture.
   e. inability to void.

13. In the presence of an extraperitoneal bladder injury, consideration for open surgical intervention should be given if:
   a. gross hematuria with clots is present.
   b. the pubic ramus is fractured.
   c. a vaginal laceration is present.
   d. a coexisting rectal injury is present.
   e. the bladder neck appears incompetent.

14. While assessing bladder function for a delayed urethroplasty, a static cystogram reveals contrast in the posterior urethra. The next step is:
   a. video urodynamics.
   b. a pudendal nerve electromyogram (EMG).
   c. MRI of the pelvis and perineum.
   d. MRI of the lumbosacral spinal cord.
   e. combined cystoscopy per suprapubic (SP) tube tract and urethroscopy per meatus.

15. A newborn has excess skin excised during circumcision, leaving a 7-mm gap between the residual penile shaft skin and the mucosal collar. The next step is:
   a. wet-to-dry dressings and antibiotic ointment.
   b. to mobilize and suture the penile shaft skin to mucosal collar.
   c. to bury the phallus in scrotal skin with planned second-stage release.
   d. a split-thickness skin graft from thigh.
   e. a full-thickness skin graft from thigh.

ANSWERS

1. **d. Hematuria disproportionate to severity of trauma.** The classic patient history that should make the physician think of a preexisting renal anomaly is that the degree of hematuria present is disproportionate to the severity of trauma. None of the other distracters have been found to be related to the presence of a preexisting renal abnormality during the evaluation of trauma.

2. **d. triphasic abdominal computed tomography (CT).** A triphasic CT study—a precontrast study, followed by a study immediately following injection, and then a 15 to 20 minute delayed study—is the most sensitive method for diagnosis and classification of renal trauma. A single-phase CT study is beneficial in determining renal perfusion and major renal fractures but may, on occasion, miss the presence of urinary extravasation and will miss the vast majority of ureteral injuries. Focused assessment with sonography for trauma (FAST) evaluations are operator and experience dependent and will miss 5% to 10% of clinically significant renal injuries. It is noteworthy, however, that a normal FAST sonographic evaluation coupled with serial normal physical examinations over 24 hours will reliably detect all clinically significant genitourinary (GU) injuries.

3. **d. grade 4.** A grade 4 renal injury is a laceration extending into the collecting system with urinary extravasation, with viable or devitalized renal fragments, or is an injury to the main renal vasculature with contained hemorrhage. (See Table 138–2 in *Campbell-Walsh Urology, 10th Edition.*)

4. **e. transportation to the emergency room by ambulance.** Approximately 25% of patients with grade 3 to 4 renal trauma managed in a nonoperative fashion will have persistent or delayed hemorrhage. Classically, delayed hemorrhage will present 10 to 14 days postinjury, but may occur up to 1 month after the insult. Delayed hemorrhage arises from the development of arteriovenous fistulas, will not spontaneously resolve, and may be associated with life-threatening hemorrhage. Management should be by ambulance transportation, remembering that shock in a child may be one of the later signs of severe bleeding. Intravenous access should be obtained by emergency

medical technicians and the patient immediately returned to the hospital for angiographic evaluation and embolization of the bleeding site.

5. **a. angiographic embolization of the functional renal fragment.** Urinary fistulas associated with a viable renal fragment that is separate from the remaining portions of a traumatically injured kidney are initially managed with percutaneous nephrostomy tube drainage and double-J stent placement. If persistent fistula drainage continues, it may be managed by angiographic infarction of the isolated functional segment, which will prevent the need for open surgical excision of the functional segment.

6. **a. continued observation.** Postembolization syndrome is well recognized and self-limiting. It is manifested by pyrexia up to 40° C, flank pain, and adynamic ileus. Symptoms should resolve in 96 hours after the embolization. When pyrexia develops, blood and urine cultures are necessary to rule out bacterial seeding of the necrotic tissue. Consideration for a repeat CT scan with possible aspiration, culture, and drainage of a perinephric hematoma/urinoma should be given if febrile response persists for greater than 96 hours or if a patient's clinical course deteriorates.

7. **c. percutaneous nephrostomy.** Post-traumatic urinomas are asymptomatic and have a spontaneous resolution rate approaching 85%; they will occasionally persist and be associated with continued flank pain, adynamic ileus, and/or low-grade temperature. Frequently, the authors will manage these patients by endoscopic intervention, with cystoscopy, retrograde pyelography, and placement of a ureteral stent. It should be noted that both percutaneous nephrostomy drainage and internal stenting are equally efficacious. The advantage of an internal stent is that it prevents possible dislodgment of the draining tube and the need for external drainage devices. The two major disadvantages of internal drainage are that both stent placement and removal, in the pediatric patient population, require general anesthesia. In addition, the small-size ureteral stents (4 to 5 Fr) placed in young children may become blocked with blood clots from the dissolving hematoma, resulting in persistence of the urinoma. In this young infant with large perinephric clots, the best way to manage the problem is with a percutaneous nephrostomy. This will allow external irrigation of the system, if the tube becomes blocked with clots.

8. **a. only if the patient develops localized signs or symptoms.** Follow-up renal imaging is not recommended for grade 1 to 2 renal injuries and for grade 3 lacerations where all fragments are viable. In patients with grade 3 renal lacerations associated with devitalized fragments and grade 4 and salvaged grade 5 renal injuries, a repeat CT scan with delayed images should be obtained 2 to 3 days following the traumatic insult. This study serves the purpose of assessing the extent of the hematoma/urinoma and will serve as a baseline evaluation in case secondary hemorrhage or infection occurs. Irrespective of the grade of the injury, repeat imaging with a triphasic CT scan is recommended for patients with a history of renal trauma who have a persistent and/or increased fever, worsening flank pain, or persistent gross hematuria greater than 72 hours following the traumatic insult. The authors recommend a 3-month follow-up triphasic CT scan in all grade 3 renal lacerations associated with a devitalized fragment and grade 4 and salvaged grade 5 renal injuries. This latter study is obtained

to verify resolution of any perinephric urinoma and to define the anatomic configuration of the residual functioning renal parenchyma.

9. **e. an MVA results in the need for emergent laparotomy due to vascular instability, and a retroperitoneal hemorrhage is found on exploration.** An MVA results in an isolated grade 4 renal injury. Retroperitoneal exploration is recommended in the setting of blunt trauma when abdominal exploration is performed for vascular instability and retroperitoneal hemorrhage is identified, even when there has not been adequate preoperative imaging. In these cases, assessment of contralateral function is necessary as well. (See Table 138–3 in *Campbell-Walsh Urology, 10th Edition*.)

10. **a. observation.** In a patient sustaining renal arterial trauma, the clinical triad of hemodynamic instability, inadequate collateral blood flow, and warm ischemic time almost invariably results in the inability to salvage renal function. Because of these facts, no attempt to repair injuries to segmental renal vessels should be considered, and repair of the traumatically injured main renal artery is seldom, if ever, indicated when a normal contralateral kidney is present. In essence, reconstruction of the main renal artery following trauma is only a primary consideration in patients who are hemodynamically stable, with an injury to a solitary kidney, or in patients with bilateral renal arterial injuries. The infrequent exception to this rule is the presence of an incomplete arterial injury where perfusion to the kidney has been maintained by flow of blood through either the partially occluded main renal artery or through collateral vessels.

11. **b. renal contusion.** Although it has been reported that preexisting hydronephrosis or a congenital ureteropelvic junction obstruction renders the patient more susceptible to a UPJ disruption, this is controversial. The vast majority of patients with a history of trauma and preexisting UPJ or hydronephrosis will be found to have a renal contusion or grade 1 renal injury on evaluation. When urinary extravasation is seen, rupture of the renal pelvis or a major laceration extending through a thinned renal cortex into the collecting system (grade 3 renal injury) is the most common finding, not a UPJ disruption.

12. **e. inability to void.** Absolute indications for bladder imaging following blunt abdominal trauma are currently limited to two indications: (1) the presence of gross hematuria coexisting with a pelvic fracture or (2) inability to void. Neither gross hematuria alone or pelvic fracture alone are absolute indications for screening. Relative indications for bladder imaging following blunt abdominal trauma are urinary clot retention, perineal hematoma, and history of a prior bladder augmentation. Bladder imaging following penetrating trauma should be performed any time concern exists that the missile could have penetrated the bladder.

13. **e. the bladder neck appears incompetent.** If concern for a bladder neck injury is present, the patient should undergo surgical exploration with opening of the bladder at the dome. Repair of the bladder neck should be performed by an intravesical approach with a multilayered closure. Great care should be given not to dislodge the pelvic hematoma to help prevent blood loss. The surgeon should be aware that anterior bladder neck lacerations are frequently associated with urethral injuries, and retrograde

urethrography or cystoscopy to rule out this possibility should be considered. If a bladder neck laceration is repaired, a voiding cystourethrogram (VCUG) is necessary at the time of catheter removal to adequately visualize the bladder neck and confirm healing.

14. **a. video urodynamics.** If the posterior urethra fills with contrast on the static cystogram, this could be due to either a poorly felt or described detrusor contraction or to an incompetent bladder neck. Because of the significant impact the latter has on the surgical prognosis, if contrast is seen in the posterior urethra, a video urodynamic study (UDS) is necessary. If the video UDS documents an incompetent bladder neck, or if the patient was unable to open up the bladder neck to allow visualization of the posterior urethra during the VCUG, we perform a simultaneous flexible cystoscopy and urethroscopy. On occasion, the physician may need to use flexible ureteroscopes for this procedure in small children. If cystoscopy and video urodynamics demonstrate an incompetent bladder neck, we discuss with the patient and his or her family the options of urethral reconstruction with the possible result of chronic incontinence or, alternatively, the performance of a continent abdominal stoma, appendicovesicostomy as first-line therapy.

15. **a. wet-to-dry dressings and antibiotic ointment.** Penile trauma in the pediatric patient population is most commonly iatrogenic and caused by circumcision. If excess penile skin is excised during circumcision, the majority of patients can be treated by wet-to-dry dressings and antibiotic ointment. Healing by secondary intention usually results in an excellent cosmetic appearance. If the penis is totally degloved, the penile shaft skin, if salvaged, can be defatted and replaced on the penis as a full-thickness skin graft.

Additional Study Points

1. Preexisting renal anomalies are commonly found in children who present with traumatic injuries of the kidney.

2. In children, there is a poor correlation between the presence of hematuria and a renal injury.

3. A single-shot IVP intraoperatively is only useful in determining the presence of a contralateral kidney when an ipsilateral nephrectomy is anticipated.

4. The vast majority of AV fistulas that occur after trauma will not spontaneously resolve, unlike AV fistulas following a renal biopsy, where spontaneous resolution is the rule.

5. Most post-traumatic urinomas are asymptomatic and will resolve spontaneously.

6. When there is a coexistence of an intra-abdominal injury adjacent to the urinary tract injury, the two should be separated by interposing tissue, often omentum.

7. Post-traumatic hypertension in children is usually due to a small poorly functioning kidney; it is renin mediated, and nephrectomy is generally the best option.

8. CT findings associated with UPJ disruption include medial extravasation, absence of parenchyma lacerations, and no visualization of the distal ureter. Immediate surgical repair is preferred.

9. Traumatic bladder lacerations in children are likely to extend through the bladder neck and require surgical exploration and repair.

10. When a urethral injury is found with a pelvic fracture, a concurrent rectal injury is present in 15%; in females, urethral injuries associated with pelvic fractures are associated 75% of the time with vaginal lacerations and 30% of the time with rectal injury.

11. A diverting colostomy is appropriate in traumatic injuries of the urethra associated with rectal injuries.

12. Penile strangulation caused by hair should be suspected when circumferential edema and/or necrosis is noted from a circumferential point distally.